The Medical Profession in 19th Century Florida

A Biographical Register

by

E. Ashby Hammond, Ph.D.

George A. Smathers Libraries
University of Florida
Gainesville, Florida
1996

Library of Congress Cataloging-in-Publication Data

Hammond, E. Ashby, 1908-
The medical profession in 19th century Florida: a biographical register / by E. Ashby Hammond.
p. cm.
Includes index.
ISBN 0-929595-08-4 (alk. paper)
1. Physicians—Florida—Biography—Dictionaries. 2. Medicine—Florida—History—19th century. I. Title.
R153.H36 1996
610'.92'2759
[B]—DC20 96-43502
CIP

CONTENTS

FOREWORD

The Medical Profession in 19th Century Florida: A Biographical Register is the product of years of research by E. Ashby Hammond, Ph.D., Professor Emeritus of History at the University of Florida. The book is similar to an earlier work coauthored by Dr. Hammond and C.H. Talbot, entitled *The Medical Practitioners in Medieval England: A Biographical Register,* published in London by the Wellcome Historical Medical Library in 1965. In this more recent work about practitioners of medicine in Florida during the state's formative years, Dr. Hammond significantly contributes to its history, adds to our knowledge about medical practice in a relatively unsettled region of 19th century America, and provides related information about advances in medicine and public health which helped make Florida a safer place to live.

Florida of the 1800s was characterized by port cities such as Key West, Jacksonville, Tampa, Cedar Key, St. Marks, Apalachicola, and Pensacola. The centers of population were principally coastal. With the exception of Key West at the southern tip of the state and Tampa on the Gulf of Mexico, settlers had inhabited the more northern regions of the state. Jacksonville was a notable commercial and transportation center where tourists migrated to escape harsh winters and to venture south on the St. Johns River to dozens of resorts situated on its banks. The St. Johns flowed through Lake George where numerous surrounding orange groves were advertised for sale as far away as the European continent. Settlers who bought them soon learned that the winter freezes could be severe enough to ruin the crops and dreams of profits in the new land of sunshine. In the next century orange groves would move further south.

Henry Flagler in the latter part of the 19th century built his railroad 200 miles beyond St. Augustine to Palm Beach, Miami, and later to Key West. To these more southern environs, the wealthy and the tourists flocked, followed by commercial and economic development unsurpassed in the southeastern United States. Florida would grow to become the fourth most populous state in the nation by 1900 with more than 13 million residents, a megatrend state setting examples in leadership, growth, and development. The origin of these accomplishments is found in the Spanish colonial period starting in 1513 and perhaps more significantly in the 19th century when the Americanization of

Florida began with Spain ceding the territory to the United States in 1819.

The early history of Florida also chronicles the diseases that plagued the early settlers—smallpox, whooping cough, dysentery, diphtheria, tuberculosis, scarlet fever, measles and typhoid. Particularly severe was yellow fever, an endemic infection in Havana, Cuba, from the earliest part of the 19th century. Over the 90 miles from Havana to Key West, and from Key West up the east coast to Jacksonville, and from Havana and Key West to the Gulf ports, ships of all types unwittingly transported the vector of yellow fever, resulting in the loss of thousands of lives. The episodes of these epidemics are well recorded; so too are the efforts of physicians to become organized to protect the public health from the scourges of yellow fever and other communicable diseases and to advance the art and science of medicine.

An initial attempt at organizing a county medical society occurred as early as 1826 in the territorial capital at Tallahassee. The first permanent county medical society was established in 1853 in Duval County. Subsequently, the Florida Medical Association was organized in 1874. Physician leaders of the Florida Medical Association and its component county medical societies led the legislative battle to create a State Board of Health authorized in the state constitution of 1885. However, it was not until 1889 when Francis P. Fleming, who had experienced the yellow fever epidemic of 1888, became governor that the state legislature created a state public health department. This enactment was the result of years of activity by the Association, spearheaded by one of its early presidents, John P. Wall, M.D., of Tampa. The first State Health Officer, Joseph Y. Porter, M.D., of Key West, also served as president of the Association in 1886.

Efforts to establish a state system for the licensure and certification of physicians occurred as early as 1821 with intermittent success and variant standards by county. Officials of the Florida Medical Association began work in 1878 to establish an effective medical practice act. Six medical examining boards were formed in major cities throughout the state in 1881, and an Association of Medical Examiners was established in 1894 for the purpose of standardizing certification. It was not until 1905, however, that a single medical examining board for physicians was created by the state legislature.

The history of efforts by physicians to organize in Florida is well chronicled. Establishment of county medical societies, the Florida Medical Association, the State Board of Health, and local and state licensing boards was directed at improving the art and science of medicine through the collective sharing of knowledge by physicians to provide better service to their communities and individual patients. Creation of the Florida State Board of Health and a statewide public health system through leadership of practicing physicians was necessarily an organized public/private partnership to combat and prevent deadly epidemics. Also there was the concomitant need to assure that only trained and competent persons could practice medicine according to the highest ethical and scientific standards of that era.

That which is not chronicled well in 19th century Florida are the lives of most individual physicians. While we know much about the achievements of organized medical activity, we know far less about the practitioners, pioneers in tending the sick in the urban ports and rural hinterlands. Dr. Hammond's book provides us with a glimpse of them—an account of where they practiced, a record of some of their accomplishments, and perhaps most importantly, their biographical summaries.

The Medical Profession in 19th Century Florida thus fulfills a large gap in the medical and public health history of Florida. Its register of physicians will provide other historians with a resource in which to pursue more indepth research. The book will serve the professional genealogist and assist families in quest of their origins and heritage. It will enlighten the medical practitioner, the teacher of medicine, the discoverer of cures, and the compassionate physician treating his or her patient in need, by increasing their knowledge about the ordeals and triumphs of their predecessors: the healers of their age to whom all are indebted for the foundation on which their successors have continued to build the miraculous achievements of today and the anticipated advances of tomorrow. Consequently, we are deeply indebted also to E. Ashby Hammond, Ph.D., for his devotion to enhancing the knowledge of his fellowman, which has remained steadfast throughout his life, and to his love for the history of medicine.

Sanford A. Mullen, M.D.
Historian
Florida Medical Association

PREFACE

The idea leading to the present work emanated from a similar effort, *The Medical Practitioners of Medieval England: A Biographical Register*, by C.H. Talbot and E.A. Hammond, published in 1965 by the Wellcome Historical Medical Library, London. It occurred to the author that a similar work setting forth all available data relating to physicians who practiced in Florida in the 19th century was a worthy enterprise. It is assumed that it will interest nineteenth century historians and all who have a general interest in medical history.

In many instances much-needed biographical data were nonexistent. Some early Florida physicians practiced in remote and sparsely settled parts of the Territory, often in towns and villages without a newspaper, and for them the searcher relied on censuses as the chief source of data. Gravestones are, of course, an invaluable source of data, although many family cemeteries have been neglected and inscriptions have become illegible.

Without the unique and splendid collection of Floridiana available in the P.K. Yonge Library of Florida History and the cooperation of its curator, Miss Elizabeth Alexander, the work would never have been attempted in the first place. Other members of the library staff who were exceedingly helpful over the years were Bruce Chappell, Archivist and Stephen Kerber, Technical Assistant. To Dr. William M. Straight, physician scholar of Florida medicine, and author, I extend my deep appreciation for his friendship and help.

First steps toward the publication of this work were taken by the Florida Medical Association (FMA). Two former presidents of the FMA, Dr. Gerald L. Schiebler, Associate Vice President for Health Affairs at the University of Florida's J. Hillis Miller Health Sciences Center and Dr. Sanford A. Mullen, historian for the FMA, both gave enthusiastic support for the project and deserve the author's gratitude. Dr. Mullen provided the thoughtful Foreword to the volume.

The author is also indebted to many others at the FMA who brought the early drafts to a camera-ready condition. These include FMA Executive Vice President, Donald C. Jones, and Director of the FMA Division of Programs, E. Russell Jackson, Jr., M.A., M.P.H. Tom R. Jarvis, Editorial Assistant for *The Journal of the Florida Medical Association*, edited the entire manuscript. He was careful to preserve the author's style and intent and his dedication to the project was exemplary. The typesetters were Lisa Gergen and Virginia E. Fetherol. A former Managing Editor of *The Journal of the Florida Medical Association*, Louise Rader, did much of the proofing and several FMA staff from the Divisions of Communications and Administration also served as proofreaders.

A very special thanks is due to Dodie M. Walker, Director of the Department of Health Policy Research and Development at the FMA, who served as project coordinator. Ms. Walker's competence and thoughtfulness assured a productive and pleasant relationship between the author and the FMA. Her team worked steadily on the project from 1991 until the transformation was complete in 1995 and they have all continued to be very helpful in the transfer of responsibilities to the University of Florida.

After the Florida Medical Association had produced the camera-ready copy, arrangements were made for publication by the George A. Smathers Libraries, University of Florida, under the direction of Dale B. Canelas. Financial support for publication comes from the University of Florida, and I owe a special debt of gratitude to Dr. Gene Hemp, Vice-Provost of the University of Florida, for his endorsement of this project. Sincere appreciation is extended to Samuel Gowan, Associate Director of the George A. Smathers Libraries, and to Dr. John Ingram, Director of Special Collections, the project coordinator.

Among many others who have been helpful, the author expresses thanks in particular to Dr. Samuel Proctor, Distinguished Service Professor Emeritus of the University of Florida and former editor of *the Florida Historical Quarterly*, for continual encouragement over the years; to Dr. Arthur L. Funk, professor emeritus of history, who helped coordinate the project in its final stages; to Kenneth Scott, Director of the University Press of Florida; to Margie Towery, for indexing the manuscript; and to Barbara Blocker of the Libraries' Department of Collection Management, for her computer expertise.

Lastly, a debt of gratitude is owed to the my wife, Margaret, for her support and lively interest in the work. Thanks also to my daughter, Peggy, for her assistance during the last phase of this publication.

EAH
Gainesville, Florida
1996

INTRODUCTION

The Florida Territory faced crises related to periodic epidemics of deadly fevers endemic to subtropical America from the beginning of the territorial period in 1821. Civil and military authorities were sensitive to the necessity of protective measures and the territorial government relied heavily upon the advice and assistance of medical practitioners, a pattern typical of the American Frontier where often physicians were among the few educated persons.

Boards of Health

In Pensacola and St. Augustine, ceded to the United States by Spain July 7 and July 10, 1821, respectively, yellow fever was a deadly contagion and public health measures could not be delayed. A matter of days after the transfer, provisional governments were established and each included a board of health headed by a reputable physician. The St. Augustine board, announced on July 16, consisted of Mayor Gabriel W. Perpall; William Travers, alderman; Francis P. Sanchez, merchant; the Reverend Michael Crosby, Roman Catholic priest; and Dr. Richard Murray, health officer. On July 19, Governor Andrew Jackson issued commissions creating a temporary government for Pensacola. Dr. James C. Bronaugh, his long-time friend and personal physician, was named resident physician and president of the board of health. He served with Jackson in the War of 1812 and became assistant surgeon-general in the American Army. Jackson chose Dr. John. V. D. Voorhees as health officer for the military post. As in St. Augustine, Pensacola's Board of Health consisted of the resident physician and members of the city council.

Within a week after establishment the Pensacola Board held two meetings, the first on July 21 with Dr. Bronaugh presiding and Dr. John Brosnaham, a native of Catskill, New York, who had settled in Pensacola late in the Second Spanish Period, in attendance. Using power conferred by Jackson, the Board assumed control of licensing physicians to practice in Pensacola and vicinity. Applications were to be submitted to the Board "and if two thirds of the members were satisfied that he (the applicant) is qualified, and that he is of correct moral character, he shall be licensed accordingly on paying to the Secretary the sum of five dollars." The Board ordained that every physician practicing in Pensacola would be subject to a $300 fine for failure to report any case of yellow, bilious, pestilential or contagious fever under his care.

Two days later the Board found itself in the somewhat awkward position, or dubious procedure, of issuing licenses to Dr. Bronaugh and Dr. Brosnaham. The local newspaper reported: "Dr. James C. Bronaugh, President of the Board of Health, being desirous of applying for permission to practice medicine, George Bowie, Esq., was called to the chair. . . whereupon James C. Bronaugh, M.D., presented his diploma from the University of Pennsylvania, which was deemed sufficient, and was thereupon issued a license to practice medicine in the City of Pensacola. Dr. Bronaugh then resumed the chair." The Board then examined the credentials of Dr. Brosnaham and licensed him to practice. He became a prominent citizen and practiced in Pensacola until his death in 1871. Similarly Dr. John V. D. Voorhees, having presented his medical diploma from the University of New York, was granted a license. Some six weeks later the Board examined the application of a fourth physician, Dr. Christopher Y. Fonda, and voted its approval.

To make certain that the people of Pensacola understood the degree of authority vested in the Board, Governor Jackson, "in order to remove all doubts respecting the power of the Board of Health," decreed that "the Board of Health possess free power to regulate the practice of medicine in the city of Pensacola, and to establish rules and regulations for that purpose, and grant licenses to such persons as may be found qualified to practice." He also approved the addition of Drs. Moses R. Elliott and Ayers P. Merrill, of the U.S. Army post, to the Board of Health.

The St. Augustine newspaper was less diligent in reporting transactions of the Board of Health. Its licensing function is not mentioned but no doubt such responsibility existed since the general ordinances of St. Augustine and Pensacola were identical. The St. Augustine Board was empowered to "make, and from time to time to alter, such laws and regulations as they may deem necessary to ensure the health of the City."

Only three references to actions of the St. Augustine Board survive. Dr. Micah Stone, a Board member, was authorized on November 23, 1821, to declare that the epidemic (yellow fever) had ended. Earlier the Board is reported to have issued two resolutions demanding the removal of the old Spanish Hospital from the center of the city. But licensed or not, some seven or eight physicians are believed to have practiced in St. Augustine and its environs in 1821.

Local Epidemics

Control of membership in the medical profession was important but the acuteness of problems arising from the periodic recurrence of yellow fever and kindred ailments superseded it. Local newspapers, inclined throughout the 19th century to minimize or even conceal the seriousness of local epidemics, provide only minimal information of the onslaughts of fevers. Evidence indicates that St. Augustine and Pensacola were hit hard in the summer and fall of 1821. Dr. Benjamin B. Strobel of Charleston, who investigated the yellow fever epidemic threatening St. Augustine in 1857, reported interviews with Dr. William H. Simmons, a native of Charleston, who was present during the 1821 epidemic. Simmons recalled St. Augustine as "a Filthy place" due in some degree to failure of the Spanish, anticipating removal to Cuba, to maintain police regulation which, combined with heavy rains and intense heat of the late summer, accounted for the severity of the epidemic.

Boards of Health in both towns implementing broad powers granted by Governor Jackson designated quarantined grounds and appointed health officers. The Pensacola Board passed an ordinance (in September) detailing quarantine arrangement of the harbor, specifying duties of the resident physician and health officer as well as fines and penalties or violation of the health code. Effective immediately the health officer would meet all incoming vessels at the quarantined area to prevent "the introduction of contagious diseases into the city." The resident physician's tasks included visiting the sick and quarantined vessels, directing disposal of rubbish, enforcing health regulations, and reporting matters which required official action regularly to the Board of Health.

The following year the appointed Legislative Council of the Territory held its first session, convening on July 22, in spite of the delayed arrival of some members of the East Florida delegation. Dr. Bronaugh was elected president the next day.

The Council's agendum was overwhelming, in many instances problems were unique and guidelines did not exist. Proceedings were interrupted by appearance of yellow fever which caused a general exodus from the city. The entire Council, removed to a presumed safer place, the plantation of Don Manuel Gonzalez some 16 miles north of Pensacola, drafted and passed an act providing "against the introduction of contagious diseases, and for the establishment of Boards of Health in the Cities of Pensacola and St. Augustine," to which Governor Duval affixed his signature on September 2, ironically the day of Dr. Bronaugh's death.

The Legislative Council repealed the 1822 act (in June 1823) and passed another empowering the boards of health in both cities to pass "all quarantine laws and to make such regulations for the preservation of health of their respective cities as may seem to them good and proper." The measure reconstituted the boards to consist of the aldermen and "a resident Physician, to be appointed annually by the Mayor and Aldermen on the first day of May. . . . *The Resident Physician shall be ex officio* President of the Board of Health." This act was the first to be passed by the Council at the session in 1823 but was vetoed by Governor Duval because he may have been reluctant to allow appointive power to be removed from his control. The veto was immediately overridden by the requisite majority in the Council.

The experiences of St. Augustine and Pensacola provided the basic patterns for public health and medical regulation as other towns sought charters of incorporation. Those for the inland towns did not specify the details of regulation and did not include provisions for quarantine. Regulation was discretionary within the town councils of Marianna, Quincy, Chattahoochee and Newnansville; on the other hand, the charters of Magnolia (Leon County), Key West, St. Joseph and St. Marks contained provisions for quarantine regulation, setting forth the councils' duties, responsibilities and powers to impose quarantines and pass ordinances for protection of the inhabitants.

Licensing

The licensing of medical practitioners could not continue exclusively with St. Augustine and Pensacola boards of health. Settlers were increasing in number and counties between the Suwannee and Apalachicola rivers were experiencing notable population growth. Gadsden, Leon, Jefferson, Madison and Jackson (west of the Apalachicola) were becoming an area of plantations and large farms owned by physicians or planters whose sons became physicians. The Legislative Council late in 1824 required persons desirous of practicing medicine to file, in the office of the clerk of the county court in the county in which he intended to practice, a diploma issued by "some college or university" and a certificate of moral character, whereupon a license would be granted.

Unable to produce a diploma, the practitioner could qualify by filing a certificate showing that he had studied physic or surgery for two years either at a college or under the supervision of a reputable physician or surgeon. That fact having been established, any two county judges at their discretion could grant a license to practice. Fraudulent certification was subject to a fine not to exceed $500.

The act of 1824 remained in force less than four years and was superseded on January 5, 1828, by legislation conceived apparently to raise certification standards and centralize controls over the medical profession. Why the previous act was deemed inadequate is unknown. It may be that conscientious physicians, especially those in the Tallahassee area, feared that clerks in less populated counties could not be trusted to maintain acceptable standards. At any rate, the new law established a medical board for the entire Territory with the responsibility for examining all candidates for practice and issuing licenses to those qualified. Named to the Board by the act were physicians: Richard Weightman and William E. Simmons of St. Augustine, Robert Lacy of Key West, William D. Price and Lewis Willis of Tallahassee, Malcolm Nicholson of Gadsden County, William P. Hort of Jackson County and Christopher T. Fonda and John Brosnaham of Pensacola.

The medical board was to convene annually in Tallahassee, commencing on the second Monday in December, *with any three members constituting a quorum.* In hindsight the effectiveness of controls is questionable since any applicant presenting a diploma from some "regularly established medical university within the United States, and a certificate of moral character, shall, in all instances" be licensed without further examination. Whenever the Board was not in session each member could examine an applicant and issue a license to practice, such action being subject to review at the next regular session of the Board. The cost of the license was $10. No provision was made for reimbursing Board members for expenditures incurred in attending meetings.

An amending act of November 1828 changed the annual meeting of the Board to the third Monday in October and added as members Alfred Guthrie of St. Augustine, Henry S. Waterhouse of Key West, Thomas Munroe of Tallahassee, John J. T. Wilson of Gadsden County, and John Porter Lockhart and Harris B. Crews of Jackson County, all physicians. The members previously appointed were retained.

In spite of the efforts of a few dedicated physicians to organize a viable professional society, and notwithstanding the apparent willingness of the Legislative Council to provide legal foundations for public health controls and a responsible licensing system for medical practitioners, the results were minimal. The hardships of travel and difficulty of communication among settlements, spread sparsely from Pensacola around the Keys and up the east coast to Fernandina, discouraged doctors from participating in the professional organization. Besides, some practitioners of dubious qualification may have been reluctant to invite close professional scrutiny. Whatever the explanation the legislative act of February 10, 1831, repealing the acts of 1828, indicated the failure of efforts toward self-regulation, and represents to some degree a retrogression into a casual and haphazard system of health and medical regulation.

Significantly the Act of 1831 stated that

". . . any individual desirous of practicing medicine and surgery in the **Territory of Florida** shall be enabled to do so by pursuing one of the following methods. . . First he [shall] file in the office of the county court of the county in which he may intend to reside, a diploma from some medical college. . . Secondly, or he shall file in the office of the aforesaid, a certificate, signed by at least two practicing physicians, residing in this Territory, who shall be regular graduates of some medical college. . . Thirdly, or he shall file in the office aforesaid a certificate signed by some Professor of a medical college, that they (sic) have attended one course of lectures in some one of the medical colleges aforesaid, and also a certificate from one of the physicians aforesaid."

The rash of medical colleges appearing in many parts of the United States during the decades of the 1820s and 1830s provides some understanding of the possible consequences of the Act of 1831.

Corporate Organization

Having terminated the state medical board composed of responsible physicians from populous areas of the Territory and committed the licensing of physicians to the caprices of county clerks or at least to the discretion of a couple of physicians residing anywhere in the Territory the Legislative Council took no other significant action in matters of health and medicine. Physicians followed the patterns of behavior characteristic of general practice in rural America in the 19th century.

Doctor-patient relationships were highly personalized. Most physicians doubtless had a humanitarian spirit dedicated to relief of suffering; it was the era of the all-night vigil at the bedside. Many physicians became civic leaders and involved in the political life of their localities. Newspapers frequently reported participation by physicians in party organization. Many engaged in church activities which included the pulpit. A few turned to intellectual pursuits as naturalists and popularizers of science, for example, Dr. John Gorrie of Apalachicola, wrote columns of medical advice.

There can be no doubt that some physicians were woefully unprepared, even by the standards of the times, to practice. They were surely insensitive to the ethical restrictions imposed upon members of their profession; yet within the milieu created by such acts as that of 1831 little could be done to disbar the incompetent or the outright quack.

For the years 1831 to 1845, legislation on medical matters was of little importance. Such subjects as inoculation for smallpox, fees for attendance upon prisoners, protection of physicians from the attachment of their professional equipment, and organization of army medical personnel emerged from time to time; little more. Physicians in some counties and towns, however, were mindful of their responsibility for observing ethical behavior and acceptable standards of practice. For example, in 1833 Tallahassee physicians published a list of fees which they regarded as reasonable, pledging themselves not to exceed these rates.

Throughout these years of apparent indifference to medical needs a few physicians recognized the necessity for a corporate organization committed to the highest ideals of their profession: advancement of medical science, protection of the public's health, decent standards of practice, and service as the advisory voice of medicine in the town councils and territorial legislature. Origin of the impetus is difficult to determine. Census schedules and professional cards among newspaper advertisements of the 1830s and 1850s show that many physicians were entering Florida each year. Some of them, recent medical college graduates, had high ideals and deep concerns for their commitment. others had been affiliated with professional associations elsewhere and were cognizant of the benefits.

State Medical Society

Whatever the motivations, the consequences were evident by early 1848 when a small group of physicians from Leon and neighboring counties gathered in Quincy on May 14 and 15 with the purpose of establishing a state medical society. Present were:

Gadsden County—Richard Jarrot, Jean H. Verdier, William Booth, James L. Shields and David L. White
Leon County—James S. Bond, George W. Betton, and James Henry Randolph
Jefferson County—John L. Call and B. Waller Taylor
Calhoun County—J. M. G. Hunter
Jackson County—E. D. Graffenreid

The Quincy *Times* of May 20 reported: "The Professors of Medicine of this State held a convention in this place on Monday and Tuesday last. The assemblage was not too large, but we think their action will have a good effect upon the profession."

At the session on the 15th Dr. Booth was elected president pro tem pending meeting of the legislature the following December when a charter was expected to be approved and a permanent organization launched. Elected as interim vice presidents were DeGraffenreid, Shields, Bond, Taylor and White who were to serve also as a correspondence committee. As a final action, the group resolved to meet in Tallahassee on the first Monday in January 1849 when it was assumed that the legislature would have authorized incorporation. It was anticipated that physicians from all parts of the state would convene for an auspicious launching of the organization upon being appraised of objectives and receipt of the proper invitations.

As time for the meeting drew near the corresponding committee appealed to colleagues by newspaper columns and personal letters. In mid-November several newspapers published the persuasive plea of Dr. White to his "professional brethren" stating the necessity for a State Medical Society. His arguments were cogent and clear.

> The subscriber, one of the Vice Presidents, and of the corresponding committee, would beg leave to call the attention of his professional brethren, and urge upon them the necessity of a State Medical Society. Convinced he is of the importance of such an institution at the present moment it would tend to elevate the profession and to vast improvement in the healing art. Far removed, as we are here, from access to large libraries, and intercourse with learned, able and practical men of high standing in the profession, we are called upon from high consideration of responsibility to unite in exertions to free from the aspersions cast upon it by charlatans and superficial men.
>
> "While it is acknowledged that European physicians do surpass, in classical education, and in variety, depth and extent of erudition, many of us—yet in acuteness of penetration and promptness of remedial resource, in the use of means that are accurately adapted to the end, in the treatment of diseases of our climate, we are perhaps not as deficient as many would suppose. . . . A large proportion of those who toil in the profession among us are so situated as to command few of the ordinary advantages enjoyed in large and populous cities by the profession, and they are hence driven mainly upon their own resources. Our minds, not enfeebled by an undue reverence for authority of system, we are, I hope, open to the reception of new impressions and eliciting new lights. It is important that we watch, interrogate and scrutinize nature as exhibited in the morbid state. Thus did Hippocrates, Sydenham, and others whose names are immortalized in the pages of medical history.

". . . Let us therefore unite our best efforts and endeavors to introduce into the study and practice of physic that high and refined degree of reason and philosophy, without which it is so far from affording useful aid that it becomes in reality a public scourge.

". . . The uncertainty and even inutility of medicine is the favorite cant among men who enjoy robust health, among incurable patients, and among that portion of our fraternity who avail themselves of it as a shelter from the reproach of their ignorance and blunders. With all the imperfections and uncertainty, medicine can still justly claim a body of principles and doctrines eminently entitled to confidence. If we could suppose it to be otherwise, and believe it incapable of being reduced to rules and principles, it would be unlike all other arts; those who practice it would degenerate into a herd of visionaries, empirics and imposters, and instead of being protected, they ought not even to be tolerated by a wise government. If it were possible, therefore, to set medicine aside as a science and art, it would still be impossible to suppress the instinctive feelings of mankind, and of consequence a much greater number of victims would be sacrificed to the pretensions of ignorance and cupidity.

"Permit me to way in conclusion, the standard of hope is planted in the citadel of death—let us, then, as a body on the first Monday in January next, in the city of Tallahassee, assemble and unite in organizing, in order to counteract the ravages of death."

This letter bearing the signature of Dr. David L. White Sr. appeared in the Tallahassee *Sentinel* of November 14, 1848.

The Florida General Assembly convened on November 27. The following day the *Sentinel* noted that application was being made requesting an act to incorporate a Medical Society for the State of Florida. The bill was drafted under the title, "An Act Relating to Practitioners of Medicine," and entrusted to Nicholas A. Long of Jackson County for presentation to the House of Representatives. It was announced on December 13 and read by Long on December 22. A second reading came the next day. Immediately following the third and final reading on December 28, a member moved for referral to the committee of the whole for consideration of a special amendment. The move was defeated 19 to 12 with Long voting against. The vote on the bill followed and it was defeated 18 to 12 with Long voting affirmatively. This occurred four days prior to the convention of physicians and if any arrived neither of the Tallahassee newspapers took notice of them nor was the bill's defeat reported.

There is no explanation for the action of the House. Reports of the Quincy meeting the previous May contain no clues as to the provisions of the proposed charter. The emphasis is upon the "great necessity of a State Medical Society. . . for the protection of the rights of the people." The bill introduced into the House of Representatives may have been drafted by members of the Quincy Group or possibly the corresponding committee in consultation with Long who, having committed himself to support the bill, was opposed to any amendments which might reduce its effectiveness or alter its contents. Perhaps they preferred to retain the lax and permissive licensing system authorized by the Act of 1831.

Then came a conspiratorial move in the Senate. The day prior to defeat of the bill in the House, Senator Robert J. Floyd of Gadsden County announced that he planned to introduce a bill entitled "An Act to Incorporate the Florida Medical Society." The day following defeat of the House bill, Floyd read a bill entitled "An Act to Incorporate the Medical Board of Florida." Waiving rules of procedure the Senate permitted immediate second and third readings, then approved the bill 13 to 1, with only Senator William A. Forward of St. Augustine opposed. It passed the House unanimously on January 3 and received the Governor's approval on January 6. Since a copy of the House bill has not been located, the two cannot be compared. Therefore, determining the bases for its defeat is not possible.

The Senate bill was unusual in several respects. The first section includes the names of ten physicians, who, with their associates and successors, constituted "a body corporate, under the name and style of the Medical Board of Florida." All licensed physicians practicing in the state apparently were eligible for membership for the fifth section of the Act states that "all licensed physicians in this State shall be entitled to admission into the said Medical Board, upon complying with the constitution and by-laws prescribing the terms of admission, unless two thirds of the whole society shall object to such admission."

Employment of the word society in this instance appears to be of some significance. The legislature created a professional association, not a mere administrative board, whatever its limitations. Five physicians present at the Quincy Convention—Jarrot, DeGraffenreid, Booth, Betton and Taylor–were omitted from the list of those specifically named to the Board. If all qualified physicians were eligible for admission, how can the omissions be accounted for?

More perplexing, however, is Section Four which empowered the "corporation" to "appoint five members of said board to examine all applicants for licenses to practice medicine" and "to perform the same duties that are required by the existing laws of the State, and who may grant licenses to such applicants, and the form of such licenses shall be adopted by a majority of said board." Then follows the astonishing proviso, "That nothing herein shall prevent any physician in this State from proceeding in the *manner now directed by law for the procuring of a license to practice medicine,"* an obvious reference to the Act of 1831 which was still in force. Notwithstanding creation of a medical board, association or society, authorized to examine applicants and issue licenses, any applicant could still obtain a license from any county clerk within the state. The new medical board was doomed from its creation.

The legislature, particularly the House, appeared indisposed to incorporate an effective medical society. In the 1850-51 session a Senate bill designed to bring the law of 1831 into consonance with the Medical Board Act of 1849 was approved 14 to 1 but tabled by the House after its second reading.

Having made it clear that examination and licensing of physicians was not to be entrusted exclusively to the Medical Board, the House proceeded to pass an act and a resolution which could not have endeared it to physicians. By that act, a special license to practice medicine was granted to George W. Andres of Benton County (later to become Hernando), who followed the Thomsonian Method, a system of botanics already in disrepute among regular physicians. Almost simultaneously both houses passed a resolution requiring the Medical Board of Florida to establish a fee bill for medical service and report the same, if practicable, to this, if not, to the next legislature. This order, which could not have been favorably received, was promptly ignored by physicians.

Divided into Factions

For the remainder of the antebellum period the Legislature displayed little interest in the medical profession nor did physicians seriously attempt to organize a professional association. The politics of the 1850s consumed their energies. The burning issues of the prewar years divided them into hostile fractions. Most had been in the Whig party but with its break-up after 1852, they gradually came to embrace the cause of secession and the Confederacy. With the coming of war many became involved in military medicine.

There is no evidence that the Medical Board of 1849 ever became a viable professional society. It seems to have languished for lack of support and from its inception to have been hopelessly moribund. Infrequently the legislature dealt with minor matters such as setting rates for physicians attending prisoners, offering testimony at coroners' inquests, and tightening the laws relating to quarantine. It was not a time for progressive legislation in public health and medical education. Aside from secondary concerns, little was accomplished.

Florida must await the arrival of another group of conscientious practitioners under the leadership of Abel S. Baldwin and R. P. Daniel of Jacksonville, George W. Betton and R. B. Burroughs of Leon County and T. P. McHenry of Marion County, who were instrumental in founding the Florida Medical Association in 1874, which marked the beginning of constructive legislation designed to improve the quality of medical practice in the state.

This introduction provides an overview of the conditions of medical practice in 19th century Florida, but in order to more thoroughly understand it, the many individuals must also be considered who dedicated their lives to the health and well-being of their fellow settlers. They were generally an independent lot who, besides their essential role as physician, often made other important contributions to their communities. No doubt there were scoundrels and scallywags among them, as there are in any population, but on the whole they should be remembered for the safety and security they brought the newly emerging state.—EAH

A Biographical Register

Abadie, Eugene Hilarian, Army Surgeon, 1814-1874

Dr. Abadie was born in France about 1814. The record of his migration to America has not been located but he was awarded the M.D. degree by the University of Pennsylvania in 1833, having presented a thesis entitled "Epilepsy."[1] He entered the Medical Corps of the United States Army in 1836 with the rank of Assistant Surgeon[2] and was assigned to service in connection with removal of the Creek Indians from their lands in Georgia. His service with the army in Mexico during the Mexican War apparently earned him promotion to the rank of Surgeon.[3] He served with the Northern Army throughout the Civil War and on July 28, 1866, was appointed Assistant Medical Purveyor,[4] an assignment which he relinquished on March 4, 1867, to return to the rank of Surgeon. He died in St. Louis, Missouri, on December 12, 1874.

Dr. Abadie's Florida practice was apparently confined to a brief period in 1846 when he was stationed in Pensacola as assistant army surgeon. In this capacity he was a member of a five-man Board of Medical Officers (Army and Navy) meeting at the Pensacola Naval Hospital on November 2.

1. University of Pennsylvania, Archives, Medical Records.
2. *The Medical Department of the United States Army from 1775 to 1873,* Washington, 1873, p. 292. The commission was issued July 4, 1836, and shows him to have been a resident of Pennsylvania.
3. Ibid., p. 288. The promotion came on July 24, 1853.
4. Ibid., p. 287.

Abernathy, J.G., Jackson County, 1860

Dr. Abernathy was born about 1830 in Tennessee. He appears to have practiced medicine in Jackson County just prior to outbreak of the Civil War. The 1860 Census lists him as a member of the household of William Miller, a farmer living outside Marianna.[1]

1. U.S. Census, 1860, Jackson County, Item 803.

Addison, Joseph, Hillsborough County, 1840

Dr. Addison has been identified as one of several persons who moved to the Tampa area of Hillsborough County following the panic of 1837 which financially ruined many families of the plantation section of Florida (Leon, Gadsden, Madison and Jefferson Counties). Since he is not listed in the census of 1850 and subsequent years, it is assumed that he did not long practice medicine in Florida.[1]

1. Karl H. Grismer, *Tampa,* St. Petersburg, 1950, p. 98.

Adkins, Isaac Leonard, Army Surgeon, Miami, 1850

Dr. Adkins, a native of Delaware, was commissioned Assistant Surgeon in the United States Army on November 23, 1849. Within a few weeks he was dispatched to Florida to become medical officer of the detachment of troops at the garrison on the Miami River. It was a small group commanded by Major

Francis Woodbridge, the total complement being 51 men. The census of 1850 designates him as "surgeon to the Garrison at the Miami River." He is presumed to have remained at this post until his resignation from military service on October 9, 1852. Nothing further is known of him.[1]

1. Francis B. Heitman, *Historical Register and Dictionary of the United States Army*, Washington, D.C., 1903, I. 154, U.S. Census, 1850, Dade County, Florida, p. 169.

Agnew, Enoch W., Marion County, 1823

Dr. Agnew, one of numerous South Carolinians who settled in Marion County in the mid-19th century, was born in Abbeville District in 1823.[1] After attending local school and serving an apprenticeship in the office of his father, Dr. Enoch Agnew, he matriculated at the Medical College of the State of South Carolina, Charleston, in the fall of 1843. He was granted the Doctor of Medicine degree in March 1845, having submitted a thesis bearing the title "Morbid Effects of Intemperance on the Animal Economy."[2]

After a few years of practice in his native state Dr. Agnew moved to Marion County, bringing with him sufficient resources for the purchase of a fairly large acreage west of Ocala in the vicinity of Juliette and Cotton Plant.[3] Subsequently he became more businessman than physician. His success in land speculation was phenomenal. More profitable, however, were certain other ventures. After rejecting an offer to invest in phosphate mining in the Dunnellon area, he was given a second chance when he was invited by George Baldwin of Savannah to form a competing company capitalized at $5 million.[4] Notwithstanding its competition the Agnew-Baldwin company was successful.

Equally important was Dr. Agnew's decision to build a railroad connecting Ocala with Homosassa via Dunnellon designed to provide rail transportation for the entire area but obviously to meet his own needs. Not content with these ventures, he proceeded to organize E.W. Agnew and Company, the principal component of which was banking. Other enterprises included a general merchandise store and Ocala Gas and Fuel, organized in 1891 in partnership with other local investors. The store had only a brief period of success.[5]

In somewhat less than a philanthropic gesture, in 1894 Dr. Agnew loaned the city of Ocala $5,133 to purchase a plot of land on which to construct a jail, a loan secured by city scrip. In September that year he revealed a trace of philanthrophy by donating "a plot of land large enough for a Church (Methodist) and a parsonage."[6]

Dr. Agnew's luck, however, was beginning to sour. In October 1894 he was listed among the county's delinquent taxpayers, although the unpaid amount was trivial.[7] Four months later the delinquent tax list included several properties belonging to him and his brother Sam.[8] In October 1895 a court action brought by D.C.W. Smith resulted in a judgment against Dr. Agnew for $11,213 plus court costs.[9] It is apparent from the columns of the Ocala *Banner* that by 1895 Dr. Agnew had become the target of widespread criticism and apparently had lost the trust of his fellow townsmen.[10]

The blow which virtually destroyed him was a court case in 1897 resulting from alleged violation of federal banking laws. The charge was misappropriation of funds. The ensuing trial resulted in conviction and a sentence of five years. He was sent to the federal prison in Columbus, Ohio.

On June 17, 1900, the Ocala *Banner* in a column headlined, "Agnew Gets a Reprieve," reported: "The ex-banker and merchant will soon be able to come home. Mrs. Agnew has been notified that her husband's sentence has been commuted to three years instead of five. This will give him his liberty and restore him to citizenship on the eighth day of next March."

The Columbus (Ohio) *Daily Citizen*, on learning that Dr. Agnew was soon to be released, commented: [11]

> Enoch W. Agnew, former president of a Florida bank but now the prison clerk at the subsistence office of the penitentiary, received word today that his five-year sentence has been commuted by President McKinley to three years. This will release him next March. Mr. Agnew was a wealthy man one evening but the next morning he was worse than a pauper, the frosts having completely ruined him in a few brief hours. His misfortune was a technical violation of the banking laws rather than a crime.

The Ocala *Banner*, reflecting the interest and anxiety of the town, made certain that the return of Dr. Agnew was well reported. After repeating the circumstances which had brought about imprisonment, it stated that he had left Columbus on Thursday morning, March 7, at two o'clock and arrived home at two o'clock p.m., Friday, March 8, over the Plant (R.R.) System. Only a few, however, knew of his coming and no one was present to grasp his hand.[12] The *Banner* further reported:

> He looks the picture of health. . .weighs fully twenty pounds more. . .the ex-banker's face had a distressed look, and to those who spoke to him and shook him by the hand he made no response. . . Mr. Agnew's family, not knowing which road he would arrive over, one daughter went to the Florida Central and Peninsular Station, the other to the Plant System station.

Finally, on March 10, the *Banner* having presumably interviewed Dr. Agnew made the following report:

> Mr. Agnew reports only the kindest treatment from his keepers at the Columbus, Ohio, penitentiary. They gave him every freedom and privilege consistent with the rules of the prison. While he was such a model prisoner, he won admiration and respect. . . .As a member of the clerical staff he was given sleeping comforts outside the prison walls. . . .When Mr. Agnew left for home he was presented with a fine suit of clothes, $5, and a through ticket.

The last years of Dr. Agnew's life were spent in semiretirement. His son, Enoch W., Jr., had shown exceptional business acumen, becoming the proprietor of a successful general merchandising establishment in Ocala. The doctor, although no longer active in either medicine or business, continued to enjoy the fellowship of his old friends in the town as well as the company of his son and grandchildren. Apparently the poor judgment he had exhibited in connection with the Ocala bank was forgiven. His tragedy was summed up in the following statement:

> It is the story of an intelligent man who was the victim of his own overweening ambition and the vicissitudes of economic change.

1. The date of this extrapolation is from the Census of 1860, Marion County, Florida.
2. Charleston *Mercury*, March 12, 1845, List of Graduates and Theses.
3. J. Lester Dinkins, Dunnellon: Boom Town of the 1890s, St. Petersburg: Great Outdoors Publishing Co., 1969, p. 45. For substantial information relating to the Agnew investments, Mr. Dinkins' book is the main source.

4. Ibid., pp. 120-121.
5. Ocala *Banner*, issue of June 29, 1891.
6. Ibid., June 4, 1894. See also ibid, June 5, 1894; also ibid., September 28, 1894.
7. Ibid., Several issues of the newspaper in February and March 1894.
8. Ibid.
9. Issues of the *Banner*, October 1895.
10. On April 2, 1895, the *Banner* reported a "fist and skull fight" which occurred on the front porch of Ocala House between Dr. Agnew and Judge W.S. Bullock. The fracas apparently had arisen out of disparaging remarks made by Dr. Agnew about the Judge. Bystanders broke up the fight before any damage was done by either party.
11. The comment of the Columbus paper, the *Daily Citizen*, was printed in the Ocala *Evening Star*, January 20, 1900.
12. Ibid., March 9, 1900. In this issue the *Evening Star* chose to provide its readers with a resume of the whole unpleasant affair. Under the headline "Free and at Home," it was reported that he was cordially received.

Agnew, Washington, Marion County, 1826

Dr. Agnew, member of a prominent South Carolina family,[1] was born in Abbeville District in 1826. He moved to Marion County in the middle 1850s, purchased land west of Ocala and settled into the life of planter and physician. He had begun his medical education in the office of Abbeville physician, Enoch Agnew, probably an uncle, who had graduated from the Medical College of South Carolina in 1830. Dr. Agnew enrolled in the same institution in the fall of 1844, and in the spring of 1846 was graduated Doctor of Medicine. His thesis topic was "Insanity."[2]

According to marriage records of Marion County, Dr. Agnew was married to Mary E. Oakes on January 12, 1857. They had two children, Elizabeth and Samuel. His property was valued at about $27,000 in 1860 and his slaves numbered 13. Nothing further is known of either him or his family.[3]

1. A search through the 1850 census of Abbeville District, South Carolina, revealed several Agnew families, all residing in the Saluda Regiment section. It is also shown that the Christian names, Enoch and Samuel, were of common occurrence in the family. Most of the families appear to have been fairly well off.
2. U.S. Census, 1860, Marion County, Florida, item 345. This lists Dr. D. Oates, a native of North Carolina, as a resident in the Agnew home. He was probably a brother of Mrs. Agnew.
3. Since Dr. Agnew is not listed in the Marion County census of 1870, it is assumed that he had returned to South Carolina.

Aiken, Edward, Tallahassee, 1831

Dr. Aiken was one of a surprising number of physicians who migrated to Florida in the early years of the Territorial Period only to fall victim to diseases of the area. He is thought to have arrived in Tallahassee in 1830 but too late to have been listed in the census of that year. In November 1830 he announced the location of his office at the southwest corner of Washington Square directly opposite the Land Office.[1] He was not long in entering public life. On January 23, 1831, he was the chairman of a meeting assembled to organize a Florida Education Society for the educational improvement of the Territory.[2]

In April 1831 Dr. Aiken announced that "in consequence of an outbreak of smallpox in Georgia he had procured some fresh vaccine matter" and was prepared to vaccinate.[3]

Nothing further is known of him until December 1831 when his wife, Jane, posted notice that she had qualified as administrix of the estate of Dr. Aiken, deceased.[4] In early January 1832 Dr. John A. Craig, physician, announced that he was moving into the office previously occupied by Dr. Aiken.[5]

Although procedures for settlement of the Aiken estate were promptly under way in early 1832, there appears to have been a lengthy delay before the matter was concluded. On May 10, 1834, Robert J. Hackley, prominent auctioneer of Tallahassee, entered legal claims against the estate.[6] Meanwhile Mrs. Aiken had sought and obtained relief through the Legislative Council of the Territory on grounds that "her husband, Edward Aiken, in his lifetime, rendered professional services to prisoners in the Leon County Jail." She was awarded $9.50.[7]

1. Tallahassee *Floridian and Advocate*, November 9, 1830.
2. Ibid., February 10, 1831.
3. Tallahassee *Florida Courier*, April 21, 1831.
4. Tallahassee *Floridian*, December 17, 1831. Lacunae in this paper, November 1, 1831-December 27, 1831, make it impossible to establish the precise date of Dr. Aiken's death.
5. Ibid., January 16, 1832.
6. Ibid., May 31, 1834.
7. This action by the Council on February 5, 1833, was approved by Governor Duval on February 9th, Ibid., April 20, 1833.

Alba, Edwin Mason, St. Augustine, 1825-1893

Dr. Alba spent only the last few years of his life in Florida. Born in Knoxville, Pennsylvania, on August 5, 1825, he was a graduate of the Vermont Medical College, Woodstock, Vermont, class of 1849.[1] After several years of practice in the North[2] he moved to St. Augustine in the 1870s accompanied by his wife, Laura; son, William E.; and nephew, George Alba,[3] who became a clerk in the drug store owned by Dr. Alba. The family resided on Hospital Street.

On recommendation of the St. Johns County Medical Society Dr. Alba was accepted for membership in the Florida Medical Association at its meeting in St. Augustine in May 1887.[4] This indicates that he had resumed practice. He continued to pay dues to the Association and was a member in good standing at the time of his death on October 29, 1893.[5] He was buried on the following day in the New Augustine Cemetery.

1. Frederick C. Waite, *The Story of a Country Medical College, History of Vermont Medical College*, 1827-1856, Montpelier, 1945, p. 157.
2. He probably practiced in New York State, his wife and son having been native New Yorkers.
3. U.S. Census, 1880, St. Johns County.
4. Proceedings, Florida Medical Association, 1887, Jacksonville, p. 3. See Ibid., Jacksonville 1893, p. 43.
5. Parish Records, Trinity Episcopal Church, St. Augustine, "Burials," p. 20.

Aldrich, Edward S., Newnansville, 1811-post 1870

Of all the physicians who practiced in 19th century Florida, none were more elusive, restless and peripatetic than Dr. Aldrich. Notwithstanding his professional skill and fine reputation which enabled him to live comfortably, he appears always to have been seeking "greener pastures" or a change of scene, often to the dismay of his gentle and patient wife. The letters exchanged among Mrs. Aldrich's family chart his continuous wanderings.

Dr. Aldrich was born in St. Mary's, Georgia, on August 12, 1811, son of Dr. Whipple Aldrich (1782-1852),[1] respected St. Mary's physician and prosperous landowner, native of Rhode Island, under whose preceptorate young Edward probably began the study of medicine. The Aldrich family lived in St. Mary's but had extensive holdings outside the town.[2] After his early education in St. Mary's Edward enrolled at the Medical College of South Carolina, Charleston, from which he was graduated in March 1833 after submitting a thesis bearing the title "Dysentery."[3] He appears to have returned immediately to St. Mary's to begin practice.

In December 1835, with little more than two years' experience, he announced that he had chosen "a permanent location in Jacksonville, Duval County, Florida," and was prepared to offer services in medicine, surgery and obstetrics from his residence and office in the home of I.D. Hart.[4] Within a few days, following a series of Indian raids on white settlements in Alachua and adjoining counties and more particularly the Dade Massacre of December 3, the Second Seminole War erupted and Dr. Aldrich interrupted his practice to join a unit of volunteer soldiers as company surgeon.[5]

Dr. Aldrich was married to Corine Brown, daughter of the Reverend David Brown of Jacksonville, on September 26, 1837. Her sister, Ellen, in announcing the wedding to her brother, Manne, wrote: "Corine has married a very clever little chap...well-off, not rich...good-looking, not splendid, and altogether a gentleman."[6]

For the next few years the Aldrichs were seldom in one location long enough to establish an address. April 1838 found them in Macon, Georgia;[7] the following December they were in Tallahassee,[8] thence to Madison, Florida, by early 1839.[9] In June of that year they had "settled" in Suwannee Springs, Columbia County, where according to Mrs. Aldrich, "Edward's business continues good." She added, however, "He was kicked by a horse, which broke two ribs, but he is better now." Scarcely had this news been transmitted to other members of the family when Ellen wrote: "Corine and Edward are about leaving (Suwannee Springs) with the intention of going to Newnansville, another squatting place in the Territory. Why leave Suwannee, I don't know..."[11]

A short while later Mrs. Aldrich wrote at length to Manne: "You see that Edward and I have again moved...Prospects much brighter here...quarters more comfortable, present business more active. Edward has been here about a month and has already booked better than $500. He expects to do better next month as the season advances (and) there is more sickness. I have been to Llangollen...[12] I am glad to get back to Newnansville with its stumps, log cabins and vegetable gardens." She then expressed concern about the growing intensity of the Indian War, hoping that it might end during the coming winter. If so "this country of Alachua with its rich hammock lands must flourish."[13] A month later, however, she wrote: "Edward's practice is excellent; indeed that is all that reconciles one to Newnansville."[14]

Dr. Aldrich and his brother, Charles, opened a mercantile business in Newnansville in January 1840, financed by the doctor and managed by Charles. Meanwhile the army was setting up a headquarters nearby which, it was expected, would provide sufficient custom to insure a profitable business. In addition, Dr. Aldrich found his medical services in great demand among the small detachments of soldiers in Alachua and Marion Counties. Corine wrote on January 26, 1840: "This is a city of logs...Edward has very sick patients...cannot leave them now. He has just returned from Ft. Clarke, twelve miles away, where there are many ill with scarlet fever. Edward is doing well."[15]

By the spring of 1840 Mrs. Aldrich was finding life in Newnansville dull, if not intolerable. Indian atrocities were a constant threat; the war was dragging on sluggishly, due, she thought, to the incompetence of the generals. She was impatient to leave the village and "return to civilization." As she expressed it, she was "tired of the woods," although the Doctor was "making money."[16] Still they remained in Newnansville through 1840 and into 1841. With the untimely death of Charles while on a buying trip to Savannah in August 1840, Dr. Aldrich persuaded his brother-in-law, George Brown, to come to Newnansville and assume management of the store.[17]

In the meantime Dr. Aldrich was encountering difficulty in collecting fees due for his army service, a problem growing out of the remoteness of the field of conflict and the slovenly procedures of the paymaster's department as well as the fact that much of the fighting was carried on by volunteer personnel. He expressed hope that his friend, David Levy recently elected to Congress, would be able to expedite action on his behalf.[18] Besides, collecting fees in Newnansville was difficult. George Brown wrote in June 1841, (Aldrich) "has a fine practice in Newnansville, but poor pay."[19] By early September the Aldrichs had moved to St. Augustine.[20]

Still restless, Dr. Aldrich left St. Augustine in early 1842, going to Thomasville, Georgia, in search of a more favorable situation.[21] Meanwhile Mrs. Aldrich returned to Newnansville to await her next move. George Brown reported on the situation in Newnansville on April 13, 1842, appending a few medical notes: "John R. Standley has paid his bill of $20 and would like to have the prescription for his lame leg...Mr. Wilson is uneasy about his 'yard,' (a medieval English term for penis)...Alex McKay complains of worms...Stephens has boils."[22] A few days later he informed Dr. Aldrich that "Wilson and other 'ghonerdeists' (those afflicted with gonorrhea) look rather blue. They report themselves well; I doubt it."[23]

Near the end of 1842 Dr. and Mrs. Aldrich went to Washington expecting to collect $2100 owed him by the government.[24] In spite of his efforts and those of Congressman Levy, the money was not forthcoming, whereupon he employed a lawyer to press for collection.[25] Without success the Aldrichs returned to Newnansville where they remained throughout most of 1843. When the Alachua County Court convened in Newnansville in December 1842, the Judge, Marshall and Attorney General found meals and lodging with the Aldrichs. There was no hotel in the village.[26]

By mid-1844 the Aldrichs were once again residents of St. Augustine, encouraged to resettle there by removal of the town's leading physician, a man named Jones, who had moved to Key West. In her letter of July 6, 1844, Corine Aldrich expressed her delight at the excellent opportunity for her husband. She also revealed something of his practice. The case of the moment: A Negro had suffered two broken legs in a sawmill accident. Dr. Aldrich was trying to save the legs; if that should fail he would amputate in days. She added: "Now such a case in the country would add nothing to his reputation, but here it will not be lost. I have known him to perform operations in Newnansville that elsewhere would have won for him a name with the best surgeons in the land."[27]

Dr. Aldrich joined Dr. John E. Peck, one of the town's most beloved physicians, in a professional partnership in August 1844.[28] This could have been an eminently successful venture but the arrangement was terminated in early 1846 when Dr. Aldrich decided to move on. After investigating opportunities in Savannah and Macon,[29] he went to Pensacola where he appears to have prospered.[30] Mrs. Aldrich wrote on July 5, 1846: "Edward's practice is excellent...he has good clientele in the Navy and among the planters."[31] A year later she wrote: "Edward has a large business; makes a handsome living."[32]

Still dissatisfied, Dr. Aldrich moved to Key West in the winter of 1848-49. To his wife, whom he had left in Pensacola, he praised the climate of Key West and expressed optimism about his future there. He spoke disparagingly about the two other Key West physicians and expressed assurance that he would receive appointment as surgeon at the Marine Hospital, a position which paid $1200 per year. He mentioned also having met a "rich and amicable Jew from Paris, Baron Rothschild" on board the ship from Pensacola. Rothschild was en route to Havana.[33]

Mrs. Aldrich joined her husband in Key West on June 8, 1849.[34] The hospital appointment had not materialized, however, and Dr. Aldrich wrote to the Washington authorities to protest. Other members of the family had learned of his failure to get the position and in July 1849 Mrs. Aldrich's brother, George, in a letter to his brother, Manne, concluded with an opinion doubtless shared by the entire family: "The doctor will do well if he will remain settled."[35] Dr. Aldrich and his wife were outraged at his failure to gain the appointment. In a letter to her brother, Manne, she expressed her disappointment and denounced Dr. James as a man "scarcely capable of spelling his own name...a man who attempted to perform the simplest operation of lancing a child's gums and slit his tongue so that he bled to death...(a man who) spells julop (sic) with a 'g' and rat with a 'w', wrat."[36]

Forthwith Dr. Aldrich decided to leave Key West. In her next letter to Manne Mrs. Aldrich wrote: "Edward has gold fever...is about to go to California...I did not tell him not to go, although I pointed out the hardships...Ellen and I are going to St. Mary's, Georgia...I shall go to New York with Edward to see him off...Edward leaves enough funds for me for six months...If he does well in California he will send for us" (i.e., Corine and Ellen, then a widow, her husband, Lt. James W. Anderson, having been killed in Mexico).[37]

In October 1850 George Brown received a letter from Dr. Aldrich who had settled in San Francisco. Reporting this to his brother, Manne, he wrote: "I do not think he will stay there. I would not be surprised to see him home any day."[38]

Dr. Aldrich lingered in San Francisco from October 1850 until the summer of 1853, toying with the idea of bringing Corine, Ellen and Ellen's children to California. George Brown wrote in June 1853: "Dr. Aldrich has sent for Corine and Ellen and wishes them to start in July, but Corine cannot go before fall."[39] This was ominous, for Corine had been suffering for some time with an incurable ailment, very probably consumption. George Brown wrote to Corine in December: "I gather you will not leave for California until spring."[40] Corine died in New York City in November 1854.[41]

It is apparent from subsequent letters that Dr. Aldrich remained in California for several years, probably until conclusion of the Civil War. In August 1865 this notice appeared in a Jacksonville newspaper: "Dr. E.S. Aldrich, physician and surgeon, late of San Francisco, may be consulted at his office at Mrs. Hadsell's

Mansion House, or at the Drug Store of Mr. J. Jones."[42] But even then he had not concluded his wandering. The Census of 1870 lists him as a resident of Lake City, Florida, "physician," alone in his household.[43]

No better insight into the life and soul of Dr. Aldrich is likely to be gained than that from his brother-in-law, George Brown, on June 3, 1849, to his brother Manne. He wrote:[44]

> He is well-known through Florida and enjoys deservedly an excellent professional reputation. Yet nature has implanted in him such a roving disposition that he has not made his talents as profitable as he could have. I wish he had a dozen children. That would act as an anchor on him...Roving runs in the Aldrich family. His brother Louis, my roommate here for some years, recently left Florida for California, abandoning a home where he commanded the good wishes of everyone and a good law practice. Had he remained he would in all probability have been one of the candidates for Congress in the next election. Save for their faults, if faults they can be called, Dr. Aldrich and his brother also, are as fine specimens of the genus MAN as one would wish to know. Kind, generous, and polite, they have ever possessed my highest esteem...

It is easy to speculate that the failure of Dr. and Mrs. Aldrich to produce children weakened the ties that bound them. Her devotion to the children of her sister, Ellen, and her brother, George, which manifests itself in many of her letters, suggests her disappointment and perhaps a bit of envy.

For all his wanderings, splendid reputation and the high social position enjoyed by his family and himself, no trace of his final years has been discovered. It can only be said that he was last sighted in Lake City, Florida.

1. Ex information, Mrs. J.W. Bailey, St. Mary's Georgia, Letter, Novemer 4, 1983.
2. These holdings included the Borrell Plantation, joining St. Mary's on the west; Harriet's Bluff Plantation, lying on the north side of Crooked River; and a large tract (2666 acres) on the south side of Crooked River; a residence in the town of St. Mary's. Ibid.
3. Charleston *Mercury*, March 13, 1833.
4. Jacksonville *Courier*, December 17, 1835.
5. Dr. Aldrich's name has not been found on any official list of medical personnel serving in the Second Seminole War. This was not unusual, however, in remote areas where services of local physicians were contracted for informally. His army service is mentioned in several letters of 1837 and later.
6. Ellen to Manne, November 12, 1837.
7. Ellen to Manne, April 1838.
8. Ellen to Manne, December 30, 1838.
9. Ellen to Manne, February 1839.
10. Corine to Manne, June 9, 1839. Suwannee Springs, usually known as White Springs, was situated on the north side of the Suwannee River in what is now Hamilton County.
11. Ellen to Manne, July 23, 1839.
12. "Llangollen," the Brown home near Jacksonville.
13. Corine to Manne, Newnansville, August 18, 1839.
14. Corine to Manne, Newnansville, September 29, 1839.
15. Corine to Manne, Newnansville, January 26, 1840.
16. Corine to Manne, Newnansville, May 23, 1840.
17. Corine to Manne, Newnansville, August 30, 1840.
18. Corine to Manne, Newnansville, May 30, 1841.
19. George Brown to Manne, St. Mary's, Georgia, June 12, 1841.
20. Corine to Manne, St. Augustine, September 3, 1841.
21. Corine to Manne, Newnansville, March 27, 1842.
22. George to Edward Aldrich, Newnansville, April 13, 1842.
23. George to Edward Aldrich, Newnansville, April 24, 1842.
24. Corine to Manne, Washington, D.C., January 1, 1843.
25. Corine to Manne, Washington, D.C., January 6, 1843.
26. Corine to Manne, Newnansville, December 29, 1843.
27. Corine to Manne, St. Augustine, July 15, 1844.
28. St. Augustine, *Florida Herald and Southern Democrat*, July 23, 1844.
29. Corine to Manne, St. Augustine, January 12, 1846.
30. Corine to Manne, Pensacola, April 18, 1846.

31. Corine to Manne, Pensacola, July 5, 1846.
32. Corine to Manne, Pensacola, November 21, 1847.
33. Edward to Corine, Key West, January 1, 1849.
34. Corine to Manne, Key West, June 8, 1849.
35. George Brown to Manne, Newnansville, July 27, 1849.
36. Corine to Manne, Key West, August 17, 1849.
37. Corine to Manne, Key West, March 21, 1850.
38. George to Manne, Newnansville, October 22, 1850.
39. George to Manne, Newnansville, June 13, 1853.
40. George to Corine, Newnansville, December 9, 1853.
41. George to Manne, Newnansville, November 30, 1854.
42. Jacksonville *Herald*, August 11, 1865.
43. U.S. Census, 1870, Columbia County, Florida, p. 13.
44. George to Manne, Newnansville, June 3, 1849.

The principal source of information relating to Dr. Aldrich are the letters exchanged by members of the family of the Reverend David Brown, who in the 1830s and later were sojourners in Duval County, Florida. The Reverend Brown was for more than a year editor of the Jacksonville *Courier* (1838-39). The Browns originated in Utica, New York, but prior to coming to Florida had lived in Portsmouth, New Hampshire. They purchased a plantation, probably of modest proportions, near Jacksonville, which they called "Llangollen," which suggests a Welsh origin. The Brown family was connected by marriage to Dr. James Hall, thought to have been the first physician to practice in East Florida. Mrs. Hall, whose first husband was Robert Pritchard, was apparently the sister of the Reverend Brown's wife. She is repeatedly referred to in the Brown letters as "Aunt Hall." Her plantation, La Grange, was situated on the St. John's River, at Beauclerc Bluff, some four miles north of Mandarin, and about 11 miles from Jacksonville. The Brown children were frequent visitors there.

The children of the Reverend Brown, who were writers and recipients of the letters, were: Mandevillette Elihu Dering Brown (affectionately known as "Manne"), an eccentric portrait painter who, after several years of study in Paris, returned to Utica, New York, where he gained considerable renown, dying there on September 1, 1896; Ellen, wife of Lt. James Anderson; Corine, wife of Dr. Aldrich; and George L., merchant of Newnansville. These letters, which span the years 1835-54, are now in the possession of Mrs. Louis Goolsby of Gainesville, Florida, for whose kindness in permitting him to examine the letters the present writer is very grateful.

Alexander, Columbus R., Hernando County, 1824

Dr. Alexander was born in Georgia about 1824. In the late 1840s he moved with his wife, Mary, and three-year-old daughter, Sara, to Benton County (later Hernando County), Florida, settling in the Annustaliga community, some 15 miles south southeast of the present town of Brooksville.[1] There he purchased land and pursued the dual occupations of farming and practicing medicine. After the death of his wife, he remarried and fathered nine children.[2]

Owing to remoteness of the Alexander residence only scant information concerning the doctor has been preserved. Nevertheless available evidence suggests that Dr. Alexander was highly regarded throughout Hernando and neighboring counties. This is amply substantiated by his selection in 1850 as one of two county representatives at the Ocala Convention called for the purpose of discussing the forthcoming Nashville Convention at which Southern leaders were to enunciate their stand on the States Rights issue.[3] In 1853 he was instrumental in promoting the building of a railroad from some point on the St. Johns River across central Florida to Tampa Bay.[4] In January 1855, C.L. Friebele, one of Tampa's most successful merchants, contracted with Dr. Alexander to manage the Friebele business at DeSoto.[5]

The renewal of hostilities between the scattered remnants of Seminole Indians and the encroaching whites, a conflict soon to become the Third Seminole War, caused alarm in many of the remote white settlements. Although numerous makeshift forts had been established, most were inadequately manned. Therefore, when a reconnaissance party en route from Lake Okeechobee to Ft.

Myers was attacked by a small party of Indians, Florida Governor James E. Broome began mobilizing the militia, augmented by volunteers, for a major encounter.

Late in December 1855 Dr. Alexander was mustered into a militia unit commanded by Col. Whit Smith as first lieutenant and surgeon.[6] He had volunteered his services.

From this time nothing is known of Dr. Alexander except for the censuses of 1870, 1880 and the special Florida census of 1885. No census was taken for Hernando County in 1860. It is not known whether he remained with the military unit until the end of the conflict, but that seems unlikely. The Census of 1870 designates him as "physician" owning property valued at $500; 10 years later he was designated "farmer and physician," while in 1885 no occupation is indicated. The agricultural survey which was part of the 1885 census provides the following: "C.R. Alexander, 35 acres of improved land; 400 acres of unimproved land. Value of land, fences, buildings: $3,000. Livestock value: $2,000." It is apparent, therefore, that in his later years he turned to cattle-raising, with fair success.[7]

1. The date of Dr. Alexander's birth is an extrapolation from the census data. Originally Benton County was named Hernando but in March 1844 it was renamed Benton in honor of the Missouri statesman Thomas Hart Benton who had in that year gained fame and a measure of popularity for his opposition to the current Democratic slogan, "Fifty-four Forty or Fight." Six years later, however, his opposition to slavery and support of the Compromise of 1850 prompted Floridians to change Benton County back to Hernando County, an act of December 24, 1850.

2. Florida Special Census, 1885, p. 2.

3. Jacksonville *News*, May 11, 1850. The other delegate from the county was Col. B.M. Pearson who became a delegate to Nashville.

4. Jacksonville *Florida News*, April 23, 1853.

5. Tampa *Herald*, January 20, 1855. Several localities in Florida have borne the name DeSoto. This one, however, does not appear on maps of the 1850s, and appears to have been the settlement to be called Cedar Tree.

6. *Soldiers of Fortune*, Board of State Institutions, publisher, Tallahassee, 1903, p. 12.

7. Special Census, Florida, 1850, p. 2.

Allen, Joe M., Leon County, 1840

The only information about Dr. Allen comes from an obituary notice and a gravestone. He died October 30, 1840, at the home of Richard Bradford in Leon County and was buried in the Bradford Cemetery. He was a native of Union County, New Jersey, and a graduate of Princeton University, then Princeton College. Although the gravestone designates him M.D., the newspaper notice makes no mention of medical education. He was 23 years old at the time of death.

1. Tallahassee *Floridian*, November 14, 1840. Here his name is shown as Job M. Allen. The notice of his death suggests that he was a victim of consumption.

Allison, William P., Suwannee County, 1820-1879

Dr. Allison was born in Alabama in 1820.[1] In the early 1850s he moved to Suwannee County, Florida. In the brief campaign to rid Florida of the Indian threat, known at the Third Seminole War (1856-1857), he enlisted as a member of Capt. Thomas Hughey's Company but no information has survived as to his actual participation in the skirmishes. He had returned to Suwannee County by 1858 and settled in the vicinity of Houstoun, a village some six miles southeast of Live Oak. Soon, thereafter, probably in early 1859, he married a young woman known only as Sarah. The Census of 1860 lists her as aged 17 and their son, William P., Jr., as aged six months.[2]

Ten years later the Allisons were still at the same location but in the meantime another son, Humphrey, had been born.[3]

About 1871 Dr. Allison began to advertise his services as physician and surgeon to the citizens of the Live Oak community.[4] These professional notices continued to appear as late as March 1876. Three years later he died and was buried in Marybelle Cemetery some four miles west of Live Oak.

If census data are to be trusted it would appear that Dr. Allison never enjoyed more than a meager income. His personal property was valued at $500 and 10 years later it was $400. He owned five slaves in 1860.

1. The dates of Dr. Allison's birth and death are found on his gravestone in the Marybelle Cemetery.

2. U.S. Census, 1860, Suwannee County, Florida, p. 775.

3. Ibid., 1870, item 555.

4. Live Oak *Times*, March 22, 1876. This does not indicate a change of residence for Dr. Allison. Houstoun lost its post office to Live Oak a year or so earlier.

Alston, Lemuel J., Escambia County, 1828

Dr. Alston, a native of Alabama, practiced medicine in Florida only briefly. He appears to have come to the state as a young physician and settled in the community of Beelersville at the mouth of the Escambia River.[1] An obituary item gives his birthplace as Live Oak Level, Alabama, where his father was postmaster.[2]

At a Fourth of July celebration in Beelersville in 1828, Dr. Alston not only read the Declaration of Independence but gave two toasts, one honoring Andrew Jackson.[3]

Dr. Alston died on August 17, six weeks later, in Pensacola where he sought medical assistance. Although he had suffered some time from a mild intermittent fever "contracted at the brick yard at the head of (Escambia) Bay," his death was said to have been "occasioned by a cramp in the stomach." The notice of his death added that Dr. Alston had, in the brief period he had resided in the neighborhood, endeared himself to a considerable circle of friends.[4]

1. Charles Beeler owned a plantation on the south bank of the Escambia River in 1822 and attempted to promote the development of a town on a portion of his land near the mouth of the river, about eight miles from Pensacola. A settlement was established but it seems not to have flourished for there is no record of a post office having been established there. Pensacola *Floridian*, February 4, 1822, advertisement.

2. The identity of Live Oak Level has not been established; perhaps it may be present-day Oaklevel, a small community in Cleburne County near Fruithurst.

3. Pensacola *Florida Argus*, July 22, 1828; Pensacola *Gazette*, July 15, 1828.

4. Ibid., August 19, 1828; Pensacola *Florida Argus*, August 19, 1828.

Ambler, Daniel C., Jacksonville, 1798-1866

Dr. Ambler has been identified as both dentist and physician,[1] but evidence that he belonged to the latter profession has not been discovered. It is known, however, that he had a substantial dental practice in Jacksonville and on occasion would become something of an itinerant, taking his practice to surrounding towns such as St. Augustine, Alligator, Suwannee Springs, and Newnansville.[2] There can be no doubt that he was a man of broad learning and enormous talent in the areas of scientific experimentation, animal breeding and horticulture. He is said to have had the best breeds of cattle and sheep from foreign countries with the purpose of improving local herds.

Dr. Ambler is thought to have arrived in Jacksonville in the late 1840s from his native home in New Berlin, Chenango County, New York. He immediately established himself as a worthy citizen of the community by joining the congregation of St. John's Episcopal Church in the building of a new sanctuary, having contributed both time and money to the effort. He was a member of the vestry for many years, serving with the well-known physician, Dr. Abel S. Baldwin. The two became close friends.[3]

Dr. Ambler's later years were saddened by two deaths. His wife, Laura, died in June 1850 while on a visit with her brother, H. Moss, in New Berlin,[4] and three years later one of his two sons, Moss Hobart Ambler, died of consumption on March 3, 1853, at the age of 20, in New Berlin.[5] Dr. Ambler's own tragic death occurred in early April 1866 when his small boat was rammed by the steamer Sylvan Shore as he was crossing the St. Johns after dark. He had taken a New York friend, Mr. Shelton, across the river to show him some of his farming interests.[6] On the occasion of his death Dr. Baldwin, a vestryman at St. John's, offered the following resolution at the vestry meeting of April 15.[7]

> Resolved, that a page in the Journal of the Vestry be set apart for the purpose of recording thereupon the deep sense of pain and sorrow the Vestry feel for the loss of those who have for so long been members—the Honorable Samuel L. Burrett and Dr. D.C. Ambler, both having taken part in founding the infant church in our city, at all times have been liberal contributors to its support and progress, and by their lives always illustrated the benevolence and integrity of the Christian character.

1. Webster Merritt, *A Century of Medicine in Jacksonville and Duval County*, Gainesville, University of Florida Press, 1949, p. 58.
2. St. Augustine, *The Ancient City*, December 28, 1850.
3. Dr. Baldwin was closely associated with Dr. Ambler as fellow members of the vestry of St. John's Episcopal Church, and as medical practitioners.
4. Jacksonville, *Florida Republican*, October 17, 1850.
5. Ibid., May 25, 1853.
6. Tallahassee *Florida Sentinel*, April 7, 1866.
7. The Burrett mentioned here was a Connecticut-born lawyer and resident of Jacksonville.

Amos, James, Pensacola, 1860

Dr. Amos, a native of South Carolina, was a resident of Pensacola in 1860.[1] He was the only member of his household; the census lists his age as 75. Nothing further is known of him. The name Amos was not uncommon in West Florida; several families of that name were residing in Escambia and Santa Rosa Counties in 1870.

1. U.S. Census, 1860, Escambia County, p. 7.

Anders, William W., Suwannee County, 1870

Dr. Anders appears in the 1870 census of Suwannee County as a resident in the home of Emilius Calhoun of Houstoun, a village a few miles southeast of Live Oak, the county seat. He was born in South Carolina and was 37 years of age in 1870. Emilius Calhoun was Florida-born, possibly a relative of Dr. Anders who presumably was unmarried.[1]

1. U.S. Census, 1870, Suwannee County, Florida, item 538.

Anderson Sr., Andrew, St. Augustine, 1839

Although his medical career in St. Augustine spanned only four years (1829-1833), Dr. Anderson's contributions, civic, commercial, and spiritual as well as medical, to the city were significant. He was a native of New England, probably New Hampshire, who had been trained in one of the colleges there and prior to moving to Florida had practiced medicine for several years. Accompanied by his wife and possibly two daughters, he arrived in St. Augustine in 1829 and entered quickly into the public life of the city.

The early years of the American occupation, beginning in 1821, were not a period of tranquility. The Spanish Administrators, in anticipation of the transfer of the territory to the United States, had relaxed their control and lawless elements of the population took advantage of the situation. Dr. Anderson, arriving from New England, was appalled at the worldliness and impiety which he found in sharp contrast to the puritanical tone of his native state. He lost no time in aligning himself with the more responsible, even more godly, elements. Not belonging to the Catholic faith, he assumed leadership in building the Presbyterian Church.[1] He expressed shock at the drunkenness he observed on the streets and sought to combat the excessive use of alcohol which was estimated to have been at least 10,000 gallons per year. He became the first president of the Temperance Society of St. Augustine.[2] In a related action of May 1830, he organized the East Florida Bible Society and served on its Board of Directors.[3]

Equally important was Dr. Anderson's interest in the civic affairs of the town. Convinced that the commercial life could be improved he led the effort to erect a proper wharf for its harbor.[4] While serving as provisional governor of Florida in 1835 William Marvin appeared in St. Augustine on a kind of inspection tour which he mentioned in his autobiography.[5]

> I also joined a party of gentlemen, among whom were...Dr. Anderson and other gentlemen of St. Augustine, to make an exploring trip up the St. John's River (early 1836). As soon as the boat left the wharf, we were all called into the cabin, and a meeting was organized by appointing Dr. Anderson chairman...

For reasons unknown, but probably related to the need for a larger income, Dr. Anderson decided in late 1833 to discontinue medical practice.[6]

While announcing his decision he graciously recommended to his patients the services of Dr. Seth S. Peck of New York recently settled in St. Augustine, "As a gentleman who has liberal attainments, long experience and extensive practice as a physician and entitled to the patronage of the public..."[7]

Having abandoned his medical career Dr. Anderson turned to a variety of business ventures, the most noteworthy having been vice president of the Southern Life Insurance and Trust Company. His presence on the staff did much to reassure the public that ethical standards prevailed in operation of the company.[8]

Dr. Anderson was twice married. His first wife, whose name and origin are unknown, had died prior to his removal to Florida. Two daughters, Emily Constance and Hannah, had been born to this marriage. Emily became the wife of Dr. George Taylor of Columbia, South Carolina, where her death occurred on October 8, 1843. Hannah, the younger daughter, was married to Claudian B.

Northrop, their wedding having occurred on April 26, 1838.[9] They had a son, Andrew, on March 3, 1839.

Meanwhile, Dr. Anderson had married a widow, Mrs. Clarissa C. Fairbanks of Boston. To this union was born one child, a son Andrew on May 13, 1839.[10] Dr. Anderson did not long survive, dying in St. Augustine on November 7, 1839,[11] leaving a widow and an eight-month-old son, Andrew, who was destined to become a St. Augustine physician.

1. Several references to the activities of Dr. Anderson are found in *Centennial of the Presbyterian Church of St. Augustine*, privately published in St. Augustine in 1924 in observance of the one hundredth anniversary of the Church.
2. St. Augustine *East Florida Herald*, November 18, 1830.
3. Ibid., May 26, 1830.
4. St. Augustine *Florida Herald*, October 30, 1834.
5. Kevin E. Kearney, ed., Autobiography of William Marvin, *Florida Historical Quarterly*, January-April, 1958, XXXVI, 1956.
6. St. Augustine *East Florida Herald*, November 28, 1833. Dr. Anderson had been elected Alderman just two weeks prior to this announcement. Ibid., November 14, 1833.
7. Ibid., November 28, 1833.
8. St. Augustine *Florida Herald*, August 4, 1838. Dr. Anderson had served earlier as a trustee of the company. The report on its condition was signed by Mr. Anderson, Vice President. There appears to have been some uneasiness on the part of investors and clients. Controversy had developed concerning the ethics of the company, whether it was out to bilk the public and the election of Dr. Anderson as vice president is thought to have allayed such fears.
9. Ibid., April 28, 1838.
10. S. Walter Martin, Flagler's Associates in East Florida Developments, *Florida Historical Quarterly*, XXVI, No. 3, p. 256.
11. See *Centennial* cited in note 1 above for date of death and eulogy. Dr. Anderson's obituary appeared in the St. Augustine *News*, November 8, 1839, in which he is designated simply as "President, Southern Life and Trust Company, of this City."

Anderson Jr., Andrew, St. Augustine, 1839-1924

The contributions of Dr. Anderson Jr.[1] to the economic and cultural development of St. Augustine in the latter part of the 19th and early part of the 20th centuries can hardly be overestimated. He stands with Henry Flagler, whose friend and adviser he was, in imparting to the city its aura of elegance and charm which made it a mecca for tourists from many parts of the world decades before South Florida developed its attractions. While Flagler's contributions were motivated primarily by business considerations, Dr. Anderson's were more humanitarian and spiritual.

Dr. Anderson was born in St. Augustine on May 13, 1839, the only son of Dr. Andrew Anderson Sr. and his second wife, Clarissa Fairbanks of Boston. He spent his early life in St. Augustine where he received his early education. As an adolescent he was sent to a preparatory school in the East where he prepared for admission to Princeton University, from which he was graduated in 1861. A year later he matriculated at the College of Physicians and Surgeons (later to become an affiliate of Columbia University) from which he received his medical degree in 1865.[2]

As a young man Dr. Anderson traveled extensively in Europe where he became acquainted with the great art collections and where his own artistic tastes were developed. His opinions in such matters were of significance in his advice to Henry Flagler in the planning of Flagler's two elegant hotels, the Ponce de Leon and the Alcazar. Not to be overlooked were Dr. Anderson's own contributions of parks and statuary in the city.[3]

Dr. Anderson Sr. owned valuable sections of land in St. Augustine, most notably the property along King Street and extending northward. When Flagler decided to spend vast sums building hotels in the city he not only purchased a portion of the property (the main source of the Anderson wealth) but he also employed Dr. Anderson to supervise construction of both the Ponce de Leon and Alcazar. The two men became close friends. Flagler was a frequent guest at the Anderson home, Markland Place, while Dr. Anderson on several occasions was a guest at the Flagler home at Mamaroneck, New York, where yachting parties were a frequent form of entertainment.[4]

Information on Dr. Anderson's medical practice is not abundant although he is known to have devoted some of his time to it. He was one of 14 physicians in 1874 who met in the office of Dr. Abel S. Baldwin in Jacksonville to inaugurate the Florida Medical Association.[5] Henceforth, however, he was an infrequent participant in its transactions although he continued to pay annual dues and remained a member until 1898. Subsequent to 1874, however, he attended one meeting, that of 1889 in St. Augustine.[6]

Dr. Anderson is best remembered in St. Augustine for his philanthropy which was expressed in numerous ways. He was donor of two parks, Anderson Circle and Ponce de Leon. He gave generously to Flagler Hospital while serving for many years as president. As a memorial to his mother he built the Nurses Home adjacent to the hospital. The Memorial Presbyterian Church, where he worshipped and for many years served as President of the Board, was the recipient of numerous bountiful gifts. A more whimsical gift to the city were two lions carved from Carrara marble in Italy which were to be placed at the approach to the bridge across Matanzas Inlet. Another significant gift was $50,000 to the University of Florida for purchase of a pipe organ to be installed in the University Auditorium upon its completion.[7]

Dr. Anderson had deep concerns for the plight of the Negro in the South, especially in the matter of educational opportunity without which he saw little hope for improving their condition. His concern was significantly expressed by a generous gift to the Florida Normal and Industrial Institute for Negroes which was established just west of the city. His concern was symbolized by allocation of considerable space in the Presbyterian Church for the seating of Negroes at his funeral and selection of young men from the Institute to serve as pallbearers. The administration building at the Institute, Anderson Hall, was his gift.

It is apparent that Dr. Anderson did not crave public acclaim. With one exception he avoided public office; in 1886 he was elected Mayor of St. Augustine, serving for the term 1886-1887.

Dr. Anderson was married somewhat late in life to Mary Elizabeth Smethurst, the wedding occurred on January 29, 1895. She was 24 years younger than her husband. The wedding which took place in the Saint Augustine Episcopal Church was attended by Mr. and Mrs. Henry Flagler. Mrs. Anderson, never in robust health, died on September 12, 1912. Dr. Anderson died on the morning of December 1, 1924.[8] Surviving him were two children, a son Andrew of Encampment, Wyoming, and a daughter Clarissa of St. Augustine.

1. Biographical data included in this sketch has been drawn largely from three sources: Thomas Graham, *The Awakening of St. Augustine*, St. Augustine, St. Augustine Historical Society, 1978; Sidney Walter Martin, *Florida's Flagler*, Athens, University of Georgia Press, 1949; and Dr. Anderson's obituary which appeared in the St. Augustine

Evening Record, December 1, 1924. For more complete biographical details the work of Professors Graham and Martin should be consulted. The former, a Professor of History, Flagler College, St. Augustine, had access to materials not previously used.

2. With the coming of the Civil War, Dr. Anderson, as Professor Graham explains, was faced with a dilemma. He had strong northern ties; yet he had been born in St. Augustine where he had many friends. St. Augustine was not in spirit a Southern City, so with impunity Dr. Anderson could return to the North having been for several years attending northern schools, and enter medical school, which he chose to do.

3. Professor Martin has explained in detail the close relationship of Dr. Anderson and Flagler, which had been mutually beneficial.

4. S. Walter Martin, Flagler's Associates in East Florida Developments, *Florida Historical Quarterly*, Vol. XXVI, No. 2, p. 257.

5. *Proceedings, Florida Medical Association*, Jacksonville, 1874.

6. Ibid., 1889.

7. A strong bond of friendship developed between Dr. Anderson and the first president of the University of Florida, Dr. A.A. Murphree. For the background negotiations which led to the Dr. Anderson gift see Orland K. Armstrong, *The Life and Works of Dr. S.A. Murphree*, privately published, St. Augustine, 1928, pp. 92-94.

8. St. Augustine *Evening Record*, December 1, 1924. Dr. Anderson having died in the very early morning of December 1, the obituary appeared in the issue of the same day.

Anderson, Daniel G., Gainesville, 1806-post 1870

Dr. Anderson, a native of Landsford, Chester District, South Carolina, was born about 1806, son of William Anderson, a plantation owner. Nothing is known of his childhood and education; however, it is probable that he "read medicine" in the office of a local physician, thereby qualifying for a license to practice.

Following the lead of many South Carolinians of the times, Dr. Anderson migrated to Florida in the 1840s, settling first on Black Creek where he established a sawmill and engaged in medical practice.[1] Being something of an opportunist and possessed of acumen in business matters, he took notice of the struggle being waged over the permanent site for a county seat in Alachua County;[2] the established towns of Newnansville and Micanopy were the chief contenders. In late December 1852 the Florida Legislature authorized an election for the following year hoping to settle the issue. In the voting which took place in May 1853 it was decided that the seat should be located as near the center of the county as feasible. Simultaneously, David Levy Yulee indicated that his Fernandina to Cedar Key railroad would run through the center of Alachua County. Shortly after the votes on the issue were counted, Dr. Anderson purchased 300 acres of land on the east side of Sweetwater Branch, extending northward to the head of the stream. It was a profitable transaction.

Later in 1853 Dr. Anderson contracted with the Finger Brothers, W.L. and Mike, to move his sawmill to a location "at the head of Sweetwater Branch."[3] According to W.L. Finger, the first timber in Alachua County was sawed at this mill.[4] On the fourth of July 1854 a public gathering assembled at Dr. Anderson's mill for two purposes: to commemorate the birth of the nation and to celebrate the selection of Gainesville as the county seat. Dr. Anderson presided at the meeting. Dr. W.H. Stringfellow, also a native of Chester District South Carolina, delivered "a fiery address" and Dr. W.H. Babcock, who resided briefly in Alachua County, read the Declaration of Independence.[5] These events were then followed by a barbecue. Finger made no mention of sobriety.

Dr. Anderson, however, did not remain in Alachua County. With the Civil War looming, he appointed an agent to handle his Florida affairs and returned to his South Carolina home. The Chester District Census of 1860 lists him as a citizen of means, owning property valued at $106,000. His slaves numbered 72.[6]

Notwithstanding his Florida property, there is no record of Dr. Anderson's ever returning to the state. There are records, however, of his having appointed agents to handle his business. In the early years after the war he disposed of his Alachua County holdings. Deed books contain records of numerous sales of parcels of land in the later 1860s, some of them to persons of prominence in the community, e.g., J.H. Roper, the town's first schoolmaster and a civic leader, Stephen McCall, eminent clergyman, and Stephen F. Harvard, physician.[7]

The ravages of war by no means had impoverished Dr. Anderson. If the data recorded by the census enumerator of Chester District in 1870 are to be trusted, his property was worth $128,400 at that time, a substantial estate.

Dr. Anderson was married in the 1830s. His wife, known only as Margaret, was also a South Carolina native. Children born to them were sons Samuel and Henry and daughters Margaret and Missouri. The date of Dr. Anderson's death has not been determined.

1. Information on the life of Dr. Anderson is not plentiful. The main facts relating to his Florida residence are derived from the material collected by early Gainesville resident, E.C.F. Sanchez, who sought to rescue the early history of Gainesville from oblivion. Unfortunately many persons from whom he had hoped to obtain data had faulty memories, or no recollections at all. One notable exception was W.L. Finger, whose response is cited here.

2. It was unthinkable to the people of both Micanopy and Newnansville that their towns were not chosen.

3. W.L. Finger's statement, preserved in "Sanchez Papers," uncatalogued manuscript, P.K. Yonge Library of Florida History, University of Florida.

4. This statement is questionable.

5. Ibid. Dr. Stringfellow had settled at Ft. Clark, some five miles west of Gainesville. Dr. Babcock, also a native of Chester District South Carolina, became one of mid-19th century Florida's most eminent citizens in his dual roles of newspaper editor and physician.

6. See Chester District, South Carolina, censuses of 1860, p. 165, and 1870, p. 52.

7. See Alachua County Deed Books, E, G, I, and J. Other well-known Alachua County purchasers bore the names Finley, Doig, Pardee, and Waits.

Anderson, D.F., On the St. Johns River, 1858-1859

Dr. Anderson,[1] a Philadelphia physician, spent the winter of 1858-1859 in Florida in the expectation that the mild climate would be beneficial to his health. With his younger brother, Everett, as his companion, he arrived in Palatka on November 23, 1858. After a few days rest the men made their way slowly up the St. Johns River, camping or finding lodging in the small settlements. They spent several days in the vicinity of Ft. Gates, situated on the west bank of the river some four miles south of the effluence of the Oklawaha into the St. Johns. Their wanderings took them up the river as far as Enterprise on Lake Monroe, thence to Lake Harvey, and on to Smyrna and southward to Ft. Pierce. Retracing their southward journey they made their way back to Palatka, whence they departed for the homeward journey on April 19, 1859.

For the entire sojourn in Florida Dr. Anderson wrote a day-by-day account, marred only by his omission of the names of places and persons he encountered on the journey. The hardships of the trip and the primitive conditions which prevailed among the scattered settlements through which they passed are described in detail as are his observations of the flora and fauna. The chief diversion of the travelers appears to have been the random shooting of alligators which appear to have been plentiful.

Although it had been Dr. Anderson's intention to avoid all medical practice throughout the journey, he found himself occasionally pressed into professional service. On January 2, 1859, he wrote: "Had a call for my professional services, but refused to act. I went, however, as a friend and prescribed." The patient was a man named Saunders, who about a week later again required the doctor's assistance. In the entry of January 9 he wrote: "I was again in demand as a doctor. No less than five messengers came to carry me to see my old patient who was worse since the Sunday previous. The medicine had not been applied as thoroughly as it should have been and the disease was still extending." Again, on January 18, Saunders once more sent for Dr. Anderson, who noted in his journal that the old fellow had imprudently exposed himself and suffered a relapse.

During a part of February the Andersons found lodgings at Ft. Gates. Here again he relented and answered an urgent call, which he recorded in his diary for February 7:

> While at breakfast I was called on by a gentleman, who had come some five miles and crossed the river besides, requesting me to visit a child that was very sick. What was I to do? I could not refuse to go. No doctor was to be had. I had no medicine. They would send for anything I would order, do anything if I would go. A horse was waiting for me across the river, and a boat at the shore. I saw the child, a bright little girl of four years, sick past recovery. A few days at most would end her life. I gave them directions but no hope. It was useless and I returned to Ft. Gates.

Such experiences were not uncommon among physicians sojourning in Florida, expecting to leave their professions behind them for the enjoyment of a holiday or for recuperation from their own illness.

1. All information contained in this sketch is derived from "The Anderson Journal: an account of the winter of 1858 and 1859 spent in Florida by Dr. D.F. Anderson and his younger brother, Everett, undertaken for Dr. Anderson's health." Photocopy of transcript (1976), in P.K. Yonge Library of Florida History.

Anderson, James, Tallahassee, 1850

Dr. Anderson, Florida native and son of Mrs. Jane Anderson of Connecticut, is thought to have practiced medicine for a short while in Leon County, possibly Tallahassee. The Census of 1860 lists him at the age of 21 living in the home of his mother. Other members of the household were his brother, Laurence, and his sister, Augusta. No other data has been discovered.[1]

1. U.S. Census, Leon County, Florida, 1860, item 122.

Andrews, George W., Hernando County, 1850

A legislative oddity appears to justify inclusion of Dr. Andrews in the list of 19th century medical practitioners of Florida. Among the acts passed by the Florida Legislature in its session of 1850-1851 was one investing George W. Andrews of Hernando County with the privilege of practicing medicine in the state of Florida. In the language of the Act Dr. Andrews was "hereby authorized and empowered to sue for and collect any amounts that may hereafter come due to him as such practitioner, *the same as any person legally licensed to practice in the State.*"[1]

The Act was passed by the Senate on January 7, 1861, by a vote of 28 to one, the nay vote having been cast by Senator W.M. Maxwell of Leon County. Six days later it was passed by the House of Representatives by the vote of 11 to seven. Among the seven opposing the Act was Dr. John L. Crawford of Wakulla County, the only physician in the House.[2]

Little is known of Dr. Andrews' earlier years. The Benton County[3] (to be renamed Hernando by legislative act of December 24, 1850) Census of 1850 lists him as a resident of the Annutaligo (Annuttelgia),[4] aged 55, and a native of North Carolina. His wife Amy was 54. Also included in the household were their sons, George W. Jr., 28; W.S., 25, a merchant; Amos, 19, and daughter, Margaret, 13, both born in Georgia.

No further information on this family has been located. It is assumed that the family had departed the state by 1860.

1. No similar permit to practice has been found in Florida Legislative records. This single exception may possibly be explained by the predominately rural nature of the county and the sparseness of its population. The Bill, an Act to permit George W. Andrews to practice medicine in the County of Hernando, was sent to Governor Thomas Brown by the Senate Secretary, Neill McPherson, on January 22, 1851. It was promptly signed.

2. It is not surprising that Dr. Crawford, one of Florida's best educated and most capable physicians of the 19th century, opposed the bill.

3. Hernando County was named in honor of Hernando de Soto at the time of its establishment in 1843. In the following year it was changed to Benton honoring Senator Thomas Hart Benton of Missouri. Then in 1850, displeased with Benton's stance regarding the Missouri Compromise, the Florida Legislature renamed the county Hernando.

4. Annutaligo, according to Allen Morris, was also known as "The Big Hammock." It extended through much of what was in the late 1840s known as Benton County. According to Morris the proper spelling was "Annuttelgia." Allen Morris, compiler, *Names Under the Florida Sun,* 1973, I., 14.

5. U.S. Census, 1850, Benton County, Florida, p. 26, Annutaligo Settlement. Two other members of the household were Benjamin Harney, planter, aged 19, and James M. Thompson, "gentleman," aged 20, both Kentucky born.

Anthony, S.W., Marianna, 1860

Dr. Anthony,[1] a native of Georgia, was graduated as Doctor of Medicine from the Medical College of Georgia, Augusta, in 1855.[2] He had removed to Marianna by 1860 and was a resident in the home of Dr. Franklin Hart. The census that year indicated that he was 24 years of age, owning personal property valued at $1500. On October 3, 1862, he was mustered into a cavalry unit recruited locally by Captain M.F. Irvin. Eight days later, however, this company was disbanded,[3] following which no further information on Dr. Anthony has been discovered. It is probable that he returned to his native state, perhaps for further military service and ultimately to resume medical practice.

1. The hand-written record of Dr. Anthony as it appears in the Census of 1860, Jackson County, Florida, p. 801, is not clearly decipherable. The first initial is possibly an L rather than an S.

2. Medical Department, University of Georgia, Augusta, *List of Graduates, 1829-1891,* Augusta, 1891, p. 13.

3. This company was assembled on October 3, 1862, and mustered out on October 11, 1862. No further military record for Dr. Anthony has been located.

Archer, Robert, Assistant Surgeon, U.S. Army, 1835

Very little is known of Dr. Archer's medical service in Florida beyond the fact that he spent much of the year 1835 at Ft. King, a few miles east of present-day Ocala. Facing the threat of the American government to remove them from the Florida Territory in 1834 the Indians had become increasing recalcitrant and a second Seminole War loomed. Brevet Brigadier General Duncan L. Clinch, having received command of the militia in Florida in November 1834, had established headquarters at Ft. King, regarded as a key defense post.[1] By April of the following year, as hostilities intensified, he was forced to make certain critical decisions concerning deployment of his numerically inadequate troops.

In a letter to Adjutant General Robert Jones he set forth his plans.[2] These included retaining four companies at Ft. King with Dr. Archer as their medical officer.[3]

In October 1835, General Clinch, in another letter to General Jones, transmitted the following information: "I have been informed by Asst. Surgeon Archer that nearly one hundred of the Command now at Ft. King have been more or less sick within the last two or three months and although many of them (are) fit for Garrison duty, and most of the others are convalescent, they cannot be relied upon for active service. . . ."[4]

No more is known of Dr. Archer's Florida practice. Army Medical Department records, however, contain the following information:

Robert Archer—
Commissioned Hospital Surgeon's Mate—May 13, 1814.
Born in Virginia; Commissioned from Virginia.
Commissioned Post Surgeon—April 18, 1818.
Promoted to Asst. Surgeon—June 1, 1821.
Promoted to Surgeon—May 9, 1825.
Resigned—August 5, 1826
Re-appointed Asst. Surgeon—August 5, 1826.
Resigned—February 29, 1840.[5]

1. For an account of the events of these critical months see John K. Mahon, *History of the Second Seminole War*, Gainesville, 1967, pp. 87-113.
2. *Territorial Papers*, XXIV, 130.
3. Ibid. Two other medical officers, Drs. Richard Weightman and Richard Clarke, also at Ft. King, were reassigned to other posts.
4. Ibid., 187.
5. *MDUSA*, pp. 287, 290, 291. There is no explanation of Dr. Archer's resignation as surgeon and his immediate reassignment to the lower rank.

Argyle, William, Leon County, 1831

Dr. Argyle (Argyll), a native of Virginia, came to Florida in the 1820s and settled on a tract of land in the community known as Tuscawilla about 12 miles east of Tallahassee on the Tallahassee-Monticello post road.[1] Like many other Territorial physicians he divided his time between medicine and farming. He first appears in the public records as bondsman for John Parkhill, a neighbor, who was appointed postmaster of Tuscawilla in 1828.[2] Subsequently on at least three occasions he served as Inspector of Elections for his district in company with the Parkhills (John and Samuel) and other prominent men of the community.[3] On one occasion he joined a group of Jefferson County citizens in petitioning President Andrew Jackson for the appointment of Charles E. Sherman to the office of District Attorney for the Middle District of Florida.[4]

Dr. Argyle's career was tragically brief, however, his death coming on October 29, 1831.[5] On December 27, administrators of his estate, Kitty Argyle, presumably his widow, and John W. Argyle, his brother, a Tallahassee merchant, posted the customary notices relative to settlement.[6] The Argyle property, both real and movable, was sold at auction on February 15, 1832. The notices of sale would establish Dr. Argyle as a man of middling means.[7] All indications are that he was highly respected as a person of cultivation and civic responsibility. Unfortunately nothing is known of his medical practice.

1. A post office was established at Tuscawilla in 1828 and discontinued in 1837. Dr. Argyle's farm was situated

in sections 14 and 15, township 1, range 2, north and east. Tallahassee *Floridian*, February 15, 1832.

2. *Territorial Papers*, XXIII, 982.

3. Ibid., XXIV, 169, 410, 519.

4. Ibid., p. 576.

5. Tallahassee *Floridian*, November 1, 1831. As late as mid-August 1831, Dr. Argyle had attended a dinner honoring Col. Joseph M. Woite, Florida's delegate in Congress. Tallahassee *Floridian and Advocate*, August 17, 1831.

6. Ibid., January 17, 1832. The 1830 Census of Leon County lists Dr. Argyle's age as between 20 and 30. Since only heads of families were listed the identities of his children cannot be established. Four males under five years of age are shown as are one female and two males between 15 and 20, age groupings which indicate a second marriage for Dr. Argyle; however, his age, under 30, seems to argue against that probability.

7. Ibid. While the 1830 Census indicates that Dr. Argyle owned 13 slaves, the notice of sale in 1832 mentions only seven. Offered for sale also were 230 acres of land, several mules, cows and hogs, a riding horse, household furniture and harvested crops. The range of these items suggests that Mrs. Argyle contemplated returning to her native Virginia.

Armistead, Latinus C., Gadsden and Jackson Counties, 1860s

Dr. Armistead was listed in the Gadsden County census of 1850 as a farmer of modest means, 24 years of age, and a native of Virginia.[1] The Jackson County census of 1860, however, indicated that he was a physician, although probably only a part-time practitioner.[2] His chief claim to prominence, however, derives not from his medical career but from his public service to Jackson County as its representative in the Florida House in the sessions of 1865 and 1867. In the latter year he was chosen as one of four delegates from Jackson County to the infamous "Carpetbagger Convention" which was convened in Tallahassee in January 1868.[3] It must be said for Dr. Armistead that in spite of the high level of emotionalism which threatened to project irrational thinking in the proceedings, he was able to maintain a moderate position. His name was affixed to the finished document.

1. U.S. Census, 1850, Gadsden County, Florida, p. 366.

2. Ibid., Jackson County, Florida, p. 97. A genealogical study of the Armistead family of Florida has not been completed. It appears that one branch migrated from Virginia, while another came from North Carolina. Several members of the family achieved prominence in Jackson, Gadsden and Leon Counties.

3. An interesting account of the mood and transactions of the Convention is that of John Wallace, *Carpet-Bag Rule in Florida*, Jacksonville, 1888. Also published in Facsimile Edition, with Introduction by Allan Nevins, by the University of Florida Press, Gainesville, 1964. John Wallace, a former slave, had been a senator from Leon County.

Armistead, Marcus L., Apalachicola and Quincy, 1847

Among earlier settlers in Gadsden County were the Armistead brothers, Latinus and Marcus A., who migrated from Petersburg, Virginia, in the 1820s and in 1827 laid out the village of Aspalaga on the Apalachicola River.[1] In the same year they were authorized by the Legislative Council of Florida to establish and maintain a ferry across the river from their newly established town,[2] which was about 12 miles from the Georgia border. Dr. Armistead was the eldest son of Marcus A. Armistead.[3] Little is known of his early life but he is presumed to have been born in Petersburg and to have been still a child when his family moved to Florida. As for his education, nothing is known.[4]

Dr. Armistead was already a young physician when he arrived in Apalachicola on February 18, 1843, aboard the steamer Oriole from Columbus, Georgia.[5] A week later he announced the opening of his professional office "over the store of T.H. and C.H. Austin."[6] In August of that year he formed a medical partnership with Dr. William Sidney Green, also a Virginian, recently arrived in

Apalachicola.[7] By the end of the year, however, the association was terminated and Dr. Armistead disappeared from the scene. About a year later he emerged as a practitioner in Quincy with the following announcement: "Dr. Armistead having resumed the practice of medicine, and heretofore accustomed to an extensive practice, both in City and Country, has consented to reside in Quincy, where he offers his professional services. . ."[8]

It is impossible to say how long Dr. Armistead remained in Quincy, although his professional notice continued to appear in the Tallahassee *Florida Sentinel* through its issue of March 2, 1847. It was probably about the first of January 1847 that he responded to the call for physicians for army service in the Mexican War. He was with General Winfield Scott's Army as assistant surgeon at the capture of Vera Cruz in March 1847. There he died, a victim of yellow fever on June 11 following.[9]

1. *Laws of the Territory of Florida*, Tallahassee, 1829.
2. Ibid. Their permit was granted for a 15-year period, provided the ferry was kept in good repair.
3. Tallahassee *Florida Sentinel*, November 14, 1843, obituary notice of Marcus A. Armistead, who died at the age of 56. It is stated that he had been a merchant of Petersburg for 25 years prior to removing to Florida. In the obituary notice for Dr. Armistead, Tallahassee *Southern Journal*, July 19, 1847, he is identified as the eldest son of Marcus A. Armistead.
4. Florida census schedules of 1830 and 1840 provide no listing for the Marcus A. Armistead family.
5. Apalachicola *Commercial Advertiser*, February 18, 1843.
6. Ibid., February 25, 1843.
7. Apalachicola *Watchman of the Gulf*, August 12, 1843.
8. This professional card first appeared in the Tallahassee *Florida Sentinel* of January 1, 1845. It appears probable that Dr. Armistead's departure from Apalachicola was prompted by the death of his father on November 3, 1843.
9. See note 3 supra. Dr. Armistead's obituary included the following: "His life was one of elevation and usefulness, the short time allotted him, during which he attached himself to many friends. His body was attended by the Chief Surgeon and Medical Department of the City (Vera Cruz)."

Arrowsmith, William L., Leon County, 1886

Dr. Arrowsmith spent the last two years of his life in Florida. A native of England, he arrived in Florida in 1884. Apparently a man of means, he purchased the Arvah Hopkins mansion near Tallahassee, furnished it lavishly, and settled into what he hoped would be a pleasant existence for the last years of his life. The Tallahassee *Weekly Tallahassean* announced on March 31, 1886, that Dr. Arrowsmith "got wet recently in a rain and had been dangerously ill since." He died shortly thereafter.

On realizing the seriousness of his illness Dr. Arrowsmith had summoned Dr. Henry R. Stout, a homeopathic physician of Jacksonville, to hurry to his bedside, Dr. Arrowsmith himself being a homeopath. Arrangements were made for a special train to bring Dr. Stout to Tallahassee but it was to no avail. Dr. Arrowsmith lived only a few hours after Dr. Stout's arrival.

Realizing that the end of life was soon, Dr. Arrowsmith directed that his body be placed in a wooden coffin for burial in the Tallahassee City Cemetery. He was said to have been between 80 and 85 years of age at the time of his death.[1]

1. All that is presently known of Dr. Arrowsmith is found in the *Tallahassean*, issues of March 31, 1886 and April 2, 1886.

Ashmead, L. Preston, Gainesville, 1850-1878

Dr. Ashmead, a man of superior intelligence and professional skill, was born in Philadelphia, Pennsylvania, on August 27, 1850. In early manhood he was graduated from the New York College of Physicians and Surgeons. So impressive were his credentials that at the age of 22 he was appointed head physician at the Brooklyn City Hospital where he remained for two years. On discovering that he was suffering from tuberculosis Dr. Ashmead resigned his position and sailed for Europe hoping that the salubrious climate of the Mediterranean would bring him back to good health. After a year he appeared to have conquered the disease, so he returned to America.[1] For reasons of health he chose to settle in Florida, and in early 1876 arrived in Gainesville and entered into a professional partnership with Dr. Newton D. Phillips who had recently begun practice in the town.[2]

Dr. Ashmead returned to Brooklyn in October 1876 where he married Caroline A. Price, daughter of the late Col. W.W. Price of Lake George, New York.[3] On arrival in Gainesville the couple were received with utmost hospitality by the citizens of the town, the local newspaper offering its congratulations with the hope "that the doctor is now a fixture in our midst."[4]

The Ashmeads entered happily into the social and religious life of Gainesville. Early in 1877 Dr. Ashmead was elected to the vestry of Trinity Episcopal Church[5] and a few days later represented the church at the Diocesan Convention in Jacksonville.[6]

The happiness of the Ashmeads was short-lived, however, for before the end of April he realized that the old illness had returned. On April 28 he announced he was withdrawing from medical practice for an indefinite period and recommended that his patients seek the services of his partner, Dr. Phillips, who "is so well known" and whose "abilities so highly appreciated" that "it is unnecessary for me to add one word in recommending him to my patients."[7]

Meanwhile, Dr. Ashmead placed his business affairs in the hands of the law firm of E.M. and Wm. W. Hampton.[8] His business interests included part ownership in the recently-built Arlington Hotel.[9] In May, accompanied by his wife and mother-in-law, he departed for the North to spend the summer. In the fall of 1877 the Ashmeads returned to Gainesville, but the mild climate was of no avail. Dr. Ashmead's health continued to deteriorate and on March 12, 1878, he succumbed to tuberculosis.[10] After a funeral service at Trinity Church his body was taken to Lake George, New York, for burial in the Price family plot. In addition to his wife, the doctor was survived by one small child.

1. Information from the Gainesville *Times*, May 13, 1878, which includes a complete obituary.
2. Ibid., July 6, 1876.
3. Ibid., October 26, 1876.
4. Ibid., November 9, 1876.
5. Ibid., April 7, 1877.
6. Ibid., April 14, 1877.
7. Ibid., April 28, 1877.
8. Ibid.
9. Ibid., March 10, 1877. It is possible that the part-owner of the Arlington Hotel was not Dr. Ashmead but instead his father. The item of *Times* simply states that "Mr. L.P. Ashmead, of Philadelphia, one of the proprietors of the Arlington, arrived this week." The Arlington, for many years one of Gainesville's largest and most popular hotels, stood at 134 W. Arlington Street (now 16 SW 4th Avenue) and continued to exist as a hostelry until 1967.
10. Ibid., March 13, 1878.

Ashurst, Josiah, Duval, Clay and Suwannee Counties, 1820

Biographical data on Dr. Ashurst (Asherst) is not abundant. He first appeared in the Florida sources in 1853 when he advertised his services through the columns of two Jacksonville newspapers, the *Florida News* of April 23, 1853, and the *Florida Republican* of April 7, 1853. His claims were not modest. He claimed to keep on hand a variety of medicines for many ailments, viz., consumption, bronchitis, asthma, piles, old ulcers, dropsy, dyspepsia, and female troubles, promising to "cure all in a few days." If not, he would "refund $10." He was also willing to "examine and prescribe for diseased slaves."[1] "Write him," he urged, "at Jacksonville, East Florida."

Although the Duval County Census of 1850 listed Dr. Ashurst's wife, Eliza, and sons, Watson and Robert, 11 and 13 respectively, the doctor himself is not included.[2] These three were residents in the home of George Stone and his wife, Martha. Mrs. Stone being presumably the sister of Mrs. Ashurst.

The Ashursts were residents of Middleburg (Clay County) by 1860. The census of that year shows that son Watson was no longer living with the family.[3] Another son, William, had been added, however; he was four years of age. By 1870 the Ashursts were residents of Wellborn (Suwannee County). The family now numbered three: the doctor, aged 50 and owning property of a total value of $550;[4] Mrs. Ashurst, 45; son, Watson, 30, an attorney owning property valued at $200.

Nothing further is known of this family. They do not appear in the Suwannee County Census of 1880.[5]

1. Jacksonville *Florida News*, April 23, 1852; Jacksonville *Florida Republican*, April 7, 1853.
2. All members of the Ashurst family were natives of Georgia, except son, William, who was born in Florida. U.S. Census, 1850, Duval County, Florida, p. 19, item 62.
3. U.S. Census, 1860, Clay County, Florida, p. 46.
4. U.S. Census, 1870, Suwannee County, Florida, item 298.
5. A search of the lists of graduates of the Georgia colleges of medicine in existence at the time when Dr. Ashurst would have attended has not yielded any information as to his medical education. It is probable that he served an apprenticeship under a practicing physician in Georgia.

Atkins, Ira, Calhoun County, 1775-post 1860

Dr. Atkins was born in North Carolina in 1775. After his marriage to Emily (family name unknown) he moved to Alabama where his seven children were born. By 1850[1] the family had settled in the Ochesee community of northeastern Calhoun, County. He was a man of above average means, his properties having been valued at more than $40,000 on the eve of the Civil War.[2] As a younger man he had practiced medicine but after settling in Florida he apparently turned his energies mostly to farming. He is known to have owned 49 slaves in 1860, only four planters in the county having owned more.[3] The date of Dr. Atkins' death has not been determined.

1. U.S. Census, 1850, Calhoun County, Florida, p. 34.
2. Ibid. The Atkins children from eldest to youngest were: Lewis, Elizabeth, Sarah, William, Samuel, Delilah, and Francis. Both Samuel and Francis served in the Confederate Army, 5th Infantry Regiment, Company B (Liberty Guards), recruited from Liberty and Calhoun Counties.
3. Slave schedule, Calhoun County, 1860.

Atkinson, C.C., Ocala, 1860

Dr. Atkinson was a resident in the home of L.H. Henderson, a Marion County planter, in 1860. He is listed as a native of South Carolina, aged 27. He was possibly a son or nephew of Shadrack Atkinson, a planter from South Carolina, who owned property near Ocala. He may possibly be identified as Camden Atkinson, who received his medical degree at the Medical College of the State of South Carolina, Charleston, in 1855. Nothing further is known of him.[1]

1. No positive identification can presently be made of this physician. Among the soldiers killed in the Battle of Olustee of February 20, 1864, was a Craven Atkinson. He is not identified as a physician, however.

Auld, Isaac, Leon County, 1818

Dr. Auld, who practiced medicine for a decade or more in mid-19th century, was born in Charleston, South Carolina, in 1818. He is thought to have been the son of an eminent physician and scholar of the same name who maintained residences in Charleston and Edisto Island.[1] Although very little is known of Dr. Auld's early education, it appears certain that he was afforded the best Charleston could provide. It is assumed that his preceptor was his father.

Isaac Auld matriculated at the Medical College of the State of South Carolina, Charleston, on November 8, 1841, and received his degree in March 1844, having submitted a doctoral thesis entitled "Scrofula."[2] Not yet ready to begin practice he enrolled for the 1844-45 term as a postgraduate student, a luxury not often afforded by medical students of that era.

Dr. Auld began his medical practice at Bradford Springs, a spa located in the northwestern part of Sumter District, which in the antebellum period attracted a fair number of visitors.[3] He was married in Charleston on December 23, 1846, to Harriet M. Hamlin of that city.[4] In the following year the Aulds moved to the village of Greenwood, then within the District of Abbeville, where the census enumerator found them in 1850. The family included a daughter, Mary, aged three, and a boy, Donald, aged 12, probably a nephew, while the doctor himself was designated "M.D. and Teacher."[5]

By the mid-1850s the Auld family had joined a number of Abbeville families in moving to Middle Florida. Dr. Auld purchased a farm outside Tallahassee and with the labor of seven slaves carried on a modest farming enterprise. His property was estimated to have had a value of $5400 in 1860.[6] By that date three sons had been born to the couple: Thomas H., six; Donald I., four; and Isaac, one (thus perpetuating the favored family name). The three were born in Florida.

No information on the latter years of Dr. Auld has been discovered. Since neither he nor any member of his family is listed in the Census of 1870, he is presumed to have left the state by that date. One Isaac M. Auld, a merchant, aged 29, was a resident of Mellonville, Orange County, Florida, in 1870. He was doubtless a cousin, possibly a nephew, of Dr. Auld.

1. The elder Dr. Isaac Auld, a native of Scotland, was a prominent figure in the medical faculty of Charleston for many years. His Edisto Island home was a summer retreat, a refuge from the heat of the Charleston summers. While there he developed an interest in the high mortality rate, mostly from fevers, of the island population. His observations were set forth in an essay published as an appendix in David Ramsay's *History of South Carolina*. See Joseph Ioor Waring, M.D., *A History of Medicine in South Carolina*, Columbia, S.C., 1964, pp. 175-176.

2. Lists of Students and Graduates, Medical College of the State of South Carolina, preserved in the Waring Historical Library, Medical University of South Carolina, Charleston.

3. Bradford Springs was situated near the main road leading from Sumterville, the county seat, to Camden, seat of Kershaw County.

4. Marriage Notice, Charleston *Courier*, December 28, 1846. The service was conducted by Reverend Mr. J.D. Auld.

5. U.S. Census, 1850, Abbeville District, S.C., p. 120.

6. U.S. Census, 1860, Leon County, Florida, p. 46. The following obituary notice appeared in the Tallahassee *Floridian and Journal*, August 9, 1853: "Died, in Madison, on March 29, 1853, aged twelve months, Harriet Ann, infant daughter of Dr. Isaac Auld." This suggests that Dr. Auld may have practiced in Madison for a brief period.

Ayers, Samuel R., Alachua Settlement, 1823

A group of New York and New Jersey speculators organized what was known as the "Florida Association" in 1822 for the purpose of settling a portion of the Arredondo Grant, a tract of some 289,645 acres lying near the center of the so-called Alachua County.[1] Dr. Ayers was employed as physician to accompany the first group of would-be settlers who left New York aboard the chartered schooner, Bold Commander, about December 21 and arrived at Picolata on the left bank of the St. Johns River on December 29.[2] A deposition made on October 30, 1824, by LeGrand Jarvis, surveyor for the settlement, indicated that after establishing a base across the River from Picolata, the settlers made their way westward into what is now the Micanopy community. Thus it appears that Dr. Ayers was probably the first qualified physician to practice in Alachua County.

Dr. Ayers' Florida sojourn was brief, however. In a deposition made by him later, he stated that he had left the settlement, "not being satisfied with his situation, and hearing a report that the Indians were opposed to the white settlement." He was replaced by Dr. James Kelly, of Charleston, who was already residing in St. Augustine.

1. Historical Records Survey, "Spanish Land Grants in Florida," 5 vols., Tallahassee, 1940-41, Vol. II, 103, 105, 108. Several years ago Dr. Webster Merritt set forth some of the background information concerning the Alachua settlement in which the much-publicized Moses E. Levy was involved. See his "Physicians and Medicine in Early Alachua County and Gainesville, Florida," *Journal of the Florida Medical Association*, XXXVII, No. 1, July, 1950, 23-27.

2. The Alachua territory of this period was a vast expanse of land extending from the St. Johns River to the Suwannee River. Its northern and southern boundaries were less well defined.

Babcock, William H., Alachua and Nassau Counties, 1827-1888

Dr. Babcock, one of the most competent physicians and enlightened citizens of antebellum Florida, was born in Chester District, South Carolina, in 1827.[1] Nothing is known of his early education but it appears to have been of sufficient quality to gain entrance for him to Yale College, from which he received a baccalaureate degree in 1849.[2] Upon his return to South Carolina he read medicine under the guidance of Dr. William M. Michel, distinguished Charleston physician, and his son, Dr. R.F. Michel.[3] In the fall of 1850 he entered the Medical College of the State of South Carolina, Charleston, from which he received his degree in the spring of 1852.[4]

In late 1852, following the lead of many other South Carolinians, Dr. Babcock made his way to Florida, settling in the village of Gainesville instead of the slightly more populous towns of Newnansville and Micanopy. According to one of the earlier Gainesville settlers, Dr. Babcock bought land on the west side of the village and built a house on the southwest corner of what is today West University Avenue and Southwest Second Street.[5] At approximately the same time (1853) he joined Col. Tillman Ingram in operating a general merchandise store on the east side of the court house square.[6]

By early 1854 Dr. Babcock had begun his medical practice in Gainesville. He could soon claim as his patients the most prominent families of the village including the Baileys, Ingrams, and Geigers. The earliest entry in his account book bears the date, February 15, 1854, "for sewing an artery and sewing up a wound for a boy." The latest entry was recorded on November 31, 1858. His services covered the range of medical practice but related preponderantly to fevers and obstetrical cases. On some occasions he resorted to cupping and bleeding and quinine was one of the most frequent prescriptions.[7]

In the meantime Dr. Babcock had responded to the call for volunteer physicians for the Third Seminole War (1855-58). The hiatus in his "Record Book" from May 30, 1857 to March 1858 appears to coincide with his term of military service, although his commission as assistant surgeon was dated August 6, 1856. The fall of 1857 found him at Ft. Myers on the Caloosahatchee, the base of operations for that segment of the war. In a dispatch of January 1858, he was addressed as "Assistant Surgeon and purveyor of Medicine."[8] In May 1858 a special order issued by Army Headquarters at Ft. Brooke named him Judge Advocate for a general court martial at which charges against six enlisted men were to be adjudicated.[9] The order was issued, however, after Dr. Babcock had returned to Gainesville and it is doubtful that he actually participated in the trial.

The data on Dr. Babcock make it clear that in those midcentury decades it was difficult for a physician to make his living by medical practice alone. Like many others he turned to supplemental sources of income. He opened his Gainesville house to boarders in 1856. An entry in his "Record Book" reads: "(David) Black & (Daniel) Reinhardt commenced boarding with me on the first day of December at the rate of twelve dollars per month & one dollar a month for ashing." On January 2, 1857, he entered: "Ben Young commenced boarding with me on the 2nd of Jan. 1857 at fifteen dollars per month." A little later this entry appeared: "Ben Young quit sleeping at my house on the 20th of May, 1857."[10]

When Joseph F. Rogers gave up editorship of the Fernandina *Florida News* in April 1859, the paper was bought, after an interval of six weeks during which E.A. Papy was editor, by Dr. Babcock, the first issue under his direction appearing on May 26 under the masthead, Fernandina *East Floridian*.[11] As an editor, Dr. Babcock was more than merely competent, exhibiting not only fine writing skill but keen insight into public issues and concern over local matters. In his columns can be discerned the growing political tensions which would lead in January 1861 to Florida's secession from the Union. Dr. Babcock, a dedicated Democrat, never veered from his secessionist point of view. As soon as Lincoln's election had been verified he inserted in bold letters at the top of the editorial page his slogan, calling for THE SECESSION OF THE STATE OF FLORIDA, THE DISSOLUTION OF THE UNION, THE FORMATION OF A SOUTHERN CONFEDERACY.[12]

Having thus established his position in the trust and confidence of the citizens of Fernandina, Dr. Babcock from his vantage point as editor of the local newspaper assumed a leadership role. At a gathering of Nassau County Democrats on March 1, 1860, assembled for the purpose of choosing delegates to the State Convention in Madison a few weeks later, he helped draft the resolutions.[13] He was secretary for a political meeting on July 2, 1860, assembled to discuss the plight of the Party following the Charleston Convention at which support for John C. Breckenridge and Joseph Lane for president and vice president respectively was declared.[14] In the spring of 1860 he was elected to the Fernandina City Council.[15]

As the political waters became more turbulent Dr. Babcock went out of town to serve his party, appearing at Callahan on September 1, 1860,[16] and at Baldwin on the 27th.[17] In October he helped organize a Vigilance Committee whose alleged purpose was to enlist "respectable, reliable persons to refute the Lincoln propaganda" being circulated in the South.[18]

In early 1861, with the secession of Florida a *fait accompli*, Dr. Babcock was instrumental in organizing a company of Fernandina Volunteers, serving as its secretary as well as its quartermaster.[19]

He gave up editorship of the *East Floridian* in December 1860, which was briefly revived in the following spring by T.J. Wombwell only to expire after the issue of May 29.[20]

Unfortunate lacunae in the military record of Dr. Babcock do not permit a complete account of his service. It is apparent, however, that he moved at an early date into the Medical Department of the Confederacy and was assigned to hospital service. In a report of an inspection tour of Confederate hospital facilities made in 1863, Dr. G. Troup Maxwell, himself a physician of the First Florida Cavalry, wrote: "The Florida Hospital (near Richmond), which is under the control of the courteous and skillful surgeons Palmer (Thomas M.) and Babcock. . .nowhere in the Confederate States is the Medical Department conducted with greater skill and ability than in this. . ."[21]

Upon his discharge from the Army, Dr. Babcock returned to his home in South Carolina and undertook the editing of the Chester *Standard*, a paper which had been a casualty of the War.[22] He found this unprofitable and soon gave it up. The Gainesville *New Era* published this item on April 20, 1867: "The many friends of Dr. W.H. Babcock, late editor of the Chester, S.C. *Standard*, will be glad to learn that he has returned to Florida with the intention of making it his permanent residence. Gainesville will be his headquarters for the present."[23]

Evidence indicates that Dr. Babcock resumed his medical practice in Gainesville,[24] at the same time engaging in the insurance business as a representative of Aetna Life although the Alachua County census of 1870 lists him as "Druggist." There can be little doubt, however, that newspaper work was his first love, so in the mid-1870s he was in Jacksonville as a member of the fourth estate writing editorials for the *Times*, while serving as Florida correspondent for the Savannah *Morning News*.[25] For two sessions (1881 and 1883) he was Secretary for the Florida State Senate.

Dr. Babcock accepted the office of Superintendent of Public Schools for Duval County in 1885 and held this position until his death[26] on October 4, 1888, at his home[27] at 90 East Duval Street. Death resulted from a heart ailment of several months duration. He was 61.[28]

Dr. Babcock was remembered by many Jacksonville citizens for his fearless and unselfish medical service in the deadly smallpox epidemic of 1883 when he volunteered to take charge of the pest house, for months isolating himself from his family and friends "in the discharge of his self-imposed task."[29] His eulogist added: "Dr. Babcock was a courteous and conscientious gentleman, kindhearted as a woman, soft of speech and slow to anger; but when he thought he was in the right, he was ready to lay down his life in defense of his opinions. As a journalist he was painstaking and discriminating. . . ."[30]

Very little information concerning Dr. Babcock's family has come to light. They seem to have been seldom in the public eye. Mrs. Babcock (Mary), whom he had married after the Civil War, was a native of Georgia and they had three daughters.[31]

1. Archives, Medical College of the State of South Carolina to be found at present in the Library, Medical University of South Carolina, Charleston. It appears that Chester was Dr. Babcock's birthplace, although the obituary in the Savannah *Herald* and reprinted in the Jacksonville *Florida Times-Union*, October 7, 1888, indicates that he was born in Charleston, where his father is said to have been a bookseller.

2. Archives, MCSSC.

3. Ibid.

4. Ibid. His thesis topic was "Natural Labor."

5. James Doig, "Reminiscent Sketches of Gainesville's Early Days." Gainesville *Sun* issues of July 15, 22 and 29, 1917.

6. Ibid.

7. "Record Book," Dr. H. Babcock, MS, Box 70, PKYLFH, University of Florida.

8. Letter, Col. S. Loomis to W.H. Babcock dated Ft. Myers, January 29, 1858. Records, U.S. Army, Continental Command, RG 393 (Florida Volunteers) 111-C, Reel 13.

9. Letter, Thoe. Talbot, Acting Asst. Adj. General, to Babcock, dated at Ft. Brook May 27, 1858. Ibid., p. 307.

10. See note 7, supra.

11. Fernandina *East Floridian*, November 28, 1860. See also Fernandina *Florida News*, April 14, 1859.

12. Fernandina *East Floridian*, November 28, 1860.

13. Ibid., March 8, 1860.

14. Ibid., July 12, 1860.

15. Ibid.

16. Ibid., September 6, 1860.

17. Ibid., September 27, 1860.

18. Ibid., October 24, 1860. Heading this committee was Ex-Governor Broome.

19. A local militia unit known as the Fernandina Volunteers had actually been organized in Fernandina on January 17, 1860 with Capt. Thomas I. Long commanding and Dr. Babcock as treasurer. Its avowed purpose was to "safe-guard Fernandina against an attack from the North." *East Floridian*, January 5 and January 19, 1860. This unit later became a part of the state militia when war became imminent in early 1861.

20. Ibid., May 29, 1861.

21. Tallahassee *Florida Sentinel*, August 25, 1863.

22. Gainesville *New Era*, May 25, 1866.

23. Ibid., April 27, 1867.

24. The list of active medical practitioners in the United States compiled by the Medical College of the University of Pennsylvania in 1869-70 lists Dr. Babcock as a practitioner in Alachua County. Gainesville *New Era*, August 10, 1867, advertisement of Dr. Babcock's Insurance Agency.

25. Jacksonville *Florida Times-Uion*, October 7, 1888.

26. Lee E. Bigelow, "Public Schools of Duval County, Florida," Library Project, WPA (Jacksonville 1939), Typescript, p. 63.

27. The data on Dr. Babcock found in *Medical Department of the Army*, 1775-1873, Harvey E. Brown, compiler (Washington: Surgeon General's Office, 1873), giving October 3, 1859, as the date of Dr. Babcock's death is obviously in error as was his place of death which is given as Gainesville.

28. Jacksonville *Florida Times-Union*, October 5, 1888.

29. See note 25, supra.

30. Ibid.

31. U.S. Census, 1880, Duval County, Florida, p. 542. See also Special Florida Census, 1885, Duval County, Duval Street (Jacksonville).

Bacon, Henry, Columbia County, 1870

Dr. Bacon, a Connecticut-born practitioner, spent much of his adult life in St. Marys, Georgia, where he was the town's leading physician for some time. Extrapolating from census information for Camden County for 1850 and 1860 the date of his birth appears to have been 1802[1] He was married to Miss Harriet Sadler, daughter of Henry R. Sadler, a wealthy resident of Cumberland Island, Georgia, about 1830. To this marriage were born five sons; two, Henry Sadler and William F., became physicians.[2] At some time between 1860 and 1870 Mrs. Bacon died and soon thereafter Dr. Bacon left St. Marys to settle in rural Columbia County near the home of his son, William, already in practice there. It is not certain that Dr. Bacon actually practiced after moving into Florida although the census of 1870 lists him as physician.[3] He died prior to 1880.

1. U.S. Census, 1850, Camden County, Georgia, p. 390; ibid., 1860, p. 21. His age in 1850 was 48, in 1860, 58.

2. See infra for brief sketches of these two sons. After serving as a physician in the Confederate Army, Dr. Henry S. Bacon settled on a plantation in Nassau County. Dr. William F. Bacon, also in army service, was discharged in 1862 because of continued ill health and settled soon afterward in Columbia County.

3. U.S. Census, 1870, Columbia County, Florida, p. 160. Here his age is erroneously stated as 64.

Bacon, Henry Sadler, Nassau County, 1832-1866

Dr. Bacon was born in St. Marys, Georgia, on November 28, 1832, one of five sons of Dr. Henry Bacon and Harriet Sadler Bacon, daughter of Henry R. Sadler of Cumberland Island, Georgia. After completing his medical education Dr. Bacon returned to St. Marys and entered practice. He was married to Anna Maria O'Neill, daughter of James O'Neill of New Hope Plantation, Nassau County, Florida, on November 28, 1855.[1]

Nassau County and its seat, Fernandina, underwent a severe economic depression about 1850, a situation which was only relieved in the mid-1850s when the cross-Florida railroad (Fernandina to Cedar Key) was begun. For several years there was no physician in the county. When ill the residents who could afford to do so sought the services of physicians living across the St. Marys River in Georgia. Among those responding to such calls was Dr. Bacon, who became the family doctor of the O'Neills of New Hope. Mrs. Isabel Barnwell (nee O'Neill), younger sister of Mrs. Bacon, recalled in an interview in 1936 that Dr. Bacon was often summoned to treat not only members of her family but their slaves as well, her father paying for the services at the rate of $600 per year.[2] The sum included payment for medicines as well, "most of which were purchased for the slaves." She cited a document in which was recorded "one operation on one negro field hand, $30." She also recalled subsequent visits by Dr. Bacon to check on the recovery of the patient.

With the coming of the War in 1861 Dr. Bacon enlisted in a Georgia regiment with the rank of first lieutenant, serving in both Virginia and Florida. He was later transferred to the Confederate Army Medical Department with the rank of captain. By the conclusion of the War he had become a major. With his military career finished he settled with his family in Fernandina. His professional career in Florida was of tragically brief duration, however, his death occurring on August 12, 1866. He was remembered as man "gentle in spirit, of a kind and amiable disposition, sincere, modest and refined," whose "many endearing qualities had drawn around him a large circle of friends. . . ."[3]

1. The greater portion of the information on Dr. Bacon is derived from two interviews with Mrs. Isabel Barnwell, younger sister of Mrs. Henry Sadler Bacon, recorded by Rose Shepard in 1936. These are found in WPA Project on the History of Fernandina and Nassau County, an unpublished manuscript a copy of which is among the holdings of the P.K. Yonge Library of Florida History. New Hope Plantation, Nueva Esperanza, as it was known in the Second Spanish Period of Florida History, had been settled by an O'Neill ancestor in the late 18th century. It was situated on the west side of the Amelia River, southeast of Yulee, its earlier existence being marked by the present-day village of O'Neill.

2. Ibid.

3. Gainesville, *New Era*, August 24, 1866. A son of Dr. Henry Sadler Bacon, also named Henry, later became a physician in Jacksonville.

Bacon, William F., Columbia County, 1834-post 1880

Dr. Bacon, son of Dr. Henry Bacon, was born in Camden County, Georgia, in 1834. Nothing is known of his medical education but by 1860 he had entered the practice of medicine in Lake City, Florida, and was living in a hotel.[1] With the Civil War already under way he enlisted for military service in the Confederate Army and was mustered in on March 8, 1862, assigned to Co. B, Fifth Florida Infantry Regiment, with the rank of first lieutenant. Although the post of regimental assistant surgeon was offered to him, he chose not to accept it.[2] His actual term of service was brief, his resignation having been tendered on August 30, 1862, presumably for reasons of poor health. His statement of resignation was presented to Justice of the Peace, W.B. Ross in Lake City on October 24, 1862.[3]

After leaving the service Dr. Bacon is presumed to have returned to Lake City for resumption of his medical practice. A short time later he acquired a tract of land outside the town on which he settled with his wife, Clementine.[4] A daughter, Annie, was born in 1870. The Bacon household by 1880 included his sister-in-law, Clifford Ross, aged 31 and her 12-year-old son, Boston.[5] As far as is known Dr. Bacon lived out his life in Columbia County; the date of his death is not known.

1. U.S. Census, 1860, Columbia County, Florida, p. 172, item 28.

2. NA, Serv. Recs. CSA, M251, Roll 59.

3. Ibid. On two muster rolls recorded during his five months of service Dr. Bacon is shown to have been absent because of illness.

4. U.S. Census, 1870, Columbia County, Florida, item 1240.

5. Ibid., 1880, p. 441.

Badger, George E., Leon County, 1838

Dr. Badger, a native of Raleigh, North Carolina, and medical graduate of Tulane University, settled in Leon County, Florida, in the late 1850s.[1] He was doubtless persuaded to do so by his half brother, Col. Joseph John Williams, who had come to Leon County more than a decade earlier and through a propitious marriage[2] and numerous shrewd business deals had accumulated vast acreage a few miles north and east of Tallahassee. His plantations included the well-known Hickory Hill and LaGrange.[3] His slaves numbered 245 in 1860 and Dr. Badger was responsible for the medical care of the personnel associated with Williams' "cotton kingdom."[4] As a consequence his services were generally unavailable to the public.

With emancipation of the slaves and collapse of the cotton economy in the postwar period Williams' fortune dwindled rapidly, and by the time of his death in 1876[5] only his town house, a mansion located at 217 North Calhoun Street, Tallahassee, was left. In the face of these changes and the loss of his retainer's income, Dr. Badger abandoned his Florida practice. In the meantime, however, he had married a young Irish girl who was visiting one of Williams'plantations. His subsequent whereabouts is not known; presumably he returned to North Carolina to resume practice there.

1. Henry E. Palmer, Physicians of Early Tallahassee and Vicinity, *Apalachee*, Tallahassee, 1944, p. 40.
2. Clifton Paisley, *From Cotton to Quail*, Gainesville, 1968, p. 7. Williams' wife was Eliza, daughter of Noah Thompson, wealthy Leon County planter.
3. Ibid., p. 7.
4. Palmer, Physicians, p. 40.
5. Williams died of a heart attack on November 19, 1876, while on a visit to his mother in Raleigh, N.C. Dr. Badger, who had gone to Florida at about the age of 21, was only 38 at the time of Williams' death.

Badger, James N., Marion County, 1815

Marion County physician, James N. Badger, was born in Barnwell District, South Carolina, in 1815.[1] As a youth he read medicine in the office of Dr. Erwin in Barnwell and in 1835 entered the Medical College of the State of South Carolina, Charleston, where he received his medical degree on May 14, 1837, having submitted a thesis entitled "Pleuritis."[2]

By 1850 Dr. Badger had established his medical practice in Marion County, Florida, west of Ocala.[3] Like many medically-trained settlers of that area he purchased land, brought slaves from South Carolina, and engaged in the dual occupations of farming and medical practice, with the former probably claiming the greater part of his time. The Marion County Census of 1860 indicated that he was successful, his real property was valued at $7,000. Other property, including 37 slaves, was worth $25,000.[4] The census enumerator designated him "Planter and M.D." A University of Pennsylvania list of medical practitioners, compiled in 1869-70, included the name, J.N. Badger of Ocala.[5]

Census data indicate that Dr. Badger had been married and widower before removing to Florida.[6] His only child of the first marriage, Edward N., educated in law, had a successful career in the Civil War, having been an enlistee in the Fifth Florida Infantry Regiment and rising to the rank of lieutenant colonel by 1863. He was wounded at the Battle of Franklin (Tenn.) on November 30, 1864.[7]

Dr. Badger's second wife, Harriet, was a Florida native; they had four children,

John, Sarah, and twins, James N., Jr., and Laura.

The date of Dr. Badger's death has not been discovered. Since he does not appear in the Marion County Census of 1870, it is possible that he died in that year or perhaps returned to his native state.

1. Dr. Badger appears to have been the only son of Elizabeth Badger, who was a widow by 1830.
2. Archives, Medical University of South Carolina, Lists of Matriculants and Graduates.
3. U.S. Census, 1850, Marion County, Florida, p. 253.
4. Ibid. 1860, p. 315.
5. Archives, University of Pennsylvania, MS. UPS. 2.3 #16.
6. Edward Badger was 20 years old in 1860, his stepmother was only 30.
7. NA. Ser. Recs., CSA.M 251, Roll 53.

Baker, Daniel, Gasden County, 1803

Vital data on the career of Dr. Baker is almost nonexistent. He is known to have been among the earlier settlers in the Philadelphia community some four miles north of Quincy, having been one of the founders of the Philadelphia Presbyterian Church whose membership included several natives of Scotland. As the Quincy community began to take on the appearance of a town, Dr. Baker moved there and became one of the founders of the Presbyterian Church of Quincy. Although no information relating to his professional activities has been discovered, he is presumed to have practiced there at least for a brief time. No gravestone for him has been discovered.[1]

1. See WPA Writers Project, Gadsden County, Florida, Historical Section by Dorothy Atkinson, p. 12. See also J. Randall Stanley, *History of Gadsden County*, revised with index by David A. Avant Jr., Quincy 1985, p. 66. Stanley lists Dr. Baker among the charter members of the Quincy Presbyterian Church, adding "many of whom had been members of the Old Philadelphia Church."

Baker, Joseph S., Duval County, mid-19th century

Notwithstanding his relatively prominent position in religious and business affairs in Jacksonville about the middle of the 19th century, Dr. Baker remains an obscure figure. Born in Georgia in 1799, he was called to Jacksonville in early 1850 as pastor of the Jacksonville Baptist Church, a charge which had not been satisfactorily filled since the resignation of the Reverend James McDonald four years earlier. He remained in this position for four years, "during which both the Church and the Sunday School prospered."[1]

Dr. Baker appears to have been a man of more than average means. In early 1851 he purchased from the Reverend McDonald a tract of land immediately west of Jacksonville, a section known as LaVilla. At about the same time his kinsman, Samuel Spencer, bought the tract immediately to the west which came to be known as West LaVilla, bringing all of the LaVilla suburb into his possession.[2]

Dr. Baker, thought to have overextended himself in August 1851 and doubtless unable to support his family on the meager salary of a Baptist preacher, advertised his services as physician to the citizens of the Jacksonville community. His qualifications for medical practice were somewhat vague.[3]

> He flatters himself that a thorough course of collegiate and medical studies, the benefit of a course of private lectures under two distinguished Professors of Surgery connected with different Medical Colleges, together

with his past experience and observation of diseases in different latitudes, while engaged for several years in active practice of his profession, will enable him to afford essential relief for the afflicted who may confide their cases to his hands. Office on his farm in the Western Suburb of the town.

Two months later Dr. Baker announced the opening of his office at the corner of Market and Forsyth Streets, "opposite the Court House."[4]

At about the same time Dr. Baker began to sell his recently acquired "lands and lots adjoining the Town of Jacksonville." His public notices emphasized the medicinal properties of "two strong Chalybeate springs which yield copious deposits of dehyrdated peroxide of iron" which, he claimed, in their medicinal properties compared favorably to Broghton and Turnbridge (sic) (i.e., Turnbridge Wells) in England. Also offered for sale were a number of building lots, timbered lots ranging in size from five to 50 acres, all in the immediate vicinity of Jacksonville.[5] Two months later he was willing to sell his Brick Yard in LaVilla.[6]

Although information relating to Dr. Baker's activities during the later 1850s is scarce, it is clear that he maintained his medical practice at his office located at the corner of Market and Forsyth, the last known notice of such activity being that of November 4, 1859, in which he assured his clients that he was continuing to offer his services in Medicine, Midwifery and Surgery.[7] The Duval County census of 1860 lists him as the sole occupant of his household "outside Jacksonville." He was then 61, his occupation, "Baptist Clergyman," his property was valued at $2,500.[8]

Since Dr. Baker's name does not appear in the Duval County Census of 1870, he is presumed to have died prior to that date. No gravestone to his memory has been discovered in any of the Jacksonville cemeteries.[9]

1. T. Frederick Davis, *History of Jacksonville, Florida and Vicinity*, St. Augustine, 1925, p. 403. The Reverend McDonald had retired in 1846. For the next four years the Church had been without a pastor until Dr. Baker arrived in 1850.

2. Ibid., pp. 43-44. Davis states that it was Dr. Baker's son, James McRobert Baker, who became a prominent business man and was elected to the Florida Senate for the sessions of 1856, 1858, and adjourned session of 1859, who remodeled the McDonald home and named the plantation LaVilla.

3. Jacksonville *News*, August 16, 1851; Jacksonville *Republican*, August 21, 1851.

4. Jacksonville *News*, October 18, 1851.

5. Ibid., September 6, 1851.

6. Ibid., December 13, 1851.

7. Jacksonville *Florida Republican*, November 4, 1859, (1st printed October 16, 1859).

8. U.S. Census, 1860 Duval County, Florida, Item 376. Since the following entry (#377) is that of James McRobert Baker, it would appear that he lived either next door to his father, or possibly in the same household.

9. Except for James McRobert the only other child known to have been born to Dr. Baker and his wife, Sara, was Richard Spencer Baker, who died on October 3, 1851, at LaVilla at the age of nine. Jacksonville *Florida Republican*, October 9, 1851.

Baker, Simmons J., Jackson County (Greenwood), 1840

Dr. Baker, a native of Gates County, North Carolina, arrived in Florida prior to 1840[1] and settled in the Greenwood community of Jackson County. There he bought land, acquired slaves,[2] and established himself as one of the more prominent citizens of the area. As a member of St. Luke's Episcopal Church in Marianna, he was a delegate to the Second Diocesan Convention at St. John's Church in Tallahassee in 1839.[3] He appears to have been more planter than physician, however; although it may be assumed that he carried on a local practice in his own neighborhood. Two of his sons, Simmons J. Baker Jr.,[4] and James

Lawrence George Baker,[5] were also wealthy planters, active in the public affairs of Jackson County. Dr. Baker died *ante* 1850.

1. A few biographical details and a photograph of Dr. Baker appear in J. Randall Stanley, *History of Jackson County*, Marianna, 1950, passim.
2. Ibid., p. 142. A survey of 1845 showed him as owner of 82 slaves.
3. Ibid., p. 77
4. U.S. Census, 1850, Washington County, Florida, Item 293, lists this son as resident of Washington County.
5. Dr. Baker's son, James L.G., was a delegate to the Secession Convention in Tallahassee in January 1861. He achieved some distinction by being the only delegate voting against the secession of Florida from the Union. Stanley, op cit., p. 157.

Baker, Simmons Jones, Jackson County, 1805-1887

Dr. Baker, a North Carolina native, arrived in Jackson County in the late 1820s, bringing his wife, Elizabeth, his sons, James L. G. and Simmons J. Jr., and daughter, Mary. They laid claim to land north of the present site of Marianna and immediately assumed a major role in the development of Jackson County. In addition to his farming interests he is presumed to have practiced medicine, but not on a very extensive scale. An Episcopalian, he was one of the organizers of St. Luke's Church in Marianna, becoming its first senior warden. His sons and daughter married into some of the county's most substantial families. His grave marker in St. Luke's Cemetery indicated that Dr. Baker was born on January 16, 1805, and died on January 9, 1887.[1]

1. Biographical data included here have been drawn from two sources: J. Randall Stanley, *History of Jackson County*, Jackson County Historical Society, 1950, p. 23 et passim, and "Cemeteries of Jackson County, Florida," vol. I, Doris E. Pamphilon, compiler, 1984.

Baker, William H., Martin County, 1836-1893

Dr. Baker[1] was born in Jefferson County, Alabama, on August 18, 1836. He is said to have studied medicine at "the medical schools of Philadelphia and Charleston," although no confirmation has been located. He removed to Florida in the 1870s seeking a more healthful climate and the restoration of his broken health. His Florida practice was limited to a small clientele in and around Waveland, Martin County.[2] He is said to have been "ever ready and willing to render gratuitous aid to any one who needed his professional service." He died at his Waveland home on June 9, 1893.[3]

1. The meager information relating to Dr. Baker is derived chiefly from his obituary in the Titusville, *The Florida Star*, June 30, 1893, p. 5.
2. Waveland was located a short distance inside St. Lucie Inlet, new Sewall's Point and south of Stuart.
3. The recently published *History of Martin County*, Janet Hutchinson, compiler, and Emeline K. Paige, editor, Martin County Historical Society, Hutchinson Island, Florida, 1975, contains occasional references to Dr. Baker. Map facing page 1 shows location of Dr. Baker's house.

Baldwin, Abel Seymour, Jacksonville, 1811-1898

Among the most eminent men ever to adorn and dignify the medical profession in Florida stands Abel Seymour Baldwin.[1] Few have labored so diligently and unselfishly for the improvement of medical practice in the state while simultaneously engaged in major political and social service. His role and influence were accurately stated by Webster Merritt.

> For six decades, almost to a day, Dr. Baldwin led the vanguard of progress in Jacksonville. At the time of his death on December 8, 1898 in his eighty-eighth year, he was the city's most distinguished citizen.

Born in Oswego County, New York, on March 18, 1811, Dr. Baldwin was orphaned at an early age. He was reared by an uncle and aunt in neighboring Madison County who provided tutoring for his elementary education. Approaching adolescence he was enrolled in Cazenovia Seminary, Cazenovia, New York, and later in Polytechnic Institute of Chittenango, New York. His hopes for attending one of New England's prestigious colleges being thwarted by the untimely death of his uncle, he enrolled instead in 1830 in Little Geneva College (now Hobart College), in Geneva, New York, from which he was graduated in 1834 with both B.A. and B.S. degrees. He leaned heavily toward the natural sciences, especially botany and chemistry. For the two years following he was employed as botanist for a geological survey of Michigan, only to find the climate too rigorous for his health. Giving up his position he returned to Geneva and entered the Medical Department of the College from which he received his medical degree in 1838, and simultaneously his Master of Arts degree.

Dr. Baldwin began his professional practice in Geneva in the summer of 1838, but as winter approached and his rheumatic symptoms reappeared he decided to go south for a more benign climate. In the meantime he had married Eliza Scott. So with his bride of a few months he made his way to Jacksonville, where he tentatively set up practice. On September 1, 1839, he announced his intention to settle permanently in the village with an office "a few rods north of the court house."[2] For Jacksonville it was an auspicious decision.

Dr. Baldwin's countless public services will not be enumerated. It is sufficient to recall that there was scarcely a project or enterprise designed to promote the welfare and prosperity of Jacksonville and Duval County to which he did not in some manner lend his support. These included harbor improvements for the accommodation of ocean-going ships,[3] railroad development to connect Jacksonville with the West and North,[4] and significant sanitation measures for safeguarding the public health of Jacksonville. While in Washington in 1852 seeking support for the harbor project he was elected to a seat in the Florida House of Representatives, and in the sessions of 1858, 1860 and 1861 he represented Duval County in the Florida Senate. For some 55 years he was a vestryman in the St. Johns Episcopal Church.

Notwithstanding such varied and demanding interests Dr. Baldwin maintained a constant and enlightened interest in the advancement of medicine. Yellow fever, the scourge of the times, had brought personal tragedy to his own household when in 1857 it had claimed the life of Mrs. Baldwin at the age of 42. In 1888 his only son, William, also a physician and professional partner of his father, was a yellow fever victim. In search of an effective treatment for the disease Dr. Baldwin devoted all the energies and acumen of his scientific mind. He even attempted to apply Dr. John Gorrie's ice-making invention to some practical solution, but to no avail. He was more successful, however, in coping with a bowel condition known as intussusception encountered in some of his patients. He succeeded in developing a procedure of pumping large amounts of tepid water into the intestines. This brought him national acclaim.

It was Dr. Baldwin's deep concern about the absence of a professional medical organization and the lack of effective regulation of medical practice, however, that brought him lasting fame. In 1848 the attempts of a small group of physicians, mostly from Gadsden and Leon Counties, to organize a statewide medical association had come to naught. In November 1873 the effort was renewed by Dr. Baldwin who invited the doctors of Florida to meet with him in Jacksonville in the following January to organize such a professional society. On January 14 nine other physicians, all except Drs. Betton and Burroughs of Leon County from northeast Florida, met with Dr. Baldwin in his Jacksonville office and launched the Florida Medical Association.[5] Twenty-one years earlier he had been chiefly responsible for the founding of the Duval County Medical Society, the first of its kind in the state. Not present, but nominated and elected to membership, were 14 other physicians. By the close of the meeting a year later—also in Jacksonville—the membership numbered 42. Much of the early success of the Association must be attributed to Dr. Baldwin, who not only initiated the organizational meeting but also served as its president for 1875 and 1876.[6]

It is not surprising, given his multifarious interests, that Dr. Baldwin did not distinguish himself as a writer on medical subjects. In his earlier years in Florida he had made careful observations and records of climatic phenomena. Meteorology was a lifelong interest. It is not particularly surprising, therefore, that his presidential address before the Association at its meeting in Jacksonville in February 1875 bore the title, "The Climatology of Florida."[7] It was a carefully documented paper, scientifically methodical, treating the relationships of climate to health. His presidential address of the following year, delivered at the meeting of the Association in Tallahassee, was noted in the Proceedings without mention of its title.[8] Although referred to the Committee on Publications, it was never published.

The year 1860 was doubtless an agonizing one for Dr. Baldwin. He was an opponent of secession. But once Florida had made the decision (January 1861) to leave the Union he offered his services to his adopted state. Soon after the War had begun he was commissioned chief surgeon of East Florida and placed in command of the General Confederate Hospital at Lake City. In February 1865 he became medical director of the General Hospitals of Florida and Quitman, Georgia. His well-kept letter-books and hospital journals are preserved in the Confederate Museum, Richmond, Virginia.

At the end of the War Dr. Baldwin returned to Jacksonville to find that his various properties had been confiscated by federal authorities. Only after lengthy litigation was he successful in recovering them. In the meantime, in 1866, he remarried, in this instance, Mrs. Mary E. Dell, a well-to-do widow some 24 years his junior.[9] To this union was born one child, a daughter, Edna Seymour,[10] who would later marry Samuel P. Holmes of Jacksonville. In November 1865 Dr. Baldwin formed a professional partnership with his son, William L., an arrangement which terminated after a year or two, but which was resumed in 1879 and continued until the death of William in 1888.[11]

Throughout his adult life Dr. Baldwin maintained his interest in matters scientific. He was for some years a meteorological correspondent of the Smithsonian Institution. In 1857 he became a member of the American Scientific Association meeting that year in Montreal. He was also a member of the Boston Natural

History Society, and a frequent correspondent with Louis Agassiz on subjects of mutual interest. And yet he never appeared to have neglected his local civic responsibilities. It is remarkable that in his 84th year he was elected president of the Jacksonville Board of Trade!

Dr. Baldwin's death came with little warning on December 8, 1898. A few days earlier he had caught a cold, which had been considered a minor illness, but complications developed and death came quickly. A Louisiana doctor, chance visitor at the annual meeting of the Florida Medical Association, May 1887, in St. Augustine, expressed the esteem in which Dr. Baldwin was generally held.[12]

> It gave us peculiar pleasure to meet the venerable Dr. A.S. Baldwin, the Nestor of Florida Medicine and the father of the State Association. . .Dr. Baldwin's presence falls ever like a benediction upon the annual gathering of Florida doctors.

It is a regrettable oversight and poignant irony that to this day in the City of Jacksonville no street, no park, no medical institution, no public place bears the name of this illustrious man who contributed so much to its development so that one must travel 15 miles westward to the very rim of Duval County to find him commemorated by the town of Baldwin.

1. The principal data included herein are found in the lengthy obituary which appeared in the Jacksonville Florida *Times-Union*, December 9, 1898. Additional details stem from the researches of two eminent Florida physician-historians, Webster Merritt, who devoted a chapter of his *Century of Medicine in Jacksonville and Duval County*, Gainesville, 1949, to Dr. Baldwin and Samuel M. Day, *Medical Leadership*, Journal of the Florida Medical Association, 52: 468-476, 1965.
2. The Baldwins arrived in Jacksonville on December 2, 1838. See Jacksonville *East Florida Advocate*, September 1839. The notice was first printed in the issue of September 1, 1839, not extant.
3. Dr. Baldwin was convinced that the harbor could be rendered adequate only by closing off Ft. George Inlet, thus eliminating the problem of constantly shifting sands resulting from the proximity of the effluence of the Inlet with that of the St. Johns River into the Atlantic. He made several trips to Washington and persuaded Congress to appropriate funds for the project only to have the money diverted for the dredging of the River by the Army Engineers.
4. Dr. Baldwin was elected president of the Florida Atlantic and Gulf Central Railroad in 1853.
5. Proceedings, Florida Medical Association, Jacksonville, 1875.
6. Ibid., 1875, 1876.
7. Ibid., 1875, pp. 21-56. This address was also printed in the same year as a separate item by the *Florida Agriculturist*, Jacksonville, 1975, 15 pp.
8. Ibid., Sessions of the 1876-77, Jacksonville 1877, p.9. Dr. Baldwin's brief paper "Artificial Disinfection," read at the 1877 meeting, is published in ibid., pp. 65-67.
9. The wedding took place in 1866. Mrs. Dell had a son, William A. Dell, Duval County Census 1870, p. 492, by a previous marriage. He too became a physician and practiced for some years in Jacksonville.
10. Although no documentation can be offered, it is apparent that Dr. Baldwin's mother's patronym was Seymour, the name given to Dr. Baldwin's daughter. He is said to have been a cousin to Thomas Hart Seymour, sometime governor of Connecticut, and Democratic candidate for the presidency at the Convention of 1864 in Chicago.
11. Jacksonville *Florida Union*, September 29, 1866. The notice first appeared in the issue of November 17, 1865, not extant.
12. The account of the meeting, written by a physician who signed himself simply "T.O.S.," was published in the *New Orleans Medical and Surgical Journal*, XIV, No. 12, June 1887, and reprinted in the *Journal of the Florida Medical Association* 53:749-752, 1966.

Baldwin, William L., Jacksonville, 1840-1888

Although his Florida career was brief and somewhat overshadowed by that of his distinguished father, Dr. Abel S. Baldwin, Dr. William L. Baldwin attained a high degree of professional respectability as a practitioner in Jacksonville where he was born on March 18, 1840.[1] He was the only child of Dr. Baldwin and his first wife, Eliza Scott Baldwin. He received his early education in the schools of Jacksonville and probably began the study of medicine in the office of his father. About 1859 he enrolled in the Albany (N.Y.) Medical College from which he was graduated.

No records which might indicate Dr. Baldwin's activities during the war years, 1861-65, have been located. In the fall of 1865, however, he joined his father in a medical partnership located at the corner of Laura and Adams Streets. They announced themselves as physicians and surgeons, promising to attend to calls "in the City and County."[2] This joint arrangement continued well into 1867. For reasons not clear the estate of Dr. William's mother (December 1857) had not been settled, and in the fall of 1865 father and son filed for letters of administration of the estate. In 1866, however, the father was permitted to transfer full responsibility for settlement of the estate to his son who completed it that year.[3]

At some undetermined date Dr. William terminated the partnership with his father, returned to the State of New York and practiced medicine there, first in Geneva his mother's home town, and later in Utica.[4] In 1879 he returned to Jacksonville and resumed practice with his father at the office on Laura Street remaining there until his own death nine years later. At the earliest opportunity he became a member of the Florida Medical Association. At the session in Jacksonville in April 1880 he was nominated by Dr. Charles J. Kenworthy and elected to permanent membership.[5] He did not attend subsequent meetings in Tallahassee and Pensacola but at the session of 1883 in Jacksonville he rose to question the legality of his election three years earlier, whereupon a new vote was taken and for the second time he was elected. He was appointed to the Committee on Accounts.[6] Dr. Baldwin was more involved in the transactions of Duval County Medical Society, having been elected president in 1887 and reelected in the following year. He held the office at the time of his death.

Dr. Baldwin was a victim of Jacksonville's deadliest yellow fever epidemic, that of 1888. His death came on September 3 at the height of its fury. As was true of all Jacksonville physicians (there were far too few), he had labored night and day as physician and nurse for his patients, reducing his own resistance and rendering himself a helpless victim. The *Times-Union* of September 4th reported.

> The whole city will learn with deep regret of the death of Dr. W.L. Baldwin yesterday from yellow fever. He had been recovering it was thought but the disease took a sudden change for the worse yesterday morning and the patient was unable to rally from it.

Dr. Baldwin was survived by his wife and two children all of whom were visiting in the State of New York at the time of his death. He was closely identified with the temperance movement in Jacksonville but aside from medicine his chief interest was Freemasonry. It was said of him at his death that he had worked at it and lived by its percepts. He was the Worshipful Master of Duval Lodge No. 18 whose members presided at his funeral held at the home of his father on September 4, 1888.

1. Included here are a few of the biographical details from an obituary notice in the Jacksonville *Florida Times-Union*, September 4, 1888.
2. Jacksonville *Florida Union* September 29, 1866. Notice first printed in issue of November 17, 1865, not extant.
3. Ibid., September 30, 1865, and subsequent issues through February 1866.
4. Lacunae in Jacksonville newspapers of this period make it impossible to construct a precise chronology of his movements.

5. Proceedings, Florida Medical Association, 1880, Jacksonville, p. 12.
6. Ibid., 1883, Jacksonville, pp. 12, 15.

Ballard, Charles Wiley, Manatee County, 1826-1901

Dr. Ballard, who spent the latter part of his life in Florida, was born in New York City on January 22, 1826, the son of Rebecca (nee' Ogden) and William R. Ballard.[1] He received his early education in private schools of Elizabethtown, New Jersey, and Newburgh, New York. He then enrolled in Baltimore Dental College, Baltimore, from which he was graduated in 1849. Simultaneously he was attending Washington Medical University in Baltimore, earning his medical degree from that institution in the same year.

Dr. Ballard practiced dentistry in New York City for several years. One of his patients was Theodore Roosevelt, then a youngster of 12. He was also the dentist for several other members of the Roosevelt family.

During these early years of practice Dr. Ballard resided in Darien, Connecticut, and enjoyed the distinction of serving for a term in the Connecticut Senate. For reasons unknown Dr. Ballard moved to Minnesota in 1870, remaining there for 14 years before removing to Bradenton, Florida, for reasons of health.

After establishing his residence in Bradenton Dr. Ballard immediately entered into the civic affairs of the rapidly growing town. Education was of primary importance to him; therefore he contributed both time and money to the development of a good school system. Basically a religious man he was a useful member of the Presbyterian Church of Bradenton.

As for family, Dr. Ballard was married on February 4, 1849, to Annie E. Harris of Frederick, Maryland. She was a niece of Dr. Chapin A. Harris, founder of the Baltimore Dental College. The Ballards were childless and appear to have enjoyed a long and happy marriage. Their golden wedding anniversary was celebrated on February 4, 1899. Dr. Ballard lived on until 1901.

1. Besides census schedules the information in the present sketch has been gleaned from two sources: Robert E. King, M.D., *A History of the Practice of Medicine in Manatee County, Florida*, Manatee Memorial Hospital, Bradenton, 1985, pp. 75-76; and Roland H. Rerick, *Memoirs of Florida*, edited by Francis P. Fleming, Atlanta, Ga., 902, Vol. II, 423-424.

Baltzell, George F., Jackson County, 1809-1877

Dr. Baltzell, a native of Kentucky,[1] was among the early settlers in Jackson County, having arrived there in 1845.[2] As a citizen of the Webbville community he supported the effort to establish the county seat there.[3] He is said to have begun the study of medicine as an apprentice to local physicians and proceeded to the Medical College of South Carolina, Charleston, for further study.[4] About 1830 Dr. Baltzell moved to Pensacola where he was elected Clerk of the Superior Court, a position he held for eight years.[5] His name was appended to several petitions requesting Congressional support for projects calculated to improve the public facilities of Pensacola and Escambia County.[6] In his spare time he read law and qualified for admission to The Florida Bar.

In the latter part of 1838 Dr. Baltzell moved to Apalachicola[7] where he was soon appointed to the clerkship of the recently established Superior Court of Franklin County while simultaneously serving as postmaster of the town.[8] He joined T.H. Thompson in July 1840 in the publication of a newspaper, Apalachicola *Commercial Advertiser*, with E.R. Boyle as editor.[9] Upon the death of Thompson soon after the enterprise was launched, Dr. Baltzell sold the paper.[10]

For reasons which are unknown Dr. Baltzell left Apalachicola in 1845 to settle in Washington County[11] where the census enumerator found him in 1850.[12] In the census of that year he was designated "medical," the only instance in which he was so labeled. He appears to have been the only properly-qualified physician practicing in Franklin County. A year or so later his restless spirit led him to Marianna in Jackson County where he was destined to live out his life. It appears, however, that having settled in Marianna he abandoned the practice of medicine completely, spending his latter years as lawyer, postmaster (1857-65), merchant, and finally as County Judge.[13]

Dr. Baltzell was twice married, first to Rebecca Long, daughter of Richard Long, and after her death, to Ann Penelope Armistad.[14] To the first marriage were born three daughters and two sons, in order of birth: Louisa, Margaret, George, Ann and Thomas.[15]

Dr. Baltzell probably was never a full-time medical practitioner but his career was not unlike those of numerous other antebellum Florida physicians who found the profession unremunerative and resorted to other enterprises or avocations for livelihoods. It is clear that he was a respected public servant, generally supportive of efforts to improve not only the judicial system but the general welfare of the communities in which he resided.

1. Rowland H. Rerick, *Memoirs of Florida*, Atlanta, 1902, I, 426-427.
2. J. Randall Stanley, *History of Jackson County*, Marianna, 1950, p. 34.
3. *Territorial Papers*, XXXIII, 947.
4. An examination of the lists of students and matriculants of the Medical College of South Carolina does not confirm that he was a student there.
5. Dr. Baltzell first appears in Pensacola as a signer of a petition bearing the date, December 1830. By December 1838, he was residing in Apalachicola. See Territorial Papers, XXV, 558.
6. Ibid., XXIV, 466, 908, 953.
7. Ibid., XXV. In December 1838, Dr. Baltzell signed a petition requesting that Congress reimburse certain private citizens for expendutures they had made toward improving the harbor of Apalachicola.
8. Stanley, op. cit. p. 34.
9. James G. Knowles, *Territorial Florida Journalism*, Deland, 1926, p. 33.
10. Ibid.
11. Apalachicola *Commercial Advertiser*, March 21, 1846: 1st printing, January 10, 1864.
12. U.S. Census, 1850, Washington County, Florida, p. 561.
13. Stanley, History, p. 34.
14. Ibid., p. 23.
15. See nolte 12, supra.

Bamber, Alexander, St. Augustine, 1824-1867

Very little information concerning the practice of Dr. Bamber, a brief sojourner in St. Augustine, has survived. He apparently settled in the town just after the Civil War. The local newspaper announced on October 13, 1866, that he had moved his office to the house of Mr. Phillip Gomez on Marine Street.[1] He died in St. Augustine on April 24, 1867, at age 43 and was buried in the Protestant Cemetery.[2]

1. St. Augustine *Examiner*, October 13, 1866.
2. Parish Register, Trinity Episcopal Church, St. Augustine, Unpublished.

Banks, Benjamin H., Jackson County, mid-19th century

The medical career of Dr. Banks is somewhat obscure, if indeed he ever practiced in Florida. A native of North Carolina, he moved to Jackson County prior to 1850[1] to become a resident in the household of Marmaduke A. Dickson, a Jackson County farmer and like Dr. Banks a North Carolina native. Also in the Dickson home was Dr. Banks' 11-year-old son, William. The Census of 1860, however, does not list the name of Dr. Banks, although his son was then a salesman employed by Marianna merchant, James G. Hearn. At some time, presently unknown, Dr. Banks abandoned the medical profession to become a Baptist minister. In 1870 he was living in the home of his son William, who was then married and the father of an infant daughter.[2] No further information on Dr. Banks has emerged.[3]

1. U.S. Census, 1850, Jackson County, Florida, p. 587.
2. William Banks was married to Lucy, an Alabama native.
3. A search through the Jackson County Census of 1880 revealed no entry for Dr. Banks.

Barnard, Thomas E.J., Tallahassee, 1837-1858

The professional career of Dr. Barnard was tragically brief. Edward Barnard and Mary Jane Hanna arrived in Tallahassee in the mid-1830s and were married in St. John's Episcopal Church on December 2, 1836.[1] He was a native of Massachusetts and a druggist by profession; she was born in Maryland.[2] Their son, Thomas E.J., was born in Tallahassee in 1837. Since they were a family of above average means the Barnards provided their son with the best education, general and professional, available in the United States. The identity of the medical school he attended, however, has not been ascertained.

Dr. Barnard had scarcely established himself in Tallahassee, if indeed he practiced there at all, when he learned of a devastating yellow fever epidemic raging in New Orleans. Eager to learn something of the nature of the disease and how it might be dealt with, he set out for the beleagured city. Upon arrival he accepted an appointment as resident student at the New Orleans Marine Hospital, where he remained through the summer of 1838. In October he came down with the ailment, and died on October 18 at age 21.[3] No notice of his funeral or burial has been located.

1. Church Records, St. John's Episcopal Church, Tallahassee.
2. U.S. Census, 1850, Leon County, Florida, p. 66.
3. Tallahassee *Floridian and Journal*, November 6, 1838.

Barrett, C.B., Jefferson County, 1838

Dr. Barrett, one of the better educated physicians practicing in Florida in the Territorial Period, was a native of Virginia. He had studied in Edinburgh, London and Paris and arrived in Florida in the latter part of 1838, settling in Monticello "with a view of making it a permanent resident."[1] He offered services in Physic, Surgery and Midwifery at his office in the home of Henry W. Bacon.

Dr. Barrett was married to Elizabeth Augusta, daughter of Jonathon Crawford, Esq., of Northumberland, New Hampshire, on March 6, 1840.[2]

During his brief residence in Monticello he shared his experience with fellow-physicians by writing a paper, "Extirpation of Aneurismal Tumor of the Os-Humeri," which was published in the *Southern Medical and Surgical Journal*, 3:581-583, 1839.

Dr. Barrett did not linger long in Florida subsequent to his marriage, having removed from the Territory prior to the Census Survey in the summer of 1840.

1. Tallahassee *Floridian*, December 1, 1838. Dr. Barrett's professional notice first appeared in the issue of November 3, 1838.

2. Ibid., March 21, 1840, Northumberland, a village on the Connecticut River in northern New Hampshire.

Barron, Charles S., Cape Florida and Key West, 1858-1893

Very little is known of the career of Dr. Barron and the few facts which have been uncovered are perplexing. The earliest reference to his Florida career is found in a Key West newspaper of November 1858 where he is identified as physician and lighthouse keeper at Cape Florida on the southern tip of Key Biscayne. On a visit to Key West he had reported the recent appearance of a small party of Seminole Indians, accompanied by their leader, Tiger Tail, at the mouth of the Miami River. Dr. Barron expressed concern that they might become a threat to that sparsely settled area especially if they should resort to piracy and prey upon the vessels which were frequently stranded along the coast. He estimated that there were still some 125 or so Indians left in Florida and that an agent should be sent to Miami to deal with them.[1]

Dr. Baron had moved to Key West by 1860. The census of that year lists him as a Virginia native, aged 59 and married to a Belgian-born woman named Margaret, aged 50.[2] Ten years later he was still residing in Key West but married to German-born Wilhelmina, aged 67.[3]

Dr. Barron next appears in the annals of the Florida Medical Association. At its annual meeting in Jacksonville in February 1875, he was proposed and accepted for honorary membership in the Association.[4] He was still living as late as 1893 when a list of members of the Association was compiled but his name does not appear in a similar list prepared in 1893 and published in a separate issue in 1898.[5]

1. Key West *Key of the Gulf*, November 6, 1858.

2. U.S. Census, 1860, Monroe County, Florida, p. 8.

3. Ibid., 1870, p. 46.

4. No explanation for such recognition is recorded. In all probability he had earned a good reputation in his profession prior to coming to Florida, and was therefore deserving of the honor. Others similarly recognized in 1875 were Dr. John T. Metcalfe of New York, Dr. Franklin Branch of Tampa, and Dr. Charles J. Kenworthy of Beverly, New Jersey, all physicians of distinction.

As for his occupation as lighthouse keeper one can only surmise that he had come to Florida because of ailing health as was true of so many of the earlier physicians. If, however, he lived until 1893-94 and if the census information of 1860 is approximately correct, he would have been in his early 90s by the time of his death, a ripe age for a man of weak constitution.

5. Proceedings of the Florida Medical Association, Jacksonville, 1893, passim, ibid., Jacksonville, 1893, p. 48. Here his name is erroneously listed as Chas. S. Bavan. See also *Catalogue of the Physicians of the State of Florida* prepared by the FMA, Jacksonville, 1898.

Barrows, Egbert S., Jacksonville and Ft. King, 1833

In the early summer of 1832 shortly after the Treaty of Payne's Landing had been negotiated with the Seminole Indians, who had been corralled in the Alachua settlement near Ft. King, it was decided that, as a measure of precaution, the entire tribe should be inoculated against smallpox. Dr. John Hamilton, citizen-surgeon at Ft. King, had accepted the task but upon learning that the compensation for the entire project would be no more than $100 he informed Governor Duval as well as the Washington authorities that he would not proceed with the project.

Dr. Hamilton's decision produced an impasse which stalled the project for more than a year. Not until November 1833 did Captain William M. Graham, commanding officer at Ft. King, revive the matter. On November 20[1] he reminded Lewis Cass, Secretary of War, that the vaccinations had never begun, restating the reasons and concluding with a recommendation of Dr. Egbert S. Barrows of Jacksonville for the job, if indeed the Secretary still thought the Indians should be vaccinated. Concerning Dr. Barrows, Captain Graham wrote: "He has been employed as the attending citizen-surgeon at this post from May 9th to the present, and has knowledge of the Indians." On the same day he wrote a similar letter to Colonel James Gadsden,[2] special Indian agent to handle their transfer out of Florida, and still another letter to Elbert Herring, Commissioner of Indian Affairs in Washington.[3]

Although the vaccination project was never actually revived, Dr. Barrows remained for at least another year as surgeon at Ft. King. He submitted a bill in late 1833 to the Office of Indian Affairs "for services rendered to the persons and families of John Hicks and Jumper, First Chiefs of the Nation, during the summer of 1833, thirty dollars."[4] The bill was paid by Capt. J.B.F. Russell, U.S. Army, with Dr. Barrows signing the receipt and designating himself "acting surgeon," Ft. King, October 22, 1833. A similar transaction occurred in late 1834 when the fee was $50 "for services rendered to Indians."[5]

No further information concerning Dr. Barrows has emerged. It is probable that he did not remain long in Florida. The Registers of Medical Officers of the United States Army do not show that he was ever commissioned in the Medical Department.

1. NA, Letters Received, Office of Indian Affairs, Microcopy 234, Roll 288.
2. Ibid.
3. Ibid., Roll 800.
4. Ibid.
5. Ibid. The experience of Dr. Barrows is a prime example of the type of irregular medical practice and uncertain compensation of physicians practicing in Florida's frontier in the early territorial period.

Bates, George M., Marion and Columbia Counties, 1815

Dr. Bates, who spent the greater part of his life in Florida, was born in Newberry District, South Carolina, about 1815.[1] He appears to have decided to study medicine at a later age than most, having matriculated at the Medical College of the State of South Carolina in the fall of 1841, receiving his degree in March 1843 after submitting a thesis entitled "Uterine Hemorrhage."[2] He is thought to have begun his medical practice in South Carolina. About 1845 he was married to South Carolina native, L. Sophia. Their first four children, Orlando B., William H., Laura, and Louisa, were born in South Carolina.[3]

At some unknown date in the 1850s Dr. Bates moved with his family to Marion County settling on a farm west of Ocala, an area which had attracted several families from the Newberry District of South Carolina. There, he appears to have devoted less time to medical practice and more to farming. In fact, the Marion County Census of 1860 lists him not as physician, but as "Planter." His slaves numbered nine which with other properties were valued at $17,000.[4]

For the Bates family the Civil War appears to have been disastrous. In addition to the loss of slaves, they appear to have been unable to make mortgage payments on their land. For whatever reason they abandoned their Marion County farm and removed to Columbia County, Florida, settling on land in the Lake City township. The Bates properties were valued at $2400 in 1870. He was still living in Columbia County in 1880 at age 65. Meanwhile, six additional children had been born. They were, in order of birth, John C., James C., Bernard Hodges, David E., Sophia C., and Margaret.[5]

As far as is known, Dr. Bates continued to live in Columbia County until his death, the date of which has not been determined.

1. This date is an extrapolation from the Census of 1860, Marion County, Florida, which gives his age as 45.
2. Charleston *Mercury*, March 18, 1843. Report of Medical College of the State of South Carolina Commencement Exercises.
3. U.S. Census, 1870, Columbia County, Florida, p. 355.
4. Ibid., 1860, Marion County, Florida, p. 22.
5. Ibid., 1880, Columbia County, Florida, p. 382.

Bates, John C., Monroe and Benton Counties, 1850

The Florida sojourn of Dr. Bates was apparently brief. The census enumerator located him in Key West on August 16, 1850,[1] a resident in the home of Mrs. Ellen Mallory,[2] the proprietress of a boarding house in the town. He was 26 years of age and a native of Ohio. Three months later, however, he was living in Benton County in the home of Bird M. Pearson, a wealthy lawyer and planter.[3] Indications are that he lingered there only briefly. Nothing further is known of Dr. Bates; he is presumed to have left the state as the war became imminent.

1. The Monroe County enumeration for Dr. Bates was made on August 16 while that of Benton County bore the date, November 26, 1850. It is unusual that a person should appear twice in different locations in the same census.
2. Mrs. Mallory was the mother of Stephen R. Mallory, U.S. Senator from Florida for two terms. He was also Secretary of the Navy in the Confederate Cabinet.
3. Bird M. Pearson, a native of Columbia, was one of the early settlers in Benton County (presently Hernando County). He laid claim to 5,000 acres of land north of Brooksville. See Richard J. Stanaback, *A History of Hernando County, 1840-1876*, Brooksville, Florida, 1976, p. 14.

Beattie, Francis Smith, Leon and Wakulla Counties, 1800

Dr. Beattie, a native of New York State, enrolled in the Medical Department of the University of Pennsylvania in the fall of 1819 and was graduated as Doctor of Medicine in the spring of 1821. His doctoral thesis was entitled "Tetanus." Subsequently he practiced in Philadelphia for a few years before joining the newly-assembled faculty of the Jefferson Medical College in 1825 in the dual capacity of Professor of the Institutes of Medicine and Professor of Obstetrics and Gynecology.[1] It is not known how long he remained at Jefferson but in the summer of 1838 he appeared in Tallahassee, advertising his services to the citizens of the town and its vicinity.[2] His office was located at the corner of Adams and Clinton Streets, "opposite the residence of James D. Westcott, Jr.," sometime Secretary and Acting Governor of the Territory.

In January 1839, Dr. Beattie was among the hundreds of signers endorsing a petition to Congress requesting that a "township of land" be granted "in aid of the Dade Institute of Florida," to be established as a memorial to Major Francis L. Dade, victim of Indian ambush in December 1835 and as an educational facility for underprivileged children.[3] He was appointed Collector of Customs for the port of St. Marks in June 1829. His tenure appears to have been terminated in the following summer, however, for on July 18, 1840, the following professional notice appeared in the Tallahassee *Floridian*: "Dr. F.S. Beattie has resumed the practice of medicine in all its branches, and tenders his professional services to the community. His office is at St. Marks, in the house of S.C. Spencer."

Very little is known of the Beattie family beyond the census data of 1840, which lists him as resident of Leon County, with a wife, aged between 40 and 50, a daughter between 15 and 20, and a son between 10 and 15.[5] Nothing further is known of the doctor and his family.

The reasons may have been many why a well-trained and highly respected physician would depart Philadelphia for the comparative obscurity of Leon and Wakulla Counties; probably a matter of health induced many to leave the north for a moderate climate. Why the Beattie family disappeared from Florida records after 1840 cannot be determined.[6]

1. Archives, University of Pennsylvania, Lists of Students, Jefferson Medical College opened for its first session in the fall of 1825.
2. Tallahassee *Floridian*, July 7, 1838.
3. *Territorial Papers*, XXV, 1834-1839, 578.
4. St. Joseph (Florida) *Times*, June 1, 1839.
5. U.S. Census, 1840, Leon County, Florida, p. 63.
6. The "Dr. Beattie" present at the July 4th celebration at Port Leon, an event reported by the Tallahassee *Floridian*, is presumed to have been the subject of this sketch. He offered the toast, "Our County, Our Home, Our All!"

Beatty, D.P., Fernandina, 1832

Details relating to the life of Dr. Beatty are meager. A native of North Carolina, he first appears in Florida records about 1858 when he was elected to the vestry of the recently organized St. Peter's Episcopal Church of Fernandina.[1] The next year on May 26 he and Dr. J.F. Lesesne announced the formation of a partnership for the practice of medicine and surgery.[2] The census of 1860 lists him as M.D., aged 28, owning property valued at $16,500, the major portion in real estate. In his house were his wife, Elizabeth, his mother, Elizabeth, both North Carolina born, and an infant daughter, Kate, born in Florida.[3]

Soon after secession of Florida from the Union on January 7, 1861, Joseph Finegan of Fernandina organized a militia unit which included Dr. Beatty as surgeon, with the rank of first lieutenant.[4] A year later, with the war already well under way, Dr. Beatty offered his services to Company K, 2nd Florida Cavalry, and was mustered in on the same day, May 16. Quite oddly, however, he entered as a private although immediately detailed as surgeon to the Company. He was then 30 years of age. Service records show him serving in that capacity through December 1862.[5] Beyond that date little is known of him and his family.

The Jacksonville *Peninsula* included this item in its issue of May 12, 1864.

Joseph Remington as United States Marshall for the Northern District of Florida advertises the property of Hon. D.L. Yulee, General J. Finegan, A.W. Cole, Jacob Cohen, Dr. D.P. Beatty, F. Clark, Jas. E. Broome, Daniel Calahan, Colonel B. Timanus and Captain Felix Livingston, in the town of Fernandina, to be sold as sequestered property.

1. W.P.A. Writers Project, Fernandina, St. Peter's Episcopal Church Records.
2. Fernandina *East Floridian*, June 2, 1859, 1st printing, May 26, 1859.
3. U.S Census, 1860, Nassau County, Florida, Item 119.
4. W.P.A. Writers Project, Fernandina, p. 67. Muster roll of officers serving under Colonel Finegan at Ft. Clinch, near Fernandina, April-November 1861.
5. NA, Service Records, CSA, M251, Roll 6. Dr. Beatty's is one of numerous Confederate service records which are incomplete.
6. This issue of the *Peninsula* is no longer extant but was cited in Mary Elizabeth Dickison, *Dickison and His Men*, Facsimile edition, Gainesville 1962, p. 169.

Beckett, J.L., Marion County, 1837

Dr. Beckett, who practiced his profession for only a few years in Marion County, was born on Edisto Island, Charleston County, South Carolina, about 1837.[1] In the fall of 1856 he enrolled at the Medical College of the State of South Carolina, Charleston, from which he was graduated on March 12, 1858, having submitted a thesis entitled "Dysentery."[2] He subsequently practiced his profession for a year or two before moving to Marion County in early 1860, where he joined his brother, William S. Beckett, who had purchased a farm west of Ocala. The date of his arrival in Florida is known through the Fernandina *East Floridian* of March 29, 1860, in which the arrival of the ship, Gordon, in Fernandina harbor was mentioned. Among its passengers was Dr. Beckett.[3]

The Marion County Census of 1860 lists Dr. Beckett as a resident in the home of his brother and sister-in-law. Dr. Beckett's property was valued at $1,000 which probably indicated the cost of his horse and medical equipment.[4] Since Dr. Beckett's name does not appear in subsequent Marion County records, it is assumed that the disruptions attending the outbreak of war in 1861 prompted his departure from the state.[5] There is no further information on him.

1. This date is an extrapolation based on the date of his graduation from medical college.
2. Charleston *Mercury*, March 22, 1858. The graduation exercises were held on March 12.
3. Fernandina *East Floridian*, March 28, 1860.
4. U.S. Census, 1860, Marion County, Florida, item 152.
5. Civil War records for Florida have yielded no information relating to the Becketts which leads to the conclusion that the doctor and possibly his brother had returned to Charleston following the surrender of Fort Sumter.

Bell, Stephen Bennett, Leon County, 1844

Very little is known of the early years of Dr. Bell. He was born in Florida in 1844 but the place of his birth has not been determined. For some unknown reason his name does not appear in the Florida Census of 1860. By 1870,[1] however, he is listed in the Leon County census as a resident of the Iamonia area and designated "physician," aged 26. His wife, Caroline (Carrie), also appears, her age being 27, her birthplace, Florida. Whatever his background, Dr. Bell was able to acquire a fairly extensive acreage. An agricultural survey made in 1885 shows him to have owned more than 400 acres of which 240 were "improved," that is, under cultivation and turned to pasturage.[2] In the same year his farm was valued at $4,400, his livestock at $1,500. He is also known to have been among the first to plant tobacco in Leon County, his tobacco acreage having been 20 acres in 1892.[3] The meager evidence about him suggests that he was actually more farmer than physician.

Regarding Dr. Bell's medical career very little is known. He is said to have attended an Eclectic Medical School,[4] there were several in the United States in the antebellum period. If indeed he did attend such an institution, it was probably the Eclectic Medical College of Cincinnati which had been founded in 1832 and was certainly the best of its kind.

Five children are known to have been born to Dr. and Mrs. Bell. In order of birth they were: Edward, Margaret, Charles, Bennett, and John. Of his descendants very little is known, and no particular effort has been made for present purposes to track them down.[5]

1. U.S. Census, 1870, Leon County, Florida, p. 603, item 1767.
2. Special Florida Census, 1885. Agricultural data, p. 15.
3. Clifton Paisley, From Cotton to Quail, Gainesville, Florida, University of Florida Press, 1968, p. 52.
4. Henry E. Palmer, M.D., Physicians of Early Tallahassee and Vicinity, *Apalachee*, Tallahassee, Tallahassee Historical Society, 1944. Dr. Palmer's complete statement is: "Dr. S.B. Bell is said to have had an office at Iamonia and a home on the Meridian Road north of Lake Iamonia. He was a graduate of Eclectic Medical College, and was the grandfather of Charles Bell of Tallahassee."
5. Dr. Bell was living as late as 1898. His name was included in *Catalogue of Physicians of the State of Florida* issued by the Florida Medical Association, January 1, 1898.

Bellamy, Edward C., Jackson County, 1801-1853

Dr. Bellamy was one of many medically trained men who migrated to Florida in antebellum days, bringing with them sufficient financial resources to enable them to purchase valuable lands and settle down to live as country gentlemen. He was granted the M.D. degree by the University of Maryland in 1825. Scion of an illustrious Huguenot family and native of North Carolina, he arrived in Jackson County in the 1830s with his wife and four sons and purchased a plantation on the Chipola River, north of Natural Bridge.[1] His property was said to have contained 2,060 acres, third largest in the county, and its slave population numbered 66.[2] The decades 1830-1850 were prosperous for most planters, especially those who had obtained the best lands. The tax records of Jackson County for 1850 show that Dr. Bellamy's holding had increased to 4,000 acres and the number of slaves to 166.[3]

Seemingly flaunting his affluence, Dr. Bellamy proceeded to build one of the most imposing mansions in all antebellum Florida. Situated on a hill overlooking the Chipola it was a two-story brick structure with a long front veranda adorned with splended Doric columns. Its interior is described by Jackson County historian, J. Randall Stanley:

> In the parlor, dining room and elsewhere the marble mantels were of colonial design. The chandeliers were elaborately decorated with cut glass prism pendants. The furnishings were luxurious and in good taste, and all the servants, standing at beck and call, wore handsome livery.[4]

During the earlier years of his Florida residence Dr. Bellamy had displayed some civic concern. He was one of the organizers of St. Luke's Episcopal Church in Marianna, a member of its first vestry, and a delegate to the second diocesan convention to be held in Florida.[5] He joined five fellow planters along the Chipola River in asking Florida's congressional delegate, Charles Downing in 1838, "to take action for improvement of Chipola river" by cutting away the natural bridge under which the river ran for about a quarter of a mile. It was their contention that such action would eliminate the flooding of portions of their plantations and, besides, make the river navigable for many miles upstream.[6]

Dr. Bellamy was elected in September 1851 to represent Jackson County at a convention of cotton planters to be held in Macon, Georgia, on October 27,[7] a meeting prompted by the concern of growers for their dwindling profits. It appears that Dr. Bellamy's farming ventures were becoming less profitable and in the meantime he had become party in court cases involving his slaves. In the November 1849 term of the Jackson County Circuit Court he was able to persuade the jury to acquit one of his slaves accused of murder. Subsequently, however, he was the defendant in a suit charging him with "keeping a slave on his plantation," that is, harboring a criminal. He was found guilty and fined $99.

By 1850 Dr. Bellamy's extravagant life-style and inept management of his assets combined with the changing status of the large slave owners began to undermine his economic well-being which had appeared secure in earlier years. He offered his plantation or a portion thereof for sale in December 1851, a tract of 880 acres for $6 per acre, 500 acres were under cultivation. Included in the offer were a gin house, a screw (ginning machinery), an overseer's house, Negro quarters, and other buildings. This property was located nine miles north of Marianna, on the main road, and 11 miles from Neal's Landing on the Chattahoochee River. Dr. Bellamy indicated a willingness to accept a mortgage for a large portion of the sale price.[9] Obviously he was in financial trouble.

Meanwhile Dr. Bellamy's relationship with his younger brother, Dr. Samuel Bellamy, had become strained. Samuel accused his brother of fraudulently attempting to gain possession of all of his property under the guise of trying to rescue him from financial disaster and was indiscreet enough to state his accusation in the Marianna newspaper.[10] His outright hatred of Edward surfaced again in his will drawn up in December 1849. Although he bequeathed his estate such as it was to Edward's minor son, Hardy, he stipulated that nothing should go to his brother.[11]

The subsequent history of the family remains obscure. Only one of Dr. Bellamy's six sons, Edward, seems to have remained in Florida in the later 1850s. Dr. Charles A. Hentz, recollecting a series of sorrowful events occurring in his family in 1856, mentioned the illness of his five-year-old nephew, Henry Keyes, suffering from a bladder stone. The family had engaged "Dr. Edward Bellamy, a very skilled young surgeon to remove the stone." Although the operation was expertly performed the child died a day or so later.[12] Five of the Bellamy sons, William, Edward, Eugene, Croom and Hardy, would have been of enlistment age during the Civil War, but there is no record of them serving in the Confederate Army. Since not one member of the family appears in the census schedules of 1860 and 1870, it is assumed that all had left the state by 1860.[13]

The Bellamy plantation with its elegant mansion was used by Mrs. Caroline Lee Hentz as the setting for her romantic novel, "Marcus Warland." Mrs. Hentz was a frequent guest in the Bellamy home; her descriptions of it are presumed to have been authentic.[14]

1. U.S. Census, 1850, Jackson County, Florida, p. 615. Dr. Bellamy's age is shown here to have been 49, his wife, Ann, was 38. Both were natives of North Carolina as were three eldest sons, William, Edward, and Eugene. The fourth

son was born in Georgia, which suggests a brief sojourn in the state by the family. The three youngest children, Hardy (8), Elizabeth (7), and George (3), were born in Florida, the youngest having been baptized at St. John's Church, Tallahassee. Dr. Bellamy's real estate was valued at $25,000.

2. J. Randall Stanley, *History of Jackson County*, Marianna, 1950, pp. 142-143.

3. Ibid., p. 144.

4. Ibid., pp. 145-146.

5. Ibid., p. 77.

6. TP, XXV, 492. The plan to destroy the natural bridge never materialized. In recent years the obstructions—an accumulation of logs and other debris—have been cleared and the bridge remains.

7. Tallahassee *Sentinel*, September 30, 1851.

8. Stanley, *History*, p. 149.

9. Tallahassee *Sentinel*, December 2, 1851.

10. Marianna *Florida Whig*, January 26, 1848.

11. I am indebted to Cecil Rhyne Jr., a native of Marianna but presently a resident of Tallahassee, for information on Dr. Samuel Bellamy's will. Mr. Rhyne has made extensive notes on the abstracts of wills from Jackson County Abstract Company and shared these with me. It cannot be explained why Dr. Samuel Bellamy singled out this particular nephew, then only aged six, as his beneficiary. The will further stipulated that in case of young Hardy's death, the estate should pass to Benjamin A. and Richard A. Bellamy, sons of Samuel's older brother, Alexander.

12. Charles A. Hentz, "Autobiography," unpublished manuscript, Southern Historical Collection, University of North Carolina, Chapel Hill. I have consulted the transcription in the P.K. Yonge Library of Florida History, University of Florida, Gainesville.

13. The Jackson County Census of 1860 includes the names of the two sons of Dr. Edward's brother, Alexander. They were B.A. and Richard A., aged 26 and 27, respectively.

14. Caroline Lee Hentz, Marcus Warland, published posthumously, Philadelphia, T.B. Peterson, c. 1869.

Bellamy, Samuel C., Jackson County, 1810

Dr. Bellamy, North Carolina-born aristocrat, followed his brother, Dr. Edward Bellamy, to Florida about 1830 settling as his brother had on the Chipola River a few miles north of Marianna. Census data suggest that he was born about 1810.[1] It would appear that both came laden with cash or credit or both sufficient to purchase plantations of considerable size. Perhaps envious of the splendor of his brother's mansion overlooking the river, and in the meantime winning the hand of Elizabeth Ann Croom in marriage, Dr. Samuel directed his interest and a not inconsiderable sum of money toward the building of a pretentious house on North Green Street in Marianna. It was completed in 1837 becoming a symbol of planter affluence and the showplace of the town.[2]

Before the house could be occupied, tragedy struck. Local legend has it that on their wedding night amid the festivities of the occasion Mrs. Bellamy's wedding dress, fluffy and inflammable, was accidentally set on fire by a candle. In her panic she ran outside and was immediately engulfed in flames dying very shortly. Overcome by grief Dr. Bellamy chose never to live in the mansion although it appears that he retained possession of it for several years. The earliest pertinent document is one of about 1850 indicating that it was sold to Chandler C. Yonge.[3] Years later it came into the hands of the William Nickels family and henceforth was known as the Nickels House, or the Nickels-Mooring House, Nickels' daughter having married Edwin Mooring. There is no record that Dr. Bellamy ever remarried. The fact that in 1850 he was living in the home of James Baker would seem to confirm this assumption.[4]

Biographical information on Dr. Bellamy is not abundant. This is due in large measure to the loss of files of the Jackson County papers and the burning of the court house in 1840. Nevertheless, it is clear that he did not withdraw from public life after the death of his wife. In 1837, for example, he was appointed appraiser for Jackson County properties being offered as security for subscriptions for stock in the Union Bank of Tallahassee,[5] although he himself had subscribed $27,710.[6] In 1838 the voters of the county elected him as a delegate to the Constitutional Convention in St. Joseph.[7] He attended the meeting and was signatory to the constitutional instrument produced there.[8] The list of executive appointees in 1841 included Dr. Bellamy as justice of the peace,[9] while in the military elections of 1842 he was assigned the rank of colonel.[10]

Meanwhile Dr. Bellamy continued to supervise his plantation beyond the famous Rock Caverns.[11] In 1843 and again in 1844 the appearance of his "first of the season" bale of cotton caught the attention of the local newspaper editor who praised its beautiful staple. But then, for reasons which may only be surmised, good fortune forsook him.[12]

For many prosperous planters between the Suwannee and Apalachicola Rivers and even farther west collapse of the Union Bank was catastrophic. Product of an era, following suspension of the Second United States Bank in 1836, during which banking regulations were lax or unenforced, the Bank was an unsound speculative venture at best, but the investment lure was tantalizing, enticing some who owned land to mortgage it for additional purchases, and many who did not, to take risks, hoping to become landed gentry. The Bellamys belong to the former class. Both came to grief not only because they had invested in the bank but because by the middle 1840s the plantations were less prosperous. Dorothy Dodd put it bluntly and accurately when she wrote ". . .times were far from good in 1845."[13]

Dr. Samuel Bellamy was faced with economic hardship in 1848. This led to a break with his brother, target of a bitter attack which he was foolish enough to print in the Marianna paper. He wrote: "The public are hereby cautioned against hiring or buying from or otherwise trading with Edward C. Bellamy for, or on account of any part or portion of the property which he pretends to have purchased from me. He has no claim to it, except what he obtained by the hypocritical pretence of trying to help me out of my difficulties, urging me over and over again that I was in no state of mind to attend to my own business."[14] In the following issue the editor made a profuse apology for his indiscretion in publishing the advertisement.[15]

Dr. Bellamy's professional card appeared in the Marianna newspaper on April 4, 1898, and continued to appear for several months afterward. It was a pitiable and unusual statement indicating his deplorable financial condition.[16]

> Dr. Samuel C. Bellamy offers his professional services to the public. He has now no other means of making his living; he therefore solicits the patronage of his neighbors, his books, and his profession.
>
> He will keep constantly on hand a supply of fresh and genuine medicines adapted to all diseases the flesh is heir to.
>
> April 4, 1848 — Rock Cave (Plantation)

Near the end of 1848 Dr. Bellamy drafted his last will and testament, naming the fifth son of his brother, Edward, as his sole heir. The boy's name was Hardy; he was only six at the time. The Doctor's animosity toward his brother is explicit in the wording of the will, in which he states that the legacy to the boy was not to be subject in any way to the claims of Edward.[17] Should Hardy die before coming of age the legacy would go to the sons of the older brother, Alexander.

By that time, however, it was well known that Dr. Samuel was given to excessive drinking. The death of his wife had been a tragic event for him. As his plantation, through neglect, gradually yielded less and less profit, he tried to turn to the practice of medicine. It was much too late although he had been educated for the profession. He had doubtless lost the confidence of his neighbors whose patronage he sought. He gained a brief respite, however, in 1851 when he was elected Clerk of the Probate Court of Jackson County.[18] But that too came too late.

During the last week of December 1852, Dr. Bellamy made a trip to Tallahassee and on his return crossed the Chattahoochee River. On the morning after the crossing he was found dead by the ferryman on or near the steps of the ferryman's station. His throat had been cut with a razor. The Marianna *Whig* of December 31, 1853, concluded the account of the tragedy by stating gratuitously: "The deceased had been exceedingly intemperate for years past, and was most probably laboring under delerium tremens at the time."

1. U.S. Census, 1850, Jackson County, Florida, p. 613. He was 40 years of age in 1850.
2. J. Randall Stanley, *History of Jackson County*, Marianna, 1950, pp. 59-60.
3. The legend of Elizabeth Croom Bellamy is told by Elizabeth F. Smith in *Magnolia Monthly*, December 1976. The facts, however, do not support this romantic story. In the Tallahassee *Floridian*, May 27, 1837, is found the following obituary: "Died, in Jackson County, on May 11 inst. Mrs. Elizabeth Jane, wife of Dr. Samuel Bellamy, aged 18 years; and on the 18th, Alexander, their son, aged 18 months." Obviously the tragedy did not occur on their wedding night although the loss of both wife and small son within a single week could account for the doctor's despair.
4. For the various transfers of the Nickels house see Stanley, loc cit.
5. T.P., XXV, 429.
6. Stanley, *History*, p. 119.
7. Tallahassee *Florida Watchman*, April 28, 1838, Tallahassee *Floridian*, January 15, 1842, Stanley *History*, p. 130.
8. St. Joseph *Times*, January 12, 1839.
9. T.P., XXVI, 262.
10. Tallahassee Florida *Sentinel*, August 26, 1842.
11. This plantation was situated close to the caverns which have been incorporated into a state park.
12. Appalachicola *Commercial Advertiser*, August 10, 1844, Tallahassee *Florida Sentinel*, August 22, 1843. The 1843 bale sold for ten cents per pound.
13. Dorothy Dodd, Florida in 1845, Florida Historical Quarterly, XXIV, No. 1, July 1945, pp. 3-27.
14. Marianna *Florida Whig*, January 26, 1848.
15. Ibid., February 2, 1848.
16. Ibid., April 12, 1848, and subsequent issues.
17. This information is courtesy of Cecil Rhyne of Tallahassee. Mr. Rhyne is a native of Marianna and quite knowledgeable of Jackson County history.
18. Stanley, *History*, p. 35n.

Bellinger, Pinckney, Jefferson County, 1813

Only a few scattered references to Dr. Bellinger have been located although he is presumed to have led an active professional life in Jefferson County. He was born in South Carolina about 1813[1] and in 1836 or thereabouts moved with his wife, Mary, to Florida settling on a farm between Waukeenah and Lloyds near the Leon County line. His plantation was a modest one valued at only $200 by the census-taker in 1850.[2] Local tradition holds that he practiced medicine throughout the county and was "a fine physician of the old school."[3]

Dr. Bellinger appears to have had more than a casual interest in politics. In the presidential campaign of 1840 he emerged as a leader of the opposition to Martin Van Buren whose term of office had been marred by the depression of 1837 and subsequent years. Dr. Bellinger and other erstwhile Democrats, calling themselves "Conservatives," campaigned actively for William Henry

Harrison, the Whig candidate, whom they regarded as having been cut in the pattern of Andrew Jackson.[4]

The Bellingers reared four children, a son and three daughters. The son, William like his father, pursued a career in medicine. The date of Dr. Bellinger's death is unknown but since he does not appear in the Census of 1860 he is presumed to have died before that date.

1. This date is an extrapolation. The Jefferson County Census of 1850 gives his age as 37.
2. Ibid., 1840. The census of this date indicates that he was the owner of two slaves.
3. Elizabeth F. Smith, *The Town of Bailey's Mill-Lloyd, Jefferson County, Florida, 1825-65*, Crawfordville, Florida, 1971.
4. Jerrell H. Shofner, *History of Jefferson County, Florida*, Tallahassee, Florida, 1976, pp. 61, 175.

Bellinger, William, Jefferson County, 1835-1883

Dr. Bellinger, son of Dr. Pinckney Bellinger, a South Carolinian of distinctive lineage, was born in Jefferson County, Florida, on September 11, 1835.[1] When, as a youth, he decided to follow his father in the medical profession, he became an apprentice in the office of Dr. Robert B. Gorman and Dr. James Lawrence Palmer, well-known practitioners in the village of Waukeenah, near where the Bellinger homestead was located.[2] In the fall of 1858 he entered the Medical College of the State of South Carolina, Charleston, from which he was graduated in March 1860. His doctoral thesis topic was "Intermittent Fever,"[3] a topic which attracted the interest of many southern medical students.

Dr. Bellinger had hardly begun his practice in Waukeenah when the Civil War began. He enlisted in the Confederate cause on March 3, 1862, and was mustered in at St. Marks, committing his services for a period of three years. In spite of his degree from a reputable medical college, he entered the army as 3rd Sergeant and was assigned to nonmedical duty in Company C, 5th Florida Infantry Regiment. In the following August, however, he was detailed as "Assistant Surgeon" on the regimental medical staff. There he remained until the following May when he was transferred to the Confederate General Hospital, Howard's Grove, Richmond, Virginia. He reported for duty on June 2 and on September 1, 1863, was relieved of his duty as hospital steward and given an officer's commission. Although the record of his service is incomplete, it appears that he remained in this position until the end of the war.[4]

Upon his return to Waukeenah Dr. Bellinger was married to Henrietta Moseley, a North Carolina native and relative of former Governor William Moseley, Florida's first governor under statehood. They had seven children, four sons and three daughters.[5]

For reasons which are not at all clear but probably because of failing health, Dr. Bellinger discontinued medical practice in the 1870s turning to running a general merchandise and drug store in Waukeenah. The census of 1880 lists him simply as "dry goods merchant."[6] He died in Waukeenah on February 14, 1883, and was buried in the local cemetery. The Special Census of Florida, compiled in 1885, indicates that his widow, listed as "H.R. Bellinger," was the owner and operator of the mercantile business.

Several of Dr. Bellinger's children continued to live in middle Florida. His youngest daughter, Eva, was for many years a secretary at the Florida State

College for Women, predecessor of the present-day Florida State University.

1. The dates of Dr. Bellinger's birth and death are found on his gravestone in the Waukeenah Cemetery.
2. Archives of the Medical College of the State of South Carolina, Lists of Matriculants, Waring Historical Medical Library, Charleston.
3. Charleston *Daily Courier*, March 14, 1860.
4. NA, Serv. Recs. CSA, M251, Roll 59. There are several unfortunate lacunae in Dr. Bellinger's war record.
5. Federal Writers Program, Jefferson County, Florida, *Waukeenah, Early Settlers*, p. 119. Ibid., *Towns and Plantations*, p. 109.
6. U.S. Census, 1870, Jefferson County, Florida, p. 478; ibid, 1880, p. 43.
7. See note 5, supra, *Towns and Plantations*, p. 109. Here it is stated that the Waukeenah post office was located in the rear of Dr. Bellinger's store and that in 1874 Dr. Bellinger was appointed postmaster in which capacity he served until his death.

Benedict, Nathan Dow, Magnolia and St. Augustine, 1815-1871

Dr. Benedict, son of Robert and Clarissa Dow Benedict, was born in De Ruyter, Madison County, New York, on April 7, 1815.[1] He attended Rutgers College, New Brunswick, New Jersey, from which he was graduated in 1837 with both A.B. and A.M. degrees. In the following year he matriculated at the Medical College of the University of Pennsylvania where he received the M.D. degree in the spring of 1840. His doctoral thesis bore the title, "Medicinal Waters." After a brief period of private practice he was appointed superintendent of the Blockley Insane Asylum of Philadelphia in 1845, a position he held for five years. In 1850 he accepted a similar position at the New York State Lunatic Asylum in Utica.

By the mid-1850s, probably for reasons of his health, Dr. and Mrs. Benedict (she was Emma Ewing Harris) and their four children moved to the resort village of Magnolia, Florida.[2] At about this time Joseph Summerlin, pioneer developer, built the Magnolia Hotel,[3] which was designed to attract winter visitors especially those suffering from pulmonary ailments. Although surviving records are not clear on the matter, it appears that as war became imminent the hotel ceased to be profitable. At any rate it passed into the hands of Dr. Benedict, either by lease or purchase, and was converted into a sanatorium.[4]

With the coming of the war in 1861 the Benedict family, in spite of their northern roots, were able to maintain an amicable coexistence with their neighbors. Dr. Benedict was put in charge of the military Post Hospital in St. Augustine in 1863, a position he held for about a year.[5] After the war the Benedicts remained in St. Augustine, and he resumed private practice.

The United States Congress extended the life of the Freedmen's Bureau in early 1866. Its Florida agents undertook a public health project by leasing Dr. Benedict's Magnolia Hotel and an adjoining building known as the "Cottage," reopening the former as a hospital into which they transferred a number of needy and ailing former slaves from a similar facility in Jacksonville.[6]

The absence of St. Augustine newspapers for the period June 1861 until September 1866[7] makes it impossible to provide a detailed account of Dr. Benedict's activities during those years while lengthy lacunae in other newspapers provoke equal frustration. A few items do permit a bare framework, however. On September 8, 1866, Dr. John E. Peck, about to leave St. Augustine for an extended absence, announced that Dr. Benedict would take care of his professional business until his return.[8] At some unknown date Dr. Benedict was appointed Judge of St. Johns County and from time to time legal notices over his signature appeared.[9] He was the successful candidate in September 1869 of the "Peoples Party" for a seat on the St. Augustine City Council (Board of Aldermen), having received more votes than any of the other nine contenders.[10]

By the winter of 1869-70 Dr. Benedict's health began to decline. On March 12, 1870, the following item appeared in the local newspaper:

> We are glad to say that Dr. Benedict, who has been more or less indisposed for some time, was able to be on his seat as Judge of the County Court on Monday last. Our citizens are always glad to hear good news of him. . .one of our most valuable and useful citizens, he has always the best wishes of us all.[11]

On November 5, 1870, appeared the following:

> We regret to state that Dr. N.D. Benedict has resigned as County Judge of this County. . .The retirement. . .is a great loss to this community, as every citizen interested in good government, the administration of justice and the laws without fear or favor, will feel that this vacancy will be hard to fill. The Doctor is so well known as an "officer" and a "gentleman" in every sense of the word, that it is unnecessary for us to say more.[12]

His life ended on April 30, 1871, in St. Augustine, at the age of 56.

In spite of the difficult years, economically and politically, of the 1860s, Dr. Benedict appears to have managed his affairs very well. In 1860 his properties were estimated to be worth $9,000,[13] while in 1870 they were valued at $40,000.[14]

1. The biographical data included in this sketch unless otherwise indicated are derived from the Archives of the University of Pennsylvania through the courtesy of the Archivist, Mr. F.J. Dallett.
2. Magnolia was located on the west bank of the St. Johns River in Clay County some three miles north of the present town of Green Cove Springs. At the time of their arrival in Florida the Benedicts had four children. Three (William H., b. 1845; Clara H., b. 1847; and Harriet N., b. 1848) were born in Philadelphia. The fourth, Mary, was born in Utica in 1850. The fifth child, Robert P., was born in Magnolia on September 18, 1859.
3. Arch Fred Blakey, *Parade of Memories, A History of Clay County, Florida*, Jacksonville, 1976, p. 65.
4. The University of Pennsylvania Archives item (note 1) identifies Dr. Benedict as "Physician and (Proprietor?), Sanatorium, Magnolia, Florida." Some of the information in the Archives was obtained in 1901 from Dr. Benedict's eldest son, William, then a resident of New Brunswick, N.J.
5. The archival material dates his tenure in St. Augustine Hospital as 1863-64.
6. Blakely, *Parade*, p. 115.
7. St. Augustine's only newspaper, the *Examiner*, suspended publication in early 1862 and resumed in August 1866.
8. Ibid., September 8, 1866.
9. An example is found in ibid., September 25, 1869.
10. Ibid., September 4 and 13, 1869.
11. Ibid., March 12, 1870.
12. Ibid., November 5, 1870.
13. U.S. Census, 1860, Clay County, Florida, p. 3.
14. Ibid., 1870, St. Johns County, Florida, p. 610. The files of the St. Augustine Historical Society include references to the marriages of two Benedict daughters: Clara H. Benedict to Caleb R. Layton, March 12, 1873, and Mary Benedict to E.K. Foster, November 18, 1874.

Benton, E.N., Monticello, Jefferson County, 1860

The Census of 1860, Jefferson County, Florida, lists Dr. Benton as a resident of Monticello. He was 32 years of age and owned property valued at $1,360. His wife, Roseanna, six years his junior and their three children, were born in Georgia as was the doctor himself.[1]

1. U.S. Census, 1860, Jefferson County, Florida, item 477. The three children were Laura, aged 12, Charles E., aged six, and John, aged two.

Benton, George W., Levy County, 1817

A single reference identifies Dr. Benton as a resident of Florida just prior to the Civil War. The Census of 1850 shows him to have been a resident of the Long Pond community in Levy County. He is designated "Physician," owning property valued at about $3,000. He was a native of North Carolina,[1] born about 1817. His wife, Ann, was a native of South Carolina while their three children, Eugenia aged six, John W. aged two, and Asberry aged two months, were born in Florida. This indicates that Dr. Benton probably arrived in Florida about 1853. Nothing further about this family has been discovered.

1. U.S. Census, 1860, Levy County, Florida, Item 103.

Benton, Washington, Duval County, 1807

Dr. Benton, a native of Connecticut, was a medical practitioner in Duval County in 1860. His age was 53 at that time. His wife, Eliza, 18 years his junior, was born in Ohio as was their eldest child, Harriet, aged 15. Two other children, Sydnia (Sidney?) aged six and Clarence aged four, were Florida natives. Dr. Benton was a man of very modest means, owning property valued at $1,000 in 1860.[1]

1. U.S. Census, 1860, Duval County, Florida, p. 432.

Best, William J., Baker and DeSoto Counties, latter 19th century

Dr. Best, a native of Virginia, received his medical degree at the University of Maryland in 1856.[1] With the outbreak of war in 1861 he is thought to have served with a Virginia unit in the army of the Confederacy. In the late 1860s he moved to Florida settling as a practitioner in Baker County.[2]

Subsequent to his arrival in Florida, Dr. Best took a wife, known only by her Christian name, Hattie. She was a native of Florida. Their first child, a daughter Willey, was born in August 1869. A few years later Dr. Best transferred his practice to DeSoto County where he was still in practice near the end of the century.[3]

1. Eugene Fauntleroy Cordell, *Historical Sketch of the University of Maryland School of Medicine, 1807-1890*, Baltimore, 1891, p. 164.
2. U.S. Census, 1870, Baker County, Florida, p. 219, item 57.
3. Florida Medical Association, *Catalogue of Physicians of the State of Florida*, Jacksonville, 1898, p. 5.

Bettes, Jerome N., Jacksonville, 1832-1895

Dr. Bettes, a native of Brighton, Ontario, was born in 1832. After completing the course of study in the local public schools he began the study of medicine in the office of a Dr. Fife of Brighton under whose preceptorate he is said to have remained for six years. He then entered the Eclectic College of Medicine in Cincinnati, Ohio, from which he was graduated in 1857. Over the next 13 years he practiced in several places including his home town of Brighton, Clinton, Ohio, and other places in the Great Lakes area. He moved to Jacksonville in 1870 where he resumed practice and continued until his death on the morning of December 21, 1895.[2]

Dr. Bettes won the affection of the citizens of Jacksonville for his gallant service during the yellow fever epidemic of 1888, when he gave freely of his professional skills at great risk to his own health.

Five children were born to Dr. and Mrs. (Ruth) Bettes. Upon his death he was survived by four children: Frederick, a resident of St. Augustine, Charles of Jacksonville, Emily (Mrs. Pratt) of Oak Hill, N.Y., and Maggie of Jacksonville. One son, William, had died in 1892; Mrs. Bettes died several years earlier.[3]

1. The data for this sketch derives principally from the obituary for Dr. Bettes, Jacksonville *Florida Times-Union*, December 22, 1895, and Wanton S. Webb *Webb's Historical Industrial and Biographical Florida*, Pt. I., New York, 1885, p. 131.

2. The Bettes grave marker in Evergreen Cemetery, Jacksonville, gives the date of his death as December 20 but it appears from the obituary that he died in the early morning of the 21st.

3. The Bettes residence was located in Jacksonville at the corner of Liberty and Monroe Streets, he had earlier lived on Newman Street, while his office was at 5½ East Bay Street.

Betton, George W., Leon County, 1824-1896

Dr. Betton, one of Leon County's most distinguished physicians, was born in Fairfax County, Virginia, on February 9, 1824.[1] He was the second son of Thurbutt Rowles and Elizabeth Lane Betton who moved to Leon County in 1825, purchased land and developed a plantation a few miles north of Tallahassee.[2] Nothing is known of young George's early education but it is assumed that he had private tutors as was true of the children of most well-to-do planters of the times. In due time he enrolled at St. John's College, Annapolis, Maryland, from which he received his Bachelor of Arts degree in 1842. In the following year he matriculated at the University of Pennsylvania School of Medicine and was graduated M.D. in 1845. His doctoral thesis bore the title, "Delirium Tremens."[3]

Within a couple of months after receiving his medical degree Dr. Betton began his practice in Tallahassee. His professional notice first appeared in the Tallahassee *Sentinel* of May 27, 1845.[4] Near the end of 1849 he moved to New Port (Wakulla County)[5] where he practiced for more than a decade. When a devastating epidemic of yellow fever struck the town in the fall of 1853 he was among those who became ill, a doubly unfortunate blow in that he was the sole physician of the vicinity. The desperate circumstances prompted the citizens of Tallahassee to organize a relief mission for the fever victims and their families. The City Council quickly voted $500 which it authorized the intendant (mayor) to spend, beyond the $300 raised by private subscription for employing physicians, nurses and medical supplies.[6] By 1859 Dr. Betton was once more in practice in Tallahassee. In May of that year he married Margaret Whitaker Holland, daughter of Dr. George W. Holland, wealthy physician-planter, whose estate lay some 10 miles north of Tallahassee.[7] The census of 1860 lists the couple as residents of the Capital, living in a house located at 321 East Park Avenue.[8] This marriage was terminated by the untimely death of Mrs. Betton on March 11, 1863, at the age of 22.[9]

Dr. Betton enlisted in the Army of the Confederacy in 1861 as Staff Surgeon of the 7th Florida Infantry Regiment.[10] Due, possibly, to his age, family responsibilities, or medical needs of the Tallahassee community, he was never actually mustered into service. For whatever reason he continued to practice in Leon County throughout the War.[11]

From the beginning of his career Dr. Betton took pride in his profession and on several occasions demonstrated his concern for improving the quality of education and professional skill of his medical colleagues. As early as 1848, when he was only three years out of medical school, he joined 11 of his colleagues from Leon and adjoining counties, meeting in Quincy for the purpose of organizing a state medical society.[12] He was elected Treasurer of the newly-formed Society which, it was assumed, would be properly chartered at the next session of the Florida Legislature. Their hopes were dashed, however, when the charter was denied (reasons for such action are not clear) and a much-altered substitute creating a Medical Board was passed instead.

Twenty-six years later Dr. Betton was one of 10 physicians who met in the office of Dr. Abel S. Baldwin in Jacksonville (January 14, 1874) to launch the Florida Medical Association.[13] Dr. Betton was chosen chairman pro tem of the session later becoming the Association's first vice president after the election of Dr. Baldwin as president. In subsequent years he held committee appointments most notably the chairmanship of the Ethics Committee. In the meeting of the Association in Tallahassee in 1881, Dr. Betton was elected president for the coming year. When the Association convened in Pensacola in 1882, however, he sent regrets that he would not be present to preside, but he did send his address which was read by the secretary. Shortly thereafter he resigned from the Association for reasons not stated in the *Proceedings* of the Association.

As a physician and citizen Dr. Betton appears to have served Leon County well. A staunch Episcopalian he was a regular communicant at St. John's Church. He was well remembered in Tallahassee for having directed his black servant, William Gunn, into a medical career. Recognizing Gunn's intelligence and aptitude Dr. Betton provided his early medical training, then saw to it that he proceed to Meharry Medical College, Nashville, Tennessee. After his graduation Gunn returned to Tallahassee as the first black practitioner of Leon County.[14] Dr. Betton died in Tallahassee on November 1, 1896.[15]

Four years after the death of his first wife Dr. Betton married Margaret McLeon, daughter of J.D. McLeon of Madison County, at whose home, Buckhall, the wedding ceremony occurred on June 5, 1867.[16] To the first marriage one son, George Holland, had been born. Three sons, John McLeon, William Lane, and Donald, were born to the second.

1. This date of birth from Dr. Betton's gravestone in St. John's Churchyard, Tallahassee, appears to be correct although it is not in agreement with the data of the University of Pennsylvania Archives which give the date of his birth as February 22, 1822. It should also be noted that his place of birth is given in some sources as Maryland, the birthplace of his father. Census schedules, however, consistently assign his birthplace to Virginia.

2. See Leroy D. Ball and John Bradford, "Map of Leon County, 1873," copy in Collection of P.K. Yonge Library of Florida History, No. 834, which shows location of Betton properties.

3. Archives, University of Pennsylvania, Lists of Matriculants and Graduates.

4. Tallahassee *Sentinel*, May 27, 1845. This issue is not extant but the card was printed in subsequent issues. See ibid., February 17, 1846.

5. New Port *Wakulla Times*, June 16, 1852, U.S. Census, 1850, Wakulla County, Florida, shows him as resident of New Port.

6. Dorothy Dodd, "The Corporation of Tallahassee, 1826-1860," *Apalachee*, 1948-50, p. 93.

7. Fernandina *East Floridian*, June 2, 1859. The wedding occurred on May 19th.

8. U.S. Census, 1860, Leon County, Florida, p. 19. See Evelyn W. Henry, "Old Houses of Tallahassee," *Tallahassee Historical Society Annual*, I, February 1934, 42, Dr. Betton is said to have lived there until 1880, when he bought the Hagner House, presently known as the Knott House.

9. Tallahassee *Florida Sentinel*, April 7, 1863.

10. NA, Service Records, CSA, M251, Roll 76. On page one of the Florida 7th Infantry Regimental Records is a list of the original enlistees (Field and Staff). Dr. Betton is designated Surgeon. No army record for him appears in the subsequent pages however.

11. In 1863 the State Treasurer was authorized to pay Dr. Betton $40 for postmortem examinations performed, Tallahassee *Florida Sentinel*, February 24, 1863.
12. Quincy *Times*, May 20, 1848. For an account of this effort and its ultimate failure see E. Ashby Hammond, "Medical Regulation and Organization in Florida, 1821-1874," *Journal of the Florida Medical Association*, January 1974, pp. 62-70.
13. *Proceedings, Florida Medical Association*, Sessions 1874-75, Charleston, Walker, Evans & Cogswell, 1875, pp. 1-5.
14. Henry E. Palmer, "Physicians of Early Tallahassee and Vicinity," *Apalachee*, 1944, p. 44.
15. Ibid., p. 43.
16. Tallahassee *Sentinel*, June 6, 1867.

Bevill, Robert John, Hamilton County, 1833

Dr. Bevill was born in Screven County, Georgia, on October 31, 1833. When he was eight years old he moved with his family to Hamilton County where they obtained land and settled down as farmers.[1] Young Robert is said to have begun the study of medicine under the guidance of a Dr. John F. Trippe about 1851, and to have graduated in 1855.[2] Soon thereafter he was married to Sarah Sutton of Lowndes County, Georgia,[3] and began a career of farming and practicing medicine near Bellville in the northwestern part of the county.

With the outbreak of war in 1861 Dr. Bevill enlisted for military service notwithstanding the domestic obligations to his wife and three-year-old daughter. He entered the army with the rank of first lieutenant in August 1861, committing himself to a period of one year and reporting for duty at Ft. Clinch, Nassau County. With the expiration of his term he promptly reenlisted for the duration of the war. His army record indicates that he remained at Ft. Clinch until March 1863 when, by order of General Braxton Bragg, he was assigned to conscription and recruitment duty.[4]

Dr. Bevill was transferred to a post in Georgia in 1864 where he became ill and was hospitalized for a time at Ocmulgee Hospital near Macon. His ailment was diagnosed as phthisis and he was sent home on indefinite sick leave. Although still technically in military service his name was placed in nomination for a seat in the Florida House of Representatives for the upcoming elections of early October. When it was clear that he had been elected to the seat he submitted his letter of resignation to the army, enclosing a statement from Judge Henry J. Stewart of Hamilton County certifying his election.[5] He answered the roll call of the House on November 22, 1864, second day of the session. Seventeen years later he was again elected to the Florida House (1881), and two years later (1883) he was once more elected to the same office.[6]

To Dr. Bevill's first marriage three children were born, Susan, Sarah, and a son, Thompson. The second daughter, Sarah, died in childhood. Upon the death of Mrs. Bevill the doctor married a widow, Mrs. Margaret D. Shiver. To this marriage were born two daughters, Julia and Rebecca, and a son, Granville.[7]

Very little information has survived concerning the latter part of Dr. Bevill's life. The Hamilton County Census of 1885 lists him as Doctor of Medicine but his name does not appear in subsequent censuses and gazeteers of Florida.[8]

In politics Dr. Bevill was in his earlier years an "Old Line Whig" but with dissolution of the party he voted the Democratic ticket in national and state elections while maintaining an independent stance in local elections. He was a member of the Missionary Baptist Church.[9]

1. Much of what is known about the life of Dr. Bevill is summarized in J.V. Drake, ed. and comp., The Florida Legislature, an Official Directory, Jacksonville 1883, p. 42. This contains brief biographical sketches of members of the Florida legislature for the 1883 session. Presumably much of the data was submitted by the members themselves.

2. Dr. Trippe has not been further identified. The Trippe family was well-known in Georgia, while there was a physician, Henry Trippe, practicing in Jackson County, Florida, in the Territorial Period. As for the medical college which Dr. Bevill may have attended we can only conjecture that it was the Southern Botanico-Medical College in Macon, Georgia, which gained considerable popularity in the 1840s and 1850s. Dr. Bevill's name does not appear among the lists of graduates of the four other Georgia medical colleges of the mid-19th century.

3. Sarah Sutton, also a native Georgian, brought to her marriage a dowry of some $10,000 which doubtless raised the economic status of the Bevill family substantially. Mrs. Cora Hinton, historian of Hamilton County, states that Miss Sutton's father, Shadrach Sutton, was the first sheriff of the county. Cora Hinton, *Early History of Hamilton County Florida*, Jasper, 1976, p. 28.

4. National Archives, Service Records, CSA, M251, Roll 46. Dr. Bevill's military unit was Company G, 3rd Florida Infantry.

5. Ibid. Dr. Bevill gave five reasons for his resignation: (1) His election to the Legislature, (2) He had been recommended for retirement on June 27th "by a proper Medical Board," (3) He had sent his papers through proper channels, (4) He was still absent from his company on sick leave, and (5) He could not take his seat in the Legislature until his resignation had been accepted.

6. Florida House Journal, 1864, 1881, 1883.

7. Granville as a Christian name occurred frequently in the Bevill family. Screven County censuses of 1840 and 1850 show that Dr. Robert J. had an uncle as well as a cousin bearing that name.

8. Hamilton County Court House records show that Dr. Bevill and his wife moved to Volusia County at some time after 1885. It is assumed that they died there although no record of their deaths has been located. Letter, Mrs. Cora Hinton to E.A. Hammond, February 13, 1982.

9. Drake, *op cit.*

Bexley, Augustus R., Lake City, 1825-1867

Dr. Bexley, a native of Georgia and graduate of the Medical College of Georgia, Augusta,[1] in 1845, began his medical practice in Alligator (later Lake City) in the late 1840s. About 1849 he married a local girl, Clarissa, by whom he had one daughter, Elizabeth, born in the early 1850s.[2] He bought a considerable amount of property in the town in July 1855.[3] Either through marriage, inheritance, or by his own enterprise and medical practice, he appears to have prospered. The census of 1860 lists him as the owner of property appraised at $20,000.[4]

After the death of his wife, Dr. Bexley married Sallie, like himself a native of Georgia. They had a son, Murray, a daughter, Eva, and another son, Robert.[5] Dr. Bexley died in the summer of 1867.[6]

1. Medical Department, University of Georgia, Augusta. "List of Graduates, 1829-1891," August 1891, p. 14.

2. U.S. Census, 1850, Columbia County, Florida, p. 81. The slave schedule of that year shows Dr. Bexley as the owner of five slaves.

3. Edward F. Keuchel, *A History of Columbia County, Florida*, Tallahassee, Florida, 1981, p. 231.

4. U.S. Census, 1860, Columbia County, Florida, p. 179.

5. U.S. Census, 1870, Columbia County, Florida, p. 418.

6. Lake City *Suwannee News*, October 2, 1867. As the administrator of her husband's estate Mrs. Bexley, by order of the Probate Court Judge of the County, placed the following notice in the paper. "(There) will be sold at auction on the first Monday in October for the benefit of creditors and all interested Fifty Town Lots lying and being situated within the Northern extension of the City of Lake City belonging to the estate of A.R. Bexley, late of the said County, deceased." September 4, 1867 (issue not extant).

Bigelow, Robert John, Duval, Lafayette, Levy, and Orange Counties, 1835-1912

Dr. Bigelow, second child and eldest son of Robert and Elizabeth Bigelow, was born on his father's estate in what is known as the Arlington section of Jacksonville in January 1835. His father was a native of Connecticut who had migrated to Jacksonville, then known as Cowford, during the second Spanish period. As a practitioner of law he had become involved in numerous land settlements at the time of the cession from Spain in 1821 and in the course of events had come into possession of valuable lands on the east side of the River.[1] On some of his land, in what is now the Mandarin area, he began a farming operation on which his son, Robert John, is known to have labored in his youth.[2] Robert John became an apprentice to a local physician and in due time was qualified for further training in medicine. In the fall of 1858 he matriculated at Jefferson Medical College in Philadelphia from which he was graduated Doctor of Medicine in the spring of 1860.[3]

Upon returning to Florida Dr. Bigelow entered practice, not in Jacksonville as would have been expected, but in the remote village of Long Pond in Levy County.[4] He obtained room and board in the home of a farmer, John J. Wester, the members of whose household numbered 17.

On September 1, 1861, Dr. Bigelow enlisted for service in the Confederate Army and was mustered in as a private in Captain William A. Sheffield's Company (D), Fourth Florida Infantry Regiment. One year later he was given the appropriate rank of Assistant Surgeon of the Regiment. For the next two years he served with his unit at various places in Alabama, Georgia and Tennessee. In the fall of 1864 he appeared before a court martial for what must have been a very minor offense, possibly insubordination. He was reduced to the rank of private but two weeks later was reinstated as Assistant Surgeon. He was mustered out of the Army on April 26, 1865.[5]

Soon after discharge from the Army, Dr. Bigelow returned to Florida, settling not in the more comfortable environs of a growing town, but at a rural settlement on a bend in the Suwannee River known as Hatch's Bend,[6] some seven miles south of Branford. Here he was married in 1872 to a girl whose Christian name was Stella.[7] To this union were born three children: a son, St. John, a daughter, Jessie Florence, and a second son, Robert C.[8] Scarcely any information regarding the lives of the Bigelow family during these years on the Suwannee has survived. Since the doctor appears on no list of public officers of the County or Village, it is assumed that this segment of his life was devoted to family and practice.

It is not known precisely when Dr. Bigelow abandoned his practice in Lafayette County. He was still there in the summer of 1885 when the special Census of that year was tabulated. He is shown to have owned 166 acres of land of which only six were cultivated. His total land value was estimated at $200, while his livestock were worth about $300.[9] The Bigelows are thought to have left Lafayette County in the late 1880s for their new location in Orange County, west of Orlando, where they were among the founders of the town of Ocoee.

In Orange County, which was becoming the citrus-growing center of Florida, Dr. Bigelow appears to have thrived. After resuming his medical practice, he opened a drug store in partnership with his son Robert C.[10] It was a successful venture. Dr. Bigelow was listed among the practicing physicians of the state in the survey compiled by the Florida Medical Association and published by the State Board of Health in 1898. He was never a member of the Association, however. He died at Ocoee in 1912 at the age of 77 and was buried in the Ocoee cemetery. His descendants have played important roles in the development of Orange County in the 20th century.[11]

1. For plats of his lands and information on certain transactions see Bigelow Papers, MSS, Box 50, P.K. Yonge Library of Florida History, University of Florida, Gainesville.
2. U.S. Census, 1850, Duval County, Florida, p. 102, item 75. Robert John is listed as a laborer aged 16.
3. *General Alumni Catalogue of Jefferson Medical College*, W.J. Maxwell, comp., Philadelphia, 1917, 67.
4. This village since virtually disappeared was situated some three miles south of the present Chiefland.
5. The Civil War record of Dr. Bigelow is incomplete. For such parts as have survived, see National Archives Service Records CSA, M251, Roll 53.
6. Holmes Melton, *Lafayette County History and Heritage*, Mayo, Florida, 1974, p. 19.
7. U.S. Census, 1880, Lafayette County, Florida, p. 167, item 17. The older son, St. John, had died prior to 1900. In the census of that year, it is shown that of the three children born to the Bigelows one was deceased.
8. Ibid., 1880 Census.
9. Special Census, Florida, 1885, Lafayette County, p. 11, "Agricultural Production."
10. The partnership of Dr. Bigelow and his son is listed in more than one *Florida Gazeteer*.
11. No effort has been made to present information on the Bigelow family which remained in Duval County. Mrs. Elizabeth Bigelow, widow of Robert, remained on the family land in the Mandarin area. The cemetery records of Duval County show that she and several of her children, brothers and sisters of Dr. Robert John, are buried in the family cemetery in the Arlington section. Mrs. Bigelow died on January 30, 1891, while the eldest daughter, Minerva (Mrs. Georgia A. Turknett,) died on December 7, 1868. The father of the family, Robert, born 1792, died on August 8, 1868. It is not known whether Dr. Bigelow maintained contact with his family.

Bird, Richard L., Gadsden County, 1832

Very little is known of the career of Dr. Bird, who practiced for a brief period in Chattahoochee, Gadsden County. A native of Georgia he was graduated from the Medical College of Georgia, Augusta, in 1854.[1] After a few years practice in his home state he moved to Florida in 1859, settling in Chattahoochee, where he formed a professional partnership with another young physician, William L. Jones. On May 2, 1859, they announced their services in "all matters pertaining to their profession." They could be found at their office "on the street leading from the Arsenal to the River."[2]

Possibly because of the disruptions of war the partnership did not endure for long. Although Dr. Jones remained in Chattahoochee for some years, Dr. Bird had left the state prior to 1870. His family consisted of wife, Margaret, and son, Richard L. Jr.[3]

1. *Medical Department, University of Georgia*, "60th Annual Announcement List of Graduates from 1829 to 1891," Augusta, 1891, p. 14.
2. Quincy *Republic*, October 15, 1859, 1st printed in issue of May 2, 1859.
3. U.S. Census, 1860, Gadsden County, Florida, p. 16, item 473.

Bishop, James W., Botanic Physician, Leon County, 1850

From earliest times man in his search for substances efficacious in the treatment of human ailments has relied heavily upon botanical products. Currently producers of medicinal products depend to a great extent on botany or botanical products. Certainly in the 19th and earlier centuries, botany was as important as chemistry in the search. Physicians advertised their services as "botanic physicians." Dr. Bishop was one of these. All that is presently known of him is that he was a Georgian by birth, born in 1824, and in 1850 a resident of Leon County.[1]

1. U.S. Census, 1850, Leon County, p. 140, item 512.

Blair, Hugh A., Ocala, 1858

Dr. Blair announced the opening of his office in Ocala on July 1, 1858. Prior to moving to Florida he had been Professor of Anatomy at Oglethorpe Medical

College, Savannah, Georgia. His practice in Ocala was apparently of brief duration for he does not appear in the Marion County Census of 1860. It is assumed that he returned to Georgia, probably to enter practice in that state.

1. *The Ocala Home Companion*, July 12, 1858.

Blake, Aaron C.F., Leon County, 1827

Dr. Blake, native of Georgia, is thought to have studied medicine in that state prior to moving to Leon County in the early 1850s. Since his name does not appear in the lists of students of any of the medical colleges of the south he is presumed to have prepared himself for practice through the apprenticeship system. He married Mrs. Virginia S. Moore, a widow and the mother of three, on May 4, 1856.[1] By the year 1870 three children, a son Edwin, daughters Sarah and Mary, had been born to this marriage. By that year, however, Dr. Blake had ceased to practice medicine as his major occupation, turning instead to farming. It is apparent that the disruptions of the Civil War had been a disaster for the family, their total wealth having been estimated at over $3,000 in 1860, and a mere $800 in 1870.[2] The various cemetery surveys for Leon County do not list gravestones for Dr. Blake or his wife; the dates of their deaths remain unknown.

1. The Leon County Census of 1860 lists Dr. Blake as physician, aged 33; his wife was 32. The three children of Mrs. Blake by her first husband, Mr. Moore, were William, 15; G.F., (daughter), 12; and C.C., (son), eight. The marriage ceremony for Dr. Blake and Mrs. Moore was performed by Dr. Blake's relative, a clergyman, E.L.T. Blake. See Leon County, Florida, records compiled by the Daughters of the American Revolution, Tallahassee, 1937, p. 78.
2. U.S. Census, 1870, Leon County, Florida, p. 568.

Blodgett, John L., Key West, 1809-1853

Dr. Blodgett, far better known as botanist than as a physician, was a resident of South Florida for about 15 years (1838-1853). Born in Connecticut in 1809,[1] where he is presumed to have received his early education, he attended the Berkshire Medical College, Pittsfield, Massachusetts,[2] from which he was graduated in 1831 having submitted a doctoral thesis entitled "The Use of Friction to the Skin." Soon thereafter he succumbed to wanderlust, making his way westward into Ohio and subsequently southward into Alabama, Mississippi and finally into Louisiana. At New Orleans he took passage on a ship about to depart for Liberia with a number of liberated slaves who were being returned to the land of their fathers. He remained in Liberia for about a year. While there he made the acquaintance of Dr. Ezekiel Skinner and his daughter, Mary, through whose influence he is presumed to have developed his interest in botany.[3]

Returning to the United States in 1838 he elected to settle in an area in which he could continue his study of tropical plants so he chose Key West since that settlement was the most southerly. There he earned a living by the practice of medicine but apparently devoting much of his time to collecting botanical specimens which he sent to his northern colleagues, most notably John Torrey of New York.

As for his medical practice, Dr. Blodgett was scarcely able to eke out a living, the result in some measure of his divided interests, but also of the presence of five of six other physicians in Key West and neighboring Keys.[4] The principal demands for physicians' services arose from military installations at Key West, Dry Tortugas, and other nearby Keys. In addition, Key West was the most convenient haven for the commercial shipping in the Caribbean. Ships often brought their ailing seamen there for treatment. Many appear to have been suffering from the fevers endemic to those latitudes. This situation doubtless explains Dr. Blodgett's contract with the United States Treasury Department through its agent, Adam Gordon, Collector of the Customs in Key West, dated September 15, 1841, stipulating that Dr. Blodgett would attend to sick seamen in the Keys. It was an unsatisfactory arrangement for him in that the contract failed to provide for the purchase of medicines required in the treatment of the sick. After protesting the terms he finally agreed to work for one quarter pending renegotiation of the contract.[5]

Soon after this difficulty had been ironed out a deadly epidemic of yellow fever beset the island and Dr. Blodgett, much concerned about the safety of his wife, suddenly left the island leaving the sick seamen to manage as best they could.[6] This departure was shocking to the islanders but within a few days he returned and set about assisting in the battle against the fever and, as time permitted, collecting tropical flora.

It is a matter of more than passing interest that after settling in Key West Dr. Blodgett reestablished contact with another well-known physician-botanist, Dr. Alvan Wentworth Chapman, a native of Massachussetts. The two men had probably known each other previously. Dr. Chapman moved to Florida prior to 1840, settling first in Gadsden County, but soon moving to Jackson County before settling permanently in Apalachicola, Franklin County. This earlier acquaintance probably explains why the Apalachicola *Commercial Advertiser* of April 27, 1848, printed a lengthy account of a meeting of Whigs on April 24, a gathering at which Dr. Blodgett was active.

Near the end of his life Dr. Blodgett returned to Massachusetts, dying in Amherst on July 15, 1853. His only close relative was his wife, Julia, also a native of Massachusetts. No children are known to have been born to them. Dr. Blodgett's estate was a modest one, his property having been valued at a mere $500 in 1850.[7] George D. Allen, of Key West, was appointed administrator. For some reason the estate was not settled until 1856. On November 3, 1855, Mr. Allen announced that "six months from date he will present his accounts for settlement of the estate of John L. Blodgett late of Monroe County Deceased."[8]

1. There is some confusion as to the place of Dr. Blodgett's birth. The Florida Census of 1850 indicates Connecticut; other sources, probably more reliable place it at South Amherst, Massachusetts. The career of Dr. Blodgett as natural scientist has been thoroughly set forth in an article by Professor R. Bruce Ledin of the University of Miami, "John Loomis Blodgett (1809-1853): A Pioneer Botanist of South Florida, *Tequesta: The Journal of the Historical Association of Southern Florida*, XXII, 1953, pp. 23-33.

2. Berkshire Medical College, Pittsfield, Massachusetts, existed from 1823 until 1867.

3. This presumption, however, is questionable.

4. Physicians known to have practiced in the Keys during Dr. Blodgett's residence were Daniel W. Whitehurst, John Wayles Eppes, C.H. Crane, John O'Hara, Samuel A. Wiltam, S.F. Jones, and J.C. Bates. Some were doubtless brief sojourners.

5. Letter, Adam Gordon, Collector of the Customs, Key West, to the Honorable Thomas Ewing, Secretary of the Treasury, September 15, 1841. Printed in House of Representative Reports, No. 396, 29th Congress, 1st Session.

6. Gordon further explained, "The other physicians rendered services, and the citizens raised $400 to aid the seamen and the poor." Then follows: "These physicians have charged one quarter the rates prescribed in your (i.e. Ewing's) circular. They say they will not continue on that basis, however."

7. U.S. Census, 1850, Monroe County, Florida, p. 293.
8. George Allen was a Key West druggist who doubtless had supplied drugs for Dr. Blodgett. See Key West *Key of the Gulf* issue of November 17, 1853. An interesting, but irrelevant item appeared in ibid., July 16, 1859, a list of unclaimed letters held in the Key West Post Office included one for Dr. Blodgett five years after his death.

Blunt, A.F., Jackson County, 1860

Dr. Blunt appears to have lived in Florida briefly. The Census of 1860 lists him as 40 years of age, born in Virginia, and married to Caroline Blunt, a native of North Carolina.[1] They were residents in the home of Margaret Ann Hearn, widow of Lawrence Henry Hearn, aged 39, also a native of North Carolina, and her daughter, Winifred, and son, Robert, aged 18 and 14 respectively. It is almost certain that Mrs. Blunt and Mrs. Hearn were sisters.[2]

With the coming of the War in 1861 a home guard, composed of older men and boys, was organized for the defense of Jackson County and particularly Marianna. They were popularly known as "The Minute Men of Marianna." Col. A.B. Montgomery was their commandant. One of their officers was Dr. Blunt who was assigned the rank of lieutenant. Early in September 1864 Union Officer Brig. Gen. Alexander Asboth, then at Ft. Barrancas, decided to attack Marianna, then a point of adamant Southern resistance. The onslaught came on September 27, a brief but bloody affair. Among the wounded was Dr. Blunt who was attended to in the home of Mrs. W.S. Wilson, wife of Dr. Wilson.[3]

1. U.S. Census, Jackson County, Florida, 1860, p. 130.
2. J. Randall Stanley, *History of Jackson County*, Marianna, 1850, p. 185.
3. Ibid., p. 193.

Boardman, Samuel, Gadsden County, 1816

English-born Dr. Boardman practiced his profession for a few years in rural Gadsden County about the middle of the 19th century. He arrived in Florida prior to 1840[1] with his wife, Elizabeth Ann Monroe Boardman, a native of Washington, D.C., settling in the Chattahoochee community in the northwestern part of the county.[2] They were the parents of two children, John and Alice who died on September 25, 1852,[3] in her ninth year. Since the Boardmans do not appear in the Florida Census of 1860, it is assumed that they had left the state by that date.

1. U.S. Census, 1840, Gadsden County, Florida, p. 94.
2. Ibid., 1850, p. 384.
3. Tallahassee *Sentinel*, October 19, 1852.

Bobo, Burrell A., Madison County, 1850

Dr. Bobo was a native of South Carolina and moved to Madison County as a youth. Upon the premature death of his father, his mother, Sarah, was left with five children.[1] In due time young Burrell began the study of medicine under the preceptorate of the prominent Madison physician Joseph Fickling Bythewood. In the fall of 1855 he entered the Medical College of the State of South Carolina, Charleston, and received his degree in the spring of 1857.[2] His doctoral thesis bore the title "Intermittent Fever."

Upon graduation Dr. Bobo returned to Madison where, on September 8, 1858, he was married to Roberta Cooper of Madison. He had probably begun his Madison practice in the previous year, however, for in October 1858 he announced that he had "removed to Mrs. A.C. Cooper's one mile south of Sandy Ford. . ." and was soliciting the continued patronage of his clients.[3]

With the coming of the War Dr. Bobo enlisted in the Confederate cause in May 1862, was given the rank of captain and assigned to command Company A, 8th Florida Infantry Regiment. Soon after its organization the Eighth Florida was ordered to Virginia and with minimal experience found itself in the second Battle of Manassas and shortly thereafter in the Battle of Sharpsburg (Md.). In one of these engagements Capt. Bobo failed to exhibit the qualities of leadership expected of him which led to a court martial in early November 1862. He was judged guilty of cowardice and cashiered out of service on November 11, scarcely seven months after his appointment.[4]

Subsequent to this personal tragedy Dr. Bobo disappeared from the records and nothing further is known of him.

1. U.S. Census, 1850, Madison County, Florida, p. 100.
2. Archives, Waring Historical Library, Medical University of South Carolina, Charleston.
3. Madison *Southern Messenger*, December 25, 1858, also Madison County Marriage Records.
4. NA, Service Records, CSA, M251, Roll 81.

Bobo, John E., St. Augustine, 1835

Dr. Bobo, a native of Union District, South Carolina, was a graduate of the Medical College of South Carolina, Charleston, in 1828. His preceptor in Union had been a Dr. Ross. His graduation thesis bore the title "Rheumatism."[1] He arrived in St. Augustine and began his medical practice there in May 1835.[2] It is assumed that since he was not listed in any subsequent Florida census he had left the state prior to 1840.

1. Lists of Matriculants and Graduates, Medical College of South Carolina, Waring Historical Medical Library, Charleston.
2. St. Augustine *Florida Herald*, May 20, 1835. The name Bobo was a fairly common one in Union District. William J. Bobo was a physician there in the mid-19th century. U.S. Census, 1850, Union District, p. 5.

Bond, John Screven, Tallahassee and Quincy, 1824-1882

Dr. Bond was born in McIntosh County, Georgia, son of Samuel H. Bond, a wealthy planter, whose lands lay near the town of Darien.[1] Of his early education nothing is known but as he approached manhood he was sent to Savannah to read medicine under the direction, first, of Dr. J.S. Sullivan and later of the eminent physician James P. Screven.[2] He entered the Medical College of the State of South Carolina in the fall of 1844, graduating as M.D. in the spring of 1846 after presenting a thesis entitled "Malaria."[3]

After receiving his degree Dr. Bond tarried briefly in Georgia before moving to Tallahassee. His professional card appearing on May 19, 1847, announced the launching of his career from his office in "Col. Fisher's Hotel."[4] His impeccable connections in Leon County as well as his aristocratic background in Georgia augured well for his future. His position was probably further enhanced by his marriage in late 1848 to Louisa M. Randolph, daughter of recently deceased Thomas P. Randolph of Quincy.[5]

At about the time of his marriage Dr. Bond transferred his practice to Quincy, taking up residence with his wife's family[6] where he remained for eight years. Returning to Tallahassee in 1858 he became a partner of Dr. William F. Robertson,[7] an arrangement which endured for less than a year, for in February 1859 he joined Dr. John B. Taylor in a partnership located "at the old stand of Dr. Taylor."[8]

Scarcely any details relating to Dr. Bond's practice during the 1850s have survived. One item relating to his fees is of interest. In his early years at Quincy he was retained by planter, Oscar Fillyaw, to care for his Negroes. In 1852 he presented his bill of "$163.25 for twenty-three visits" for the year. This included prescriptions and mileage to and from the plantation. For night visits and bad weather he charged more. A notation on one of his bills shows that 25 bushels of corn were accepted as part payment for the bill.[9]

During the early years of his professional career Dr. Bond manifested interest in organizing a state medical society through which the quality of practice in the state might be improved. He was an active participant in the much publicized State Medical Convention which met in Quincy on May 15-16, 1848,[10] for the purpose of organizing a state association and drafting a charter to be presented at the Legislative Assembly which would meet in the coming December. He was chosen as one of the vice presidents of the society and at the same time was selected as Orator for the first annual meeting scheduled for Tallahassee on the first Monday in January 1849. The Legislature, however, failed to grant the charter, but instead established a Medical Board whose chief function would be to examine prospective practitioners in Florida and issue licenses to those judged to be qualified. Dr. Bond was one of the 10 physicians named to serve on the board.[11]

Of Dr. Bond's war service it is only known that he volunteered his service and was assigned to the staff of General Braxton Bragg as surgeon.[12]

With the organization of the Florida Medical Association in Jacksonville in January 1874, a professional society was at last established. At its second annual meeting in Jacksonville in 1875, Dr. Bond although not present was nominated and elected to membership and simultaneously appointed to serve on an important committee. There is no indication, however, that he ever attended a meeting nor is there a record of his having ever paid the $5 annual dues.[13]

Dr. Bond in failing health in 1881 moved with his family to Jacksonville where he died the following year.[14] His residence was situated on East Adams Street near its intersection with Market Street.[15]

Dr. Bond's domestic life was marred by a series of misfortunes.[16] His wife, Louisa, died in September 1865 giving birth to a daughter who was christened Louisa. A son, Claude Houston, died in 1863 at age two. Another child, John Screven Bond Jr., born February 9, 1872, died at age seven months.

Dr. Bond married Ellen Augusta Smith, a native of Burlington Vermont[17] in 1866. They had five children: Julia Frances, Ashley, John Screven, who died at age seven months, John Sanford, and Edward Screven, the latter two becoming prominent business and civic leaders in Jacksonville.[18] Numerous descendants of Dr. Bond still reside in Jacksonville.

1. U.S. Census, 1840, McIntosh County, Georgia, p. 84. "Catalogue of Students, Medical College of the State of South Carolina," p. 167.

2. Ibid. Although I have been unable to establish the degree of kinship, it appears likely that Dr. Bond was a close relative of Dr. Screven, possibly a nephew. It is also intresting that Dr. Bond's eldest child, a son named Thomas Spalding, born in 1850, bore the name of one of South Carolina's wealthiest and most distinguished citizens, Thomas Spalding, 1774-1851 or Thomas Spalding of Sapelo as he was known, the entire Island of Sapelo having once been his domain. See E. Merton Coulter *Thomas Spalding of Sapelo*, Baton Rouge, Louisiana, 1940.

3. "Catalogue of Students. MCSSC," p. 167.

4. Tallahassee *Floridian*, May 29, 1847.

5. Tallahassee *Sentinel*, January 9, 1849. The marriage occurred on December 21, 1848.

6. U.S. Census, 1850, Gadsden County, Florida, p. 390.

7. Tallahassee *Florida Sentinel*, March 2, 1858.

8. Tallahassee *Floridian and Journal*, January 12, 1861, first printing February 1, 1850.

9. Julia Floyd Smith *Slavery and Plantation Growth in Antebellum Florida, 1821-1860*, Gainesville, 1973, pp. 97-98.

10. Quincy *Times*, May 20, 1848. Here is published a complete acocunt of the two-day session.

11. *Acts and Resolutions, General Assembly of the State of Florida, 1848-49*, 4th Session, Tallahassee, 1949, pp. 74-75,

12. *Soldiers of Florida*, Board of Institutions, published Tallahassee, 1903, p. 320. The record is far from complete, giving only the date of Dr. Bond's commission, 1861, his organizational assignment, and place and year of death, the last item being incorrect.

13. *Proceedings, Florida Medical Association*, Jacksonville, 1875, p. 8.

14. Jacksonville *Times-Union*, April 25, 1923. The obituary notice of Dr. Bond's widow states that the family moved to Jacksonville in 1881 and that Dr. Bond died in 1882.

15. The address on East Adams Street is found in several editions of the Jacksonville City directory beginning in 1883.

16. See "Parish Records, St. John's Episcopal Church, Tallahassee, Florida," typed copy in P.K. Yonge Library of Florida History, for these and other details relating to the Bond family.

17. See note 14. supra.

18. U.S. Census, 1880, Leon County, Florida, p. 324, lists in the Bond household in addition to those named two daughters, Nannie and Louisa, by Dr. Bond's first marriage.

Booth, Robert C., Gadsden and Liberty Counties, 1834

Dr. Booth, son of Dr. William Booth, was born in Gadsden County in 1834 some three years after his father had migrated from Virginia and settled in the Mt. Pleasant community about eight miles northwest of Quincy. His mother was Sarah Coe, daughter of Jesse Coe, one of the wealthier planters of Jackson County. By the measure of the times the Booth family was one of affluence. Although they owned two plantations,[1] Dr. Booth elected to establish his practice in Quincy and the four Booth children were reared there.[2] Under the preceptorate of his father young Robert read medicine and observed surgical techniques. He was enrolled at the Medical College of the State of South Carolina and was graduated in 1856. His doctoral thesis was titled "Pneumonia."[3]

On returning to Florida Dr. Booth entered a medical partnership with his brother-in-law, Dr. Charles A. Hentz, who had moved from Marianna to Quincy to assume the practice of the elder Dr. Booth who had died in May 1854.[4] This arrangement was mutually satisfactory; however, chiefly, according to Dr. Hentz, due to Robert's incurable alcoholism and undisciplined behavior, the partnership was dissolved, probably to the immense satisfaction of both parties, by the onset of war.

Dr. Booth was among the first Quincy citizens to enlist in the Confederate cause. He was mustered in on April 19, 1861, by Capt. (Dr.) John H. Gee and assigned to Company G, First Florida Infantry, without military rank. At the end of a year's service he reenlisted, this time in the Second Florida Cavalry, with the rank of Third Lieutenant. He became Second Lieutenant in 1863 and for some months served as Commander of Company H. He was among the troops who surrendered at Baldwin, Florida, in early May 1865. His service record described him as five feet seven inches tall, dark hair, blue eyes and fair complexion. He was paroled on May 15.[5]

Upon his release Dr. Booth resumed practice in Quincy. He married Mary Smith of Attapulgus in 1866,[6] daughter of Thomas Smith who was violently opposed to the marriage and, according to Dr. Hentz, "properly so, on account of Bob's habits and poor record."[7] They lived for a brief time with his mother in Quincy, but in 1867 moved to Bristol where Mary died of fever on July 18.[8]

Little is known of Dr. Booth's latter years. The Liberty County Census of 1870 lists him as a medical practitioner of Bristol, living alone and owning property valued at only $200.[9] He was one of only three physicians practicing in the county at the time. His life can be described as tragic: born into a wealthy family, son of over-indulgent parents, early victim of excessive use of alcohol, and bereft of his wife after only a few months of marriage.[10]

1. At the time of his death in 1858 Dr. William Booth's assets had dwindled to almost nothing. He left debts estimated at $40,000. Upon their release from the Confederate Army in 1865, his sons, Robert and James, faced a dire situation. Numerous references to Dr. Robert Booth appear in Charles A. Hentz "Autobiography," 2 vols., MS, Southern Collection, University of North Carolina Library, Chapel Hill. Dr. Hentz spent the later years of his life in Jackson and Gadsden Counties, was married to Dr. Booth's sister Bettie. Being something of a moralist he had small patience with Dr. Booth. Dr. Hentz is known to have written candidly of many persons of whom he disapproved. He did not spare his brother-in-law.

2. Besides Bettie and Robert, the other Booth children were Jesse who later settled in Liberty County, married and reared a family, and Sarah, who was married to James Evans of Quincy, Ibid. p. 292.

3. Archives, Waring Medical Library, Medical University of South Carolina, Charleston, Lists of Students and Graduates.

4. Hentz, Op. Cit. I. 304.

5. NA, Service Records, CSA, M151, Rolls 25 and 26.

6. Attapulgus was a village in Decatur County, Georgia, 12 miles north of Quincy.

7. Hentz, Op. Cit. II, 19.

8. Dr. Hentz went to Bristol to offer his medical assistance, remaining there for eight days. Judging the patient to be recovering, he returned to Quincy. Her condition worsened. She was removed to her father's home in Attapulgus, where she died.

9. U.S. Census, 1870, Liberty County, Florida, item 234.

10. The date of Dr. Booth's death remains undetermined; it is thought to have occurred at some time in the 1770s.

Booth, William, Gadsden County, 1800-1858

Dr. Booth, one of the pioneer settlers of Gadsden County, was born in Virginia about 1800, son of William Fitzgerald Booth. He arrived in Florida about 1831 and purchased a plantation northwest of Quincy in what came to be known as the Mt. Pleasant community. He was among the founders of the Mount Pleasant Methodist Church said to have been one of the first Protestant churches established in the Territory.[1] About 1833 Dr. Booth married Sarah Coe, daughter of the Reverend Jesse Coe, a wealthy plantation owner of Jackson County, whose lands lay on the west side of the Apalachicola River. It appears to have been through this marriage that he came into possession of additional acreage which added considerably to his total wealth. According to his son-in-law, Dr. Charles A. Hentz, Dr. Booth was inept in the management of his plantations and consequently relied on overseers to look after his farming interests while he moved with his family to Quincy and carried on an extensive medical practice.[2]

Dr. Hentz, from whom much of the information on Dr. Booth is derived, held him in highest esteem. Although Dr. Hentz was often given to censure and condemnation in judging his colleagues and acquaintances, he had only praise for his father-in-law. After an overnight visit with the Booths in 1851 he wrote in his journal: "The good Doctor was then in the full tide of his practice; a mild, benevolent, excellent man who looked as if he could not speak a harsh or unkind word."[3] Elsewhere he revealed his intense annoyance and impatience with Dr. Booth's sons Dr. Hentz's brothers-in-law, Robert and Jesse. After an overnight visit he wrote:

> As for the former (Robert), about twenty-two or twenty-three, slight and slender of build, dark hair and large prominent eyes...with lids always red and sore-looking from chronic dissipation, but an alcoholic...frequent attacks of dèlerium tremens...Jesse, the younger, was also very slender, sandy, almost red hair, was expecting to become a lawyer. But Jesse too was a hard drinker. Dr. Booth was too gentle to discipline them. Meanwhile they ran up large bills at shops, bills which Dr. Booth was expected to pay. The doctor paid the bills without complaining. But the cost was great. Disaster loomed. The expense of his family was compounded by crop failures, inept overseers, inability to collect his professional fees and pay the mortgage on his two plantations.

In early 1858 Dr. Booth's health broke. A stomach ailment developed, probably cancer, and in March 1858 he was forced to give up his practice. He died on May 1, 1858. The funeral was held on the following Sunday at the Presbyterian Church, the Methodist Church was being repaired. Old Dr. David L. White preached the funeral sermon. Mrs. Booth survived her husband by 23 years, dying on June 22, 1881.

1. J. Stanley Randall, *History of Gadsden County*, Quincy, 1948, pp. 62-63.
2. Charles A. Hentz, "My Autobiography." A typed transcript is found among the manuscripts of the Southern Collection, Library, University of North Carolina, Chapel Hill. Having married the daughter of Dr. Booth, Dr. Hentz made frequent remarks concerning members of the Booth family, including candid and often unflattering remarks about the two brothers of his wife.
3. Ibid, I, 217.

Bozeman, James, Calhoun County, 1850

Dr. Bozeman, a native of Georgia, practiced medicine in Calhoun County about the year 1850. Apparently unmarried, he was a boarder in the home of Almerin P. Wood.[1]

1. U.S. Census, 1850, Calhoun County, Florida, p. 40, item 129.

Bradford, Edward, Leon County, 1798-1873

Dr. Bradford,* one of Leon County's most beloved physicians and eminent citizens, was born in Halifax County, North Carolina, on August 25, 1798, and died at his plantation home, Pine Hill, some 10 miles north of Tallahassee on August 28, 1873.[1] He was a descendant of the renowned Bradford family of Massachusetts. After receiving his basic education at home, he enrolled at the University of Maryland, Baltimore, from which he was graduated in 1822.[2] Soon thereafter he began medical practice at Enfield, North Carolina, near the place of his birth.[3] A short time later, apparently desirous of further study, he entered the recently-established Jefferson Medical College in Philadelphia where he received a second degree. Family tradition holds that he then spent a year or more as an intern under the well-known Dr. Charles Delucena Meigs of Philadelphia.

Upon his return to North Carolina Dr. Bradford married Martha Lewis Branch on November 10, 1825, daughter of John Branch of Enfield, at that time U.S. Senator from North Carolina and previously (1817-1820) Governor of that state. The Branches were a wealthy and socially-prominent family and after they moved to Florida in 1836 John Branch continued to be politically active, being appointed Governor of the Territory in 1844 and serving until it became a state in the following year.

Meanwhile Dr. Bradford's older brother, Henry, had migrated to Leon County, purchased land and settled down to the life of a planter.[4] When the doctor found himself failing in health in 1829-30 he too decided to move to Florida. The precise date is uncertain but it was either in late 1830 or early 1831. With ample resources at his disposal he purchased two large tracts of land north of Tallahassee, one he named Pine Hill, the other he called Horseshoe, which lay further north on the south shore of Lake Iamonia. While his slaves and overseers were busy clearing these tracts for cultivation and building residences, Dr. Bradford settled in Tallahassee and continued his medical practice. He had offered his services to the citizens of the community on April 10, 1832. His office was located on Jefferson Street "next door to Wilson's Printing Office," while his residence was on the west side of Market Square.[5]

The spacious but unpretentious house at Pine Hill was completed about 1836 and with the outbreak of a yellow fever epidemic in Tallahassee in that year he moved his family to the plantation for a brief stay before sending them back to North Carolina for greater safety. In the meantime he remained in Tallahassee helping to combat the fever and earning the gratitude and respect of the town.[6]

By mid-1832 two other Bradford brothers had arrived in Florida and purchased land which they developed into profitable plantations. They were the eldest, Thomas who owned Walnut Hill, and the youngest, Richard who named his place Water Oak. All these families were to play important roles in the social, political and economic life of Leon County.

Dr. Bradford had virtually ceased to practice medicine by 1840, instead devoting his energies to the running of two plantations. In addition to the cultivation of cotton, corn, and forage crops, he built at Pine Hill a sawmill, shingle mill, brickyard, blacksmith shop, tannery, grist mill, a soapmaking apparatus, and most important of all, a cotton gin and compressor.[7] He enjoyed success; by 1850 his slaves numbered 110 and ten years later, 142.[8]

In view of his wealth, education, and social position, it was inevitable that Dr. Bradford would also become a political leader. He and his brothers were active in the struggle for statehood for Florida.[9] About 1850, as the pressure for abolition of slavery began to mount, he was among those involved in the Nashville Convention called to plan opposition strategy.[10] In the following year he participated in the meeting of the Southern Rights Association at Centreville (Leon County) to counter the "threats of the non-slavery states to impose their will on the South."[11] Early in 1854 Governor Broome, newly-elected, announced his military staff which included Dr. Bradford as Surgeon General with the rank of Colonel.[12]

With the exception of Dr. Bradford's son-in-law, Junius Taylor, husband of Sarah Bradford, the entire Bradford family supported secession when the decision came in January 1861. Taylor had hoped the South would remain in the Union but when war came later in the year the whole clan, including Taylor, supported the Confederate Cause. Dr. Cushman wrote: "The younger men enlisted; food supplies from the plantations were sent to the front; Dr. Bradford ran a hospital, started a saltworks, and used his tannery to make shoes for the Army." The Bradford women also did their part, sewing, knitting, and nursing the wounded who came to Pine Hill. But the war took its toll in many ways, and life on the plantations, as they had known it, was over. Dr. Bradford's health began to fail. His son-in-law, Francis Eppes, took over the operation of the plantations and tried to hold the pieces together but not very successfully.[13]

Dr. Bradford never recovered his health. He died in 1873 at Pine Hill and was buried in the family cemetery nearby. Mrs. Bradford lived on until 1892.

Dr. Bradford was a man of high moral and professional standards. He placed great store by education and saw to it that his five daughters had the best governesses and tutors that could be employed. His own intellectual interests were profound and varied. When well along in life he became interested in the ideas of the great Swedish philosopher and theologian, Emanual Swedenborg, which he appears to have embraced. His eulogist summed up his splended qualities: "Generous, hospitable, benevolent, bountiful in deeds of kindness to the needy, charitable in his judgements of others, pure in his own life, he was deservedly esteemed a model Christian gentleman."[14]

*The biographical data on Dr. Bradford are fairly abundant but the present sketch is a condensation charting only the main features of his career. He played an important role in the early development of Leon County and for 20 years or so of his active medical practice he was a highly regarded physician. Anyone interested in a personalized treatment of Dr. Bradford and his family should consult the book written by his daughter, Susan Bradford Eppes, *Through Some Eventful Years*, Macon Georgia, 1926, or the facsimile edition published in Gainesville, Florida, in 1968. The latter contains an excellent introduction and index by Professor Joseph D. Cushman Jr. Citations below are from the 1968 edition.

1. Tallahassee *Floridian*, November 18, 1873, obituary notice.
2. Eugene F. Cordell, Historical Sketch of the University of Maryland School of Medicine, 1807-1890, Baltimore, 1891, p. 165.
3. Henry E. Palmer, "Physicians of Early Tallahassee and Vicinity," *Apalachee*, Tallahassee Historical Society, 1944, p. 37.
4. U.S. Census, 1830, Leon County, Florida, sheet 118. Henry was the only Bradford name listed in the Florida Census of 1830 although the other male (age between 20 and 30) could have been Dr. Edward, residing with his brother temporarily. This, however, seems unlikely.
5. Tallahassee *Floridian*, May 1, 1832, 1st printed April 10, 1832.
6. Palmer, "Physicians," p. 37.
7. There is considerable evidence that Dr. Bradford ceased to practice medicine after moving to Pine Hill. Ibid., p. 38. Dr. Palmer shows that the slaves on Dr. Bradford's plantations received their medical care from Dr. William H. Bradford, a nephew of Dr. Edward. See also Eppes, *Through Some Eventful Years*, p. xiii.
8. Slave Schedules, Leon County, Florida, 1850 and 1860.
9. Among the trivia and chitchat of Mrs. Eppes book the increasing anxiety of the Bradfords concerning the impending struggle is reflected. Interestingly, Mrs. Bradford held antislavery convictions. See pp. 56, 58, 61, 112 et passim.
10. Tallahassee *Sentinel* March 26, 1850.
11. Tallahassee *Floridian and Journal*, March 22, 1851.
12. Ibid., January 24, 1854.
13. Eppes, *Through Years*, p. xvi.
14. Tallahassee *Floridian*, November 18, 1873.

Bradford, James H., St. Augustine, 1859

Except for the fact that he died in St. Augustine on April 10, 1859, nothing is known of Dr. Bradford. The Trinity Parish Register of St. Augustine, in the section headed "Burials," lists him as M.D. and resident of Westchester, Pennsylvania. He was buried in the Protestant Cemetery.

Bradford, Samuel A., Madison County, 1850

Nothing is known of Dr. Bradford beyond the data included in the Florida Census of 1850, where he is shown to have been a resident in the home of Dr. Theodore Hartridge, aged 24, and a native of South Carolina.[1]

1. U.S. Census, 1850, Madison County, Florida, p. 160.

Bradford, Thomas A., Leon and Alachua Counties, 1830

Dr. Bradford, who spent his mature years in Florida, was born in Tennessee in 1830. His father, Thomas A. Bradford Sr., was one of four brothers who migrated to Florida in the 1830s and 1840s from Halifax County, North Carolina,[1] acquiring large tracts of land in Leon County just north of Tallahassee which, with numerous slaves, they developed into profitable plantations and assumed their proper places among Florida's aristocracy. The senior Bradfords prior to moving to Florida, however, had sojourned briefly in Tennessee and thence to Alabama, probably in the Huntsville vicinity, before moving to Leon County, in the mid-1840s.[2]

Nothing is known of the early education of Thomas A. Bradford Jr. but given his family's resources it must be assumed that he enjoyed the advantages of a private tutor. It may be speculated but not shown that he attended the prestigious military academy which flourished in Tallahassee in the antebellum period. In the fall of 1848 he matriculated at the Jefferson College of Medicine in Philadelphia, from which he was graduated in the spring of 1850.[3] He returned to Tallahassee and began the practice of his profession. A short time later, however, he moved to Newnansville, Alachua County, where his brother, Henry, two years his senior, and brother-in-law, Jesse T. Bernard, both attorneys-at-law and solicitors-in-chancery, soon joined him.[4] The Tallahassee *Floridian and Journal* announced Dr. Bradford's marriage to Miss Frances V. Dell of Huntsville, Alabama, on November 22, 1851.

The extent of Dr. Bradford's medical practice cannot be determined but it appears to have been somewhat limited, probably due to the presence of four other physicians in the Newnansville community at the time. The 1860 census designates him only as "Merchant," owner of property valued at about $10,000.[5] There is other evidence that he was also engaged in farming, probably on a small scale, with the labor of four slaves.[6]

With the coming of the War in 1861, Dr. Bradford enlisted for service on May 1, 1862, giving his occupation as "farmer" and committing himself for the duration of the conflict; this in spite of the fact that he was leaving his wife and five small children, aged nine to less than one. He entered the service as a private and was assigned to Captain W.E. Chambers' Independent Company (Co. B), 2nd Florida Cavalry. He furnished his own horse. He was transferred on June 12, 1863, for unknown reasons, to the Milton Light Artillery, Company A, commanded by Captain J.L. Dunham. For the greater part of his service he was stationed in East Florida. His unit surrendered to the enemy at Thomasville, Georgia, on May 23, 1865, and on the following day he was paroled.[7]

It appears that Dr. Bradford returned home in broken health. Although he lived for a year or so after the end of the war, he died prior to 1870. His youngest child, a son named Clement, was three years of age in 1870.[8] His last years were marked by despair, cheered only by the devotion of his wife, Frances, and that of his five sons and one daughter, a tragic contrast to his childhood and youth which were spent in the carefree environs of an antebellum plantation.

1. The first Bradford to arrive in Florida was Henry, who came in time to be included in the Census of 1830. He was followed in the early 1830s by Edward, also a physician, who developed Pine Hill Plantation; then by Richard, owner of Water Oak Plantation. All were men of good breeding and comparative wealth. The chief source for Bradford family history is Susan Bradford Eppes, *Through Some Eventful Years*, Macon, Ga., J.W. Burke and Co., 1926. A facsimile edition reproduction of this work was published by the University of Florida Press, 1968, with Introduction and Notes by Joseph D. Cushman Jr. Mrs. Eppes, wife of Nicholas Ware Eppes, was the youngest of the five daughters of Dr. Edward Bradford. This work, in diary form, is chatty and intimate. She usually designated the Thomas A. Bradfords, father and son, as Uncle Tom and Cousin Tom, respectively.

2. The first child of Thomas A. Bradford Sr. to be born in Florida was William, aged 18 in 1850. U.S. Census, 1850, Leon Colunty, Florida, p. 72.

3. Jefferson Medical College, *List of Dead or Lost Graduates: Classes from 1826 to 1879*, Philadelphia, 1917, p. 68.

4. Jesse T. Bernard, a Virginian, was married to Dr. Bradford's sister Mary about 1853. A few years later, probably in 1858, he moved from Leon County and settled in Newnansville and began the practice of law. In June 1859 he began publication of a weekly newspaper, *The Florida Dispatch*, editing it himself, with S.W. Burnett as Proprietor. Only two issues, those of May 11, 1860 and June 1, 1860 have survived. Both Henry Bradford and Bernard were much involved in civic matters as well as fraternal organizations.

5. U.S. Census, 1860 Alachua County, Florida, p. 92.

6. Newnansville *Florida Dispatch*, June 1, 1860. In this issue Bernard included an item calling attention to Dr. T.A. Bradford's success in growing an early variety of corn. He added: "Dr. Bradford now has the fine roasting ears from the common gourd seed (variety), which is something unusual for the month of May."

7. NA, Service Records, CSA, M251, Roll 6.

8. No gravestone for Dr. Bradford has been discovered nor has any newspaper account of his death. The Alachua County Census of 1870 lists his widow, aged 45, and their eight children (seven sons and one daughter) as: Thomas A., 17; Samuel B., 15; Frank, 13; Henry, 11; Ida, nine; Leonidas (Lee), seven; Oscar, five; and Clement, three. From the age of the youngest child is extrapolated the probable date of Dr. Bradford's death.

Bradford, William Henry, Leon County, 1829-1883

Dr. Bradford, eldest child of Richard and Nancy Bradford and nephew of Dr. Edward Bradford, was born in Halifax County, North Carolina, in 1829. When still a small child he moved with his parents and two younger brothers, John B. and Edward, to Leon County where his uncles, Henry and Edward, had settled earlier.[1] His father purchased land north of Tallahassee near the present village of Bradfordville and developed a plantation to which they gave the name, Water Oak. After gaining his basic education under the guidance of tutors, William entered Harvard University from which he was graduated and then went on to earn a medical degree at the University of Pennsylvania.[2]

On returning to Florida Dr. Bradford settled on a portion of the family land which came to be known as Edgewood Plantation and subsequently devoted much of his time to farming, but at the same time maintained a steady medical practice. In fact, the Leon County Census of 1860 designated him only as "Planter,"[3] while the slave schedule of that year shows him as owner of 16 slaves. His property value, including the slaves, was estimated at $9,000.

One of Dr. Bradford's professional ledgers has survived. It contains numerous entries relating to his practice in the 1850s, in several instances recording his treatment of the slaves of his Uncle Edward at nearby Horseshoe Plantation. Between January 12 and September 19, 1852, he visited Horseshoe on 10 occasions, "the usual charge being $2.50 per visit." His practice involved the customary treatments: bleeding, cupping, extraction of teeth, et cetera, while his prescriptions included iron and gentian pills, calomel, squill, digitalis, opium, croton oil, and quinine.[4]

When the war came in 1861 Dr. Bradford was one of many of his class and kin to enlist in the Army of the Confederacy, this notwithstanding his responsibility for a young wife and daughter. His unit was known as the Dixie Yeomen. When the day came to be sworn into service, however, a number of his fellow enlistees vigorously protested his leaving the community without the services of a physician. His cousin, Susan Bradford (Eppes) made the following entry in her diary under the date September 15, 1861:[5]

> Cousin William (as she called him) has been practicing in this county for twelve years and everybody loves and trusts him. When the men composing the Dixie Yeomen came forward to be sworn into the Confederate service, first one man and then another, until nearly all had spoken, said he could not take the oath nor sign the Roster unless Dr. William Bradford would consent to resign and stay home. . .They said they could not leave their wives and children unless the doctor would stay with them. "I should be obliged to desert," said one man, "if Dr. Bill was not in call when my folks got sick." So after much discussion he consented to resign.

Mrs. Eppes then mentioned the delight of her own mother and father that their nephew had made the decision. "He is their adopted son, you know. They love him as if he were their very own, and no brother could be dearer to me." So Dr. Bradford remained in Leon County.

Life during and after the war was not without hardships for Dr. Bradford. His practice was heavy and his remuneration often skimpy. Medical supplies, such as could be found, were collected and sent to the battlefields and hospitals of Virginia and Tennessee. Then came the economic disasters of Reconstruction and the loss of slave labor. Added to Dr. Bradford's woes was the death of his wife in the late 1860s, leaving him with two small daughters. His properties were valued at $3,640 in 1870.[6]

Dr. Bradford continued his practice in the Bradfordville community for another decade or more. In 1880, still master of Edgewood Plantation, he was designated "physician and farmer,"[7] while his daughters, Nannie and Emily, aged 12 and 17 respectively, were still members of his household, as was his plantation overseer, J.E. Grice.

The Tallahassee *Weekly Floridian* on August 29, 1882, included this item: "Dr. W.H. Bradford, of Bradfordville, proposes to remove to this City." A week later his professional card appeared with the announcement that his office would be located at Elliott's City Drug Store. His career was ended a little more than a year later, his death coming on December 11, 1883, at his home near Bradfordville. A few lines from his obituary invite inclusion here:[8]

> By his death not only the community in which he lived, but Leon County, is deprived of one of her best citizens. Dr. Bradford was a gentleman of exemplary character, a good neighbor, ever faithful to oligation and duty, and esteemed by all who knew him. It may be truly said of him that he went about doing good, and those who were the objects of his benevolence have lost a friend indeed.

1. U.S. Census, 1850, Leon County, Florida, p. 137.
2. Henry E. Palmer, "Physicians of Early Tallahassee and Vicinity," *Apalachee*, 1944, p. 38.
3. U.S. Census, 1860, Leon County, Florida, p. 42.
4. Palmer, "Physicians," loc. cit.
5. Susan Bradford Eppes, *Through Some Eventful Years*, Facsimile Edition, Joseph D. Cushman, ed., Gainesville, 1968, p. 159.
6. U.S. Census, 1870, Leon County, Florida, p. 597.
7. U.S. Census, 1880, Leon County, Florida, p. 282.
8. Tallahassee *Weekly Floridian*, December 18, 1883. The reduced value of Dr. Bradford's estate is indicated in the Special Florida Census of 1885 for Leon County, section on "Agriculture," p. 14. "Estate of W.H. Bradford."

Acres: Improved land, 250; unimproved, 150	
Value of Land and Buildings	$1,500
Value of Machinery	50
Value of Livestock	675
Total	$2,225

Bradley, Thomas, Taylor County, 1870

Dr. Bradley is presently known only through an entry in the Taylor County Census of 1870[1] in which he is designated "Physician," owning property valued at $500 and a resident of the Rose Hill community.[2] In his household were a son, Henry, and a daughter, Nellie, and also a 10-year-old "Black boy who worked on the farm." The four persons were natives of Alabama. Dr. Bradley appears to have practiced only briefly, if at all, in Florida.

1. U.S. Census, 1870, Taylor County, Florida, p. 715.
2. Rose Hill's location has not been identified. The only place of that name known to have existed in Florida in the 19th century was in Citrus County. There was, however, a locality known as Rose Head in Taylor County.

Bradwell, Daniel, Gadsden County, 1850

Very little information has been found on Dr. Bradwell, a resident of Gadsden County about the middle of the 19th century. The Census of 1850 lists him as a farmer of modest means, 50 years of age, and father of nine children. Both he and wife, Jane, were born in South Carolina and moved to Georgia about 1833. They appear to have arrived in Florida about 1845 settling on a farm outside Quincy.[1] Only his two youngest sons were born in Florida.

The following announcement appeared in the Tallahassee *Floridian and Journal* on August 28, 1852: "Married at the residence of Dr. Daniel Bradwell on August 12, 1852, Mr. Samuel B. Love and Miss Matilda C. Bradwell, all of Gadsden.[2]

1. The Bradwells of South Carolina were a family of prominence in the 18th and early 19th centuries. Particularly notable was one Nathaniel, an officer in the American Revolution. He was one of the first to chart the lands along Goose Creek and parts of the Ashley River.
1. U.S. Census, 1850, Gadsden County, Florida, p. 197.
2. One may speculate that Matilda Bradwell was actually Mary Bradwell, eldest daughter of Dr. Bradwell. She would have been 22 in 1852.

Bradwell, Washington, Liberty County, 1815

Dr. Bradwell was born in South Carolina about 1815.[1] He migrated to Florida in the 1840s, settling first in Gadsden County, later moving to the Blue Creek community of Liberty County.[2] The census of 1860 indicates that he had acquired substantial properties, his real estate having been valued at $10,000 and personal property at $15,000.[3] He was designated physician and farmer. His wife, Louisa, whom he appears to have married about 1856, was 20 years his junior and a native of Florida. Three children, two daughters and one son, were born to the union.[4]

Dr. Bradwell was doubtless a beloved citizen of his community. The earliest reference to his civic activities relates to his participation in a Fourth of July celebration in Quincy in 1847.[5] In his later years he was elected to the Florida

House of Representatives serving in the sessions of 1868, 1869 and 1870.[6]

1. This date of birth is an extrapolation from the Gadsden County Census of 1830 in which his age was given as 35. He was unmarried at that date.
2. U.S. Census, 1860, Liberty County, Florida, Item 1. Blue Creek, a Liberty County settlement, was situated on the Gadsden County line about 17 miles from Quincy. It had a post office from 1858 till 1970.
3. Ibid.
4. U.S. Census, 1870, Liberty County, Florida, p. 23.
5. Tallahassee *Floridian*, July 17, 1847.
6. Allen Morris, *The People of Lawmaking in Florida, 1822-1977*, Tallahassee, 1977.

Branch, Darwin A., Tampa, 1832-1858

Dr. Branch, eldest son of Dr. Franklin Branch, distinguished Tampa physician and clergyman, was born in Abbeville, South Carolina, the birthplace of his mother, Matilda Vashti Branch (nee Wilson), in 1832.[1] After receiving his early education in the schools of Abbeville he moved with his family to Tampa where he is presumed to have served a medical apprenticeship in the office of his father. In 1851, doubtless influenced by his father who was graduated from Castleton Medical College, Castleton, Vermont, in 1825, young Darwin matriculated at that school in the fall of 1851 and was graduated at the conclusion of the spring term in 1853.[2]

Following graduation Dr. Branch returned to Tampa and began his professional practice. A year or so later the municipal government of Tampa underwent a reorganization, with a mayor-council plan being instituted in December 1855.[3] Elections were held in February 1856 with Judge Joseph B. Lancaster being elected Mayor and Dr. Branch winning one of the Council seats.[4]

Meanwhile in mid-1857 Dr. Branch had joined his father in a professional copartnership.[5] His reputation as doctor and public servant was being established and his future appeared bright, but it was not to be. His life was cut tragically short when he fell victim to yellow fever which beset the city in 1858 and he died on August 16 that year at age 26.[6] His sister, Mrs. Helen Clarke, also died during the epidemic.

1. U.S. Census, 1850, Hillsborough County, Florida (Manatee Settlement), p. 265.
2. Frederick Clayton Waite, *The First Medical College in Vermont*, Montpelier, Vermont, Historical Society, 1949, p. 200.
3. Karl H. Grismer, *Tampa*, St. Petersburg, 1950, p. 324.
4. Ibid., p. 217.
5. Tampa *Florida Peninsular*, February 27, 1858. Notice first appeared in issue of July 25, 1857 not extant.
6. Grismer, *Tampa*, p. 324.

Branch, Franklin, Hillsborough County, 1802-1882

Dr. Branch, whose career in Hillsborough County spanned more than 40 years, was born in Orwell, Vermont, on November 28, 1802.* After an early education in the common schools of Orwell, he matriculated at Castleton Medical College, Castleton, Vermont, located 15 miles from his home. He was graduated as Doctor of Medicine at the end of the session of 1823.[1] Soon thereafter he moved to Abbeville District, South Carolina, where he practiced for about 20 years. He was married in Abbeville on December 16, 1830, to a local girl, Matilda Vashti Wilson. To this marriage were born three sons: Darwin A., who like his father was a graduate of Castleton Medical College (1850), Franklin A. and James

O., both of whom became Methodist ministers, and three daughters, Frances Levonia, Helene and Lucy.[2]

Arriving in Florida in the late 1840s Dr. Branch resumed medical practice while operating a drug store and on occasion filling a Methodist pulpit. Just prior to 1850 he purchased a tract of land on the Manatee River, at that time within the boundary of Hillsborough County, with the intention of establishing a sanitarium. He constructed two buildings, but the project was soon abandoned. He also launched a timber business but this too proved to be unprofitable. He then returned to Tampa as physician and druggist where he spent the balance of his life.

Tragedy struck the family in the summer of 1857 when a yellow fever epidemic claimed the life of Mrs. Branch. The following year Dr. Branch's granddaughter, Clara Clarke, daughter of Edward and Helene Branch Clarke, was a victim of the disease as were Dr. Darwin A. Branch and his wife.

Dr. Branch married his second wife, Martha Turnbull, daughter of Richard Turnbull of Monticello on January 16, 1860.[3] A son, Henry Lee, was born to this union. He is remembered by Tampans as the man who built the town's first opera house.

Although it was removed from the center of military action during the Civil War, Tampa, with its fine harbor and military installation, could not escape the attention of Union forces. Blockade runners in the earlier stages of the war were fairly successful in penetrating the entrance to Tampa Bay. As the war dragged on, however, the town suffered repeated bombardment and in 1864 was occupied by Union troops. Because of their ages or occupations none of the Branch sons was involved in military service. In the 1864 seizure nearly all business houses were looted, only Dr. Branch's store escaping. As Karl Grismer related it:[4] "Only one business establishment remained open throughout the war. That was the apothecary shop of Dr. Franklin Branch. His stock of priceless drugs and herbs was valueless to those who did not know how to fill prescriptions and consequently it was not looted. . .Besides even the Federals found it convenient to have a drug store in operation."

Dr. Branch remained as both physician and druggist until the end of his life. His death occurred on August 24, 1882, just three months short of his 80th birthday. The 1880 census still designated him "physician and druggist."[5]

*The biographical data included in the present sketch were drawn chiefly from Karl H. Grismer, *Tampa, A History of the City of Tampa and the Tampa Bay Region of Florida*, D.B. McKay, ed., St. Petersburg, Florida, 1950, pp. 324, et passim.

1. Frederick Clayton Waite, *The First Medical College in Vermont*, Montpelier, Vermont, Historical Society, 1949, p. 200.
2. U.S. Census, 1850, Hillsborough County, Florida, p. 265.
3. Monticello *Family Friend*, February 4, 1860.
4. Grismer, *Tampa*, p. 150.
5. U.S. Census, 1880, Hillsborough County, Florida, p. 405.

Brevard, Ephraim A., Leon County, 1839

Notwithstanding eminent family connections which included the Call and Long families, the brief career of Dr. Brevard remains obscure, even somewhat mysterious. He was born in Macon, Alabama,[1] in 1839, the second son of Theodore Washington Brevard, a North Carolinian of distinction. The family moved to Leon County, settling near Tallahassee in 1847.[2] Young Ephraim and his four brothers no doubt received their basic education in the common schools of Tallahassee. As for Ephraim, since he does not appear among the matriculants and graduates of any of the Southern medical colleges it is assumed that he received his professional training as an apprentice to a local physician. The Census of 1860 lists him simply as "Physician," aged 21, residing in the home of his father.[3]

During the unquiet days of 1860 Leon County and other counties of Middle Florida became obsessed with national politics as the antislavery movement gained support. This was especially true after withdrawal of the Florida delegation from the Democratic Convention in Charleston, South Carolina, in April 1860. Dr. Brevard was soon drawn into the tumult. At a meeting of Leon County Democrats in Tallahassee on May 26 he served as secretary with Col. John Miller as chairman. The discussions centered on the reasons for the withdrawal from the Charleston gathering. It was reported that the arguments for secession as formulated by the dissident Democrats drew wild applause. Having been thus thrust into a major role within the party he was chosen as one of Leon's delegates at the State Democratic Convention meeting in Quincy of June 4.[4]

Having allied himself with the Florida secessionists Dr. Brevard was among the first Floridians to respond to the call to arms. He enlisted for service in the Army of the Confederacy in early June 1861 and a few weeks later was mustered into the unit being organized by R.B. Hilton, Company D., 1st Florida Infantry Regiment. He entered without military rank.

Subsequent developments related to Dr. Brevard are unclear. He was discharged "by order of General Bragg" with "pay due from the date of enlistment"[5] on July 6, 1861. Equally puzzling is the fact that nothing further is known of this apparently capable and personable young man.[6] His brother, Theodore Washington Brevard Jr., whose wife was Mary Call, daughter of General Richard Keith Call, became one of Florida's most eminent lawyers, while another brother, Richard, became a successful physician. His nephew, Ephraim Mays Brevard, born in 1871 was an outstanding physician.

1. U.S. Census 1850, Leon County, Florida, p. 131. See also the biographical sketch of Ephraim Mays Brevard, M.D., nephew of Dr. Ephraim A. Brevard, in Harry G. Cash, *History of Florida*, 3 vols., Vol. III, Chicago, Lewis Publishing Co., 1923, pp. 140-141,

2. U.S. Census, 1860, Leon County, Florida, Item 261. Although Theodore W. Brevard was listed as "farmer" in the previous census, he was in this instance designated "lawyer". Mrs. Brevard prior to her marriage was Carolina E. Mays.

3. There is, of course, some doubt that Dr. Brevard ever actually practiced medicine.

4. Tallahassee *Floridian and Journal*, June 2, 1860, ibid., June 16, 1860.

5. National Archives Service Records CSA, 1st Florida Infantry.

6. It is strange indeed that no public record of Dr. Brevard appears to have survived. Cemetery and church records of Leon County have been examined to no avail.

Brinson, William A., Madison, 1820-1857

Although the professional career of Dr. Brinson was terminated by his untimely death, he achieved a position of eminence in the town of Madison where he resided for scarcely a decade. He appears to have arrived in the county about 1847. In 1850 his property was valued at $6,000, while his slaves numbered 26. As early as April 1850,[1] he joined a group of Madison physicians endorsing P.P. Lewis, a dental surgeon, to open a practice in Tallahassee.[2] He was married in May 1853 at Madison Court House to Miss Aurelia Miller, a resident of Madison.[3]

The absence of Madison newspapers makes it impossible to trace the medical career of Dr. Brinson, but there can be no doubt that he was a respected and active physician. He was nominated in 1854 by the Democrats of Madison County for a seat in the Florida Senate which he won by a comfortable majority over the Whig candidate.[4] After serving in the legislative session of 1854 as well as the adjourned session of 1856,[5] he died in October 1857 at age 37 leaving a widow and young son William A. Jr.[6]

Records show that on at least two occasions the Florida Legislature authorized payments to Dr. Brinson for medical services (postmortem examinations), once in the amount of $25 for examining the bodies of two slaves of one James W. Foy and later another $75 for similar services.[7]

1. U.S. Census, 1850, Madison County, Florida, p. 159. Among the members of the Brinson household were brothers George M., who later became a Judge of Probate for the County (see U.S. Census 1860, Madison County, Florida, p. 148) and Columbus.
2. Tallahassee *Sentinel*, April 9, 1850.
3. Tallahassee *Floridian and Journal*, June 4, 1853.
4. Jacksonville *Florida News*, August 24, 1854, Tallahassee *Florida Sentinel*, October 10, 1854.
5. *Florida Senate Journal*, 7th session, 1854, Ibid, Adjourned Session 1855. Ibid., 8th Session 1856.
6. Tallahassee *Floridian and Journal*, Brief notice, reprint from the Madison *Messenger*, not extant.
7. *Acts and Resolutions General Assembly of Florida*, 7th Session, 1854, p. 91.

Bronaugh, James Craine, Pensacola, 1788-1822

When Dr. Bronaugh died of yellow fever at Pensacola on September 2, 1822, the Territory of Florida lost one of its most gifted and popular young leaders. Andrew Jackson, to whom Dr. Bronaugh had been for several years military comrade, secretary, personal physician, and confidant, was visibly touched. In words uncommon for a man who had lived so close to death on many battlefronts and whose toughness of spirit had earned for him the sobriquet "Old Hickory," he expressed his deep sorrow. On being apprised of Dr. Bronaugh's death by their mutual friend Col. George Walton, Jackson wrote from the Hermitage on November 26, 1882:

> I sincerely thank you for the circumstantial account you have given me of the death and sufferings of my ever to be lamented friend Dr. Bronaugh. How I wished I could have been with him in his sufferings to have endeavored to soothe and comfort him and to have endeavored to have saved him as Dr. Brosenham (sic) has well expressed. "Men of his noble spirit ought not to die." Few men know of the worth of Dr. Bronaugh. I well knew it and knew how to appreciate it. He was my bosom friend, he was in every way worthy of that confidence I reposed in him. He was incapable of violating confidence, or departing from the true principals of friendship. He was noble and brave and his exit from life notices (?) what I always expected and what I thought of him. He has gone the way of all the earth, he has done his duty here below, and I have fond hope that he is changed to a better, happier clime where his spirit is blessed and is at rest.[1]

Obviously Dr. Bronaugh was a man of uncommon intelligence and splendid character.[2] He was born on July 14, 1788, in Loudon County, Virginia, son of William and Rebecca Craine Bronaugh. He entered the Medical Department of the University of Virginia in 1806 from which he was graduated M.D. in the spring of 1808 after submitting a doctoral thesis entitled "Hepatitis."[3] His pursuits for the next three years are unknown but in 1812 when a war with England appeared imminent he offered his skills to the United States Army and on April 28, a few weeks short of his 24th birthday he was commissioned surgeon and assigned to the 12th Infantry Regiment.[4] Two years later, on April 15, he was promoted to Hospital Surgeon and shortly thereafter joined the staff of General Jackson.[5] Four years later on April 18, 1818, he became Assistant Surgeon General (the Surgeon General was James Tilton) and was attached to the United States Army, Southern Division. His military career ended on June 1, 1821, with the disbanding of the Southern Division and a reorganization of the Army.[6]

Although the records are not totally clear on the matter, Dr. Bronaugh was apparently surgeon to the 12th Regiment when it was engaged in the campaign against the British along the Canadian border in late 1812. This phase of the War was a virtual disaster for the Americans due in large part to the incompetence of General James Wilkinson. The hardships endured by the troops were rigorous. Wrote the Surgeon of the 12th (presumably Dr. Bronaugh) on November 27, 1812: "Many men are sick. Forty men are sick in hospital tents at Camp near Buffalo. No room for more. Some have measles, others fever. . .situation alarming."[7]

Two years later Dr. Bronaugh was with General Jackson in defense of the City of New Orleans when the British launched their campaign to gain control of the Gulf of Mexico and ultimately the Mississippi River. The brilliant victory for Jackson ended the threat. Dr. Bronaugh was present as hospital surgeon. It was the close association with Jackson at this juncture that appears to have sealed the friendship of the two men and established Dr. Bronaugh as one of the General's most trusted aides as well as his personal physician. Henceforth for the remainder of his all-too-brief life, he was never out of Jackson's presence for long. With other Jackson favorites including Sam Houston, Richard K. Call and James Gadsden, he was much at the Hermitage from which Jackson preferred to conduct his military affairs.[8]

In late 1817 the Seminole Indians, restless under the threatened encroachments on lands in southwest Georgia and north Florida which had been allocated to them in the Treaty of Ft. Jackson in 1814, warned General Edmund P. Gaines that they would not tolerate further disregard of the Treaty, and if such occurred a bloody encounter would result. Gaines proceeded to burn their principal settlement, Fowltown (Foultown) in Georgia. This brought revenge from the Indians, who attacked a boatload of Americans ascending the Apalachicola River, killing almost the entire lot, including four children. Thus began the First Seminole War on November 21, 1817.[9] Jackson was, of course, quick to act, having a long standing suspicion that the Indians had been receiving aid and encouragement from the Spanish settlements in Pensacola and St. Marks as well as British agents, notably Alexander Arbuthnot and Robert Armbrister. Also present was the poorly concealed desire to rid Florida of the Spanish. Jackson proceeded with his customary rashness to achieve his objective with little or no regard for the proprieties of international law regarding the rights and properties of the subjects of the King of Spain. He ordered the execution of British agents. His actions brought repercussions in Washington, including a congressional investigation. Among those from whom depositions were required was Dr. Bronaugh whose opening statement was "I was attached to General Jackson's staff during the whole Seminole campaign."[10]

Jackson accepted the governorship of Florida in January 1821 but not until June 14 did he arrive in Pensacola where three days later on June 17 the formal transfer of West Florida to the United States took place. Having been commissioned by the Secretary of State, John Quincy Adams, to establish a territorial government Jackson lost no time in exercising his authority. His first appointments included the membership of the Pensacola Board of Health, with Dr. Bronaugh as Chairman and Resident Physician, and Dr. John V.D. Voorhees as Health Officer.[11] Less than two weeks later Dr. Bronaugh announced his association with Dr. Voorhees in a professional partnership.[12]

Notwithstanding Dr. Bronaugh's intentions with regard to private medical practice in Pensacola he was much too valuable to Jackson's purposes to be left to pursue it. On finding the Spanish Governor of West Florida, Jose Callava, not at all amenable to Jackson's wishes with respect to the technicalities of the transfer to the United States, Jackson relied on Dr. Bronaugh to deal with Callava. Dr. Bronaugh was also charged with making an inventory of the Archives, Public Buildings and other Properties involved in the transfer.[13] In the latter part of 1821 he was sent on numerous missions as Jackson's agent and courier,[14] ultimately arriving in Washington for the winter of 1821-1822.[15] He was doubtless the bearer of Jackson's letter of resignation from the Territorial Governorship of Florida.[16]

Dr. Bronaugh remained in Washington until May 1822 or at least until the appointments were made for the newly organized government of Florida. He then made his way to Florida, going as far as Louisville, Kentucky, in company with appointee Governor William P. Duval who went to Bairdstown to visit relatives. Dr. Bronaugh continued down river to New Orleans and thence to Pensacola.[17]

When appointments to the Territorial Legislative Council were announced in May 1822, Dr. Bronaugh's name led the list followed by Henry M. Brackenridge and Richard K. Call, both close associates of Jackson.[18]

No sooner was Dr. Bronaugh back in Florida than it was announced that he was a candidate to represent Florida in Congress.[19] This decision was almost certainly made in Washington and doubtless had the blessings of Jackson, Call and Brackenridge. Nevertheless it touched off a furor in Florida. Although there was little doubt that he was an exceptionally well-qualified candidate there was rancor over the method by which his candidacy had been advanced. He was obviously "Jackson's man" as well as a close friend of Governor Duval. Citizens of East Florida were especially incensed and vented their anger in the columns of the St. Augustine *East Florida Herald*.[20] They threw their support to Col. William Barnet (Barnett) a Pensacolian who had been appointed to the City Board of Aldermen in July 1821.[21] The main issue, however, was whether or not the soldiers would be allowed to vote in the elections scheduled for October 1822.[22]

Meanwhile the Legislative Council met in Pensacola on July 22, 1822, and by unanimous vote chose Dr. Bronaugh to preside. But alas, on August 10 yellow fever in its most virulent form made its appearance in the city.[23] Dr. Bronaugh as Resident Physician and President of the Board of Health, published a lengthy statement on August 17 emphasizing the seriousness of the situation with suggestions as to precautions which all citizens should observe. He did not minimize the dangers.[24] A few days later, as fear engulfed the city, the Legislative Council abandoned Pensacola and retreated to the plantation of Don Manuel (Emanuel) Gonzales, some 15 miles to the north where it planned to reassemble. Dr. Bronaugh, however, fell ill and was not among those repairing to Gonzales' place.

Instead, he was taken into the home of his dear friend of many years, Col. George Walton;[25] several members of whose family were also sick. On August 29 realizing that his death was imminent, Dr. Bronaugh summoned his host to his death bed and dictated his last will and testament.[26] Thus was lost to fledgling Florida a man of unusual ability whose talents and experience were sorely needed in the struggles of the next few decades.

Dr. Bronaugh's estate was a modest one which included three slaves and money owed him which when and if collected was to be sent with the slaves to his aging mother in Loudon County, Virginia. A gold watch he left to Mrs. Walton, while his bookcase and library he bequeathed to Col. Walton. His wardrobe was to be given to those who had attended him in his final illness.

A fine portrait of Dr. Bronaugh in military regalia hangs in the Hermitage near Nashville.

1. P.K. Yonge Library of Florida History, MSS, Box 8, No. 10. Dr. Brasenham mentioned herein was Dr. Juan (John) Brosnaham for many years a Pensacola physician.

2. Webster Merritt, West Florida: Three Centuries Under Four Flags, Conquest, and Disease, *Journal Florida Medical Association*, XXXIX, No. 10, April 1953, pp. 749-765. Pages 762-765 contain a brief biographical treatment of Dr. Bronaugh.

3. Archives, University of Pennsylvania, Lists of Matriculants and Graduates.

4. MDUSA 1775-1873, pp. 266-268.

5. Ibid.

6. Ibid.

7. ASP Military Affairs, Class V, Vol. I, Washington, 1832, p. 501.

8. Robert V. Remini, *Andrew Jackson and the Course of American Empire*, New York, 1977, p. 321.

9. Ibid., p. 346.

10. ASP Military Affairs, I. 751.

11. Pensacola *Floridian*, August 18, 1821.

12. Ibid., September 1, 1821.

13. TP, XXII, Letter, Jackson to John Quincy Adams, Secretary of State, Pensacola, July 30, 1821, pp. 147-149.

14. House Documents Nos. 28-53, 17th Congress, 2nd Session, 1821-1822. Record of travel pay for Dr. Bronaugh for travel to New Orleans, Mobile, Balkeley (Ala.), Baton Rouge and Nashville.

15. TP, XXII, 298, Letter, Acting Governor George Walton to Jackson, dated at Pensacola, December 19, 1821. "I take it for granted that since your arrival at home you have been busily engaged in arranging your papers preparatory to Dr. Bronaugh's visit to Washington."

16. Ibid., p. 335.

17. Pensacola *Floridian*, June 9, 1822.

18. Ibid. Neither Brackenridge nor Joseph M. White actually served in the Legislative Council, both having accepted other appointments.

19. Pensacola *Floridian*, June 22, 1822.

20. St. Augustine *East Florida Herald*. See copy printed in *Territorial Papers*, XXII, pp. 542-546.

21. Ibid., p. 131.

22. Ibid., p. 473. Letter, Col. Duncan L. Clinch to President Monroe, June 24, 1822. Col. Clinch clearly set forth his objections to extending the franchise to officers and soldiers only temporarily in the Territory.

23. Ibid., p. 531.

24. Pensacola *Floridian*, August 17, 1822.

25. TP, XXII, 557, Letter, Acting Governor Walton to John C. Calhoun, Secretary of War, November 4, 1822. "The sickness of my family and of an esteemed friend (Dr. Bronaugh) who was confined at my house detained me a considerable time in the city after the Legislative Council adjourned to Emanuels." Governor Duval was also ill at Walton's house. (See letter, Duval to President Monroe, September 10, 1822.) "I lived with my friend Dr. Bronaugh in Col. Walton's family during the epidemic. It is almost a wonder that I escaped for every member of my family has been down with the fever except himself (Walton) and his venerable mother. . . ." Ibid., p. 531.

26. Last Will and Testament of Dr. Bronaugh, Escambia County Court House, Old Will Book, No. 3, p. 35. Typed copy in P.K. Yonge Library of Florida History was consulted.

Bronson, Oliver, St. Augustine, 1860

Dr. Bronson, a regular winter resident of St. Augustine, apparently devoted only a small part of his time to the practice of medicine. The earliest reference to his Florida existence is found in the Fernandina *East Floridian* of November 14, 1860, in which the list of passengers on the Schooner *Carolina* from Charleston included "Dr. O. Bronson, wife, two attendants, and Master Bronson." A native of New York and practitioner in New York City, he was able to accumulate considerable wealth, some of which he spent in building "an elegant and commodious mansion" on the Plaza in St. Augustine.[1] In spite of adversities brought on by the Civil War Dr. Bronson's estate was estimated at almost $60,000 in 1870.[2]

Dr. Bronson was without doubt socially prominent both in New York and Florida. He was a close friend of Thomas Buckingham Smith and was named executor of Smith's estate in 1871.[3] The wealthy society belle, Julia Newberry, when advised by her New York physician to go to Florida for her health, made this entry in her diary: "The doctor now strongly advises Florida. Sister has written to Dr. Bronson to enquire about rooms, and we have nearly decided to go & take John, Marie, a phaeton & croquet box."[4] In another entry she saucily penned a list of "My Particular Male Friends as they stand at the present time." Included among "Old or Married Gentlemen" was Dr. Bronson.[5]

It is evident that Dr. Bronson took an active interest in the beauty and welfare of St. Augustine. His civic concern is apparent in his having been the organizer and first president of the Buckingham Smith Benevolent Association.[6] He was cited in 1866 for having "ornamented" the Plaza by planting water oaks.[7] He accepted the position of Superintendent of Schools in 1868, an office he held as late as 1873.[8] His home noted for its charm and attractiveness was described by a real estate agent who offered it for sale in 1879 as "fronting the Plaza bounded by St. George Street, Artillery Lane and Trinity Church. . .commodious, surrounded with piazzas". . .whose gardens "are filled with tropical trees, shrubs, etc."[9]

Since no record of Dr. Bronson's death has been found in St. Augustine, it may be assumed that he was in New York at the time of his death. His son, Oliver Jr., a lawyer, was married on June 2, 1870, to Julia F. Colt, a native of Massachusetts. The ceremony took place in Trinity Episcopal Church, St. Augustine.[10]

1. St. Agustine *Examiner*, December 5, 1868.
2. In the St. Augustine Census of 1870, p. 606, Dr. Bronson's age was 71, while that of his wife, Joanna, was 56. She was also born in New York.
3. He was so named in the will of Buckingham Smith, a copy of which is in the biographical file of Smith in the P.K. Yonge Library of Florida History.
4. Julia Newberry's Diary, New York 1933, p. 37. Julia Newberry was the daughter of Walter L. and Julia Butler Newberry. The Newberry family was among Chicago's most illustrious in the last half of the 19th century.
5. Ibid., p. 81, Miss Newberry seems to have known most people of social importance wherever she traveled. She enjoyed dropping their names about.
6. This Association provided for in the will of Smith was established for the benefit of the Negroes of St. Augustine and was charged with administering a fund also provided for in the will.
7. St. Augustine *Examiner*, October 27, 1866.
8. Oliver Bronson biographical file, St. Augustine Historical Society.
9. St. Augustine *Florida Weekly Press*, August 23, 1879.
10. Trinity Parish Records, St. Augustine, "Marrriages."

Broome, J. Harris, Live Oak, 1870

Dr. Broome, a native of Georgia, is thought to have migrated to Suwannee County shortly after the Civil War. Nothing is known of his educational background but it is assumed that he had studied medicine as an apprentice to a Georgia physician. His wife, Annie, was also a native of Georgia. They were the parents of two children, Mary, aged four, and Joseph, aged 11 months in 1870.[1] The Broomes lived in Live Oak.

1. U.S. Census, 1870, Suwannee County, Florida, p. 694.

Brosnaham, George Othman, Pensacola, 1835-1933

Dr. Brosnaham, second son of Dr. Juan and Isabella Eugenia Sierra Brosnaham, was born in Pensacola, Florida, in 1835.[1] After receiving his basic education in Pensacola he enrolled at the New Orleans School of Medicine[2] from which he was graduated in 1859. Soon thereafter he returned to Pensacola and began medical practice. With outbreak of war two years later, Dr. Brosnaham enlisted for military service, not as a medical officer but as an ordinary soldier with Captain E.A. Perry's Rifle Rangers, a unit recruited primarily from the Pensacola area. Soon thereafter, however, he joined an Alabama company participating in at least two major battles, Shiloh and Chicamauga. After being wounded at Chicamauga he was transferred to a military hospital at Greenville, Alabama. Upon his recovery he was appointed assistant surgeon and assigned to the 12th Louisiana Infantry, but finally completing his military career in a Mississippi unit under the command of Captain Putnam Darden.[3]

Soon after his discharge from the militry service Dr. Brosnaham returned to Pensacola and resumed medical practice. At about the same time he was given a part interest in his father's drug store in Pensacola in which enterprise he was later joined by his brother, John Alfred, who was also a physician.

In spite of the economic hardships inflicted by the War and its aftermath the elder Dr. Juan Brosnaham had managed to retain possession of his various properties. According to the Census of 1870 his real estate was worth $69,000 while his personal property was valued at $10,000. Upon the death of Dr. Juan in 1871 his entire estate was bequeathed to his wife, Isabella.[4] Juan Brosnaham had wisely invested in Pensacola real estate and upon his widow's death in 1889, her two sons inherited valuable real estate in the city. Dr. George Brosnaham was named executor of her will.[5]

At some date in the late 1860s Dr. Brosnaham was married to Cynthia McKee of Haynesville, Alabama. Several children were born of whom three, John, George and Mary, survived to adulthood.

According to Rerick, Dr.Brosnaham retired from medical practice in 1892.[6] He died in Pensacola in 1933. Mrs. Brosnaham had died on February 1, 1895.

1. The vital data on Dr. Brosnaham and his family are derived for the greater part from the U.S. Census Schedules, Escambia County, Florida, for the years 1850, 1860, 1870, 1880, and the Special Florida Census of 1885 and also from gravestones in St. Michael's Cemetery, Pensacola.

2. Numerous schools of medicine made their appearance in the two decades prior to the Civil War. Many were closed during the course of the War; some never reopened. The New Orleans School of Medicine became defunct in 1870.

3. Rowland H. Rerick, *Memoirs of Florida*, Vol. I, Atlanta, 1902, pp. 454-455. See also *Soldiers of Fortune*, Tallahassee 1903, p. 80.

4. It is the good fortune of anyone interested in the Brosnaham family of Pensacola that the Pensacola Historical Society has brought to light the will of Isabella Brosnaham published with annotations by Virginia Parks. See *The Echo*, Vol. I., No. 2, 1980, pp. 8-10. At the time of her death Mrs. Brosnaham was living at the family home at the corner of Palafox and Romana Streets, Pensacola.

5. Ibid., p. 9.

6. Rerick, *op. cit.* Several members of the George O. Brosnaham family were buried in the new family plot in St. Michael's Cemetery.

Brosnaham, John Andrew, Pensacola, 1830-1905

Dr. Brosnaham was the eldest child of Dr. Juan and Isabella Sierra Brosnaham. He was born in Pensacola on August 31, 1830.[1] As a youth he began the study of medicine with his father as preceptor, and in the fall of 1851 matriculated at the Medical College of the University of New York, from which he was graduated in the spring of 1853. On his return to Pensacola he is presumed to have begun the practice of medicine but soon succumbed to the lure of the California gold rush which was still attracting scores of adventurers. He had little luck in the gold mines, however, and returned to the East, making his way eventually to New York, where according to his obituary, he was graduated from "a celebrated dental college."

On February 2, 1856, he announced to the citizens of Pensacola and vicinity that he had just returned from New York, "with all the latest improvements of his profession and has opened his office one door above the Custom House on Palafox Street," thus launching his practice as a dentist.[2] But this does not appear to have signaled the cessation of his medical practice.

Dr. Brosnaham was married to Mary Eleanor (Nenna) Walker on December 24, 1856, a union to which three children were born.[3]

As the War Between the States became imminent Dr. Brosnaham moved with his family some 20 miles up the Escambia River to the town of Moline, a move prompted by the vulnerability of Pensacola and the struggle for possession of Ft. Pickens. Although Dr. Brosnaham is listed among the Confederate veterans buried in St. Michael's Cemetery, Pensacola, there is no evidence that he was ever inducted into the Confederate Army. His brother, George Othman, did have a distinguished career as a member of the Pensacola Rifle Rangers, Co. A., 2nd Florida Infantry Regiment. It is assumed, therefore, that Dr. John served in a civilian capacity.

After the War Dr. Brosnaham resumed his regular practice of medicine and dentistry with considerable success. He took his family to California with the intention of settling there, but reconsidered and returned to Pensacola, purchasing Gull Point and living there for a few years until he built a fine house on Stoddard Street in Pensacola.

Mrs. Brosnaham died on July 17, 1894. Two years later Doctor John married Miss Sallie Moseley of Richmond, Virginia. This marriage produced one son, John Andrew. Dr. Brosnaham lived until January 9, 1905. A portion of his eulogy merits inclusion:

> He was much beloved by all classes of people—was given to charity—gave freely of both his means and his services. Often did not charge for his services. The poor for miles around knew him as a friend. As a humanitarian he knew no equal. . . Hardly a home among old Pensacola families where he had not at some time administered as physician and friend.

Dr. Brosnaham was survived by his widow, his daughter, Mrs. Isabella Ingraham, his sons, Henry A. (child of his first wife), and John Andrew.

1. In consideration of space it is here stated that the greater part of the information included in this sketch is drawn from the obituary for Dr. Brosnaham published in the *Pensacola Daily News* of January 9, 1905, a lengthy statement. Vital dates are found in "Records of St. Michael's Cemetery at Pensacola, Florida, 1810-1938." Comp. by Pensacola Chapter, D.A.R., 1938, Typescript. Copy in P.K. Yonge Library of Florida History, University of Florida, Gainesville.
2. Pensacola *Gazette*, February 2, 1856.
3. Ibid., December 22, 1856.

Brosnaham, Juan, Pensacola, 1781-1871

Dr. Brosnaham, for more than 50 years a member of the medical faculty of Pensacola, was born in Catskill, New York[1] on April 1, 1791, of an Irish family. Nothing is known of either his early education or medical training, although it is in New York in the early 19th century. It is fairly certain, however, that he did not complete the work for his medical degree. From New York he moved to New Orleans where he appears to have begun medical practice and where he remained for only a brief time before settling in Pensacola where he would remain for the rest of his life. He is thought to have arrived in Pensacola prior to 1821.

The conflict between Spain and the United States over possession of Florida ended in 1821 with the signing of the Adams-Onis Treaty. Soon thereafter President Monroe appointed Andrew Jackson to the office of Governor of Florida. One of Jackson's first official acts was to appoint his personal physician, Dr. James C. Bronaugh, Resident Physician of Pensacola. Dr. Bronaugh was a physician of distinction who had earned his medical degree at the University of Pennsylvania. His immediate concern was the poor quality of medical practice in the town of Pensacola. He sought to improve the situation by establishing a Board of Health which was convened on July 23, 1821, for the purpose of examining the credentials of physicians practicing in the town. Several presented their medical diplomas and were immediately licensed to practice. In Dr. Brosnaham's case, however, it is recorded that "Dr. Brosnaham presented his credentials, which were deemed sufficient and was thereupon deemed qualified to practice in the City of Pensacola."[2]

The occasional glimpses of Dr. Brosnaham's activities, civic and professional, found in the columns of the Pensacola newspaper, indicate that he was a highly esteemed citizen and physician, although in the latter role he divided his time between medicine and pharmacy, tending in his later years to abandon medical practice almost completely. Arnold Rosenbleeth, who made a study of Pensacola's early pharmacies, wrote: "Dr. Juan Brosnaham. . .was probably one of the first drug store owners, along with Dr. J.O. Smith."[3] His first drug store, incidentally, was located in the basement of his house on Palafox Street. He moved his pharmacy to the corner of Palafox and Intendencia Streets in November 1845. Henceforth, for a long time, his drug store was prominently advertised in the Pensacola *Gazette*,[4] the notices claiming almost miraculous cures for a variety of pills and tonics. By the standard of the times Dr. Brosnaham was a successful practitioner and businessman. Many of his investments were in Pensacola real estate. He was able to leave to his wife substantial properties in the town.[5]

Dr. Brosnaham was twice married. His first wife was Maria Josepha Martinez whom he married in New Orleans in 1816. To this marriage were born three daughters: Margaretta Sinvestra, Clotilde Santiago, and Angelina Petronia. Clotilde became the wife of William Louis Shuttleworth who after her death married her half-sister, Amanda Brosnaham. Dr. Brosnaham's second wife was Isabella Sierra, daughter of Dr. Eugenio Antonio. She was born in St. Marks, Florida, on March 6, 1799. To this union were born four children, John Andrew, who became a physician; Amanda, who married William L. Shuttleworth; Georgianna, who married, first, E.B. Renshaw, and second, William Kirk; George

Othman, also a physician, who married Cynthia Gingles.[6]

Dr. Brosnaham died in Pensacola on June 11, 1871; Mrs. Brosnaham died in Pensacola on May 13, 1899. Both were buried in St. Michael's Cemetery, as were several other members of the family.

1. Much of the biographical data included in the present brief sketch is derived from two brief articles, "Isabella Brosnaham" and Isabella's "Will" published in Pensacola Historical Society Quarterly, *The Echo*, Pensacola, Winter, 1980, pp. 8-10. These were presumably prepared for publication by Editor, Virginia Parks. The several pertinent censuses were also consulted, as was the St. Michael's Cemetery survey.

2. Pensacola *Floridian*, August 18, 1821. Dr. Bosnaham was also appointed to the Pensacola Board of Aldermen by Governor Jackson.

3. Arnold Rosenbleeth, Pensacola's Early Pharmacies, *The Echo*, Winter 1980, p. 16.

4. For months on end the advertisements of Moffat's Vegetable Life Pills and Phoenix Bitters containing fantastic claims for their curative powers were printed in the Pensacola *Gazette*. These wonder drugs could be bought at the Drug Stores of Dr. John Brosnaham and John O. Smith. See Pensacola *Gazette* issues of 1845.

5. Dr. Brosnaham wisely invested heavily in Pensacola real estate. Many of his properties, which he willed in their entirely to his widow, are specifically named in the Will of Isabella Brosnaham. See note 1, supra.

6. Both Brosnaham sons, John Andrew and George Othman, were successful physicians in Pensacola.

Brown, A.C., Ocala, 1824

Dr. Brown, a native of Georgia, was a medical practitioner in Ocala in the early 1850s. He appears in the Census of 1850 at age 26 as a resident of the Ocala boarding house of Josiah Paine. His property was valued at a mere $500.[1] His professional card first appeared in the Ocala *Conservator* on June 4, 1851.[2] He continued to advertise his services to the citizens of Marion County as late as October 1853 after which date no further information about him has been located.[3]

1. U.S. Census, 1850, Marion County, Florida, p. 220.

2. Ocala *Conservator*, November 19, 1851.

3. Ocala *Florida Mirror*, October 7, 1853.

Brown, C.J., Leon County, 1860

Dr. Brown was the eldest son of S. Willard and Elizabeth Brown who had moved from their native Georgia in the late 1830s and settled in rural Leon County. As of 1860 they were a family of above average means, their property having been assigned a value of about $30,000 in 1860.[1] Dr. Brown although a native of Florida is thought to have left the state at about the time the Civil War began. His name does not appear in the Civil War records of Florida, but it is quite possible that he served in the Georgia regiment. There is no reason to believe that he ever returned to practice medicine in Florida.

1. All that is known of Dr. Brown is derived from the U.S. Census, State of Florida, 1860.

Brown, John W., Ft. Gaines, 1844

Except for his obituary notice which indicated that he died at Ft. Gaines in Gainesville on March 17, 1844, nothing is known of Dr. Brown. He was in the 40th year of his age at the time of his death.[1]

1. Apalachicola *Commercial Advertiser*, March 30, 1844. The fact that Dr. Brown's death was noted in the Apalachicola newspaper seems to indicate that he had been a resident of Franklin County. Any further mention of this man would be only speculation. Incidentally, he is not mentioned in Frances B. Heitman, *Historical Register and Dictionary of the United States Army*.

Brush, Nehemiah, St. Johns and Alachua Counties, 1787-1843

Dr. Brush of Fishkill, Dutchess County, New York, came to Florida in the early 1820s as a land speculator and developer and it is doubtful that he was ever a regular medical practitioner after his arrival in the Territory. He was one of the original investors in the Florida Association, a joint stock enterprise organized by a small group of business and professional men in New York and New Jersey.[1] It was the design of the group to purchase at low cost vast acreage in the interior of Florida west of St. Augustine in what was vaguely known as the Alachua District, whose eastern boundary was the St. Johns River and western boundary the Suwannee. In the center of the District lay the well-known Arredondo Grant, which in 1817 had been granted by Alexander Ramirez, Intendent (agent of the Spanish Crown) of Cuba and the Floridas, to Fernando de la Maza Arredondo. After the cession by Spain in 1821 this land was sold through an agent, B.H. Betts, attorney, to various purchasers, the chief being the Florida Association.

Subsequently advertisements appeared in New York newspapers in an attempt to lure settlers into the Florida Wilderness. Dr. Brush and two other members of the Association constituted the committee to enlist "families of good character" to settle in Alachua. The committee chartered a schooner on December 21-22, 1822, which with the would-be settlers aboard sailed from New York arriving at Picolata on the St. Johns on December 29 to begin opening the Alachua District for settlement.[2] Dr. Brush did not go as physician to the settlement but instead employed one Dr. Samuel R. Ayers in that capacity.

It is impossible to determine the acreage in Alachua owned individually by Dr. Brush. In one deposition he stated that he had on April 15, 1821 bought 1,000 acres for $5,000 through attorney Betts. In another deposition he claimed 10,000 acres in Alachua and "an undivided part of 289,645 acres" in the Arredondo Grant.[3] Besides he purchased in 1826 1,200 acres on the west side of the St. Johns River on which the City of Palatka is now situated. The purchase price was $1,500. He is also known to have owned a tract of unstated dimensions on the east side of the River, directly across from Palatka,[4] while there is record of an unconfirmed claim to a tract near Matanzas in what was then known as Mosquito County.[5]

There is some evidence that Dr. Brush built a modest house on the west bank of the River thought to have been the first to be built in Palatka. That he resided there and supervised the clearing of land to the west is fairly certain. In the Territorial Papers there is a letter from the Post Master General to Dr. Brush dated December 4, 1826, in which reference is made to a letter from Dr. Brush requesting that the postal route from St. Augustine to Tallahassee be changed (presumably to pass through Brush's property) and that a post office be located at Pilitica (Palatka).[6] Still there is no evidence that Dr. Brush's sojourn in any one Florida locality was of long duration. His mail was addressed to him at St. Augustine,[7] that being the only urban settlement in East Florida. His business activities appear to have been conducted from New York City. His eldest son, Ansel J. Brush, died at Jacksonville on October 10, 1832,[8] at the age of 17. Dr. Brush died at his rural home near the village of Fishkill, New York, on September 3, 1843. The obituary notice, however, identified him as a resident "of the City of New York,"[9] age 56.

The Florida properties of Dr. Brush at the time of his death were extensive. In the Arredondo grant alone the most authentic map of the area (drawn in 1846 by surveyors David H. Burr and Henry Washington) shows some 15 sections belonging to the heirs of Dr. Brush.[10]

1. The basic structure of the Florida Association can be determined by examining the numerous depositions taken in 1824 by Richard Riker, Recorder, Civil and Criminal Court Judge, New York City. These are printed in *Spanish Land Grants in Florida*, Tallahassee, 1940-41, 5 vols., II, 103ff.
2. Ibid., p. 108.
3. Ibid., I, p. 34.
4. Ibid., p. 24. This information is incidental to a claim by Francis J. Avice that he owned a section of land on the east side of the St. Johns River between lands of Juan B. Entralgo and Dr. Brush, nearly opposite Palatka.
5. Ibid., p. 206. This was a claim for 1,800 acres on the Matanzas River.
6. Kenin E. Kearney, ed., "Autobiography of William Marvin," FHO, XXXVI, pp. 197-198.
7. St. Augustine, *East Florida Herald*, April 2, 1825.
8. Ibid., October 11, 1832.
9. St. Augustine *Florida Herald and Southern Democrat*, October 3, 1843. It is an interesting coincidence that the same issue carried an obituary notice of one of Florida's most notable pioneers, Zephaniah Kingsley, resident of Duval County, who died on September 13 in New York at age 78.
10. This map, a copy of which is located in the P.K. Yonge Library of Florida History, depicts the sectional subdivisions of the Arredondo grant with the names of owners as of 1845. No effort has been made in this connection to determine the identities of Dr. Brush's heirs. One possible heir was Charles W. Brush, Judge Probate, born in New York State, resident of St. Augustine in 1850, U.S. Census, 1850, St. Johns County, Florida, p. 200. Another was possibly Dr. John Brush, who died in St. Augustine, May 26, 1846, at age 36, Parish Register, Trinity Parish, St. Augustine, 1821-1904, Section on "Burials."

Bulson, Henry V., Fernandina, 1860

Dr. Bulson appears to have been a brief sojourner in Fernandina about 1860. A native of Prussia, he was in his 60s in that year. His property was valued at $500. He was the only member of his household. No further information concerning this man has been found.[1]

1. U.S. Census, 1860, Nassau County, Florida, p. 407.

Burke, Christopher C., Marianna, 1860s

Dr. Burke was born in Georgia about 1837. By 1860 he had established his medical practice in Marianna and was residing in the household of James C. Coker, a Marianna merchant.[1] Apparently a political activist, he was chosen as a delegate from Jackson County to the State Democratic Convention meeting in Quincy during the first week of June 1860, a particularly turbulent session reflecting the emotional tensions of the times.[2]

Provoked by the Federal attack on Ft. Sumter in April 1861 Jackson County, along with other Florida counties, responded by mustering into service its militia, in Jackson County the 4th Infantry Regiment. This was done on July 1. In the process Dr. Burke was mustered in as regimental adjutant with the rank of second lieutenant.[3] A part of the regiment saw early service in Tennessee and the muster rolls indicate that Dr. Burke was with his regiment from January through July 1862. A few weeks later he was in Fernandina under arrest charged with disrespect toward his commanding officer. However serious the offense, he was soon cleared and returned to his regiment and is shown to have been present at their headquarters near Murfreesboro from August through December 1862. In an encounter with the enemy at Stone River December 31, 1862-January 2, 1863, Dr. Burke suffered a foot wound which would almost end his army service. Out of this mishap there ensued a lengthy correspondence between the regiment and the Office of Adjutant and Inspector-General in Richmond concerning the disability suffered by Dr. Burke. In one instance Lt. Col. Edward N. Badger of 4th Infantry Headquarters in a letter to General Sam Cooper, Adjutant and Inspector General, unequivocally accused Dr. Burke of malingering. The issue was finally resolved, however, when surgeon Henry H. Robinson attested that Dr. Burke had indeed suffered a permanently disabling wound of the instep which rendered him unfit for further active service. Robinson's letter was dated at Marianna on September 18, 1863. Seven days later Dr. Burke's letter of resignation was accepted by General Cooper's office.

With a clear conscience and all blemish removed from his record Dr. Burke returned to Marianna. A short time thereafter he assisted Dr. Henry Robinson in operating a military hospital which had been established there.[4]

At the end of the War Dr. Burke married Elmira McNealy of Marianna whom according to Stanley he had met while treating her father, Adam McNealy. The couple later moved to Texarkana, Texas, where they settled permanently.[5]

1. U.S. Census, 1870, Jackson County, Florida, item 495. Here Dr. Burke's age was given as 23.
2. Fernandina *East Floridian*, June 21, 1860.
3. All military information included here may be found in NA, Service Records, CSA, M. 251, R 53. The service record of Dr. Burke, as filmed from the National Archives sources, is somewhat confusing due to the fact that there was also a Charles C. Burke in the 4th Infantry Regiment. In some instances only initials of the two men were recorded, rendering it difficult to distinguish between them.
4. J. Randall Stanley, History of Jackson County, Marianna 1950, p. 187.
5. Ibid., p. 193.

Burrough, M., Explorer in Southern Florida, 1821

In the summer of 1821 an expedition fitted out in Philadelphia "by a patriotic association under the protection of government, for the most laudable and meritorious purpose—that of exploring the interior part of the Peninsula below the 27th degree of latitude" arrived in St. Augustine in late July. The expedition was directed by Peter S. Chazotte and accompanied by Dr. Burrough as physician. The group included a surveyor, a chaplain, four volunteers and five laborers.[1]

1. St. Augustine *Florida Gazette*, July 28, 1821. As the expedition departed for the unknown area of South Florida, the editor wished them well in their enterprise expressing the hope that great economic advantage would accrue to such efforts.

Burroughs, Richard Berrien, Leon and Duval Counties, 1832-1901

Dr. Burroughs, one of Florida's most distinguished physicians and civic leaders, was born in Savannah, Georgia, on January 19, 1833, son of Joseph H. Burroughs. His mother was the daughter of John McPherson Berrien, attorney general in Andrew Jackson's first cabinet and on two occasions a member of the United States Senate. He was grduated from the University of Georgia in 1853. He then enrolled at Jefferson Medical College, Philadelphia, where he became Doctor of Medicine in 1856.[1]

Upon receiving his medical degree Dr. Burroughs returned to his native state and set up practice in Camden County.[2] Within a matter of weeks, however, he moved to Tallahassee where he remained in practice for the next 24 years.

He appears to have achieved a high degree of success; his services were in great demand from townspeople and planters alike. One of his medical bills which has survived in the James Whitehead Estate Papers reveals something of the medical customs of the antebellum period. The bill, rendered for the treatment of Negroes on the Whitehead plantation in the year 1857, amounted to $265.27 of which $17.77 was for interest charged for delayed payment. Julia Lloyd Smith discovered that "Burroughs charged from four to six dollars a visit, this including medicine, mileage, and treatment, and there was an additional fee for inclement weather."[3] One item in the bill for treatment of a Whitehead slave reads: "Visit in rain, mileage, and medicine to Henderson $5.50."

As one of a small group of Florida physicians concerned about the dubious quality of medical practice in the State Dr. Burroughs responded to the invitation of Dr. Abel S. Baldwin to meet with others of the profession in Jacksonville in January 1874 for the purpose of organizing a state medical association. He and Dr. Geroge W. Betton were the two representatives from Leon County. At this meeting Dr. Burroughs emerged as a leader in his profession, serving on two important committees.[4] In the following year he was elected first vice president of the Association. The published proceedings of this and subsequent meetings abound in references to the activities of Dr. Burroughs as a dedicated and progressive member. In 1875 he delivered "an eloquent address on the 'Origin and Progress of Medicine'." In 1884, in the absence of President E.T. Sabal, because of illness, Dr. Burroughs gave the presidential address and in the following year he read a paper entitled "Diagnosis of Bilious Dengue and Yellow Fevers."

By the mid-1850s there was strong sentiment within the Association for the establishment of a state board of health. Dr. Burroughs and Dr. Joseph Y. Porter of Key West were among the most vocal advocates, the former heading a committee to draft a bill to be forwarded to the State Legislature for action. Dr. Burroughs went to Tallahassee in 1888 to lend his support to the passage of the bill. To his delight the bill found little opposition in the House but came to grief in the Senate on what he considered to be trivial objections. Upon discovering that the defeat of the bill was attributable in part to the meddling opposition of a member of the Medical Association Dr. Burroughs forthwith tendered his resignation from the Association. The presiding officer, however, tabled the matter in the hope of persuading Dr. Burroughs to reconsider. He appears to have been successful, for Dr. Burroughs was once more an active member in 1889 and continued as such almost to the time of his death.

With the onset of the Civil War in 1861 Dr. Burroughs had entered the Confederate Army as a surgeon, being assigned at first to the 63rd Georgian Infantry Regiment but in the latter part of the War serving under the command of the heroic Col. J.J. Dickison in his Florida campaigns.

Dr. Burroughs gave up his practice in Tallahassee in 1880 and settled permanently in Jacksonville in a home on West Ashley Street. Here he continued to be an active practitioner for several years and, in addition, found time for public service. He was elected to the City Council in 1889. He is said to have been responsible for changing the name of the city's downtown plaza from St. James Square to Hemming Park. The Seaboard Airline Railroad retained him for several years as the chief surgeon of its Florida division. He was a trustee of Jacksonville's Confederate Soldier's Home and an able supporter of Jacksonville's two major hospitals, Duval and St. Lukes.

Dr. Burroughs was twice married first to Ella J. Burroughs,[5] who died on August 13, 1868, then to Florida Lewis, who died on April 14, 1895. There were six children from these marriages, one daughter and five sons.

Dr. Burroughs health began to fail in 1899 whereupon he was taken to Norfolk, Virginia, to live with his son, Joseph Hallett. He died there on September 11, 1901. His body was brought to Savannah for burial in Laurel Grove Cemetery.

1. Jefferson Medical College, Philadelphia, List of Graduates. A substantial portion of the information included in this sketch may be found in Rowland H. Rerick, *Memoirs of Florida*, Atlanta, 1902. I. 464-465. Additional data are found in Dr. Burroughs obituary, Jacksonville *Evening Metropolis*, September 12, 1901.

2. The stay in Camden County was brief, probably a matter of only a few weeks. His notice of practice in Tallahassee first appeared in the Tallahassee *Sentinel*, June 24, 1856, his graduation from medical school having occurred the previous March.

3. Julia Lloyd Smith, *Slavery and Plantation Growth in Antebellum Florida*, Gainesville, 1973, p. 98.

4. This and other information relating to Dr. Burroughs' activities in the Florida Medical Association are recorded in the annual publication of the Association's Proceedings. See also Webster Merritt, *A Century of Medicine in Jacksonville and Duval County*, Gainesville, 1849, pp. 73, 78. For Dr. Burroughs involvement in the founding of the ill-fated Florida University Medical School, ca. 1883-1885, see ibid., p. 143.

5. Marriage to Miss Burroughs occurred in late April or early May 1857, "Genealogical Records of Leon County, Florida," typescript, P.K. Yonge Library of Florida History, p. 80.

Burst, Henry, Newnansville, 1870

Nothing is known of Dr. Burst except information in the census schedule of 1870, where he is listed as a native of Georgia, aged 22 and the sole resident of his household.[1] Since his name does not appear in the Census of 1880, it is probable that he resided in Florida only briefly.

1. U.S. Census, 1870, Alachua County, Florida, p. 377.

Burton, William H., Madison, 1830

Dr. Burton, native of Virginia, and graduate of the Jefferson Medical College of Philadelphia in the class of 1856, moved into Florida soon after the Civil War, settling in the town of Madison. He was a man of modest means, owning property worth less than $1,000 in 1870.[1] His family consisted of wife, Mary L., and son, William M., age seven that year. Also there was Martha Pilcher, a woman of 26 who "helps in the home." Nothing further is presently known of this family.

1. U.S. Census, 1870, Madison County, p. 10.

Butler, L.M., Fernandina, 1860

Dr. Butler was one of five brothers residing in Fernandina in 1860. They were a family of considerable means, their combined properties being valued at more than $50,000. Except for the youngest, who was still a minor in 1860, they were a professional family, two being attorneys and the third an engineer, and except for the youngest all were born in South Carolina.[1]

In the fall of 1858 Butler was a matriculant at Jefferson Medical College in Philadelphia from which he received his medical degree in the spring of 1860.[2] Immediately after graduation he returned to Fernandina. On April 5 he announced the opening of his professional office in Dr. Lesesne's Building on Fourth Street.[3]

During the mid-1860s Fernandina was enjoying an economic boom. The Florida

Railroad Company had been chartered and the construction of the railroad which would eventually link Fernandina with the Gulf of Mexico was begun in 1855. Many jobs were created and engineers were needed for the building of bridges and surveying the route to be followed. In short, Fernandina appeared to be a promising locality for a professional man, but the war clouds were gathering. Dr. Butler had scarcely begun practice when actual conflict appeared likely and Florida's secession from the Union was imminent.

In mid-December 1860 a local militia unit known as the Fernandina Volunteers was organized. Joseph Finegan, later to become a Confederate General, was elected to command while Dr. Butler was surgeon to the outfit. His younger brother, W.B., was given a commission as second lieutenant.[4] Seven months later the Fernandina Volunteers were mustered into the Confederate Army as Company K 2nd Florida Infantry Regiment.[5] As for Dr. Butler, he was mustered in on July 13 as first sergeant and promoted to a lieutenancy (whether 1st or 2nd not specified) on August 21.

Dr. Butler's further war record has not survived but it is assumed that he was with the 2nd Florida when it moved to Richmond in September 1861. If so, he saw action at Yorktown, near which the Regiment was encamped for the winter of 1861-62, and later at Williamsburg when General McLellan launched an attack on the post. It is regrettable that beyond this point nothing is known of Dr. Butler. Having lost two of his brothers, William B., who was killed at Chancellorsville and C.A., who was a casualty at the Battle of Seven Pines, the War was a particularly bitter experience for him. If he did indeed survive the struggle there is no evidence that he ever returned to Fernandina.

1. U.S. Census, 1860, Nassau County, Florida, p. 91. Here the youngest Butler brother aged 15 is shown to have been a native of Florida. Since there is no further evidence that the family lived in Florida prior to the 1850s this is not accepted as evidence to the contrary.
2. Jefferson Medical College, *List of Dead or Lost Graduated in Classes from 1826 to 1879*, p. 69.
3. Fernandina *East Floridian*, April 5, 1860.
4. Ibid., December 19, 1860.
5. N.A. Service Records, CSA, Roll 35. There were five Fernandina men, all bearing the name Butler, in the 2nd Florida Regiment. Of these, four belonged to Company K. It is a sad statistic that four of the five were casualties of the War.

Butler, M.A., Jackson County, 1841-1864

Dr. Butler, whose life ended tragically at the age of 23, was a native of Greenwood, Jackson County. Nothing is known of his youth and education. As a member of the Greenwood Home Guards, he was on duty in Marianna when the town was attacked by a detachment of Union soldiers in September 1864 and was among those who had taken refuge in the Episcopal Church to which the attackers set fire. In their effort to escape through the front door, Dr. Butler, 23, and Frank Allen, 76, were shot and killed. This unfortunate event took place on September 27, 1864.[1]

1. A full account of the Battle of Marianna by the late Mark F. Boyd was published in the *Florida Historical Quarterly*, XXIX, No. 4, 1951, pp. 225-242. Since Dr. Butler's name does not appear in the Florida Census of 1860, it is assumed that he had been a resident of Florida for only a short time. Another account of the incident is found in Charlotte Corley Farley, *Florida's Alamo*, Marianna, 1980, p. 30.

Butler, Ready S., Palatka, 1834

The Florida career of Dr. Butler was brief, spanning scarcely two years. He was born in Lawrenceville, Georgia, in 1834.[1] In the fall of 1857 he entered recently-established Oglethorpe Medical College in Savannah from which he was graduated in the spring of 1859 after presenting a thesis entitled "Inflammation."[2] Soon thereafter he settled in Palatka and began medical practice.[3]

Dr. Butler responded to the call for volunteers for Confederate service on May 23, 1861, enlisting in a Putnam County Company called the St. Augustine Rifles, organized by local planter, E.C. Simkins. A few weeks later, on May 23, the Company was mustered into service at Camp Virginia near Jacksonville, becoming Company H 2nd Florida Infantry regiment.[4] Dr. Butler entered without military rank notwithstanding his mature age (27) and medical degree. He was transferred with his unit to Richmond, Virginia, in September 1861 and some weeks later to winter encampment near Yorktown.[5]

During the winter of 1861-62, when Company H was without a medical officer Dr. Butler was assigned to special duty as company surgeon, but without advancement in rank.[6] As spring arrived in 1862 the Florida Second came under fire at both Yorktown and Williamsburg in the first stages of McLellan's Peninsular Campaign. It is unlikely, however, that Dr. Butler saw action in either of these engagements for in February he was granted a furlough because of a serious ailment, amaurosis, producing a loss of eyesight. He was granted a discharge on May 13, 1862, signed at Chicahominy and paid the $98.68 due him. Presumably he returned to his Georgia home since there is no indication that he ever returned to practice medicine in Florida. His discharge papers provide the following descriptive details. He was five feet, six inches tall, of dark complexion and dark hair. His eyes were gray. By occupation he was a physician.[7]

1. NA Service Records, CSA, M251, Roll 35.
2. Oglethorpe Medical College, Lists of Graduates. Records preserved by Georgia Historical Society, Savannah.
3. U.S. Census, 1860, Putnam County, Florida, p. 84. Dr. Butler was the sole member of the household. See Tampa *Florida Peninsular*, March 19, 1859.
4. *Soldiers of Fortune*, published by State Board of Institutions, Tallahassee, 1903, pp. 77, 91.
5. Ibid., p. 78.
6. See note 1, supra.
7. Ibid.

Butler, Robert Hays, Leon County, 1813-1873

Dr. Butler, a minor figure in the history of Florida medicine, could hardly have been born under more favorable auspices. His father, Colonel Robert Butler, a Pennsylvania native, had been an early military associate of Andrew Jackson serving under his command in the War of 1812 and in the Seminole campaign of 1818 as adjutant general. His mother was Rachel Hays of Tennessee, niece of Mrs. Andrew Jackson. The Colonel had been appointed commissioner to relieve St. Augustine of its dependencies in East Florida from the hands of the Spanish in the summer of 1821 and to occupy the town until further dispensations should be made. Having discharged these responsibilities he returned to Tennessee. In 1824 he returned with his family to Florida to assume the office of surveyor-general of the Florida Territory.[1]

Upon his arrival in Tallahassee to assume his office, Colonel Butler took full advantage of the opportunity to acquire valuable property at low cost. He purchased lots in the town, but more important large acreage on the southwest shores of Lake Jackson which with the help of his gifted wife he developed into a plantation renowned for its beauty. There with half a hundred slaves, the family is said to have lived in "baronial splendor." There also young Robert Hays spent the formative years of his youth.

Robert Butler's older brother, Thomas, after an apprenticeship in 1834 under Dr. John McLemore of Tallahassee, entered the newly-organized Medical College of the State of South Carolina[2] (formed as a protest against the South Carolina Medical Society's rigid control of the hiring and firing of professors in the older Medical College of South Carolina). He died before the term ended in 1835. In the fall of 1835 Robert Hays entered the new college,[3] remaining there for a full term. He had also studied under the preceptorate of Dr. McLemore. For reasons unknown he did not return for the second term, but instead returned to his home on Lake Jackson where, it is thought he remained for the greater part of his life.

Practically nothing is known of Dr. Butler's medical practice. In the absence of evidence one hesitates to suggest that he was without ambition. Surely the death of his brother, four years his senior, had been a crushing blow. It is a reasonable assumption that his father, who retained his position as surveyor-general until 1845, and whose duties demanded frequent and lengthy absences from home, had little time for managing a large plantation, leaving that responsibility on the shoulders of his only surviving son, Robert Hays.

The Butler household in 1850[4] included not only the aging parents, both 63, but also the eldest daughter, Sarah Jane, and her husband, Alexander Patton, and two children, Robert and Rachel, in addition to the second Butler daughter, Ellen Mary, and her husband, James Henry Hawkins, and two unmarried sisters, Eliza and Rachel. Ten years later, his father having died on January 13, 1860, Dr. Butler assumed headship of the family with an estate valued upwards of $100,000 and 55 slaves.[5] Obviously his burdens were not light. Still he is said to have continued the practice of medicine though on a limited scale. In a paper read in March 1939, Dr. Henry E. Palmer wrote: "Dr. Robert Butler, son of Robert Butler, first surveyor-general of Florida, was. . .a practicing physician at Lake Jackson about 1851."[6] In his only known venture into politics he was one of six Leon County physicians chosen to represent the County in the State Democratic Convention to be held in Tallahassee on April 9, 1860.[7]

Of Dr. Butler's later years very little is known. When the Civil War began in 1861 he was 46 years old; therefore military service was not required of him. At about that time he was married to Lula Parham. They had one daughter, Lula, on February 12, 1862 in Tallahassee.[8] It may be assumed that war and reconstruction brought disruption and ultimate disaster to the Butler Plantation. Dr. Palmer could only remark: "Dr. Butler is said to have moved to Bainbridge, Georgia, after the Civil War."[9] However, an examination of the Decatur (Ga.) Census of 1870 does not reveal his presence in Bainbridge. Family history provides the date of his death as October 12, 1873. Of his widow and child nothing has been learned.

Before the end of the 19th century the Butler lands on Lake Jackson had passed out of the family's hands. In the early part of the 20th century they were owned by the Florida Planting Company, headed by A.P. McCaskill. In 1911 a portion of the property was purchased for Florida Pecan Development Company.[10]

1. TP XXII, 32n.
2. List of Matriculants and Graduates, MCSSC, Waring Historical Library, Medical University of South Carolina, Charleston.
3. Ibid.
4. U.S. Census, 1850, Leon County, Florida, p. 106, item 205. A genealogical table of the Butler Family is found in *The Butler Family in America*, William David Butler, John Cromwell Butler, and Joseph Marion Butler, compilers, St. Louis, Shallcross Printing Co., 1913, pp. 221-227. Assistance in gaining access to this material from Mrs. Winifred Shine Frysel, great, great granddaughter of Col. Robert Butler, and Mrs. T.O. Bruce, both of Key West is greatly acknowledged.
5. U.S. Census, 1860, Leon County, Florida, p. 43, item 125.
6. Henry E. Palmer, Physicians in Early Tallahassee and Vicinity, *Apalachee*, Tallahassee, 1944, p. 36.
7. Tallahassee *Floridian and Journal*, March 24, 1860. In the newspaper account of the meeting in Tallahassee on April 9 there is no indication that Dr. Butler actually attended.
8. See *Butler Family*, p. 227.
9. See note 6 supra.
10. Clifton Paisley, From Cotton to Quail, *An Agricultural Chronicle* of Leon County Florida, 1860-1967, Gainesville, 1968, pp. 5, 9, 67, 69.

Butler, Thomas P., Leon County, 1809-1835

Thomas P. Butler, eldest son of Colonel Robert Butler, early Leon County settler and from 1824 to 1848 surveyor-general of Florida by appointment from President Andrew Jackson, was born in Tennessee in 1809. His mother was Rachel Hays, niece of Mrs. Andrew Jackson. He read medicine in Tallahassee under the direction of Dr. John McLemore and in 1834 matriculated at the Medical College of South Carolina, Charleston.[1] He died in Charleston on January 30, 1835, before completing his first term as a student.[2]

1. List of Matriculants, MCSC, Waring Historical Library, MUSC, Charleston, South Carolina.
2. *The Butler Family in America*, William David Butler, John Cromwell Butler and Joseph Marion Butler compilers, St. Louis, Shallcross Printing Company, 1913, p. 226.

Butt, Zephaniah, Levy and Marion Counties, 1812-1883

Dr. Butt or Dr. "Ze" Butt as he was familiarly known was a native of New Jersey. He attended the Jefferson Medical College, Philadelphia, from which he was graduated in the spring of 1841.[1] Of the years following his graduation very little is known beyond the fact that he practiced medicine in Philadelphia "and other large cities of the United States."[2] He moved to Florida a few years prior to the Civil War establishing himself on Atsena Otie, one of the larger islands of the Cedar Key group. The Census of 1860 lists him as 48 years of age, a resident in the household of Street Thompson.

Due in large measure to the efforts and faith of two men, Augustus Steele and David L. Yulee, the commercial potential of Cedar Key was beginning to be realized during the 1850s. The prevailing wisdom of Steele, jurist and newspaper editor, brought a measure of stability to the little community while the dream of Yulee, builder of the Fernandina-to-Cedar Key railroad, encouraged a number of people to settle there. Among them was Dr. Butt who is said to have invested heavily in the lumber business. According to a contemporary account he also built a costly residence "surrounded with choice fruits and flowers." But with the capture of Atsena Otie by Federal troops early in 1862 he lost his entire investment.[3] In the meantime he continuned to carry on his medical practice, albeit without authorization of a proper license to practice.[4]

Somewhat discouraged by the turn of fate Dr. Butt moved to Ocala where he soon achieved a good reputation as a physician. F.E. Harris, editor of the Ocala newspaper, wrote of him: "Dr. Butt is the oldest practitioner in the vicinity and has long earned the reputation that places him at the top of his profession. . . He has been eminently successful in his practice in this community."[5]

Notwithstanding the implications of this statement, it would appear that the exigencies of war and reconstruction had not been totally calamitous for Dr. Butt. The Census of 1870 indicates that he was the owner of real property valued at $3,000 and personal property worth $500, while his servants, three blacks and two mulattos, numbered five.[6] His spacious orange groves and flower gardens were one of the scenic attractions of the city.

Too advanced in years for military service Dr. Butt carried on an extensive medical practice in Ocala through the later war years. Among his better-known patients were members of the John Morgandollar Taylor family, erstwhile residents of Sumter District, South Carolina, who migrated to Marion County and bought a plantation some five or six miles southwest of Ocala. Mrs. Taylor, nee Maria Baker, in her diary for the years 1864-67, included many entries relating to Dr. Butt's attendance at the bedside of ailing members of her family. Their faith in his medical skills was apparent.[7]

Dr. Butt entered into a professional partnership in May 1876 with young Dr. Eaton O. Paschall, a recent medical school graduate, who had grown up in Waldo. In announcing the association of the two men the Ocala newspaper remarked: "Dr. Paschall is a young physician and has recently moved to our village. He is studious and energetic and has very high testimonials as to his proficiency in his profession."[8] The arrangement lasted for about two years after which Dr. Paschall returned to Waldo to practice there.

Dr. Butt's concern for the advancement of the medical profession is indicated by his leadership in the founding of the Marion County Medical Society in February 1873 when he presided over the organizational meeting.[9] Although he never became a member of the State Association, which was founded the following year, it is certain that he had its best interests at heart.

Very little is known of the private life of Dr. Butt. His wife, Annie, was a native of Delaware and some 10 years his junior.[10] They were members of the Episcopalian Church. Dr. Butt died in Ocala in November 1883.[11]

1. General Alumni Catalogue of Jefferson Medical College, Philadelphia 1917, p. 69. Pennsylvania is here listed as the state of his residence, although he is known to have been born in New Jersey.

2. Ocala *East Florida Banner*, May 27, 1876.

3. Ibid., May 8, 1875.

4. The enterprising local historian, S.E. Gunnell, while searching the court records of Levy County, discovered the following item dated 1860: "Zephaniah Butt(s) and John W. Beonton were indicted for practicing medicine without a license. Witnesses were E.M. Graham and Simeon Edwards. W.M. Rogers was city marshall at Atsena Otie." *Search for Yesterday, A History of Levy County*, Bronson, Levy County, Archives Committee, 1977, chap. 6, p. 3.

5. See note 3.

6. U.S. Census, 1870, Marion County, Florida, p. 203.

7. The Diary of Maria Baker Taylor, January 1864-December 1867, Typescript copy, P.K. Yonge Library of Florida History, MSS, Box 26.

8. See Note 3.

9. Jacksonville *Florida Republican*, February 5, 1873.

10. U.S. Census, 1880, Marion County, Florida, p. 14, item 176.
11. Tallahassee *Weekly Floridian*, November 6, 1883.

Bynum, William Forsyth, Lafayette and Suwannee Counties, 1832-1904

Dr. Bynum, physician and public servant, was born in North Carolina in 1832.[1] Of his education and medical training nothing is known. He appears to have begun his medical practice in Georgia in the mid-1850s where he was married and his two older children, Forsyth and Troup, were born. About 1859 he moved to Florida settling first in the village of New Boston which lay on the Suwannee County side of the Suwannee River some five miles upstream from Branford.

With the outbreak of war in 1861, Dr. Bynum volunteered for service in the Confederate Army and was assigned to Company E, 4th Florida Infantry Regiment, with the rank of First Lieutenant. His company was known as the "La Fayette Rangers." His various assignments included Ft. Brooke (at Tampa Bay), Chattanooga, Tennessee, and Manatee County, Florida. He was overcome by illness in August 1862, took sick leave, and upon the advice and recommendation of two army physicians, Drs. J.H. Randolph and I. Dubose, members of the Board of Medical Examiners of the Florida District, he tendered his resignation which was accepted by the Office of the Adjutant General effective January 8, 1863.[2]

Prior to the War Dr. Bynum had been elected Assistant Clerk of the Florida House of Representatives for its 1860 session.[3] For the session of 1864 he was unopposed for the position and for a total of 15 subsequent sessions he was to serve in this capacity, his last being the session of 1903 only a year prior to his death.[4]

At some unknown date the Bynum family moved into Live Oak. The Census of 1870 lists him as a resident of the town with the occupation of druggist. It is evident that he prospered in spite of the hardships of war and reconstruction. In 1860 his real estate was valued at $1,000, in 1870 at $10,000.

Dr. Bynum died in Live Oak in 1904. He was buried in Antioch Cemetery some five miles north of Live Oak.[5]

1. It is fairly certain that Dr. Bynum was a native of Chatham County, North Carolina, where the Bynum family was one of prominence. A village called Bynum with a population of some 300 still exists.
2. The information relating to Dr. Bynum's military career is found in NA Service Records, CSA, Microcopy 251, Roll 53.
3. *Journal of the Proceedings of the House of Representatives of the General Assembly Florida*, Tenth Session, November 26, 1860, Tallahassee, 1861, p. 5.
4. Allen Morris, *The People of Lawmaking in Florida*, Tallahassee, 1977, unpaginated.
5. The dates of Dr. Bynum's birth and death as well as his burial place are found in WPA Project, Veterans Graves Registration, Florida, Suwannee County, No. 61, p. 11.

Byrd, Edward C., Monticello, 1839

In 1839, Dr. Edward Caldwell Byrd, a surgeon and dentist who had practiced for 10 years in New York City, moved to Monticello. It is obvious that he had made the move for reasons of health. He seemed to be developing a sound practice until his untimely death in 1841.[1]

1. This entry is taken almost verbatim from Jerrell H. Shofner, *History of Jefferson County, Florida*, p. 61.

Byrd, Flavius Augustus, Leon County, 1822-1874

Dr. Byrd was born in Fayetteville, North Carolina, on April 16, 1822.[1] At about age five he was brought to Florida by his parents who obtained land on the west side of Lake Miccosukee where they settled and where Flavius spent his youth. After graduation from the University of Alabama with the A.B. degree he studied medicine at Jefferson Medical College in Philadelphia, where he became Doctor of Medicine.[2] On his return to Florida about 1843 he began practice in the Miccosukee community. In March 1845, however, he moved to Tuscaloosa, Alabama, "partially," he said, "for reason of health."[3] He opened a professional office there two months later. At the end of that summer he returned to Florida on business and for unstated reasons decided to stay. He remained in Miccosukee until his death on December 26, 1874, a victim of pneumonia.[4]

Dr. Byrd was married on March 3, 1853, to Catherine D. Lloyd of Leon County, a union to which two sons and three daughters were born.[5]

Although he was never a man of more than modest means Dr. Byrd was a highly esteemed citizen and a trusted physician. Politically he allied himself with the Democratic Party. In July 1846, as one of Leon County's delegates to the state Democratic Covention, he emerged as a party leader serving on at least two important committees.[6] Two years later he was his party's nominee for the House of Representatives, losing along with other Loco-Focos, as they were still derisively designated by their Whig opponents, in the Whig sweep in Leon County.[7]

Dr. Byrd was a popular man in the Miccosukee area. His death notice included the following eulogy: ". . .in his death that neighborhood loses a most excellent man. He stood high in his profession and was esteemed by a wide circle of friends. He will be sadly missed by the people of the country, but mournfully so by his large family to whom he was very dear and who were dependent upon him for support."[8] The level of his learning as well as his literary skill are demonstrated in a nine-page article on general conditions in Leon County in 1873, a discourse on the economy, growth, society, and health published in 1875.[9]

Dr. Byrd was an active member of the Masonic Order and the Methodist Church. He was buried in Tallahassee following a funeral service at the Tallahassee Methodist Church.[10]

1. Henry E. Palmer, Physicians of Early Tallahassee and Vicinity, *Apalachee*, 1944, p. 41.
2. Ibid.
3. This brief segment of his career was revealed by Dr. Byrd himself in response to Whig claims that he was ineligible to run for the Florida House of Representatives because he had lost his Leon County citizenship by his brief residence in Tuscaloosa. Tallahassee *Southern Journal*, September 1, 1846. He declined the nomination but made it clear that he had no doubts as to his eligibility to run for office.
4. Tallahassee *Weekly Floridian*, December 29, 1874.
5. DAR, Records Survey, Leon County, Florida, 1937, p. 70, U.S. Census, 1870, Leon County, Florida, p. 794, lists the Byrd children as William, age 12; Thomas, age 10; Eliza, age five; Fanny, age three; Lina, age seven months. Mrs. Byrd was born on July 27, 1820 in Flatbush, Long Island, and died in Tallahassee on October 28, 1874.
6. Tallahassee *Floridian*, July 25, 1846.
7. Ibid., August 19, 1848. For tabulated results of that election see Ibid, October 7, 1848.
8. See note 4 supra.
9. *Journal Proceedings of the Assembly of the State of Florida*, Tallahassee, 1875, 8th Session, 1875, Appendix, pp. 55-64.
10. See note 4 supra.

Byrne, Bernard Myles, East Florida, 1806-1860

Dr. Byrne, who spent the greater part of his professional life as a military surgeon, was born in Wicklow, Ireland, about 1806.[1] When still a small child he was brought to America by his family who settled in Baltimore, Maryland. There he received a classical education and served an apprenticeship preparatory to entering the University of Maryland School of Medicine from which he was graduated with highest honors in 1828. In recognition of the excellence of his doctoral thesis, which incidentally was written in Latin, he was awarded the gold medal.[2] Immediately after receiving his medical degree he was employed as Prosector to the Professor of Anatomy at Washington University School of Medicine in Baltimore[3] where it is said he acquired the accurate anatomical knowledge which enabled him to pass with distinction the severe examination required of applicants for admission into the medical staff of the United States Army.[4]

Meanwhile Dr. Byrne had entered medical practice in Baltimore. He was commissioned Assistant Surgeon in the Army on May 20, 1836,[5] and assigned to Ft. Monroe at Old Point Comfort near Hampton Roads, Virginia. Within a few weeks, however, he was transferred to Florida where the Second Seminole War was under way. For the next seven years he was to spend the greater part of his time in Florida serving four of those years "in the field" as he later stated in the preface to a series of articles describing his experiences and observations there.[6] The St. Augustine newspaper reported occasional glimpses of him as, for example, on November 3, 1837, when it noted that he had been assigned to duty "in the field" with the Second Dragoons and a few months later when he sailed out of St. Augustine aboard the Schooner *Medium* "for a leave of absence."[7]

A man of superior intellect and keenness of observation, Dr. Byrne undertook to record his views of the Florida scene as he moved with troops throughout much of East Florida. His notes formed the substance of a series of nine articles signed "A Physician" which were accepted for publication by the *National Intelligencer*.[8] Dr. Byrne strongly felt that Florida had been much maligned by several writer-visitors who had found its climate insalubrious and its soil unproductive. Such unfavorable publicity he blamed on military personnel who were there "to deal with the Indians and who saw little, if any, of the productiveness potential." He concluded the preface to the series with the following:

> I shall simply state the fact that in the early part of the War it was a common expression among them that the whole Peninsula was not worth the medicine it would cost to conquer it, meaning thus to imply in one pithy sentence both the insalubrity and sterility of the soil.

Dr. Byrne was transferred to Texas in 1846 where preparations for the war with Mexico were well along. There he was assigned as surgeon to an artillery battery under the command of the heroic Major Samuel Ringgold who like Dr. Byrne was a veteran of the Florida conflict. As medical officer he found himself in the thick of the battle on May 5 when Ringgold fell mortally wounded. It is recorded that he bore the stricken officer off the field and attended him until his death three days later. Dr. Byrne continued with the troops at the battles of Monterey, Saltillo and Buena Vista.[9]

Dr. Byrne was soon to be involved in the western phase of the war which took him to the Pacific, presumably under the command of Col. Stephen W. Kearny. At the conclusion of the War in early 1848 he returned to Florida where his assignments appear to have allowed him freedom to move about and leisure for his writing.[10] He was promoted to the rank of surgeon on March 31, 1853.[11] Meanwhile, on November 18, 1851, he was married to Louisa, daughter of Col. J.J. Abert, Chief of Topographical Engineers, U.S. Army, the wedding having taken place in Washington.[12]

During this phase of his career Dr. Byrne found more time for writing. He revised the Florida series in 1851 which had appeared in the *National Intelligencer*, offering them to Dr. Charles Byrne, editor of the Jacksonville *News*, who published them between April 20 and June 8, 1851.[13] These revisions reveal a greater range of knowledge and experience than earlier versions.

In 1857 Dr. Byrne became post surgeon at Ft. Moultrie, Sullivan's Island in Charleston Harbor, certainly one of the more desirable assignments. He apparently established a cordial relationship with the medical fraternity in Charleston. What was no doubt a pleasant tour of duty was marred in early 1858 by charges preferred against him by his young colleague, Assistant Surgeon William J. L'Engle, who accused him of deserting his post during a fever epidemic, leaving Dr. L'Engle to cope with the situation alone. Trial by a court martial was arranged, the court itself being composed of a distinguished panel of army officers headed by General Stephen Churchill and including several officers with whom Dr. Byrne had served in Florida and Texas.[14]

Dr. Byrne's defense was built principally on the facts of his own illness and that of his wife, who lay near death of yellow fever at the time in question. It was a brilliant and cogent statement prepared by Dr. Byrne himself and read before the court by his attorney, William E. Martin, a Charleston lawyer. The trial had begun on March 26, 1859 and was concluded with the defense statement on April 15. Dr. Byrne was readily acquitted by the court apparently to the immense satisfaction of the majority of those present including representatives of the press.[15]

Dr. Byrne died at Ft. Moultrie on September 6, 1860, a victim of a virulent type of typhoid fever. He was survived by his widow and three small children.

1. Sources are in disagreement as to the date of Dr. Byrne's birth. The Charleston *Courier* in its obituary notice of September 8, 1860, states that he died in his 46th year while the Charleston *Mercury* of the same date claimed that he was in his 48th year. Since he received his medical degree in 1828 the latter date appears to be more acceptable. Both appear incorrect, however.

2. Eugene F. Cordell, *Historical Sketch of the University of Maryland School of Medicine*, 1807-1890, Baltimore, 1801, pp. 162, 212.

3. The prosector's duty was to prepare dissections for anatomical demonstrations. The Washington University School of Medicine existed from 1827 till 1877 except for the years 1852-1867. It was during this time that Dr. Byrne wrote a treatise on cholera, *An Essay to Prove the Contagious Character of Malignant Cholera With Brief Instructions for its Prevention and Cure*, Baltimore & Philadelphia, 1833, 156 pp. This was considered a veritable textbook on the subject and widely used.

4. *Charleston Mercury*, September 8, 1860.

5. Harvey E. Brown, comp., *The Medical Department of the Army from 1775 to 1873*, Washington, Surgeon General's Office, 1873, p. 292.

6. Jacksonville *News*, April 20, 1851.

7. St. Augustine *News*, November 3, 1838, ibid., July 13, 1839.

8. *National Intelligencer* periodically between May 1 and December 2, 1843. These articles elicited immediate refutations from a reader who signed himself "Physician Second" in a series of letters published in ibid between May 18 and December 25, 1843. A casual reading of these items convinces one that both "Physician" and "Physician Second" overstated their convictions.

9. Charleston *Courier*, September 8, 1860.

10. Random notices in the newspapers of St. Augustine and Jacksonville between 1849 and 1853 indicate Dr. Byrne's occasional presence in Florida. The latest of these, Jacksonville *Florida News*, May 7, 1853, stated, Col. W.W. Loring and Dr. B.M. Byrne, of the U.S. Army, passed up the river on Wednesday (May 4th) in the *Florida* for St. Augustine.

12. Jacksonville *News*, December 6, 1831. The marriage was an event of November 18 in Washington.

13. The two Doctors Byrne were closely related, probably brothers, but the precise relationship has not been estblished.

14. Charleston *Mercury*, April 19, 1859. Officers serving on the court martial were Capt. Sam Jones, Major Wm. A. Nichols, Col. Crittenden (son of famous Kentucky Senator John J. Crittenden), Col. Edward J. Steptoe, Col. W.H.J. Walker, Col. Daniel J. Chandler, Col. Justin Dimmick, Col. Carlos A. Waite, Col. Charles A. May and General Stephen Churchill.

15. Both the *Mercury* and the *Courier* were represented among the spectators. On April 22, 1860 the *Mercury* published an extra edition giving the full text of the Byrne defense.

Byrne, Charles, St. Augustine, 1803-1853

Dr. Byrne, a man of exceptional intelligence and ability, was one of the more eminent physicians to practice in Florida in the 19th century. His interests were varied. As a writer and journalist he was courageous and perceptive; as a politician, fearless, and as a physician, knowledgeable and skillful. His death at the age of 50 was untimely, depriving the Jacksonville community in which he abided at the time of one of its most enlightened citizens.

Dr. Byrne was born in Wicklow, Ireland in 1803.[1] At the age of 13 he was brought to America by his family settling in Baltimore, Maryland, where he began preparation for a career in medicine. He was graduated from the Medical School of the University of Maryland in Baltimore in February 1825,[2] and soon thereafter entered medical practice in Baltimore. A short time later he was married to an estimable lady by whom he had three children.[3] After the death of his wife in 1838 he left Baltimore for St. Augustine where on November 29, 1838 he announced the opening of his practice from an office in Florida House.[4]

Dr. Byrne emerged into the public life of St. Augustine through his appointment in August 1839 to the post of Port Physician by the City Council.[5] In this capacity he appears to have vigorously enforced the quarantine laws of the City.[6] He held the position until July 1841 when he was replaced by S.F. Jones. Almost immediately an altercation developed when Jones reported to the City Council that he had discovered two cases of fever aboard steamers in the harbor, cases which had been "grossly perverted and exaggerated," presumably by his predecessor.[7] Dr. Byrne responded with a scorching denunciation of Jones' slipshod diagnostic methods, saying the Jones examinations were perfunctory at best.[8]

Soon thereafter Dr. Byrne purchased a farm and orange grove on the St. Johns River near the mouth of Julington Creek, about two miles from the Mandarin post office. To the place he gave the name Wicklow. There he appears to have permitted himself a fairly tranquil existence with his family which had arrived from Maryland in the meantime. Although he was not a political activist he was a declared supporter of Whig principles and a keen observer of political developments. He was outraged in 1844 to receive from a Pennsylvania acquaintance a copy of a recently launched Philadelphia newspaper, *The Native American*, a jingoistic journal antiforeign as well as antipapist in tone and policy.[9] His response published in the St. Augustine newspaper is an eloquent condemnation of the *Native American* and its sponsors, followed by his own definition of true Americanism. He concluded: "I am and have been a Whig but if your statement has the endorsement of the Whig Party, I shall immediately become a Democrat."[10] A short time later he switched to the Democratic party.

Dr. Byrne moved into Jacksonville in 1848 and resumed full-time medical practice. Already well-known in the city he was cordially accepted as a member of its medical faculty and joined the eminent Dr. Abel S. Baldwin as a partner.[11] Although he continued medical practice it was somewhat overshadowed by other interests and pursuits. Early in 1849 in the waning days of President Polk's term of office Dr. Byrne, then a staunch Democrat, received appointment as Collector of Customs, Port of Jacksonville, only to be removed soon after inauguration of Zachary Taylor, a Whig. This event provoked a lengthy editorial in the Jacksonville *Florida Republican* on the evils inherent in the "Spoils System."[12]

With achievement of statehood in 1845 East Floridians were more than ever aware of the inaccessibility of the capital in Tallahassee. In late 1850 a group of Jacksonville citizens met for the purpose of promoting the building of a plant road connecting Jacksonville with Alligator (Lake City). Dr. Byrne was present and addressed the group.[13] About a year and a half later he was chairman of a meeting in the Duval County Courthouse called to arrange for the sale of stock in the enterprise.[14] In addition to such interests he was active in the local affairs of the Democratic Party having been chosen as an East Florida delegate to the party's national convention in Baltimore in 1852.[15]

Not to be overlooked is Dr. Byrne's venture into the newspaper business. He purchased the Jacksonville *News* in early 1851 from its retiring owner and editor, Augustus C. Gillett. The first issue under his new management was that of April 19, 1851, which carried the information that its editor would be Felix Livingston, a Jacksonville attorney and sometime Judge of the County Probate Court. The paper was, of course, the local voice of the Democratic Party, standing in opposition to the Jacksonville *Florida Republican*, the voice of the Whigs, edited by the capable Columbus Drew. For almost two years the people of Jacksonville enjoyed the luxury of two newspapers of opposing points of view, each edited by a man of superior intelligence and editorial skill. In spite of their differences they respected each other and remained friends.

Death came suddenly for Dr. Byrne who suffered a cerebral hemorrhage while enroute to Charleston aboard the *Carolina*.[16] Physicians among the passengers made every effort to revive him, but to no avail. On arrival in Charleston the ship's captain turned his body over to a local priest under whose direction his corpse was prepared for shipment to Jacksonville. On arrival in the city it was moved to St. Patrick's Cathedral for the funeral. He was buried in the Old City Cemetery.

Among the many tributes paid Dr. Byrne, none was more fitting than that of Columbus Drew who wrote: "In the death of Dr. Byrne, an aged surviving mother has lost a devoted son, a fraternal circle a devoted brother and several children a kind parent. He was a man of generous feelings and social disposition. He was valued as one among the best medical practitioners in this part of the State."[17]

1. Jacksonville *Florida News*, March 12, 1853.

2. Eugene F. Cordell, *Historical Sketch of the University of Maryland School of Medicine*, 1807-1890, Baltimore 1891, p. 166. See Webster Merritt *A Century of Medicine in Jacksonville and Duval County*, Gainesville 1949, pp. 20-21, photographs of his medical certificate and his portrait.

3. See note 1, supra.
4. St. Augustine *News*, November 29, 1838. On his visit to St. Augustine in 1838, Dr. Benjamin B. Strobel of Charleston, who was preparing a treatise on Yellow Fever, consulted with Dr. Byrne concerning his observations on the disease during his residence in the town. Dr. Byrne's opinions on the subject are to be found in B.B. Strobel *An Essay on the Subject of the Yellow Fever Intended to Prove its Transmissibility*, Charleston, Asa J. Muir, 1840, pp. 165-66.
5. St. Augustine *News*, August 30, 1839.
6. St. Augustine *Herald* and *Southern Democrat*, October 31, 1839.
7. Ibid., July 23, 1841.
8. Ibid., July 30, 1841.
9. *The Native American* had only a brief existence, first appearing in April 1844, and expiring before the end of the year.
10. St. Augustine *Florida News* and *Southern Democrat*, October 1, 1844.
11. In the Jacksonville *Florida Republican*, February 8, 1849, appeared a report of a postmortem examination performed by Drs. Byrne and Baldwin on a slave who had suffocated from a piece of beef lodged in his throat. In another instance Dr. Byrne announced receipt of a fresh supply of smallpox vaccine with which he was prepared to vaccinate, Jacksonville *Florida News*, August 26, 1852.
12. Jacksonville *Florida Republican*, May 3, 1849. The editor was Columbus Drew, a man of fine intellect.
13. Ibid., November 7, 1850.
14. Jacksonville *Florida News*, January 15, 1853.
15. Tallahassee *Floridian and Journal*, May 22, 1853.
16. His death occurred on March 1, 1853. See Jacksonville *Florida News*, March 12, 1853.
17. Ibid., a reprint from the Jacksonville *Florida Republican*.

Byrne, Charles C., St. Johns and Duval Counties, 1837

Only brief notice is taken of the career of Dr. Byrne, son of Dr. Charles Byrne, distinguished physician and newspaper editor. He was born in Baltimore, Maryland in 1837 and was brought to Florida the following year. His youth was spent first in St. Augustine, later at his father's country place near Mandarin and finally in Jacksonville.[1] He attended the Medical School of the University of Maryland from which he was graduated in 1859.[2] He was commissioned Assistant Surgeon in the United States Army on June 23, 1860.[3] After serving throughout the Civil War in the Medical Department of the Union Army, he was promoted to Surgeon effective July 28, 1866, and on December 4, 1893, became Assistant Surgeon General, a post he held until his retirement on May 7, 1901.[4] The date of his death has not been determined.

1. See sketch of Dr. Charles Byrne.
2. Eugene F. Cordell, *The University of Maryland School of Medicine 1807-1890*, Baltimore 1891, p. 166.
3. Francis B. Heitman, *Historical Register and Dictionary of the United States Army, 1789-1903*, 2 vols., Washington, Government Printing Office, 1903, p. 271.
4. Ibid.

Byron, Edward L., Quincy, 1850

The 1850 Census of Gadsden County includes the following entry: "Byron, Edward L., 35, physician, born in Virginia." He was a resident in the household of Jacob Bradwell, a resident of Quincy, whose occupation was "farmer." In addition to the Bradwell family, which included Mrs. Bradwell and five children, there were seven other residents in the house including Samuel Love, Sheriff of the County. No further information concerning Dr. Byron has been discovered which suggests that his sojourn in Florida was brief.[1]

1. U.S. Census, 1850, Gadsden County, Florida, p. 342.

Bythewood, Joseph Fickling, Madison County, 1822-1890

Dr. Bythewood, son of Benjamin F. and Sarah Bythewood, was born in Beaufort County, South Carolina, November 12, 1819.[1] He began medical studies under the preceptorate of two Beaufort physicians, Dr. Thomas Fuller and his son, Dr. Henry Fuller.[2] He entered the Medical College of the State of South Carolina in 1841 from which he received his medical degree in the spring of 1843 having submitted a thesis entitled "Quinine."[3] He subsequently returned to Beaufort where for a few years he practiced medicine, living in the home of his parents.[4]

Meanwhile Dr. Bythewood's sister, Isabel, had married Eldred James Simkins, who with their three children, Martha Isabel, William Stuart and Eldred James Jr., had moved to Florida and purchased a plantation in the western part of Madison County on the Aucilla River.[5] About 1850 Dr. Bythewood was indued to move to Florida and assume management of the Simkins property. Simkins had died at a fairly early age. Dr. Bythewood also bought property nearby in the Sandy Ford (later Greenville) community and soon became a well-to-do plantation master and physician.[6] Being unmarried he also assumed the responsibility for his niece and nephews. When the boys became of age he transferred them to his portion of land, estimated at about 1,250 acres, a transaction of September 1, 1865.[7] The Simkins plantation was known as Blythe Wood.

Although Dr. Bythewood was never married he was seldom the lone occupant of his household. His mother and father spent their last years with him, the former alive in 1870 at the age of 76. Then there were other nieces, nephews and kin.[8]

Living as he did in the comparative obscurity of the country town of Greenville very few of Dr. Bythewood's professional and social activities are matters of record. Scattered evidence, however, clearly indicates that he was a trusted and popular physician. The mortality schedules of Madison County for the year 1884-85 indicate that his services were much in demand. About 1880 he joined Dr. Henry J. Parramore in a professional partnership in the town of Greenville, an association which endured for only two or three years. Their professional card, published in 1882, assured the public that "in case of necessity the attention of both will be given without extra charge."[9] In the same issue of the newspaper it was stated that Dr. Bythewood had gone to Texas to attend a nephew who was reported to be very ill. Extant Florida Gazetteers for the years 1884-87 list him as physician and landowner of Greenville. In January 1889 he was called to assist Dr. A.M.R. Sessions in repairing the damage done to the hand of a Negro laborer, Clem Perry, in a cotton gin accident.[10] Finally there was a social note: Mr. and Mrs. P.S. Coggins, Mr. and Mrs. J.W. Smith, Dr. Bythewood, and Mrs. A.J. Dozier are in New Orleans attending Mardi Gras."

Dr. Bythewood died on June 2, 1892. He was buried in Roseland Cemetery, Monticello, where his mother had also been buried.

1. The dates of Dr. Bythewood's birth and death are found on his gravestone in Roseland Cemetery, Monticello. He was the grandson of Daniel Bythewood, a well-known sea captain who, in his later years, commanded a schooner plying the waters between Charleston and Beaufort, South Carolina. See "The Autobiography of William John Grayson," Samuel G. Stoney, ed., *South.*

2. Archives, Matriculants and Preceptors, Medical College of the State of South Carolina, Waring Historical Medical Library, Charleston.

3. Ibid., See Charleston *Mercury*, March 18, 1843.

4. U.S. Census, 1850, Beaufort Dist., S.C., p. 9. Both Drs. Fuller are listed in ibid, loc cit.

5. Terry B. Zeigler: "A Madison County Plantation, 1865-1900." Typed MS, P.K. Yonge Library of Florida History.

6. Ibid.

7. Ibid.

8. U.S. Census 1870 and 1880, Madison County, Florida.

9. Madison *Recorder*, November 4, 1882.

10. Ibid., January 25, 1889.

11. Ibid., March 8, 1889.

Cadwell, Edward C., Monticello, 1841

The Florida career of Dr. Cadwell was brief. He was a native of New York State and is known to have practiced for several years in New York City prior to moving to Monticello, Jefferson County, about 1839. Shofner states that Dr. Cadwell "had practiced for ten years in New York City...where he seemed to be developing a sound practice until this untimely death in 1841..."[1] The Jefferson County Census of 1840 gives his age at between 30 and 40. Mrs. Cadwell was about the same age. Their only child, a daughter, was under five years of age. The Cadwells owned 11 slaves.[2] After her husband's death Mrs. Cadwell is presumed to have returned to New York.

1. Jerrell H. Shofner, *History of Jefferson County,* Tallahassee, Sentry Press, 1976, p. 61.
2. U.S. Census, Jefferson County, 1840, p. 44.

Caldwell, Andrew C., Seminole County, 1821-1895

Dr. Caldwell was born in Greensboro, North Carolina, in 1821. In the fall of 1846 he matriculated at the Medical College of the State of South Carolina, Charleston, from which he was graduated in March 1848,[1] having submitted a thesis entitled "Prophylactic Treatment of Hydrophobia." Immediately thereafter he returned to Greensboro where he launched his practice and where he married Julia. The couple continued to reside in Greensboro for several years. The first six of their eight children, Sallie, David, Charles, Anne, Letitia and Andrew, were born there. The two youngest, Alice and Ernest, were born in Sanford.

In 1867 Dr. Caldwell became concerned about his deteriorating health.[2] After some hesitation he decided to move to Florida, which by then had become a retreat for people suffering from a variety of ailments, especially pulmonary problems. He chose to settle at Fort Read, at that time located in Orange County but later to lie within the borders of Seminole County, on the shore of Lake Monroe. He is said to have had no intention of returning to the practice of medicine but, according to one account, "was forced to practice because he was the only physician in that part of the State."[3]

Dr. Caldwell, being an educated man, which could not be said of most settlers in the area, soon found himself drawn into local politics and civic affairs of Orange County. At a meeting of citizens of the county at the Court House on December 11, 1869, assembled for the purpose of organizing a Board of Public Instruction, he responded to pressure and accepted membership on the Board.[4] The other members were W.C. Roper and Zelotes A. Mason, the latter also a physician.

Dr. Caldwell's arrival in Orange County coincided with the arrival of General Henry S. Sanford, a man of considerable means, who purchased more than 12,000 acres and began the cultivation of oranges which resulted in a period of prosperity for the area. Dr. Caldwell was most certainly a beneficiary of this development. He died at his home in Sanford in 1895 and was buried in Lake View Cemetery.

1. Charleston *Courier,* March 23, 1848. The graduating class of 1848 was one of the largest ever, 78 degree recipients.
2. Sources relating to the early settlement of the Sanford area are by no means plentiful. One invaluable reference is an unpublished "Account of Belair," also of the City of Sanford, with a brief sketch of founder, Sanford, 1889, photocopy,

p. 124, P.K. Yonge Library of Florida History, University of Florida, Gainesville.
3. Ibid.
4. William Fremont Caldwell, *History of Orange County, Florida*, The Mickler House, Chuolota, 1973, p. 49.

Calhoun Jr., John Caldwell, Putnam County, 1823-1855

John C. Calhoun Jr., third son and seventh child of the great South Carolina statesman, spent only the last four years of his life in Florida. He was born in Washington, D.C., on May 17, 1823,[1] and as was true of several of his brothers and sisters he never enjoyed robust health. He suffered a severe illness in the summer of 1826 and for several days lingered between life and death.[2] His youthful years were divided between Georgetown, D.C., and the family home near Pendleton, South Carolina.

In his earlier years young Calhoun exhibited little interest in or aptitude for learning. He entered the University of Virginia in the spring of 1843[3] but did not return for the following year. From 1844 until 1847 he seems to have drifted rather aimlessly, spending much of his time with his eldest brother, Andrew, but in 1847 he began to show some interest in scientific subjects and enrolled for courses in Charleston. Among these were lectures in medicine. He went to Philadelphia in March 1848 and within a short time had completed requirements for a medical degree, coming home in July of that year with a diploma, an occasion for rejoicing within the family.[4]

In the summer of 1849 Dr. Calhoun was married to Anzie Adams, daughter of the Calhouns' South Carolina neighbor, Mrs. Jasper Adams. She died on September 15, 1850.[5] There were no children.

Before his marriage Dr. Calhoun had become ill with what proved to be consumption. He had gone to Milledgeville, Georgia, to submit to a new "water treatment" which had been much publicized and had learned the technique of administering it. When his father came down with the disease in early 1849, he was able to treat him according to the Milledgeville principles. As Senator Calhoun described it, the process consisted of wrapping the patient in a damp sheet and covering him heavily with blankets, thereby producing a sort of vapor bath. The ultimate effect was only to arrest the disease temporarily for both father and son would eventually succumb.[6]

Later in 1850, Dr. Calhoun, grief-stricken and depressed by failure to throw off the illness, decided to remove to a more benign climate. He was among the guests arriving at the Magnolia Hotel in St. Augustine on December 18, 1850.[7] At about this time the lands of George Kingsley, recently deceased, were offered for sale and among these was Drayton Island near the north outlet of Lake George into the St. Johns River. The island contained approximately 17 acres and a portion of it had been under cultivation for several decades. Groves of oranges, lemon and lime were well-known.[8] Dr. Calhoun bought the island and proceeded to build an imposing home. A visitor in January 1859 described it as "a snug residence. . .for a southern gentleman fond of a retired home."[9]

The mild climate of Anzie Island appeared to favor Dr. Calhoun's health. He took an active interest in building the house as well as producing fruit for the market. The lime and lemon trees were severely damaged by a freeze in the winter of 1851-52, but he reported that the orange trees were undamaged and that he expected a bountiful crop the following year.[10] Beyond such domestic concerns Dr. Calhoun resumed his interest in politics. He was chosen in December 1851 as one of Florida's two representatives at a dinner in New York honoring Louis Kossuth, currently on a visit to America. Dr. Calhoun delivered a speech "on behalf of sundry citizens of Florida."[11] In May 1852 he was appointed secretary of the American legation to either France or Spain but there is no record of his having served in such a post.[12]

Dr. Calhoun was married in a service at the Episcopal Church of St. Augustine on January 27, 1853, to Katherine Kirby Putnam, daughter of socially and politically prominent Benjamin A. Putnam of St. Augustine.[13] According to the Census of 1860 three children were born to this union,[14] but such bliss as may have attended this marriage was of brief duration. The ravages of consumption were once more gnawing away at Calhoun's health by 1855. In the summer it was decided that he should return to Pendleton where the higher altitude might be beneficial. In spite of his weakened condition the journey was undertaken but arriving at Winnsboro, still more than a hundred miles from his destination he was too feeble to go any further and was taken to the residence of Major J.H. Rion, a family friend, where he died on July 31. His body, accompanied by his brother William L. Calhoun and Major Rion, was taken to Ft. Hill, the Calhoun family estate and buried in the family burial ground.[15]

Except for his attendance at the bedside of his father there is no record of Dr. Calhoun's medical practice. It appears unlikely that he ever offered his professional services to the public after his arrival in Florida.

1. Vast literature exists on the Calhoun family. For the purposes of the present sketch only these items were used: Charles M. Wiltse, *John C. Calhoun*, 3 vols., New York, 1944-1951, and A.S. Salley, The Calhoun Family of South Carolina, *The South Carolina Historical and Genealogical Magazine*, Vol. II, No. 3, July 1906, p. 163.

2. Wiltse, op. cit., I, 340-41. Although a namesake of his father, young Calhoun was never known as John C. Calhoun Jr. In family documents he was invariably known as "Johnny."

3. Ibid., III, 435.

4. Ibid., III, 439-40.

5. Ibid., III, 445.

6. Ibid., III, 443.

7. St. Augustine *The Ancient City*, December 21, 1850. After taking stock of available properties, Dr. Calhoun apparently returned briefly to South Carolina. He was among the arrivals at the Jacksonville Hotel on January 21, 1851. Jacksonville *Florida Republican*, January 23, 1851.

8. Ibid.

9. Journal of Dr. D.F. Anderson of Pennsylvania. Photocopy of MS which provides details of his brief sojourn in Florida, 1858-59, P.K. Yonge Library of Florida History.

10. Letter, J.C. Calhoun to Col. J.E. Calhoun, an uncle, Anzie Island, Lake George, June 27, 1852, MS, St. Augustine Historical Society, Calhoun Files.

11. St. Augustine *The Ancient City*, December 27, 1851. The full text of his remarks are here printed.

12. Jacksonville *Florida Republican*, May 12, 1852.

13. This marriage, linking two very prominent families, was widely publicized. Benjamin Alexander Putnam, father of the bride, was one of St. Augustine's most eminent citizens. He had served in both houses of the Florida Legislature, having been Speaker of the House in 1848. He later moved to Palatka, seat of the county which bears his name, where he died on January 25, 1869.

14. The Census of 1860, Putnam County, Item 222, is probably in error. Mrs. Calhoun is listed as a resident in the home of Benj. A. Putnam. The full entry is: K.P. Calhoun (no age given); J.C. Calhoun, aged six, B.A. Calhoun, aged four, and Wm. L. Calhoun, aged two. But if Dr. Calhoun married Miss Putnam on January 27, 1853 and died July 31, 1855, the existence of a third child, aged two in 1860, is impossible. Since Dr. Calhoun's youngest brother, William Lowndes, had died in 1858, a possibility of mistaken identity must be discarded.

15. Jacksonville *Florida Republican*, August 9, 1855.

Call, George W., Tallahassee, 1795-1867

George W. Call, member of the distinguished Leon County family, was born about 1795 near Petersburg, Prince George County, Virginia, son of William and

Helen Walker Call. After the death of her husbnd in 1795 Mrs. Call, doubtless persuaded by her brothers who had previously migrated to Kentucky, bundled up her four sons, Jacob, George, Richard Keith and William, with all their family belongings and made the long trek across the mountains to Nicholasville (Jessamine County), Kentucky. After a brief stop they moved on to Barren River and finally to the home of her brother, David Walker, near Russellville in Logan County. David Walker and his brothers, George, Andrew and Wyeth, were gentlemen of learning and political influence, and their devotion and assistance in the upbringing of their sister's children had much to do with shaping their careers. David Walker donated a small farm in Kentucky to Mrs. Call. His son, David Shelby Walker, later to become governor of Florida, was a youthful companion of the Call brothers.[1]

With the death of their mother in 1810, the Call sons were separated into the homes of their Walker relatives. Young George, lacking a formal education but through his mother's efforts well-grounded in Biblical and classical literature,[2] was accepted for matriculation by the Medical Department of the University of Pennsylvania in 1816. Two years later he was granted a medical degree[3] and returned to Russellville to begin practice. There he would remain for about 18 years. Virtually nothing is known of this segment of his career beyond the fact that, like his brother Richard Keith, he developed great admiration for Andrew Jackson. He wrote Jackson in 1827 urging him to endorse the Henry Clay principles of an "American System," whch included a protective tariff and a program of internal improvements. He concluded with the statement, "I have embarked my political all in your cause."[4]

Dr. Call married Lucinda Lee, daughter of Lt. John Lee of Logan County, about 1821. They had three sons, John L., George Jr., and Wilkinson, usually known as "Wilk," who became a United States senator from Florida. Dr. Call moved with his family to Tallahassee about 1836,[5] joining his brother, Richard, who in that year was appointed Governor of Florida. In addition to his medical practice, which appears to have been extensive, Dr. Call entered vigorously into the political and civic activity of the city and territory. He was elected president of the Tallahasse Temperance Society in 1842 and the following year was named head of the Total Abstinence Society.[6] Disillusioned by what he considered the unsound policies of President Van Buren, Dr. Call abandoned the Democratic Party and threw his support to the Whigs. He presided over the Leon County and Middle District (of Florida) Whig Conventions in 1844.[7]

In the meantime Dr. Call's eldest son, John L., returned to Tallahassee as a fledgling physician and in early 1845[8] joined his father in a medical partnership. This association lasted for only about two years when the younger Dr. Call opened his office in Wakulla County.[9] Very little is known of the elder Dr. Call's activities for the remainder of his life. The sudden death of son, Dr. John L., in Monticello on May 1, 1850, was a shocking event for the entire family but the father's public life does not appear to have been curtailed. In July 1852, for example, Dr. Call and his brother, Richard, were still active in the rapidly disintegrating Whig Party, both serving as delegates from Leon County at the State Whig Convention.[10] Dr. Call was still a practitioner in Tallahassee in 1860.[11] His death occurred, however, not in Leon County but in Putnam County on August 7, 1867. The obituary notice read, "Dr. George W. Call, an old and esteemed citizen of Florida, died at his residence, Orange Mills. . . .[12] No explanation as to when and why he chose to reside in rural Putnam County has come to light.

1. Research on the career of Dr. Call has been negligible. Overshadowed by his brother, Governor Richard Keith Call, and son, Senator Wilkinson Call, he has been generally overlooked. Occasional items appear in biographies of his more famous kinsmen, however. These include Herbert J. Doherty, *Richard Keith Call, Southern Unionist*, Gainesville 1961, and Edward C. Williamson, Wilkinson Call: A Pioneer in Progressive Democracy, unpublished M.A. thesis, University of Florida, 1946. See also Albert H. Roberts, "Wilkinson Call, Soldier and Senator," *Florida Historical Quarterly*, XII, 95. A casual perusal of the Call Papers, Southern Historical Collection, University of North Carolina, Chapel Hill, Library, revealed little information on Dr. Call.
2. Doherty, *Richard Keith Call*, pp. 4, 52, 86, 129, 132, 135, 144, 146; Williamson, "Wilkinson Call," Ch. I.
3. Archives, University of Pennsylvania, Lists of Graduates.
4. Call Papers, Letter, Geo. W. Call to Andrew Jackson, July 11, 1827.
5. This date is undocumented but appears to be a reasonable conjecture.
6. Doherty, *Call*, p. 129.
7. Ibid., p. 132.
8. Tallahassee *Florida Sentinel*, December 26, 1846. This notice, first printed in the issue of April 1, 1845 (not extant), continued through the issue of April 20, 1847.
9. Newport *Gazette*, July 20, 1847.
10. The senior Call was the presiding officer at both conventions. Doherty, *Call*, p. 132.
11. U.S. Census, 1860, Leon County, Florida, p. 20. In this census schedule Dr. Call's age was recorded as 65, that of his wife, 64. Included also are George W. Call Jr., 29, and E.M. (female), 25, probably wife of George W., Jr. Also shown are two boys, William, 12, and John, 10, apparently sons of Dr. John L. Call, deceased, 1850.
12. Gainesville *New Era*, September 7, 1867.

Call, John L., Tallahassee, St. Marks and Monticello, 1823-1850

Dr. Call, eldest son of Dr. George W. and Lucinda (Lee) Call, was born in Logan County, Kentucky, about 1823. When still a youth he was brought to Tallahassee at about the time his uncle, Richard Keith Call, was beginning his first term as governor of the Florida Territory in 1836.[1] After completing his medical education (at an unidentified medical school), young Call returned to Tallahassee where in early 1845 he joined his father in partnership, their office being located near their residence on Monroe Street, "nearly opposite the Episcopal Church."[2] This association continued for approximately two years. In the meantime, on December 17, 1846, John Call was married to Mary Jane Long,[3] a Tennessee native, whose lawyer-brother, Medicus A. Long, had married Ellen Call, the governor's daughter.

Existing records offer no clue as to why the Call partnership was dissolved but by March 1847 young Dr. Call had located "at the Railroad Terminus near St. Marks," and was offering "professional services to citizens of Newport, St. Marks, and Wakulla County generally."[4] He appears to have been cordially received in the coastal community for in September 1847[5] he was elected to the City Council and appointed Health Officer with the responsibility of enforcing the quarantine laws for the busy harbor.[6]

By the early summer of 1848 Dr. Call had left St. Marks and established a practice in the more tranquil town of Monticello in an office over Puleston's Drug Store.[7] Within a matter of a few weeks he had joined Dr. Henry G. Wirt in a professional partnership,[8] an arrangement, however, which continued only briefly. Dr. Wirt, already in poor health from a bronchial ailment, soon retired to the family plantation, Wirtland,[9] where he died on June 26, 1850. Dr. Call, however, had died suddenly some weeks earlier, on May 1, at age 27.[10] His widow and two-year-old son, William, survived.[11]

Thus an untimely death cut short a promising career. There were many indications that Dr. Call was on the threshold of a notable career. He had been a member of the State Medical Board in 1845. In 1848 he was prominently involved in the effort of a group of middle Florida physicians to establish a meaningful state medical association, an effort thwarted at the last minute by a capricious legislature. At the preliminary meeting in Quincy on May 15, 1848, Dr. Call had been chosen secretary pro tem, as well as nominee for the presidency.[12] His role as a leader in a group whose objectives were laudable suggests that he was a young man of good character and intelligence.

Dr. Call was buried with the ceremony of the Masonic Order at the Grove Cemetery in Tallahassee.[13]

1. John L. Call's maternal grandmother, after the death of her husband, William Call, in Virginia, moved to Kentucky with her four sons, Jacob, George, Richard Keith, twice governor of Florida, and William. She was born Helen Meade Walker and her nephew, David S. Walker, was Florida's governor from 1866 to 1868. Dr. Call, perhaps due to an early death and overshadowed by eminent relatives, brother Wilkinson, or "Wilk," was a U.S. Senator and brother George W., Jr., a Confederate hero with the rank of major killed in action in May 1862, has gone unnoticed by historians. It is odd that Ellen Call Long in her book of reminiscences, *Florida Breezes*, makes no mention of Dr. Call, her first cousin, nor his father, Dr. George W. Call, her uncle. Nor does Caroline Mays Brevard, granddaughter of Governor Call, mention either of these physicians in her two-volume *History of Florida*. Dr. Henry E. Palmer in his "Physicians of Early Tallahassee," *Apalachee*, Tallahassee, 1944, devoted four lines to Dr. John Call and slightly more to his father, Dr. George W. Call.

2. Tallahassee *Florida Sentinel*, December 26, 1846. This notice, first printed in the issue of April 1, 1845 (not extant), continued through the issue of April 20, 1847.

3. Ibid., December 22, 1846.

4. Newport *Gazette*, July 20, 1847; first printed March 23, 1847.

5. Ibid., September 14, 1847.

6. Ibid. Here the provisions of the quarantine law are specifically stated.

7. Quincy *Times*, May 20, 1848. See also Tallahassee *Floridian*, July 22, 1848.

8. Tallahassee *Floridian and Journal*, August 5, 1848. See Jerrell H. Shofner, *History of Jefferson County*, Tallahassee, 1976, p. 202, for further information on this partnership.

9. Ibid.

10. Tallahassee *Florida Sentinel*, May 7, 1850. Dr. Call died unexpectedly after an illness of a few hours. He was said to have been "a young man of high character and great promise."

11. U.S. Census, 1850, Jefferson County, Florida, p. 4.

12. Tallahassee *Southern Journal*, May 29, 1848.

13. Tallahassee *Floridian and Journal*, May 11, 1850.

Cameron, James G., Alachua County, 1865

Only minimal information has been discovered concerning the life of Dr. Cameron, a native of South Carolina, who settled in Micanopy in the 1840s. County records show that on February 21, 1849, he purchased two sections of land, 1,280 acres, within the Arredondo Grant near the town of Micanopy. Within a few months, however, he sold the property to John P. Feaster, his future brother-in-law, through a transaction concluded on February 5, 1850, the price being $1,280.[1] The 1850 census lists Dr. Cameron as 24 years of age, a farmer, sharing his house with John P. Feaster, aged 21, listed probably erroneously as physician.[2] On August 7, 1854, he was married to Feaster's sister, Drusilla K.[3]

Nothing further is known of Dr. Cameron's activities until the late summer of 1860 when he and Dr. Augustus H. Mathers of Micanopy announced formation of a partnership for the practice of medicine and surgery.[4] This joint venture included operation of a drug store, therefore the two physicians referred to themselves as "druggists and apothecaries."[5] The arrangement was doubtless terminated when Dr. Mathers enlisted in the Confederate Army in June 1861.

Only an isolated item of evidence suggests that Dr. Cameron remained in Micanopy throughout the war.[6]

Dr. Cameron died in the fall of 1865. Evidence of this derives solely from a legal notice appearing in the Gainesville *New Era* of September 7, 1865, in which his widow, as administratrix of his estate, made the customary representation. In the same issue she announced the forthcoming sale of certain chattels to be held at the residence of John M. Feaster[7] (her father?) a week hence. Finally, on September 17, 1866, Mrs. Cameron sold at public auction the balance of her husband's property consisting of "one unimproved lot in Micanopy and a dwelling house near the residence of John M. Feaster." She added, "I will also apply at the same time to have my dower set apart from the estate."[8]

1. Alachua County, deed book A, p. 230.
2. U.S. Census, 1850, Alachua County, Florida, p. 20. Information on the two men appears to have been erroneously reversed. Feaster was doubtless the farmer and Cameron the physician.
3. Alachua County, Book of Marriages, II, 40.
4. Micanopy *Cotton States*, September 28, 1861; first printing, September 7, 1860.
5. Ibid.
6. Franklin A. Doty, ed., The Civil War Letters of Augustus Henry Mathers, *Florida Historical Quarterly*, XXXVI, No. 2, October 1957, pp. 107, 113. These letters contain only two references to Dr. Cameron, who, from the context, seems to have been in Micanopy.
7. John M. Feaster, listed in the 1860 Census, Alachua County, item 545, was 53 years old, owning property with a combined value of $44,600, is not to be identified as the John P. Feaster of note 2 above.
8. Gainesville *New Era*, August 17, 1866.

Campbell, Daniel L., Walton County, 1833-1922

Dr. Campbell,[1] for more than half a century a medical practitioner in Walton County, was born on August 28, 1833, in Euchee Valley, that portion of the county which had been settled in the 1820s by a cluster of Scottish Highlander families. His father, Daniel Douglass Campbell, was born on the Atlantic Ocean when his parents were on their way to America. Along with many other Scots the Campbells settled in Richmond County, North Carolina.[2] In the spring of 1820, young Daniel Douglass Campbell joined his sturdy pioneer neighbor, Neill McLendon, and a small band of fellow Scots on the long trek to Walton County where they sought out the fertile Euchee Valley and settled as thrifty and often prosperous citizens.[3]

Daniel Douglass Campbell was married to Nancy McLean in February 1828 and among the numerous children born to this marriage was Daniel L. Campbell. These Scottish Presbyterians for the most part adhered rigidly to the tenets of their sect. They also placed a high value on education; thus the children of Daniel Douglass and Nancy Campbell were reared with a firm hand and exposed to the best education available. It is quite likely that young Daniel Campbell received his basic education under the guidance of the most notable teacher of the area, the Reverend John Newton, a Pennsylvanian and graduate of Amherst College.[4] As for Daniel Campbell's medical training nothing is known, but it appears quite likely that he served an apprenticeship under Dr. Angus D. McKinnon, Euchee Valley's most prominent physician.[5]

Dr. Campbell began practice in Eucheeanna in the mid-1950s. The year 1860 found him a resident in the home of Alexander Monroe, a local merchant.[6] Soon thereafter he was married to Annie Curry, daughter of Col. John L. McKinnon, one of the Valley's earliest settlers. To this marriage were born six children,

McKinnon, Leonidas, Cleopatra, Douglass, Daniel Curry, and Patillo.[7] Mrs. Campbell died on December 5, 1875, at age 44.[8] A few years later Dr. Campbell married Elizabeth Anne Bowers, also of Eucheeanna. Of the several children born to this marriage three died in infancy or early childhood.

About 1883 the Campbells moved from Eucheeanna to DeFuniak where Dr. Campbell continued practice for a few years. He died there on January 27, 1922, at age 88.[9]

There can be no doubt that Dr. Campbell was a man of considerable influence in Walton County. In 1871 and again in 1872 he represented the county in Florida's Legislative Assembly (House). As for his medical practice, little information has survived. It is assumed that he was an ideal country doctor, a man of compassion and common sense, serving the community to the best of his abilities. Through marriage or blood he was related to many of the foremost families of West Florida.

1. Census data relating to Dr. Campbell are confusing. In the 1870 census he appears as David L. Campbell, while in the censuses of 1850, 1880 and 1900 he is listed as Daniel L., the latter being correct. To complicate the matter further, his gravestone in the Euchee Valley Cemetery is inscribed "Daniel McLean Campbell." Is one to assume that "Macks" were so common that the initial "L" is sufficient?

2. Information concerning these early settlers is found in John L. McKinnon's *History of Walton County*, Gainesville, facsimile ed., original published in Atlanta, 1911, pp. 21, 41, et passim.

3. Ibid., pp. 43-47.

4. Ibid., pp. 181ff. McKinnon devoted several pages to John Newton and his significant contributions to the cultural development of the county.

5. Records of the Medical College of the State of South Carolina list D.A. Campbell as the recipient of a degree in March 1854. This date agrees chronologically with date at which Dr. Campbell might have received a degree (he was 21 in 1854) but the D.A. Campbell, recipient of the degree, had entered the College from Troy, North Carolina. Charleston *Mercury*, March 15, 1854.

6. U.S. Census, 1860, Walton County, Florida, p. 1.

7. Ibid., 1880, p. 18.

8. Patillo was the middle name of the Rev. William P. Harrison, a popular Presbyterian minister of the Euchee Valley Church. Incidentally, Patillo Campbell had a successful career as a lawyer in Pensacola.

9. A survey of grave markers in the Euchee Valley Cemetery, made under supervision of the Daughters of the American Revolution, Pensacola Chapter, and distributed in typescript under the title, "Walton County, Florida," (1951), has been a valuable aid in determining dates and family relationships.

Carn, Francis Elvin, Leon and Alachua Counties, 1822

Dr. Carn was born in Orangeburg District, South Carolina, in 1822.[1] After serving an apprenticeship in the office of local physician, Dr. B.F. Johnson of Orangeburg,[2] he matriculated at the Medical College of the State of South Carolina, Charleston, in the fall of 1844. He was graduated in March 1846 after submitting a doctoral thesis entitled "Hysterotomy."[3]

Within a year after receiving his degree Dr. Carn moved to Leon County, settling in the Centerville community which had already attracted numerous settlers from South Carolina[4] including his kinsman, Dr. Julius Marcellus Carn. He was married to Mary Ann Hall, a Georgia native, on April 7, 1847.[5] Their first child, a son, David, was born the following year and in time two other children, Edward and Margaret, were born.[6]

At some unknown date in the later 1850s Dr. Carn moved to Micanopy, probably anticipating a more lucrative practice. This could hardly have been a propitious move for five other physicians were already in practice in the community. The only known record of his activities in Micanopy relates not to his profession but to his politics. When the issue of whether to incorporate the town of

Micanopy was presented to the voters on September 15, 1858, Dr. Carn cast a "no" vote, the only physician to oppose incorporation.[7]

Beyond that date nothing further is known of Dr. Carn. Since his name does not appear in the Florida Census of 1860, it is presumed that he had left the state by that year, possibly returning to South Carolina.

1. U.S. Census, 1850, Leon County, Florida, p. 127. Dr. Carn is not to be confused with Francis E. Carn, a prosperous planter of Orangeburg District, whose wife was also Mary A. See U.S. Census, 1850, Orangeburg District, S.C., p. 285.

2. *Catalog of Students*, Medical College of the State of South Carolina, 1845-46, p. 167. See also Charleston *Courier*, March 21, 1846.

3. Ibid.

4. This is indicated by Leon County censuses of 1850 and 1860.

5. Marriage Records, Leon County, Florida.

6. See note 4 supra.

7. A handwritten report of his voting is found in the Glunt Papers, P.K. Yonge Library, University of Florida. Physicians voting for incorporation were: George B. Payne, A.H. Mathers and J.A. Stewart.

Carn, Julius Marcellus, Leon County, 1845-1911

Dr. Carn, who spent the greater part of his professional life in Leon County, was born in Orangeburg County, South Carolina on August 5, 1845.[1] His father, David N. Carn, moved with his family to Florida prior to 1850, purchased a plantation in the Centerville community some 12 miles northeast of Tallahassee and settled in to the life of a gentleman farmer. Of the several children born to David Carn, Julius was the youngest.[2] By 1870 he had completed his professional training, thought to have been acquired through the apprenticeship system, and launched his career as a physician. He was married to Laura E. Braswell (1852-1925) in 1871, a union to which several children were born, at least six of whom died in infancy or early childhood.[4]

With the mobilization of troops following the fall of Ft. Sumter in April 1861, Dr. Carn offered his services to the Confederacy and was mustered into the Third Infantry Regimental staff as Assistant Surgeon on July 23. Not until March 1862 was the Regiment assembled. The various units of the Regiment were brought together at Midway, Gadsden County, in May 1862; soon thereafter elections for field officers were held and Dr. Carn was confirmed in his post as surgeon. In this capacity he was with the Regiment when it moved to Chattanooga, Tennessee, in August 1862, encamping at the foot of Lookout Mountain near the Tennessee River. Shortly thereafter the Regiment was assigned to the Brigade of General John C. Brown, a part of General Patton Anderson's Division. From this point the military record of Dr. Carn is missing. It is known that on April 30, 1862, he was paid $139 for one month's service.[5]

Although he was not present at the inaugural session of the Florida Medical Association held in the office of Dr. Abel S. Baldwin in Jacksonville, Dr. Carn was elected to membership on the recommendation of Dr. George W. Betton of Tallahassee.[6] The date was January 14, 1874. He was present, however, at the annual meeting held in Tallahassee in the Capitol Building in 1876, his only appearance. Although not present at the Jacksonville meeting in 1878, he was chosen as a delegate to the annual meeting of the American Medical Association. He did not attend. At about this time he resigned from the Florida Medical Association.[7] One can only speculate as to his reasons. It is known that family responsibilities had been burdensome and doubtless there were also monetary considerations.

For the remainder of his life Dr. Carn appears to have devoted his energies to his practice in the Centerville community where he was a beloved citizen. He also served for a brief time as postmaster of Centerville, his appointment dating from January 30, 1882. He lived on until August 3, 1911.[8] His only survivor was his wife, Laura who lived until March 24, 1925.

Within a few days after his death his long-time friend, Thompson B. Lamar, of Leon County, and officer in the United Confederate Veterans, Camp No. 161, of which Dr. Carn had been a member, wrote the following tribute to his departed friend:[9]

> We, the surviving United Confederate Veterans, do deeply mourn the death of our comrade, Dr. J.M. Carn, which occurred at his home in Centerville, Leon County, on August 3, 1911. He was buried on August 5, 1911, which was the 67th anniversary of his birth. Dr. Carn was a good soldier; a good and valuable citizen; was very highly respected by all who knew him, and was a Christian gentleman. We extend our deepest sympathies to his family.

1. Gravestone, Pisgah Methodist Church Cemetery, near Centerville.
2. U.S. Census, 1850, Leon County, Florida, p. 74.
3. Ibid., 1870, p. 140.
4. See Floreda Duke Varick and Phyllis Rose Smith, *Tallahassee and Leon County Cemeteries*, Tallahassee, 1979, p. 56. Two of the Carn children died in the same year, 1882.
5. National Archives, Service Records, CSA, 3rd Florida Infantry Regiment.
6. *Proceedings, Florida Medical Association*, 1874-77.
7. It is probable that Dr. Carn could not in good conscience abandon his wife and small children for a lengthy and expensive trip to an eastern city to attend the American Medical Association meeting.
8. Gravestone, Pisgah Methodist Church Cemetery, Centerville.

Carn, Lewis M., Alachua County, 1860

Dr. Carn, a native of Orangeburg District, S.C.,[1] practiced medicine only briefly in Florida. A graduate of Jefferson Medical College, Philadelphia,[2] class of 1859, he arrived in Micanopy in mid-1860 and announced his services as "resident physician." His office was located at the Post Office. He added, "Special attention is given to surgery and diseases of children."[3] Although his Confederate service record is incomplete it appears that by early 1862 he had volunteered as a medical officer in the Third Florida Infantry Regiment. A pay voucher of April 30, 1862, lists him as surgeon, while a regimental return of July 1862 shows him as surgeon, stationed in Chattanooga, Tenn.[4]

No record has emerged which might verify Dr. Carn's return to Florida after the war. It may be speculated that he either died in service or elected to practice elsewhere. Information from the Census of 1860 shows him living in Micanopy with his wife, Leonora, a native of Florida. Both were 22 years old.[5]

1. Orangeburg, S.C., Census schedules for 1850 include several Carn entries. It seems likely that Dr. Carn was a son of one Lewis D. Carn, age 54, planter, p. 283, item 162. His relationship to Dr. Francis E. Carn, physician in Leon County in 1850 and Micanopy in 1858, has not been established.
2. Archives, Jefferson Medical College, List of Graduates.
3. Micanopy *Cotton States*, September 28, 1860.
4. NA, Service Records, CSA, M251, Roll 46.
5. U.S. Census, 1860, Alachua County, Florida, Item 212.

Carroll, William J., Jefferson County, 1830

Dr. Carroll was born in Duplin County, North Carolina, in 1830, son of James Carroll, a man of prominence in his community.[1] Nothing is presently known of his youth and medical education. He first appeared in Florida records in early 1856 when he announced his professional services to the citizens of the Waukeenah community of Jefferson County, Florida, with the assurance that he could be found when needed at his "office in the Front Room of Mr. W.T. Carpenter's New Building."[2]

By 1860 Dr. Carroll had taken as his wife a South Carolinian, known only as Mary R. Carroll, three years younger. The Census of 1860 lists also their first child, James D., born in 1859.[3]

With the Civil War intensifying in November 1861 and probably confronted with a lagging medical practice, Dr. Carroll offered his services to the Confederacy by joining a company being organized locally by Capt. William Bailey Jr., the outfit being designated the Aucilla Guards, named for the river which is the boundary line between Jefferson and Madison Counties. His enlistment was dated November 28. With formation of the Fifth Florida Infantry Regiment in early 1862, the Aucilla Guards became Company G of the Regiment.[4] Notwithstanding his family responsibilities, Dr. Carroll committed himself to serve for the duration of the war. He joined the Regiment on March 3, 1862. He entered as a private but in May or June 1862 he was detailed "physician to attend the sick of his company" by order of the Medical Director of the Regiment with approval of General Joseph Finegan, commanding officer of military operations in East and Middle Florida.

In the latter part of 1862 Dr. Carroll accompanied his unit to Virginia, encamping in the vicinity of Richmond. His actual service was destined to be brief, however. Within weeks he became ill, seriously enough to be sent to the Florida Hospital at Richmond, the facility under the direction of Dr. Thomas M. Palmer, of Jefferson County. His ailment was diagnosed as "hemiplegia," paralysis in one side of his body. He was examined by Dr. Palmer himself who wrote in his report: "I certify that I have carefully examined the said William J. Carroll and find him incapable of performing the duties of a soldier because of paralysis of the whole left side. . .I recommend his discharge."[5] Dr. Palmer's recommendation was followed and Dr. Carroll was at home again by early 1863.

In spite of the apparent seriousness of his ailment Dr. Carroll soon recovered and was able to return to medical practice. From this point very little is known of his activities. The 1870 Census indicates that his wife, Mary, was no longer living; he had remarried, in this instance a native Floridian, Jane E. Also five additional children had been added to the family since 1860. They were, in order of birth, Flenza (sic), aged nine; Rebecca, aged seven; George W., aged five; Mary E., aged three; and Jesse, a son of five months,[6] an indication that his sexual activity had not been seriously impaired.

Whether Dr. Carroll lived out his last years in Florida has not been determined. Since he does not appear in the census records of 1880, it is assumed that he was deceased by that date.

1. The greater part of the information contained in this sketch is derived from Dr. Carroll's Confederate service record where it is learned that he was 32 years old in 1862; that he was five feet, ten inches tall; of fair complexion,

with blue eyes and dark hair; and by profession a physician. See NA, Service Records, CSA, M 251, Roll 60.

2. Tallahassee *Floridian and Journal*, April 19, 1856, 1st printed, April 12, 1856.
3. U.S. Census, 1860, Jefferson County, Florida, item 201.
4. See note 1, supra.
5. Ibid.
6. U.S. Census, 1870, Jefferson County, Florida, p. 436. Several members of the Carroll family of Duplin County, N.C., moved to Florida in the 1850s. The Census of 1860 lists two in Leon County and one in Marion County. It merits mention that the Christian name, Jesse, was common in the family.

Carson, Lewis David, Liberty County, 1834-1894

Dr. Carson was born in St. George's Parish, Colleton District, South Carolina, on August 11, 1834.[1] He matriculated at the Medical College of the State of South Carolina in 1858 and was graduated in the spring of 1860.[2] He is said to have served with distinction in the Confederate Army as a regimental assistant surgeon. When the war was finished he moved to Florida and by 1870 had settled in Liberty County a short distance south of Bristol. His wife, Virginia, to whom he was married in 1869, was a native of Georgia. Their first child, a son named Lucius, was born in 1870.[3]

Never short on energy Dr. Carson managed in a comparatively short time to acquire a large tract of land and henceforth was both physician and farmer.[4] As was the situation with most rural doctors of Florida in the 19th century, his practice imposed many hardships. Regardless of his medical skills,[5] which may have been suspect, he endeared himself to many families over a wide area along the Apalachicola River. Their trust was evident in 1885 when the voters of the county chose him as their delegate to the State Constitutional Convention.[6] In 1891 he was a Liberty County member in the Florida House of Representatives.[7]

Dr. Carson died in 1894 leaving a widow and five children. He was buried in the Lake Mystic Methodist Cemetery three miles south of Bristol.[8]

1. Whitfield, J.W.: *Florida State Government, 1885*, Tallahassee, 1885, p. 17.
2. Archives, Waring Historical Library, MUSC, Charleston, Lists of Matriculants and Graduates.
3. U.S. Census, 1880, Liberty County, Florida, p. 19.
4. Special Florida Census, 1885, Liberty County, p. 11. Here Dr. Carson is shown to have owned 1,750 acres of land, of which 50 acres were under cultivation.
5. Dr. Charles A. Hentz, well-known Quincy physician and author, a man not averse to criticizing his medical colleagues for what he deemed to be their ignorance, ineptness and immorality, had nothing favorable to say about Dr. Carson. He related one incident in which he was summoned from Quincy to Ricoes Bluff, some 15 miles down river from Bristol, to attend one of Dr. Carson's patients suffering from fistula in ano. Dr. Hentz reported it as a simple case requiring only the most elementary surgery which he promptly performed with success. In committing this to his journal, he wrote: "Dr. Carson, his physician. . .a poor chance for an M.D. . . .full of gas and chat." C.A. Hentz, "My Autobiography." Typed transcription of an original MS, Southern Historical Collection, University of North Carolina, Chapel Hill, II, 26.
6. Whitfield, Florida State Government, loc cit.
7. Morris, Allen, *People of Lawmaking in Florida, 1822-1877*, Tallahassee, 1977.
8. Veterans' Graves Registration Project, Liberty County, Florida, St. Augustine, 1940-41, p. 9.

Carter, Thomas W., Columbia County, 1823-1880

Information on the life of Dr. Carter is sparse. A native of South Carolina (according to the Census of 1860; the Census of 1870 gives Georgia as his native state), he was living on a farm outside Lake City in 1860.[1] Unmarried, he was a member of the household of his sister-in-law, Julia A.H. Carter, a widow, and her four children. The Carters were a family of more than average means. In 1860 Dr. Carter owned property valued at $4,000, while Mrs. Carter owned 23 slaves and other properties valued at $20,000.

There can be no doubt that Dr. Carter was a respected member of his community. He was also concerned about the sorry state of medical practice in Florida in mid-century. In 1874 he was one of a small group of Florida physicians who responded to the call of Dr. Abel. S. Baldwin of Jacksonville to join him in organizing a medical association calculated to eliminate some of the quackery by raising the standards of licensing and providing a forum for the exchange of ideas. Of the 10 men present at the initial session on January 14, two, Dr. Carter and Dr. M.M.T. Huchingson, were from Columbia County, both members of the county medical society.[2] There is no evidence, however, that Dr. Carter ever attended another session. He was listed as a member in 1878 but thereafter was dropped from membership for "non-payment of dues."[3] Since his name does not appear in the Columbia County census of 1880 it is assumed that he had died by that date.[4]

1. U.S. Census, 1860, Columbia County, Florida, p. 77. Since Mrs. Carter's youngest child, Julia, aged three, was born in Florida while the next youngest, aged five, was Georgia-born, it would appear that the family had moved to Florida about 1856. This is possibly the date of Dr. Carter's arrival in Florida.

2. *Proceedings, Florida Medical Association, 1874-5,* Charleston, S.C., 1875, p. 4.

3. *Proceedings, Florida Medical Association, 1893,* Jacksonville, 1893, p. 43.

4. There is a probability that Dr. Carter's latter years were plagued by ill-health but this has not been verified.

Casey, J.L., Jackson County, 1832-1869

Except for the inscription on his gravestone in the Campbellton Cemetery nothing is known of Dr. Casey. Since he is not listed in the Jackson County censuses of 1850 or 1869, it can only be said that he practiced medicine in Jackson County briefly in the 1860s.

Cato, Philip W., Alachua County, 1818-1882

Dr. Cato was born in the Charleston District, South Carolina, on October 31, 1818. About 1848 he arrived in Florida, settling in the Newnansville community of Alachua County.[1] Since he does not appear in the student listings of the Medical College of the State of South Carolina, Charleston, it is assumed that he was trained as an apprentice to a local physician. Soon after settling in Florida he purchased a parcel of land which he farmed as a secondary occupation.[2] He joined the Reverend Jesse M. Valentine, M.D., in a professional partnership for medical practice in 1858. The following year Dr. Valentine in his clerical role performed the wedding ceremony for the marriage of Dr. Cato's daughter, Ophelia, to Joseph J. Warren.[3]

Random evidence suggests that Dr. Cato took an active interest in the civic affairs of both county and state. He was one of the chief supporters of the effort in April 1860 to build a railroad from Fernandina to Tampa by way of Newnansville.[4] He served on a committee charged with drafting to that purpose and putting pressure on Governor Perry to support the effort. His sudden death from apoplexy occurred while attending a political gathering in Newnansville and listening to a speech by General Jesse J. Finley, Democratic candidate for Congress in the fall of 1882 (October 10). It was reported that he had risen from his seat to put a question to the Speaker when he fell to the floor dead.[5]

Dr. Cato was twice married. His first wife, Eliza, was a native of Georgia. To this marriage were born nine children, the elder five in Alabama where Dr. Cato had practiced medicine for a few years. The younger four were Florida-born. His second wife, Carrie, was a native of South Carolina. Three of the Cato sons served in the Army of the Confederacy, the eldest, Homer, enlisting in May 1862, at age 21.[6] A wound received in battle in Virginia required amputation of his left hand in the summer of 1864. The second son, Tamberlane, erroneously spelled Tamblin in Confederate Records, enlisted on January 1, 1862, at age 18, also saw action in Virginia. He was among those surrendered at Appomattox by General Lee. The third son, Charles, enlisted for service in April 1864, at age 18 and died of pneumonia in the Confederate General Hospital, Richmond, on January 16, 1865.[7] The three served in Co. F, 10th Florida Infantry Regiment. Besides these sons there were Ophelia, previously mentioned, a second daughter, Serepta, and the youngest of the children, William.

1. U.S. Census, Alachua County, Florida, Schedules of 1850, 1860, 1870 and 1880. The 1870 Census, Suwannee County, shows sons Homer, Tamberlane and William as residents of Wellborn.

2. Ibid., Schedule of 1860. Here Dr. Cato's real estate was appraised at $2,000, personal property at $29,900.

3. Alligator, Lake City, *Columbia Democrat*, March 27, 1858.

4. Fernandina *Florida News*, May 5, 1860. The proposed route for the railroad appeared to have pleased only a few people, becoming a major political and economic issue in Alachua, Marion and Sumter Counties. It received extensive newspaper coverage.

5. Gainesville *Weekly Bee*, October 13, 1882. Dr. Cato was buried in Newnansville Cemetery.

6. This and subsequent military information is derived from NA, Service Records, CSA, M251, Roll 93.

7. Upon the death of son Charles, Dr. Cato, stricken with grief, wrote a touching eulogy to the departed young man. Lake City *Columbian* March 22, 1865. Incidentally, he gave the birthplace of his son as Russell County, Alabama (county seat, Phenix). It is assumed that Dr. Cato had practiced there for a few years.

Chapman, Alvan Wentworth, Franklin County, 1809-1899

Dr. Chapman, son of Paul and Ruth (Pomeroy) Chapman, was born in Southampton, Mass., on September 28, 1809. He was graduated from Amherst College in 1830 with the A.B. degree, having displayed special interest and talent in botany. The following year he moved to Georgia where he spent the next four years teaching, first as a private tutor with a Savannah family and later as the principal of an academy in Washington, Georgia. In the latter place he began the study of medicine under the preceptorate of a local physician. He is said to have then proceeded to Louisville, Ky., where in 1835 he was awarded his medical degree.[1]

Dr. Chapman arrived in Florida prior to 1840, settling in Gadsden County where he purchased land and engaged in farming as well as medical practice. It appears, although documentation is lacking, that between his medical study and appearance in Florida, he had traveled about the South pursuing his botanical interests. At some juncture he met and married Mrs. Mary Ann Hancock (nee Simmons) of New Bern, N.C., a widow with at least two children.[2] As early as 1838 Dr. Chapman had begun to collect botanical specimens indigenous to Florida some of which he sent to Asa Gray and John Torrey.

In the early 1840s the Chapmans are said to have lived for a brief time in

Jackson County but by late 1845 they had moved to Apalachicola where Dr. Chapman would spend the last 54 years of his life. His professional notice first appeared in the local newspaper on January 10, 1846, announcing that he would occupy an office over the Drug Store of B.S. Hawley, while his residence was that previously occupied by Dr. Baltzell.[3]

Dr. Chapman took more than a passing interest in the politics of the area. While in Gadsden County in 1840 he was elected to represent the conservative element of the county at the forthcoming meeting of the state's Conservative Party in Tallahassee on August 22, 1840.[4] Later, in Apalachicola, he served a term on the City Council.[5] Although he had become a slaveholder after coming to Florida he later rejected the arguments of the plantation owners and the secessionists and took a firm stand for preservation of the Union, a decision which provoked a temporary separation from his wife who remained adamantly secessionist.

It is impossible to fathom the reasons for Dr. Chapman's move to Apalachicola but one is led to speculate that with the virtual destruction of neighboring St. Joseph by tidal wave and yellow fever in 1841, Apalachicola suddenly enjoyed a business boom. The great number of business notices in the local newspaper about 1846, relating to the marketing of cotton; the mercantile establishments doing business with plantations to the north along the Apalachicola River, not only in Florida but in Alabama and Georgia as well, show an optimism and an almost frantic commercial activity. Also there was a scarcity of doctors; only Dr. William Sydney Green practiced there until Dr. Chapman arrived. Quincy and Marianna, however, were well staffed with medical practitioners.

With the onset of the Civil War Dr. Chapman decided to remain in Apalachicola in spite of the separation from his wife and the probable hostility of his fellow townsmen. It is a tribute to his medical skills and a test of the esteem in which he was held that no harm came to him. So fine was his reputation that his neighbors protected him from wanton mischief or bodily harm by overzealous rebels. The state Treasurer paid him in 1863 for performing postmortem examinations for the sheriff's office.[6]

Notwithstanding the stresses of the time and the many distractions Dr. Chapman devoted much time to his botanical interests. He published the results of his researches in Gadsden County in an article in 1845 titled "A List of the Plants Growing Spontaneously in the Vicinity of Quincy, Florida."[7] His major work, *Flora of the Southern United States*, which was to become the standard text on the botany of this region appeared in 1860. It went into some 10 or 11 editions and, of course, brought him international acclaim.[8]

After the war Dr. Chapman was reconciled with his wife who returned to Florida; henceforth his medical practice consumed less of his energies as his botanical searches claimed the majority of his time. His fame brought a flood of inquiries from botanists far and wide. Many, including Gray and Torrey, made the difficult trip to remote Apalachicola to observe at first hand the rare species he had discovered and identified. Several plants, e.g. the *Rhododendron Chapmanii*, bear his name. Along with such recognition came honors. The University of North Carolina conferred upon him the honorary degree of Doctor of Laws in 1866. Other honors came from the New Orleans Academy of Sciences (1854), Philadelphia Academy of Natural Sciences (1861), Buffalo Society of

Natural Sciences (1866), American Academy of Arts and Sciences of Boston (1866), and the Botanical Society of America (1895).

Dr. Chapman was a man of commanding presence and splendid physique, possessed of courtly manners, and "the old-time deferential courtesy," but he suffered the misfortune of losing his hearing as he grew older. Communication with others became increasingly difficult. He gave up medical practice completely because, he explained half in jest, that he could no longer hear the groans of his patients, and in his last years became a virtual recluse. He never lost the love and admiration of the people of Apalachicola.

The only child born to Dr. Chapman and his wife died in infancy. He died in Apalachicola on April 6, 1899, a few months short of his 90th birthday. After his death they preserved his memory by naming the new high school after him.[9]

In the 10 years during which their lives overlapped in Apalachicola Dr. Chapman and Dr. John Gorrie were close friends. It is a notable coincidence that these two exceptional men, perhaps the most widely known of all Florida practitioners of the 19th century, lived at the same time in the small town of Apalachicola and that the fame of each rests not on medical achievements but on mechanical genius for Dr. Gorrie and on contributions to the science of botany for Dr. Chapman.

1. Some material in this sketch is from the entry on Dr. Chapman, *Dictionary of American Biography*, New York, 1937, IV, 16-17, by Donald C. Peattie. Other sources are "Obituary Notice," *Apalachicola Times*, April 15, 1899, and a letter, R.M. Harper to *New York Times*, January 2, 1910, in *New York Times Saturday Review of Books*, January 8, 1910, p. 21.

This date, 1835, from the item in the *New York Times*, is apparently in error. There was no medical school in Louisville prior to 1837 although the Medical School of Transylvania University, Lexington, Ky., had been in operation since 1817. John H. Ellis, *Medicine in Kentucky*, Lexington, 1977, pp. 8-16.

2. Peattie states that Dr. Chapman moved to Gadsden County in 1838, the year of his marriage.

3. Apalachicola *Commercial Advertiser*, March 21, 1846. First printing, January 10, 1846. By this date Dr. George Baltzell had moved to Washington County. It appears that Dr. Chapman bought an interest in the Drug Store of Hawley, for the census of 1850, Franklin County, lists him as druggist not physician.

4. Quincy *Sentinel*, August 21, 1840.

5. Apalachicola *Commercial Advertiser*, November 4, 1847.

6. Tallahassee *Sentinel*, February 24, 1863. The payment of $40 had been authorized by the State Legislature.

7. Published in *Western Journal of Medicine and Surgery*, III, No. 6, new series.

8. The first edition was published in 1860 by Ivison, Phinney & Co., New York.

9. A more commodious building has been erected for the Apalachicola High School. The older building is the Chapman Elementary School.

Chittenden, E., Apalachicola, 1838

A single reference to Dr. Chittenden, who practiced for a brief period in Apalachicola, identifies him as a member of a committee responsible for arranging a dinner honoring Benjamin Hurd.[1] The committee chairman was Dr. John Gorrie. Hurd was said to have deserved this honor for his role in developing Apalachicola Harbor and other services relating to the growth of the town. No further information relating to Dr. Chittenden has been discovered.

1. Apalachicola *Gazette*, April 20, 1838.

Christian Jr., William M., Calhoun and Sumter Counties, 1825

Census schedules of 1850 and 1860, the only source of information on Dr. Christian, leave room for much speculation. In the 1850 Census for Calhoun

County, p. 57, he is listed as physician, aged 25, and native of Alabama. In his household were a female, Leona J., aged 17, presumably his wife, Florida-born, also two young men, N.W., and N.D. Williams, aged 23 and 16 respectively, both native to Florida, and possibly brothers of Leona.[1]

Ten years later Dr. Christian was a resident of Adamsville, Sumter County. He is shown to have been a native of Mississippi, with a wife, M.A., Georgia native, and seven-month-old son, Samuel, born in Florida. By 1870 the Christians had moved from Florida.[2]

1. U.S. Census, 1850, Calhoun County, p. 57.
2. Ibid., 1860, Sumter County, p. 811.

Churchill, Charles C., Gainesville and Cedar Key, 1880

The Florida sojourn of Dr. Churchill was brief. From the limited information surviving it appears that he arrived in Gainesville in the late 1870s with his wife, Elizabeth, and son, Charles. The census of 1880 gives his age as 52 and his place of birth Ohio.[1] Mrs. Churchill was 39 and a native of New York while his son, aged 19, was born in Tennessee. Within the next two years he departed for Cedar Key, his professional card having appeared in the local newspaper in July 1882,[2] when he announced his service to the community as physician and surgeon with residence and office at the Suwannee Hotel. The special Florida Census of 1885 lists him as 59.[3]

Nothing is known of Dr. Churchill's Levy County practice except that it was terminated in early 1886. His departure was announced in the following notice: "Dr. and Mrs. Churchill have left for Santiago, California, where the doctor has family connections and a ready-made practice awaiting him. Cedar Key society sustains a loss in their departure."[4]

1. U.S. Census, 1880, Alachua County, Florida, p. 108.
2. Bronson *Levy Enterprise*, February 23, 1883; earlier issue not extant.
3. Special Florida Census, 1885, item 46.
4. Bronson *Levy County Times*, April 1, 1886.

Clark, Richard, Surgeon, U.S. Army, 1839

Dr. Clark, a native of New York State was commissioned Assistant Surgeon in the United States Army on March 2, 1833.[1] After serving as post surgeon at two army posts in Michigan Territory, Fort Gratiot and Fort Brady,[2] the latter at Sault Ste. Marie, he was ordered to Florida, arriving there in the spring of 1835. His first station was Ft. King, a short distance east of Ocala, whose commanding officer was General Duncan L. Clinch. In the assignment of some of his newly-arrived troops in April 1835, Dr. Clark became surgeon of Company C, 3rd Artillery Regiment, which meant that he would remain at Ft. King, at least temporarily.[3]

Later in the year and probably for the convenience of General Clinch, a new army post was established on a part of Clinch's plantation, some 20 miles north and west of Fort King. It was called Ft. Drane, thus honoring its builder, Capt. Gustavus D. Drane. Upon its completion Clinch and a part of the Ft. King garrison moved to the new location.[4] Among the group was Dr. Clark.

When the news of the massacre of Captain Francis L. Dade's company, enroute from Ft. Brooke, Tampa Bay, to Fort King, at the Withlacoochee River arrived in Ft. Clinch, a small detail of soldiers led by Clinch himself hurried to the scene of the tragedy. Among them was Dr. Clark. It was a precipitate move touched off by shock and anger. The expedition was doomed to fail. The Indians were grouped on the south bank of the Withlacoochee. It was only with great difficulty that Clinch and his soldiers were able to cross the stream. Although their courage was laudable, the result was a disaster. Four men were killed and 59 wounded. Clinch himself escaping with bullet holes in his clothing, while Dr. Clark's horse was shot from beneath him.[5] The foray occurred on December 31, 1835, three days after Dade's encounter of the 25th.

For the next two years or so Dr. Clark's activities are impossible to follow. For some time he remained at Fort Clinch, but at some point he was reassigned to posts across the Suwannee River in Middle Florida, probably serving at more than one place over the more than two years. It was without doubt a dreary existence as the war dragged on. On July 7, 1838, he was rewarded by promotion to the rank of surgeon.[6] During this period his problems were not those imposed by Indian threats but by the fevers endemic to the undrained marshlands along the coast from Cedar Key to St. Marks.

Fever appeared among the troops at recently-established Fort Roger Jones on the Aucilla River in May 1839. Of the company of 42 men nearly all were ill including the commander of the post, Capt. Enos Mitchell, and the other officer, Lt. Pew. The surgeon of the post, Dr. Charles McCormick, alarmed at the seriousness of Capt. Mitchell's condition, summoned Dr. Clark to come for consultation.[7] While there trying to save the life of Mitchell, he was seized by an attack of the fever and moved to the nearby plantation home of Col. Robert Gamble, known as Welaunee, for nursing care. It was unavailing; he died 15 days later on June 29, 1839.

1. Harvey E. Brown, comp., *Medical Department, from 1775 to 1873*, Washington, D.C., Surgeon General's Office, 1873, p. 288.
2. *American State Papers*, Vol. V, Washington, 1860, pp. 279, 608; ibid., Vol. VI, Washington, 1861, p. 36.
3. *The Territorial Papers of the United States*, Clarence Edwin Carter, comp. and ed., Vol. XXV, Washington, 1960, p. 130.
4. Mahon, John K.: *History of the Second Seminole War, 1835-1842*, Gainesville, 1967, p. 107.
5. Ibid., pp. 108-112.
6. See note 1, supra.
7. See note 1, supra, p. 162. See also *Statistical Report on the Sickness and Mortality in the Army of the United States*, Surgeon General's Office, Washington, 1840, pp. 306, 307.

Clarkson, Samuel B., U.S. Navy, Pensacola, 1829

Dr. Clarkson, a native of Pennsylvania, entered the naval medical service as surgeon's mate on August 8, 1826.[1] He was assigned to sea duty aboard the Sloop Natchez.[1] By late 1828 or early 1829 he was transferred to the Schooner Grampus with a change of title to assistant surgeon.[2] His death occurred aboard the Grampus on May 16, 1829, as the ship lay in Pensacola harbor.[3]

Dr. Clarkson's death and those of other members of the Grampus' crew touched off an acrimonious exchange of words when a certain Captain Reeves of the Schooner James Star, who left Pensacola at about the time of Dr. Clarkson's death, arrived in New York and reported serious epidemics of smallpox and yellow fever in the Florida town. The *Gazette* was quick to defend the salubrity of Pensacola acknowledging that Dr. Clarkson and a few others had indeed died but from smallpox, not yellow fever. He also stated that all the sick aboard the Grampus had been transferred to the hospital at Barrancas, "nine miles from Pensacola."[4]

1. ASP Nav. Aff., III, 102. Register for year, 1828.
2. Ibid., p. 253. Register for year, 1829.
3. Pensacola *Gazette*, May 19, 1829.
4. Ibid., July 21, 1829.

Clay, Eleazer G., Fernandina, 1819-1879

Dr. Clay, one of Fernandina's most esteemed physicians, was born in Chesterfield County, Virginia, in 1819.[1] After early schooling in local schools he entered the University of Virginia from which he was graduated in both medicine and law in 1840.[2] He began his professional career in medicine in Richmond near his ancestral home. In 1857 he moved to Fernandina and except for brief intervals remained there until his death on July 9, 1879.[3]

Soon after the beginning of the Civil War Fernandina, owing to its strategic location as a gateway to Florida and fairly good harbor, found itself a target for Union occupation. Aware of the vulnerability of Fernandina and Amelia Island, Governor John Milton named Joseph Finegan, a Fernandina lawyer, to head the state's military forces. He established headquarters at Ft. Clinch near the mouth of the St. Mary's River. In the earlier stages of its organization the post was without a medical staff, relying instead on local physicians. Dr. Clay was one of those who offered his services, actually enlisting on July 23, 1861, and serving as acting surgeon during the month of September. There is no evidence that he was ever mustered into the Confederate Army although he continued to lend his help in emergency situations as, for example, during the measles epidemic which struck Camp Davis on Amelia Island in the winter of 1861-62.[4] It is assumed that Dr. Clay's age, 42 in February 1862, and family, wife and four children ages two to 13, relieved him of any military obligation beyond that which could be fulfilled locally.

With the occupation of Amelia Island by Union troops in March 1862, Dr. Clay is presumed to have departed with his family for the interior of the state, as did nearly all who were loyal to the Southern cause. The meager evidence points to the probability that he spent the next three years in Gainesville.[5] The following notice appeared in the Gainesville *New Era*, December 9, 1865:

> All persons indebted to me for medical services in Gainesville and its vicinity are requested to make payment to Col. L. Dozier, who is fully authorized by me to collect and receipt for the same. (Signed) E.G. Clay, M.D.

Once more in Fernandina in early 1866 Dr. Clay presented himself as a candidate for a seat on the City Council. As a member of the Union Party he won handily as did all Union Party candidates.[6] Henceforth he was an active practitioner and citizen of the town. His professional card appeared regularly in the local newspaper.[7]

Dr. Clay was among the small group of Florida physicians who responded to the call of the Duval County Medical Society in 1874 to meet in the Jacksonville office of Dr. Abel S. Baldwin on January 14 for the purpose of organizing a Florida Medical Association.[8] He became a charter member, maintaining his membership until his death, having attended the session of April 1878 held at the Florida Yacht Club in Jacksonville.[9]

A few months later Dr. Clay was beset by illness which ended his medical career. The Fernandina *Florida Mirror* announced on March 8, 1879, with pleasure that the doctor was able "to appear again on our streets after a lingering illness of nearly two months." He died on July 9.

Of Dr. Clay's three sons and one daughter, two sons preceded him in death. The eldest son, John L., survived him and in 1880 was a druggist in Fernandina.[10]

1. Archives, University of Virginia, Lists of Students and Graduates.
2. Ibid. The obituary notice for Dr. Clay states that, after receiving degrees at the University of Virginia, he enrolled at "the Philadelphia Medical College" from which he received a second M.D. This has not been verified, however, and since he does not appear among the graduates of either the University of Pennsylvania or Jefferson Medical College, he may have received such a degree from Pennsylvania Medical College which existed from 1839 until 1861.
3. Fernandina *Florida Mirror*, July 12, 1879, obituary notices. Some statements are not to be trusted without further verification. For example, his date of birth is stated as 1829, while University of Virginia records show him as a graduate in 1840. Also the assertion that the town of Fernandina consisted of only two houses in 1857 is an obvious error. The statement that he was born on the same Virginia plantation as Henry Clay is open to question.
4. Franklin A. Doty, ed., "The Civil War Letters of Augustus Henry Mathers, Assistant Surgeon, Fourth Florida Regiment, CSA," Florida Historical Quarterly, XXXVI, No. 1, July 1957, p. 119.
5. With cessation of publication of most Florida newspapers after the war began we are deprived of a most useful source. Although the Fernandina *Peninsula* began publication in April 1863 and continued for several months, it was little more than an organ for the local command post of the Union Army supplying information on events in the North as well as developments on the battlefronts. Besides, only 212 white persons, i.e., civilians, a third of them children, remained there. See ibid., April 30, 1863.
6. Gainesville *New Era*, March 31, 1866.
7. See, for example, Fernandina *Observer*, June 28, 1873.
8. *Proceedings, Florida Medical Association*, 1874, Jacksonville.
9. Ibid., 1878, Jacksonville.
10. U.S. Census, 1880, Nassau County, Florida. No information has emerged concerning the fate or whereabouts of Dr. Clay's widow, Anna, and his daughter, Letty.

Clements, Joel B., Marianna, 1812-1834

Dr. Clements, a native of Fayetteville, Tennessee, began the practice of medicine in Marianna in the fall of 1832 at age 21. What appeared to be a promising career was terminated by his untimely death on September 19, 1834. Obituary notices identified him as the son of Major Benjamin Clements. According to the Pensacola *Gazette*, he "obtained a considerable business and practiced his profession with such success. His amiable manners and upright conduct obtained for him the goodwill and confidence of all who became acquainted with him."[1]

1. Tallahassee *Floridian*, October 4, 1834; Pensacola *Gazette*, October 11, 1834. At the Fourth of July celebration in Marianna in 1834 Dr. Clements offered a toast to General Jackson, "the hero of New Orleans." Tallahassee *Floridian*, August 2, 1834.

Clopton, J.A., Monticello and Tallahassee, (unknown)

Dr. Clopton was probably typical of the itinerant physicians who from time to time offered their services to the people of North Florida. It was their custom to establish a contact in the town which they expected to visit and use that person as a reference in gaining the confidence of local citizens. Dr. Clopton, based in Huntsville, Alabama, visited Florida in the winter of 1865, stopping first at Monticello and proceeding from there to Tallahassee. His public notice first appearing in the Tallahassee *Semi-weekly Floridian* on December 5, 1865, announced that he would be at the City Hotel, Tallahassee, from December 10 to 17, after finishing his stint in Monticello. He professed expertise in "treating piles, fistula, fissures, strictures, polypus, tumors, hydrocele and sarcocele." He further stated that he had operated on "the worst cases in the State—one case of forty-one years standing, Mr. W.H. Berry, of Monticello." He assured his prospective patients that he "has never lost a patient, never had an accident happen."

Coe, William E., Jackson, Gadsden and Franklin Counties, 1831

Dr. Coe was born about 1831 in Alabama, son of Major Jesse Coe, one of north Florida's wealthiest planters. Major Coe had migrated to Florida in the 1830s and purchased extensive acreage on the Apalachicola River a few miles north of the Ochesee settlement.[1] The plantation was known as Ioney Place. William's early interest in medicine was nurtured by Dr. Charles A. Hentz who became a friend of the Coe family during his brief residence in Ochesee.[2] Young Coe went to Quincy where he continued to "read medicine" under the direction of Dr. William Booth,[3] then entered the Medical College of South Carolina in the fall of 1853 and was graduated as M.D. in the spring of 1855 after writing a doctoral thesis on "Dysmenorrhea."

Returning to Florida Dr. Coe apparently felt no particular urgency about practicing his profession until he met and married Mary McClay of Apalachicola sometime in 1857. In March 1858, he announced the opening of his office in Apalachicola "over J.I. Griffin's Drug Store."[4] Two years later, however, he had transferred his practice to Quincy where he bought what was known as the Boling Baker Place just south of the town.[5] In the meantime his father and older brother Jesse, had died, and Dr. Coe inherited the bulk of the family estate. He escaped war service probably because of his profession or possibly, thought Dr. Hentz, by employing a substitute.[6] At any rate, he divided his time from about 1860 until the end of the war between his Quincy home and the plantation on the river. Soon after the war Dr. Coe sold the plantation and used the initial payment from the purchaser to enter the mercantile business in Apalachicola in partnership with James Evans. Neither partner, however, seems to have been endowed with much business acumen and this, combined with economic disruptions following the war, proved disastrous. Their business failed.[7]

Dr. Coe, even prior to his marriage, had survived some skirmishes with alcoholism. Dr. Hentz, who certainly had great affection for Dr. Coe, tells of an earlier encounter with death as the result of an extended "spree."[8] Discouraged by the business failure, Dr. Coe turned again to drink. This time it proved fatal, although Dr. Hentz, never one to hide his disdain for the skills of certain of his colleagues and surely not one to minimize his own, asserted that Dr. Coe was killed by the "insane medication" administered by the two physicians in attendance in total disregard for the pleadings of his distraught wife.[9]

After Dr. Coe's death, which occurred prior to 1870, Mrs. Coe moved from Apalachicola back to Quincy. Two children had been born to the marriage, a son, John McClay Coe, and a daughter who died at an early age. The son later moved to Pensacola where he opened a successful book and stationery shop. Some of his descendants are prominent citizens of Pensacola today.[10]

1. Julia Floyd Smith, *Slavery and Plantation Growth in Antebellum*, Gainesville, 1973, p. 216. The slave schedule, in the census of 1860, Jackson County, p. 38, lists for William E. Coe 26 slaves and for the "Estate of Jesse Coe" 34. Major Coe had been born in Maryland and had lived in Alabama before coming to Florida. His two sons, Jesse Jr. and William, were born in Alabama. U.S. Census, 1850, Jackson County, Florida, p. 550.

2. Chas. A. Hentz, "Autobiography," typed transcription of manuscript in the Southern Collection, University of North Carolina, Chapel Hill, Library. Dr. Hentz wrote in intimate detail of his close relationship with the Coe family during his stay in Ochesee.

3. Ibid., p. 243. Here Dr. Hentz states that young Will Coe "entered a course of reading under me." The Medical College record, however, cites Dr. Booth as Coe's preceptor. Archives, Medical College of South Carolina, List of Matriculants and Graduates.

4. Apalachicola *Commercial Advertiser*, March 10, 1858.

5. Hentz, "Autobiography" I. 244. The home was later purchased by a Mrs. McFarlin and subsequently called the "McFarlin Place."

6. Ibid.

7. Ibid., I, 245-6.

8. Ibid., I, 244-5. The pages of Dr. Hentz's "Autobiography" abound in strictures against excessive use of alcohol which he observed among both his patients and his colleagues. If we may accept his accounts, intemperance was not an uncommon weakness even among the well-to-do males of his acquaintance. His remarks, however, were more often compassionate than censorious.

9. Ibid., I, 246. The physicians were Drs. J.M.G. Hunter and F.B. Wakefield.

10. U.S. Census, 1860, Gadsden County, p. 57. Here the son John's age was two.

Cohen, Jacob, Nassau and Madison Counties, 1818-post 1880

Dr. Cohen was born in Georgetown, South Carolina, in 1818, the son of a father of the same name. He appears to have spent his childhood in Georgetown. After choosing medicine as a profession he went to Charleston, where he had relatives, and in due time began an apprenticeship in the office of Dr. Benjamin B. Strobel, one of the city's more reputable, though sometimes controversial, practitioners. In the fall of 1837 Cohen matriculated at the Medical College of the State of South Carolina from which he was graduated on March 13, 1839, after submitting a thesis on the subject "Rubeola, or Measles."[1]

After practicing for about 20 years in South Carolina Dr. Cohen and his wife, Leah, then aged 42 and 43 respectively, moved to Fernandina, arriving there in the summer of 1859. They found lodging in a boarding house along with 19 others, including another physician, Dr. Daniel Catchen.[2] The census enumerator found them there the following June. Meanwhile, in November 1859 Dr. Cohen opened a drug store in the town, a notice of which appeared in the local newspaper on November 17.[3] A week later the editor called attention to Dr. Cohen's presence with the following testimonial.[4]

> The doctor is a regularly educated physician, has had twenty years of practice in his profession, and therefore his goods may be relied upon as being pure and well selected. Moreover, the Doctor is a first rate fellow and those who deal with him will be certain to find out.

Dr. Cohen's practice in Fernandina was abruptly terminated three years later when Union forces besieged the town in early March 1862. The Cohens were among the Confederate sympathizers who hurriedly evacuated the town, many of whom—especially the merchants—had little time for removing their belongings.[5] Most of the people fled into the interior of Florida, among them Dr. Cohen who settled in the village of Ellaville, in Madison County.[6] As far as is known the Cohens spent the rest of their lives there. The Census of 1880 includes the following entry: "J. Cohen, 62, practicing medicine, born in S.C.; Leah Cohen, 64, wife, b. S.C."[7] One additional item bears inclusion. In its issue of May 20, 1879, the Tallahassee *Weekly Floridian* listed the signers of a petition urging the rebuilding of the Leon County Court House. Included among the signers was Jacob R. Cohen.

1. Archives, Waring Medical Historical Library, Medical University of South Carolina, Charleston. See also Charleston (S.C.) *Courier*, March 21, 1839.
2. U.S. Census, 1860, Nassau County, Florida, p. 69. This entry indicates that Dr. Cohen was a man of moderate means, owning real estate valued at $3,000 and personal property worth $35,000.
3. Fernandina *East Floridian*, November 17, 1859. Dr. Cohen advertised Fresh Drugs, Genuine Chemicals, Imported and Domestic Perfumes, to be sold only for cash. He added that he would not be undersold in any Southern market.
4. Ibid., November 24, 1859.
5. For an account of the siege and evacuation see John E. Johns, *Florida During the Civil War*, Gainesville, 1963, pp. 62-63.
6. Ellaville, Madison County, is located on the Suwannee River about 13 miles southeast of the town of Madison. Several Cohen families are listed in the Florida Census of 1870. Dr. Jacob Cohen was not among them.
7. U.S. Census, 1880, Madison County, Florida, item 374.

Colbert, Thomas M., Gainesville, 1865-1866

Dr. Colbert, a brief sojourner, arrived in Gainesville in late 1865 and offered his services in medicine and surgery to the people on December 21.[1] His professional card claimed for him "fourteen years of constant practice in the South," an obvious effort to rid himself of the label of "carpetbagger." His specialty was diseases of women; his residence and office at the Suwannee Hotel.

If the citizens of Gainesville and vicinity had any reservations as to the professional skill and dedication of Dr. Colbert, they were totally dispelled during the onset of a smallpox epidemic in the spring of 1866. In his account of the sickness, W.H. Robertson, editor of the Gainesville *New Era*, wrote that the work of "Dr. Colbert should not be unnoticed; a stranger, it is true, but he cast his all with those who mostly needed professional service." This statement was followed by a paragraph of lavish praise for his efficient and unselfish attention to his patients.[2] This was followed by the letter of a subscriber who had survived the disease, thanks in great measure to the attention he had received at the hands of Dr. Colbert. In part, he wrote, "Prominent among those who have stood forward in this Christian and noble duty is Dr. T.M. Colbert (now down with the disease himself), Col. Spencer,[3] and Lt. M.R. Cooper.[4] These three, though strangers, disregarded the danger to themselves and courageously attended to the needs of the afflicted."[5]

With the epidemic under control and his reputation as a trustworthy citizen firmly established, Dr. Colbert entered into other areas of community activity. He was one of a small group which included Dr. Gabriel P. Thomas and the Honorable J.C. Gardner, Mayor of Gainesville, who met on May 25, 1866, and organized the Gainesville Literary Association, which provided a forum for the discussion of challenging issues and topics of the times.[6] Their first regular meeting a short time later featured a debate on the question, "Is Military or Literary Fame Preferable?" A later meeting would address the topic, "Is Monarchical or Republican Government Preferable?"

Dr. Colbert's professional card continued to appear in the *New Era* until it ceased publication after the issue of November 23, 1866. Beyond that date nothing is known of this highly-regarded citizen.

1. Gainesville *New Era*, December 9, 1865.
2. Ibid., April 20, 1866.
3. Mayor of Gainesville.
4. An officer of the Gainesville Post, U.S. Army of Occupation.
5. The compassion of these men helped reduce the hostility of local residents toward the federal troops occupying the town.
6. Gainesville *New Era*, June 1, 1866.

Cole, Algernon S., Leon County, 1823

Dr. Cole, a native of North Carolina, was the son of Charles Cole, a successful planter who settled in Leon County in the 1830s.[1] The Cole plantation is thought to have been located near Dawkin's Pond, five miles south of the Georgia border just off the Thomasville Road.[2] The 1840 Census indicates that only the elder Cole and his son were members of the household. Records of the Jefferson Medical College, Philadelphia, list Algernon Cole as a graduate of the College in the spring of 1846, with the added note that he had matriculated from Florida.

After receiving his degree Dr. Cole returned to the home of his father and began medical practice. Two entries in the diary of a neighbor, planter Charles Bannerman, show that Dr. Cole was the family doctor in 1857.[3] No record of military service of Dr. Cole has been found. On November 2, 1865, after the death of his father, he married Miss Fannie E. Barksdale of Blakely (Early County) Georgia. They had two sons, Charles and Willis. Dr. Henry E. Palmer of Tallahassee writing about Dr. Cole in 1939, and depending upon information supplied by persons who recalled Dr. Cole, mentioned him as "a very fine man" and "a great hunter." The date of Dr. Cole's death has not been located.

1. His earliest appearance in Florida records is thought to have been that found in the Leon County Census of 1840.
2. Henry E. Palmer, "Physicians of Early Tallahassee and Vicinity," *Apalachee*, Tallahassee, 1944, p. 42.
3. "Journal of Charles Bannerman, Leon County, Florida." Typescript, 1930, P.K. Yonge Library of Florida History. This document is included in James D. Glunt, "Plantation and Frontier Records of East and Middle Florida, 1789-1868," unpublished, doctoral dissertation, University of Michigan, 1930. Entry of March 10, 1857: "Our little son, George, is very ill; sent for Dr. Cole." The entry of April 13, 1857: "Death of Bannerman son, Thomas. Attended by Dr. Cole."
4. Tallahassee *Semi-Weekly Floridian*, November 10, 1865.

Coleman, Allen W., Leon and Gadsden Counties, 1820s, 1830s

Although nothing is known of his origin and ultimate fate, Dr. Coleman was a fairly prominent practitioner and citizen of Florida for at least 20 years. He appears to have arrived in Leon County in 1825, at least in time to participate in the town election held on the first Monday of January 1826 in which he served as one of three supervisors.[1] He was present at the town's celebration of the occasion where he proposed a toast on July 4, 1826, to John MacPherson Berrien, United States Senator from Georgia, famous for his firm stand on states' rights and at one time President Jackson's attorney-general.[2] A few weeks later, on August 24, he announced the continuation of his medical practice from his residence at the northeast corner of the Capitol Square.[3] From this it may be inferred that he had been practicing in Tallahassee for some time and had moved to a new location. In December of that year he sought to retrieve his copy of the *Edinburgh Depository* by publishing a plea that the borrower "not having thought proper to return it, oblige him by leaving it at the office of the *Florida Intelligencer*."[4]

Earlier in 1826 Dr. Coleman had joined four other Tallahassee doctors in publishing a schedule of fees agreed upon as compensation for attendance, performing operations, and for medicines.[5] After the platting of the town in 1828 and 1829, Dr. Coleman entered the real estate market, purchasing, all told, 10 lots, the first transaction occurring in February 1828, the last in the summer of 1829.[6] The total price for the 10 lots was $819.[6]

There are indications that before the end of 1829 Dr. Coleman's fortune began to wane. Two of his lots were sold by the Sheriff of Leon County, presumably to satisfy the tax collector.[7] At approximately the same time he advertised opening of a bathing house "where GENTLEMEN can take a cold or hot bath any time of day or until 10 o'clock at night."[8]

Further evidence that things were not going well for Dr. Coleman may be inferred in his decision to leave Tallahassee in 1830 and take over operation of a Quincy hotel formerly run by a Dr. Wilson. In a weakly-worded announcement of February 16, 1830, he promised "To those who may favor him with a call, he only pledges himself to do the best he can."[9] This also appears to have been an unprofitable venture for in late 1831 or early 1832 he had returned to practice medicine in Tallahassee. Among his patients was David S. Rogers who languished in the Tallahassee jail for several months after being arrested for murder. Dr. Coleman's bill for $65 was finally paid in 1833 by authorization of the Florida Legislative Council.[10]

Beginning in June 1832 Dr. Coleman's professional card appeared regularly for nearly a year then ceased altogether; however, on December 31, 1836, there appeared in the Tallahassee newspaper an advertisement somewhat typical of the medical notices of the times. It offered for sale at the drug store of E. Barnard Jr. & Co. Dr. A.W. Coleman's Soldier's Pills for which the following claim was made: "They have been used in private practice for the last twelve years, and have been found highly beneficial in fever, influenza, liver affections, colds and measles. They act with certainty on the Bowels and Skin."[11] Does this suggest a last effort at professional success or the beginning of a profitable enterprise?

Information on the private and family life of Dr. Coleman has not been forthcoming. The Gadsden County Census of 1830 indicates a wife and three sons, while in the Leon County Census of 1840 only the doctor and his wife are listed. In both instances there are two slaves. Dr. William S. Coleman, a medical practitioner of the 1840s and 1850s in Leon, Wakulla and Gadsden Ccounties, may have been a son of Dr. Allen W. Coleman; however, proof is lacking.[12]

1. Bertram H. Groene, *Ante-Bellum Tallahassee*, Tallahassee, 1971, p. 26.

2. Tallahassee *Florida Intelligencer*, July 22, 1826.

3. Ibid., September 1, 1826.

4. Ibid., December 3, 1826. "Depository," as shown here, is an error for the *Edinburgh Dispensatory*, an extremely popular pharmaceutical handbook or *Vade Mecum* of the times. Between 1699 and 1841 it went through 12 editions and is said to have had more than 50 printings, including six in America.

5. Ibid., April 14, 1826. The other signers were: C.A. Watkins, M.D.; Edmund Tucker, R.S.R. Wilson, M.D.; and Lewis Willis, M.D. It is significant that neither Coleman nor Tucker claimed a medical degree, made obvious by the fact that the other three did.

6. "Leon County, Florida." Records compiled by the Tallahassee Chapter, Daughters of the American Revolution, typed copy, 1937, pp. 105-110.

7. Ibid.

8. Tallahassee *Floridian and Advocate*, September 1, 1829. Incidentally the Edinburgh Medical Faculty favored

frequent and careful bathing.

9. Ibid., March 2, 1830. The notice bears the date, Quincy, February 16, 1830.

10. *Florida Legislative Council*, 11th Session, Acts, February 6, 1833. Also included in *Proceedings* of same session, p. 49.

11. Tallahassee *Floridian*, December 31, 1836.

12. If this surmise should be valid we may conclude that Dr. A.W. Coleman was born in South Carolina, Dr. William having been a native of that state and an 1840 alumnus of the Medical College at Charleston.

Coleman, George E., Volusia County, 1839-1883

Dr. Coleman, the first physician to settle and practice medicine in Volusia County, was born in Towanda (Bradford County), New York, on January 4, 1839. He was the son of Joseph H. and Sarah (Roberts) Coleman.[1] He is said (probably on the basis of information provided by his daughter) to have attended a medical school in Fond du Lac, Wisconsin.[2] He was married on January 17, 1867, to a Wisconsin girl, Ella E. Johnson, some four years his junior. She was the daughter of Alfred E. Johnson, who moved to Volusia County in 1867, purchased a large portion of land known as the Heriot Tract located on the west bank of the Halifax River and embracing a large part of what is now Daytona Beach (west of the river).

In late 1867 the Colemans came to Florida for a visit with Mrs. Coleman's parents. They were pleased with the area, decided to settle there, where they would spend the rest of their lives. From this time on Dr. Coleman appears to have devoted less time to medical practice and more to other pursuits. He purchased a substantial part of the Heriot property from his father-in-law. Within a few years, however, probably because of the "Panic of 1873" and the general economic collapse of the country, Dr. Coleman sold about half his Heriot holdings to George W. Kingston, a sale of 1875. A short time later he sold a portion of the remainder to his older brother, Silas, who had decided to settle in Florida.

Subsequent events further indicate that times were indeed hard. With incorporation of the town of Daytona Beach in 1874, Dr. Coleman ran for the office of Tax Assessor which he won. He also served for a brief period as postmaster of nearby Port Orange during the illness of the incumbent, his friend, James Sawyer. At about the same juncture he purchased a mule, said to have been the first such creature in Volusia County. With a mule and a buggy he brought the mail from St. Augustine to Daytona. He is also known to have run a livery stable. Still, there is evidence that he continued to practice medicine.[3]

Dr. Coleman died at his home in Daytona Beach on January 4, 1883,[4] his 44th birthday, and was buried in Greenwood Cemetery. He was survived by his wife, who lived on until 1919, and his only child, a daughter named Harriet (Hattie), who became the wife of Doty Hobart of Daytona Beach.

1. Except for census data this biographical sketch has been drawn from two sources: Pleasant Daniel Gold, *History of Volusia County*, Biographical Section, Deland, E.O. Painter Printing Company, 1927, pp. 316-317, and T.E. Fitzgerald, *Volusia County: Past and Present*, Daytona Beach, The Observer Press, 1937, pp. 98, 111, 113.

2. This medical school apparently existed for only a brief period.

3. In the Volusia County Censuses of 1870 and 1880 Dr. Coleman is designated "Physician." Other census data are not to be trusted, however. The 1870 census indicates that he was a native of Wisconsin while that of 1880 states his birthplace was New Jersey.

4. Iantha Bond Hebel, "Cemetery Records of Pinewood and Greenwood, in Daytona Beach, Florida," 1958, typed copy.

Colley, William J., Marianna, 1860

Dr. Colley, a native of Georgia and graduate of the Medical College of Georgia in 1858,[1] was a brief sojourner and practitioner in Marianna. The Census of 1860 lists him as a resident in the home of Franklin Browne, whose wife is thought to have been Dr. Colley's sister.[2] He appears to have left Marianna with the outbreak of war in 1861, and there is no evidence that he ever resumed practice in the state.

1. Medical Department, University of Georgia, Augusta, "List of Graduates from 1829 to 1891," Augusta, 1890, p. 15.
2. U.S. Census, 1860, Jackson County, Florida, p. 50.

Colman, William S., Leon, Wakulla and Gadsden Counties, 1840-1850

Florida sources yield very little information about the life of Dr. Colman. He was a native of South Carolina[1] and in the spring of 1840 received his medical degree from the Medical College of the State of South Carolina.[2] About a year later he arrived in Florida and announced his intention to practice medicine in Port Leon, situated in what was then Leon County.[3] The announcement had a tentative ring, however, in that he committed himself to practice only for the summer. In April 1842 the following notice appeared:[4]

> Dr. Colman, being about to leave Port Leon and St. Marks for the present year would offer the citizens of those places and surrounding country due acknowledgements for past favors, and would inform those who are indebted to him for professional services, that the opportunity for settlement will be offered personally at the above place Quincy during the present month.

It may be inferred that Dr. Colman's experience with the devastating yellow fever epidemic of 1841, especially deadly in the ports of the Gulf Coast, dictated that he leave before the onset of the following summer or perhaps the economic blight following the fever had rendered it impossible to make a living in Port Leon as a physician.

By 1850 Dr. Colman was again a Florida resident, this time in rural Gadsden County. The Gadsden Census of 1850 shows him married to a South Carolina native, aged 20. He had become the father of three children, aged five, three and one. The latter two were Florida-born, so it may be assumed that he had returned to Florida not later than 1847. The eldest child, aged five, was born in South Carolina. The doctor himself was 28 and the owner of real estate valued at $4,500.[5]

Except for published endorsement of a patent medicine, Dickinson's Sarsasparilla and Queen's Delight, in a Tallahassee newspaper on April 2, 1850,[6] no further information concerning Dr. Colman has been located. Since he does not appear in subsequent censuses he is presumed to have left Florida by 1860.

1. U.S. Census, Gadsden County, Florida, 1850, p. 375.
2. *Centennial Memorial, Medical College of the State of South Carolina*, Charleston, 1924, p. 119.
3. Tallahassee *Florida Sentinel*, June 18, 1841. Port Leon was located on the east bank of the St. Marks River two miles downstream from the present town of St. Marks and had been established as a picket station or lookout post for protection of St. Marks. It was destroyed in a great tidal wave of the fall of 1843 and never rebuilt.
4. Ibid., May 13, 1842, 1st printed April 15, 1842.
5. See n.1 above.
6. Tallahassee *Florida Sentinel*, April 2, 1850. This notice had been submitted by Dr. Colman on August 23, 1848.

Conover, Simon B., Lake City, Tallahassee, and Eustis, 1840-1908

Of all the so-called "carpetbaggers" who entered Florida in the aftermath of the Civil War none enjoyed greater success in both medicine and politics than Dr. Conover. Assigned to serve in a hostile environment he managed through moderation and common sense to survive the turbulence of Reconstruction in North Florida and become a trusted citizen and practitioner. He was born in New Jersey on September 23, 1840, attended medical school in the East and in 1863 entered the medical service of the United States Army. For the next three years he was surgeon in hospitals in Philadelphia, Cincinnati and Nashville. In 1866 he was assigned to the General Hospital in Lake City where he remained for about a year.[1] In September 1867 he entered private practice in Lake City in partnership with Dr. Edward S. Aldrich.[2]

With reorganization of the state government of Florida and implementation of "Radical Reconstruction," Dr. Conover was inevitably drawn into the vortex of Reconstruction politics. His stance was conservative, his party Republican. In November 1867 he was chosen to represent Columbia and Baker Counties in the constitutional convention scheduled for January.[3] Here he participated in the drafting of a constitution along more or less moderate lines and for his work was appointed to membership on the Committee of Permanent Reorganization.[4]

In the fall of 1868 Dr. Conover entered the cabinet of newly-elected Governor Harrison Reed as State Treasurer, a position he held throughout Reed's term.[5] In the meantime, having established his residence in Tallahassee, he was elected to represent Leon County in the Florida Assembly for the session beginning January 7, 1873.[6] While still there he was drawn into the contest for a seat in the United States Senate which he won by a single vote over Col. Thos. W. Osborn and Gen. S.H. Sanford.[7] When his term in the Senate came to an end in 1878 he was nominated for the House of Representatives from the First Florida Congressional district.[8] He lost to Col. R.H.M. Davidson of Gadsden County. In 1880 he was nominated for the governorship of Florida only to be defeated by William D. Bloxham.[9] This ended Dr. Conover's political career except for a brief mission as Leon County's delegate at the constitutional convention of 1885.[10]

Dr. Conover returned to his medical practice in Tallahassee in 1879 and appears to have remained there for some three or four years. By 1886, however, he had transferred his practice to Eustis in Lake County.[11] In that year he was elected to membership in the Florida Medical Association. It is recorded that he paid his dues which amounted to $5.[12] There is no record of his having ever attended a meeting of the Association and in 1892 his membership was discontinued for nonpayment of dues.[13]

It is not known just when Dr. Conover left Florida nor why he spent his last year or years in Washington State. An obituary item reveals only the following:

> Many Tallahasseeans remember ex-Republican U.S. Senator Simon B. Conover and his excellent wife kindly and will regret to read the following: "Port Townsend, Wash., Apr. 19, 1908. Dr. Simon B. Conover, who during the administration of President Hayes was U.S. Senator from Florida, died at a hospital today of infirmities resulting from old age."[14]

1. Basic information concerning Dr. Conover may be found in J.B. Whitfield, comp., *Official Directory of State*

Government, Florida, Tallahassee, 1885, pp. 35-36. See also Harry G. Cutler, *History of Florida*, Chicago, 1923, I, 157.

2. Lake City *Suwannee News*, October 2, 1867.

3. Richard L. Hume, "Membership in the Florida Constitutional Convention of 1868," FHQ., LI, No. 1, July 1972, p. 19, et seq.

4. John Wallace, *Carpet-Bag Rule in Florida*, Facsimile Edition, Gainesville, 1964, p. 50.

5. Whitfield, *Official Directory*, p. 35.

6. Ibid.

7. Cutler, *History of Florida*, I, 157. See also Jerrell H. Shofner, "Political Reconstruction in Florida," FHQ, XLV, October 1966, 162-163.

8. Whitfield, *Official Directory*, p. 36.

9. Ibid.

10. Cutler, *History pf Florida*, I, 157.

11. *Proceedings, Florida Medical Association*, Session of 1886, Jacksonville, 1886.

12. Ibid., Session of 1887, Treasurer's Report.

13. Ibid., Session of 1892.

14. Tallahassee *Weekly True Democrat*, April 24, 1908, p. 10, col. 2. Ft. Townsend is a small town located on Admiralty Inlet some 40 miles northwest of Seattle. Dr. Conover and his wife, Elizabeth, a native of Pennsylvania, were the parents of two sons, Carroll D. and Leonard W. Conover. See U.S. Census, 1880, Leon County, Florida, p. 366.

Coon, Isaac S., Bradford County, 1831-1907

It is unfortunate that some of the biographical data relating to the career of Dr. Coon (Cone) are of questionable accuracy. There can be no doubt, however, that he was a man of superior intelligence and adequate professional skill. A native of Georgia, he matriculated at Oglethorpe Medical College in Savannah in the fall of 1857 and was graduated Doctor of Medicine on March 1, 1859, having submitted a doctoral thesis entitled "Gastritis."[1] He began his practice in Savannah and had hardly established himself when the Civil War loomed. Responding to the need for professional skills in the Confederate Army, he enlisted as a private in Company H, Ninth Georgia Infantry,[2] in which he is presumed to have served for the duration of the War. Prior to entering Confederate service, however, he had married, his wife known only as Georgia. She was 10 years his junior. To this marriage were born two sons, William and Harold, aged 10 and eight years respectively in 1870.[3]

There is some doubt that Dr. Coon ever returned to medical practice after the War. The Florida Census of 1870 lists him at age 34 as a resident of Bradford County, occupation, "preacher," living with his wife, Georgia, and two sons.

The remainder of Dr. Coon's career is somewhat obscure. It is apparent from the census data of 1880 that, subsequent to the War's end, he retired from active medical practice. The Bradford County census of 1880 designates his occupation as "farming." Meanwhile the first Mrs. Coon had died and he had married Eliza, a Georgia native. The Census of 1880 lists the following members of the family: Thomas, aged 22, probably a son of Mrs. Coon by her previous husband, Ada, Ann, Isaac, John and George, the latter two apparently twins being only two months old.

It is doubtful that, subsequent to the Civil War, Dr. Coon ever returned to full-time medical practice. In fact, the Census of 1880, designates him only as farmer.[4] He lived on until 1907.[5]

1. Savannah *Daily News*, March 3, 1859.
2. Confederate Records, Ninth Regiment, Georgia Infantry Volunteers, 1831-1907.
3. U.S. Census, Bradford County, 1880, p. 247.
4. See note 2, supra.
5. Dr. Coon was buried in Crosby Lake Cemetery located on State Highway 48 north of Starke.

Cooper, James A., Madison and Alachua Counties, 1797-1883

Dr. Cooper, who spent the greater part of his professional career in Florida, was born in Georgia on January 18, 1797.[1] Of his early education and professional training nothing is presently known. It is assumed, however, that he read medicine and observed medical procedures in the office of a practicing physician, thus qualifying him for a license to practice.

Dr. Cooper was a resident of Madison County in 1850. By that date he was apparently a widower, sharing his home with his daughter, Mary, and her husband, Dr. Augustus H. Mathers. Soon after their marriage Dr. and Mrs. Mathers left their Madison County home, moving to Alachua County and availing themselves of the cheap land then available in and around Micanopy. Dr. Mathers opened an apothecary shop, an enterprise in which Dr. Cooper joined him in 1853. Their place of business after a few years came to be known as The Old Reliable Drug Store. The Cooper house was located at the corner of Main Street and Ocala Road.[2]

Dr. Cooper appears to have taken an active interest in the public affairs of the village. When the issue of incorporation of Micanopy was presented to the citizens for their consideration, Dr. Cooper was one of eight voters opposing incorporation.[3] Presumably he assumed that incorporation would soon entail regulation regarding the use of property. Besides incorporation would surely lead to imposition of taxes for the support of various civic requirements such as laying out streets, providing fire and police protection, and stipends for town officials.

Dr. Cooper enjoyed a fairly long and pleasant life in Micanopy.[4] His death came on March 24, 1883. Survivors included his wife, Mary Ann, who died on December 8, 1892, a daughter, Mrs. Mathers, and son James (1852-1904).

1. U.S. Census, Madison County, Florida, item 30.
2. Carolina B. Watkins, *The Story of Historic Micanopy*, Gainesville, Alachua County Historical Commission, 1976, p. 76. Mrs. Watkins has been able to identify the location of the Cooper house with information provided by Dr. Cooper's granddaughter, Mrs. A.H. Simpson of High Springs, Florida.
3. A record of this vote has been preserved in the James D. Glunt Collection, P.K. Yonge Library of Florida History, University of Florida. Interestingly, five of the six physicians of Micanopy voted against incorporation, only Dr. F.E. Carne voting affirmatively. Other physicians voting against were Drs. A.H. Mathers, George B. Payne, L.B. Montgomery, and James A. Stewart.
4. The dates of birth and death of members of the Cooper family are from gravestones in the Micanopy Cemetery.

Copland, Alexander, Leon County, 1830-1831

Information concerning Dr. Copland is meager, but it is known that for at least a short time he was a medical practitioner at Tuscawilla. In July 1830 he announced his presence by means of a professional card which read: "Dr. Copland, having fixed himself at Tuscawilla, at the residence of Mr. John Parkhill, offers his professional services to the public."[1]

For at least another year Dr. Copland resided in Tuscawilla. When Joseph M. White, Florida's delegate in Congress, visited the community in August 1831 he was honored at a dinner. Among those offering toasts was Dr. Copland, whose flattering words were addressed to President Andrew Jackson.[2] Nothing moreis known of Alexander Copland.

1. Tallahassee *Floridian and Advocate*, July 6, 1830. Tuscawilla, a settlement about 12 miles from Tallahassee

on the Tallahassee-Monticello post road. Its post office was established in 1828 and discontinued in 1837. For several decades the Parkhill family were politically and socially prominent in Leon County.

2. Tallahassee *Floridian and Advocate*, August 17, 1831. Dr. William Argyle, also a resident of Tuscawilla, also gave a toast.

Cornick, William F., Key West, 1862

In spite of the prevailing Southern sympathies of most Key West residents the island remained in Union hands throughout the Civil War. Among those serving the medical needs of the Union soldiers garrisoned there was Assistant Surgeon William F. Cornick, who in 1862 was the health officer of the city. He had been commissioned in the Medical Department of the United States Army on October 31, 1860. He was born in Virginia and had enlisted from that state.[1] Dr. Cornick was transferred to Hilton Head, South Carolina, in August 1862 being replaced by Dr. Edward S. Hoffman, hitherto a medical officer at Ft. Jefferson, The Tortugas.[2] Dr. Cornick resigned his commission on October 9, 1865.[3]

1. MDUSA, p. 295.
2. Key West *New Era*, August 16, 1862.
3. MDUSA, p. 295.

Cousins, William E.M., Hamilton, Columbia and Suwannee Counties, 1814

Although biographical data are sparse, there is evidence for designating Dr. Cousins as physician-politician, a not uncommon dual role for medically trained men in the 19th century when medical practice was not always a full-time occupation. Born in Virginia about 1814,[1] Dr. Cousins was graduated from the Medical Department, University of Georgia, in the class of 1845.[2] There is some evidence that he had previously lived in Butts County, Georgia, possibly "reading medicine" with a local doctor. No preceptors have been identified, however.

On completion of his medical degree or shortly thereafter Dr. Cousins established a medical practice in Hamilton County. He is thought to have been one of the earliest physicians in the area.[3] He was doubtless a man of moderate means. The 1860 census enumerator valued his real estate at $1,600 and other properties at $7,575.[4] A list of guests at Buffington House, Jacksonville's best hotel, in late December 1851 includes Dr. Cousins and servant.[5] Men of meager means did not normally travel with servants. Further evidence of Dr. Cousin's financial competence is seen in his assumption of leadership of the Whig Party in Hamilton County in the critical year, 1852. In Florida this was the party of the planter and well-to-do business and professional men in whose company Dr. Cousins felt comfortable.

Dr. Cousins first came into political prominence at a meeting of Whigs from the Middle District of Florida in Tallahassee on May 29, 1852. He was named Hamilton County delegate to the national convention of Whigs scheduled for Baltimore in June.[6] Simultaneously he was appointed corresponding secretary for his party in Hamilton County.[7] After his return from Baltimore and the disappointment of the Southern Whigs at their failure to nominate Millard Fillmore, Dr. Cousins was Hamilton County's delegate to a convention of Florida Whigs in Tallahassee on July 14, its purpose being to evaluate the Baltimore proceedings and chart a future for the rapidly disintegrating party.[8]

Dr. Cousins was among the leaders who kept the party alive in Florida for an additional two years. In July 1854 he presided over a Whig caucus at Providence, Columbia County,[9] a dying gasp for the party which had already fallen apart nationally. But Dr. Cousins was not finished. In 1856 he was elected to a seat in the Florida Legislature representing Columbia County in the House.[10]

The year 1860 found Dr. Cousins living alone in Suwannee County, which had been organized in 1858.[11] Beyond this nothing more is known. Since he does not appear in the Florida Census of 1870, he is presumed to have died by that time.

1. This date is based upon information in censuses of 1850 and 1860. In the former he was 37 years old, in the latter, 46.
2. Medical Department, University of Georgia, *List of Graduates from 1829 to 1891*, August 1791, p. 15.
3. Cora Hinton, *A Brief History of Hamilton County*, Jasper, 1976, p. 51.
4. U.S. Census, 1860, Hamilton County, Florida, p. 460.
5. Jacksonville *Florida Republican*, January 8, 1852.
6. Ibid., June 8, 1852.
7. Ibid.
8. Ibid., July 29, 1852. The nomination went instead to General Winfield Scott who lost to Democrat Franklin Pierce in the November general election.
9. Ibid., July 20, 1854. Providence is now located in Union County which was organized in 1921.
10. *House Journal*, 8th session, Tallahassee, 1856, p. 4.
11. U.S. Census, 1860, Suwannee County Florida, p. 44.

Cowgill, Clayton A., Putnam County, 1826-1893

Of the numerous Northerners who yielded to the charm of the St. Johns River and chose to settle on its banks in the early years after the Civil War none possessed more laudable qualities nor fitted more congenially into the local scene than did Dr. Cowgill. He was born in Kent County, Delaware, on January 21, 1826, grew up in Dover, where he attended the common schools until he was 14. He then enrolled at Dickinson College, Carlisle, Pennsylvania, where he prepared himself for medical study. According to his own statement he then attended medical college in Philadelphia, graduating in 1846.[1] He then returned to Dover where he practiced medicine until 1861, when he entered the Federal Army as surgeon to a volunteer regiment.

While in Dover Dr. Cowgill became involved in local politics, accepting the principles of the old Whig Party. In 1852, in spite of the imminent demise of the Party, he was appointed Clerk of the Delaware House of Representatives. As a matter of course he allied himself with the emerging Republican Party to which he remained faithful for the remainder of his life.[2]

In 1862, with the Civil War well under way, Dr. Cowgill was sent to New Bern, North Carolina, which had fallen to the Union troops of General Burnside on March 14. He occupied the post of chief medical officer of the hospital there, which he held until the end of the War. When a deadly epidemic of yellow fever swept through the town in 1864, he was said to have performed heroic service at great personal risk. His unselfish devotion to duty, notwithstanding his own serious illness and near encounter with death, came to the attention of President Lincoln at whose order he was breveted Lieutenant Colonel in 1865.[3]

Dr. Cowgill moved to Florida in 1867, settling in Putnam County on the east bank of the St. Johns River some eight miles down river from Palatka. To the site he gave the name Penn. There he built a house and planted an orange grove of about a thousand trees on some 20 acres of his total holding of more than 200 acres. It appears to have been a moderately successful enterprise.[4]

After a couple of years, and being fully recovered in health which had been seriously impaired during the last year of the War, Dr. Cowgill gave in to the lure of politics, running successfully for a seat on the Putnam County Commission. From this position he became the prime organizer of the Republican Party in the County. It is quite probable that his deliberate and restrained approach to the public issues of difficult times contributed much to the peaceful transition out of the explosive situation created by radicals of his party. His moderation was shared by Ossian B. Hart who became Governor of Florida in 1873. Dr. Cowgill was County Commissioner from 1869 to 1873.[5] His good sense and devotion to the Party were rewarded by appointment to the office of Comptroller in Hart's cabinet. His wisdom and restraint during his term as Commissioner had not been overlooked.

With the untimely death of Governor Hart only a year and three months after taking office, and the subsequent elevation of Marcellus L. Stearns from Lieutenant Governor to acting Governor, Dr. Cowgill was retained as Comptroller. His presence there in 1876 thrust him into the midst of the bitter controversy following the presidential election of that year. According to Florida law the State Canvassing Board was composed of the Secretary of State, Attorney General and Comptroller. So Dr. Cowgill was joined on the Board by Samuel B. McLin, Republican, and William Archer, Democrat. It was their responsibility to canvass the disputed Florida election. Dr. Cowgill is said to have regarded his role in the deliberations as a balancing element between the strongly pro-Hayes-McLin and the equally staunch pro-Tilden supporter, Cocke. It was a vexatious experience for Dr. Cowgill. The election had been close and feelings were intense. He could not escape censure in spite of efforts to maintain a nonpartisan posture.[6] He was accused of equivocation and outright weakness. When the equally controversial gubernatorial election was finally decided by the State Supreme Court in favor of George F. Drew, the Democratic candidate, Dr. Cowgill's Tallahassee days appeared to be numbered. He was not yet finished with public life, however for in 1882 he won the Putnam County seat in the Florida Legislature and served, with somewhat diminished influence, (it had become a predominantly Democratic body) in the session of 1883.

Meanwhile, on October 7, 1873, Dr. Cowgill was married to a widow, Mrs. S.T.M. Babb, of Boston, the marrige having taken place in that city.[7] It was probably with some feeling of escape and relief that the couple returned to their home on the St. Johns River. There is evidence that Dr. Cowgill resumed the practice of medicine in his later years. The mortality schedule for Putnam County in the special Florida Census of 1885 shows him to have been the attending physician of a patient, Charles Clark, who died in November 1884.[8]

So far as is known, Dr. Cowgill lived out his life at his rural home. A post office was established at Penn in 1881 and Mrs. Cowgill was named postmistress. The only clue to the possible date of Dr. Cowgill's death comes from the fact that on January 28, 1893 the name of the post office was changed to

Clayton, perhaps a memorial to the doctor, but if true it was a brief one for on Januaryh 15, 1900, it was discontinued, being replaced by Orange Mills.

1. The biographical data relating to Dr. Cowgill are derived from two main sources: A biographical sketch written on the occasion of his becoming a member of Governor Hart's cabinet in 1873 and printed in the Jacksonville *Weekly Florida Union*, January 23, 1873, and two days later in the Tallahassee *Sentinel*; J.V. Drake, *The Florida Legislature*.
2. Drake, *The Florida Legislature*.
3. Dr. Cowgill was mustered out of the Army as Lieutenant Colonel.
4. Special Census, Putnam County, Florida, 1885; Precinct 7. Dr. Cowgill's acres numbered 210 of which only 20 were under cultivation. Its total value was $5,900.
5. Dr. Cowgill was said to have been exceedingly skillful in the management of the County's public revenues which prepared him for the Comptroller's post.
6. The entire controversy has been thoroughly explored by Professor Jerrell H. Shofner and is the subject of two excellent articles: "Florida in the Balance: The Electoral Count of 1876,"*Florida Historical Quarterly*, XLVII, October 1868, pp. 122-150, and "Florida's Courts and the Disputed Election of 1876," ibid, XLVIII, July 1969, pp. 24-46.
7. Tallahassee *Weekly Floridian* October 14, 1873.
8. See note 4, supra, Mortality Schedule.

Cox, James, St. Augustine, 1830-1831

Dr. Cox of Philadelphia arrived in St. Augustine in the late summer of 1830 apparently in search of a more benign climate. In November of that year the local newspaper, in its report on sailing vessels in and out of the harbor, noted that "a cargo of merchandise and sundries for Dr. Cox" had arrived in the schooner *Charles Millard* from Philadelphia."[1] In the same issue the report of Dr. Cox on the health of the City appeared. If indeed he were in poor health (it is assumed that he was suffering from tuberculosis), the move to Florida availed little; he died on December 21, 1831, at age 35.[2] It is doubtful that he practiced in St. Augustine.

1. St. Augustine *East Florida Herald*, November 24, 1830.
2. Ibid., January 12, 1832.

Craig, John A., Leon County, 1831-1834

Only sparse data concerning the medical career of Dr. Craig have survived. His Florida residence appears to have spanned only a few years. He was graduated from the University of Maryland School of Medicine in 1830,[1] the records of the School listing Maryland as his native state. Late in the following year he arrived in Tallahassee where on November 22 he announced his services to the citizens of the community. His office was located on Jefferson Street, "next door to Mr. Perkins' Apothecary Shop."[2] A few weeks later he removed to "the office formerly occupied by Dr. Aiken, recently deceased," which was situated at the southeast corner of Washington Square.[3]

It is evident that Dr. Craig quickly established himself as a respected member of the Tallahassee medical faculty. Early in 1833 he was among the small group of local physicians who drew up and published a "fee bill" announcing the fees agreed upon for a variety of medical services. In addition to Dr. Craig, the proponents were Drs. Lewis Willis, John B. Taylor, J.H. Randolph and John McLemore, all prominent professionally as well as socially.[4] When the bill set off a storm of protest among the few remaining physicians and other local citizens who regarded it as a move to discontinue all charity practice, Dr. Craig responded with a lengthy letter explaining the bill and assuring the public that indigent patients would still be treated without charge. The letter reveals a high degree of intelligence and literacy on the part of the writer.[5]

Among Dr. Craig's first Tallahassee patients was David S. Rogers, accused murderer, languishing in the Tallahassee jail awaiting outcome of his appeal that his death sentence be revoked. An itemized bill prepared for presentation to the Florida Legislative Council requested compensation for his services to the prisoner in a series of visits from November 3 to November 15, 1831, and another from June 3 to June 6 in the following year.[6]

Dr. Craig continued his Tallahassee practice at least throughout 1834 but he appears to have subsequently moved to lands owned by himself and his brother, William Pinckney Craig, in the Lake Hall area some five miles north of Tallahassee. The Census of 1840 lists him as owner of 37 slaves.[7] No further information on Dr. Craig's career has emerged; it appears probable that he returned to Maryland to live out his life.

1. Eugene F. Cordell, *Historical Sketch of the University of Maryland School of Medicine, 1807-1890*, Baltimore, 1891, p. 169.
2. Tallahassee *Floridian*, January 3, 1832, First printing, November 22, 1831.
3. Ibid., January 17, 1832.
4. Ibid., February 2, 1833.
5. Ibid., February 9, 1833. Dr. Craig's letter follows a similar statement by Dr. Taylor.
6. The Rogers affair created much excitement throughout Florida. Governor William P. Duval, prior to leaving Florida for an extended absence, had denied the prisoner a stay of execution. In his absence another plea for clemency was made to Secretary of the Territory James D. Westcott, then Acting Governor, but Westcott disclaimed the authority to grant such a request. Other efforts were made to delay the execution pending the next meeting of the District Court of Appeals. This too was unavailing. Rogers was publicly hanged on July 27, 1832. The questionable nature of the official proceedings created a furor which was aired in several Florida newspapers; especially the Tallahassee *Floridian*, August 14, 1832.

For more than a year after the death of Rogers Dr. Craig sought compensation from the Territory for his services in the amount of $105.50. The Legislative Council, however, rejected the request on two flimsy grounds: the record of Dr. Craig's visits to the jail had been compiled by the jailer but lacked the signature of the Judge of the District, and Rogers had friends who could well afford to pay his medical expenses. Proceedings of the Legislative Council, Rept. of James Riz, Chairman of Claims Committee. Tallahassee *Floridian*, March 1, 1834. For records of Dr. Craig's visits to the Tallahassee jail to attend David S. Rogers, see Glunt, James D., Papers, Box I, "Miscellaneous Legal Papers, 1821-1831," MSS PKYLFH, University of Florida, Gainesville.

7. U.S. Census, 1840, Leon County, Florida, p. 11. Dr. Craig, unmarried, was the sole resident of the household. His brother William P. (see ibid., p. 15) owned 73 slaves. John A. Craig, pioneer horticulturist of the Lake Hall community in the last half of the 19th century, was apparently the son of William P. Craig.
8. The statement is conjectural. Dr. Craig disappears from Florida records subsequent to 1840. William P. Craig died in Tallahassee on August 12, 1862, at age 55. Tallahassee *Sentinel* August 19, 1862.

Crawford, John C., Columbia County, 1833

Dr. Crawford, a native of South Carolina, arrived in Florida in the late 1850s,[1] settling in the village of Ellisville, a few miles north of the Santa Fe River. The year 1860 found him residing in the home of Dr. Samuel T. Day. His properties were valued at about $9,000.[2]

Dr. Crawford enlisted at Newnansville for three years' service in the Army of the Confederacy on May 20, 1862, and was assigned to Company "F", 2nd Florida Cavalry. About one year later, April 23, 1863, he obtained a discharge, having provided a substitute, a man named Green Hill.[3]

Less than a year later Dr. Crawford, then living at Cedar Keys, went aboard the Union craft, S.S. Sagamore, and took an oath of allegiance to the government of the United States. He also contracted his professional services to Union military personnel stationed at Cedar Keys. The correspondence of the U.S.

Army, Continental Command, contains a letter addressed to Surgeon A.E. Stockton, Army Medical Director at Key West, ordering him to furnish the medical supplies requisitioned by "Dr. John C. Crawford, contract physician for the Military Post at Cedar Keys, Florida." The letter was signed by H.W. Bowden, Assistant Adjutant General.[4]

Nothing further is known of Dr. Crawford. It is unlikely, however, that he would have resumed medical practice after the war in either South Carolina or Florida.

1. The earliest known reference to Dr. Crawford's presence in Florida is found in the list of arrivals at Whitfield House, Fernandina, in June 1859. His residence is shown as Ellisville, Fernandina *East Floridian*, June 9, 1859.

2. U.S. Census, 1860, Columbia County, Florida, item 323. Here Dr. Crawford's age is given as 27, which is in agreement with the age given in his military record.

3. NA, Service Records, CSA, M251, Roll 7.

4. Records, U.S. Army Continental Commands, Vol. I, 1821-1920. 111-C, Reel 4, PKYLFH.

Crawford, John Lovick, Wakulla and Leon Counties, 1816-1902

Very few public figures of Florida have enjoyed the esteem and love of their fellowmen in the measure accorded Dr. Crawford. Although his medical career was overshadowed by a long and distinguished service in public office, he is remembered as one of Florida's more eminent 19th century physicians.

Dr. Crawford was born in Greene County, Georgia, on April 17, 1816, son of David and Fanny (nee Crawford; she was a cousin of her husband) Crawford. He came from a notable family. His uncle on his mother's side was William H. Crawford, United States Senator and sometime Secretary of the Navy and Secretary of the Treasury.[1] The Crawfords were rural people, engaged in farming. When he was still a small boy, his family moved to nearby Covington, Georgia, seat of Newton County, where he spent his youth and received a basic "literary" education. With the early death of his father young John Crawford's hopes for a college education were thwarted. Instead he went to work and by 1841 had earned sufficient funds to enable him to matriculate in the Medical Department, University of Georgia, Augusta. At age 25 he was some five or six years older than most matriculants. In the spring of 1843 he was graduated with high honors.[2]

Soon after graduation Dr. Crawford entered medical practice at Bainbridge but with the admission of Florida to statehood in 1845 he moved, settling for a time in Newport, the early county seat of Wakulla County. Although Newport was at the time a thriving commercial town, Dr. Crawford, after sizing up the situation, moved inland to the village of Shell Point[3] where he purchased land and began a farming venture. He prospered as both physician and farmer, and by 1850 had accumulated a fairly large tract of land and acquired 13 slaves. In 1848 he was married to Elizabeth E. Walker, daughter of one of the county's wealthiest planters.

Inevitably Dr. Crawford's qualities of leadership were recognized and in 1847 he began a long career in public service when he was elected to the Florida House of Representatives, an office which he exchanged in the following year for a seat in the Florida Senate. In 1850 he was again elected to the Senate. In the mid-1850s, after the birth of their second child, the Crawfords left Shell Point and for several years lived in Bainbridge, it was said, so that his children might have better educational advantages than those available in Wakulla County. Upon their return to Florida as the War appeared imminent, Dr. Crawford resumed medical practice. He was again elected to the Florida Senate in 1865, continuing in office until 1875. He was returned to the Senate for the last time in 1881[4] and was there when Governor William D. Bloxham appointed him Secretary of State, the position he held until his death.

Dr. Crawford was a man of noble and steadfast principle, unwavering in time of stress. Although a slave owner he still opposed secession and deplored the South's decision to go to war. He obviously preferred emancipation of slaves to the dreadful alternative. Even after hostilities had begun he declined to support the Confederacy and yet, stated the *Weekly Tallahasseean*, "his honesty of purpose and purity of character won the confidence of his neighbors; he was unmolested."[5]

For several weeks prior to his death Dr. Crawford was in declining health. A week before Christmas 1901 he suffered a fall which resulted in a hip fracture and this hastened his death at 7 a.m. on January 24, 1902, less than three months after the death of his wife which had occurred on November 11.

His last official act was one of generosity. It had been a matter of concern to him that no portrait of Territorial Governor Richard Keith Call had ever been displayed in the State Capitol. Two days before his death Dr. Crawford donated an oil portrait of Governor Call, a treasure which had belonged to his family for many years, in the name of Ellen Call Long, "with the wish of Mrs. Long and myself that the portrait of the illustrious man be suspended in the Executive Chamber." This message was signed by Dr. Crawford above the date January 22, 1902.[6]

Of the several children born to Dr. and Mrs. Crawford, only three survived them, Henry Clay Crawford, 1856-1929, who succeeded his father as Secretary of State; Mrs. Julia Crawford Adams, wife of J.W. Adams Jr., of Crawfordville; and Charles Y. Crawford, a merchant of Arcadia, Florida.[7]

1. Of the numerous sources for the life of Dr. Crawford the most important are: Rowland H. Rerick, *Memoirs of Florida*, Francis P. Fleming, ed., I, 498-500; Elizabeth F. Smith, "A Man For All Seasons," *The Magnolia Monthly*, VI, No. 1, January, 1968, unpaginated, and Tallahassee *Weekly Tallahasseean*, issues of January 24 and 31, 1902. Much of the detail of Dr. Crawford's political career has been omitted from the present sketch.

2. Medical Department, University of Georgia, "List of Graduates from 1829 to 1891," Augusta 1891, p. 15. Rerick, loc cit, gives 1844 as the date of Dr. Crawford's graduation. The date supplied in the University List is probably the correct one.

3. In territorial times Shell Point was a rural village situated near the center of Wakulla County. In 1866, when the county seat was moved from Newport to Shell Point, its name was changed to Crawfordville in honor of Dr. Crawford who had been instrumental in effecting the change. Meanwhile Shell Point came to designate a small portion of Florida's Gulf Coast lying immediately west of the outlet of the St. Marks River.

4. Allen Morris, comp., *The People of Lawmaking in Florida*, Various editions.

5. Tallahassee *Weekly Tallahasseean*, January 24, 1902.

6. Ibid.

7. U.S. Census, 1900, DeSoto County, Florida, p. 317.

Creswell, Pickens, Marion County, 1860

The career of Dr. Creswell remains obscure. Born in South Carolina about 1830 into a family of social and political prominence, Butler and Pickens,[1] he moved to Marion County prior to 1860. His holdings were located in the Orange Springs community northeast of Ocala and near the Putnam County line. The census of 1860 lists him as planter and physician, living alone, his properties being valued at $18,000, but managed by an overseer named Robert Harper.[2]

Dr. Creswell enlisted for service in the Confederate Army on May 2, 1862, and was assigned to Company H, Seventh Florida Infantry Regiment.[3] He entered service without military rank but soon was promoted to Brevet 2nd Lieutenant. He spent more than two years at Camp Lee near Savannah, Georgia,[4] but in mid-1864 saw action in the fighting near Atlanta where he was wounded. Meanwhile he had been promoted to a first lieutenancy. He was paroled at Greensboro, North Carolina, on April 28, 1865.

Subsequent to parole nothing further is known of Dr. Creswell. He may have become incapacitated by his war wounds. No evidence has been discovered which would indicate that he returned to Florida.

1. For the family connections see Theodore D. Jervey, "The Butlers of South Carolina," *South Carolina Historical Magzine*, IV, p. 308.
2. U.S. Census, 1860, Marion County, Florida, item 167.
3. NA, Service Records, CSA, M 251, Roll 77. Dr. Creswell's military record is garbled and incomplete.
4. Of several camps named Lee, that at Savannah seems likely.

Crill, Edward S., Putnam County, 1843-1915

Dr. Crill, one of Putnam County's most eminent physicians and a public figure of distinction, was born in Oneida County, New York, on December 25, 1843. He spent his early years on the family farm, receiving his elementary education in the local school. He then attended a seminary in the area from which he gained what might be called a secondary education. In 1863 he was enrolled at the Physio-Medical Institute of Cincinnati[1] from which he was graduated as Doctor of Medicine in 1865. Following graduation he began a professional practice in Iowa Falls, Iowa, but within a year or so moved to Memphis, Tennessee, where he was practicing when the city suffered a devastating yellow fever epidemic.

In 1874 Dr. Crill, with his wife, Josie, and daughter, Carrie, arrived in Putnam County and settled at Georgetown, a village on the St. Johns River near its exit from Lake George. He practiced there for two or three years before moving to Palatka in 1877. From the very beginning of his Florida practice Dr. Crill was successful, earning the trust and devotion of his many patients. Inevitably he was drawn into public life, which after a few years completely overshadowed his medical practice. A staunch Democrat, he was persuaded to run for a seat in the State Senate in 1880. He won handily and was in Tallahassee for the opening of the session on January 4, 1881.[2] He was returned to the Senate for the sessions of 1883 and 1885. At the end of the 1885 session he was appointed State Treasurer by Governor Edward A. Perry and held this office throughout Governor Perry's administration.

After a lapse of 10 years during which he was busy with medical practice and certain business interests, Dr. Crill was returned to the Senate in 1899 and subsequently reelected for the sessions of 1901, 1903, 1905 and 1907. As a legislator he provided effective, progressive leadership, having been responsible for creation of the State Geological Survey and enactment of a much-needed Pure Food Law. As leader of the Putnam County Democrats he was, on at least one occasion, chairman of the Florida delegation to the National Democratic Convention.

As a businessman Dr. Crill was both shrewd and benevolent. Having founded the East Florida Savings and Trust Company, one of the state's leading financial institutions, he was considered an exceptionally capable financier. He was said to have been a splendid judge of the worthiness of applicants for loans and was known to have helped dozens of deserving persons through financial crises.

Dr. Crill was twice married, first on April 1, 1866, his wife dying in April, 1874. He married again in 1877, this time to a Tallahassee lady. To the first union one daughter was born and to the second two daughters.[3]

At the end of the legislative session of 1909 Dr. Crill retired to private life, resisting the urging of his friends to return to politics in 1910.[4] By that date he was already in failing health, having contracted Bright's disease (nephritis). His death came on the early morning of October 23, 1915. He was buried with full Masonic rites.

1. This college existed only from 1859 to 1885 and like its rival Cincinnati institution, the American Eclectic Medical College, lost favor with the medical profession.
2. *Florida Senate Journal*, 1881, Tallahassee, 1881.
3. The Crill daughters as listed in their father's obituary were Mrs. William H. Markham of Tallahassee, Mrs. John H. Randolph Jr. of Savannah and Mrs. Charles P. Cooper of Jacksonville.
4. *The Palatka News*, October 27, 1911.
5. A complete obituary for Dr. Crill appeared in *The Palatka News* of October 29, 1915.

Crichton, John P., Newnansville, Brooksville and Tampa, 1816-1888

Dr. Crichton, who spent the greater part of his adult life in Tampa, was born in St. Mary's, Camden County, Georgia, in 1816.[1] He was the son of John Crayton (as it was spelled by the census enumerator), a man of Scottish origin. Nothing is known of either his basic or professional education, but it is thought that he qualified for medical practice as an apprentice to an established physician, as was common procedure of the times.[2] He began his professional practice in Newnansville, Alachua County, in the 1830s. There he met and married Margaret Townsend, daughter of James L. Townsend.

After a brief residence in Newnansville, Dr. Crichton removed to Benton (later renamed Hernando) County, settling in the Chocochatta community,[3] which encompassed Brooksville, where he continued his practice for about four or five years.

About 1856 he moved to Tampa where he immediately established a fine reputation as both physician and public servant. When Tampa suffered its first major yellow fever epidemic in the fall of 1858, Dr. Crichton joined Dr. John A. Rice and Dr. S.B. Todd in addressing this statement to Tampa Mayor, Madison Post:[4]

> As members of the Board of Health we consider it our duty to inform you that there are some cases of fever in the town, which we believe to be yellow fever, though in a mitigated form. We do not believe there is any danger that it will become epidemic.

The statement found its way into the office of the Tampa *Peninsular*, whose editor published it, followed by his opinion that although the situation did not warrant alarm concern should be expressed. He urged precautionary measures such as "a guarded diet" and followed with a suggestion found in a Charleston, S.C., newspaper: "Take half a teaspoonful of *pulverized* charcoal, mix it in a glass of water, and drink it every morning or before going to bed." He also called attention to a common bugaboo about miasma rising from undrained ponds as probably causing the spread of the disease.[5]

The fever did reach epidemic proportions, however, claiming Dr. Crichton's wife as one of its many victims.

In 1860 Dr. Crichton ran successfully for Mayor of Tampa, winning the post over the other candidate, attorney O.B. Hart.[6] He did not run a year later when the office was won by Captain H.V. Snell over John Darling.[7] But Dr. Crichton was not finished with public life. When the election of President Lincoln in November 1860 and assumption of office in 1861 sent shock waves throughout the South, a mass meeting was held in Tampa. Fiery speeches were made and a strong protest was drafted to which the first signature was that of Dr. Crichton.[8] It was a declaration of determination to resist national policy with regard to slavery.

Dr. Crichton continued his medical practice in Tampa throughout the Civil War.[9] At some unknown date, but probably before the end of the War, Dr. Crichton married Jane Kennedy, daughter of Thomas Pugh and Adelaide (nee Christy) Kennedy, an accomplished musician and graduate of the New England Conservatory of Music. Family tradition holds that it was she to whom the composer J.A. Butterfield, her teacher, dedicated his popular song, "When You and I Were Young, Maggie."[10]

In 1868 Dr. Crichton inherited valuable property in Scotland and went there to assume possession. Soon after his return he moved from Tampa to Atlanta where he spent the last years of his life, dying there in 1888.

To Dr. Crichton's first marriage were born four children, John P. Jr., James, Thomas and Mary Eliza (who became the wife of James McKay Jr.). By his second wife he had four children. Eugene, Logan, Mrs. Callaway, and Mrs. John Giddings, all of whom were reared in Atlanta.

1. Biographical data on Dr. Crichton is not abundant. Important is the brief sketch by Charles E. Harrison in his "Genealogical Records of the Pioneers of Tampa," unpublished copy in P.K. Yonge Library of Florida History, University of Florida, Gainesville, p. 125. See U.S. Census, 1830, Camden County, Georgia, p. 182.

2. Dr. Crichton's name does not appear in lists of students and graduates of any of the major medical schools in existence during the time of his youth. There is the possibility that since he was of Scottish extraction he may have attended one of the Scottish medical schools which were among the best in Europe.

3. James L. Townsend is shown in the U.S. Census of 1840, Alachua County, Florida, as the only head of family by that name in the County.

4. Tampa Florida *Peninsular*, October 2, 1858. Dr. Crichton's professional card was first printed in ibid., June 12, 1858.

5. Particular attention was directed to the stagnant waters in and about Jackson Street.

6. Tampa *Florida Peninsular*, February 4, 1860.

7. Ibid., Issues of January 26, February 2 and 9.

8. Ibid., December 1, 1860. The statement was signed by 66 men and 26 women of Hillsborough County.

9. The publication of the Tampa newspaper was suspended from the summer of 1861 until May 5, 1866. Dr. Crichton's professional card reappeared in the issue of April 27, 1867, and continued to appear until March 7, 1868

10. C.E. Harrison, "Genealogical Records," loc cit.

Dake, David Merit, Walton County, 1814-1891

Dr. Dake, a native of Saratoga Springs, New York, was born on April 14, 1814.[1] He was graduated in 1863 as Doctor of Medicine at Castleton Medical College, a school which called itself "The First Medical College of Vermont." Nothing is known of his professional career beyond the fact that at some point he moved to Walton County, entering into medical practice in the village of DeFuniak Springs. He died there on March 17, 1891.[2]

1. Frederick Clayton Waite, *The First Medical College in Vermont*, Vermont Historical Society, Montpelier, 1949, p. 306.
2. Ibid. This date is accepted as correct. Historical documents for Walton County for this period are not abundant.

Dame, William A., Columbia County, 1860

Dr. Dame was a resident of Lake City in 1860. He was 38 years old at the time and his property was valued at $25,000. With him in the household were his wife, Anda, aged 24, and their four-year-old son, Marsa. All three were born in Georgia and appear to have been recently arrived residents of the town.[1]

1. U.S. Census, 1860, Columbia County, Florida.

Daniel, Richard Potts, Duval County, 1828-1915

Dr. Webster Merritt has included a scholarly biographical sketch of this distinguished Jacksonville physician in his *A Century of Medicine in Jacksonville and Duval County.*

Dr. Richard Potts Daniel,[1] son of James M. and E. Jaqueline H. Daniel,* was born in Pineville, Charleston District, South Carolina, August 19, 1828. Soon after Richard's birth his father moved to Columbia, South Carolina, to take charge of the Male Academy in that city, and it was there that the boy received the first impressions of his childhood. In later years he wrote with feeling that his mother sang "those dear old Scotch melodies while she played on the queer old spindle legged piano" and that his father played the flute and could dance "Fischer Hornpipe" splendidly. One of Dr. Daniel's earliest recollections was of riding behind his father on a horse "...tied on with a handkerchief for I was a very small boy...when I was almost four, I remember being lifted upon the bed...to look at a brand new little baby brother, Jacquelin—he...was a twin."**

When very young, Richard fell from a fence and fractured his right collar bone. In later years he wrote: "...they must have been careless about my recovery—because I have been *left handed* through my life—a serious inconvenience to say the least." Young Richard was every inch a boy. On one occasion "...my stepbrother, John,†...was building a pigeon house. I kept meddling with his tools although he charged me not to do so—finally whilst trying to chop with a spade I chopped one of my great toes off it merely hanging by the skin on sole of foot....It grew together all right... ."

*Formerly E. Jaqueline H. Murdoch, mother of Dr. John Smith Murdoch.
**Colonel J. J. Daniel, later an important figure in the medical history of Duval County.
† Dr. John Smith Murdoch.

Richard's father was a strict disciplinarian and used the hickory rod freely on both Richard and the boys of the academy. Nevertheless, Mr. Daniel was a talented teacher, tireless in both mind and body, and was popular with the boys.

Richard attended high school in Columbia and after graduating began to teach in the schools. Early in the year 1847 his father decided to move South. Leaving a comfortable home in Columbia, the family set out for a rough and primitive section of Florida. In later years Dr. Daniel wrote:

"I was about...eighteen years old and preceded the rest by a few weeks—coming on ahead with a wagon and four or five negro men to prepare things somewhat. Mother and the smaller children, as well as an aunt...rode in the family coach. Father had rented from Captain Wm. Haddock a small farm in Nassau County in the fork of the Mills' and Thomas' creeks, which two, united, form Nassau River....The farm was some twenty-two or three miles northwest of Jacksonville...a clearing of ten or twelve acres in the midst of a magnificient virgin forest of yellow pine, which then covered most of Duval and Nassau Counties, held a little group of shanties...the living house was a log pen with rough piazzas front and rear.... The floor was of great wide boards cut from logs with a whip saw...clapboards were the shingles...and formed the weather-boarding....The chimney was built of mud and sticks with a huge fireplace that one could sit inside of when there was only a small fire.

"A hole about eighteen or twenty-four inches, cut in a log near the chimney, served as a window outside of which was a rough, swinging shutter with wooden hinges."

Mrs. Daniel was an invalid with a chronic cough. She found life on the frontier hard, but never complained. The rough, free living held charm for young Richard, and in later years he wrote with considerable warmth and feeling, describing the primitive life:

"The...people in this sparsely settled region lived simply and roughly...but never wanted...or went into debt...all had cattle and hogs (some sheep). In the woods cane, corn, and sweet potatoes gave sugar, syrup, cornbread and hominy...a small patch of long-staple cotton ginned on a simple roller handpin and picked by hand too, gave enough cash to buy their coffee, simple clothing and other outside needs...cattle always represented a cash asset, too....Everybody ground their corn for meal or grits at home—either with a small pair of stones set upon a block and worked by hand or with a small steel mill also turned by hand."

Mr. Daniel, aided by a crew of Negroes, did the logging, which was tedious and risky work, while Richard, assisted by his brother, worked zealously in the field making the crop. Toward the end of the summer the boys were stricken with malaria and were seriously ill. Mr. Daniel, concluding that this life was too rigorous, moved his family into Jacksonville in the fall of 1847 and rented a small cottage which stood on Market Street at the corner of Duval—many years later the site of the Telfair Stockton residence. This location, now in downtown Jacksonville, was then in the heart of a pine grove in which wire grass and cockspur abounded. There was an occasional narrow boardwalk; the streets were sandy; the houses were scattered.

Becoming interested in medicine, Richard studied in the office of Dr. H.D. Holland and in 1848 entered the Medical College of South Carolina at Charleston. In 1849 he transferred to the University of Pennsylvania School of

Medicine in Philadelphia, where he was graduated on April 5, 1851, choosing for his thesis, "Dengue As It Appeared in Jacksonville in 1850." Returning to his home to practice medicine, Dr. Daniel was elected the first treasurer of the Duval County Medical Society.

In the fall of 1854 Dr. Daniel was commissioned Assistant Surgeon in the United States Navy and was assigned to the frigate *Columbia,* then lying in the Navy Yard near Pensacola. En route from Virginia, where he had been visiting relatives, Dr. Daniel passed through Augusta, Georgia, and Birmingham, Alabama, where epidemics of yellow fever were raging, and was actively exposed to the disease in each of these cities. This was Dr. Daniel's first contact with yellow fever, but he did not contract the disease until later. He arrived safely in Pensacola and reported for duty on the frigate.

Ordered to St. Thomas Island a few weeks later, his ship reached that destination about the first of February, 1855. After sailors had been allowed shore leave, it was discovered that a malignant type of yellow fever was prevalent on the island. In the course of a few days two or three cases of fever occurred among the crew, whereupon urgent orders were issued for the ship to sail for Norfolk, Virginia. The uncertainties incident to weather at that time of the year made the voyage tedious. Nearly every day a member of the crew died of yellow fever and was buried at sea. Dr. Daniel was at great disadvantage in treating the patients properly for the man-of-war was crowded, the quarters were poorly ventilated, and he could not get competent nursing help. Many years later he wrote:

"We had an old Son-of-a-Gun of a Fleet Surgeon who seemed imbued with the therapeutic ideas of the eighteenth century in regard to the treatment of yellow fever and went recklessly on shovelling in scruple doses of calomel with other drastic and depleting measures regardless of direful results. Providentially, I myself was not taken ill with the fever until the morning of the day we anchored in Chesapeake Bay; and a few hours afterwards I was carried ashore to the Naval Hospital at Portsmouth where, under the kind and judicious care of the Surgeon in charge at the place, I was but mildly ill."

After Dr. Daniel recovered from his illness he was assigned to the *San Jacinto,* a flagship in the United States Navy. On October 25, 1855, the ship set sail and for forty-four months did not return to the United States. During a major portion of this time Dr. Daniel sailed the seas of the Orient. "A Medical Journal" with notes on the voyage of the *San Jacinto* written by Dr. Daniel is in the possession of his nephew, Richard P. Daniel of Jacksonville. This record shows an orderly, careful observation of the sick on board the vessel and offers entertaining reading to the layman as well as to the physician.

In 1859 Dr. Daniel resigned from the United States Navy and during the summer of that year returned to Florida. With the exception of three years spent in serving the army of the Confederacy, he devoted his long life to the practice of medicine in Jacksonville. Later pages of this history will bring out in more detail the life and activity of Dr. Daniel. Born seventeen years after Dr. Baldwin, he survived his senior by almost the same number of years. At the time of his death in 1915, in his eighty-seventh year, Dr. Daniel was recognized as the outstanding leader of the medical profession in Duval County.

1. This sketch is reprinted from Dr. Webster Merritt's book, *A Century of Medicine in Jacksonville and Duval County,* Gainesville, University of Florida Press, 1949, pp. 45-49.

Daniel, William Augustine, Duval County, 1834-1909

Dr. Daniel, familiarly known as Dr. Gus Daniel, a member of one of Jacksonville's most illustrious families,[1] was born in Columbia, South Carolina, in 1834. In his early childhood his parents, James M. and Edward (sic) Jaquelin Daniel, removed to Spartanburg, South Carolina, where they remained for only a few years before migrating to Florida in 1842.[2] They settled in Nassau County where the elder Daniel engaged for a year or so in logging and lumbering, then moved into Jacksonville where he became a successful lumber processor and dealer. He built the old St. John's Mills situated on the River in east Jacksonville. The family home was located at Talleyrand Place.

Dr. Daniel's career has been somewhat overshadowed by those of his two older brothers, Richard Potts, a physician who had a long and successful practice in Jacksonville, and James Jaquelin, a Civil War hero and for many years one of Jacksonville's most prominent lawyers and civic leaders. All were privileged to have had a firm-handed father and more important a mother of cultivation and refinement who assumed most of the responsibility for the education of her sons. Young William especially benefited from her tutelage. In addition the sons had the advantage of association with the city's wealthiest and best educated families particularly the L'Engles.

Notwithstanding his family's position, very little is known of Dr. Daniel's adolescent years. He is assumed to have worked in his father's lumbering business until the outbreak of war in 1861. When his brother, James Jaquelin, assumed responsibility for a company of local volunteers for Confederate service, William was one of the first to enlist. He was mustered into Company G, 2nd Florida Infantry Regiment on July 1. The Company encamped in the suburb of Springfield. When the full complement of companies had been formed the regiment encamped at Burch's Brick Yard, La Villa.[3]

The lacunae in Dr. Daniel's military record make it impossible to follow his military career. It is fairly certain, however, that he was assigned to a Field and Start position in charge of the Regimental commissary, that he was with his unit in Virginia during a part of the War, and involved with the campaign around Williamsburg and Yorktown. Also he is assumed to have remained in the service until the end of the War.

On his return to Jacksonville Daniel, not yet a physician, was married to Anna Margaret L'Engle. The wedding took place in Lake City[4] to which the family had fled when Union troops occupied Jacksonville. Miss L'Engle was the third daughter and seventh child of Capt. John Claudius and Susan Fatio L'Engle of Jacksonville.

Daniel enrolled at the Savannah Medical College in Savannah in 1867 from which he was graduated in the spring of 1869. Upon his return to Florida he and his wife bought a tract of land in Mandarin, said to have been a lovely location on the St. John's River. Henceforth for several years the doctor carried on an extensive practice throughout much of Duval County. As Miss Gertrude L'Engle recalled:[5]

> When a call came for a doctor, Dr. and Mrs. Daniel would immediately make ready to answer the summons which was often brought by some country neighbor on horseback. The doctor would make sure that his satchel was complete with scales and needed drugs, calomel, castor oil, niter, cholagogues (?), sulphur, cream of tartar, quinine, but alas no capsules. Meanwhile his wife packed mustard and flaxseed, plenty of clean white cloth and turpentine. They never failed to take a clean bucket to water the horse and a good bundel of hay.

Prematurely aged by his strenuous life, Dr. Daniel retired from practice in the early 1880s. The couple bought a parcel of land in the Palermo section where they lived until 1888 when they moved into a house in East Jacksonville one block from the river at Hill and River Streets. Mrs. Daniel died there on February 10, 1901. Dr. Daniel lived on until 1909. Having no children of their own, the couple adopted a son and a daughter. The son, William Augustine Daniel Jr., studied law and spent his professional career in Jacksonville. He resided at 1853 Swift Street near the river where he died in 1919.[6]

1. Much of what is known of Dr. Daniel's early life is derived from the obituary of his more famous brother, James Jaquelin Daniel, who died on October 2, 1888. A concise history of the family is included in this death notice and eulogy. See *Florida Times-Union*, October 4, 1888.
2. Ibid.
3. Ibid.
4. Extensive information on the L'Engle family and its connections was published by Miss Gertrude N. L'Engle of Jacksonville. See especially her published work, *A Collection of Letters, Information and Data on Our Family*, Jacksonville, 1951, pp. 171-173 provides a sketch of the life of Mrs. Daniel, nee Anna Margaret L'Engle.
5. Ibid., p. 171.
6. A scattering of data on the son, William A. Daniel Jr., has been gleaned from Jacksonville city directories of various years as well as gravestones in Jacksonville's Evergreen Cemetery. No information on the adopted daughter has been located.

Dansby, George W., Alachua County, 1827-1851

Dr. Dansby was born in South Carolina on April 20, 1827.[1] In the fall of 1848 he enrolled at the Medical College of the State of South Carolina, Charleston, giving his place of residence as Shelby County, Texas. In early April 1850 he was graduated as Doctor of Medicine after submitting a thesis bearing the title, "Chemistry."[2] Soon after graduation he is presumed to have departed for Florida settling in the village of Windsor a few miles east of Gainesville.[3] He died on January 15, 1851, and was buried in the Windsor Cemetery. He is thought to have moved to Florida for reasons of health.

1. The dates of Dr. Dansby's birth and death are found on his gravestone in Windsor Cemetery.
2. See Charleston *Courier*, April 8, 1850.
3. Dr. Dansby apparently arrived in Alachua County too late to have been included in the Census of 1850.

Dantzler, M.J., Confederate Surgeon, Civil War, 1863

The total knowledge of Dr. Dantzler is derived from his military service record as Assistant Surgeon assigned to Field and Staff duty with the Tenth Florida Infantry Regiment with the military rank of Captain.[1] His appointment was dated February 11, 1863. In July-August of that year he was assigned to Camp Scott, Florida, located in Jackson County. For a portion of that period he was away for a few weeks attending the sick (it is not shown where), after which he was granted a leave of absence for 30 days.

Dr. Dantzler was at Camp Thunderbolt located five miles east of Savannah in November-December 1863, where he is presumed to have been throughout that year, remaining there as late as February 7, 1864, when he signed for hospital supplies. At a later date not indicated in his record he was transferred to Petersburg, Virginia, where he was assigned to Field Hospital duty.

Dr. Dantzler was mustered out of the Army on April 9, 1865. No further information has been located.

1. Service Record, Tenth Florida Infantry Regiment. It is somewhat odd that a physician holding the military rank of Captain was never promoted to the medical rank of Surgeon.

Darby, Charles Thomson, Jefferson County, mid-19th century

Only minimal evidence establishes Dr. Darby as a Florida physician. A native of St. Matthews, S.C., he received his medical degree from the Medical College of the State of South Carolina on March 14, 1842.[1] He presumably practiced in his native state before moving to Jefferson County in the spring of 1849.[2] His professional notice, first appearing on May 5, 1849, stated that he had settled permanently in Monticello. The Census of 1850 shows him as the sole member of his household at age 48.[3] In addition to his medical practice he was an ardent supporter of the Temperance Movement in Monticello, having affiliated with Sons of Temperance, Jefferson Division, No. 22.[4] Since his professional notice ceased to appear after November 30, 1850, he is presumed to have left Florida at about that date.

1. Charleston *Mercury*, March 17, 1842.
2. It is calculated that Dr. Darby was about 40 years of age at the time of his graduation from medical school.
3. U.S. Census, 1850, Jefferson County, Florida.
4. Jerrell H. Shofner, *History of Jefferson County*, Tallahassee, 1976, p. 192. See also Tallahassee *Floridian and Journal*, March 9, 1850.

Davidson, John Edward A., Gadsden County, 1829-1892

Dr. Davidson, eldest of the five sons of Dr. John M.W. Davidson, was born in 1829 soon after his parents moved from Mecklenburg County, North Carolina, and settled in the Philadelphia community of Gadsden County a few miles north of Quincy.[1] When he became of school age the family moved into Quincy where he received his early education. Arriving at adolescence he began reading medicine under the guidance of his father[2] and observing the surgical procedures in which his father and other physicians were involved. By the fall of 1848 he was sufficiently qualified for admission to the Medical College of South Carolina from which he was graduated in the spring of 1850. His doctoral thesis bore the title "Alteratives."[3]

Soon after graduation Dr. Davidson returned to Quincy and began practice in partnership with his father, an association which continued until the outbreak of war in 1861. Meanwhile he had married in the mid-1850s and before the end of the decade his two sons, Walter E. and John E., were born. Another son, William, was born in 1863.[4]

The election of Lincoln in November 1860 and the subsequent secession of six Southern states removed all possibility of closing the widening breach between North and South. The attack on Fort Sumter by Southern gunners on April 12, 1861, signaled the start of the War. Mobilization of troops followed quickly. Dr. Davidson received his appointment in August 1861 as surgeon in the Medical Department of the Confederate Army from President Jefferson Davis, following which he was assigned to the 3rd Florida Infantry Regiment then being mustered in at Fernandina.[5] A month later, on September 10, he received his first army pay: $280.80 monthly wage, $23 for forage for two horses, and $22 as an allowance for his quarters, a total of $325. In March 1862, however, he was transferred to the 4th Florida Regiment as surgeon,[6] but a short time later was ordered to return to Quincy as Medical Purveyor of the district of Middle Florida.

In spite of the considerable advantage of living in Quincy with his family the position was no sinecure. Upon him fell the responsibility of procuring medical and hospital supplies for Confederate Hospitals in Lake City, Madison (where two were maintained), Tallahassee, Quincy and Marianna and as the war dragged on supplies were increasingly difficult to obtain. His correspondence with Confederate Surgeon General Samuel Preston Moore from October 1862 until March 1865 is a chronicle of frustration and disappointment.[7] In many instances the requisitioned medical supplies were only partially available while hospital needs were met in large part by women of the towns in which the hospitals were located.

When the War was finished Dr. Davidson returned to civilian status and resumed practice in Quincy. Inevitably, however, he was soon drawn into the political turbulence of the Reconstruction era. The altered status of the Negro called for constitutional adjustments which would bring legal systems of the Southern states into harmony with the federal system. This could only be met by bringing into session a constitutional convention. Factional strife was rampant in Florida in 1867; nor were the factions motivated by the noblest of intentions. The Convention began in Tallahassee on January 20, 1868, in disarray. Among the Radical members were several without proper credentials; some were not citizens of the state. Soon, however, a conservative element gained control and several of the Radicals were ousted. When the military commander of the Third District (Georgia, Alabama and Florida), General George Gordon Meade, refused to intervene, the ousted members were replaced by conservatives, among them Dr. J.E.A. Davidson.[8]

The constitution which emerged from the Convention was not totally acceptable to any of the factions,[9] but under the circumstances it was about the best that could have been produced and its ratification was really never in question. In the state election which followed Dr. Davidson was chosen to represent the Sixth Legislative District in the Florida Senate. The Legislature (Florida's 15th) was convened on June 8 and adjourned on August 6, with instructions to reassemble on November 3 for an adjourned session. The *Senate Journal* for the regular session reveals Dr. Davidson as a legislator of responsibility and sound judgment. At one juncture he served as President pro tem for the body. When the readjourned session sat on November 3, however, Dr. Davidson was not present, having sent his letter of resignation. It may be assumed that his business or professional duties were to him of greater importance than the four day session in Tallahassee.

For the next 15 years Dr. Davidson continued an active medical practice. The *Florida Gazetteer* for 1884-85 lists him as druggist and physician. He and his colleague, Dr. Charles A. Hentz, attended the annual meeting of the Florida Medical Association in 1876 in Tallahassee and both were elected to membership. Dr. Hentz resigned from the organization in 1877 as did Dr. Davidson the following year. No reason for their actions was recorded in the *Proceedings* of the Association. In his voluminous "Autobiography" Dr. Hentz recalled: "On Jan. 19th I attended the meeting of the State Medical Association in Tallahassee in company with Dr. Ed Davidson...I met Dr. Wellford there...the Secretary; a very polished and agreeable gentleman."[10]

For the last few years of his life it is appearent that Dr. Davidson devoted very little time to medical practice, preferring instead to assist in the operation of his Quincy drug store which he eventually turned over to his sons, John and William. The notices and advertisements of the store appeared frequently in the columns of the Quincy newspapers of the postwar era. It appeared to have carried on a thriving business in patent medicine so much in demand in that period. Dr. Davidson's name does not appear in a list of practicing physicians appearing in the Quincy Herald of March 28, 1885, although he was listed in the *Florida Gazetteer* of 1884-85 as "physician and druggist."

Death came for Dr. Davidson on October 9, 1892.[11]

1. J. Randall Stanley, *History of Gadsden County*, Quincy, 1848, p. 66.
2. Archives, Waring Historical Library, Medical University of South Carolina, Charleston. Lists of Matriculants.
3. "Alteratives," i.e., medicines or treatments which gradually induce change and restore healthy functions of the body. Examples are iodine, arsenic, iron, mercury compounds, etc.
4. U.S. Census, 1870, Gadsden County, Florida, p. 831.
5. NA, Service Records, CSA, M251, Roll 47.
6. Ibid., M251, Roll 54.
7. Important information on Dr. Davidson is found in MSS, Box #16, PKYLFH, University of Florida, Gainesville. The Davidson folder contains 119 items, the majority of which are bills for household purchases, etc., but included are letters to Dr. Davidson from Samuel Preston Moore, Surgeon General of the Confederacy. They cover the period from October 1862 to March 1865. They contain valuable information on army hospital administration and the difficulties encountered in procuring the needed supplies.
8. For a complete and scholarly treatment of this subject see Jerrell H. Shofner, "The Constitution of 1868," *Florida Historical Quarterly*, XLI, 356-374.
9. Ibid.
10. Charles A. Hentz, "My Autobiography," typed copy of MS in Southern Collection, University of North Carolina, Chapel Hill, II, 128. Dr. Wellford, President-Elect of the Association for 1877-78, died in Fernandina while ministering to those suffering with yellow fever in September 1877.
11. Ibid., II, 353.

Davidson, John M.W., Gadsden County, 1801-1879

Dr. Davidson, one of Gadsden County's most eminent citizens, was born in Mecklenburg County, North Carolina, in 1801.[1] His grandfather, Major John Davidson, had been active in colonial politics, serving in the Colonial Council under Governor John Martin and also in the North Carolina Assembly.[2] His great uncle, Ephraim Brevard, was a signer of the controversial Mecklenburg Declaration of Independence.[3] A year or so prior to departure for Florida, Dr. Davidson married Mary J. Sylvester, member of a prominent South Carolina family. Their eldest child, a daughter named Martha, was born in North Carolina in 1827 and taken to Florida by her parents in the following year.

No part of Middle Florida could have been more attractive to prospective settlers intent upon agriculture than Gadsden County, whose topography and natural resources were considered to have been the finest in the Territory. In the 1820s many families from the Carolinas staked their futures among its hills and valleys. Among them were the Davidsons and Sylvesters. Census data suggest that Dr. Davidson settled first in rural Gadsden County as a physician and farmer, his land being located north of Quincy in the vicinity of the Old Philadelphia Church, Presbyterian, thought to have been the first church established in the County.[4] In 1830 his slaves numbered 30, sufficient to have carried on substantial farming operation. His professional card appeared for the first time in January 1832, offering his services "in the several departments of his profession to his friends and the citizens of Gadsden County."[5] He promised "punctuality and faithfulness in every application, and his charges will be made to correspond with the hardness of the times." His residence, so the notice indicated, was located at Woodville, Gadsden County.[6]

Dr. Davidson by 1840 had moved into Quincy, which had attracted a host of settlers in the 1830s. Already well-known he had no difficulty attracting a substantial number of patients and, as Dr. Charles A. Hentz was to recall, "he did a large practice and made much money."[7] He did not abandon his farm, however, but continued to operate it profitably for several years.

It is not surprising that Dr. Davidson entered actively and effectively into the public life of the county and town. As early as 1829 his signature appeared on petitions addressed to the President calling for federal judicial action to clarify the somewhat beclouded titles to lands which had been a part of the "Forbes Purchase."[8] As a staunch supporter of schools and specifically as a trustee of the Quincy Male and Female Academies, he was among the petitioners requesting that Congress donate one township toward endowment of the Quincy Female Academy.[9] He served Quincy as mayor in 1839-40.[10]

From an early date Dr. Davidson was a supporter of the movement to obtain statehood for the Florida Territory.[11] In the 1840s and early 1850s he was an ardent Whig, attending the party's regional meetings and assisting in planning its campaign strategies.[12] At a Fourth of July celebration in 1847 he filled the role of orator. With demise of the Whig Party Dr. Davidson became a Democrat and in 1860 was elected a delegate to its convention in Baltimore.[13] He was also involved in unrelated public activities, having been a strong supporter of the Temperance movement, serving as president in 1860.[14]

In the meantime the Davidsons were rearing a large and multi-talented family. In addition to Martha, there were three other daughters, Sarah F.A.; Mary J.L.; and Alice (the elder Davidsons were given to three Christian names), and five sons: J. Edward A., who became a successful physician; Joseph J.M., later a Quincy druggist; Robert H.M., law graduate of the University of Virginia, Florida legislator, and Congressman for three terms; William M., who, after a distinguished military career, turned to railroading, ultimately becoming general manager of the Florida Central and Western System and later superintendent of the Jacksonville Terminal,[15] and finally Edgar Lee, about whom very little is known. The family was saddened by the death of Mrs. Davidson on April 24, 1855.

With the coming of the Civil War all five sons saw action. J. Edward A. became medical purveyor to the Confederate Army. Robert H.M. rose to the rank of Lt. Colonel in the 6th Florida Infantry and was seriously wounded in the fighting north of Atlanta in May 1864. Captain William M. was Adjutant in the 1st Florida Infantry, later becoming aide to General Patton Anderson. Joseph S.M., commissioned as Captain in the Quartermaster Corps, finished his military career as a Major. Meanwhile the youngest son, Edgar Lee, near the end of the War was sent to the Everglades to assist in containment of the Seminole Indians, although he was a mere boy at the time.[16]

Throughout the War Dr. Davidson continued medical practice in Quincy. With the resumption of newspaper publication in 1865-66 he was able to announce publicly that his services were still available.[17] By 1870, however, he had retired. His death came on November 16, 1879, the event prompting Dr. Hentz to remark upon his long time acquaintance and association with his departed colleague. He wrote:[18]

> On the 16th of November old Dr. Davidson died-; one of the oldest citizens of the county; many years ago he did a large practice, and made much money-; but now for many years his practice had gradually retired from him; he had not practiced for a long time. When I first came to Quincy, when he was still practicing, and in his prime, he roused me with jealous suspicion, and was under very unfriendly feeling towards me in several cases in which he fancied that I had not treated him with due professional courtesy; but I was almost always careful and punctilious in all such matters, and paid no attention to his unfriendly manners & they wore off. We were very good friends for many years. For the last years of his life he devoted himself entirely to religious reading and conversation, and visited about trying to do good and I trust that he passed away to a better world. He died at the home of his son, Honorable R.H.M. Davidson; I acted as one of the pallbearers together with Mr. Wm. Munroe, E.P. Dismukes, W.B. Malone, A.W. Smith, S.B. Stephens, F.B. Mathews and A.K. Allison.

1. Rowland H. Rerick, *Memoirs of Florida*, Atlanta, Southern Historical Association, 1902, I, 504.
2. Major John Davidson's public activities are recorded passim in several volumes of *The Colonial Records of North Carolina*, collected and edited by William L. Saunders, et al, see especially Vol. IX, 384, 389 and 1263.
3. The original Mecklenburg Declaration was destroyed by fire. At a later date it was rewritten from memory, presumably by one of its authors. Among many historians the extant copy is regarded as spurious. There is no reason to believe, however, that the list of signers is not accurate. Incidentally, Dr. Davidson's name is not among them. See ibid., IX, 1263-1264
4. J. Randall Stanley, *History of Gadsden County*, Quincy, 1948, p. 64.
5. Tallahassee *Floridian*, January 10, 1832.
6. Since Woodville appears on no map of the period and never had a post office, it is presumed to have been the name given to Dr. Davidson's modest plantation. It is not to be confused with Leon County's Woodville, a village located a few miles south of Tallahassee.
7. Charles A. Hentz, 1827-94, "My Autobiography," 2 vols. Microfilm of a transcription of the original manuscript in the Southern Historical Collection, University of North Carolina, Chapel Hill.
8. *Territorial Papers*, XXIV, 158-159; ibid., XXV, 269-270.
9. Ibid., XXVI, 340-341. The petition bears the date, June 19, 1841.
10. Stanley, *History*, p. 33.
11. Quincy *Sentinel*, December 4, 1840.
12. Jacksonville *Florida Republican*.
13. Tampa *Florida Peninsular*, April 28, 1860. The Democratic Convention meeting in Charleston, S.C., on April 23 broke up in factional strife. One faction, supporting the presidential candidacy of Stephen A. Douglas, adjourned to reconvene in Baltimore on June 18. It was to this meeting that Dr. Davidson was delegated.
14. Jacksonvile *Florida Republican*, December 13, 1849.
15. Rerick, *Memoirs*, I, 505-506.
16. Information from National Archives, Service Records, CSA, and from Stanley, *History*.
17. Quincy *Commonwealth*, May 15, 1866; 1st printing January 12, 1866.
18. Hentz, "Autobiography," II, 178.

Davis, Enos Adam, Confederate Army, 1838-1864

Except for his military career, which spanned little more than two years, data on Dr. Davis are scarce. Born in Georgia about 1838 he attended the Medical College of Georgia, Augusta, from which he received his medical degree in the spring of 1860.[1] He is presumed to have moved to Florida later that year, too late to have been included in the census. No record of his medical practice in the state has been discovered.

With the War Between the States already in progress Dr. Davis enlisted for military duty in the Confederate Army on April 5, 1862, at Station No. 4 on the Florida, Atlantic and Gulf Central Railroad.[2] He was mustered in on May 24, committing himself for the duration. At this juncture the Ninth Florida Infantry was being organized. Company A, the first in the Regiment, was assembled by John C. Chambers, a wealthy farmer of Long Pond, Levy County, who became its commanding officer with the rank of Captain. Regimental headquarters of the Florida Ninth was located in Tampa, and Dr. Davis is presumed to have joined it there in the summer of 1862 with the rank of 1st Lieutenant.

It appears to have been the primary responsibility of the Ninth Regiment to secure the Gulf coast of the Peninsula against enemy attack at its more vulnerable points: Bay Port, Homosassa and Crystal River. Meanwhile Capt. Chambers, bothered by serious health problems, resigned his commission on the recommendation of Dr. John P. Wall of Tampa[3] and on July 22, 1863, Dr. Davis assumed command with the rank of Captain, also acting in the role of company assistant surgeon. His outfit remained at Bay Port through much of the summer of 1863. Before the end of the year, however, he had moved with the Company to Camp Finegan, located some eight miles west of Jacksonville near the railroad.[4]

The move to Camp Finegan was part of the build-up of troops as a counter measure against Union control of both Jacksonville and Fernandina; however, it was unavailing. On February 8, 1864, Union troops overran the camp, scattering the defenders. In his company returns to regimental headquarters for March-April, 1864, Capt. Davis wrote: "Having lost all Rolls and Company Records at the evacuation of Camp Finegan, Florida, on the 8th of February, 1864, it is impossible to give the date of enlistment of all members of the Company." Signed E. A. Davis, Capt., Commanding.[5]

By early 1864 the plight of Confederate forces in Virginia necessitated removal of certain Southern units into the Army of General Lee in Virginia. An entry in the Confederate Army record covering the months June, July and August 1864 was submitted from "Trenches, near Petersburg, Virginia." It included data on the bitter battle at Cold Harbor. Capt. Davis was there. A day or so later he fell ill "from exposure at Cold Harbor" and was taken to the Confederate General Hospital in Richmond, where he died a few days later. No record of his family or survivors has been located.[6]

1. Medical Department, University of Georgia, "60th Annual Announcement," List of Graduates, 1820 to 1891, Augusta, 1890, p. 16.

2. The Florida, Atlantic and Gulf Railroad, extending from Jacksonville to Alligator (later Lake City), a distance of 60 miles, was begun in 1853 and completed in March 1860. Since there were no villages of much size between the two termini, the scheduled stops were designated by numbers. Hence the fourth stop from east to west, later called Sanderson, was known as Station No. 4. For further information on this railroad see Geroge W. Pettengill Jr., *The Story of the Florida Railroads,* The Railway and Locomotive Historical Society, Boston, 1952, pp. 20-21.

3. National Archives, Service Records, CSA, 9th Florida Infantry, Record of Capt. John C. Chambers. Dr. John P. Wall had a distinguished war record as Assistant Surgeon and later Surgeon in the Ninth Infantry Regiment. For the latter part of service he was on the staff of a Confederate Hospital (probably the Chimborazo) in Richmond, Va. He had doubtless returned to field duty, however, at the time he examined Capt. Chambers. His diagnosis was continual inguinal hernia and repeated attacks of "billious colic and tonsilitis."

4. Union troops occupied Jacksonville on more than one occasion, but each time chose to abandon it as their troops were required for more ungent purposes elsewhere. Their 1864 occupation, however, was followed by the raid on Camp Finegan, a staging area for Confederate recruits in Florida and South Georgia.

A vivid account of the third occupation of Jacksonville by Union troops in March 1863 was written by T.W. Higginson, a Union solider who participated in the action. His remarks on the reaction of the Northern soldiers and the liberated blacks toward each other make it a valuable document. The article, "Up the St. John's River," was published in the *Atlantic Monthly,* September, 1865, pp. 311-326.

5. See note 3, supra.

6. Ibid. It is unfortunate that so little information has survived to throw light on Dr. Davis. There is some hint that he might have settled in the village of Sanderson when he came to Florida in 1860. It is stated in his army record that on one occasion he was dispatched to Sanderson for the purpose of procuring food from the local populace, which

fact may indicate that he was acquainted with people in the community. Baker County, in which Sanderson is located, had been a part of New River County until February 1861.

Davis, William, Leon County, 1855

Very little is known of Dr. Davis, for a short time a resident of Tallahassee. It is known that he died on January 14, 1855, and was buried in St. John's churchyard.[1] Another entry, this one for October 19, 1856, records the death of William, "1 yr. 7 mo., son of late Dr. Wm. Davis." Since Dr. Davis' name does not appear in the Leon County Census of 1850, it may be assumed that he was a relative newcomer to the county.[2]

1. Parochial Records, St. John's Episcopal Church, Tallahassee, Burials, p. 40.
2. In the List of Students, Archives, University of Virginia, is this entry: "Wm. Davis, born 1813, Lynchburg, Va., M.D., d. Florida, 1832"(?). He received his premedical education at the University of Virginia but had gone elsewhere for medical study.

Day, Alexander Hamilton, Pensacola and Key West, 1834

Dr. Day, a native of Louisiana, arrived in Pensacola in 1830. His professional notice appeared in the Pensacola newspaper on November 27, 1830, giving the location of his office as four doors west of the Collins Hotel.[1] In less than two years he moved to Key West, doubtless in the hope of finding a more salubrious climate—he was in poor health—and also because his sister, wife of army officer Lt. F.D. Newcomb, was residing there.[2] Apparently ignoring his frail condition Dr. Day entered immediately into the civic life of the island city. He lent his support to a petition, dated March 26, 1832, calling for annulment of an act of the Florida Legislative Council regulating Spanish fisheries, an act directed toward the fisheries of the lower west coast of the Territory which some Key Westers found repugnant to their commercial interests.[3]

Dr. Day's rise in public esteem was rapid. In early 1832 he was appointed Clerk of the Superior of the Southern (Florida) Judicial District in place of Joel Yancey, resigned.[4] Less than a month later, in elections of May 3, he was chosen alderman on the Town Council.[5] It was not until August 15, 1832, that he offered his medical services to the community, having located in the store of P.J. Fontaine, in quarters currently occupied by Dr. B.B. Strobel.[6] In the following month it was announced that "Dr. A.H. Day has been elected Health Officer of the Port of Key West."[7]

Due to discontinuation of the Key West newspaper with departure of its editor, Dr. Strobel, in late 1832,[8] little more is known of Dr. Day and his career in Key West. His health having continued to deteriorate, he left the island sometime in 1834 hoping that the waters of a Kentucky spa might prove beneficial. This was to no avail, however, for he died on September 29, 1834.[9] The notice of his death, which had appeared in the Maysville (Ky.) *Republican*, was printed in the Key West *Enquirer* of December 13, 1834. He was said to have been returning south (either to Louisiana or Florida) but upon arriving in Washington (Mason County, Ky.) he had stopped at the home of Baker Wood where he died a short time later. He was buried there with military honors arranged by the Maysville Light Infantry Company.

Key West mourned the death of Dr. Day in a manner reserved only for those held in highest esteem. Eulogies were spoken and resolutions were passed by the City Council, copies of which were sent to Dr. Day's aging father in Louisiana.[10] Concerning his medical skills not much is known, but there can be no doubt that he was an honorable and beloved man.

1. Pensacola *Gazette*, November 27, 1830.
2. Key West *Enquirer*, December 13, 1834.
3. *TP.* XXIX 681. Dr. Day's name also appeared on a recommendation put forth by Key West citizens in support of Theodore Owens for the post of U.S. Marshal for the Southern District of Florida. Ibid., p. 701.
4. Key West *Gazetter*, April 11, 1832.
5. Ibid., May 9, 1832.
6. Ibid., August 29, 1832. 1st printing, August 15, 1832.
7. Ibid., September 8, 1832.
8. Dr. Strobel discontinued the paper with the issue of September 5, 1832.
9. Key West *Enquirer*, December 13, 1834.
10. Ibid.

Day, James M., Gainesville, 1866

Dr. Day appeared in Gainesville soon after the end of the Civil War. Nothing is known of his origin, education, or medical practice. The earliest known reference to his presence in the town is the announcement in May 1866 that he was assuming proprietorship of the Suwannee House (Hotel) following the failures of at least two previous proprietors.[1] W.H. Robertson, editor of the Gainesville *New Era,* greeted the undertaking with approval, stating:[2]

> This Hotel is now under a better management than has characterized it for a long time and we can conscientiously recommend it to the patronage of the public. Dr. James M. Day is a gentleman and good fellow, and will spare nothing to make his guests at home.

Dr. Day entered actively into the affairs of the community. As a member of the recently-organized Gainesville Literary Association he participated in a debate on the question: "Monarchy versus Republic?" arguing for the advantages of monarchy.[3] Soon thereafter he was elected to the Association's Committee for Choosing Future Speakers for the organization.[4]

Dr. Day soon disappeared from the Gainesville scene, probably moving to another state to resume medical practice. His name did not appear in the Florida Census of 1870.

1. In spite of its location hard by the railroad track, which assured the traveler "a ready communication...to any part of the United States," the hotel under the management of Capt. I.B. Nichols and his successor, C.F. Thone, was apparently losing its customers to the competing hotel, Cannon House, Gainesville *New Era,* May 25, 1866.
2. Ibid.
3. Ibid., August 10, 1866.
4. Ibid., August 31, 1866.

Day, Samuel T., Columbia County, 1828

Dr. Day, far better known for his luckless encounter with Reconstruction politics than for his medical practice, was born in Virginia in 1828.[1] He arrived in Florida in the early 1850s, settling in the village of Ellisville, where he entered medical practice.[2] He married Celetta (Seleta) Weeks, only daughter of Theophilus Weeks, a farmer of average means in the Ellisville community, on May 25, 1854, and to this union were born a son, DeMotte, and two daughters, Gabriella and Nina (Nana?).[3,4]

Dr. Day's first venture into politics came to nought when, as the Democratic candidate to the Florida House of Representatives in 1856, he lost to Garrett VanZant, a well-to-do planter, the Know Nothing candidate.[5]

There is no indication that Dr. Day was ever in military service during the Civil War, although it is quite probable that he served in a civilian capacity at the Confederate hospital in Lake City. With a wife and three small children, as well as medical skills which were needed on the home front, there was probably no pressure on him to enlist. He appears to have remained in good favor, however, for in 1866 the Receivership of the Land Office in Tallahassee was offered to him. He declined, preferring to remain on his farm near Lake City.[6]

About 1868 Dr. Day was appointed assistant marshal of Columbia County and in 1870, notwithstanding his allegiance to the Democratic Party during the Republican administration of President Grant, he was appointed census enumerator for the County, his signature appearing on all the schedules of that year.[7]

As early as 1865 Dr. Day was drawn into the vortex of Reconstruction politics. Two months after the close of the War, with general confusion prevailing and the status of Southern public officials in doubt, he joined a delegation of East Florida Unionists, 12 in number, in a journey to Washington to attempt to convince President Andrew Johnson of the urgency of appointing a level-headed and nonpartisan provisional governor for the state of Florida. The trip was unnecessary. Judge William Marvin of Key West was Johnson's choice and, all things considered, a proper one.[8]

When the election for lieutenant governor of Florida was held in 1870, Dr. Day, then a Republican, was the party's candidate. His Democratic opponent was William D. Bloxham, a man of fine capability. In a close election Dr. Day was declared the winner, although with passions running high and fraudulent tactics suspected, the outcome was obviously tainted.[9] Two years later, when Florida politics sank to an all-time low with impeachment of Governor Harrison Reed, Dr. Day became a central figure in a struggle for power between opposing factions. While Reed was awaiting trial by a strife-torn legislature, Dr. Day was appointed Acting Governor, Reed having retired to his farm near Jacksonville. A short time later Dr. Day went to Jacksonville on business. Reed, hearing of his absence from office, hurried to Tallahassee and by fraudulent means had himself declared rightful Governor of Florida. His action was finally confirmed and Dr. Day resumed the office of Lieutenant Governor. Exhausted by the odious business he resigned the office on May 27, 1872, and returned to his farm near Lake City.[10]

Of the last years of Dr. Day's life nothing is known. It is doubtful that, subsequent to his brief but unhappy adventure in politics, he ever returned to the practice of medicine. Actually he had probably given up medicine prior to 1870. A list of medical practitioners of Lake City in the year 1870-71 was included in a gazetteer of the latter year. Dr. Day's name was not among them.[11]

1. The date of birth is an extrapolation from census data 1860 and 1870 for Columbia County, Florida. Nothing is known of his early education and medical training.

2. Ellisville, named for a wealthy planter, Giles M. Ellis, was situated some three miles north of the Santa Fe River and about 12 miles due south of Lake City.

3. Ocala *Southern Sun*, June 10, 1854.

4. U.S. Census, 1870, Columbia County, Florida, p. 420.

5. Tallahassee *Floridian and Journal*, August 2, 1856.
6. Tallahassee *Sentinel*, January 16, 1866.
7. Dr. Day's responsibility for the compilation of the Census may have derived from his position as Columbia County Judge at the time. See J.M. Hawks, M.D., ed., *The Florida Gazetteer*, New Orleans, 1871, where he is listed among the Columbia County officials.
8. This turbulent and spectacular period of Florida history has drawn the interest of several recent scholars, notably Jerrell R. Shofner and Ralph L. Peek. For an interesting contemporary account see John Wallace, *Carpet-Bag Rule in Florida, the Inside Working*, Jacksonville, 1888, pp. 127ff. See also William Watson Davis, *The Civil War and Reconstruction in Florida*, Columbia University Studies in History, Economics and Public Law, New York, 1913, pp. 355 *et passim*.
9. Wallace, *Carpet-Bag Rule*, pp. 133-139.
10. Ralph L. Peek, "The Election of 1870 and the End of Reconstruction in Florida," *Florida Historical Quarterly*, XLV, No. 4, April 1967, p. 364.
11. Hawks, *Gazetteer*, p. 22.

Day, Warren E., Dry Tortugas, 1868-1870

Dr. Day served for a short time as civilian contract surgeon[1] at the Post Hospital, Ft. Jefferson, Dry Tortugas, during the time when Dr. Samuel Appleton Storrow was the Army Medical Officer of the post. Returns from the post for 1869 indicated that he began his service there on May 12, 1868, continuing into the following year. He returned for another stint in 1870 and was listed in the Census of 1870 as a native of New York, 28 years of age.[2]

1. Post Returns, U.S. Army; 1800-1916, Roll 543, Ft. Jefferson, Returns for January 1869.
2. U.S. Census, 1870, Monroe County, Florida, p. 308, item 3.

Day, William, St. Augustine, 1834

Only an obituary notice identifies Dr. Day as a resident, though not a medical practitioner, in St. Augustine. He died of consumption on December 28, 1834, at age 29. He had come to St. Augustine from Newark, N.J., presumably for reasons of health. He was a Presbyterian and was survived by his wife and three small children.[1]

1. St. Augustine *Florida Herald*, January 10, 1835.

Dean, David, Calhoun County, 1860

A single reference identifies Dr. Dean, a Georgia native, as a medical practitioner living in the home of T.H. Yon, a farmer of the Blountstown community of Calhoun County in 1860. Since he is not listed among the students at any of the four medical colleges existing in Georgia in the 1850s, his medical education probably was limited to an apprenticeship in the office of an established practitioner.[1] He does not appear in the Florida Census of 1870 nor is he listed among the Florida soldiers serving in the Confederate Army.

1. U.S. Census, 1860, Calhoun County, Florida, p. 119, item 98.

deGraffenreid, E.D., Jackson County, 1848

Dr. deGraffenreid was a brief sojourner in Jackson County in the mid-19th century. He is known because of his participation in a convention of physicians held in Quincy on May 14 and 15, 1848,[1] to discuss their concern for the lack of a professional organization to regulate the licensing of physicians in the state. They had hoped to present a united front as petitioners at the next session of the Legislature and thereby obtain a charter for establishment of a state medical society. Dr. deGraffenreid was elected vice president of the convention. In plans drawn up for the organization his name was proposed as one of the vice presidents.

Two months later Dr. deGraffenreid was present at a meeting of Jackson County Democrats at which he was selected as a delegate to the forthcoming State Convention of the Democratic Party.[2]

Nothing further is known of Dr. deGraffenreid. He is presumed to have been a member of the well-known Swiss family whose first American settler was the Landgrave, Baron Christopher de Graffenreid (1661-1743), who had received an enormous grant of land in North Carolina and settled the town of New Bern, named for his beloved Swiss city of Bern.[3]

1. Quincy *Times*, May 20, 1848.
2. Tallahassee *Floridian*, July 1, 1848.
3. It is regrettable that no further information relating to Dr. deGraffenreid and his brief Florida residence has been discovered. There is small doubt that he belonged to the famous Swiss family of that name. A search through *The DeGraffenreid Family Scrap Book*, Charlottesburg, Va., University of Virginia Press, 1958, yielded no information on him. One must wonder how and why he happened to be in Jackson County and whither he may have departed.

Delavan, B., Pensacola, 1823-1824

Dr. Delavan, surgeon in the U.S. Army, served only briefly in the Florida Territory. An army register for the year 1823 lists him as a member of the staff at Pensacola,[1] although there is no indication whether his station was Cantonment Clinch or Barrancas. There is a similar entry for the year 1824.[2] By 1825, however, he is shown to have been assigned to the 7th Infantry Regiment,[3] five companies of which were located in the Arkansas Territory with the other five in Louisiana.[4] Dr. Delavan appears to have been the medical officer for the companies at Cantonment Jesup, near the town of Nachitoches, Louisiana, where his death occurred on November 26, 1827.[5]

Medical Department records provide the following details of Dr. Delavan's professional career:[6]

Born in New Jersey, appointed from New Jersey.
Commissioned surgeon's mate, April 15, 1814; assigned to 16th Infantry.
Commissioned hospital surgeon's mate, May 1816.
Commissioned post surgeon, April 18, 1818.
Commissioned assistant surgeon, March 2, 1821.
Commissioned surgeon, January 27, 1823.

1. ASP., Mil. Aff., II, 515.
2. Ibid., II, 614.
3. Ibid., II, 838.
4. Ibid., III, 625.
5. MDUSA., p. 287.
6. Loc. cit.

Dell, James Gadsden, Alachua and Duval Counties, 1825-1857

Several members of the Dell family migrated into Florida from Georgia during the latter years of the Second Spanish Period and obtained lands in various locations but principally in the northern part of Alachua County where they became successful farmers and political leaders whose influence extended far beyond the boundaries of the county. One of these was James Dell who stated in a deposition regarding the Arredondo Grant that he had come to Florida in 1807 on what appears to have been a scouting expedition, going as far as "Alligator Pond or Lake."[1] He stated further that he had returned later and since 1824 had resided in Alachua County.[2] A post office known as Dell's was established in the vicinity of the Dell properties on June 7, 1826, with James Dell as its first postmaster.[3] Here James Gadsden Dell, youngest child of James Dell, was born in 1825.

The details of Dr. Dell's general and professional education have not been ascertained. It is known, however, that the Dell family placed a high value on education and it may be assumed that young James was provided with the best instruction available. It is also known that as a young physician he had returned to Alachua County by 1848 and entered practice in Newnansville, although the earliest data relate not to his medical but to his political activities. In May 1848 he was an active participant in a meeting of Alachua County Democrats in Newnansville.[4] A month later he was secretary at a similar meeting called for the purpose of choosing a Democratic nominee for the State House of Representatives.[5]

With recurrence of Indian problems provoked by continued encroachments onto lands designated for their occupancy, Florida whites geared themselves for war. The summer of 1849 saw preparations under way in several counties. On August 11, a Jacksonville paper announced that "A company of Alachua County Volunteers has left Newnansville under the command of Capt. James G. Dell for Pease Creek, and another from Marion County will follow shortly" to stem the Indian uprising in lower Florida.[6] While on this expedition Dr. Dell met, wooed and married Mary C. Harn of Hillsborough County, the wedding taking place on October 15.[7] Dr. Dell chose to remain in or near Ft. Brook after his marriage, the census schedule listing him as a resident in the home of his father-in-law, William Harn, his occupation "doctor," and his property valued at $3,000.[8]

By 1852 the Dells were residents of Alachua County where he entered vigorously into the affairs of the Democratic Party. On April 20 at the State Democratic Convention in Madison, he was one of 14 men chosen to represent Florida at the National Convention of Democrats in Baltimore on June 1.[9] Incidentally four of the delegates were physicians.[10] Dr. Dell's support of the ultimate nominee, Franklin Pierce, was rewarded shortly after Pierce's inauguration by appointment as Collector of Customs at the Port of Jacksonville, an appointment which provoked the following comment from a local newspaper:[11] "We only have the general objection to Dr. Dell's appointment, that it might be equally as well filled here on the spot," i.e., by a local applicant.

In the remaining years of his life Dr. Dell was primarily concerned with collection of customs and improving the commercial facilities of the port. His medical practice had apparently become an avocation. He performed his duties efficiently and gained the respect of the community. Among the internal improvements for which he labored was the project to build the railroad, known as the Florida Atlantic and Gulf Central headed by his colleague, Dr. Abel S. Baldwin.[12] Other interests included establishment of a school for the teaching of the Classics and English which opened in 1854 "in a room adjoining the Customs House."[13]

After inauguration of James Buchanan as president in 1857, Dr. Dell quickly received notice of his reappointment to the Customs Office[14] but his remaining days were few. He died suddenly on the evening of September 20, having only that afternoon returned from a visit to New York and seemingly in the best of health. The cause of death was said to have been "a disease of the heart."[15] His death brought shock and deep sorrow to the many people who knew him. The editor of a Jacksonville paper, J.F. Rogero, in a touching lament praised him for his exceptional service in the community as a Democrat, Mason, Presbyterian, and Supporter of Internal Improvements. In his death, Rogero continued, the social circle had lost "one of its liveliest companions, the poor and distressed an ever ready hand, the mariner and seafaring man a good protector, the Government an efficient and valuable officer..."

Dr. Dell, 32 years old at the time of his death, was survived by his wife, Mary Catherine, son, James G., aged six; and daughter, Mary, aged two.[16] His firstborn child, a daughter, had died in infancy.[17]

1. *Spanish Land Grants in Florida*, Tallahassee, 1940, II, 58-59, Alligator Lake is located near Lake City, Columbia County.
2. James Dell Sr. was one of Alachua County's most eminent citizens. Though possessing less wealth than his brother, Bennett M., he was singled out for positions of trust in the Territory, having been appointed to the Legislative Council by Governor Duval in 1825 and then winning his seat in the Council by election for four additional terms, 1826-1831. He was the first postmaster of Dell's, later to be called Newnansville, in Alachua County. In the 1830s he was Collector of Customs for the Port of St. Johns (Jacksonville). He was born in Georgia on March 3, 1784, and died in Alachua County on November 12, 1845. See his Will, Alachua County, Wills, Book A., p. 35,for additional information. His letters to the Secretary of the Treasury during his tunure as Collector of Customs reveal a high degree of literacy.
3. TP, XXIII, 978.
4. Jacksonville *News*, May 13, 1848.
5. Ibid., June 10, 1849.
6. Ibid., August 11, 1849.
7. Ibid., November 10, 1849.
8. U.S. Census, 1850, Hillsborough County, Florida, p. 490.
9. Tallahassee *Floridian and Journal*, May 22, 1852.
10. The other physicians were John Westcott and W.S. Spencer of Mid-Florida, and Charles Byrne of East Florida.
11. Jacksonville *Florida Republican*, March 24, 1853.
12. Ibid., May 3, 1855. The first part of this railroad, Jacksonville to Lake City, although projected much earlier, was not begun until the summer of 1857. It was completed in 1860.
13. Jacksonville *Florida News*, March 18, 1854.
14. Ibid., April 11, 1857.
15. The most complete obituary notice of Dr. Dell appeared in ibid., September 26, 1857. This was, as is obvious, a Democratic journal.
16. The ages of the children are those given in the Alachua County Census of 1860. It appears that the younger child was born posthumously. After her husband's death Mrs. Dell returned to the family lands near Newnansville, sharing her home with her mother and father. U.S. Census, 1860, Alachua County, Florida, p. 50.
17. Jacksonville *Florida News*, February 25, 1854.

DeSaussure, Gabriel Edward, St. Augustine, 1800-1821

Dr. DeSaussure, native of Charles, South Carolina, and son of Judge Henry William and Eliza DeSaussure of that city, arrived in St. Augustine aboard the Schooner *Florida* on July 24, 1821.[1] About a week later he announced the opening of his office "opposite Don Fernando Arredondo's storehouse" from which he offered his services as physician and surgeon.[2] His presence in Florida was a mere sojourn, however, for within a few weeks he had moved to Savannah where he resumed medical practice. There his work was tragically terminated by his untimely death of yellow fever on October 10, 1821.[3]

His obituary, which appeared in the Savannah *Georgian* of October 11, indicated that he had elected to practice in Florida in order to study at close range yellow fever in which he had presumably become interested while still a medical student.[4] The disease made its appearance in St. Augustine in August of that year, and it is likely that Dr. DeSaussure had become infected prior to departure from Florida although the fever was by no means uncommon in Savannah. His death notice, a panegyric, written in the style generally employed in the period, indicates that he was a young man of exceptional endowments and nobility of spirit.

1. *South Carolina Historical and Genealogical Magazine*, XXXIII, 308. Here is printed an excerpt from the Register of the Independent Congregational (Circular) Church of Charleston in which the following entry occurs: "Friday Feb. 9, 1800, baptised, Gabriel Edward, son of Henry William and Eliza DeSaussure." For his arrival in St. Augustine see St. Augustine *Florida Gazette*, August 4, 1821. See "shipping news" Charleston *Courier*, July 19, 1821, for departure from Charleston.
2. St. Augustine *Florida Gazette*, August 4, 1821.
3. Charleston *Courier*, October 15, 1821. Reprint from Savannah *Georgian*, October 11, 1821.
4. Interest is mentioned in the obituary notice.

de St. Charles, Dr., Jacksonville, 1868

Although homeopathy, i.e., treatment of a disease by administering drugs which produce a condition similar to the disease, had been introduced into Europe as early as 1810 by the German physician, Samuel Hahnemann, it was not until mid-19th century that it gained a modest following in the United States. The Hahnemann Medical College and Hospital were established in Philadelphia in 1848. Twenty years later, in January 1868, Dr. de St. Charles arrived in Jacksonville and announced that he was launching his practice in that branch of medicine. He claimed to be "thoroughly educated in the school of medicine which he follows."[1]

The editor of the Jacksonville *Florida Union* called the attention of the public to Dr. de St. Charles' presence, recommending his services "to those of our citizens who believe in the same theory and practice," which hardly constituted an endorsement. Since Dr. de St. Charles is not listed in the Florida Census of 1850, it is assumed that he did not long remain in practice in Florida.

1. Jacksonville *Florida Union*, January 11, 1868.

Dewitt, William R., Putnam County, 1828-1891

Dr. Dewitt, born in Pennsylvania, settled in San Mateo, Putnam County, shortly after the Civil War. In addition to his medical practice which was apparently not extensive he operated an orange grove of about 15 acres in the vicinity.[1] He died on Anastasia Island, St. Augustine, on May 31, 1891, and was buried in the Palatka Cemetery.[2] His only survivors were his wife, Susan, and a 23-year-old son, William,[3] both natives of Pennsylvania.

1. U.S. Census, 1885, Putnam County, Florida, Precinct 6, p. 12.
2. Ibid., Agricultural Production Statistics, Precinct 6.
3. Parish Register, Trinity Episcopal Church, St. Augustine, "Burials."

Dickson, James R., Suwannee County, 1870

Dr. Dickson, born in Alabama about 1830, practiced medicine at Wellborn in Suwannee County after the Civil War. The census schedule of 1870 lists him as a householder sharing his home with a family named Sevier.[1]

1. U.S. Census, 1870, Suwannee County, Florida, item 307. Wellborn lies at about the halfway point between Live Oak and Lake City.

Dixon, James R., Hamilton and Suwannee Counties, 1860-1870

Information relating to Dr. Dixon, (Dickson) is derived from the censuses of 1860 and 1870. In the former he is listed as a member of the household of Dixon F. Cross, a North Carolina-born farmer of moderate means living near Jasper in Hamilton County. Dr. Dixon was then 33 years of age, owning property valued at $2,000.[1] Ten years later, however, he was a resident of the town of Wellborn in Suwannee County and his age was shown to be 43. In this instance the state of his birth was shown to have been Alabama. He was head of his household, which he shared with one Frank Seever, and Seever's wife and child. His wealth was estimated at a mere $500.[2]

1. U.S. Census, 1860, Hamilton County, Florida, p. 589, item 199.
2. Ibid., 1870, Suwannee County, Florida, p. 682, item 307.

Dozier, Albert John, Monticello and Madison, 1809-post 1870

Dr. Dozier, physician and planter, was born in Abbeville District, South Carolina, in 1809. As a youth he read medicine in the office of Drs. Calhoun and Geddings of Abbeville. In March 1829 he was graduated from the Medical College of South Carolina, having submitted a thesis titled "The Functions and Sympathies of the Liver."[1]

About 1831 Dr. Dozier joined a number of relatives and neighbors in moving to Middle Florida,[2] the doctor himself settling in Monticello where he appears to have enjoyed a successful practice. He also entered actively into the civic life of the community. He was a member of the Board of Trustees of the Jefferson Academy in 1832[3] and supported the two major political causes of the times—nullification and statehood for Florida. He also signed a petition in 1832 urging Congress to appropriate funds for rendering the Aucilla (Ocilla) River navigable from the Gulf of Mexico to the Georgia border.[4] He was also among a small group of prominent young men of Monticello who were arrested for betting, the charges for which were later dropped.[5]

Dr. Dozier twice served in the legislative body of the Territory. In 1838 he represented Jefferson County in the Legislative Council, and after adoption of the new constitution later that year he was elected as a representative to the House.[6]

With the failure of governmental agents, military and civil, to bring the Florida Indians under control and the breakdown of treaty negotiations, scattered remnants of Seminoles resumed sporadic raids on some of the white settlements of Middle Florida, the area between the Suwannee and Apalachicola Rivers. The outcry prompted renewed efforts on the part of the military not only to contain the Indians but to eliminate them from the area. One result was the establishment of several makeshift camps or forts out of which small detachments of troops could operate. One of these was Ft. Industry near St. Marks to which Dr. Dozier was assigned as medical officer with the rank of assistant surgeon in the summer of 1839. His letter to Col. William Davenport, commander of the area, reveals something of the dismal lot of soldiers assigned to duty along the Gulf coast of Jefferson and Wakulla Counties.[7]

Upon completion of his service with the military Dr. Dozier appears to have settled in Madison County, where he purchased a modest plantation and undertook a farming operation, an enterprise in which he was moderately successful.[8] Since the census schedules of 1850, 1860 and 1870 designate him as planter and in the two latter instances as farmer, it may be assumed that he abandoned the practice of medicine. His lands lay in the Moseley Hall community, some 15 miles southwest of Madison.[9] Scant evidence suggests that he was among the many farmers of Middle Florida for whom the Civil War and Reconstruction meant disaster. His death occurred sometime between 1870 and 1880.[10]

1. Archives, Medical University of South Carolina, Lists of Matriculants and Graduates, Medical College of South Carolina.
2. Notable among these migrants was Judge John C. McGehee, whose wife, Charlotte, was Dr. Dozier's sister.
3. Jerrell R. Shofner, *History of Jefferson County, Florida*, Tallahassee, 1976, pp. 43, 49.
4. TP., XXIX, 699.
5. Shofner, *History*, p. 155.
6. Tallahassee *Floridian*, October 14, 1837; Ibid., October 13, 1838.
7. Davenport Papers, MS, No. 203, PKYLFH, University of Florida, Gainesville. This letter, written at Ft. Industry, Dr. Dozier to Col. Wm. Davenport, September 23, 1839, is one of several in the Davenport Collection bearing witness to the hardships and suffering endured by the soldiers assigned to ferret out the few Indians remaining in the area. Scarcity of physicians and lack of medical supplies was a frequent complaint.
8. U.S. Census, 1850, Madison County, Florida, p. 215. Here Dr. Dozier's real property was valued at $4,000 while the slave schedule shows him owning 16. Ten years later his real property was valued at $3,600 and personal property at $11,700. His slaves numbered 20.
9. Dr. Dozier's son, John, married with two children, was living on the farm in 1880. U.S. Census, 1880, Madison County, Florida, p. 554.
10. This assumption is based on the fact that Dr. Dozier's name does not appear in the Census of 1880. He was shown to be living with his 17-year-old son, John, in 1870. No effort has been made to establish his numerous family connections in Jefferson and Madison Counties.

Drake, Castilian J., Santa Rosa County, 1805-1884

There remains some doubt that Dr. Drake should be included in a register of 19th century Florida physicians. He was so considered, however, by the people of Santa Rosa County. Born in Virginia in 1805,[1] he apparently departed his native state at a fairly young age. No record of his attending a medical school has been found, but the same could be said of dozens of practitioners who learned their craft as apprentices. At a fairly early age he made his way to Georgia where he met and married a woman five years his junior, known through census schedules as Nica, or possibly Nicy. By 1845 the couple had settled in Milton where their first child, Mary, was born in 1846. The Census of 1850, Santa Rosa County, designates him "Druggist,"[2] his age, 45. By this date two additional children had been born, Albert and Virginia.

The Census of 1860 adds little regarding Dr. Drake. It designates him "Teacher," however.[3] It also includes the names of daughters, Matilda, Carolina and Margrett (sic), aged 11, 10 and nine, respectively. Also in the household was G.A. Lounsberry, female, Florida-born, whose occupation was doubtless that of servant. Having given birth to six children in six years, all single births, Mrs. Drake doubtless required some domestic assistance. In neither census is he called "Doctor" or "Physician."

The gravestone of Dr. Drake in the Milton cemetery, however, bears the following inscription: "Dr. Castilian J. Drake, 1804-1884," "Milton's First Physician." Are we to doubt, then, that he was a recognized and competent physician?

1. Dates of birth and death are shown in Richard Earl Jernigan, Compiler and Editor, *Santa Rosa Cemeteries*, The West Florida Genealogical Society, Pensacola, 1987.
2. U.S. Census, Santa Rosa County, Florida, p. 294.
3. Ibid., 1860, p. 22.

Drew Columbus, Jacksonville, 1846-1922

Dr. Drew, one of Jacksonville's most capable medical practitioners and beloved citizens, was born in Richmond, Virginia, on December 1, 1846.[1] He was the eldest son of Columbus Drew Sr., who had settled in Jacksonville in 1846 and begun the publication of a newspaper, the *Florida Republican.* The elder Drew later became a partner in the M. and W.B. Drew Company, a general store which dealt in building materials, ice and marine equipment. Too young for military service at the beginning of the Civil War, Drew is said to have served as a drummer boy. If this be true, it would doubtless have been with Company B, First Florida Cavalry, a unit recruited largely from Duval County.

Dr. Drew probably attended the College of Physicians and Surgeons in Baltimore, matriculating in 1865, and receiving his degree in 1869.[2] Although the date of his return to Jacksonville is not known, it was probably late 1869. He was destined to remain there for the rest of his life.

Although Dr. Drew was not present at the organizational meeting of the Florida Medical Association in the Jacksonville office of Dr. Abel S. Baldwin on January 14, 1874, he was among the small group of local physicians nominated for membership and forthwith became charter members. He had previously established his professional status by becoming a member of the Duval County Medical Society.[3]

Dr. Drew approached medical practice with a scientific bent, carefully recording case histories of many of his patients from which he could draw rational conclusions. The various fevers endemic to the area were of particular interest to him. In 1880 he was elected Chairman of the State Society's Committee on Endemic Diseases, at the same time serving as a member of the Committee on Vital Statistics. In 1883 he was assigned to the Committee on Credentials, a proper assignment, given his concern for proper qualifications for persons entering the profession.[4] In the following year he became a member of the Committee on Ethics. At the same time he was elected to represent the State Society at the annual meeting of the American Medical Association.

Throughout his professional career Dr. Drew maintained a constant interest in the quality of medical practice and the integrity of its practitioners. In 1889, at the meeting of the Association in St. Augustine, he read a paper in which he proposed creation of a State Board of Health empowered to impose quarantines to curb the spread of contagious diseases.[5] In subsequent years Dr. Drew did not attend Association meetings held in towns other than Jacksonville, although at the meeting in Key West in 1892 he was elected First Vice President. While not in attendance at the annual meetings, he maintained his membership, however.

After a lapse of several years the Florida Medical Association held its annual meeting in Jacksonville. At its opening session on April 6, 1910, Mayor W.S. Jordan gave the welcoming address. This was following by an address by Dr. R.P. Daniel of Jacksonville. In the course of his remarks he harked back to the organizational meeting in 1874, calling attention to three members who had been present.

> My old friend, Dr. A.J. Wakefield, resting and waiting, my equally dear friend, Dr. Columbus Drew, who doubtless you all know, and obviously to know him is to appreciate him and value him, and third, Dr. J.D. Fernandez.

As for family, Dr. Drew married Marion T. Carr of St. Augustine in 1872 and a son, Stanley, was born in September 1887 and died in 1906. Mrs. Drew died in 1919 and was buried in the family plot in Evergreen Cemetery.

Dr. Drew lived on for several years at his home at 42 West Monroe Street, dying there on December 13, 1922, at the age of 76. His funeral was held at St. John's Episcopal Church. His obituary noted:[6]

> Dr. Drew was a man of firm integrity, a type of the old school gentleman, a devout member of St. John's Episcopal Church. With a heart responsive to all claims for sympathy and comfort, he was intimately associated for more than half a century with the history and growth of the City that he loved, and in his removal Jacksonville suffers a distinct loss and hundreds stand in the shadows of great grief.

Dr. Drew was survived by his sister, Alice T. Drew, three brothers, Horace J., Graeme, and William B., and a large number of nieces and nephews.

1. Vital statistics are drawn chiefly from his obituary which appeared in the Jacksonville *Florida Times-Union*, December 13, 1922.
2. There is a some doubt as to the identity of the medical school. The Baltimore medical school known as the Baltimore College of Physicians and Surgeons was not established until 1872. There were two other medical colleges in that area.
3. The year-by-year activities of Dr. Drew regarding his affiliation with the Florida Medical Association are chronicled in the *Proceedings*. These begin with his admission as a member in 1875, in which it is stated that he was admitted and was already a member of the Duval Society.
4. Ibid, 1884. At this meeting Dr. Drew was elected as a delegate to the American Medical Association. He also published a paper, "Endemic Diseases in East Florida."
5. It seems unnecessary to cite references from subsequent annual reports on the *Proceedings of the Association*.
6. Jacksonville *Florida Times-Union*, December 14, 1922.

Drinker, John Henry, Magnolia, 1821-1859

Although he died in Magnolia,[1] it is doubtful that Dr. Drinker actually practiced medicine in the state. He was born on March 28, 1821, in Philadelphia, was graduated as Doctor of Medicine from Harvard University in 1844, and spent the greater part of his professional life in New Bedford, Massachusetts. He is presumed to have moved to Florida for health reasons, seeking a more benign climate. His death occurred on May 16, 1859, probably from tuberculosis.[2]

1. Magnolia, which was situated in Leon County about seven miles north of St. Marks in Wakulla County, has ceased to exist as an incorporated community. Its name was revived when Elizabeth F. Smith began the publication of a monthly magazine, *The Magnolia Monthly*, in 1963. The magazine, devoted chiefly to local history and personalities, unfortunately ceased publication with the death of Mrs. Smith in 1977.
2. The biographical data included here were derived from two sources: *Transactions of the Medical Society of Pennsylvania*, 1860, pp. 134-135, and *Boston Medic al and Surgical Journal*, Vol. LX, 368.

Dudley, Dr., Key West, 1858-1859

Dr. Dudley, whose Christian name is unknown, was a mere sojourner in Key West. On November 6, 1858, he announced to the people of Key West that his services were available. In quaint fashion he added: "As he is an entire stranger it may not be amiss to say that he has been practicing in Southern and tropical regions more than a quarter of a century." He could be found at "Mr. Russell's Hotel."[1] In October of the following year he was still in Key West but residing at Mr. Brightman's Boarding House.[2] Since he does not appear in the Florida Census of 1860 it is presumed that he had departed the state.

1. Key West *Key of the Gulf*, November 6, 1858. William A. Russell was proprietor of a Key West Hotel at the time.
2. Ibid., October 29, 1859.

Dunn, Lewis P., Hamilton County, 1860

Dr. Dunn was a resident of Hamilton County about 1860. The census of that year lists him as a householder, aged 37, and owner of property valued at $2,500. Other members of the household were Rowena Dunn, aged 44, and William Dunn, aged 32, probably his sister and brother. All were natives of North Carolina.[1]

1. U.S. Census, 1860, Hamilton County, Florida, p. 61, item 397.

Dunn, William A., Columbia County, 1860

Dr. Dunn, native of Georgia, settled in Lake City just prior to outbreak of the Civil War. He is thought to have been a graduate of the Medical College of Georgia, Augusta, in 1844.[1] Whatever his background and education, he was a man of far above average means, having owned real estate valued at $10,000 and personal property at $15,000 in 1860.[2] That year his family included wife, Anda, and a four-year-old son, Marsa. His Florida residence was of short duration, however, doubtless terminated by disruptions of the Civil War. His name does not appear in the Florida Census of 1870. He is assumed to have moved from the state.

1. This is an assumption based on the fact that among graduates of the Medical College of Georgia in 1844, there was a William G. Dunn, possibly the doctor presently under consideration.
2. U.S. Census, 1860, Columbia County, Item 260.

Dupont, E.P., St. Augustine, 1830

Aside from the fact that he was a student of medicine at the Medical College of the State of South Carolina for the term 1828-29, very little is known of Dr. Dupont.[1] Records of the college show that he was a resident of St. Augustine and that his preceptor was Dr. F. Porcher. He is thought to have been the son of Abraham Dupont, prominent landowner, and slaveowner, Mayor of St. Augustine in the 1840s. He was among the signers of a petition from St. Johns County citizens in 1831 addressed to Congress urging the reappointment of Judge Joseph L. Smith to the East Florida Judicial District. Another signer was Abraham Dupont.[3] No evidence has been located which would establish him as a Florida physician.

1. The Dupont family, whose South Carolina origins extend well back into the 18th century, were prominent in the public affairs of Charleston and Colleton Districts. They were apparently descended from the early Huguenot settlers.

2. Abraham Dupont lands are thought to have been located west of the Matanzas River, some four miles due west of Crescent Beach, where there is a community known as Dupont Center.

3. *Territorial Papers*, edited by Clarence E. Carter, Washington, 1959, XXIV, 602.

Durr, Joseph E., Gadsden County, 1860

Very little data exist concerning the life of Dr. Durr. In 1860, at 19, he was a medical student living in the home of his father, Ralph E. Durr, a fairly well-to-do farmer of Gadsden County. The family had migrated from South Carolina where young Durr was born.[1] Six years later the Quincy newspaper printed the following item: "Dr. Durr of Gadsden County left this place on Sunday last for Mexico to try his fortune in that country. We wish him success." The editor added, however, that the doctor would probably have difficulty in departing from New Orleans where General Sheridan was enforcing a ban on emigration.[2]

1. U.S. Census, 1860, Gadsden County, Florida, p. 9.

2. Quincy *Commonwealth*, as reprinted in the Tallahassee *Semi-Weekly*, March 23, 1866. No military record for Dr. Durr has been located.

Duval, Benjamin F., Madison County, 1860-1870

Dr. Duval, who practiced medicine in Madison County in the latter half of the 19th century, remains an obscure figure. The Census of 1870[1] lists him at the age of 55 residing in Madison County with his wife Josephine, a South Carolina native some 20 years younger. He was a native of Virginia, a fact which would indicate that he was a relative of two well-known Leon County physicians, John Pope and Lucien Spence Duval. The surname Duval was not uncommon, however, it is mere conjecture to link Dr. Duval as a kinsman of William Pope Duval, Territorial Governor of Florida. A single reference shows him to have had agricultural interests to which he probably devoted the greater part of his time and energy.[2] The date of his death has not been learned.

1. U.S. Census, 1870, Madison County, Florida, p. 75.

2. Elizabeth H. Sims, *A History of Madison County, Florida*, Madison County Historical Society, Madison, 1986, p. 106.

Duval Jr., John Pope, Leon and Wakulla Counties, 1820-1866

Dr. Duval was born in Virginia, probably Buckingham County in 1820. His father, John Duval, and uncle, William Pope Duval, first Territorial Governor of Florida, after a sojourn of a few years in Kentucky, moved to Florida in the early 1820 settling in Leon County where they soon achieved prominence in the rapidly growing Tallahassee community. Dr. Duval's father had purchased land and become a fairly prosperous planter. He is best remembered, however, for having contracted to complete the construction of the unfinished Territorial Capitol in 1828, a plum which had doubtless fallen into his hands through the influence of his brother, the Governor.[1] Records of Dr. Duval's childhood and youth are virtually nonexistent. Student lists of the University of Virginia, preserved in the University Archives, show him to have been a matriculant for the term 1839-40,[2] but there is no record of his having received either an arts or medical degree. By the mid-1840s he had returned to Tallahassee and begun medical practice.

A single reference to his political activities appeared in the summer of 1846 when, at a meeting of the Leon County Democrats, he was chosen as a representative to the State Convention which met at Suwannee Springs on the second Monday in July.[3]

In early February 1848 there appeared in a Tallahassee newspaper two professional cards which in juxtaposition were unusual.[4] In the first Dr. Duval offered his medical services to the community from his office located in the William Wilson Building "over Hayward's Bookstore." In the second, as an attorney-at-law, he offered his legal services from the same offices![5]

The Leon County Census of 1850 lists Dr. Duval, aged 28, sharing his house with his younger brother, Lucien, also a physician. Nothing is known of Dr. Duval's activities for the next five years but on February 21, 1855, the following announcement appeared in the Tallahassee *Floridian and Journal:* "Married, on February 15, 1855, at the residence of Capt. William Fisher, Wakulla County, Dr. J.P. Duval of Tallahassee and Miss Mary S. Fisher of Wakulla."[7] Meanwhile it is assumed that Dr. Duval was about his professional duties as physician and lawyer.

In March 1859 the following item appeared in a Tallahassee newspaper:[8]

> Dr. John P. Duval, of this City, was yesterday commissioned by the Secretary of the Treasury as Surgeon of the Marine Hospital at St. Marks. This is an appointment worthily bestowed. Dr. Duval is a thoroughly read physician and has filled the responsible post of Surgeon in the United States Army.

The Wakulla County Census of 1860 supports the assumption that he had moved to St. Marks, where he resided with his wife, Mary, and their one-year-old daughter, Anna.

The Confederate Service record of Dr. Duval is incomplete. He was 40 years of age when the War began and there is no evidence that he served outside Florida. Newly-elected Govenor John Milton on October 13, 1861, appointed him assistant surgeon of the military districts of St. Marks and Suwannee.[9] Two entries in the records of the Tenth Florida Infantry (May and June 1862) list him as Staff Surgeon for the Regiment. In the second of these it is known that he was stationed at Ricco's Bluff where a recruitment post had been established.[10] No further data have been discovered.

University of Virginia student lists preserved in the University Archives show that Dr. Duval died in Tallahassee in 1866.[11] Two years before his death his second child, a son named John Pope Duval II, was born. This son is said to have spent his youth in Tallahassee where he "mastered the art of telegraphy" and later moved to Jacksonville where for a number of years he was identified with the Mutual Life Insurance Company. He was later employed by the Western Union Telegraph Company who transferred him to its office in Augusta, Ga. He died there in 1897.

1. This contract availed Dr. Duval little or nothing, however, in that the public funds allocated for the building were mismanaged and a long delay ensued. Meanwhile he withdrew from the commitment. See Bertram H. Groene, *Ante-Bellum Tallahassee*, Tallahassee, 1871, p. 27.

2. Archives, University of Virginia, Lists of Students.
3. Tallahassee *Floridian,* issues of June 20 and 27, 1846.
4. Ibid., February 26, 1848.
5. It was not uncommon for physicians in those early times to operate drug stores, carry on farming operations, and fill pulpits. Dr. Duval's dual occupations of medicine and law, however, were unusual.
6. U.S. Census, 1850, Duval County, Florida, p. 71. Lucien's age in 1850 was 24. Neither was married at that date.
7. William Fisher was a Virginia-born planter of modest means.
8. Tallahassee *Floridian and Journal,* March 19, 1859. St. Marks Hospital was situated a few hundred yards north of the confluence of the St. Marks and Wakulla Rivers. It was built in 1857-58 in response to demands for a facility to care for ailing seamen who might be put ashore there in those days when St. Marks was a thriving seaport. It was abandoned in 1867. See J. Richard Shenkel and William Westbury, *The Marine Hospital of St. Marks,* Tallahassee, 1865, pp. 2-6.
9. Report of the Adjutant and Inspector General, Francis L. Dancy, Tallahassee *Florida Sentinel,* February, 11, 1862.
10. NA, CSA Service Records, M251, Roll 94. Ricco's Bluff was situated on the east bank of the Apalachicola River in Gadsden County.
11. Additional information on John Pope Duval II and his son, John Pope Duval III, may be found in Harry G. Cutler, *History of Florida, Past and Present,* 3 vols., Chicago, 1923, II, 78.

Duval, Lucien Spence, Leon and Wakulla Counties, 1826-1883

Dr. Duval, son of John Pope Duval and nephew of Governor William Pope Duval, was born in Virginia about 1826.[1] While still an infant he was brought to Leon County where his family purchased land and established themselves as members of the planter aristocracy. Lucien Duval entered Jefferson Medical College, Philadelphia, in 1848 and was graduated in the spring of 1850.[2] He returned to Leon County in time to be counted in the Census of 1850 in which he is shown to have shared a residence with his older brother, John Pope Duval Jr., also a physician, practicing in Tallahassee.[3] After the death of his father, Dr. Duval moved into the home of his mother where he was living in 1860. Meanwhile, on September 22, 1859, he had married Cornelia O. Tebbs of Fauquier County, Virginia, daughter of Col. Samuel J. Tebbs.[4]

In the 1850s Dr. Duval, a stalwart Democrat, entered vigorously into the political affairs of Leon County. In early June 1856,[5] he attended a Democratic meeting in Centreville and was among those chosen as representatives to the State Democratic Convention scheduled for Tallahassee on June 21. Throughout that summer he was active in the Democratic cause, speaking to Democratic clubs and helping organize local support for the national ticket headed by James Buchanan. For his labors he was nominated for one of Leon County's four seats in the State House of Representatives to which he was duly elected, the Democrats having swept the election.[6] Dr. Duval took his seat in December.[7] This, however, was his only venture into public office.

As the Civil War took on an increasingly grim aspect in the summer of 1862, Dr. Duval, like most Southern physicians, offered his services to the Confederate Army. As was too frequently the case, however, his assignments were nonmedical. He enlisted at Lake City on August 14, 1862.[8] Within a few days he was commissioned second lieutenant and assigned to the First Battalion, Tenth Florida Infantry. A year later, on August 12, 1863, he became a first lieutenant. He spent his last year of military service as commander of Company G and was among those surrendering at Appomattox.[9]

After the War Dr. Duval returned to Leon County to join wife and family. Soon thereafter he moved to Wakulla County to become one of the early settlers in Crawfordville where he resumed his medical practice.[10] At about this time Mrs. Duval died leaving him with three small children, two daughters and a son. It may be inferred from some of the sources that from this time to the end of his life Dr. Duval found life difficult. His older daughter, Nena, married James Wright and moved to Texas. The second daughter, Nannie, who had been afflicted since early childhood, thought to have been the result of severe fevers, suffered from disfiguring burns. Before her father's death she went to live with her sister in Texas. The son, Douglass, was in his early teens at the time of his father's death. He had apparently received no professional education or training for a trade and was a source of worry in Dr. Duval's final days.[11]

Dr. Duval died about the first of December 1883. He had recently returned from a visit to Texas where he had contracted a lingering illness. Depressed over his condition and fearing that his mental faculties were becoming impaired he carefully planned suicide, which he accomplished. His letter to his brother Sheffield of Tallahassee specified disposal of his effects which included little more than $1,200 which he had converted into money orders to be sent to his beloved daughter, Nannie, in Texas. The letter also expressed deep concern for Douglass, with the hope that Sheffield would assume the responsibility. He wrote: "I shall bear in mind your promise to take care of the boy, if anything happens to me."

Dr. Duval then wrote a brief letter to his friend, Wright Walker, of Crawfordville, enclosing $10 to be used for his burial expenses including the digging of his grave and the purchase of "a plain pine coffin." He expressed the hope that at some future time his remains might be removed to Tallahassee to "be laid beside my wife" adding that "her grave is just east of my father's." Another letter was addressed to his nephew, John, asking him to make certain that Uncle Sheff receives his instructions. And finally, there was a letter to his dear Douglass, brief but heart-rending. It begins: "Dear Doug, Your father is about to die, my boy. Your Uncle Sheff will take care of you, if I do...God bless you."[12] Thus ended the career of an intelligent, well-educated physician and public figure, scion of one of Florida's most distinguished families.

1. U.S. Census, 1850, Leon County, Florida, p. 71. His age was 24.
2. Jefferson Medical College, Philadelphia, Archives.
3. See note 1, supra.
4. Tallahassee *Floridian and Journal*, October 15, 1859.
5. Ibid., June 14, 1856.
6. Ibid., June 28, 1856.
7. Ibid., October 11, 1856. Of the five Leon County representatives, three were physicians, Duval and George W. Parkhill in the House, and Thompson B. Lamar in the Senate.
8. NA, CSA, Service Records, M251, Roll 94. Certain vital data from Dr. Duval's record are missing but in spite of a young wife and a small daughter, he enlisted for a term of three years.
9. Ibid.
10. Upon removing to Crawfordville, Dr. Duval offered for sale his place in Leon County. Tallahassee *Semi-Weekly Floridian*, October 9, 1866. The notice reads, in part: "For Sale: My place, two miles south of Tallahassee. The dwelling, situated on a high hill, is new, 5 rooms, 3 of which are nearly 20 x 20. Cost before the War, about $1700. New fence and ditch. Well, 64 feet deep. Also a good cistern on premises...Convenient to City, lying on the railroad."
11. Nearly all that is known of Dr. Duval's last years is derived from a series of letters published in the Tallahassee *Weekly Floridian*, January 1, 1884. The circumstances of their publication were unusual. Upon learning of his brother's death in Crawfordville, Sheffield Duval requested that the newspaper not publicize the matter until he had an opportunity to investigate the facts relating to the tragedy. The newspaper complied with his wishes. Later in December Sheffield place in the hands of the editor his own account of the matter, describing his brother's state of mind prior to the suicide, enclosing therewith four letters written by the deceased shortly before his death.
12. The letter to Douglass was apparently the last of those written by Dr. Duval.

Eastin Jr., Thomas Pensacola, 1837-1860

Dr. Eastin, whose tragic death occurred in Pensacola when he was only 23 years of age, was the son of a newspaper editor whose restless disposition did not permit him to remain in any one location for more than a year or so. He is known to have edited newspapers in Natchez, Mississippi; Alexandria, Alabama; and Key West, Florida, prior to settling in Pensacola. It is not known whether his son was born in Key West or Pensacola. It is known, however, that his all-too-brief professional life was spent in Pensacola. He met his death by drowning in Pensacola Bay, whether while swimming or boating is not known, on July 6, 1860. His epitaph indicates that he was an only son.[1] It states that:

> "All the hopes and dreams of his aged Parents lie buried here."

Soon after the death of their son, Mr. and Mrs. Eastin left Pensacola to spend their last years in Mt. Vernon, Alabama.[2]

1. Dr. Eastin was buried in Pensacola's St. Michael's Cemetery.
2. For a brief biographical sketch of Thomas Eastin Sr., see James Owen Knauss, *Territorial Florida Journalism*, Deland, The Florida State Historical Society, 1926, pp. 68-69. Professor Knauss did not hold Eastin in high regard. He wrote: "Of Eastin as an editor, nothing complimentary can be said, if the extant copies of the Key West *Register* are any criterion."

Eastlake, Samuel, St. John's River Settlement, 1790s

Dr. Eastlake took his oath of allegiance to the Spanish crown in 1798. The record shows him to have been American-born, Protestant, married, and owner of two slaves. He resided in the St. John's settlement and is listed as planter and physician.[1] Earliest references indicate that he had settled in Florida as early as 1791[2] when he was engaged as surveyor for the Spanish government. There are numerous references to his surveying services in the records of Spanish land grants, often in company with Pedro Marrot, another surveyor. In spite of his professional designation as physician, in only one instance does he appear in land grant records as a member of that profession,[3] and in this case as Dr. Eslick.

Other land grant records show him to have been in possession of land called "Montpellier" east of the St. Johns River, a holding which he lost for failing to comply with conditions stated in the grant.[4] Here it is revealed incidentally that Dr. Eastlake had a daughter, Anna, who was married to Juan Salon (John Salome) but who apparently died soon after her marriage.

The last reference to Dr. Eastlake, January 22, 1800, is included in a petition for certificate of a grant to Governor White, which was approved.[5]

1. E.F.P., Bundle 350 U4, Reel 163.
2. *Spanish Land Grants*, I, G.8. Here Dr. Eastlake is identified only as a surveyor who on November 27, 1791, certified the occupancy of a tract of land, a plantation known as San Frederico, on the St. Johns River.
3. Ibid., T22.
4. Ibid., IV, P. 53.
5. Ibid., V, S. 3.

Edgar, Richard C., Key West, 1820s

Dr. Edgar appears to have been the first American surgeon to practice in Key West. From the time of the Louisiana Purchase from France by the United States in 1803, the maintenance of safe commercial lanes between the eastern United States and the newly acquired Louisiana Territory was a problem. Pirates based in several of the West Indies flourished and ships plying the lanes to and from Louisiana were a prime target. Not much could be done to ensure safe passage until annexation of Florida in 1821. In early 1822 a naval presence in Key West was established with assignment of a squadron to the Island. It was known as the West Indies Station.

The medical needs of the squadron were met by one surgeon, Dr. Edgar, and five Surgeon's Mates. A Report on Surgeons of the Navy, bearing the date January 16, 1823, shows Dr. Edgar as recipient of $50 per month and two rations per diem, or a total annual income of $782.50.

Nothing is known of Dr. Edgar's origins or educational background.[1]

1. See U.S. Government, Executive Papers, No. 27, 17th Congress, 2nd Session, Vol. I, Washington, 1823.

Edwards, Thomas H., Jefferson County, 1837-1892

Dr. Edwards, son of Captain James B. and Mary Turnbull Edwards, was born in Georgia in 1837.[1] At the age of two he was brought to Florida by his parents who settled first on Amelia Island but later moved to the Bailey's Mill (later to be renamed Lloyd) community in Jefferson County, purchased land and engaged in farming.[2] Thomas was the eldest of five children. Nothing is known of his early education but he is presumed to have attended the common school of the district, and very probably began his medical education under the preceptorate of a Jefferson County physician, thought to have been Dr. Theodore Turnbull, the elder, a relative of his mother. Subsequently he earned his medical degree at the Medical College of the University of Pennsylvania.[3]

Dr. Edwards began his medical practice at the village of Waukeenah several miles south of Monticello but later transferred to Lloyd where he remained until the outbreak of war in 1861. He was among the first to respond to the call for troops in Jefferson County, enlisting as a private in a company being organized by Capt. George E. Call, Co. K, 2nd Florida Infantry Regiment. He joined the company on July 13, 1861, at Camp Virginia, a staging area on the outskirts of Jacksonville. Two months later he was ordered to Richmond on detached service as physician.[4]

Dr. Edwards' military career was, however, brief and beset by misfortune. Shortly after arriving in Richmond he became ill and was admitted to the Chimborazo Hospital, a Confederate facility in Richmond. The Regimental return for December 1861 listed him simply as "Physician, in Richmond" but the return of February following stated that he had been discharged. This was confirmed by the hospital report, "Admitted, Dec. 10, 1861; ailment, organic heart disease. . .discharged, Dec. 16, 1861."[5]

After returning from Richmond Dr. Edwards gradually regained more or less normal health, although he seems never to have become robust. He resumed medical practice, probably at Lloyd, where he earned a splendid reputation. His last years were spent at Waukeenah,[6] where he died in 1892. The Special Florida Census of 1885 indicates that his professional services were much in demand.

1. Reliable information on the career of Dr. Edwards is not abundant. Although incomplete, the best sources are

Elizabeth F. Smith, "The Town of Bailey's Mill-Lloyd," *Magnolia Monthly*, Vol. VII, October 1971, and WPA, Writers' Project, Jefferson County, Florida, "Towns and Plantations," p. 7.

2. Smith, op. cit.

3. WPA, Writers' Project.

4. National Archives, Service Records, CSA 2nd Florida Infantry.

5. Ibid.

6. Mrs. Smith in the previous citation stated that only a few years prior to his death, Dr. Edwards married a Miss or possibly Mrs. Bellinger. This has not been verified.

Eichelberger, John B., Marion County, mid-19th century

Very little is known of the Florida career of Dr. Eichelberger. He was a native of Newberry District, South Carolina,[1] who came to Florida in the 1850s and settled in the Ocala community. In the renewal of the Third Seminole War in the winter of 1855-56, Dr. Eichelberger was among the physicians called into service. On March 18, 1856, he was appointed Assistant Surgeon for the company of volunteer troops commanded by Captain Abner D. Johnson, then stationed at Camp Carter.[2] With final suppression of the Seminoles in 1858 Dr. Eichelberger returned to his Marion County farm. The Census of 1860 lists him as "Planter and M.D.," aged 36, living with his wife, Mary, 10 years his junior. His properties were valued at $14,000.[3] Nothing further is known of him.

1. Dr. Eichelberger is thought to have been the son of Col. John Eichelberger, a man of considerable wealth, who was the father of seven sons and whose slaves numbered 47 in 1840. See U.S. Census, 1840, Newberry District, S.E., p. 232. For further information on the Eichelbergers see Thomas H. Pope, *The History of Newberry County*, South Carolina, Columbia, S.C., 1973, pp. 114, 222, et passim.

2. Journal, Florida Senate, 8th Session, 1856, Tallahassee, 1856, p. 77. Camp Carter is thought to have been located on Bay, Sumter County. It apparently existed for only a few months.

3. U.S. Census, 1860, Marion County, Florida, p. 213. Dr. Eichelberger's name does not appear in the Marion County Census of 1870.

Elliott, Jacob, Leon County, 1856

Very little information concerning Dr. Elliott has emerged. A native of North Carolina, he is known to have practiced briefly at Centreville in Leon County in the early 1850s. The Leon County Census of 1850 lists him as physician sharing a household with his mother, Susan, and three young girls named Moseley, presumably his nieces.[1] He was 44 years of age at the time and possessed property valued at $8,000. He appears to have died in early January 1856 in that notices of his death and settlement of his estate first appeared on January 19.[2] On February 16, 1856, Dr. R.N. Gardner advertised that he would henceforth be occupying rooms at the home of John R. Crump "formerly occupied by the late Dr. Jacob Elliott."[3]

1. U.S. Census, 1850, Leon County, Florida, p. 125.

2. Tallahassee *Floridian and Journal*, January 19, 1856.

3. Ibid., February 16, 1856.

Elliott, Moses H., Escambia County, 1822

Dr. Elliott, a native of Massachusetts, entered the Army's Medical Department as surgeon on March 11, 1814.[1] When his unit, the 40th Infantry Regiment whose headquarters were in Boston, was disbanded in June 1815, he retired briefly to private life. On November 7, 1816, however, he was recommissioned but at the lower rank of surgeon's mate. He was promoted to the rank of surgeon on October 31, 1817, and assigned to the 4th Infantry Regiment which, after the successful campaign of Andrew Jackson through West Florida, was ordered to occupy several posts in that territory and to establish its headquarters in Pensacola. Dr. Elliott, the regimental surgeon, was destined to remain in Florida and become the victim of yellow fever on September 8, 1822.

In those troubled years between 1818 and 1822, at least in frontier areas, when there was a general scarcity of medical practitioners, no sharp distinctions were apparent between civilian and military practice. Especially was this true when epidemics occurred. Dr. Elliott performed in a dual capacity. While still an army surgeon, he advertised his professional services for the citizens of Pensacola "from his office on Intendant Street, opposite the residence of Mayor (George) Bowie."[2] In the meantime he had been named a member of the Board of Medical Censors, whose responsibility was to examine applicants for license to practice in Pensacola and determine their qualifications.[3] At the same time a recommendation was drafted and forwarded to Governor Jackson requesting that Drs. Vorhees, Elliott and Merrill, the latter two army surgeons, be appointed to the Board of Health. This resolution bore the signature of Dr. James C. Bronaugh.[4]

Dr. Elliott's reputation as physician and citizen among army personnel as well as the citizens of Pensacola was above reproach. It is evident that he enjoyed the trust and friendship of Dr. Bronaugh. When in late 1821 an army inspection team visited Pensacola and subsequently filed an approbatory report but failed to mention the good work of Dr. Elliott, the editors of the Pensacola *Floridian* were moved to take the inspecting officers to task for their oversight.[5]

An Army Medical Department report for the third quarter of 1822, later printed by Surgeon General Thomas Lawson, includes an account of the death-dealing yellow fever epidemic of that year in Pensacola. It began on August 7 when "a young lady, who had recently arrived from New Orleans, died of black vomit. Her physicians, Drs. Elliott and Bronaugh, had no suspicion of the real character of the disease, until this last harbinger of death made its appearance."[6]

Within a month both physicians were victims of the disease. Dr. Bronaugh died on September 2, while Dr. Elliott's death came on September 8. Wrote Dr. Lawson, "Among its first victims was Dr. Elliott, an officer whose loss cannot be too much regretted; his amenity of manners and correctness of conduct entitle him to the lasting esteem of all who knew him."[7]

1. MDUSA, pp. 270, 284, 287.
2. Pensacola *Floridian*, May 4, 1822.
3. Ibid., September 8, 1821. Report of action of the Board of Health on September 6, 1821.
4. Ibid.
5. Ibid., February 11, 1822.
6. Lawson, SRSM, p. 37.
7. Ibid., p. 38.

Ellis, Robert W., Wakulla County, 1850

Dr. Ellis, a native of Georgia, practiced medicine for a brief period in Wakulla County. The 1850 Census lists him as a resident of Shell Point, a remote fishing village on the Gulf of Mexico some 15 miles south of Tallahassee. This census indicates that he was a resident in the home of Dr. John L. Crawford, prominent citizen of the County and like Dr. Ellis a native of Georgia.[1] There is no indication that Dr. Ellis was more than a brief sojourner in the state. He does not appear in the Florida Census of 1860.

1. U.S. Census, 1850, Wakulla County, Florida, p. 513, item 166. Dr. Ellis' name does not appear in the lists of graduates of the Medical College of Georgia in Augusta nor does he appear in the lists of either of the medical schools in Savannah.

Elwes, Alfred W.H., Surgeon, U.S. Army, 1800-1842

Dr. Elwes, a native of Pennsylvania, was a graduate of the Medical School, University of Maryland, Baltimore, in 1820.[1] After a few years of private practice he offered his services to the Medical Department of the United States Army and on May 9, 1825, was commissioned Assistant Surgeon. He was promoted to Surgeon on July 4, 1836.[2]

At an unknown date he was married to Miss Adelaide Brent of Virginia. Soon thereafter Dr. Elwes was assigned to duty at the Pensacola Navy Yard where his wife joined him in the summer of 1825.[3] Soon after her arrival she became ill, probably of one of the fevers common to the area, and died on October 12. Newspaper accounts indicate that she was the daughter of Colonel Daniel Carroll Brent, a graduate of West Point, and a woman of charm and intelligence.

The latter months of the Second Seminole War found Dr. Elwes on duty with the troops along the St. Johns River where he died on June 12, 1842, the actual place of death being Palatka.[4]

1. Eugene Fauntleroy Cordell, *Historical Sketch of the University of Maryland School of Medicine*, 1807-1890, Baltimore, 1891, p. 173.
2. Medical Department, U.S. Army, from 1775 to 1873, Harvey E. Brown, compiler, Washington, D.C., Surgeon General's Office, 1873, pp. 288, 291.
3. Pensacola *Gazette*, October 15, 1825.
4. See note 2 supra.

Ely, Horace, St. Joseph and Marianna, 1788-1860

Dr. Ely was born in Massachusetts about 1788.[1] Upon reaching manhood he migrated to Plymouth, North Carolina, where he is said to have amassed a fortune in shipping and other business ventures.[2] It was there that he married Mary Jane Roulhac and a son, Francis, was born.[3]

Dr. Ely moved to Florida in the 1830s, settling in the town of St. Joseph where he established his medical practice. Mrs. Ely died in St. Joseph in 1835.[4] For reasons that are not clear Dr. Ely appears to have suffered serious financial losses. At the time of his wife's death only her property remained, this having been due to a marriage contract which stipulated that the doctor was not to have access to her assets. It is probable that the general depression or panic of 1837 was in part responsible for the losses.

Dr. Ely moved to Marianna in the early 1840s where his son, Francis, had entered the mercantile business. Soon thereafter he married his second wife, Charlotte Maria Daffin of a prominent Jackson County family.[5] Here he entered upon a regular medical practice, but in order to recoup his fortune he also opened a hotel which became a fairly prosperous enterprise. Among the residents of

"Dr. Ely's Hotel," as it was called, in 1850 were three Marianna lawyers, Wm. E. Anderson, James F. McLellan, and Jesse J. Finley who would become a distinguished judge and renowned Civil War general. Among other residents were Dr. John W. Keyes and family.[6] In 1849 the Marianna newspaper published an account of a dinner at the hotel hosted by Dr. Ely and attended by "notables, as a part of the Fourth of July celebration."[7]

Dr. Ely lived past age 70.[8] In his last years, however, he and his son were beset by financial disasters no doubt resulting in part from disruptions of the War but probably also from extravagant living and poor business management. The Ely debacle has been summarized as follows:

> Even the fabulous Ely fortune had vanished, and creditors filed more claims against the estate of Francis R. Ely, prominent Marianna merchant noted for his extravagance and hospitality, than could be paid on the basis of reconstruction values. Dr. Horace Ely's property had been attached in 1867 (probably the year of his death) by innumerable creditors who had reduced their claims to judgments, several dating back as far as 1860. The property of John R(andolph) Ely, son of Francis and grandson of Dr. Ely, was advertised on the delinquent tax list of 1869. . . .[9]

1. This date is an extrapolation from the Jackson County Census of 1850 in which his age is shown as 63 and the 1860 Census in which it is shown to have been 71.
2. J. Randall Stanley, *History of Jackson County*, Marianna, 1950, p. 58. This well-documented book is the best available source on the subject. It is used extensively in this brief sketch.
3. Ibid., Francis R. Ely, born ca. 1812, became one of Marianna's leading merchants. His splendid home was considered to be the town's most elegant and pretentious.
4. Ibid.
5. Ibid. It is something of a genealogical oddity that Charlotte Maria Daffin was a sister of Wm. R. Daffin, who in 1840 had married Dr. Ely's daughter, Mary Jane. St. Joseph *Times*, July 7, 1840.
6. 1850 Census, Jackson County, p. 320. Stanley's statement that Dr. Ely died in 1850 is obviously in error.
7. Marianna *Florida Whig*, July 8, 1848.
8. Census, 1860, Jackson County, item 53. Here his age is shown to have been 71 and that of his wife as 50.
9. Stanley, *History*, p. 201.

Emery, Chandler S., Duval County, 1814

Dr. Emery, born in Maine about 1814, was among the early settlers of Mandarin, Duval County, having arrived there about 1835.[1] Except for the fact that he was designated "physician" in the Census of 1850 and that he was usually accorded the title "Doctor" in printed sources, there is no evidence that he was ever a full-time medical practitioner after his removal to Florida. According to the census schedule of 1840 he was the owner of nine slaves which would indicate that he was at least a part-time farmer or citrus grower.[2]

It appears that Dr. Emery as well as other Mandarin settlers found life difficult. The winter of 1835-36 brought destructive freezes, severely damaging the young groves. This was followed immediately by a series of Indian raids marking the beginning of the Second Seminole War. Then came an infestation known as purple scale which further discouraged citrus growers. But with cessation of the War in 1842, Mandarin entered a period of recovery and Dr. Emery opened a general store in the village.[3]

Life continued to be rigorous, however, and in December 1843 Dr. Emery sought the increased security of a federal appointment as customs collector of the Port of Jacksonville. In a lengthy dispatch to the Secretary of the Treasury, J.C. Spencer, he called attention to the flagrant neglect and mismanagement of the office under the incumbent collector and deputy collector resulting in substantial loss of revenue for the Treasury Department. He then requested that his name be added to the list of applicants for the position, appending as referees some of the most distinguished citizens of East Florida including Generals Duncan L. Clinch and Joseph M. Hernandez, Judge I.H. Bronson, and the Reverend David Brown of Jacksonville.[4] Nothing came of his effort.

In spite of such setbacks, however, Dr. Emery's fortunes began to improve when he received appointment as a justice of the peace.[5] A short time later he moved into Jacksonville which was entering a period of growth and prosperity. In May 1855, he was among the citizens urging the building of the Atlantic and Gulf Railroad, projected to connect Jacksonville with West Florida.[6] Meanwhile his civic status was recognized by election by unanimous vote to the office of "Worshipful Master of the Masonic Lodge of Jacksonville," Solomon Lodge No. 20, in December 1857.[7]

Dr. Emery became probate Judge of Duval County in 1860,[8] an office he held for one term. This was apparently his last venture into public service. In the meantime he was appointed by Judge B.A. Putnam to assist in the settlement of the estate of James Winter, deceased, who had extensive holdings in Duval and Alachua Counties.[9] He continued to be active in Masonic affairs, representing the Solomon Lodge at the annual meeting of the Grand Lodge of Florida at its January 1866 meeting in Tallahassee where he was appointed to several committees.[10]

Meanwhile Dr. Emery's eldest son, Samuel C., also a physician, had established practice in the village of Aucilla, some 10 miles southeast of Monticello in Jefferson County. His father joined him there in the late 1860s, apparently having retired from his own practice. He was there in 1870 to be included in the census enumeration of that year.[11] A few years later, however, he returned to Duval County to live in the home of his daughter, Anna (Mrs. James S. Turknett), whose husband, a farmer, owned land located in what is presently the Wesconnett section of Jacksonville. He is presumed to have died there date unknown.[12]

1. Jacksonville *Courier*, December 24, 1835. Letter held, Jacksonville Post Office.
2. U.S. Census, 1840, Duval County, Florida, p. 145.
3. Mary B. Graff, *Mandarin on the St. Johns*, Gainesville, 1953, pp. 30-31.
4. Clarence E. Carter, ed., *Territorial Papers of the United States*, Vol. XXV I, Washington, 1962, Letter, December 14, 1843, pp. 808-810.
5. Jacksonville *Florida Republican*, December 12, 1850.
6. Ibid., May 3, 1855.
7. Jacksonville *Florida News*, December 19, 1857.
8. U.S. Census, 1860, Duval County, Florida, p. 251. See also Jacksonville *Standard*, April 5, 1860. List of Duval County administrative officers.
9. Jacksonville *Standard*, March 3, 1899.
10. *Proceedings, Grand Lodge of Free and Accepted Masons of the State of Florida, A.D. 1860-1866*, Tallahassee, 1866, p. 279, et passim.
11. U.S. Census, 1870, Jefferson County, Florida, p. 317.
12. U.S. Census, 1880, Duval County, Florida, p. 471. Here Dr. Emery is designated "Retired Physician, aged sixty-six." James S. Turknett (d. December 2, 1901, at 77) and his wife, Anna (d. May 5, 1899, at 64) are buried in the Turknett Cemetery, located in southwest Jacksonville. No date of death nor place of burial for Dr. Emery has been found.

Emery, Samuel Chandler, Jefferson County, 1838-1886

Dr. Emery, son of Dr. Chandler S. Emery, Duval County physician, was born in the county's Mandarin community on June 28, 1838.[1] After a medical apprenticeship, thought to have been served in the office of his father, he enrolled in the Atlanta Medical College, Atlanta, in the fall of 1859 and was graduated as

Doctor of Medicine in the spring of 1861.[2] Soon after receiving his degree Dr. Emery was married to a Florida native one year his senior known only as Charlotte. Soon thereafter the couple settled in the village of Aucilla, earlicr known as Williamsburgh,[3] situated 11 miles southeast of Monticello. He is said to have been the first physician to practice in Aucilla as well as the owner of the first drug store.[4]

Very little is known of Dr. Emery's civic activities during his 25-year residence in Aucilla. Only a few Jefferson County newspapers of the period have survived.[5] There is no record of his having served in the Army of the Confederacy, although he was of an age to have been eligible for recruitment. Possibly his marriage in 1862 and birth of his first child, christened William, in March 1863 accounts for his exemption. He was appointed justice of the peace in 1876,[6] and in 1882 was one of 10 delegates from Jefferson County selected to attend a State Democratic Convention.[7] Otherwise he is assumed to have lived quietly and usefully in Aucilla practicing medicine and operating his drug store. A mortality schedule of 1885[8] indicates that he continued his practice almost to the time of his death, which occurred on July 18, 1886.

Two children are known to have been born to Dr. Emery and his wife. They were William (d. May 8, 1896) and Maud (August 23, 1872-May 8, 1896). Mrs. Emery died on June 28, 1885, at the age of 48.

1. The dates of birth and death included here are found in a cemetery survey of Jefferson County. Members of the Emery family were buried in the Emery Cemetery located a mile east of Aucilla.
2. "Annual Announcement, Atlanta Medical College, Atlanta, Georgia," 1872, p. 15, Archives, Georgia Historical Society, Savannah. This publication includes rosters of earlier graduates. Although he is erroneously listed as L.C. Emery of Florida, it is clear that it should have been S.C.
3. Mary Oakley McRory and Edith Clarke Barrows, *History of Jefferson County, Florida*, Monticello, 1935, p. 102. With completion of the Tallahassee, Pensacola and Georgia Railroad about 1858, the village was known as Station 4.
4. Ibid.
5. The Monticello *Family Friend* ceased publication in December 1861.
6. Jerrell H. Shofner, *History of Jefferson County*, Tallahassee, 1976, p. 331.
7. Ibid., p. 342.
8. Special Florida Census, 1885, Jefferson County, Florida, Mortality Schedule, 1884-85.

Emswiler, George W., Jefferson County, 1850

By the time of his arrival in Florida in 1849 Dr. Emswiler was a well-traveled physician. A native of Virginia, born about 1813, he was married in 1840-41 to Lucy A. (cognomen unknown), also a native of Virginia. Soon after their marriage the couple migrated to Missouri where their eldest child, a son named Edwin, was born. A few years later the family moved to Louisiana where two additional children, a daughter Fanny and son named Charles, were born.[1]

The Emswilers were residents of Monticello by 1850, where the doctor resumed his medical practice. He appears to have been a gregarious type, quickly affiliating with the Masonic Order,[2] and also joining the congregation of Christ Church, Episcopal.[3] Subsequent to 1851, however, no further trace of Dr. Emswiler has been discovered. His name does not appear in the Florida census of 1860.

1. U.S. Census, 1850, Jefferson County, p. 4.
2. Jerrell H. Shofner, *History of Jefferson County*, Tallahassee, Sentry Press, 1976, p. 191.
3. Ibid., 197.

English, Charles G., Tallahassee, 1810-1872

Available contemporary records do not convey a clear picture of the career of Dr. English. In at least two instances he appears unmistakably to have been a medical practitioner. More frequently, however, he was found in other professional capacities, notably secretary to the surveyor of the Florida Territory and bookkeeper in a bank. He first appeared in Tallahassee about 1835-36 as correspondence clerk in the Office of the Surveyor-General, Robert Butler,[1] a position he continued to occupy until the early 1840s when Butler came under suspicion of irregularities in the management of funds accruing to his office. Lest they be implicated in the matter Dr. English and his colleague, Col. Robert W. Williams, hastened to establish their innocence in the alleged fraud.[2] For the protection of their reputations both men filed formal charges against Butler.[3]

On leaving the Office of the Surveyor-General, Dr. English appears to have entered, or returned to, the practice of medicine in 1842-43. On November 17, 1843, as Secretary of the Medical Faculty of Tallahassee, he was present at a special meeting called for the purpose of planning a suitable memorial for Dr. William W. Waddel, a highly-respected physician of the city, recently deceased.[4]

Dr. English was once more engaged in clerical work by 1850, this time as bank clerk.[5] The Census of 1850 gives his age as 40 and his birthplace as the District of Columbia. It also includes his wife, Martha, a North Carolina native, aged 25.[6] Ten years later he was apparently a widower with a nine-year-old son, Charles D.[7] His property was valued at $18,600. To confuse matters New Jersey is given as the place of his birth and to further compound the uncertainties the Census of 1870 indicates that he was born in Virginia.[8] His occupation is physician.

Beyond the age for military service in the War Between the States, Dr. English contributed his services to the effort on the home front. At a gathering of citizens of Tallahassee on February 11, 1863,[9] he served on a committee for the relief of citizens of St. Augustine who had been banished from their homes by the Union Army following capture of the city on March 11, 1862. Later in the year he acted as secretary for a meeting of citizens called to discuss the critical shortage of food and other essential commodities.[10]

Dr. English still resided in Tallahassee as late as 1870, sharing his home with Kate Madison, aged 17, and Lennie Maxwell, aged 13, probably relatives. Meanwhile his son, Charles Daniel, had departed Tallahassee and taken up residence in St. Louis where he died on February 8, 1872, at the age of 21.[12] Only four days later, on February 12, Dr. English died near Charleston, West Virginia, at the residence of D.E. Henderson.[13]

1. TP., XXV, 318-319. Robert Butler, Surveyor General of Florida, to E.A. Brown, Commissioner, General Land Office, Washington, D.C., June 27, 1836. See also Ibid., p. 461. In 1934 Mrs. Evelyn Whitfield Henry, Tallahassee historian, published her findings on many of the historic homes of the city. Included were some data on Dr. English, whom she identified as a "professor of mathematics from Harvard, who had come to Tallahassee for his health." It was her claim that Governor Duval had appointed him as a commissioner to supervise the erection of the Capitol. She identified the house at 217 N. Calhoun Street as having been the residence of Dr. English. Unfortunately Mrs. Henry's article was published without documentation and her facts remain unverified. Evelyn Whitfield Henry, "Old Houses in Tallahassee," *Tallahassee Historical Society Annual*, Vol. I, February, 1934, 39-55.

2. TP., XXVI, 383.

3. Ibid., 445.

4. Tallahassee *Sentinel*, April 2, 1843. If indeed Dr. English had abandoned the medical profession for the less rigorous occupation of clerk, it was probably because of his poor health. See note 1, supra.

5. U.S. Census, 1850, Leon County, Florida, p. 36.

6. Ibid.
7. U.S. Census, 1860, Leon County, Florida, p. 15. Martha English is thought to have been buried in the Bradford Cemetery, north of Tallahassee. No grave marker has remained, however. Joyce Smith Paisly, *The Cemeteries of Leon County, Florida*, Tallahassee, 1978, p. 34.
8. U.S. Census, 1870, Leon County, Florida, p. 50.
9. Tallahassee *Florida Sentinel*, February 17, 1863.
10. Ibid., November 17, 1863.
11. See note 8, supra.
12. Tallahassee *Weekly Floridian*, February 20, 1872.
13. Ibid.

Eppes, John Wayles, Leon, Jefferson and Madison Counties, 1825-1908

No resident of antebellum Florida could claim a more illustrious ancestry than Dr. Eppes. He was born at Ashton, Albemarle County, Virginia, in 1825.[1] His father, Francis Eppes, was the grandson of President Thomas Jefferson, while his mother, Elizabeth, was the daughter of Thomas Eston Randolph of Virginia, who in 1829 settled in Leon County. A year earlier, however, Francis Eppes had made the long journey to Florida to explore the possibilities of settling there and, finding the lands around Tallahassee fertile and well-drained, returned with his wife and three children the following year.[2] John Wayles was the second child and eldest son.[3] Their modest plantation was known as L' Eau Noir.

After the death of his wife in April 1835, at 34, Francis Eppes moved to Tallahassee where young John Wayles received his early education and developed an interest in medicine.

John Wayles entered the Jefferson College of Medicine in Philadelphia in 1847 and received his medical degree in the spring of 1849. The subject of his doctoral thesis was "Malaria."[4] Returning to Tallahassee in the summer of 1849 he did not enter straightway into medical practice but instead sought an army appointment.[5] His effort was given a boost by Governor Thomas Brown who recommended him to Major General David E. Twiggs, Commander of the 2nd Division, U.S. Army, with headquarters at Tampa Bay.[6] An army contract was soon forthcoming and within weeks he was commissioned acting surgeon with artillery units stationed on the Caloosahatchee River at the site later to be known as Ft. Myers. He was to remain there for a year.[7]

Upon fulfillment of his army commitment in the spring of 1851 Dr. Eppes returned to Tallahassee and on May 12 advertised his professional services to the citizens of the community.[8] He married Josephine Bellamy on November 14, 1854, in a ceremony at St. John's Episcopal Church.[9] Thus were joined two of Florida's most aristocratic families, Josephine was the daughter of Abram Bellamy, one of the area's wealthiest planters who upon his death had left his widow and children well endowed.[10] Upon receiving her inheritance about 1855, John and Josephine Eppes settled on her lands in Jefferson County where they apparently lived comfortably and quietly until the outbreak of war in 1861. The Census of 1860 shows them as owners of property valued at more than $40,000.[11] In the household also were the three-year-old daughter, Eliza, and George Dawkins, overseer of their farm. There were 33 slaves. Significantly Dr. Eppes was designated not as physician but as farmer.

The Civil War record of Dr. Eppes is marred by numerous lacunae but indicates that he enlisted for Confederate service in Tallahassee on August 20, 1861, for a period of three years. He was mustered in a week later as surgeon with the rank of 1st lieutenant and assigned to Company M, 2nd Florida Infantry. Before the end of 1861 he resigned his commission but on September 8, 1862, he was again commissioned as surgeon and assigned to the 5th Battalion, 2nd Florida Cavalry. He appears to have served with this unit at Camp Finegan, near Jacksonville, until April 1864, when he was transferred to hospital service at the Confederate Hospital, Georgetown, South Carolina.[12] The date of his discharge is unknown.

When the War ended Dr. Eppes did not return to Jefferson County but settled instead in the northwestern part of Madison County in the Hickstown community where he lived out his life as physician and farmer. In the meantime two other children were born, Mary and Frank.[13] The family appears to have lived in comparative obscurity during the postbellum period. Perhaps they, like so many other Southern plantation owners, found themselves in reduced circumstances through loss of slaves and farm income. Dr. Eppes died in 1908 at age 83.[14]

1. Dr. Eppes was the namesake of his paternal grandfather, John Wayles Eppes, 1773-1823, whose first wife was Maria Jefferson, daughter of President Thomas Jefferson. Grandfather Eppes represented his Virginia district in the U.S. House of Representatives for several terms and was later a United States Senator from Virginia. For further genealogical information on the Eppes family see W.G. Stanard, "Abstracts of Virginia Land Patents," Virginia *Magazine of History and Biography*, III, No. 4, April 1896, 396-397.

2. For an account of these migrations to Florida by the Eppes and Randolph families see the useful genealogical study of these families by Dr. John Chipman and Randolph Whitfield under the title, "The Florida Randolphs." It exists in typescript and photocopy. The third edition was produced in Tallahassee in 1978.

3. Three additional children were born to Francis and Elizabeth Eppes. Upon her death in 1835 he married a widow, Susan Margaret Ware Crouch, and they had seven children.

4. Archives, Jefferson College of Medicine, Philadelphia, Lists of Graduates.

5. Tallahassee was over supplied with physicians about 1850, a situation which probably prompted Dr. Eppes to seek opportunity elsewhere.

6. Florida *Senate Journal*, 5th Session, 1850-51, App., p. 22. This letter also contained a commendation for Dr. S.B. Todd praising his professional skill and unselfish service with the army on the Caloosahatchee.

7. The Monroe County Census enumerator found Dr. Eppes there in September 1850, attached to Co. B, 3rd Artillery Regiment. He had the distinction of being listed also in the Leon County Census of that year.

8. Tallahassee *Sentinel*, September 23, 1851; 1st pr. May 12, 1851.

9. DAR, Parochial Records, St. John's Episcopal Church, Tallahassee, 1832-80.

10. "Old Plantations Near Monticello," typescript, PKYLFH, p. 49. Section on Lyndhurst Plantation. Mrs. Abram Bellamy later married William J. Bailey, also a man of wealth and social position, who built a splendid mansion on Lyndhurst Plantation, some 15 miles northeast of Tallahassee.

11. U.S. Census, 1860, Jefferson County, Florida, p. 48.

12. NA, Service Records, CSA, M251, Rolls 8 and 36.

13. Frank Eppes became a merchant in the town of Madison. His gravestone in the Madison Cemetery gives the date of his birth as 1863, his death as 1929. Dr. Eppes' wife, Alberta Wharton Eppes (1867-1945), is also buried there. This information, courtesy of William Goza. Dr. Eppes' daughter, Mary, was married on November 20, 1889, to J.B. Morrison of Tallahassee, "one of Tallahassee's most prominent young men." Madison *Recorder*, November 29, 1889.

Farrington, John S., Pensacola, 1827

The only available information concerning Dr. Farrington has been derived from his professional card which was published in four consecutive issues of the Pensacola newspaper in July 1827. Its quaintly formal language bears citing here.

PHYSIC AND SURGERY

John S. Farrington, M.D., Respectfully informs the citizens of Pensacola that he has commenced the practice of his profession in this City, and may be consulted on all occasions at the house of Mr. J. Smith, Water Street, where all applications in his professional business will be promptly obeyed and diligently attended to. Pensacola. 5th July 1827.[1]

1. Pensacola *Gazette*, July 6, 1827, a weekly newspaper also had the notice in the issues of July 13, 20, and 27. Note that the medical degree is included.

Feaster, John P., Alachua and Marion Counties, 1850

Dr. Feaster, a native of South Carolina, was a resident of the southwestern part of Alachua County in 1850.[1] The census of that year lists him as physician, aged 21, a resident in the home of a farmer, James G. Cameron. Ten years later he was residing in adjoining Marion County with his wife and two small children, a son and a daughter. In this instance he is designated "Planter," owning property valued at $8,000.[2] He was probably one of many early Florida settlers who had served a brief internship in the office of a physician, electing to attempt medical practice, but abandoning it in favor of a more rewarding occupation.

1. U.S. Census, 1850, Alachua County, Florida, p. 20. Dr. Feaster's name does not appear in the lists of students and gradutes of the Medical College of the State of South Carolina.
2. U.S. Census, 1860, Marion County, Florida, p. 278.

Ferguson, Christopher C., Alachua and Marion Counties, 1832

Very little is presently known of Dr. Ferguson, medical practitioner, who was living at Newnansville, Alachua County, in 1880. He was 48 years of age at the time. Both he and his wife, Elizabeth, were natives of Kentucky.[1] They had moved to Marion County by 1885 and meanwhile had adopted a daughter, Anna L., who was eight years of age that year.[2] Nothing further is known of the family.

1. U.S. Census, 1880, Alachua County, Florida.
2. Special Florida Census, 1885, Marion County, p. 29.

Ferguson, John A., Marion County, 1851-1877

Dr. Ferguson, a native of Marion County and highly respected physician of Ocala, was born in January 1851 in the Cotton Plant community west of Ocala. His father, Neill Ferguson, a well-to-do planter, owner of property valued at $28,000 in 1860, was a native of Scotland while his mother, Nancy, was born in Georgia.[1] Following an early education in local schools John A. entered the Savannah Medical College, Savannah, in the fall of 1868 and on March 1, 1870, was graduated Doctor of Medicine. His doctoral thesis was entitled "Tetanus."[2]

Although only 19 years of age Dr. Ferguson returned to Florida and entered practice in Ocala. A short time later he joined the highly-respected Dr. Thomas P. Gary and W.P. Trantham in establishing a general merchandise business, a portion of which was allotted to the sale of drugs. In late 1874 this partnership was dissolved by mutual consent. The notice of dissolution was accompanied by the following statement: "The undersigned will continue the Drug Business in Ocala and solicits patronage. Signed, Dr. J.A. Ferguson, M.D."[3] In January 1875 Dr. Ferguson notified the public that the "Drug Business in Ocala heretofore conducted by J.A. Ferguson, M.D., will, after January 1, 1875, be carried on under the name and style of J.A. Ferguson & Co."[4]

In the summer of 1874 Dr. Ferguson made his only known excursion into local politics when he came to the support of his partner, Dr. Gary, candidate for the office of mayor of Ocala. In a heated contest Dr. Gary won the office but was accused by his opponents of having switched to the Republican Party in order to win the Negro vote. Dr. Ferguson responded to the charge with a letter, branding the charge as false and assuring the public that Dr. Gary "is still a good Democrat."[5]

For reasons quite unknown Dr. Ferguson announced in the spring of 1876 that he was giving up his Ocala business and departing for Scotland. The local newspaper, the Ocala *East Florida Banner*, stated: "Our esteemed friends, Dr. Jno. A. Ferguson and wife, left here on last Wednesday for Scotland where they will permanently reside."[6] Whether or not they actually made the trip has not been determined. If indeed they did go their sojourn was brief, for on March 18, 1877, the doctor died at his Ocala home at age 26 years and two months. He was buried in Ocala's Evergreen Cemetery.[7]

There is evidence that Dr. Ferguson may have suffered from a congenital weakness of constitution, possibly a susceptibility to pulmonary ailments. It is known that his sister, Margaret, wife of John M. Dye of Sanford, North Carolina, died in 1874 at age 27.[8] She was said to have been a person of frail health. Furthermore, their father, Neill Ferguson, died also in 1874 at age 54.

1. U.S. Census, 1860, Marion County, Florida, p. 291, item 333. This census lists John's age as nine. The other children of Neill and Nancy Ferguson were: Margaret, 13; Sarah, 11; James, five; C.A. (daughter), three; and an infant, three months.
2. Savannah (Ga.) *Morning News*, March 2, 1870.
3. Ocala *East Florida Banner*, January 8, 1876, 1st printing December 4, 1874 (issue not extant).
4. Ibid., March 13, 1875, 1st printing, January 16, 1875.
5. Ibid., August 8, 1874, reprint of letter appearing in Savannah *Morning News*, July 25, 1874.
6. Ocala *East Florida Banner*, April 15, 1876.
7. Ferguson Gravestone, Evergreen Cemetery, Ocala.
8. Ocala *East Florida Banner*, June 13, 1874.
9. Ibid., January 31, 1874. Legal notice regarding settlement of Neill Ferguson's estate naming Dr. John A. Ferguson as administrator.

Fewgate, William M., Marion County, 1870

Of Dr. Fewgate it is known only that he was a medical practitioner in Marion County shortly after the Civil War and probably for some years prior to the war. His residence appears to have been located in the agricultural area northwest of Ocala. The Census of 1870, the only known source of information on the doctor, lists him as a native of Virginia, 43 years of age and the owner of property valued at a mere $500. His wife, Sarah, a native of Florida, was 20 years younger.

Two other members of the household were Carolina, probably his sister-in-law, and two-year-old George, his son.[1]

1. U.S. Census, 1870, Marion County, Florida, p. 279, item 1173.

Finlayson, John L., Jackson County, 1869

Except for the fact that he was born in Georgia about 1840, nothing is known of the early life of Dr. Finlayson. He was a resident of Marianna living in the home of Dr. R.A. Sanders in 1860. The census of that year lists him as 20 years of age and a medical student,[1] presumably under the preceptorate of Dr. Sanders.

Two years later Dr. Finlayson enlisted as a private in Company "B" (the Marianna Dragoons), Fifteenth Confederate Cavalry Regiment, a unit recruited from Florida and Alabama. His enlistment date was March 4, 1862, and his term of enlistment three years or the duration. By order of General John H. Forney on September 15, 1863, he was placed on detached service at Moore General Hospital in Mobile, still with the rank of private. In 1864 he was admitted to Ross Hospital in Mobile suffering from ophthalmia, an inflammation of the eyeball, but he was with his Company at Quincy when it surrendered to the Union commander in Tallahassee on May 11, 1865. He was discharged on May 22.[2]

Dr. Finlayson returned to Marianna as a medical practitioner at the conclusion of the War. Unfortunately he found himself caught up in the emotional stress which accompanied implementation of reconstruction policies in what had been a planter-controlled society. Governor Harrison Reed, a Republican, in an effort to placate some of his most unyielding foes, made several appointments calculated to bring them around, but to no avail. One was the appointment of Dr. Finlayson as Circuit Court Judge of Jackson County which had been announced in early 1869. Dr. Finlayson's lineage as a Southern-born white man did not save him, however, nor did it allay local passions. In March 1869, while walking home from his office with Major William Purman, agent in the Freedmen's Bureau Office in Marianna, about 10 o'clock in the evening, he was killed by an assassin's bullet. The assassin was never apprehended.[3]

1. U.S. Census, 1860, Jackson County, Florida, p. 737. This approach to becoming a certified physician, i.e., "reading medicine" under the guidance of a practicing physician or preceptor, who in time would recommend that his pupil be licensed, was widely used in Florida until the Florida Medical Association was organized in 1874.

2. The details of Dr. Finlayson's military service, i.e., pay vouchers, special orders, etc., are found in NA, Confederate Service Records, Microcopy No. 258, Roll 30.

3. J. Randall Stanley, *History of Jackson County*, Marianna, 1950, pp. 36, 164, 206, 208. Mr. Stanley noted that the bullet which killed Dr. Finlayson and wounded Purman was fired from behind the fence around John Davis' residence, which was later the home of Dr. Theophilus West.

Fisher, George Doughty, Escambia and Santa Rosa Counties, 1814-1862

Dr. Fisher,[1] a native of Hillsboro, North Carolina, was brought at an early age to Alabama. His family settled in Hayneville, Lowndes County, where he received his early education and began the study of medicine under the preceptorate of Dr. Merriweather L. Gilmer, a local physician. In the fall of 1834 he matriculated in the Medical Department of Transylvania University, Lexington, Kentucky, where in the spring of 1836 he received his medical degree, having submitted a doctoral thesis entitled "Cynanche Trachealis."[2]

Shortly after graduation Dr. Fisher married Lauretta Virginia Grimes, a Lexington girl, whom he brought as a bride to Camden, Alabama, where he began his professional practice.[3] After a brief sojourn in Camden, where his two older children, Ann and Marshal, were born, the Fishers moved to Escambia County about 1839 and the doctor practiced briefly in and around Pensacola. The mid-1840s, however, found him in the village of Ucheeanna (Eucheeanna), Walton County.[4] There he ventured into politics, running successfully for the Florida House of Representatives as a Whig[5] in 1846, but his wanderings were not finished. By the end of 1847 the Fisher family had settled in the village of Milton, Santa Rosa County.

In Santa Rosa County Dr. Fisher immediately assumed a position of leadership in the Whig Party. At the county meeting of April 15, 1848, he served as secretary and member of the resolutions committee[6] and later in the year, as the presidential election approached, his influence was apparent in the organization of the local "Rough and Ready Club" in support of the candidacy of war hero, Zachary Taylor.[7] When his beloved party had virtually disintegrated in 1856, he refused to follow some of his fellow Whigs into the rapidly expanding Democratic Party, choosing rather to remain with the fragmentary group calling itself the American Party but known as Know Nothings by their opposition. In his candidacy for the state Senate that year he won handily over his Democratic rival for the District Two seat.[8] Nor was he yet finished, for in 1858 without substantial party backing he was returned to the Senate, retaining his seat through the adjourned session which was convened on November 28, 1859.[9]

The slender available evidence suggests that Dr. Fisher was a man of intelligence, pleasing demeanor, and exceptional energy, with an element of restlessness in his nature. He was never a man of wealth although he appears to have been able to provide adequately for his large family which in 1850 included his wife, seven children, and Mrs. Fisher's sister, Susan Grimes. An eighth child, Georgetta, was born in 1853. His real property was estimated to have been worth $3,000 in 1850 but was valued at $4,000 10 years later. His farming interests seem to have been of minor importance since he owned a single slave in 1850 and only seven in 1860.[10]

The Fisher family did not escape the tragic consequences of the War Between the States. Somewhat too advanced in years to be eligible for conscription into the Confederate Army, Dr. Fisher became a member of the Milton Home Guard while continuing his medical practice. In March 1862, however, when Union troops approached, residents of Santa Rosa were ordered to destroy all materials which might be of use to the enemy. This meant destruction of the entire lumber business, lifeblood of the area. When the troops arrived in early June, they found desolation in Milton and other settlements, much of the population having fled, while such Confederate troops as had been located there were fragmented into small units attempting a guerrilla-type resistance.[11] Dr. Fisher and his family had fled to Marianna, thence to Geneva, Alabama, some 50 miles distant. There he was shot by deserters from the Confederate Army a short time later.

1. Unless otherwise indicated the biographical data included in this sketch were provided by Miss Dena Snodgrass, of Jacksonville, a great-granddaughter of Dr. Fisher. Her assistance is gratefully acknowledged.

2. Archives, Transylvania University, Lexington, Kentucky, courtesy, Prof. Eric H. Christianson, University of Kentucky, Lexington. "Cynanche Trachealis," illness of the tonsils, throat or windpipe.

3. Camden, county seat of Wilcox County, is located south of Selma.
4. Dr. Fisher's residence in Ucheeanna as early as the fall of 1845 is established by the Pensacola *Gazette* of October 4, 1845, which named him as the paper's agent through whom subscriptions might be obtained.
5. Ibid., October 17, 1846. See also *Florida House Journal*, 1846, passim, for his participation in House proceedings and committee assignments.
6. Marianna *Florida Whig*, April 26, 1848.
7. Pensacola *Gazette*, October 14, 1848.
8. Although the Democrats returned a solid majority to the Legislative Assembly, the Know Nothings of Santa Rosa County scored majorities in all contests on the ballot, due in part no doubt to the leadership of Dr. Fisher. In the course of the upcoming legislative session a bill "for the relief of George D. Fisher" came up for consideration. It dealt with his claim for $26 for attendance at a coroner's inquest on the body of Hustes Gonzales in 1854. Dr. Fisher asked to be excused from voting. His request was honored; the vote of the Senate was unanimous for the bill. *Florida Senate Journal*, 1856, p. 66. See also *Laws of Florida*, 1856, p. 65.
9. *Florida Senate Journal*, Adj. Session, 1859, p. 3. Dr. Fisher was present at the opening session but three days later, on December 1, Senator T.J. Eppes made the motion that Dr. Fisher be granted leave of absence for 10 days. The Senate agreed. No explanation for his absence was recorded although he never appeared again throughout the session which adjourned on December 22.
10. U.S. Census, 1850, Santa Rosa County, Florida, p. 448; Ibid., 1860, p. 29.
11. *The War of the Rebellion*, Ser. I, Vol. XV, pp. 108-109.

Fisher, Robert Westwood, Leon County, 1823-1879

Dr. Fisher, a native of Virginia, spent the greater part of his life in Leon County. He was the son of George Fisher Sr., who had moved with his family to Florida in the late 1820s and settled north of Tallahassee in the Centreville vicinity. Young Fisher matriculated at the New York University College of Medicine in the fall of 1845 and was graduated M.D. in the spring of 1847.[2] Proceeding soon thereafter back to his home in Florida, he announced publicly his professional services, stating that he was locating at Hickory Hill, the rural home of his brother, George Henry Fisher.[3] Four years later the partnership of Dr. Fisher and Dr. William F. Robertson was given public notice. This arrangement with Dr. Robertson, a few years senior to Dr. Fisher, lasted for about three years and was terminated in 1851 when Dr. Robertson decided to move into Tallahassee to become the partner of Dr. John W. Eppes.[4]

Dr. Fisher was married in 1855 to Henrietta Bembry, member of a well-to-do Leon County family which had moved from North Carolina to Florida. Her family had accumulated substantial properties, a considerable portion of which passed by inheritance to Mrs. Fisher.[5] Two children, Hunter and Mary, were born to this marriage.[6] The Fisher family, like most Southern planter families, was much reduced by the economic disasters stemming from war and Reconstruction. Their material wealth, estimated at more than $50,000 in 1860, was said to have been worth slightly more than $5,000 in 1870.[7]

Unlike many planters, however, Dr. Fisher had a profession to which he could return. In his earlier professional years he had enjoyed a steady practice and built up a good reputation This he had virtually abandoned in the mid-1850s as he turned increasingly to farming, indeed to such a degree that the census enumerator in 1860 designated him not "physician" but "farmer." In 1870 he was once more "physician."

The latter years of Dr. Fisher's life were apparently uneventful. He died on January 30, 1879, in what could have been the prime of his life. Although he had never been affiliated with the Florida Medical Association, his demise was brought to the attention of the group. At its annual meeting in Jacksonville in April 1879 at the conclusion of the report of the Necrology Commitee, its

President, Dr. R.D. Murray, added the following remark:[8]

> One other death has occurred in our profession that I am impelled, from the worthy character of the man, to note. I refer to R.W. Fisher, M.D., of Leon County. . . .resident of Florida for fifty years. He was well known, and had the entire confidence of all who knew him.

The Tallahassee newspaper offered similar praise: "Died on January 30, 1879, Dr. R.W. Fisher, aged about fifty-five, at his residence in the County. He was one of our most estimable citizens. . .widely known through the County as a physician, and greatly esteemed for his high character."[9]

1. Several members of the Fisher family appeared in the Florida census of the years 1830-1880. That the doctor was the son of George Sr. is established by the entry in the Leon County Census, 1850, p. 128., which shows him as a member of the household of William E. Fisher, the other members of which were his brothers, George H. and Westwood, and sister, Landonia, all unmarried at the time.
2. *Proceedings, Florida Medical Association*, Jacksonville, 1879, p. 30. It was unusual for the Association to take notice of nonmembers in such laudatory manner.
3. Tallahassee *Floridian*, July 17, 1847.
4. Tallahassee *Sentinel*, September 30, 1851.
5. Tallahassee *Florida Sentinel*, January 2, 1855. Leon County Court House Records show the date as December 29.
6. U.S. Census, 1870, Leon County, Florida, p. 132.
7. U.S. Census, 1860, Leon County, Florida, p. 81; Ibid., 1870, p. 571.
8. See note 2, supra.
9. Tallahassee *Weekly Floridian*, February 4, 1879.

Fitzpatrick, Valentine, St. Johns County, 1800

Oaths of allegiance to the Spanish crown sworn by settlers in East Florida include one by Dr. Valentine Fitzpatrick ante 1799. Born in Ireland, he was of Catholic faith, married with one child, and a practicing physician in St. Augustine. The record indicates that he was employed in the government hospital.[1]

On July 23, 1803, he petitioned for land for himself and eight slaves in the amount of 400 acres at a place known as Sam's Hammock in Graham's Swamp on the Matanzas River some 15 miles south of St. Augustine.[2] The petition was granted by Governor White four days later.[3] This land came into dispute years later when it was argued that Dr. Fitzpatrick had failed to settle it according to the terms of the grant.[4]

Although Dr. Fitzpatrick had died prior to December 1825, it appears that possession of the land had been secured to the Fitzpatrick family. On December 23, 1825, Charles W. Clark deposed that Dr. Fitzpatrick built houses on the property, then claimed by his heirs.[5] In 1829 the St. Augustine newspaper carried a public notice warning against trespassing on a tract of land. . .called "Sam's Hammock, formerly granted to Dr. Valentine Fitzpatrick and now claimed by his widow, Mrs. John L.K. Holsterdorf, at present residing in Georgia."[6]

1. EFP, Bundle 83 E7, Reel 31. Papers of the Comptroller of the Royal Hospital, 1776-1816.
2. SLG. III, F.49 (2).
3. Ibid.
4. Ibid., IV, P 29; III, F. 50 (3).
5. Ibid.
6. St. Augustine *Florida Herald*, April 1, 1829. This notice was first printed on March 11, 1829, when the paper was still called the *East Florida Herald*.

Flake, William, Live Oak, late 19th century

Dr. Flake, a native of Alabama, practiced medicine in Live Oak in the latter part of the 19th century. The Tallahassee newspaper, *Land of Flowers*, noted his visit to that city in June 1882 with the remark, "Dr. Flake of Live Oak made us a pleasant call. The Doctor looks cheerful and happy, and thinks that Live Oak is about as near heaven as any town in Florida, and her citizens the best in the world."[1] The 1880 Census gives his age as 40 and that of his wife, Isla, as 34.[2]

1. Tallahassee *Land of Flowers*, July 1, 1882.
2. U.S. Census, 1880, Suwannee County, Florida.

Flake, William M., Gainesville, 1838-1899

Dr. Flake was born in Eufaula, Alabama, in 1838,[1] the son of William and Sarah Flake, both natives of Georgia. His father was also a physician as was his brother, Benjamin, a graduate of the Medical College of Georgia in 1853.[2] Very little is known of William Flake's educational background but he is presumed to have begun his medical study as an apprentice in his father's office. He began his medical practice in Gadsden County about 1860. He was married to Ida Gregory, daughter of Jason Gregory, a successful farmer and businessman of Ochesee, a village in the southeastern corner of Jackson County near the Apalachicola River. Dr. Charles A. Hentz, who had boarded for some time in the Gregory home, referred to Dr. Flake unflatteringly as "an unsettled, dissipated man,"[3] an appraisal which was probably not quite justified.

It is not known exactly when Dr. Flake moved to Gainesville but he is thought to have been there by the early 1880s. The register of physicians of Florida compiled under auspices of the Florida Medical Association in 1892 and published in the following year lists him as a Gainesville practitioner, although he was never a member of the Association. He died in Gainesville in 1899, his wife having died 11 years earlier.[4]

1. Date from Dr. Flake's gravestone, Evergreen Cemetery, Gainesville.
2. *List of Graduates from 1829 to 1891*, Medical Department, University of Georgia, Augusta, 1890, p. 17. For information on other members of the Flake family see U.S. Census, 1850, Barbour County, Alabama, p. 196.
3. Dr. Hentz was a man of superior education, his father having been a professor of French at the University of North Carolina, Chapel Hill. He appears to have looked with some disdain on many of his professional colleagues. One wonders if he may have been a suitor for the hand of Miss Gregory. See C.A. Hentz, "Autobiography," transcript of unpublished manuscript, Southern Collection, Library, University of North Carolina, Chapel Hill.
4. See note 1, supra.

Fleming, George Claudius, Duval County, 1822-1857

Dr. Fleming was born on October 30, 1822, in St. Augustine,[1] son of Lewis Michael and Agustina Cortes Fleming, and grandson of George Fleming who had settled on the west bank of the St. Johns River in the late 18th century and married Sophia Fatio, daughter of the well-known Francis Philipe Fatio.[2] The Fleming properties lay on the north side of Black Creek (Duval County) at its confluence with the St. Johns and encompassed the communities later to be known as Hibernia and Magnolia. The Flemings, Lewis Michael and brother, George Jr., were prosperous planters and slaveowners, and young George Claudius doubtless enjoyed such advantages as would normally accrue to children of a well-to-do frontier family.

George Claudius entered the medical division of the University of Pennsylvania in the fall of 1844 and was graduated with the degree of doctor of medicine in the spring of 1846. His graduation thesis bore the title "Masturbation."[3]

Dr. Fleming appears to have returned soon after graduation to the Black Creek area to establish his medical practice.[4] At some point either before or after graduation he was married to Mary, a native of New York.[5] To this union two children were born.

In the summer of 1851 Dr. Fleming, somewhat suddenly and doubtless to the amazement of his family and friends, decided to give up the practice of medicine and embark on a theological career. To this purpose he entered the Princeton Theological Seminary.[6] In August 1851, he made a formal announcement of his decision appointing Capt. O. Buddington as his agent, and urging all persons indebted to him to make immediate settlement.[7] The reaction of at least one of his cousins, Dr. William J. L'Engle, has been preserved in the following letter:

> Have you heard that Dr. George Fleming has given up his profession and gone to Princeton, N.J. to study Divinity? He should have done that four or five years ago and he would have been better off than he is now. He had entirely too much conscience to make a successful physician; he left his son, Edwin Williams, with Mrs. Holloway and his wife has taken the other child and gone to live with her relatives. . . .[8]

After receiving the Bachelor of Divinity from Princeton in 1853, Dr. Fleming returned home to Florida where he was ordained in the Presbyterian Church. He served briefly as a missionary at Woodstock Mills in Nassau County but about 1855 became pastor of the Presbyterian Church in St. Mary's, Georgia. His ministry was cut short by his untimely death in 1857 at the age of 35.[9]

1. University of Pennsylvania, Archives, List of Graduates.
2. For important information on the Fleming family see Arch Fredric Blakey, *Parade of Memories, A History of Clay County, Florida*, Jacksonville, 1976, pp. 13-14, et passim. Dr. Fleming's father, Lewis Michael Fleming, was married twice, first to Agustina Cortes of Havana, Cuba, and second to Margaret Seton of Fernandina. Dr. Fleming was the second son of the first marriage.
3. University of Pennsylvania Archives, List.
4. Ibid.
5. U.S. Census, 1850, Duval County, Florida, p 212.
6. *Biographical Catalogue*, Princeton Theological Seminary, Princeton, 1909.
7. Jacksonville *Florida Republican*, August 21, 1851.
8. "L'Engle Letters, 1843-1863," collected by Gertrude L'Engle and Tracy L'Engle, typescript, p. 30. The letter cited here, Dr. William Johnson L'Engle to his aunt, Miss Leonis L'Engle, was dated at Raleigh, N.C., August 25, 1851. PKYLFH.
9. University of Pennsylvania Archives, List. Here his death is said to have occurred in 1857. Church Records, Presbyterian Church, St. Mary's, Ga., however, indicate that his ministry there extended from 1856 to 1858. This note **ex info** of Miss Dena Snodgrass, Jacksonville, Fla.

Fletcher, Lionel, Leon County, 1798

Census data indicate that Dr. Fletcher spent the greatest part of his life in the comparative obscurity of rural Leon County. A native of Virginia, he migrated to Mississippi as a young man and there he met and married his wife, Phoebe, and there also his eldest child, Amanda, was born.[1] By the mid-1820s the Fletcher family had moved to Leon County, settling on the Ochlockonee River, some seven miles west of Tallahassee. He appears to have been a respected citizen of the community, enjoying local prominence as inspector of elections,[2] and later as justice of the peace.[3]

Nothing is known of Dr. Fletcher's medical education. His earliest professional notice was that which appeared in the Tallahassee *Floridian* of March 9, 1833, in which he announced that he had "resumed the practice of medicine" and that his residence was located "seven miles west of Tallahassee, near Murry's Ferry. . .on the Ochlockonee River."[4] According to the census of 1850, he had become the father of six children, four sons and two daughters.[5] Dr. Fletcher was a man of modest means, possessing real property valued at $800 in 1850, total property, i.e., real and personal, valued at $2,800 in 1860, and $1,800 in 1870.[6]

Dr. Fletcher lived on into the 1870s. The 1870 Census lists him as head of family in a household which included his wife, Phoebe, his son Richard, and daughter, Amanda. The 1880 census, however, shows Mrs. Fletcher as "widow."[7]

1. U.S. Census, 1850, Leon County, Florida, p. 103. Dr. Fletcher first appears in Florida records for the year 1829. He appears in the Florida census of the following year.
2. TP, XXIV, 169, 410; ibid., entries dated March 19, 1829, and May 11, 1830.
3. Ibid., p. 815; ibid., XXV, 105.
4. Tallahassee *Floridian*, March 9, 1833.
5. The ages of the children suggest that Dr. Fletcher was twice married.
6. U.S. Census, 1850, Leon County, Florida, p. 103; ibid., 1860, p. 38.
7. Ibid., 1870, p. 557; ibid., 1880, precincts 10 and 11, p. 305.

Flowers, Andrew J., Columbia County, 1870

Dr. Flowers, a graduate of the Medical College of Georgia, class of 1858, and a native of that state, spent the earlier years of his professional career in Georgia. Judging from the ages of his five children, the youngest aged two in 1870, perhaps he did not migrate to Florida until about 1869-70.

He settled in a rural area but there is no indication that he was ever engaged in farming. In 1870 his property was estimated to have been worth $1,560.[1]

1. U.S. Census, 1870, Columbia County, Florida, item 558.

Floyd, Henry, Ocala, 1860

Dr. Floyd's[1] Florida career appears to have been brief. A native of North Carolina, he had entered medical practice in Ocala in the late 1850s and in 1860 he was a resident at the hotel operated by E.J. Harris. It is interesting that three other Ocala physicians, J.A.S. Todd, George Wilson, and R.T. Morris, were living at the same hotel. With the outbreak of war in the following year it appears likely that Dr. Floyd returned to his native state for military service. He does not appear in subsequent records.

1. U.S. Census, 1860, Marion County, Florida, item 33.

Folker, William H., Leon County, 1831

Dr. Folker announced his professional services to the citizens of Tallahassee and vicinity on January 13, 1831. His office was at the home of his father "one door west of the Clerk's Office."[1] He was still in Tallahassee as late as the following summer[2] but did not remain much longer. The Folkers are not listed in the Leon County Census of 1830.

1. The Tallahassee *Floridian and Advocate*, January 13, 1831.
2. The Tallahassee *Floridian*, July 7, 1831.

Folsom, Lewis A., Hamilton County, 1860

Although he is designated in the Census of 1860 as "physician," it is doubtful that Dr. Folsom ever offered his professional services to the public. He had moved into Hamilton County in the 1850s from his native Georgia, acquired a large tract of land, and settled down as a planter. In 1860 his property, real and personal, was valued at about $40,000.[1] His slaves numbered 44.[2] Only two citizens of the county appear to have owned more property than Dr. Folsom; they were the Marions and the Staples. Dr. Folsom does not appear in the Florida census after the Civil War. It must be assumed that for some reason, financial or otherwise, he departed the state.

Evidence, although flimsy, points to the probability that the Folsoms came to Florida from either Lowndes or Brooks County. Census records of both include numerous families bearing the name.

The household of Dr. Folsom included an E.V. Folsom (female), aged 43, 10 years the doctor's senior, and Sarah Folsom, aged 73, presumably his mother. She was a native of Massachusetts. In addition, there were four residents named Wyche, ages 12 to 21, probably nieces and nephews, or cousins, of the doctor.[3]

1. U.S. Census, 1860, Hamilton County, Florida, p. 22, it. 150.
2. Slave Schedule, 1860, Hamilton County, Florida.
3. Lacking further evidence it is assumed that E.V. Folsom was the sister of Dr. Lewis and daughter of Sarah. The Wyche children were Virginia, aged 21; L.E. (female), aged 17; C.V. (female), aged 14, and J.S. (male) aged 12.

Fonda, Christopher Y., Pensacola, 1820s

Dr. Fonda arrived in Pensacola in the summer of 1821. Shortly thereafter, on September 6, he presented his professional credentials to the Board of Health of the City whereupon it was ordained that he "having complied with the ordinance of the Board of Health 'regulating the practice of medicine', and upon examination being found duly qualified to practice medicine and surgery and being of correct moral character, be licensed accordingly."[1] Henceforth, at least for the next nine years, he was actively engaged in the practice of his profession in Pensacola.

Dr. Fonda was appointed Health Officer of the City by Governor Duval in April 1823,[2] serving on the Board of Health with Dr. J.P.C. McMahon who was Resident Physician. At least one of Dr. Fonda's periodic health reports has been preserved. For the week of July 12-18, 1823, he reported:[3]

> Miss Simpson—bilious fever; Miss Howie—bilious fever; Christopher Kenzee—intermittent ditto; George Brown—intermittent ditto (since dead), who was of an unacclimated consititution.

He was mentioned as the attending physician in a case of yellow fever during the epidemic of 1827.[4]

In addition to his medical practice Dr. Fonda was involved in other community activities and personal services such as administering the estates of deceased persons,[5] selling real estate,[6] and most notably as a lay leader of the Pensacola Methodists struggling to build their first church in the City.[7] The Reverend Isaac Boring, a Methodist missionary sent to Pensacola by the Conference of South Carolina to lend spiritual and moral support to the project, was lodged in Dr. Fonda's home.[8] Dr. Fonda himself was chairman of the building committee and a contributor to the building fund.

Available records provide no information on Dr. Fonda. The Census of 1830 lists him as the head of a household which included one woman between 40 and 50 years of age (Fonda's wife?) and one male child between 10 and 15[9] (his son?). Fonda's age is shown as between 30 and 40.

1. Pensacola *Floridian*, September 8, 1821. It appears that the ordinance creating the Board of Medical Censors which consisted of the Resident Physician of the City, Health Officer of the City, and Drs. Moses H. Elliott and Ayers P. Merrill, both of the U.S. Army, was actually drafted at this meeting.
2. Ibid., April 26, 1823.
3. Ibid., July 19, 1823.
4. Pensacola *Gazette*, September 7, 1827.
5. Pensacola *Floridian*, March 29, 1823.
6. Pensacola *Gazette*, April 27, 1827.
7. F.W. Hoskins, *The History of Methodism in Pensacola, Florida*, Nashville, 1928, pp. 41, 47, 111, 112, 114.
8. Ibid.
9. 5th U.S. Census, Escambia County.

Foreman, Jacob, St. Augustine and Jacksonville, 1806-1856

The medical career of Dr. Foreman remains obscure. Born in Pennsylvania, he settled in St. Augustine in the late 1830s and was included in the Census of 1840 in which he is shown to have owned two slaves.[1] By 1850 he was a resident of Jacksonville, living in the home of the well-known physician, Dr. Henry D. Holland.[2] In this instance, however, he was designated "merchant," his age, 45, owning property valued at $1,000. Dr. Foreman died in Jacksonville on the morning of March 27, 1856,[3] at the age of 50. His place of residence in the city was not identified nor was his place of burial.

1. U.S. Census, 1840, St. Johns County, Florida, p. 129. The two slaves, one male and one female, were obviously household servants.
2. U.S. Census, 1850, Duval County, Florida, Entry No. 35.
3. Jacksonville *Florida Republican*, March 27, 1856.

Foreman, William B., Gadsden County, 1840

Dr. Foreman, the only son of A.J. and Mary Foreman, was born in Quincy in 1840. The elder Foreman, a Maryland native, was a Quincy merchant whose properties were estimated to have been worth $50,000 in 1860.[1] According to the census of that year William B. was a military student, but whether at a local academy or elsewhere is not indicated.

With the Civil War already in progress Foreman enlisted in the Confederate Army on January 11, 1862, for a 12-month stint which he extended a few months later to a three-year commitment. It was doubtless his previous military training which enabled him to enter the service as a second lieutenant. He was assigned to Company F, 6th Florida Infantry Regiment, with Captain James C. Evans as his commanding officer. When Captain Evans became ill in the summer of 1862 and declared unfit for further service, Foreman was promoted to a first lieutenant. In that rank he remained with his unit while it was stationed at Apalachicola Arsenal and later at Chattahoochee Arsenal, moving with it into Tennessee in early 1863. He saw action in the defense of Chattanooga where heavy fighting took place. The command moved into northwest Georgia on September 1, 1863, and on September 19 and 20 engaged the enemy at Chickamauga, a battle which resulted in heavy losses on both sides. On the second day Foreman was seriously wounded.

Out of action, Foreman spent the next several months in hospitals, first at Marietta, Georgia, and later in his home town of Quincy. As the War neared its close he was sufficiently recovered to be returned to active duty but apparently not into combat. He was paroled on April 26, 1865, along with other members of his unit.

Foreman entered medical school in the fall of 1865, presumably at the Washington University School of Medicine in Baltimore, from which he was graduated in March 1867.[3] On March 26, 1867, the Quincy *Commonwealth* printed the following item: "In the list of recent graduates at Baltimore Medical University was the name W.B. Ferman (sic) of this place."

Upon graduation Dr. Foreman returned to Quincy, probably to the home of his father, but in 1870, however, the census enumerator located him at the home of John C. Walker, a well-to-do farmer residing outside the town.[4] He is thought to have remained there engaging in medical practice until 1878 when he became chief physician in the recently-established State Asylum for the Insane in Chattahoochee.[5] For the first few years of its existence the Asylum did not have a hospital. Dr. Foreman met this need by setting up a "sick-room" in one of the original barracks of the old Chattahoochee arsenal. Several years passed before a reluctant Legislature appropriated funds for an adequate hospital.

The first superintendent of the Asylum was the well-regarded Dr. D.H. Allison. He and Dr. Foreman seem to have been compatible, but at the end of a year Dr. Allison retired. Dr. Foreman continued to work under a succession of superintendents—Dr. S.T. Overstreet, Dr. J.H. Randolph, Mr. W.D. Moseley, and Dr. J. Newton Smith. Although he was judged to have been a very able physician under whom the medical facilities of the institution were greatly improved, he resigned his position on May 1, 1892.[6] The reasons for his action are not clear, but the possibility of his having been pressured to resign has been explored.[5] Evidence points to the probability that on occasion he had extended his medical services beyond the asylum, thereby earning additional income. Also it appears that his reports to the Committee of the State Board of Institutions had not pleased that body.[7] There is no evidence however, that he was ever less than ethical and professional.

No further information on Dr. Foreman has been discovered.

1. U.S. Census, 1860, Gadsden County, Florida, p. 47, item 329. Other children in the family were two daughters, Ella and Ann, aged 18 and 16 respectively in 1860.

2. Foreman's military career is traceable in National Archives, Service Records, CSA, M251, Rolls 69 and 70.

3. Two medical colleges existed in Baltimore during the period under consideration, viz, Washington University School of Medicine (1827-77) and the School of Medicine of the University of Maryland (1807-). Since Dr. Foreman's name is not found in the lists of graduates of the latter institution it is assumed that he was a graduate of the former,

records of which have not been located. No school bearing the name Baltimore Medical University ever existed.

4. Walker's farm was located in the so-called Cross Roads community south of Quincy on the Lake Talquin Road.

5. Richard B. Chardkoff, "The Development of State Responsibility for the Care of the Insane, 1830-1950," M.A. Thesis, Florida State University, 1964. Microfilm in PKYLFH, University of Florida, p. 44, et passim.

6. Ibid., p. 57.

7. *Minutes of the Board of Commissioners of State Institutions*, 1892, MS in Florida State Library, p. 57, shows that on April 30, 1892, the Board passed two resolutions affecting Dr. Foreman's duties. The first was designed to tighten the Board's controls over the asylum's physician, while the second demanded that the physician submit quarterly reports to the Board on all his activities. On May 1 Dr. Foreman submitted his resignation.

Forry, Samuel, East Florida, 1811-1844

Some would question inclusion of Dr. Forry among the physicians who practiced in Florida in the 19th century. He was indeed not a regular practitioner; nevertheless, his scientific observations on climate and disease in East Florida in the 1830s are the statements of an exceptionally well-educated man of medicine. Dr. Forry was born in Berlin, Somerset County, Pennsylvania, on June 23, 1811[1]. He received his medical degree at the Medical College of the University of Pennsylvania in 1836. Immediately thereafter he was appointed Assistant Surgeon in the United States Army.

With the Second Seminole War already under way Dr. Forry was soon assigned to duty at Ft. Taylor on Lake Winder, located some 12 miles due west of Cocoa Beach. The sharp contrast of that locality when compared with the scenes of his childhood must have been a shocking experience for the young physician. He obviously regarded it as a challenge and proceeded to record his impressions which became the substance of his book, *The Climate of the United States and Its Endemic Influences*, New York, 1842. Of equal importance were frequent letters to General J.W. Phelps and others in which he described many aspects of the Florida scene as well as the misery which he endured from the Florida heat and insects.[2]

Dr. Forry's life was brief. He died on November 8, 1844, at the age of 33.[3] It is regrettable indeed that a physician-scientist of his intellect and literary skill could not have lived for a few more decades.

1. Vital Records, Library, University of Pennsylvania, Philadelphia.

2. Professor John K. Mahon, in his *History of the Second Seminole War*, Gainesville, 1967, p. 240, has quoted Dr. Forry's description of the scene: "Our position here at Ft. Taylor is indeed melancholy. After each rain we resemble Noah on top of Mt. Ararat. Clouds of crows and blackbirds hover around, waiting for the waters to subside, to resume their daily vocation of picking up corn... .Now a mosquito buzzes in your ear, and next a flea bites you between the shoulders... .We are almost eaten up by fleas, ants, cockroaches and all manner of vermin, etc."

3. Dr. Forry carried on an extensive correspondence with Lt. John W. Phelps between 1837 and 1839. Copies are preserved in the P.K. Yonge Library, University of Florida, Gainesville. These cover a variety of subjects. Their literary style is flamboyant, showing off Dr. Forry's erudition. Their medical content is minimal. He does express his annoyance with the questionable practice of medical personnel in the Seminole War who presented "trumped-up" accounts to the Surgeon-General's Office. He mentions one hospital steward, a Tennessean, who transmitted an account of nearly $19,000, regularly made out, "for services rendered in the absence of the Regimental Surgeon." Letter, Forry to Phelps, February 8, 1839. These letters were published, 3 parts, in the *Quarterly of the Florida Historical Society*, Issues, Part 1, Vol. VI, No. 3, January 1928, pp. 133-148; Part II, ibid., April 1928, pp. 206-219, Part III, ibid, VII, No. 1, July 1828, pp. 88-105.

Foster, Charles G., Pensacola, 1821-1822

Only brief notices bear testimony that Dr. Foster practiced medicine in Pensacola at the beginning of the territorial period. The Pensacola newspaper of November 5, 1821, carried the following item: "Dr. Foster has received from New Orleans an invoice of Medicine, which he offers for sale to country practitioners and others on accommodating terms for cash or produce."[1] The following April he announced that he "was resuming the practice of medicine and would be happy to attend his former patients and friends," giving no hint as to the reason for his having suspended practice.[2] If he were indeed among the few who had remained in Pensacola during the terrible yellow fever epidemic of the fall of 1822, he apparently survived, for the list of grand jurors attending two sessions of the U.S. Superior Court held at Pensacola in January and September 1823 includes the name of Dr. Foster.[3]

Pensacola records provide no trace of the fate or whereabouts of Dr. Foster beyond 1823.[4]

1. The Pensacola *Floridian*, November 5, 1821. One may be tempted to find a link of kinship between Dr. Foster and one E.B. Foster, a prominent attorney and judge in Pensacola, who died in early September 1822. This attorney was born in the West Indies but had resided in Conecuh County, Alabama, prior to coming to Pensacola. No verification of such an assumption has been discovered, however.

2. Ibid., February 1, 1822. This advertisement continued to appear until June 1 of that year.

3. TP, XXII, 613. Since the professional notices of Dr. Foster do not provide a Christian name, one must look to post office notices of letters being held in which he is mentioned as Dr. Charles G. Foster. The Pensacola *Floridian*, April 13, 1832, and subsequent issues.

Frayser, B.F., Marion County, 1850

Dr. Frayser was a mere sojourner in Florida. The Marion County Census of 1850 lists him and his wife, Elizabeth, as residents in the home of George Morton Payne.[1] They were natives of Virginia as were the Paynes. No other information has been discovered.[1]

1. U.S. Census, 1850, Marion County, Florida, p. 243, it. 123. The Payne plantation was located in north Marion County along the southwest shores of Orange Lake. It was known as "Lochbie."

Gaillard, Edwin Samuel, Jefferson County, 1827-1885

Dr. Gaillard,[1] one of the most erudite and accomplished physicians to practice in 19th century Florida, was born in St. John's Berkeley Parish, Charleston District, South Carolina, on January 16, 1827. He was the son of Dr. Edwin and Mary Gaillard who were of French Huguenot extraction and related by blood or marriage to several of Charleston's aristocratic families such as the Gourdins, Porchers and Peyres.

At about the age of 16, young Edwin matriculated at South Carolina College (later to become the University of South Carolina) in Columbia from which he was graduated in 1845 at age 18. He did not immediately begin a medical education but returned to the family plantation near Charleston to assist his widowed mother and sister, Mary, in managing the family estate, which included 81 slaves.

In the fall of 1852 Gaillard entered the Medical College of South Carolina, Charleston, from which he was graduated on March 9, 1854, with first honors.[2] Immediately after conclusion of graduation exercises Dr. Gaillard presided over a meeting of graduates assembled to draft a statement of gratitude to the faculty. His doctoral thesis bore the title, "An Essay on Intermittent and Bilious Remittent Fever with Relation to Ozone," a fitting topic for a medical student who had spent his youth in an area in which such fevers were endemic.

For reasons not discovered but possibly because of the migration of many South Carolina families to Middle Florida, Dr. Gaillard made his way almost immediately to Jefferson County, settling in the village of Waukeenah, where he began medical practice. He was not long in building up an adequate practice in that area of plantations whose owners in those final antebellum days were fairly prosperous. With his professional career launched, he returned to Charleston in 1856 for his marriage to Jane Marshall Thomas.

From the beginning of his Florida residence Dr. Gaillard was aware of the poor quality of available medical service, a condition attributable in large measure to the inadequate professional training of many practitioners compounded by the casual licensing procedure. Dr. Gaillard saw little hope of improvement without the organization of a state medical association and a county medical association in each well-populated county. Efforts as early as 1848 by a small group of physicians of Middle Florida to form a state association came to naught when the Legislature of 1849 rejected the plan.[3] In a lengthy letter addressed "To the Physicians of Florida Regarding the Absence of either County or State Associations of Physicians," he made a strong statement of his opinions.[4] Among other questions, he asked:

> Who amongst us can read the Proceedings of the American Medical Association, lately assembled (on its eighth anniversary) in Philadelphia, without a blush and a conscious shame for Florida? Every State but this represented. States Which were Territories long after Florida became a State! Territories having at present little more than a geographical existence. Societies, Associations, Army and Navy, all represented by delegations, sat upon the floor. But where was Florida? Disregarding her own welfare, independence and importance she has, for the eighth time been publicly ignored by the convened representatives of the profession throughout the land.

In mingled despair and hope Dr. Gaillard left Florida in March 1857 for New York where he resumed practice in the stimulating company of many of the country's most capable physicians. He made new friends, some of whom had studied under noted physicians of Europe. He was persuaded to continue training and spent a year in Europe where he became acquainted with a number of the more celebrated doctors.

Back in New York Dr. Gaillard enjoyed gratifying success. He was awarded the Fiske Fund Prize for his essay, "Ozone: Its Relation to Health and Disease."

Dr. Gaillard's happiness was marred by the death of his wife in 1860. Shortly afterward the election of Lincoln as president and the growing hostility between the North and the South further distressed him. In early 1861 he abandoned New York for the more congenial climate of Baltimore and in May entered the service of the Confederacy as assistant surgeon in the 1st Maryland Regiment. He was soon promoted to Regimental surgeon and two months later to surgeon of the Brigade. He was present at the Battle of Fair Oaks (or Seven Pines) and attended the seriously-wounded General Wade Hampton. Before the battle was over Dr. Gaillard received a wound in the arm which necessitated amputation. Notwithstanding the injury and loss of an arm he continued in Confederate service as general inspector of Confederate hospitals until the end of the conflict.

At the close of the war Dr. Gaillard settled in Richmond, Virginia, resumed medical practice, and on October 5, 1865, married Mary Elizabeth Gibson, granddaughter of the eminent Philadelphia surgeon, William Gibson.

In subsequent years Dr. Gaillard did not remain in one place. In 1867 he became Professor of General Pathology at the Medical College of Virginia in Richmond. He accepted a similar position at the Kentucky School of Medicine in Louisville in 1868. He joined the faculty of the Louisville Medical College in the capacity of Dean in 1879 while continuing to serve as Dean of the other Louisville institution.

Of equal importance to his practice was Dr. Gaillard's contribution to medical literature. He was a prolific writer and able editor. Prior to departure from Florida in 1857 he had written a series of articles which were published in the *Charleston Medical Journal and Review* in 1856 and 1857. In one of these he exposed the medical quackery which he found so common in Florida, but his diatribes were not limited to the state. One of his prime targets was Samuel Thomson, originator of so-called Thomsonianism. He also aimed his fire at the purveyors of Homeopathy, Hydropathy, Isopathy, Oinopathy, Kinesipathy and other methods. The disciples of Christian F.S. Hahneman (d. 1843), patron saint of Homeopathy, also felt Dr. Gaillard's sting. "Florida," he contended, "in common with most Southern States, is polluted with nostrums.[5]

As editor of medical journals Dr. Gaillard achieved national recognition. During his brief residence in Richmond he established the *Richmond Medical Journal* and upon moving to Louisville in 1868 continued its publication as the *Richmond and Louisville Medical Journal.* After moving to New York he changed the name to *Gaillard's Medical Journal*. He did not hesitate to use the journals to expound his own theories or to attack those of others with whom he found reason to disagree.

Dr. Gaillard died at his residence in Ocean Beach, New Jersey, on February 2, 1885. He was survived by his wife and two sons, the older, Edwin White Gaillard, was also a physician.[6]

1. Dr. Gaillard, educated in the classical tradition, had acquired an amazing knowledge of the medical literature of the ancient and medieval world from Hippocrates and Galen down to his own contemporaries. He did not hesitate to denounce the members of his profession whose knowledge was limited or those who were led astray by the imposters

of the times. Some 46 years ago Dr. Emmet Field Horine of Louisville made a thorough study of the life and career of Dr. Gaillard. The results were published under the title, "A Forgotten Medical Doctor, Edwin Samuel Gaillard (1827-1885)," in *Annals of Medical History*, 3rd. Series, Vol. II, 1940, pp. 375-382. A large portion of the present sketch was derived from Dr. Horine's article.

2. Charleston *Courier*, March 15, 1854.

3. A small group of doctors of Middle Florida met in Quincy (Gadsden County) in December 1848 for the purpose of organizing a professional association. Their proposal was presented to the Florida Legislature with a request that they be granted a charter. It was denied by a very narrow vote in the lower House.

4. This letter was published in the Jacksonville *Republican* of August 16, 1855. It was an eloquent and persuasive statement.

5. E. S. Gaillard, "Medical Topography of Florida," *Charleston Medical Journal and Review*, 1856, p. 202 installment 5, of series.

6. New York *Times*, February 3, 1885, obituary. In this notice it was mentioned that in 1873 the University of North Carolina, in recognition of Dr. Gaillard's contribution to medical science, had awarded him the honorary degrees of Master of Arts and Doctor of Laws, a testimony to the esteem in which he was held.

Galphin, George, Leon County, 1811

Existing sources permit only an incomplete sketch of the career of Dr. Galphin, although he appears to have been a person of prominence in Leon County. While the Census of 1850 lists him as a native of Georgia, the schedule of 1860 shows him to have been born in South Carolina.[1] The former appears to have been correct in that the records of the Medical College of South Carolina where he received his medical degree in 1831 indicate that he was a resident of Augusta.[2] Shortly after becoming a physician he returned to Georgia where he married Matilda Maxwell, daughter of John Jackson Maxwell of Bryan County. They had three children, Mary Elizabeth, Sarah Jane and John Maxwell.[3]

By 1840 Dr. Galphin had moved with his family to Leon County, settling in a community known as Bel Air a short distance south of Tallahassee.[4] As was true of many physicians of the times he seems to have been more farmer than doctor. His real estate was valued at $14,000 in 1860,[5] while other property was estimated to have been worth $30,000, which combined established him among the well-to-do. On at least one occasion he served as a livestock judge (boars and sows) at the Leon County Agricultural Fair.[6] Nevertheless he was definitely a medical practitioner. His professional card, printed in a local newspaper on May 6, 1845, announced that "Dr. Galphin is resuming practice of medicine in Tallahassee."[7]

Mrs. Galphin died in 1855[8] and the following year Dr. Galpin married Virginia Parkhill, a native of Virginia and member of a socially prominent Leon County family.[9] Two children, George and Ellen, were born to this marriage.[10] At some time, probably in the postbellum period, Dr. Galphin moved to Fernandina and is said to have spent the remainder of his days there.[11]

1. U.S. Census, 1850, Leon County, p. 108. Here he is designated "planter." U.S. Census, 1860, Leon County, item 530. In this case he is listed as "Dr. and farmer." The elder daughter, Mary Elizabeth, born in Georgia, aged 18 in 1850, was married that year on June 27 to T.N. Whitner Jr., Tallahassee *Sentinel*, July 2, 1850.

2. Archives, Medical University of South Carolina, Lists of Students. His doctoral thesis bore the title, "Dysentery."

3. The second daughter, Sarah Jane, aged 10 in 1850, was also born in Georgia. The son, John Maxwell, aged eight in 1850, was born in Florida. Matilda Maxwell was a first cousin of Dr. George Troup Maxwell, also a Leon County physician.

4. Dr. Henry E. Palmer in his essay, "Physicians of Early Tallahassee and Vicinity," *Apalachee*, 1944, has identified Bel Air as a settlement on a sandy ridge south of Tallahassee, attractive to settlers because of its higher elevation and good drainage. The U.S Census of 1840, Leon County, lists Dr. Galphin, his wife and two daughters.

5. See note 1, supra.
6. Tallahassee *Sentinel*, October 26, 1852.
7. Tallahassee *Florida Sentinel*, March 3, 1846, but first printed in issue of May 6, 1845.
8. Palmer, "Physicians," p. 35
9. Marriage Records, Leon County, Florida, comp. by D.A.R. Typed copy. PKYLFH, p. 79.
10. George, born 1857, and Ellen, born 1859.
11. Dr. Palmer, op. cit., states this as a matter of local knowledge. An examination of the Census Schedules for Nassau County for 1870 and 1880 did not reveal their presence there. The Galphin son, John Maxwell, served for three years in the Confederate Army, achieving the rank of first lieutenant in the 2nd Florida Infantry Regiment.

Gamble, Cary Breckenridge, Leon County, 1825-1921

Dr. Gamble, son of Robert Gamble and grandson of Robert Gamble of Revolutionary War fame, was born on September 25, 1825, at the home of his maternal grandfather, General James Breckenridge, in Botetourt County, Virginia.[1] At the age of one he was brought to Florida. His uncle, John Grattan Gamble, had migrated to Florida in 1823, purchased extensive acreage in Jefferson County, and established a plantation which he called Waukeenah. Dr. Gamble's father arrived three years later, purchased land and developed a plantation to which he gave the name, Weelaunee, where Cary spent his childhood. At adolescence he was sent to Richmond, Virginia, for basic schooling. At about this juncture his father and uncle bought homes in Tallahassee where they continued to live for several years.

In the fall of 1844 Cary Gamble matriculated at the University of Virginia[2] where he remained for the 1844-45 term. He enrolled at the University of Maryland Medical School, Baltimore, in October 1845, from which he was graduated the following spring.[3] Immediately thereafter he returned to Tallahassee and began his professional career in partnership with the highly-regarded Dr. James H. Randolph.

As the outbreak of war appeared imminent in early 1861, Dr. Gamble volunteered his services in the Confederate cause, being among the first Florida physicians to make such a move. His army contract, which was negotiated at the Pensacola Navy Yard on April 15, 1861, stipulated that he would perform the duties of a medical officer "agreeable with army regulations...at or near the Navy Yard, near Pensacola...for $100 per month, his full compensation, in lieu of all allowances and emoluments."[4]

As the conflict ensued, however, the provisions of Dr. Gamble's contract were soon overlooked; instead of remaining in or near Pensacola he was soon to see service in Georgia and Tennessee.[5] The year 1863 found him in Ringgold, Georgia, a senior surgeon in charge of the hospital located there. Later that year he was ordered to reopen the Army Hospital in Newnan, Georgia. In May 1864 he was chief surgeon on the staff of General James Patton Anderson and before the end of the conflict held a similar position on the staff of General John K. Jackson. He was medical officer in the Army of Tennessee by February 1865, under the command of General Braxton Bragg, and in this capacity was captured while treating soldiers wounded at the Battle of Shiloh. He was paroled by General Edward M. McCook on May 25 following.

Dr. Gamble was married on October 24, 1849, to Frances Edwarda Shaw of

St. Augustine.[6] Among numerous children born to them were twins, Cary and Edward, the former followed in his father's footsteps, received a medical degree from the University of Maryland[7] and settled down to practice in Baltimore for a few years prior to joining the faculty of the Johns Hopkins School of Medicine.[8]

Soon after conclusion of the Civil War Dr. Gamble moved to Baltimore and practiced there until retirement in 1901. He lived to an advanced age, dying in the home of his daughter, Mrs. Robert Lowndes, near Baltimore, on November 8, 1921, aged 96.

1. The Gamble family played major roles in the public affairs of Florida and as a consequence attracted the attention of several writers. Two brief biographical sketches of Dr. Cary Breckenridge Gamble worthy of note are Henry E. Palmer, "Physicians of Early Tallahassee," *Apalachee*, 1944, p.33, and Marjorie Fain, "Some Extracts from the History of the Gamble Family in Florida," Tallahassee, Tallahassee Historical Society Annual, Vol. I, February 1934, pp. 28-31. See also Michael G. Schene, "Robert and John Grattan Gamble: Middle Florida Entrepreneurs," *Florida Historical Quarterly*, LIV, No. 1, July, 1975, pp. 61-73.
2. Archives, University of Virginia, List of Matriculants and Graduates.
3. E.F. Cordell, *Historical Sketch of the University of Maryland School of Medicine*, 1807-1890, Baltimore, 1891, p. 175.
4. NA, Service Records CSA, M 251, Roll 27. The list of military appointments announced by Governor M.S. Perry on January 14, 1861, included "Cary B. Gamble, Surgeon-General, Rank of Colonel." This appointment was superseded by order issued by Confederate authority. Tallahassee *Florida Sentinel*, February 11, 1862.
5. Dr. Gamble had established a residence for himself and his family in Pensacola. It was there on October 30, 1861, that his daughter Eliza Shaw, aged six, died of diphtheria. See "Parochial Records, St. John's Episcopal Church, Tallahassee, Florida," a compilation made by the Tallahassee Chapter, DAR, 1936-7.
6. Parish Records, Trinity Episcopal Church, St. Augustine.
7. See note 3, supra.
8. Llewellyn F. Barker, M.D., "The Early Days of the Johns Hopkins Hospital," *Maryland Historical Magazine*, XXXVIII, March 1943, p. 10.

Gamble, George B., St. Augustine, 1849

The name, George B. Gamble, M.D., appears in the Register of Trinity Episcopal Church, St. Augustine, where it is recorded that on October 23, 1849, he married Frances Edwarda Gamble, the Reverend Benjamin Wright performing the ceremony. Neither the bride nor bridegroom is listed in the St. John's County Censuses of 1850 or 1860 which suggests that they were probably residents of another state, although both surnames were not uncommon in 19th century Florida.[1]

1. Trinity Episcopal Church, St. Augustine, Register.

Gamble Jr., John Grattan, Leon County, 1816-1856

In spite of an illustrious ancestry and the social prominence of his family only meagre information relating to the career of John Grattan Gamble Jr. has been preserved. He was born in Richmond, Virginia, in 1816, son of Col. John Grattan and Nancy Greenup Gamble.[1] At age nine he was brought to Jefferson County where his father bought large acreage some 10 miles southwest of Waukeenah.[2] With the depredation wrought by Indians during the Second Seminole War (1835-1842) the Gambles moved into Leon County, settling on a plantation a short distance east of Tallahassee which they called Neamathla after the Miccosukee chief whose village had been located on the land.[3]

It is doubtful, however, that young John Grattan ever spent much time at either Waukeenah or Neamathla for in the early 1840s he enrolled in the Medical

School of the University of Maryland and was graduated in 1843.[4] He returned to Tallahassee immediately and in November announced the opening of his practice there. His professional notices continued to appear in a local newspaper for more than three years, being discontinued after the issue of March 6, 1847.[5]

After the death of his brother-in-law, Thomas H. Hagner, husband of sister Catherine Jane, at 31 on March 27, 1848, Dr. Gamble shared the Hagner residence with his sister and her two small children.[6] He continued to practice medicine until his own untimely death on February 1, 1856.[7] The medical faculty of Tallahassee met to pay their respects to their departed colleague, issuing a resolution lamenting his death as a great loss to their profession and praising him as "gifted with an intellect of the highest order, ardent in the pursuit of science, a judicious physician and skillful surgeon."[8]

1. Dr. Gamble's family connections were of high order. They included his maternal grandfather, Governor Christopher Greenup, of Kentucky; an uncle, Governor William H. Cabell, of Virginia; another uncle, William Wirt, Attorney General under President Monroe.

2. Jerrell H. Shofner, "History of Jefferson County, Florida," Tallahassee, 1976, p. 26 et passim.

3. This statement is based on local legend. See Marjorie Fain, "Some Extracts from the History of the Gamble Family in Florida," Tallahassee Historical Society Annual, Tallahassee, 1934, I, 28.

4. E.F. Cordell, *Historical Sketch of the University of Maryland School of Medicine, 1807-1890*, Baltimore, 1891, p. 175.

5. Tallahassee *Floridian*, November 1, 1845, 1st printed, November 18, 1843.

6. U.S. Census, 1850, Leon County, Florida p. 82.

7. Tallahassee *Floridian and Journal*, February 2, 1856.

8. Ibid.

Gantt, Jose, Fernandina, 1814-17

Dr. Gantt, probably an American citizen, practiced medicine in Fernandina during the latter years of the Second Spanish Period. His name has been preserved through a series of communications between Francisco Ribera, military commandant of Fernandina, and the Spanish authorities of East Florida in St. Augustine. These dispatches reveal some of the problems relating to medical practice during this unsettled period.

Smallpox was a major medical problem. Although the first vaccination in America had been performed by Benjamin Waterhouse in 1800, and although the procedure was known to doctors as remotely situated as Dr. Gantt, the vaccine was not readily procurable. An order for inoculation equipment was authorized by Governor Sebastian Kindelan on April 14, 1814,[1] but two months elapsed before he communicated with Ribera enclosing the vaccine to be used "in inoculating residents."[2] A month later Ribera reported that Dr. Gantt had received the shipment and was proceeding with the vaccinations.[3]

By midsummer of 1814 Fernandina was beset by an epidemic of fever, the precise nature of which was not described. Ribera informed the Governor of the outbreak on July 29, suggesting that it had been introduced by crews from the ships in the harbor, and asking whether Dr. Gantt should board the vessels as they put into the harbor.[4] A week later the Governor timidly agreed that it should be done.[5]

Soon thereafter came the problem of paying the doctor. On September 24 Ribera reported that Dr. Gantt would no longer treat the Spanish troops in Fernandina unless he were paid.[6] Payment was authorized by the Governor on October 4.[7]

Nothing further is known of Dr. Gantt until July 1816 when the matter of remuneration for his services was once more in arrears. This impasse prompted another appeal to the Governor, in this instance, Juan de Estrada, to which he responded.[8] Dr. Gantt is last heard from a few days later (July 19) when he negotiated a contract with the Spanish government for continuing service in treating government personnel in the town.[8]

1. East Florida Papers, Reel 64, Bundle 155L12, Doc. 1814-117. This and all subsequent references to Dr. Gantt are derived from the East Florida Papers, now in the Library of Congress, Washington. Microfilm of these Papers has been used in these researches. The author is indebted to Bruce S. Chappell, Research Scholar, P.K. Yonge Library of Florida History, University of Florida, Gainesville.
2. Ibid. Doc. 1814-196
3. Ibid. Doc. 1414-222
4. Ibid. Doc. 1814-256
5. Ibid. Doc. 1814-261
6. Ibid. Doc. 1814-298
7. Ibid. Reel 65 Bund. 155L12 Doc. 1814-305
8. Ibid. Reel 65 Bund. 157A13 Doc. 1816-156
9. Ibid. Doc. 1816-161

Gardner, James H.M., Gadsden, Leon and Jefferson Counties, 1820

The medical career of Dr. Gardner was somewhat unusual in that he spent the first 16 years or so of his adult life as a minister of the Methodist Church before deciding to enter medical school. He had moved into Gadsden County from his native Georgia[1] about 1848, settling in a rural area north of Quincy. A few years later the Florida Methodist Conference assigned him to Pisgah Church near Centreville where he served as pastor in 1853 and 1855.[2] In the following year, however, doubtless motivated by the necessity to obtain a larger income for by this time five daughters had been born to him and his wife, he left Leon County and the ministry to enter Atlanta Medical College from which he was graduated in the spring of 1858. On September 25, 1858, the following item appeared in the Tallahassee *Floridian and Journal:*

> Among those who received the degree of M.D. at the recent commencement of the Atlanta Medical College was the Rev. J.H.M. Gardner of Centreville, Leon Co. We know Mr. Gardner well, and predict for him a high position in the medical profession.

Two weeks later the same paper printed the following:[3]

> Dr. JHM Gardner—This gentleman, as will be seen from our advertising columns, has located himself at "Lloyd" on the Pensacola and Georgia Railroad. He graduated (after pursuing a course at the University of Louisiana) at the Atlanta Medical College with distinguished promise of future usefulness in the medical profession.

Two years later Dr. Gardner had moved to Gadsden County once more, this time settling in the village of Concord in the northwestern corner of the county. The Census of 1860, Jefferson County, lists him as a resident of Concord, owning property valued at $2,000. By this date his children numbered seven, all daughters.[4] At this juncture the Gardners disappear from the Florida scene; they do not appear in the Jefferson County Census of 1870 nor has any trace of them been found in Censuses of other Florida counties. Conceivably the exigencies brought on by the War and Reconstruction dictated their removal to another state.

1. The Census of 1850 gives his birthplace as Georgia; the 1860 Census indicates South Carolina.
2. "Records, Leon County, Florida," comp. by DAR Tallahassee, 1937, mimeographed copy, p. 116.
3. The village of Lloyd was in antebellum days supported by a number of prosperous plantations which surrounded it. Its railroad stop was an important commercial facility for the area. It is located west southwest of Monticello one mile from the Leon County line.
4. U.S. Census, 1860, Jefferson County, Florida, p. 99. The names of the daughters are, from eldest to youngest, Rebecca, Mary, Emily, Susan, Sarah, Amelia and Martha.

Gardner, Richmond N., Leon County, 1832-1875

Dr. Gardner, son of Methodist minister Thomas Gardner, was born in Georgia on December 31, 1832. In his middle teens he began the study of medicine in the office of Dr. Miles Nash of Tallahassee. The Leon County Census of 1850 indicates that he was a resident in the home of Dr. Nash, his age was 17, and he was designated "clerk." In the fall of 1850 he is said to have matriculated at the University of Virginia School of Medicine from which he was graduated in the spring of 1852.[1]

After a sojourn of two or three years in Alabama, Dr. Gardner moved to Leon County, settling in the Centreville community. His professional card, which appeared in the Tallahassee *Floridian and Journal*, September 29, 1855, advertised his services to the citizens of the area from his office at the "Parsonage." The following year he announced that he would be residing in the home of John Crump and assume the situation "formerly occupied by the late Dr. Jacob Eliot."[2]

From the beginning of his residence in Florida Dr. Gardner manifested an interest in politics. With the Whig Party in a state of disintegration he was among those who switched to the ranks of the Democrats.[3] He was a Leon County delegate to the State Democratic Convention in Quincy in early June 1860, a session notable for its acrimony and general boisterousness.[4]

Dr. Gardner enlisted in the Army of the Confederacy on February 20, 1862, with a captain's commission and charged with recruiting a company of volunteers. His command became Company K, Fifth Florida Infantry Regiment.[5] Soon after its organization the regiment was ordered to Virginia where it was assigned to Pryor's Brigade and with only minimal training joined the 2nd Florida Regiment in the Army of Northern Virginia. It participated in the Battle of Gettysburg where on July 2, 1863, Dr. Gardner was wounded and taken prisoner. He was sent to the Union Hospital in Gettysburg on August 10 where his left arm was amputated. He remained a prisoner for the duration of the War, receiving his parole on May 23, 1865.

Back in Leon County Dr. Gardner resumed medical practice in the Pisgah community near Centreville. Notwithstanding loss of an arm he appears to have become an active and highly respected physician. Although not present at its organizational meeting in Jacksonville in January 1874, he was nominated and elected to membership in the Florida Medical Association.[6]

Soon after returning to Leon County Dr. Gardner married Sarah Elizabeth Cromartie, daughter of planter John Cromartie of North Carolina who was among the earlier settlers. The Gardner home was located on the Thomasville Road about four miles north of Bradfordville. The land is now a part of the Horseshoe Plantation.[7] Plagued by serious illness in late 1875 Dr. Gardner sought medical assistance in Montgomery, Alabama. It was to no avail for he died there on

December 28, 1875, just three days prior to his 43 birthday. His body was returned to Florida for burial in the Cromartie family plot. He was remembered for his "clear judgment, his generous disposition, and his high moral character."[8] At the Florida Medical Association annual meeting in Tallahassee in January 1876, his death was properly noted with a tribute of respect to his memory.[9]

1. A few biographical data on Dr. Gardner are found in his obituary notice, Tallahassee *Weekly Floridian*, January 18, 1876, and in ibid., February 8, 1876.
2. Tallahassee *Floridian and Journal*, May 3, 1856. See an earlier notice in ibid., September 29, 1855.
3. Jacksonville *Florida News*, March 29, 1856.
4. Fernandina *East Floridian*, June 21, 1860.
5. NA, Service Records, CSA, M251lm Roll 62.
6. *Proceedings, Florida Medical Association*, Jacksonville, 1874, p. 4.
7. Joy Smith Paisley, comp. and editor, "The Cemeteries of Leon County, Florida," Tallahassee, 1978, Mimeographed copy.
8. See note 1, supra.
9. *Proceedings, FMA*, Jacksonville, 1877, p. 7. Mrs. Gardner survived her husband by many years, dying on October 31, 1930. The Leon County Census of 1870 lists as a member of the Gardner household, Sally Gardner, aged 15. Since Mrs. Gardner was then only 25, it is assumed that Sally Gardner was a niece of Dr. Gardner.

Gary, Thomas Porter, Hernando and Marion Counties, 1835-1891

Dr. Gary , who spent the latter half of his life in Florida, was born in Cokesbury, Abbeville District, South Carolina, on April 10, 1835. His father, Thomas Reeder Gary, was also a physician but after his marriage to Mary Ann Porter, a woman of wealth, he appears to have discontinued medical practice devoting his time to managing his plantation. In 1850 his slaves numbered 45.[1]

Dr. Gary received his early education in a local Cokesbury school, very probably the Cokesbury (Methodist) Conference Academy. He is thought to have become interested in medicine through the influence of his brother, Franklin, who had become a physician. On January 1, 1853, he was enrolled at the Citadel in Charleston[2] where he remained for two terms. In the fall of 1855 he matriculated at the Medical College of South Carolina, Charleston, from which he was graduated in March 1857, having submitted a thesis entitled "Medical Delusions."[3]

Following graduation Dr. Gary spent a year traveling before settling down to practice in Brooksville. His professional card first appeared on February 5, 1859, in the Tampa *Florida Peninsular*[4] announcing a partnership with Dr. John P. Wall, an arrangement terminated the following July when Dr. Gary advertised the end of their partnership and Dr. Wall announced the opening of his practice in Fernandina.[5] The dissolution of the partnership was mentioned in the Tampa paper as follows:[6]

> We call attention of our Hernando readers to the card of Dr. T.P. Gary...Dr. Gary has been practicing for some months past in conjunction with Dr. Wall and, during that time has established an enviable reputation for skill in his profession. We sincerely hope that he may receive the support his abilities merit. Aside from his profession Dr. Gary is a clever gentleman, a prince of good fellows. Success to you, Doc!

Dr. Gary continued to practice in Brooksville until the outbreak of war in 1861. Unfortunately his war record is incomplete. It appears, however, that he had married a Brooksville girl, Tommie Howell, just prior to beginning of the War and had moved to Ocala before enlisting in the Confederate Army. He was commissioned Assistant Surgeon but was soon promoted to Regimental Surgeon of the Seventh Florida Regiment, a unit composed of recruits from Marion and Alachua Counties. For the greater part of his army career he was engaged in field and hospital with the Army of General Braxton Bragg in Kentucky and Tennessee. Of his military service Capt. J. J. Dickison wrote:[7]

> ...Dr. Thomas Gary, of Ocala. The devoted service rendered by him during the Civil War as a skillful surgeon, will ever be gratefully remembered. This eminent physician, after careful and patient research, has discovered a remedy for the cure of a painful disease, once thought incurable, that will be a great blessing to the suffering. May his useful life be prolonged...to bless the people he so kindly and faithfully ministers to...

Dr. Gary settled in Ocala in 1867 and soon established himself as a leading citizen as well as a trusted physician. Given his intelligence and pleasing personality he could not avoid involvement in politics, soon becoming mayor, a position to which he was elected for eight consecutive terms.

In connection with the election of 1874 an incident occurred which at present appears amusing but was not a laughing matter at the time. The Ocala newspaper, in reporting the coming elections, inadvertently placed Dr. Gary's name on the Republican ballot (essentially a Negro ballot). This error was brought to the attention of the Tallahassee *Floridian* in a letter of outrage from Dr. Gary himself. The Tallahassee paper made public notice of Dr. Gary's letter but refused to publish it claiming that "it is too personal for our columns." It did not hesitate, however, to attack the Ocala *Banner* for having implied that Dr. Gary was a Republican! The incident, as later revealed, resulted from an action by Anderson Woods, a Negro, who had presented the Republican ticket to the *Banner* editor, substituting Dr. Gary's name for that of a black man, Watson Murphy.[8] Dr. Gary won the election by a comfortable margin.

This contretemps was brought to the attention of the Savannah *Morning News* which congratulated Dr. Gary for winning, praising his integrity, and reassuring the people that Dr. Gary was still a good Democrat. It was later revealed that the Savannah paper had obtained the information from Dr. John Ferguson, an Ocala physician, whose popularity was not enhanced by the incident.

Professionally Dr. Gary enjoyed the respect and trust of Marion County citizens as well as that of his colleagues throughout the state. In 1888 he was elected to membership in the Florida Medical Association.[9] And at the meeting the following year he read a paper, "Malarial Haemoturia," which was referred to the Publications Committee.[10] The Association met in Ocala in 1890 where, as mayor, Dr. Gary gave the welcoming speech. As host he had planned trips to places of interest, including Homossassa. He also read a splendid paper entitled "Selecting Medicines," designed primarily as a guide to beginning or inexperienced practitioners. At the next session he was elected president of the Association.[11]

The following year the Association met in Pensacola, and in spite of the hardships of travel Dr. Gary honored his obligation to be present. The session, as it turned out, was poorly attended, only 13 members answering the roll call. Dr. Gary read a scholarly paper, "Animal Alkaloids," after which he was requested to prepare his remarks for publication. At the same meeting he was selected to represent the Association at the annual meeting of the American Medical Association. He was also reelected president. He then presented what was destined to be his last speech, in essence a message of hope for the future of medicine, reminding his audience of the advances recently made in the conquest of disease. He noted particularly the success in dealing with smallpox by vaccination and similar progress in the use of Peruvian bark against malaria. He held out hope for the struggle against cancer, yellow fever, consumption and cholera. He emphasized the roles of county medical societies and medical examining boards in coping with the influx into the state of quacks and humbugs. His remarks were eloquent and succinct, consuming in their delivery not more than 10 minutes. Little did he realize that this was his valedictory.[12]

Dr. Gary died less than two months later, apparently from complications growing out of the stress and fatigue experienced on the Pensacola trip. His death occurred at 5 a.m. on June 10, 1891.[13]

His survivors included a son, Charles, and daughter, Anna (Mrs. Alexander) of Brooksville. Other relatives were a brother, Major William T. Gary of Augusta, Georgia, a sister, Mrs. Ryan, of Edgefield, South Carolina, and numerous nieces and nephews.

1. Census, 1850, Abbeville District, Slave Schedule.
2. Ex infor., James D. Moody, Charleston, S.C. Mr. Moody is preparing a history of the Citadel.
3. Records, Medical College of South Carolina, Waring Historical Medical Library, Charleston, S.C.
4. Tampa *Florida Peninsular*, June 18, 1859.
5. Ibid.
6. Ibid., July 16, 1859.
7. Mary Elizabeth Dickison, *Dickison and His Men*, Facsimile Edition, Jacksonville, 1971, p. 232.
8. An account of this absurd affair was printed in the Ocala *East Florida Banner*, August 8, 1874.
9. *Proceedings, Florida Medical Association*, p. 8. At this session Dr. Gary was named chairman of the Committee on Medicine.
10. Ibid., 1889. This meeting was held in St. Augustine.
11. Ibid., 1890, pp. 51-58.
12. Ibid., 1891.
13. Dr. Gary met an agonizing death. His diminishing strength was further drained by the activities and strain at Pensacola. Already committed to attend the meeting of the American Medical Association in Washington the following week, Dr. Gary boarded the train in Tallahassee for the trip but reaching Atlanta he was too sick to continue. He was taken to the Kimball Hotel and regained sufficient strength to visit friends in Edgefield, South Carolina, where he suffered another seizure of la grippe. He returned to Ocala and showed slight improvement but at 2 o' clock on the morning of June 10 he suffered a severe lung hemorrhage. Dr. Robert P. Izlar was summoned and he died in Dr. Izlar's arms. A lengthy obituary appeared in the Ocala *Banner* of June 12, 1891.

Gatlin, John Slade, Assistant Surgeon, 1835

Dr. Gatlin, whose tragic death occurred on December 28, 1835, was born in Kinston, North Carolina, son of John Gatlin. Nothing is known of his early years and education. He is thought to have served an apprenticeship under a local Kinston physician prior to entering military service.

By 1834 the influx of white settlers into Florida had aroused the hostility of Indians in the central portion of the state whose hunting grounds and other sources of food appeared to be in jeopardy. Their resistance was expressed by occasional ambush and murder of white settlers in isolated places. The response of the United States government was to strengthen military outposts such as Ft. King in Marion County and Ft. Brooke on Tampa Bay and dispatch companies to guard against the stealthy Indians. One of these companies from the Fourth Infantry Regiment was commanded by Brevet Major Francis L. Dade, whose staff medical officer was Assistant Surgeon John Slade Gatlin, who was ordered to proceed from Ft. Brooke northward to Ft. King, a short distance east of Ocala. Leaving Ft. Brooke on December 23, 1835, the detachment made its way through swamps and brush, crossing the two prongs of the Hillsborough River. Four days later on Sunday December 27 the party had crossed the Withlacoochee River encamping about two miles north of the crossing.

On Monday morning, December 28, Major Dade awoke early, exhilarated by the realization that their destination could be reached by nightfall. Frank Laumer, relates the episode:[1]

> By daybreak, however, the sky was dark, the temperature was a chilling forty-four. By seven the rain had begun to fall. By eight o'clock the drip of rain had ended. The sky brightened...spirits lifted with the sun, as every mile brought them farther from the low land of danger, and closer to Ft. King.

It was not to be, however, the Indian ambush was well concealed. They were well aware of the movement of the detachment and at the opportune moment attacked. Several members of the Dade group fell under the onslaught. As Laumer relates it, Dr. Gatlin was heroic, he "worked carefully, dealing in death as methodically as he had dealt with life...stationed himself against the barricade...his powder was nearly gone. He loaded both of his double-barreled weapons, commented, 'Well, I've got four barrels for them,' and was cut down before he could squeeze the triggers." Thus ended the life of Dr. Gatlin at dawn on Monday, December 28, 1835.

1. The data are taken from Frank Laumer, *Massacre*, Gainesville, 1968.

Gee, Charles Alston, Gadsden County, 1833-1867

Dr. Gee, sixth son of Henry Gee, was born on the Gee Plantation near Quincy on November 20, 1833. His father, a native of Fayetteville, North Carolina, had moved to Georgetown, South Carolina, where he married Agnes Forrester. One son, John Henry, was born and Mrs. Gee died shortly thereafter. Henry Gee married the sister of his first wife, Martha Elizabeth Forrester, in 1823 and to this union were born eight sons and one daughter. Soon after his second marriage Henry Gee removed with his family to Gadsden County.[1]

Family tradition maintained that as a youth Charles Gee seriously considered becoming a clergyman but "finally decided to study medicine."[2] He began his professional training in the office of Dr. William Booth, considered Quincy's most eminent doctor. After completing an apprenticeship he entered the Medical College of the State of South Carolina in the fall of 1854 and was graduated in March 1856 after submitting a thesis entitled "Menorrhagia."[3] Soon after receiving his degree he returned to Florida and married Elizabeth Walton Dismukes of a prominent Tennessee family and settled in to practice his profession in Quincy.

With the onset of war in 1861 Dr. Gee followed the lead of his eldest brother, John Henry also a physician, and volunteered for military service. He was accorded the rank of captain and assigned command of Company A, 4th Florida Infantry Regiment. His military career was, however, of little note and short duration. On April 28, 1862, he wrote the following note to Colonel Edward Hopkins, Regimental Commander: "I have the honor herewith to tender my resignation...to take effect from 1st May, 1862. After the restoration of my health, rendered feeble by nearly one year's service. I shall again enter service and will continue it as long as my country is engaged in war."[4] His resignation was accepted.

Dr. Gee never actually returned to serve in an official capacity. When the long expected attack on St. Marks occurred in March 1865, posing a threat to Tallahassee and other middle towns, several physicians, among them Dr. Gee, offered their medical services. They were especially helpful in taking care of the dead and wounded after the Battle of Natural Bridge. Dr. Charles A. Hentz, a Quincy colleague of Dr. Gee, has written vividly of their experiences during the aftermath of battle, which included attendance upon several Negro soldiers of the Union Army left wounded on the field.[5]

Upon his return to Quincy Dr. Gee resumed medical practice in partnership with his brother, John Henry. This association was of brief duration, however. Dr. Gee died from meningitis on April 24, 1867, at age 34. The widow and four small children survived. A fifth child, Elisha, was born just four days after Dr. Gee's death.[6]

1. A complete history of the Gee family was written by a collateral member, W.J. Fletcher. See his *The Gee Family*, Rutland, Vt., 1937, a work which includes genealogical tables as well as a narrative treatment of family lore. As has been true of most works of its kind, no information which might reflect unfavorably upon any member of the family has been included. See note 6, infra.

2. Flether, op.cit. p. 131

3. Archives, University of South Carolina, Charleston, S.C. Lists of Matriculants and Graduates. Menorrhagia: abnormally profuse menstrual flow.

4. NA, Service Records, CSA, M 251, Roll 54. No element of Florida's population viewed the election of Lincoln with more anxiety than did the landowners of Gadsden County, nor was there a more zealous secessionist than Charles A. Gee. Personally he raised a company of volunteers from his own community and became its commanding officer. Dr. David A. Telfair said of his zeal, "he acted as if he would like to be rammed into a cannon or mortar and fired at the Yankees." This statement was quoted by Dr. C.A. Hentz, "Autobiolgraphy," I, 332. Once in the military, however, his life appears to have been miserable, probably from boredom, possibly from the wretched conditions prevailing in the makeshift army camps. His war record shows him to have been arrested for drunkeness in January 1862 and to have faced court martial on February 12 following. Although the complete account of the incident is not available it is inferred that the offense was inconsequential in that he was able to collect back pay due him from January 1 1862, until retirement on May 1.

5. Hentz, "Autobiography," II, 354-365.

6. Dr. Gee's death was a shocking event for the people of Quincy. Dr. Hentz wrote: "Dr. C.A. Gee died very suddenly from meningitis...a very sudden and alarming case...on the 28th (April)...only four days after his death his widow gave birth to a son, Elisha, now (1892) a promising young man." Ibid. II, 33 The death of her husband placed an enormous burden on Mrs. Gee. Her eldest child, John H., was only 12, while Susan, Charles, and Sally, were 10, eight, and six, respectively. The posthumous son, Elisha, became an exceptionally successful business man in Colorado.

Gee, John Henry, Gadsden County, 1819-1876

Dr. Gee, eldest son of Henry Gee, was born in Georgetown, South Carolina, in 1819. Within a year his mother, Agnes Forrester, died and about 1823 his father married her younger sister, Martha, and moved with his family to Gadsden County. He purchased a plantation a short distance from Quincy and soon became one of the county's wealthier and more influential citizens.[1]

Not much is known of John Henry Gee's early education but no doubt he was exposed to the best instruction available at the time. His later efforts in writing verse, much of which was published in newspapers and journals, indicate an affinity for literature as well as a sensitivity of spirit.[2] Dr. Gee's medical preceptor was the eminent local physician, Dr. William Booth. Family tradition holds that about 1838 young Gee attended medical lectures in Philadelphia, although no documentation for this has been discovered. He was in attendance at the Medical College of South Carolina for the session of 1839-40 at the end of which he received the M.D. degree, having submitted a doctoral thesis on "Dysentery."[3] He returned to Quincy where he eventually set up practice with a Dr. Weatherly, whose identity remains obscure.[4]

For the next few years the activities of Dr. Gee are not, for the most part, matters of record. In the early part of the present century an Atlanta newspaper published an account of the Gee family which included a brief sketch of Dr. John H. Gee.[5] It stated that he had served as "surgeon to the Florida Troops in the Seminole War" and that he later "went to California, Mexico and South America, and when the Mexican War broke out was appointed surgeon to the 1st Alabama Regiment."[6] Some credence for this statement is supported by his professional notice which appeared in the Tallahassee paper of September 14, 1852, to the effect that Dr. J.H. Gee "has resumed the practice of medicine in Quincy."[7]

Four days after Florida's decision to secede from the Union, January 7, 1861, Dr. Gee offered his services to Governor Perry, not in a medical capacity but as a military aide. His first mission took him to Montgomery, Alabama, to consult with the Governor concerning the taking over of military installations in the Pensacola Navy Yard.[8] On April 5, after having organized a company of local volunteers, he entered the military service as Captain of Company G, 1st Florida Infantry, for a 12-month enlistment, which he terminated on April 6, 1862.[9] Shortly thereafter he was appointed Inspector General of the Army at Mobile and subsequently campaigned in Kentucky. He was present at the Battle of Perryville (Ky.) where he was said to have displayed exceptional valor.[10] Returning to Florida, later he raised a battalion of volunteers mostly from Gadsden County which he commanded with the rank of major in a campaign near Petersburg, Virginia.

Dr. Gee was nominated in June 1864 by the Secretary of War as battalion cammander in the 11th Florida Regiment. This he declined in a long letter to General Samuel Cooper, stating as his reason the desire to return to the practice of medicine.[11] But his will did not prevail. Before the summer was gone he was ordered by General Braxton Bragg to assume command of a Confederate prison in Salisbury, North Carolina.[12] Given the presence on his staff of several former officers of higher rank than himself, frequent attempts at escape by the prisoners and, most important of all, the generally poor conditions of prison life, it was a difficult assignment indeed. Most of the grievances and gripes were directed at Dr. Gee. Not surprising soon after Appomattox he was arrested on charges of cruel and inhumane treatment of prisoners. After spending months in confinement at the Old Capital Prison in Washington he was brought to trial in Raleigh, North Carolina, on February 21, 1866.[13]

The trial stirred the wrath and indignation of citizens throughout the South and elicited letters and newspaper editorials by the score defending Dr. Gee as a man of honor and human kindness who could not possibly have committed the crimes with which he was charged. Their anxiety about a possible conviction had been intensified by the outcome of the recent trial of Major Henry Wirz, the officer at Andersonville prison, on similar charges. Wirz had been found guilty and was hanged on November 10, 1865. Due in part to the growing revulsion in both North and South against the execution of Wirz, but perhaps more to the subsiding emotional fervor for conviction, Dr. Gee was acquitted. On July 6, 1866, President Johnson ordered his release from prison.[14]

A short time before the beginning of the War Dr. Gee had entered into a medical partnership with his younger brother, Charles. In late 1866 they resumed practice in Quincy but the partnership was soon terminated by Charles' untimely death in 1867. Henceforth until his death Dr. John Gee continued practice alone, although he was frequently called into consultation by colleagues. He appears to have enjoyed a fine professional reputation in the community, although it cannot be said that he was universally admired. Dr. Charles A. Hentz, who had transferred his practice from Marianna to Quincy just prior to the War, found him surly and disagreeable. Dr. Hentz also disapproved of Dr. Gee's private life which he judged to have been immoral.[15] Dr. Hentz also wrote disapprovingly of Dr. Gee's medical techniques. In one case a Quincy citizen, George Dismukes, was dying of dysentery. Dr. Hentz wrote, "The doctor, who stuck to his old-time remedy routine of calomel and opium, mistreated the case lamentably...and told me that he was giving George *Veratrum*[16]...the idea of such an absurd and miserable blunder...outrageous." These harsh words are hardly to be taken at their face value, however, for doubtless the animosity was mutual.

The life of Dr. Gee came to an abrupt and tragic end on the early morning of August 13, 1876, while he was attempting to extinguish a fire in the Quincy business section. It was Dr. Gee's idea to explode a keg of gun powder in an adjoining store hoping that the explosion would arrest the flames. This he undertook to accomplish on his own. After lighting the fuse and waiting outside a reasonable time for the explosion he decided the fuse was faulty and reentered the building. He approached the keg just as it exploded and was blown to bits.[17]

Dr. Gee was a resolute man. He appears to have been courageous and straightforward, able to inspire confidence and trust among associates both military and civilian. His success in persuading the young men of Gadsden County to enlist in his battalion of "Young Guards," even before the urgency of the situation was generally understood, is a testament to his leadership. His audacity in declining a top office in the 11th Florida Regiment, an appointment which would have made him a colonel and one recommended by Jefferson Davis, suggests an independence of mind and a bold spirit. Yet he was not without blemish. Perhaps encouraged by loneliness (he was never married), he drank to excess and his close relationship with a certain woman of the town appears to have been public knowledge. For such indiscretions, however, he should be forgiven.

1. A complete genealogical study of the Gee family was published some years ago by W. J. Fletcher, a collateral descendant of Henry Gee. Much of the data of this sketch is derived from this source. See his *The Gee Family*, Rutland, Vt., 1937.

2. Ibid., pp. 137, 152-3.

3. Archives, MUSC, List of Students. See also Charleston *Mercury*, March 27, 1840.

4. Tallahassee *Florida Sentinel*, June 6, 1843, 1st printed January 20, 1843.

5. NA, Service Records, CSA, M251, Roll 27. Included in the war record for Dr. John H. Gee is a half-page clipping from the *Hearst Sunday American*, Atlanta, date unknown, which contains biographical information on Dr. Gee, who, said the author, "had the most colorful career of the Florida Gee Family."

6. Ibid.

7. Tallahassee *Sentinel*, September 14, 1852.

8. Fletcher, *Gee Family*, p. 141. Letter, John H. Gee to General Samuel, Adj. and Insp. Gen., in Richmond, July 20, 1864.

9. Service Record, See note 5, supra.
10. Ibid.
11. Ibid.
12. Fletcher, *Gee Family*, pp. 142-3. General Bragg's order was dated August 24, 1864.
13. Ibid., p. 144
14. Ibid., p. 151.
15. Dr. Hentz appears never hesitant in speaking his mind about acquaintances in Marianna, Quincy, and elsewhere. He frequently recorded impressions of medical colleagues, even those held in low regard. His impatience with alcoholism is revealed repeatedly in the pages of his "Autobiography." Charles A. Hentz, "Autobiography," microfilm of transcript, PKYLFH. Original MS in Southern Collection, University of North Carolina, Chapel Hill. See Dr. Hentz's estimate of Dr. Gee, Vol. II, p. 78.
16. Ibid., II, 129. Veratrum, a cardiac and muscular sedative.
17. Ibid., II, 131. Other accounts of the fire and the death of Dr. Gee are found in the Tallahassee *Sentinel*, August 19, 1876, and the Savannah *News*, August 14, 1876.

Geiger, Washington Whitfield, Micanopy, 1808-1855

Dr. Geiger was born in Edgefield District, South Carolina, on April 1, 1808.[1] Nothing is known of his early years and education. As he approached manhood he began the study of medicine as an apprentice to a relative, probably his brother, Dr. David Geiger, who had received his medical degree from the Medical College of South Carolina, Charleston, in 1827.[2] In the fall of 1829 he matriculated at the Medical Department, Transylvania University, Lexington, Kentucky, from which he was graduated in the spring of 1831, after having submitted a doctoral thesis entitled "Congestive Fever."[3]

After receiving his degree Dr. Geiger returned to Edgefield District where he practiced his profession for 20 years. In early 1851 he joined the virtual procession of upstate South Carolinians who migrated to Florida, many of whom settled in the northern part of Marion County. Dr. Geiger chose to settle in nearby Micanopy (Alachua County). On May 15, 1851, the Jacksonville *Florida Republican* noted that he was among the passengers arriving aboard the steamer St. Matthews, three days earlier.[4] He was soon joined by his wife, Sarah (she was actually his second wife), and his five children.[5]

In addition to medical practice Dr. Geiger entered actively into the civil affairs of the community. He was especially interested in improving the transportation facilities of his section of the state, which he regarded as essential to development of the citrus industry. In 1853 he organized a "Board of Managers" to promote development of a canal connecting Orange Lake with the Oklawaha River, which would provide water transportation into the St. Johns River and the port of Jacksonville.[6] Later that year he presided at a meeting in Micanopy called to discuss the building of a plank road from Micanopy to Palatka.[7] An ardent Democrat, he was present at a gathering of County Democrats in Micanopy at which he was elected president of Alachua County Democrats.[8]

Dr. Geiger's life was tragically brief, however. He died on September 8, 1855, at the age of 47. He was survived by his wife and children, ranging in ages from nine to 17.[9]

1. The dates of Dr. Geiger's birth and death are found on his gravestone in the Micanopy Cemetery.
2. Archives, Medical College of South Carolina, Charleston. Lists of Matriculants and Graduates, Waring Historical Medical Library, Charleston.
3. Archives, Transylvania University, Lexington, Ky., Lists of Matriculants and Graduates.
4. Several members of the Geiger family were buried in the Micanopy Cemetery. Several members of the family are listed in the Censuses of 1860 and 1870 of the counties of northeast Florida.
5. The 1850 Census of Edgefield County, S.C., lists the following members of the Dr. Geiger family: Dr. W.W.,

42; Mrs. Sarah E., 23; Emma M., 12; William H., 10; Esther (possibly Hester), 8; Anna, 5; and Mary, 3. It is noted that Mrs. Geiger was only 11 years of age at the time of Emma's birth. From these data it is deduced that Sarah was Dr. Geiger's second wife.

6. Jacksonville *Florida News*, May 7, 1853. The other members of the Board were George Morton Payne, physician, of Orange Lake; Chapman Gordon, Orange Lake; Abner H. McCormick, Orange Lake, and Colonel J. W. Bryant, of Jacksonville.

7. Ibid., June, 18, 1853.

8. Ibid., September 16, 1854.

9. The Census of 1860, Alachua County lists Emma M. (Geiger) as the wife of Micanopy merchant, B.W. Powell. Their daughter, Mary, was five years of age. Powell is listed as the trustee for the minor children of the deceased Dr. Geiger.

Germany, William, Leon and Wakulla Counties, 1811-post 1870

Dr. Germany, son of John and Eleanor Germany, was born in Columbia County, Georgia,[1] in 1811. Records of the Georgia Medical College, Augusta, indicate that he was a student there for the term 1832-33.[2] In the fall of 1833 he transferred to the Medical Department, University of Pennsylvania, from which he was graduated in the spring of 1834.[3] Later in the year he appeared before the Board of Physicians of Georgia and after examination was licensed to practice. For the next few years his whereabouts are unknown, although he is assumed to have practiced medicine in Georgia.

In the later 1840s Dr. Germany arrived in Florida and purchased land in the northeastern part of Leon County where he settled into the life of planter-physician. Census data show him to have been comparatively well off. In 1850 he was the owner of 41 slaves while his combined properties were estimated to have been worth $70,000.[4]

Dr. Germany was married to Elizabeth M. Powell of Leon County on February 13, 1849. This appears to have been his second marriage, however, since his daughter, Felicia, aged five, was then living with Dr. Germany's sister, Sarah Germany, but by 1860 was a member of the doctor's household. Census schedules further indicate that to this marriage were born two daughters, Sarah and Mary, and three sons, William, Reid and John.[5]

The vicissitudes of war and reconstruction appear to have brought financial disaster to Dr. Germany. He was living in the village of St. Marks, Wakulla County, in 1870 earning his living by medical practice. His wife had apparently died a year or so earlier. Since he does not appear in subsequent censuses of either Leon or Wakulla Counties it is probable that he died prior to 1880.

1. *Abstracts from Columbia County, Georgia, Court Records*, compiled by Pearl Baker. Information contained therein transmitted by Mrs. Perry S. Clapp, Cantonment, Fla.

2. Early Records, Medical Department, University of Georgia, Augusta. Information courtesy of Mrs. Dorothy Mims, Special Collections Librarian.

3. Transactions, Board of Physicians of Georgia, Ninth Annual Session, 1834.

4. U.S. Census, 1850, Leon County, Florida, p. 82. Ibid., 1860, p. 19.

5. Daughters of the American Revolution, Tallahassee Chapter, Records, Leon County, Florida, 775.

Gibbs, Robert J., St. Augustine, 1810-1830

Dr. Gibbs,[1] scion of a renowned South Carolina family, was born in Charleston about 1810. When he was still a lad in his teens his family moved to St. Augustine where his father, George Gibbs, Esq., was elected Clerk of the St. John's County Court. Having shown an unusual aptitude for learning, young Gibbs was sent to New York City for his professional education and in 1828 was graduated "with merit," i.e., with honors. The medical school he attended is identified only as "the Medical College of New York" but it is thought to have been the College of Physicians and Surgeons of Columbia University, one of only two medical colleges in New York City at that time. The other was King's College Medical Faculty.

Soon after receiving his degree Dr. Gibbs returned to St. Augustine where in April 1829[2] he announced his professional services to the people. His ability was quickly recognized both as physician and citizen. He delivered the oration at the Fourth of July celebration on July 4, 1829.

Dr. Gibbs had scarcely begun what would no doubt have been a brilliant career when, as the local newspaper announced, "disease struck him." He died on September 12, 1830, after a very brief illness. His eulogy took into account his superior qualities, both as medical practitioner and citizen.

1. Information relating to Dr. Gibbs is derived almost entirely from his obituary, St. Augustine *East Florida Herald*, September 16, 1830. The Gibbs Family of Charleston was one of eminence.

2. His professional card first appeared in the *Herald* on April 15, 1829. His office was opposite that of John Rodman.

Gibson, Edward R., St. Augustine and Tallahassee, 1800-1841

Dr. Gibson, one of the more capable public figures to appear in Florida at about the beginning of the Territorial Period, was born in Maryland about 1800. Nothing is known of his early education and professional training but there can be no doubt that he was a man of exceptional learning and intelligence. It is tempting to associate him with the Medical School of the University of Maryland but he is not listed as a graduate. That he was a man of well above average education is suggested by the fact that prior to coming to Florida he had joined Duff Green, editor of the Washington newspaper, *The United States Telegraph*, as a member of the editorial staff.[1]

Dr. Gibson first appeared in Florida in the spring of 1821, having been sent to St. Augustine to take charge of the Spanish Archives upon the formal exchange of flags and completion of the act of ceding the Territory of Florida to the United States in July 1821.[2]

He was on hand to receive appointment as an alderman of the city of St. Augustine under the mayoralty of James Grant Forbes. On May 15, 1822,[3] he was commissioned Justice of the Peace of St. Johns County and shortly thereafter was appointed Judge of the County Court by Governor W.G.D. Worthington.[4] According to John Rodman, a notable public figure of the times, "The gentleman at first accepted, but without doing one act as Judge, the next day thought proper to resign."[5] A month or so later he was appointed to the seven-member Legislative Council which was to meet in Pensacola in July 1822. For reasons not known—probably distance and difficulty of travel—he chose not to attend. This failure annoyed Governor Duval who concluded his letter of July 17, 1822, to Secretary of State John Quincy Adams with the lament: "I have not heard a word from Messrs. Gibson, Macon (Edgar), or Lytle (Thomas)—a great inconvenience is felt here for want of a Council. There are but three of the Council members here, and seven are required to make a majority."[6]

In other areas of service Dr. Gibson was more active. Of prime importance at the moment was transfer by Florida to the United States of the Spanish Archives which included all records of property ownership and claims. These documents were forcibly seized from the Spanish Secretary's Office at the time of cession. A commission had been appointed to examine them and select those items which were claimed by the United States under terms of the cession treaty. These papers were stored in the basement of a building later to become the Court House. In 1823 these archives were placed in the custody of William Reynolds, who had been named Keeper of the Public Archives by Governor Duval and the Legislative Council. Some of these papers, however, had been delivered by Reynolds to Dr. Gibson and Dr. W.H. Simmons. A conflict of authority ensued between the Territorial Government of Florida and federal agents, a dispute which ended in 1824 when Drs. Gibson and Simmons were officially named Keepers of the Archives.

During these months of controversy it is doubtful that Dr. Gibson carried on a very active medical practice. He had, however, taken advantage of association with territorial authorities to lay claim to considerable lands, viz., 300 acres of a plantation previously belonging to Governor James Grant (Governor of Florida, 1763-1770); 200 acres on Guano Creek, and 300 acres on the south side of the Nassau River.[6]

Meanwhile Dr. Gibson was a member of the legislative branch of the Territorial Council. He was appointed clerk of the St. Augustine City Council in 1823 and later Treasurer of the city of St. Augustine. He received other appointments of less importance.

By 1825 much of the confusion attending the transfer of Florida to the United States had been cleared and a more orderly future seemed assured. On learning that a keeper of the archives of East Florida was about to be appointed Dr. Gibson hastened to apply for the position. His letter of application addressed to John Quincy Adams, Secretary of State under President James Monroe, set forth two impressive qualifications, viz., his fluency in the Spanish language and his "intimate acquaintance with the Archives, acquired by five months of constant and persevering examination of the Archives."[7] His hopes were shattered, however, when President Adams on March 5, 1825, announced the appointment of William Reynolds as Keeper of the Public Archives in East Florida.[8]

His failure to obtain the appointment was, of course, a dire disappointment to Dr. Gibson. He and Dr. Simmons understandably did not hurry to turn over the archives. Reynolds, in provocation, complained to the recently appointed Secretary of State, Henry Clay. Meanwhile, on May 9, 1825, Reynolds wrote to Dr. Gibson and Dr. Simmons: "Having been appointed by the President of the United States Keeper of the Public Archives...I should be pleased to know at what time it will suit you to place me in possession of that part of the Archives now under your charge, as I am now ready to receive them."[9] To this request Drs. Gibson and Simmons replied: "...We have to state that we do not think ourselves authorized to let them go from under our charge until we receive directions to do so by the President of the United States, or the Secretary of State."[10]

The failure of Dr. Gibson to obtain appointment virtually terminated his residence in St. Augustine. On June 6, 1825, Daniel Brent of the State Department wrote a gentle but firm letter to Drs. Gibson and Simmons, concluding it with: "The President directs me to request you to deliver over these Archives to Mr. Reynolds, accordingly, with such Books and Papers in relation to them as may likewise be in your possession..."[11]

Notwithstanding his failure to gain the archivist position, Dr. Gibson was still a major figure in local politics and social life. He was a member of the Florida Legislative Council in 1823.[12] A month later he was elected to the vestry of Trinity Episcopal Church in St. Augustine. In December he was elected to the City Council.[13] In 1824 he was a Justice of the Peace in St. Johns County.[14] In the same year he was clerk to the Board of Aldermen of St. Augustine.[15] In early 1825 he was appointed to the Legislative Council of the Territory by order of President John Quincy Adams.[16] Just two weeks later Governor William P. Duval's list of appointments included Dr. Gibson as Associate County Judge of St. Johns County.[17]

At some undetermined date between 1825 and 1830, probably as early as 1827, Dr. Gibson moved to Leon County, purchasing a tract of land just outside Tallahassee where he began a farming operation with the assistance of a number of slaves.[18] He did not, however, abandon either medicine or journalism. In late December 1830 he launched a newspaper, the Tallahassee *Florida Courier*, of which a single issue (April 21, 1831) is known to have survived. Among the professional notices on the front page is the following: "Edward R. Gibson, Practitioner of Medicine. Office next door to R.J. Hackley and E.W. Dorsey's Auction Room."

The entire editorial page of the one surviving issue of the *Courier* is devoted to denunciations of Colonel Joseph M. White, Florida's delegate in Congress and to what he deemed to be the rascality of the Tallahassee *Floridian*. White had been Florida's representative for 12 years (1825-1837), and Dr. Gibson could find little more than incompetence and self-service in his record. Naturally, the *Floridian* responded in kind. In its retort it never deigned to call Dr. Gibson by name, referring to him instead as "the Courier," or "the Editor of the Courier," or in one instance derisively as "Mr. Courier."[20]

For his remaining years Dr. Gibson lived quietly outside Tallahassee apparently devoting his energies to medicine and farming. In the meantime he had settled his family in St. Joseph; the reasons for which are not known.[21] In early September 1841, he went to St. Joseph preparatory to bring them back to Tallahassee to live. Arriving in Apalachicola he found the town besieged by a yellow fever epidemic and was prevailed upon to lend his assistance to the sick. By the time he arrived in St. Joseph a few days later he was seriously ill with the disease and died a few days later. His obituary notice appeared in the Tallahassee *Star of Florida* on September 8, 1841.[21]

1. Dr. Gibson's connection with the *United States Telegraph* is mentioned in his obituary, Tallahassee *Star of Florida*, September 8, 1841, in which it is stated that "many of the most able articles in that print, advocating the South Carolina doctrines, and denunciatory of the Jackson Proclamation are from Bigson's pen."
2. *Spanish Land Grants in Florida*, IV, vii-viii.
3. Territorial Papers of the United States, XXII, "Territory of Florida," p. 438.
4. Ibid., p. 443.
5. Ibid.
6. *Spanish Land Grants*, IV, p. 96.
7. *Territorial Papers*, XXIII, 198-199.
8. Ibid., p. 260.
9. Ibid., p. 247.
10. Ibid.
11. Ibid., pp. 260-261.

12. Ibid., pp. 225-26. Letter, March 21, 1825, President John Quincy Adams to Members, Florida Legislative Council. Dr. Gibson was one of 13 appointed to the Council.
13. St. Augustine *East Florida Herald*, December 6, 1823.
14. *Territorial Papers*, XXII, 438n.
15. *East Florida Herald*, March 13, 1824.
16. Ibid., April 2, 1825.
17. Ibid., April 16, 1825.
18. U.S. Census, 1830, Leon County Florida, p. 122.
19. Tallahassee *Courier*, April 21, 1831. The principal feature of this issue was a bitter diatribe directed toward Joseph M. White, at that time a resident of St. Augustine as well as United States Attorney. Dr. Gibson had known him in his (Gibson's) St. Augustine years. A second target of Dr. Gibson's wrath was Dr. Banks Meacham, who had been in charge of the poll books in a recent Gadsden County election. Dr. Gibson accused him of fraudulent mismanagement of the books. This provoked a stinging editorial by the editor of the Tallahassee *Floridian*. It is an eloquent defense of Banks, sprinkled with Latin phrases, Dr. Gibson was never mentioned by name, but always as "the Courier," or "the editor of the Courier."
20. Tallahassee *Star of Florida*, September 8, 1841.
21. Several children were born to Dr. Gibson and his wife, Jeanette (Janette?). The Leon County Census of 1830 lists four sons and two daughters, their Christian names are not given, however, it is known that the elder daughter, Emily, became the wife of the well-known Gadsden County lawyer, Pleasants Woodson White. Of the other daughter, Lydia Maria, it is only known that she was baptized at Trinity Episcopal Church, St. Augustine, on November 14, 1824.

Gibson, James H., Gadsden County, 1850

Dr. Gibson, a resident of Gadsden County, about the middle of the 19th century, was enrolled at the Atlanta Medical College for the 1856-1857 term.[1] In the fall of 1857, however, he transferred to the Medical College of Georgia at Augusta from which he received his degree in the spring of 1858. His preceptor had been Dr. D.P. Hines of Quincy.[2] There is no evidence that he ever returned to Florida to practice his profession.

1. "Annual Announcement of the Atlanta Medical College," Atlanta, 1857, p. 11.
2. Medical Department, University of Georgia, "List of Graduates from 1829 to 1891," Augusta, 1891, p. 17.

Gillis, Angus A., Pensacola, 1862-1894

Dr. Gillis, who spent his brief professional career in Pensacola, was born on a farm in Walton County in 1862. His Scottish-born parents instilled in him the virtues generally attributed to devout Scottish Presbyterians: honesty, integrity and concern for the poor and needy. Beginning medical study under guidance of a local physician in DeFuniak Springs, he proceeded to the Medical Department, Tulane University, New Orleans, from which he received his medical degree in the spring of 1891.[1] Soon thereafter he began practice in Pensacola.

Dr. Gillis soon earned the confidence and esteem of the people of Pensacola and became in a short time a popular physician much in demand. He gained a good reputation not only for professional skill but also for human kindness, willing to attend to the needs of the poor and needy in total disregard for their ability to pay for his services. Wrote his eulogist: "He was truly the kind physician to the poor and needy, and by his death will be sincerely mourned in many humble homes in which he ministered."

Dr. Gillis died at 1:45 a.m., Sunday, December 31, 1893. On Christmas Day, he was making rounds on the streets of Pensacola; that night he was called to the suburb of Millview. Although ill, he responded to the call but did not return until the early hours of the morning. By that time pneumonia had developed and although given the best nursing care death came five days later.[2]

He was taken back to DeFuniak Springs for burial. The funeral service was attended by a group from each of the brotherhoods to which he belonged: Knights of Pythias, Woodmen of the World, and Knights of Honor.

Dr. Gillis was never married. He was survived by his aged mother, Christian, a native of South Carolina, and several brothers and sisters.[3]

1. *Alumni Catalog of the Medial Department*, Tulane University of Louisiana, New Orleans, 1901, p. 18.
2. Pensacola *Daily News*, January 2, 1894.
3. A list of members of the Gillis family is found in the Walton County Census, 1870, p. 791.

Godfrey, Joshua T., Hamilton County, 1834-1903

Dr. Godfrey was born in South Carolina on June 13, 1834,[1] and was graduated from Jefferson Medical College, Philadelphia, in 1857.[2] Soon thereafter he moved to Florida and appears to have settled in Madison County just across the Withlacoochee River from the village of Bellville in Hamilton County.[3] Here he began medical practice while carrying on a small scale farming operation. With the coming of the Civil War Dr. Godfrey enlisted in the Confederate Army as regimental surgeon in the Fifth Florida Infantry and was mustered in sometime in March 1863.[4] Soon after its organization the Fifth was ordered to Virginia. Dr. Godfrey had been ordered to report to the Army Medical Board for examination in October 1862[5] but he declined on grounds of ill health which he explained to the Surgeon General, Samuel P. Moore, in a letter of resignation dated November 16. He asked that future communications be addressed through Thomas M. Palmer, Chief Surgeon, Florida Hospital, Richmond, where it is suggested that he was a patient. Two days later, on the 18th, he appeared before a notary public in Richmond to make a sworn statement regarding pay due him at the time of his resignation.[6]

At a later unknown date, Dr. Godfrey rejoined the military service, this time with the 6th North Carolina Regiment with which he remained until the surrender at Appomattox on April 9, 1865.[7]

After release from military service Dr. Godfrey returned to private practice, locating in Bellville, where he was to spend the rest of his life practicing among the rural inhabitants of four counties, Lowndes and Brooks in Georgia, Hamilton and Madison in Florida. He built a large house in which he set aside the upstairs rooms for use of sick patients, the arrangement being regarded as the first hospital in the county.[8] He was considered an able physician; there is no doubt that he was a much beloved humanitarian.

Census schedules indicate that Dr. Godfrey was twice married. The schedule of 1860 lists a wife Theresa,[9] who was also South Carolina born. Ten years later Mrs. Godfrey does not appear in the schedule but a 10-year-old son, Forest J., does appear.[10] In 1885, Dr. Godfrey's wife is identified by the initials, S.M., and five children of that marriage are shown.[11]

Dr. Godfrey continued to practice until approximately two years prior to his death which occurred on April 12, 1903.[12] He was a Presbyterian and a Mason and was buried in the Bellville-Methodist Cemetery.

1. U.S. Census, 1860, Hamilton County, Florida, item 31, p.4.
2. Jefferson Medical College, Archives, Lists of Graduates.

3. The address Dr. Godfrey provided for the Surgeon General's Office was Madison County, Florida.
4. NA, Service Records, CSA, 5th Florida Infantry Regiment M251, Roll 62.
5. Ibid.
6. Ibid.
7. Ibid.
8. Cora Hinton, comp., Early History of Hamilton County, Jasper, 1976, p. 76.
9. See note 1, supra.
10. U.S. Census, 1870, Hamilton County, Florida, "outside Jasper," p. 31.
11. Special Census, 1885, Hamilton County, Florida, item 49.
12. Jasper *News*, April 17, 1903, obituary.

Godfrey, Thomas P., Jackson County, 1793-1838

Dr. Godfrey, a native of South Carolina, practiced medicine in Jackson County from the time of his arrival there in 1826 until his untimely death on January 15, 1838.[1] He was born in Marion County, South Carolina, on December 7, 1793,[2] son of Richard and Rachel Ann (Davis) Godfrey. The Godfrey family had settled in Marion County prior to the American Revolution on a site near the Great Pee Dee River across which they ran a regular ferry service. Richard Godfrey held public office in the county and is known to have been sheriff in 1804-1805.[3]

Before leaving South Carolina Dr. Godfrey was married to Elizabeth Wilton who was also a South Carolinian. The Jackson County Census of 1830 listed four of the five daughters of the Godfreys. Mentioned also were four slaves presumably property of the family before they came to Florida.[4] Dr. Godfrey's Florida land was located some three miles northeast of Marianna on the Blue Springs road.

As customary with many medical practitioners of the time, Dr. Godfrey was both farmer and physician. His career was tragically brief. His wife and five daughters survived and Mrs. Godfrey chose to remain in Florida notwithstanding the enormous responsibility thrust upon her.[5] Family legend has it that Dr. Godfrey was given to excessive drinking which possibly accounts for death at age 45.

Mrs. Godfrey moved into Marianna in 1841 and built a house on Madison Street, the foundations of which still exist. All five of the Godfrey daughters married and two of them had children whose descendants still live in west Florida.[6]

1. I am indebted to Cecil Rhyne of Tallahassee for extensive accounts and genealogical tables of the Godfrey family. Mr. Rhyne is a great-great-grandson of Dr. Godfrey while his mother, Mrs. Cecil Rhyne Sr. (deceased), a great-granddaughter of Dr. Godfrey, was well known as a local historian of Jackson County. A batch of letters written to Dr. Godfrey by relatives in South Carolina has been preserved and is now in Mr. Rhyne's possession.

2. U.S. Census, 1830, Jackson County, Florida, item 546. Dates of Dr. Godfrey's birth and death are from gravestones in the cemetery on what was Godfrey land.

3. W.W. Sellars, *History of Marion County, South Carolina,* Marion, 1902.

4. Census Schedule cited supra.

5. See Marianna *Jackson County Floridian,* December 4, 1936, for the account of Mrs. Godfrey's difficulties by Mrs. Cecil Rhyne Sr. (Mrs. Janie Smith Rhyne).

6. The eldest daughter, Susan, was married to the Reverend R.C.B. Lawrence, and they had 13 children. The second daughter, Mary, was the wife of Oliver Rostrum. They had no children. The third daughter, Ann, was married to James Lawson Robinson, while another, Carrie, was married to Eli Moore, a Marianna merchant Neither had children. The last daughter, Harriet Elizabeth, was the wife of Dr. Thaddeus Hentz, widely known Jackson County dentist. They were the ancestors of the Rhyne Family.

Goodson, George W., Liberty County, 1870

Dr. Goodson, a native of Georgia, practiced medicine in Bristol, Liberty County, in 1870. Except for the listing in the census of 1870, at age 38, nothing is known of him. His wife, Tabitha, was a year younger, while his children, Joseph, aged 12; Susan, aged eight; and Frederick, aged six, completed the household. The three were born in Florida and considering Joseph's age, one assumes that the family had arrived in Florida prior to the Civil War.[1]

1. U.S. Census, 1860, Liberty County, Florida, item 232.

Gordon, William M., Starke and Jacksonville, 1824-1877

Dr. Gordon was born in Rhode Island in 1824. About 1850 he moved to Georgia where he began medical practice and married Elizabeth. The Census of 1860 gives her age as 28.[1] Their daughter, Virginia, known familiarly as Jennie, was born in Georgia in 1854. By 1860 the Gordons had moved to Florida and settled in Starke, the seat of what was then known as New River County, later to be renamed Bradford.[2] By 1870 Dr. Gordon had moved to Jacksonville. The Census of 1870 lists him as "retired physician," age 45, and the owner of property valued at more than $10,000. This census also lists a second daughter, Nellie, born in Rhode Island, which would indicate that the Gordons had returned there during the Civil War. Dr. Gordon died in Jacksonville on November 13, 1877, and was buried in Evergreen Cemetery.[3] Since surviving members of the family are not listed in the Census of 1880, it is assumed that they departed the state, probably returning to Georgia.

1. U.S. Census, 1860, New River County.
2. The name Bradford was chosen to commemorate Captain Richard Bradford who was killed in military action on Santa Rosa Island, Florida, on October 9, 1861.
3. Evergreen Cemetery Survey. It is unfortunate that the issue of the Jacksonville newspaper has not survived in which the obituary of Dr. Gordon appeared.

Gorman, Robert B., Jefferson County, 1828

Dr. Gorman, eldest child of William Gorman,[1] a Jefferson County farmer whose land was situated near Waukeenah, was born about 1828. He was graduated from the University of Maryland School of Medicine in 1852,[2] and soon after returned to Waukeenah to begin practice. In the summer of 1857 he joined Dr. James Lawrence Palmer in a professional partnership which was terminated when they enlisted for military service in Florida's Fifth Infantry Regiment in early 1862.[3] Dr. Gorman's military record indicates that he was not assigned to medical service but instead was ordered to join an ordnance unit with the rank of sergeant. Since he does not appear in Florida records subsequent to the War, it is assumed that he did not return to Florida.

1. U.S. Census, 1850, Jefferson County, Florida, p. 12, Dr. Gorman's father, William Gorman, a Georgia native, was a man of moderate means, owning property valued at $8,000 in 1850.
2. Tallahassee *Floridian and Journal,* August 15, 1857. Dr. Gorman is listed in E.F. Cordell, *Historical Sketch of the University of Maryland School of Medicine, 1807-1890,* Baltimore, 1891, p. 176.
3. NA, Service Records, CSA, M251, Roll 62. Dr. Gorman enlisted on February 27, 1862, and was mustered into service as a private on March 1. On May 15, he was appointed Ordnance Sergeant in Capt. C.A. Bryan's Ordnance Company, 5th Florida Infantry Regiment, a position he held for the duration of the War. His station was Camp Leon, near Tallahassee.

Gorrie, John, Apalachicola, 1803-1855

Dr. Gorrie was a well-known and much-honored physician who lived in Apalachicola from the early 1830s until his death in June 1855.[1] The 1850 census identified four family members, Dr. Gorrie, his wife, son John age 12 and daughter Sarah age seven.[2]

Dr. Gorrie spent his early years in Charleston, South Carolina, and was graduated from the Western College of Physicians and Surgeons in Fairfield, New York, sometimes referred to as Fairfield Medical College, in the late 1820s.[3] After graduation he practiced medicine in Abbeville, South Carolina, and opened his practice in Apalachicola between 1831-1833.

Although he was a highly reputable practitioner, his fame largely rests on his invention of an ice-making apparatus, the first to successfully produce artificial ice. On July 14, 1850, for the first time in history, artifically made ice was used at a public meal. It was used to cool wines at the old Mansion House in Apalachicola for guests gathered to celebrate Bastile Day. It was soon recognized as having important therapeutic application. In addition to his medical practice and role as inventor, Dr. Gorrie was an important civic figure in Apalachicola, holding various public positions including mayor.[4]

A necrology written in the New Orleans Medical and Surgical Journal of November 1855 called Dr. Gorrie "a distinguished physician," "an acute thinker and a classical writer."[5]

Only a minimal amount of information is provided here since there exists considerable biographical literature on Dr. Gorrie. He was memorialized by the erection of a statue in Statuary Hall, The Capitol, Washington, D.C., in 1924.

1. V.M. Sherlock, *The Fever Man, A Biography of Dr. John Gorrie,* Medallion Press, Tallahassee, 1982.
2. U.S. Census, 1850, Franklin County, Florida, p. 171.
3. Raymond B. Becker, *John Gorrie, M.D., Father of Air Conditioning and Mechanical Refrigeration,* Carlton Press, New York, 1972, p. 28.
4. Rowland Rerick, ed., Francis P. Fleming, *Memoirs of Florida,* Vol. 2, The Southern Historical Association, Atlanta, 1902, pp. 158-159.
5. Raymond B. Becker, *John Gorrie, M.D., Father of Air Conditioning and Mechanical Refrigeration,* Carlton Press, New York, 1972, p. 144.
6. Ibid., p. 178.

Gould, Francis James, Tampa, Jacksonville, 1828-1888

Dr. Gould was born in Charlestown, Massachusetts,[1] on January 24, 1828, son of James Gould who in his later years ran a successful fertilizer manufacturing business in Jacksonville.[2] He was graduated from nearby Harvard University in 1850 and three years later received his degree from the medical school. Possessed with an adventurous spirit he set out for San Francisco by yacht in 1854. The craft was wrecked in the Straits of Magellan but he managed to survive and make his way to Valparaiso, Chile, where he remained for two years as a teacher of English at the local university. He then went to Rio de Janeiro and began a medical practice. While there he is said to have acquired valuable experience in the treatment of yellow fever.[3]

By about 1857 Dr. Gould had returned to the United States. After a sojourn of a year in Ft. Myers, where he practiced medicine and ran a drug store, he moved to Tampa and joined Dr. John A. Rice in a professional partnership.[4] This relationship led in 1859 to his marriage to Martha Anne, eldest child of Dr. Rice, who was only 15 years old at the time. The following year their first child, a daughter, Caroline, was born and two years later a son, Charles F., was added to the family.[5]

With the outbreak of war Dr. Gould offered his services to the Union Army but no record of army service has been located. It is a matter of record that from July 1864 until June 1865 he was contract surgeon for Union troops stationed at Cedar Key, the town having fallen into Union hands in January 1862. Dr. Gould was put in charge of the post hospital.[6] At the conclusion of the War he rejoined his family in Tampa and resumed medical practice. During this period he served for one year as sheriff of Hillsborough County (1868-1869) at a time when the turmoil of Reconstruction was at its worst and violence was not uncommon.

Dr. Gould returned to military service in 1872, prompted no doubt by the need to provide an income for his growing family. There was bound to have been some hostility at that time toward a doctor who had served as physician to Union troops and perhaps for this reason Dr. Gould was sent to Ft. Jefferson on the Dry Tortugas, a lonely outpost, where he spent about one year. Subsequently he resided for brief periods at other locations including Middleburg and Gainesville before settling finally in Jacksonville in 1879.[7]

Dr. Gould's last years were by no means spent in idle retirement. In Jacksonville he assumed management of Gould & Company, "Manufacturers and Dealers in Fertilizer," Number 27, East Bay Street, using his scientific knowledge to improve the chemical quality and effectiveness of the product.[8] The elder Mr. Gould had returned to the place of his birth to live out his last years. In addition to management of the fertilizer plant, Dr. Gould appears to have continued to offer his medical services to the Jacksonville community but doubtless on a limited basis. He also operated a drug store "in the northwestern part of the city." Meanwhile he was active in the affairs of the local post of the Veterans of the Grand Army of the Republic, serving as post surgeon.

In September 1888 Jacksonville was visited by one of the deadliest onslaughts of yellow fever ever to attack a Florida community. Dr. Gould was a victim of the disease on September 21. He was survived by his widow, one son and four daughters.[9]

1. Unless otherwise indicated the biographical data are dervied from an obituary for Dr. Gould which appeared in the Jacksonville *Florida Times-Union*, September 23, 1888. Charlestown, an early Massachusetts settlement, was an independent municipality until 1874 when it was incorporated into Boston. Bunker Hill is located in Charlestown.

2. James Gould had settled in Jacksonville in the antebellum period and established the fertilizer business which enjoyed considerable success.

3. It is ironic that yellow fever caused Dr. Gould's death.

4. See sketch of the career of Dr. John A. Rice.

5. U.S. Census, 1870, Hillsborough County, Florida, p. 389.

6. National Archives, Returns from Military Posts, Roll 1502, Cedar Keys, July 1864-June 1865.

7. No dates for the various changes of residence of Dr. Gould have been located. They are listed without dates in his obituary.

8. Wanton S. Webb, *Historical, Industrial and Biographical Florida*,Part I, New York, W.S. Webb & Co., 1885, p. 148.

9. Mrs. Gould lived on to an advanced age, dying in Jacksonville on May 19, 1937, at age 93. She was survived by a son, Charles, a bookkeeper for a Jacksonville business firm, and daughters Nellie (Mrs. Garcia); Mrs. Kate Crook, herself a widow, Miss Lena Gould, all of Jacksonville, and Mary (Mrs. F.B. Scott) of Summit, N.J. No information has been forthcoming on the first-born of the Gould family, a daughter named Caroline, who was 10 years of age in 1870. See note 5, supra.

Grant, John H., Suwannee County, 1841-1925

Dr. Grant, a Virginian by birth, practiced medicine in Suwannee County during the latter part of the 19th century. He was a resident of the village of Wellborn, located only a few miles southeast of Live Oak. With the Civil War already under way he enlisted in the Confederate Army on May 10, 1862, and was assigned to Company C, 8th Florida Infantry. He was with this unit in Virginia in early 1863 and saw action in the battles of Fredericksburg and Chancellorsville. In the latter he suffered a severe wound in his right arm and was sent to the Chimborazo Hospital in Richmond for recovery. He had been hospitalized in General Hospital, No. 12, in Richmond in the fall of 1862 for another ailment. He was captured near Farmville, Virginia, on April 6, 1865, and mustered out a short time later.[1]

Soon after his return to Florida he was married to a widow, Mrs. Celestia McLellan, who had two sons, Philbin and George, by her first marriage. A son, DeSoto, was born to her marriage to Dr. Grant.[2] Although he lived for several decades after returning to Florida, very little information about his career has been preserved. He died in 1925 and was buried in the Grant Cemetery,[3] some four miles east of the town of Luraville. Although he was said to have owned property valued at $2,300 in 1870, there is no evidence that he was ever a man of more than modest means.

1. NA, Service Records, CSA, M251, Roll 83.
2. U.S. Census, 1870, Suwannee County, Florida, p. 692.
3. WPA, Veterans' Graves Registration Project. Suwannee County, Florida, St. Augustine, 1940-1941, p. 14. The dates of Dr. Grant's birth and death are found on his gravestone.

Green, William Sydney, Apalachicola, 1840

Dr. Green, native of Virginia, first appeared on the Florida scene in 1843 when he and Dr. M.L. Armistead, also Virginia-born, formed a professional partnership in Apalachicola.[1] This joint venture was of brief duration, however, as indicated by Dr. Green's announcement of December 25, 1843, thanking his customers and promising "continued good service" but making no mention of Dr. Armistead.[2]

By the summer of 1844, Dr. Green had begun to make his presence felt in the nonmedical life of the city. In June he assisted in the organization of a debating society known as the Apalachicola Lyceum[3] and was its first president. Later at a Fourth of July celebration he gave an "Ode" after which he proposed the following toast: "To the Literature of Our Country—may it be as exalted in its character as our institutions are lasting."[4]

At some undetermined date in 1844 Dr. Green was appointed City Physician, and in a City Council proceeding of late December a payment of $100 was authorized for his services for two quarters.[5] By early 1846 he was also serving as Hospital Physician for a stipend of $37.50 per quarter.[6] This probably explains why, at a meeting of the City Council in March 1864, he reported that a claim against the United States for support of sick seamen stranded in the city in the summer of 1845 had been rejected by the Collector of Customs.[7]

As in most coastal towns of Florida, Apalachicola witnessed a general exodus of its citizens with the advent of the "sickly season," i.e., during the summer months. In June 1846 the City Council announced the election of Dr. Green as Mayor pro tem during the absence of Mayor E.C. Roberts. The *Commercial Advertiser* applauded the choice. Its editor wrote: "With Doctor Green presiding over the City during the summer, we may expect her interests to be upheld in every respect. All measures our finances will allow...to be employed to remove every cause of disease, and to keep in a state of preservation the public health."[8]

Dr. Green won a seat on the City Council in January 1847 as a Whig candidate although he had probably not wished to be nominated for the office.[9] At about the same time he was reappointed City Physician and member of the Hospital Commission. Within a week after election he resigned from the Council, doubtless in order to devote more time to other duties. The Council, reluctant to accept his resignation, delayed action until February 10 when for the second time Dr. Green tendered his resignation. This time, it was accepted.[10] In April following he was named to the three-member Board of Health.[11] Finally in August he announced that he was leaving the city for an indefinite period.[12]

Beyond this date very little is known of Dr. Green. He was married on October 24, 1844, to Virginia Rogers, daughter of Charles Rogers, Esq., of Columbus, Ga. The 1850 Census lists Dr. Green as a resident of Apalachicola, aged 34 and his wife, also born in Virginia, as 28. One child, Charles, aged one, is also listed.[13] Nothing further is known of this family.

A case history of one of Dr. Green's patients has been preserved and is of sufficient medical interest to warrant inclusion here.[14]

1. Apalachicola *Watchman of the Gulf*, August 12, 1843.
2. Apalachicola *Commercial Advertiser*, January 8, 1844.
3. Ibid., June 22, 1844.
4. Ibid., July 6, 1844.
5. Ibid., December 21, 1844.
6. Ibid., April 11, 1846. Only a few issues of the Apalachicola paper of the year 1845 have survived, creating lacunae which make it impossible to trace Dr. Green's activities during most of that year.
7. Ibid., March 28, 1846.
8. Ibid., June 23, 1846.
9. Ibid., January 16, 1847.
10. Ibid., February 27, 1847.
11. Ibid., May 15, 1847.
12. Ibid., August 28, 1847.
13. U.S. Census, 1850, Franklin County, Florida, p. 318.
14. Apalachicola *Commercial Advertiser*, July 27, 1844. This was the tragic case of Lt. Charles Russell, aboard a Coast Guard Cutter assigned to the Mobile area. While on a pleasure excursion into St. Andrew's Bay his right hand was shattered by a powder flask explosion. He was brought to St. Joseph and thence to Apalachicola, arriving there three days after the accident. The hand was already mortifying and amputation was necessary. It was performed by Dr. Green with good hopes for recovery. But the next night the bandages were torn off several times after having them reapplied, and rubbing his raw arm against the bedding he produced mortification in the stump which the doctor was then unable to arrest. Owing to hot weather, the previous indisposition of the patient, his accustomed use of hard liquor, and want of constant attention, the doctor thought a second operation would result in certain death. Little hope. (Presumably he died of the wound.)

Gregory, Thomas G., Wakulla County, 1860

Dr. Gregory, a brief sojourner in Florida, arrived just prior to the Civil War. He was a native of Pulaski County, Georgia.[1] He and his wife, Mary, settled in Newport where they found living quarters in the home of Thomas Swearingen, a local farmer, also from Pulaski County. The census enumerator located them in the summer of 1860.[2] Their ages of that date were 28 and 22 respectively. Mrs. Gregory is designated "school teacher." Their property was valued at a mere $300. Since they do not appear in subsequent censuses it is assumed that they left the state as the war began.[3]

1. U.S. Census, 1850, Pulaski County, Georgia, p. 250, item 329.
2. U.S. Census, 1860, Wakulla County, Florida, item 251.
3. There is no evidence that Dr. Gregory was a member of any Confederate military unit organized in Florida.

Griffin, James, Columbia County, 1870

All that is presently known of the career of Dr. Griffin is derived from the Census of 1870 which lists him as a resident of rural Columbia County. He was a native of North Carolina, while his wife, Martha, aged 25, was born in Alabama. They were the parents of three children, Bell, James and Lola, aged 10, seven and five respectively. All were Florida-born, which indicates that the elder Griffins had been residents of the state for about 10 years.[1]

1. U.S. Census, 1870, Columbia County, Florida.

Gunnels, George M., Marion County, 1820

Dr. Gunnels, son of William C. Gunnels, was born in Greenville District, South Carolina, about 1820.[1] The elder Gunnels was a planter of considerable means, owning numerous slaves and extensive acreage.[2] After reading medicine under the preceptorate of a Dr. Leek, George Gunnels entered the Medical College of the State of South Carolina from which he received his medical degree in 1840 after submitting a thesis titled "Syphilis."[3]

After graduation young Dr. Gunnels returned to Greenville District where he settled down to the life of planter-physician as a neighbor of his father and other relatives.[4] Census data of 1870 suggest that he remained there until about 1850 when he moved to Georgia for a sojourn of a few years where two of his six children were born.[5] By 1860 he had returned to South Carolina where his two youngest children were born.

It is not known when Dr. Gunnels migrated to Florida, but indications are that he arrived just after the Civil War,[6] doubtless prompted to make the move by the collapse of the slave-based economy. He settled in the northwestern part of Marion County, an area already populated by many former South Carolinians. There he was able to purchase a small farm, 260 acres, and once more settle down to planting cotton and raising cattle.[7] There is no evidence that he ever practiced medicine as a primary occupation after settling in Florida although the University of Pennsylvania list of practitioners, compiled in 1869-70,[8] includes him as a physician in Marion County. In the special census of Florida, prepared in 1885, his designation is "farmer."

Lacking evidence to the contrary, it is assumed that Dr. Gunnels lived out his life on the farm in northwest Marion County. The date of his death remains undetermined.[9]

1. This date is an extrapolation based on later census data.
2. U.S. Census, 1830, Greenville District, S.C., p. 298; Ibid., 1840, p. 27. In the latter schedule his slaves numbered 57, which would have established him as one of the wealthier planters of the area.
3. Archives, Medical University of South Carolina, Charleston, Lists of matriculants and graduates.

4. U.S. Census, 1840, Greenville District, S.C., p. 28. Here Dr. Gunnels is listed as married but without children and owning 22 slaves.

5. U.S. Census, 1870, Marion County, Florida, p. 412. Here Dr. Gunnels is designated "physician," aged 52, with wife Jane, aged 47, and six children ranging in ages from 22 to five. Lewis and Susan, aged 18 and 15 respectively, were born in Georgia. The Gunnels' properties were valued at a modest $1,480.

6. Dr. Gunnels is not listed in the Florida Census of 1860.

7. The "Agricultural Production Schedule" included in the Census of 1885 includes the following data on Dr. Gunnels: Improved Land, 50 acres; Unimproved Land, 210 acres; Implements, $100; Farm Animals, $550; Value of Products produced in year, $585.

8. Archives, University of Pennsylvania, "List of Medical Practitioners in 1870," MS. UPC 2.3, No. 16.

9. Dr. Gunnels' age, recorded in the 1885 Census, was 68, but census information on ages is frequently unreliable.

Guthrie, Alfred, St. Augustine, 1830

Dr. Guthrie, whose birthplace is unknown, arrived in St. Augustine[1] in 1821 soon after cession of the Territory to the United States. Biographical information relating to his brief Florida career is limited to a few random remarks contained in the "Journal" kept by the Methodist clergyman, the Reverend Joshua Nichols Glenn, the first Protestant clergyman to move into the Florida Territory after its cession by Spain. The entry for February 10, 1823, includes the following: "Dined with Dr. Guthrie; his wife is a fine little woman."

A few months after his arrival the Reverend Glenn came down with an illness which appeared to require the attention of a physician. Dr. Guthrie was called to his bedside. After examination Dr. Guthrie prescribed "a poltice (sic) of mustard." He soon recovered from the ailment.

Dr. Guthrie appears to have quickly gained the respect of the St. Augustine community. Among the Acts passed by the Florida Legislative Council at its seventh session was one authorizing creation of a State Medical Board to which Dr. Guthrie was named a member.[2]

Dr. Guthrie's career came to a sad and untimely end in April 1830. No information has been located concerning the nature of his illness. On April 20 Reuben Long, administrator of the Guthrie estate, announced that he would soon apply to the presiding judge of St. Johns County for letters of administration of the estate of Dr. Guthrie.[3]

1. J.N. Glenn, "Journal of the First Part of My Life." Microfilm copy, P.K. Yonge Library of Florida History, University of Florida, No. 161-E.

2. *Acts of the Legislative Council, Florida*, 7th Session, 1828, pp. 258-60.

3. St. Augustine *East Florida Herald*, May 5, 1930.

Hackney, James S., Suwannee, Marion, Hillsborough Counties, 1822-1888

Dr. Hackney, a native of North Carolina, arrived in Florida at about the time Suwannee County was formed (1833) from portions of four other counties, Alachua, St. Johns, Columbia and Duval. Accompanying him were his wife, Mary, and three children, Thomas, Robert and Henrietta, and four slaves.[1] They are thought to have settled near the center of the county in the settlement later to be named Live Oak. Dr. Hackney's brother, Bradley J., arrived at about the same time, acquired land and began a farming operation. Dr. Hackney practiced his profession in Live Oak until the Civil War was well under way.

In 1864, responding to the urgent call for physicians, Dr. Hackney offered his services to the Confederacy and was commissioned Acting Assistant Surgeon.[2]

Beyond the fact that he was assigned to Ft. Reed in what was then Orange County some three miles south of Lake Monroe near the present city of Sanford, very little is known of Dr. Hackney's military service. His unit had been hurriedly assembled, designated First Battalion, Special Florida Cavalry, Company D, commanded by Captain William B. Watson, a Volusia County farmer, whose primary role appears to have been recruitment of men for "the Rebel Army." Even before the end of the war the unit had virtually lost its identity with the capture of its commander and the scattering of its personnel.[3]

When the war ended Dr. Hackney appears to have practiced his profession in Ocala for a short while. On March 10, 1866, he was one of 25 citizens who signed a testimonial commending the deportment of Union troops stationed in Ocala at the end of the war.[4] Within a few months Dr. Hackney moved to Hillsborough County, settling in the Tampa community, where he spent the remainder of his life. He died there in 1888 at age 66.[5]

Four other children were born to the Hackneys after they moved to Florida, Sally, James, Mary and Charlie. Later censuses for Hillsborough County show that several of the children continued to live in the county.[6]

1. U.S. Census, 1860, Suwannee County, Florida, p. 779, item 139. See also Suwannee County Slave Schedule, 1860. Dr. Hackney is thought to have been born in Chatham County, North Carolina, where the name Hackney was not uncommon.

2. NA, Service Records, CSA, M251, Roll 5.

3. This Special Cavalry Battalion, not to be confused with the First Florida Cavalry Regiment, was composed of four companies. Its commanding officer was Lt. Col. Charles J. Munnerlyn. Capt. Watson was taken prisoner at some time in 1863 and held at Hilton Head, South Carolina, temporarily, before being removed to the old Capitol Prison in Washington.

4. Gainesville *New Era*, March 10, 1866.

5. U.S. Census, 1870, Hillsborough County, Florida, p. 546. This entry indicates that Dr. Hackney was a widower at that date.

6. The Hillsborough County Census of 1880 lists the Hackney sons Thomas L., Robert, and James B. as Hillsborough County farmers.

Haire, Charles, Tallahassee, Pensacola, St. Joseph, 1839

Dr. Haire, native of Waterford, Ireland, came to Florida in the mid-1820s in all likelihood searching for a salubrious climate.[1] He was without doubt a man of cultivation and intelligence, whose talents found expression in a variety of public offices. The earliest notice of his presence was in the St. Augustine *East Florida Herald* of November 29, 1825, a news item concerning a quarrel between two Tallahasseans which culminated in a duel. It was said that Dr. Haire had delivered the challenge to one of the principals.[2] The editor added that Dr. Haire was "a name we have not heard before."

Dr. Haire was soon to enter public life. In late 1825 or early 1826 he was elected intendant (mayor) of Tallahassee but he declined reelection the following year.[3] In the meantime he had entered into the social life of the city and on March 16, 1826, married Maria E. Betton, member of a socially prominent family.[4] In addition to his duties as intendant he was chairman of a committee to plan a suitable Independence Day celebration in 1826,[5] and at about the same time he was appointed Leon County Auctioneer.[6]

Other public offices claimed his services, notably, justice of the peace,[7] and agent to investigate depredation of public timberlands especially live oaks.[8] In his recommendation of Dr. Haire to Secretary of the Navy Samuel L. Southard, Governor DuVal praised him as a man "of information, good judgment, strict honor, and persevering activity."[9]

It is impossible to document Dr. Haire's activities for the succeeding years, but it appears he settled briefly in Pensacola. An item of July 1828 in a newspaper there shows him participating in a Fourth of July observance in Beelersville, a suburb of Pensacola, near the mouth of the Escambia River. Here he offered toasts to "the inhabitants of Escambia Bay" and later in the program another to "Pensacola and her suburbs."[10] No doubt he lived in Beelersville.

In the mid-1830s Dr. Haire was once more in Tallahassee, this time employed as clerk and draftsman in the office of Robert Butler, Surveyor-General of Florida.[11] While working in this capacity he prepared a plan for expansion of the city of St. Augustine, which evoked praise from Butler.[12] Probably for reasons of health, however, he resigned this office in 1836. Butler lamented his loss in a letter to Ethan Brown, Commissioner in the General Land Office in Washington, adding that it would be almost impossible to find a suitable replacement.[13]

From such income as he earned Dr. Haire was able to make modest investments. He was among the stockholders of the Tallahassee Railroad Company, who in 1834 petitioned Congress for certain concessions in building the railroad from Tallahassee to St. Marks.[14] He was also a stockholder in the Central Bank of Florida, owning 20 shares valued at $11 each.[15]

In failing health Dr. Haire moved to St. Joseph, probably in late 1836. In September 1837 he joined other citizens of St. Joseph and Apalachicola in petitioning Levi Woodbury, Secretary of the Treasury, for establishment of separate customs offices for the two towns.[16] He died on July 4, 1839, a victim of tuberculosis. An extremely laudatory death notice stated that he was much traveled in the United States and "latterly in Europe seeking rest from the fatal pursuer."[17]

1. Obituary notice, St. Joseph *Times*, July 9, 1839.

2. The challenge was issued by George W. Ward, Register of the Land Office in Tallahassee, to David B. Macomb, prominent lawyer and jurist in Tallahassee.

3. Pensacola *Gazette*, February 9, 1827.

4. Tallahassee *Florida Intelligencer*, March 24, 1826. Mrs. Haire died 10 months later. The Pensacola *Gazette*, February 9, 1827, noted briefly that "Mrs. Maria Haire, consort of Dr. Charles Haire, Intendant of Tallahassee," had died on January 20, 1827. Given the time span of the marriage one might speculate that her death resulted from the complications of childbirth.

5. Tallahassee *Florida Intelligencer*, May 5, 1826; May 19, 1826.

6. Ibid., March 11, 1826; TP., XXIII, 469.

7. Ibid., 779.

8. Ibid., 731n., 1065n.

9. Ibid., 387. Letter of December 15, 1825.

10. Pensacola *Florida Argus*, July 22, 1828.
11. TP., XXIV, Letter, Robert Butler to General Land Office, May 8, 1833.
12. Ibid., XXV, 143. Letter from same to same, June 11, 1835.
13. Ibid., 318.
14. Ibid., 77.
15. Ibid., 47.
16. Ibid., 421.
17. St. Joseph *Times*, July 9, 1839.

Hall, James, Duval and St. Johns Counties, 1760-1837

Dr. Hall, the first white man known to have practiced medicine in Florida, was born in Keene, New Hampshire, on October 8, 1760. He was the sixth of eight children born to Benjamin and Meletiah Hall, both members of prominent New England families.[1] At age 17 he enlisted in the Third Regiment, New Hampshire militia, and in the course of the Revolutionary War participated in several important engagements including the Battle of Yorktown in October 1781. From that point onward for the next 17 years nothing is known of his whereabouts and activities. It must be assumed, however, that for part of that period he was engaged in the study and practice of medicine.

In 1790 Dr. Hall, having followed the course of events in Spanish Florida, decided to participate in the land-grabbing going on there. He made his way to the Territory and, after surveying the scene, laid claim to 16,000 acres along Julington Creek, which today forms the line between Duval and St. Johns Counties. From that time until the end of his life Dr. Hall was a major figure in public matters such as verification of land grants for which he was a trusted arbiter.

Dr. Hall could not or would not avoid involvement in the struggle for control of Florida, a matter in which England, France and Spain, as well as the United States, had an interest. His activities as a member of the Patriots, a group devoted to liberation of Florida from Spain, led to arrest and banishment from Florida from 1810 until 1812. He returned in 1813, his intransigence was forgiven after taking the oath of allegiance to Spain. Apparently his banishment had aroused great curiosity among St. Augustine residents who were eager to know the reasons for such action and 14 years later he succumbed to their entreaties, making a statement which was published in the St. Augustine *East Florida Herald* October 16, 1824. The statement revealed little about his banishment but suggests a certain arrogance of personality as well as modicum of erudition. He deposed:

> Mr. Editor: Being repeatedly asked by my new acquaintance in St. Augustine the cause of my being banished from Florida during the year 1810, the reign of the petty tyrants of the Spanish Government in this Territory. To prevent such inquisitive Gentlemen hereafter troubling me on the subject, I now through the medium of your paper give them the following short answer.
>
> In all great convulsions in nature the mountains and lofty trees suffer more than the little (trees) and scrub below them; this is the case of human nature. In all revolutions the malice, envy and wickedness of petty tyrants fall on the great, the good, and the wise, whilst the little vulgar falls harmless to the ground.
>
> In England Saint Thomas Becket had to flee for his life and was afterwards murdered by villains while he offered up prayers at the altar of Almighty God. Henry, Duke of Bedford, was banished by the tyrant, Richard II, and was afterwards King of England by the name of Henry the 4th. In later time the Dukes of Ormond and Oxford, Lord Bolingbroke and others were also banished. The great Duke of Marlborough who commanded the combined armies of England and her allies for ten years in Germany, who never lost a battle or laid siege to a fort that he did not gain, was disgraced by a set of combined Cowards who dared not shew their heads in the field of battle at Blenheim. In France thousands of shining lights of the world were exiled for their wisdom. The great and renowned Bonaparte who made the petty kings and little tyrants

> of Asia, Africa and Europe tremble on their thrones, died in exile. If you are not satisfied with these great characters, you may add that of your obedient, humble servant of East Florida.

There is ample evidence that Dr. Hall held strong antislavery convictions. One week after publication of the statement there appeared in the same paper a full column obviously written by a nonwhite man in which the discrimination prevailing in the Ordinances and Courts against nonwhites, i.e., free men who were nonwhite, was set forth. It is a literate and cogent statement. In the subsequent issue of October 30 appeared Dr. Hall's letter endorsing the sentiment and logical protest. The essence of his argument is expressed in the following paragraph:[2]

> It is no part of my purpose, Mr. Editor, to inquire into the rights of the honorable Council to levy fines, nor the extent of such fines. My question is: Whence did this Body, or any other legislative body of this Territory impose different penalties for different complexions of free men?

Dr. Hall, by one design or another, came into possession of immense acreage along the St. Johns River. As an early settler he became acquainted with the whole area of northeast Florida and knew where the best land lay. His first major acquisition was a grant from the Spanish Governor, Juan de Quesada, of 777 acres.[3] A few years later by marriage to Eleanor, widow of Robert Pritchard, he came into possession of 16,000 acres on which there already was a sawmill. In short he became a man of considerable wealth; his property included nearly all the land from Julington Creek northward encompassing the area on which the present city of Jacksonville is located.

Dr. Hall was twice married. His first wife, Eleanor, was the widow of Robert Pritchard, who had died in 1804 at age 42. They were parents of seven children, of whom four were living in 1804. She and Dr. Hall had a daughter, Eleanor, who became the wife of Oliver Wood, a prominent figure in Jacksonville's earlier years. He became the mayor in 1847.

It is apparent that Dr. Hall, as he became a man of comparative wealth, abandoned medical practice. Only occasionally is he referred to in existing documents as "Doctor."[3]

After the death of Eleanor in 1832, Dr. Hall returned briefly to New Hampshire where in 1833 he married Dorothy Deering of Portsmouth. He was 73, she was half his age. This marriage was terminated by his death on Christmas Day 1837. He was buried in a graveyard in what was formerly known as LaGrange, presently Mandarin.[4]

1. The major portion of this sketch is drawn from the excellent and authentic biography of Dr. Hall by Jacksonville historical scholars, Mary M. Dupree and G. Dekle Taylor, M.D., "Dr. James Hall, 1760-1837."

2. St. Augustine *East Florida Herald*, August 30, 1824.

3. The five-volume compilation, "Spanish Land Grants in Florida," prepared by the Historical Records Survey, Division of Professional and Service Projects, Work Projects Administration, State Library Board, Tallahassee, 1841, contains abundant information relating to Dr. Hall's land transactions. This work has been frequently consulted in the preparation of the present sketch.

4. Dr. Hall's gravestone, erected in 1926 through efforts of the Daughters of the American Revolution, still stands partially enclosed by an iron fence. It bears the inscription:

ERECTED
IN MEMORY OF
JAMES HALL, M.D.
A SOLDIER OF THE REVOLUTION
Born in Keen (sic) N.H.
8th Oct. 1760
Died at LaGrange E.F.
25th Dec. 1837
Aged 77 Years

Hamilton, John, Alachua County, 1831-1833

It appears that Dr. Hamilton arrived in Florida about 1831 and settled in Alachua County. The earliest indications of his presence in the territory appear in two memorials or petitions to President Jackson of which he was a signatory. The first was an endorsement of Joseph L. Smith for reappointment as head of the judicial department, East Florida judicial district,[1] and the second, a request that a company of troops be transferred from Cantonment Brooke at Tampa Bay to some suitable location in Alachua County.[2] The former bears the date December 1831, the latter January 1832. Also in January he joined several other Alachua citizens in recommending Col. James Gadsden for Governor of Florida, "in case Governor DuVal should resign, as it is rumored that he intends."[3]

With reactivation of Cantonment King in the latter part of 1832 under the designation, Ft. King, Dr. Hamilton was employed as citizen-surgeon for the troops stationed there.[4] At about this time the Seminoles of East Florida, uprooted and harassed, found themselves in dire circumstances. Facing starvation as an alternative, their leaders met with Col. Gadsden at a place on the Oklawaha River known as Payne's Landing and agreed to consider removal to the West.[5] In the meantime the Indian Agency for East Florida had been established a short distance from Ft. King. It was decided, probably by the Indian agent, John Phagan, and Capt. William M. Graham, commander of the military detachment at Ft. King, that all Indians should be vaccinated and that Dr. Hamilton should be employed for the task.[6]

Dr. Hamilton informed the Secretary of State, Lewis Cass, on August 4, 1832, that he was accepting the job of vaccinating the Indians "under the act of Congress extending the benefits of vaccination for the prevention of smallpox." He added, "As soon as I shall have received the necessary Instructions from Governor I shall commence vaccinating." On receipt of instructions a day or so later, however, he found the compensation totally unacceptable. Under the terms stated by the Governor he would receive $6 for every hundred Indians vaccinated while the total expenditure should not exceed $100. He stated his dissatisfaction to John Phagan and Capt. Graham and made known his objections to Secretary Cass in a letter dated August 14, 1832, at Ft. King. The compensation, he said, was too little; besides it would require some time to overcome the prejudices of the Seminoles.

Meanwhile other physicians were recommended for the vaccination project including Drs. Egbert S. Barrows of Jacksonville and William D. Price, then living at Aspalaga on the Apalachicola River. Because of worsening relations with the Seminoles the vaccination project was postponed indefinitely. More than a year later, on November 20, 1833, in his "General Report on the Indian Situation," Capt. Graham informed Secretary Cass that the order for vaccinating the Seminoles had yet to be obeyed because "$100 is not enough to employ doctors." He stated further, "Dr. Hamilton would not accept the job for so little money. No other physician would undertake it." He explained that there were about 4,000 Indians and suggested that for $400 or $500 the job might be accomplished. He calculated that it could not be completed in less than three months.

Two days later, November 22, 1833, Capt. Graham wrote to Col. Gadsden recommending Dr. Barrows and reminding him that Dr. Hamilton would not vaccinate so many for so little money. Besides, Dr. Hamilton "is about leaving the territory to reside in Maryland." Presumably he had moved by the end of 1833.

1. TP., XXIV, 599.
2. Ibid., p. 645.
3. Ibid., p. 646.
4. No date has been discovered for the actual contracting of Dr. Hamilton services. The earliest reference to the arrangement is found in the letter, Dr. Hamilton to Lewis Cass, Ft. King, August 4, 1832. A letter, Governor Duval to Lewis Cass, April 25, 1832, indicates that the project was already under consideration. He wrote, "If you have not already appointed a physician to vaccinate the Indians, I recommend Dr. Wm. D. Price."
5. A full account of the Indian problem and the roles of various government officers is found in John K. Mahon, *History of the Second Seminole War*, pp. 69-86, et passim.
6. This and subsequent information is documented in NA. Letters Received, Office of Indian Affairs, 1824-81, Microfilm 234, Roll 288. This material is arranged more or less chronologically although the items are unnumbered.

Hampton, Benjamin Wade, Madison County, 1830

Dr. Hampton was one of several members of the Hampton family who migrated from Georgia into Madison County in the 1850s. They obtained fairly large holdings in what was known as the Sandy Ford[1] section, later called Greenville, located about 14 miles west of Madison Court House. He appears to have been recently widowed at the time of the census enumeration of 1860.[2]

In August 1861 Dr. Hampton enlisted as a private in the Howell Guards,[3] organized by Captain George W. Parkhill, committing himself for three years service. Before the end of the year, he joined a few other members of his unit in signing a petition addressed to Florida Governor John Milton requesting that "His Excellency use his best exertions to have them recalled from the Army for Virginia to protect and assist in the defense of their State and homes." The request was granted and Dr. Hampton received his discharge on December 21, 1861, after four months service.[4]

The Civil War and Reconstruction proved disastrous for Dr. Hampton as well as other members of the Hampton family. From his position as a man of considerable means in 1860 (property valued at more than $25,000 including 15 slaves) he was reduced to virtual poverty by 1870 when his holdings were negligible. He was living alone near Station Five,[5] west of Madison and designated only as "farmer." The census of that year indicated that other members of the Hampton family had suffered similar losses.[6]

1. The U.S. Census, 1860, Madison County, Florida, p. 25, indicates that the five Hampton householders were men of moderate means, all owning a few slaves.

2. Ibid. The entry lists two members of the household, Dr. Hampton and a one-year-old daughter, Clara.

3. National Archives, Service Records, CSA, M251, Roll 37. The Howell Guards became Company M, 2nd Florida Infantry Regiment.

4. Ibid. Dr. Hampton is thought to have returned to his home near Sandy Ford and remained there for the duration of the War.

5. U.S. Census, 1970, Madison County, Florida, p. 121.

6. Since Dr. Hampton does not appear in the Census of 1880 it is assumed that he had died prior to that date. The list of physicians practicing in Florida in 1869-70, compiled by the Medical College of the University of Pennsylvania, includes Dr. Hampton of Madison County. University of Pennsylvina, MS, UPC 2.3, No. 16.

Hankins, Joseph S., Suwannee County, 1829

Dr. Hankins, who practiced medicine in various locations in Florida, was born in Georgetown, South Carolina, in 1829. The Hankins family, of English origin, had established its roots in the Georgetown section about the middle of the 18th century.[1] They were apparently a family of considerable wealth and social position. Dennis Hankins, the father, was the first to migrate to Florida. He settled in Madison County, acquired land, and began a farming operation. The census of 1850 lists him at age 58, owning real property valued at $10,000. Joseph, aged 21, was the second of his four children.[2]

Prior to entering medical school Dr. Hankins began the study of medicine as an apprentice to Dr. Thomas Hartridge who, prior to moving to Jacksonville in 1853, had been a practicing physician in Madison. In the fall of 1852 he enrolled in the Medical College of the State of South Carolina, Charleston, where he apparently remained for only one term, leaving without obtaining his degree.[3] By 1855 he was practicing medicine in Jacksonville when the City Council chose him to replace Dr. Henry Balsam as Port Physician.[4]

Dr. Hankins had moved to New Boston by 1860, a village on the Suwannee River in Suwannee County, although he actually resided across the river in Lafayette County.[5] The census of that year lists him as the head of his household, aged 30, married to an 18-year-old wife named Elizabeth. His real property was valued at $5000, his personal property at $12,210.[6]

As was true of many mid-19th century physicians in Florida, Dr. Hankins divided his time between farming and medical practice. His activities, social and professional, remain unchronicled, however.

At some juncture, probably in the 1870s, Dr. Hankins moved to Live Oak where he found lodging for a while in a local hotel.[7] He became a member of the Suwannee County Medical Society and in 1897 joined other members in declaring publicly that they would not continue to answer to calls from those who do not pay doctor bills.[8]

Dr. Hankins was still living in 1900 at the age of 69. He was twice married, first to Elizabeth H., a native of South Carolina. They had no children. The date of her death is not known but is assumed to have occurred about 1870. In 1872 he married a woman 26 years his junior, known to us only as Emma. She was a native of Georgia.[9] The date of Dr. Hankins' death has not been ascertained.

1. Numerous references to the Hankins Family of the Georgetown District of South Carolina are found in various issues of the *South Carolina Historical Magazine*; noteworthy are III, 136; IV, 71; IX, 98; XII, 89, et passim.

2. U.S. Census, 1850, Madison County, Florida, p. 381.

3. Archives, Medical University of South Carolina, Waring Historical Medical Library, Charleston. Lists of Matriculants and Graduates.

4. Jacksonville *Florida Republican*, June 14, 1855.

5. U.S. Census, 1860, Lafayette County, Florida, p. 976.
6. A fairly large portion of this personal property represents the value of Hankins' slaves. He was also responsible for the care and use of seven additional slaves belonging to his brother, Dennis, a minor, whose guardian he was.
7. Special Florida Census, 1885, Suwannee County, p. 139.
8. Live Oak *Suwannee Democrat*, November 20, 1897.
9. U.S. Census, 1900, Suwannee County, Florida, p. 29.

Hansford, Thomas, Calhoun County, 1870

Dr. Hansford appears to have been a sojourner in Calhoun County about the year 1870 although the census schedule that year lists him as a native Floridian, aged 55.[1] He has not been located in earlier censuses nor is he listed in the Census of 1880. Sharing his household were his wife, Ann, and their five children, Joanna, 19; Charles, 17; Peter, 15; Mary, 13; and Sarah, 11. All were Florida natives. There were other Hansfords in Calhoun and adjoining counties, notably L.T. Hansford, a Baptist minister, and his family.[2]

1. U.S Census, 1870, Calhoun County, Florida, p. 299.
2. Ibid., 1860, p. 107.

Hardee, Charles, Nassau County, 1830-1917

Dr. Hardee, descendant of a well-known family of Pitt County, North Carolina, was born in Camden County, Georgia, in 1830.[1] After receiving his early education in local schools he studied medicine at one of the Philadelphia medical colleges from which he was graduated in 1856.[2] Soon thereafter he settled in Brooksville where he later recalled that his only competitors were Dr. Thomas P. Gary, later of Ocala, and Dr. John P. Wall of Tampa. His Brooksville practice spanned the years 1856-1861.

With outbreak of the Civil War in 1861 Dr. Hardee enlisted in the Confederate Army on July 23 and was inducted without military rank in the Third Florida Infantry Regiment.[3] In May the following year he was promoted to 3rd Lieutenant and a short time later became Assistant Surgeon assigned to hospital duty. In 1864 he was promoted to the rank of surgeon and put in charge of the Army Hospital at Montgomery with four other physicians as his assistants.[4] He remained at this post until the end of the war.

With military service behind him Dr. Hardee returned to St. Mary's in Camden County where he practiced for 13 years before moving to Chester, Florida, a Nassau County village about seven miles due west of Fernandina.[5]

It is reasonably clear that Dr. Hardee had never gone through the formality of obtaining a license to practice medicine in Florida and in 1892 he apparently felt some pressure to do so for on July 12 he went to the offce of Jacksonville physician, Dr. Juan Domingo Fernandez, expecting to appear before the Board of the Florida Medical Association, and certainly expecting the procedure to be a mere formality. There, to his surprise, he found that the "Board" consisted of only Dr. Fernandez. On the following day (July 13) the Florida *Times-Union* reported that "Charles Hardee of Chester appeared before the Florida Medical Board, and after an hour's labor, withdrew."[6]

Upon being apprised of this notice Dr. Hardee, obviously incensed, responded at length, his statement appearing in the *Times-Union* of July 23. It contained not only an account of the "examination" but also extensive biographical details.[7]

> On the 13th inst. I appeared at the office of the examining board in Jacksonville, Dr. Fernandez officiating, and being the only member present...Nearby was another gentleman, a supposed M.D. answering questions propounded in writing. Dr. Fernandez gave me a sheet containing a series of questions which I read through and answered laconically. Dr. Fernandez then handed me another sheet of questions, all simple enough, but coming so suddenly under the observation of a general practitioner calculated to require some thought in the replies. I therefore remarked that on these I was a little rusty, and asked what percentage of answers would be required. Dr. Fernandez told me that if I missed twenty percent I could not pass.

Subsequently an argument ensued between the two physicians on the proper response to a question relating to proper treatment for irreducible hernia. Dr. Fernandez held that strangulated hernia was irreducible hernia and that the only treatment was the knife (i.e., surgery). At this point Dr. Hardee told Dr. Fernandez that he would "just waive the examination." Dr. Fernandez replied: "Sir, you cannot practice until you pass this Board;" thus ended the encounter.

Dr. Hardee concluded his letter with a review of his medical career, stating that he had practiced his profession "for nearly thirteen years before coming to Chester, where my interests lie." He concluded, "Submitting now to the kingly mandate to lay aside my scalpel and other things medical that have been my means of support for nearly forty years, I am still gratified to know that many will recognize me as no imposter."

It is clear that Dr. Hardee continued his practice, with or without license, for several years. He died in Chester in 1917.

As for the Hardee family, Dr. Hardee was married to Florida native, Mary G., a woman of intelligence and substantial means. They had six children: Elizabeth, Charles, John, Mary, Sarah and Noble (male), aged 15, 12, nine, six, four and one, respectively (in 1880). Due to the remoteness of Chester from the main stream of Florida commerce and social activity, information relating to the Hardee family is not abundant.[8]

1. U.S. Census, 1870, Camden County, Georgia, p. 679. See also ibid., 1880, p. 12.
2. There were several medical colleges in Philadelphia at mid-19th century. It is not known from which Dr. Hardee was graduated.
3. National Archives, Civil War Records, Third Florida Infantry Regiment.
4. Ibid.
5. See note 7, infra.
6. To Dr. Hardee this casual remark was an insult. His immediate response was: "Now if talking to Dr. Fernandez for much of that hour is termed 'labor,' then we say it was no arduous task."
7. In addition to his report on the examination in Dr. Fernandez' office Dr. Hardee proceeded to outline his career: "In conclusion I will say that I am sixty-two years old; that I graduated in Philadelphia in 1856, that I had a lucrative practice in Brooksville for four years previous to the War, with Dr. Wall (John P.) and Dr. Gary (Thomas P.) of Ocala as competitors; that early in the War I was made Assistant Surgeon on duty in hospitals; that in 1864 I was promoted to full surgeon and placed in charge of a hospital in Montgomery, Alabama, with four assistants, which post I held until the City's surrender, and that I practiced my profession in St. Mary's, Georgia, for nearly thirteen years before coming to Chester, where my interests lie."
8. A few items of interest relating to the Hardee family are found in Jan H. Johannes Sr., "Yesterday's Reflections, Nassau County, Florida, A Pictorial History," published by Thomas O. Richardson, edited by E.S. Pedrotti and printed by the Florida Sun Printing Co., Callahan, Florida, 1976. It is stated that "Dr. Hardee came from a family long established in Pitt County, North Carolina, and was directly descended from John Hardee of Revolutionary War fame. It is thought that Dr. Hardee was also related to William Joseph Hardee, who was born in Camden County, Georgia, Brigadier General in the Confederate Army and sometime Commandant of Cadets at West Point." See *Dictionary of National Biography*, Vol. VIII, 239-40.

Hargis, Robert Bell Smith, Pensacola, 1818-1893

Dr. Hargis, unquestionably Pensacola's most renowned physician of the 19th century, was born in Hillsborough, North Carolina, on June 7, 1818, son of Thomas S.N. Hargis.[1] At a fairly early age he entered the University of North Carolina at Chapel Hill from which he was graduated in 1837 with what, to judge from his writings, appears to have been a sound classical education. Soon thereafter he moved to Fayetteville, North Carolina, where he began medical studies under the preceptorate of Dr. T.J. Jordan. He then enrolled in the Medical College of Louisiana, later to become the Medical Department of Tulane University,[2] from which he received his degree, with high honors, on March 22, 1844.

For the next seven years Dr. Hargis practiced in Alabama, first in Mobile (1844-45) and later (1846-51) in the rural village of Mt. Pleasant (Monroe County). He located in Pensacola in 1851 where he would spend the balance of his life.

Dr. Hargis' presence in Pensacola was soon felt. Shortly after arrival he was appointed Port Physician, a vulnerable position which demanded frequent visits aboard ships coming into the harbor. He was constantly alert to the possibilities of yellow fever and fevers of other types among the seamen coming in and going out of the area. He had a personal encounter with yellow fever in 1853 which left him seriously debilitated, but at the same time afforded an opportunity to observe its characteristics first hand. Out of this experience as well as the innumerable cases which came to his attention he developed an intense interest in the disease and in due time gained a reputation throughout the country as an authority on the diagnosis, treatment and prevention of the dreaded scourge.

Following his own bout with the ailment Dr. Hargis retired temporarily to Milton in adjoining Santa Rosa County where he spent several months in recuperation, returning to Pensacola in 1854. Forthwith he accepted appointment as Surgeon of the Marine Hospital housed temporarily in a rented building about a mile east of the city. At about the same time he established a private hospital facility nearby, which is said to have been the first of its kind in Pensacola.[3]

As the Civil War developed in 1861 Dr. Hargis offered his services to the 17th Alabama Regiment of Volunteers (Infantry)[4] which had been organized in Montgomery earlier in the year and sent to Pensacola in the late summer. It was present there at the time of the Union bombardment of the city on October 9 at about the time of Dr. Hargis' enlistment. He moved with the outfit for field duty around Mobile, remaining with it through the Battle of Shiloh in April 1862, after which he was ordered into hospital service where he continued until the surrender in 1865.[5]

Even before he returned to practice in Pensacola in 1865 Dr. Hargis had shown a willingness to share his discoveries, procedures and professional ideas with his colleagues. He prepared a series of articles, the first known one being a potpourri entitled "Medical Olla Podrida" published in 1857.[6] This was followed by "Communicability of Yellow Fever" published in the *New Orleans Medical News and Hospital Gazette* in 1859. Other scientific items were "History and Origin of Yellow Fever—Its Cause, Communicability and Prevention" read before the American Public Health Association in 1879 and later published by the Association, and in 1880 "The Nautical Origin of Yellow Fever" in Letters to the *Sanitarian*, New York, and "The Ship — Origin of Yellow Fever," both intended to bolster his conviction that the unsanitary holds of ships were the breeding places of yellow fever.[7] As late as 1881, with the conquest of yellow fever by Carlos Finlay, Walter, James Carroll and other notables still a couple of decades away, Dr. Hargis continued to set forth his convictions.[8]

In 1882 Pensacola suffered another deadly onslaught of the fever. It is reported that nearly all persons able to travel fled the city but not Dr. Hargis, who remained to care for as many patients as possible or as his strength permitted. This act of courage and humanitarianism gained for him the undying love of citizens of every class and condition.[9]

Dr. Hargis was in the vanguard of his profession in the struggle for improvement in the quality of medical training and practice, particularly in Florida which lagged behind most states in the establishment of professional medical associations. He was instrumental in founding the Pensacola Medical Society whose early history appears to have been overshadowed by the Escambia County Board of Health of which he was also an active member. In 1878 he was elected to membership in the Florida Medical Association[10] and two years later became its vice president. Unable to be present at its meeting the following year he sent his regrets along with an invitation to the Association to meet in Pensacola in 1882. The invitation was accepted, and at this meeting Dr. Hargis was elected president. Unable to be present at the meeting in Jacksonville in 1883, he sent his presidential address to Vice President Charles J. Kenworthy, who presided. Dr. Hargis' paper, "The Natural History of Plagues," was read by Dr. Kenworthy and "was listened to with close attention by the Association," and referred to Committee on Publications.[11] The following year he was again scheduled to read a paper, but once more unable to attend, he sent it to be read by a colleague. It was entitled "Malaria and the Relations of Micro-Organisms to Disease." The paper, which was printed in the Association's Proceedings, reveals an impressive knowledge of the history of the ancient world as well as the more recent eras.[12]

Lest frequent absences from meetings of the Association be judged remissness on his part, it should be stated that Dr. Hargis was deeply involved in many more pressing matters. The virulent siege of yellow fever in 1882 had imposed heavy demands on his waning strength. The long distances involved in traveling from his Pensacola home to the meeting places were burdensome. More important he was busily engaged in scientific research and writing. A member of the American Public Health Association, beginning in 1878, he presented a paper entitled "The History and Origin of Yellow Fever: Its Cause, Communicability and Prevention" in 1879.[13] His "Sketch of the History of Quarantine at Pensacola" was published in 1881 in the *National Board of Health Bulletin*. Then, too, there were appointments which could not be shunned, as for example, his attendance at the Gulf States Quarantine Convention in New Orleans as Florida's delegate in 1885, and in the same year appointment as Acting Assistant Surgeon at the United States Marine Base in Pensacola and finally in 1889 four years before his death, appointment as Medical Examiner for Pension Claimants for the First Judicial District of Florida.[14] His routine daily practice cannot be overlooked.

Soon after coming to Pensacola in 1851 Dr. Hargis was married to Modesta Sierra, granddaughter of Dr. Eugenio Sierra. They had several children including three sons of whom one, Joseph Sierra, died in early childhood.[15] The other sons, Robert W. (the eldest Hargis child) and John Whiting, became prominent Pensacola physicians. Dr. Hargis died in Pensacola on November 30, 1893.

1. The biographical data contained in this sketch is derived for the most part from three printed sources: Elizabeth Dwyer Vickers and F. Norman Vickers, M.D., "Notations on Pensacola's Medical History, 1873-1923," *Journal of the Florida Medical Association*, January 1974. This is an extremely valuable article based on thorough research. It is flawed only by omission of footnotes due to limitations of space. Rowland H. Rerick, "Memoirs of Florida," Francis P. Fleming, editor, Atlanta, Southern Historical Association, 1902, I, 561-562. Obituary, *Pensacola Daily News*, December 1, 1893.

2. The obituary notice states that prior to entering the Louisiana College Dr. Hargis had studied medicine in New York City. This has not been verified. The Alumni Catalogue of the Medical Department of Tulane University 1834-1901, lists Dr. Hargis.

3. Vickers and Vickers, "Notations," p. 86.
4. Obituary, Pensacola *Daily News*, December 1, 1893.
5. Ibid.
6. Rerick, *Memoirs*, I, 561.
7. Vickers and Vickers, "Notations," p. 86.
8. Ibid., p. 87.
9. Obituary.
10. Proceedings, *Journal of the Florida Medical Association*, 1881.
11. Ibid., 1883.
12. Ibid., 1884, pp. 38-57.
13. This was published in the *Journal of the American Public Health Association, 1870.*
14. Vickers and Vickers, "Notations," pp. 86-87.
15. St. Michael's Cemetery, Pensacola, Gravestone.

Harlan, Harmon G., Marianna, 1860

Dr. Harlan was a brief sojourner in Marianna about 1860. The Census of that year lists him as an Ohio native, aged 65. His wife, Missouri, Georgia-born, is shown to have been 35. He apparently possessed no real property and his personal property was a paltry $200. It may be conjectured that he had moved to Florida for reasons of health and possibly left as the Civil War began.[1]

1. U.S. Census, Jackson County, Florida, 1860, p. 27.

Harris, John Junius, Orange and Seminole Counties, 1834

Of numerous Florida physicians who served in a public capacity probably none was more worthy or served with greater distinction than Dr. Harris who spent the last decades of his life in Sanford which until 1913 was situated within Orange County. Although he continued medical practice until very late in life and was without doubt a competent physician, he is best remembered for his public career which included legislator, editor, mayor, and educational leader. Nor should his success as a citrus farmer be overlooked.

Dr. Harris was born in Washington County, Georgia, on January 11, 1834,[1] son of Daniel and Vashti (Franklin) Harris. He received his earliest education in the common schools of the county, then entered Emory College, Oxford, Georgia. He read medicine in the offices of Drs. Henry and Robert Campbell in Augusta and in the fall of 1853 enrolled at the Georgia Medical College in Augusta and received his medical degree on March 4, 1855. He began practice in Rome, Georgia, where on November 1 of that year he was married to Miss Roxie Mitchell, daughter of the Honorable Daniel P. Mitchell, said to have been founder of the town. His practice was interrupted in 1862 when he enlisted for military service and was assigned to the Eleventh Battery, Georgia Artillery, commanded by Captain Allen S. Cutts. The unit, which earned the designation the Seventh Flying Artillery, was later cited for exceptional bravery in battle. His military career was cut short by illness which necessitated discharge prior to the end of the war.

Soon after the war Dr. Harris moved to Brunswick, Georgia, where he remained for several years, serving for two terms as mayor. In 1874 he moved to Florida, settling first in Titusville in Brevard County where he remained for about a year before moving into neighboring Orange County where he purchased a large tract of land on Lake Jesup[2] and settled into the dual roles of fruit grower and physician. In fact the 1880 Census designated him only as "fruit grower."

Dr. Harris, as a staunch Democrat, was persuaded to become politically active and emerged as a public-spirited man, dedicated to the development of a prosperous and enlightened community. In 1878 he ran for a seat in the House of Representatives, handily winning election. He was returned to the House in 1880 and again in 1882. In the second instance he was chosen Speaker. An examination of the minutes of the three sessions shows clearly that he was an effective leader,[2] a man of good judgment.

Meanwhile Dr. Harris continued to labor on the home front. He was organizer of the local Democratic Club of which he was president in 1882.[3] Always a person who recognized the importance of public education, he served as a member of the Orange County Board of Education.

Dr. Harris moved to Sanford in 1882, purchasing a house on Magnolia Avenue where he lived the remainder of his life. In November that year he purchased the local newspaper, the *South Florida Journal,*[4] from D.C. Brown and immediately set about improving its size and quality. His achievements were recognized and applauded by journalists throughout the state. It was a striking coincidence that he assumed ownership of the paper just days after he had been elected for a third term in the Legislature. Lest his subscribers be concerned that the paper would suffer during his absence in Tallahassee, he announced that his daughter, Lula,[5] apparently an exceptionally bright young woman, would carry on the editorial work with frequent consultations with him as to policy. She was one of six children, only two were living in 1900, according to the census. It did not escape the notice of the State Assembly that Dr. Harris was the only representative of the newspaper fraternity in the state Legislature. Incidentally, two changes were made in the newspaper during Dr. Harris' editorship. In January 1883 its title was changed to the Sanford *Journal* and in May 1884 Dr. Harris announced that John H. Banta of Tipton, Indiana, had joined him as coeditor and half owner.

In the succeeding years Dr. Harris continued to fill the role of man-for-all occasions in Sanford. Seldom was there a public gathering at which he was not called upon to make an introduction, preside, or give the major address. After a brief interlude in 1884 when he gave up his editorial chores because of failing eyesight[6] Dr. Harris remained at the editorial desk of the Sanford *Journal,* even after appearance of a second newspaper in the town, the Sanford *South Florida Argus.* As far as can be determined the rivalry between the two editors remained friendly, free of acrimony.

1. Information about Dr. Harris[1] early life is drawn principally from the autobiographical sketch which he submitted for inclusion in the official directory of the Twelfth Session of the Florida Legislature, compiled and edited by J.V. Drake, and published in Jacksonville in 1883, p. 57.

2. Ibid.

3. Sanford *South Florida Journal*, September 14, 1882.

4. Ibid., issues of November 9 and 23, 1882.

5. Ibid., December 7, 1882.

6. Sanford *Journal*, November 6, 1884. At this juncture Dr. Harris, obviously somewhat depressed by the advice of his ophthalmologist, offered his interest in the *Journal* for sale. No sale resulted, however, and he eventually returned to its editorship.

Hart, Franklin, Jackson County, 1824

Dr. Hart, a native of North Carolina, arrived in Marianna about 1847[1] with his wife and eldest daughter. His professional announcement first appeared in the local newspaper on January 12, 1848.[2] It stated that he was locating his office "in one end of Bryan and Horne's Drug Store." One of the infrequent notices relating to his activities suggests that he was readily accepted into the civic life of the town. As Marianna prepared for the forthcoming July 4th celebration in June 1848, Dr. Hart was secretary for the public meeting called for the purpose. He was also a member of the committee to select an orator and reader for the celebration.[3]

Dr. Hart's medical practice was doubtless routine and without distinction. At some unspecified date in 1850 he was called to assist another local physician, Dr. John T. Rascoe, in a postmortem examination of the body of one James Durden, "lately murdered in Jackson County." For this service the two doctors were authorized to receive $100 from the State Treasury.[4]

Dr. Charles A. Hentz, who presumed on several occasions to make judgments on the professional competence and intelligence of his medical colleagues, was of two opinions about Dr. Hart. When his mother, Mrs. Caroline Hentz, came down with a serious illness in January 1856, shortly after her arrival from St. Andrews, he sent to Greenwood[5] for Dr. Hart, "in whom I had great confidence," although there were several other physicians in Marianna.[6] On the other hand Dr. Hentz recalled taking over "a hopeless case...Mrs. Adam McNealy...a long time invalid," suffering from a prolapsed uterus. He wrote: "Dr. F. Hart had had her under his care for a year or two; promising relief all the time, but doing no good...He was a very intelligent physician, but lacked judgment...sometimes made grievous blunders, as he did in this case. When I examined the case I was astonished that a man of his experience had made so great mistake."[7]

It is apparent that at some time in the 1850s Dr. Hart had moved to Greenwood or at least was devoting a day or so each week to practicing there. The Census of 1860 lists the seven children of the Harts ranging in age from 14 to two.[8] Since the name does not appear in the Census of 1870, it appears that the family had left Florida by that date.

1. U.S. Census, 1850, Jackson County, Florida, p. 619. The eldest daughter, Mary B., was born in North Carolina in 1856. The other children, all Florida natives, were in order of birth, Olivia, Margaret, Emily, Henry, Frank and Julia, the last being two years of age in 1860.

2. Marianna *Florida Whig*, January 12, 1848.

3. Ibid., June 14, 1848.

4. General Assembly, Florida, Senate Journal, 1850-51, p. 340. See also General Assembly, Acts and Resolutions, 5th Session, 1850-51, p. 172.

5. Greenwood, a village seven miles north of Marianna.

6. In the case of Mrs. Hentz the efforts of the two physicians were unavailing. She died of pneumonia early in January 1856, the illness apparently having been induced by exposure to the bitter cold on the journey from St. Andrews. See C.A. Hentz, "Autobiography," II, 282.

7. Ibid., I, 277. Dr. Hentz concluded his account of the McNealy case by recalling that he had been successful in his treatment; so successful, in fact, that Mrs. McNealy soon became pregnant and gave birth to a daughter whom she gratefully christened Bettie Hentz.

8. U.S. Census, 1860, Jackson County, Florida, item 496.

Hartridge Theodore, Madison and Jacksonville, 1816-1893

Dr. Hartridge, who for the greater part of his life was a resident of Florida, was born in Savannah, Georgia, on September 5, 1816. His parents, John Earle and Leah Sandwich Hartridge, were English-born and soon after the birth of their son returned to England. In 1817, however, after the untimely death of her husband, Mrs. Hartridge and her small son returned to Savannah.[1] They subsequently moved to Augusta where young Theodore received his early education. In 1834 he entered the University of Georgia, or Franklin College as it was then called, and upon examination was judged to be adequately prepared to enter the sophomore class. Upon completing his second year at Athens he was offered a tutorial position in mathematics. This he declined, electing instead to enter the Georgia Medical College in Augusta, from which he was graduated as Doctor of Medicine in the spring of 1838.[2] In the fall of that year he entered the University of Pennsylvania School of Medicine from which he received a second medical degree in the following year.

Dr. Hartridge began his medical practice in Stewart County, Georgia, but after a short time moved to Madison, Florida, where he practiced his profession for some 15 years, simultaneously operating a mercantile business and a sawmill. He also purchased land in the county and became a part-time planter.

On July 29, 1846, Dr. Hartridge was married to Susan Ariana Livingston, daughter of Madison Camillus and Ariana Bird (nee Griffin) Livingston. The Livingstons were a Virginia family (Spotsylvania County), which had moved to Abbeville District, South Carolina, where Susan was born on August 5, 1829. Several children were born to this union, of whom the two eldest, Madison L. and John Earle, were born in Madison.[3]

In 1853 the Hartridges moved to Jacksonville. He had apparently contemplated this move for some time for the Jacksonville *Florida Republican* of June 26, 1850, listed him as a guest at the Jacksonville Hotel.

It is an item of Hartridge family lore that the Secession issue which intensified greatly in 1860 caused Dr. Hartridge much anguish. Intellectually he opposed it, a stand shared by many prominent Floridians, including elder statesman Richard K. Call. But when the Secession Convention, meeting in Tallahassee in early January 1861, voted overwhelmingly to leave the Union, Dr. Hartridge did not further oppose it. He did, however, remove his family to Columbia County where he had purchased land.

There is no evidence that, subsequent to his removal to Jacksonville in 1853, Dr. Hartridge ever publicly practiced medicine. It was by no means unusual in antebellum Florida for physicians to abandon practice, wholly or in part, for more lucrative undertakings. Medicine simply did not pay well. Many such as Dr. Hartridge, gifted with business acumen, turned to merchandizing. He had acquired land in both Madison and Columbia Counties and for several years led the life of a planter. Soon after his arrival in Jacksonville he entered the world of business in which he soon found success, not only in his own enterprises but in the business community. He was among the Jacksonville businessmen promoting the building of the Florida, Atlantic and Gulf Central Railroad, designed to connect Jacksonville with the interior of the state. He presided at their meeting in Jacksonville on April 14. 1855.[4] He was one of the early presidents of the Jacksonville Board of Trade.[5]

By the year 1855 Dr. Hartridge was an established merchant of the city. About 1855 he joined Col. H. Timanus in a partnership for the retailing of a variety of merchandise from their store at 14 North Bay Street. In numerous advertisements appearing in the Jacksonville newspaper of the year they brought their wares (flour, pork, brick, etc.) to the attention of the public. The arrangement was presumably terminated when a fire, originating in their warehouse, consumed their entire business, in addition to other properties in the area, the disaster occurring on January 29, 1860.[6] Within months, however, Dr. Hartridge had rebuilt and by early June was once again in business. On June 6, 1860, the Jacksonville *Standard* reported that "heavy cargoes of goods are being discharged at the wharves of Messrs Bisbee & Canova, Dr. T. Hartridge, and C. L. Roninson, whose stores are presenting a very business-like appearance and offering well-assorted stocks of new goods." The Hartridge residence was located at 87 East Forsyth Street[7] where the family continued to live until the great fire of 1901.

The Civil War brought disastrous consequences for Dr. Hartridge's business. At its conclusion he is said to have owed $40,000 to his New York creditors who offered to settle with him at 50 cents for each dollar he owed. Dr. Hartridge, however, being a man of rigid principle, refused the offer and eventually paid off the debt at its contracted value. He continued in business until 1885 when his failing eyesight forced him into retirement.

Dr. Hartridge's entire career was marked by an unselfish devotion to what he deemed his civic responsibilities. In his Madison years he was among the town's leaders in establishing a "Seminary of Learning," serving on its first Board of Trustees (1849), and in 1850 donating $200 to its support while serving as treasurer of the School.[8] In Jacksonville he was one of the founders of St. Paul's Methodist Church, later known as the McTyeire Memorial Methodist Church, located at the northeast corner of Duval and Newnan Streets. In 1902 his memory was honored by the placing of a stained glass window in the west front of the church.[9]

Although not an active medical practitioner, Dr. Hartridge, by virtue of his medical training and experience, was on more than one occasion pressed into the service of the city of Jacksonville to advise on health problems. Such was the case in 1877 when he was a member of the Board of Health.[10] In the following year as a trustee of the $250,000 Sanitary Improvement Bond issue, he had a voice as to how the money was to be allocated.[11] Still Dr. Hartridge, probably for reasons of modesty or conscience, never chose to affiliate with the medical fraternity of the town, which organized itself into the Duval County Medical Society in 1853. Nor was he ever a member of the Florida Medical Association, organized in Jacksonville in 1874. Yet one detects a certain deference on the part of his medical acquaintances to his knowledge and judgment.

In politics Dr. Hartridge was in his earlier years a member of the Whig Party, but with its dissolution in the 1850s he became a staunch Democrat which he remained for the rest of his life.

Upon his death on May 20, 1893, after a brief illness, Dr. Hartridge was survived by his wife who died on March 22, 1910, two sons, John Earle and Augustus Griffin, both distingushed lawyers in Jacksonville, and a daughter, Susan Martha. Other Hartridge children had preceded their father in death.

Through the kindness of Miss Dena Snodgrass of Jacksonville I was apprised of the work of Mr. and Mrs. Walter C. Hartridge of Savannah on the history of the Hartridge family. In response to my inquiry to Mrs. Hartridge (her husband had recently died) she graciously made available to me abundant genealogical material on the subject of the present sketch. Her assistance is gratefully acknowledged. Unless otherwise indicated the information contained herein derives from that source.

1. Jacksonville *Florida Times-Union*, May 21, 1893. Here is printed a complete obituary for Dr. Hartridge.
2. Medical Department, University of Georgia, Augusta, List of Graduates, Augusta 1891, p. 18.
3. It is a matter of some interest that the Hartridge household in Madison in 1850 included, in addition to the immediate family, Mrs. Hartridge's widowed mother, Mrs. Livingston, one Rachel Westcott, attorney Francis Wheaton, Shadrach Flowers, and two physicians, Samuel A. Bradford (b. S.C.) and Leddy McLeod (b. Ga.). U.S. Census, 1850, Madison County, Florida, p. 159.
4. Jacksonville *Florida Republican*, May 3, 1855. Nothing more is known of Col. Timanus.
5. T. Frederick Davis, *History of Jacksonville*, St. Augustine, 1925, p. 432.
6. Fernandina *East Floridian*, September 9, 1860.
7. W.S. Webb, comp., *Webb's Jacksonvile and Consolidated Directory*, Jacksonville, 1866.
8. Proceedings, Madison Lodge (Masonic), No. 11. "Minutes." Deed Book, K, pp. 7-15.
9. Jacksonville *Florida Times-Union*, September 2, 1902. The McTyeire Church has since been razed to make way for other buildings.
10. Webster Merritt, *A Century of Medicine in Jacksonville and Duval County*, Gainesville, 1949, p. 118. Dr. Hartridge was also a member of the Jacksonville Board of Aldermen. Ibid., p. 119.
11. Ibid., p. 120.

Harvard, Stephen F., Gainesville, 1825-1871

Dr. Harvard was born in Georgia on November 25, 1825.[1] Nothing is known of his childhood and education. When he arrived in Gainesville in 1854 he was accompanied by Latitia, his recent bride, who was younger by eight years. His decision to settle in Gainesville was doubtless influenced by the fact that Hardy Harvard, a relative, had purchased land and settled in Alachua County several years earlier.[2] Besides Gainesville had recently been declared the seat of the county and would appear to offer opportunities for a young physician just entering practice.

Since Gainesville could boast of no newspaper before 1861 Dr. Harvard's activities for the first years of his Florida residence have gone unrecorded. We may assume, however, that he was active in the public life of the community. On May 12, 1860, he was among the group of local citizens who met at the Court House to organize an Independent Volunteer Company of militia, calling themselves the "Gainesville Southern Guard," and installing Thomas A. McDonnell as Captain and Dr.Harvard as 1st Sergeant.[3] When the Confederacy was formed the following year the Company was disbanded, some of the members enlisting in the Confederate Army, others remaining on the home front.

Dr. Harvard, probably because of his age and family responsibilities, was among the latter group.

In his politics Dr. Harvard was a Democrat. On May 17, 1860, he attended the Alachua Democratic Convention at the Court House, a gathering at which six physicians were present.[4] He was elected to the town's board of aldermen in May 1866.[5] Somewhere along the way Dr. Harvard entered the real estate market, buying and selling lots and farmland in and around Gainesville. The Gainesville *New Era* reported on November 6, 1866, that he sold a town lot next to that of the Rev. Wm. J. McCormick for $1499.[6] This was followed by numerous other sales and purchases, all recorded in the county records.[7] So much did he become involved in farming that the Census enumerator of 1870 accorded him the following entry: "Harvard, S.F., 45, physician-planter $10,000-$20,000."[8]

Tragedy struck the Harvard family early, however. In one of the last major yellow fever epidemics to attack Gainesville,[9] three of the four members of the Harvard family succumbed to the disease. Mrs. Harvard died on November 13, 1871, while her son and husband died four days later, on November 17th. The three were buried in Gainesville's Evergreen Cemetery where their gravestones still stand.[10]

1. Grave marker, Evergreen Cemetery, Gainesville.

2. See entry for Hardy Harvard and family, U.S. Census, 1850, Alachua County, Florida, item 265. In the U.S. Census, 1860, Alachua County, Florida, item 605, it is shown that in Dr. Harvard's household in Gainesville there abided a Hardy Harvard, aged 22, whose occupation was deputy postmaster. He was probably a brother of the doctor.

3. McDonnell went on to achieve distinction in the Confederate cause, being seriously wounded at Shiloh, Tennessee, but later returning and being promoted to the rank of lieutenant colonel. Fernandina *East Floridian*, May 17, 1860.

4. Ibid., August 23, 1860.

5. Gainesville *New Era*, June 1, 1866.

6. Ibid., November 9, 1866.

7. See Alachua County Deed Books: E, p. 710; G, pp. 131, 524; H, pp. 90, 566.

8. U.S. Census, 1870, Alachua County, Florida, real property $10,000; personal property $2,000.

9. The disease appeared in Cedar Key in late summer, 1871, whence it was said to have been brought into Gainesville, the first case appearing in Gainesville in August. See Charles H. Hildreth, "A History of Gainesville, Florida," Ph.D. dissertation, University of Florida, June 1954, p. 94. Issues of the Gainesville *New Era* which described the Gainesville epidemic have not survived, but excerpts from those issues were reprinted in some other Florida papers, although names of fever victims were not recorded.

10. No information on the fourth member of the Harvard family, a daughter, Christina, aged 11, in 1870, has been located.

Hawes, George E., Putnam and Orange Counties, 1816-1896

Dr. Hawes, much beloved and highly respected physician, was born in South Carolina in August 1816. After finishing his medical education at an unidentified school he practiced for a few years in his native state before moving to Palatka in 1846.[1] In the next year he negotiated a contract to dig a canal or haulover connecting Mosquito Lagoon with Indian River in what was then Orange County. Finding life agreeable and professional opportunity promising[2] Dr. Hawes remained in Orange County for some three or four years. In 1848 and again in 1850 he was elected to represent the county in the House of Representatives.[3] He was a devoted Democrat throughout his life.

During his Orange County sojourn Dr. Hawes lived in the home of John J. Marshall, a native South Carolinian, and by far the wealthiest man in the county, whose lands lay in the vicinity of Mellonville.[4] At about this juncture the remnants of the Seminole Indian tribe in Central Florida once more became a threat to encroaching white settlers. Dr. Hawes was among the concerned citizens—another was Arthur Ginn—who met in Mellonville in July 1850 for the purpose of organizing resistance to the threat, bringing their plight to the attention of the state Legislature[5] and demanding the removal of all Indians.

By 1852 Dr. Hawes was again a resident of Palatka where he would reside for the rest of his life. The voters of the county soon returned him to the Legislature, this time as senator.[6] He was again their choice in 1854, 1856, and for the adjourned session of 1859. In 1860 and 1861 he was elected to the House. By the latter session, however, he had already enlisted in the Confederate Army but was granted the unusual privilege of a furlough to allow him to attend the legislative session.[7]

Although he was 44 years old at the time, Dr. Hawes enlisted in the Confederate Army as a private in July 1861 for a period of 12 months.[8] In January 1862, notwithstanding his rank, he was made Acting Regimental Surgeon of the 2nd Florida Infantry, but on the 18th of April he received a commission as captain and continued with the Regiment as Assistant Commissary of Subsistence, a rank which was abolished before the end of the War. He continued to serve with the 2nd Infantry in Virginia until the end of the conflict.[9]

Except for the war years, Dr. Hawes' life after his return to Palatka appears to have been uneventful. In the realm of community service he earned the esteem of his fellow citizens. He was one of the founders of St. Mark's Episcopal Church and for almost 50 years served as senior warden.[10] Either through inheritance or medical practice he was able to accumulate a substantial amount of property, his real estate having been valued at $23,000 in 1860.[11] Although he never married he maintained his own household for many years.

Dr. Hawes was not among the small group of Florida physicians who met in Jacksonville in early 1874 to establish the Florida Medical Association nor is there evidence that he ever attended any of its meetings except that held in Palatka in May 1886 at which time he became a member.[12] He did, however, continue to pay his annual dues up to the time of his death. At the 1897 meeting of the Association held in Palatka, his death was brought to the attention of the members, and the Necrology Committee presented a fitting tribute to the memory of their highly-regarded colleague.[13]

Dr. Hawes died at the home of Mrs. E.M. Haughton in Palatka on October 27, 1896, after a brief illness, at the age of 80 years and two months.[14]

1. Obituary notice, Jacksonville *Daily Florida Citizen*, October 30, 1896.
2. Only one other qualified physician was practicing in Orange County at the time, Dr. Algernon Speer.
3. Allen Morris, *The People of Lawmaking in Florida*, Tallahassee, 1977.
4. U.S. Census, 1850, Orange County, Florida, p. 376.
5. Jacksonville *News*, August 3, 1850.
6. Putnam County, established in 1849, was for legislative purposes designated Senatorial District No. 7.
7. See note 3, supra.
8. NA, Service Records, CSA, M251 Reel 37.
9. Ibid.
10. *A History of St. Mark's Church, Palatka, Florida*, author, date and place of publication not given, p. 3 et passim.
11. U.S. Census, 1860, Putnam County, Florida, Item 95. In 1860 Dr. Hawes is shown as the owner of 35 slaves, 1860 Slave Schedule, Putnam County, Florida, p. 3. The Putnam County Census, 1885, p. 149, lists him as a resident in the household of a Palatka lawyer, Eugene C. Nichols.
12. *Proceedings, FMA, Session of 1886*, Jacksonville, 1886, p. 6. Here Dr. Hawes is listed as a representative of the Putnam County Medical Society.

13. Ibid., 1897, p. 27. Incidentally, this meeting was also held in Palatka.

14. See note 1, supra, George R. Fairbanks, "Early Churchmen of Florida," *Semi-Centennial*, 1888, *Diocese of Florida*, Jacksonville 1889, p. 13. Discussing St. Mark's Parish, Palatka, Dr. Fairbanks wrote, "St. Mark's, Palatka, was the first offshoot for many years, owing its establishment to Judge Bronson, and subsequently to the faithful work of Dr. George E. Hawes (at whose baptism in St. Augustine I stood as witness), Dr. Moragne, and others..."

Hawkins, Alexander Boyd, Tallahassee, 1825-1921

There is no evidence that Dr. Hawkins[1] ever practiced medicine in Florida. His role as an educated and enlightened citizen and holder of a degree in medicine from one of the nation's finest schools, however, demands that he be included in any register of 19th century Florida physicians. Born in Franklin County, North Carolina, on January 25, 1825, at the home of his parents, John Davis and Jane A. (nee Boyd) Hawkins, he enjoyed the advantage of growing up in a family of cultivation, affluence, and concern for the public good. His education was the best available. Taught by a private tutor and later spending a year under the strict guidance of John H. Bobbitt of Louisburg, N.C., he was accepted for admission by the University of North Carolina at the age of 16. He was graduated as Bachelor of Arts in 1845 and a few months later enrolled at Jefferson Medical College, Philadelphia, from which he was graduated in 1847. Recognizing the need for some practical experience he remained in Philadelphia for several months of work in hospitals before returning to his native state.

Dr. Hawkins began a regular practice in Warren County, North Carolina, where he had purchased the practice of the popular physician, Dr. John Malone. He remained in practice there for several years, residing in the community of Shocco Springs.

Except for the fact that rural Leon and Jefferson Counties had been settled by numerous North Carolina families, some of them known to Dr. Hawkins, there is no other explanation for his decision to remove to Florida. At any rate, he made the move and there he met and married Martha L. Bailey, daughter of General William Bailey of Jefferson County, one of Florida's most distinguished citizens. Dr. Hawkins purchased land north of Tallahassee and settled in to the life of a gentleman farmer. The Leon County Census of 1860 designates him "Planter," with property valued at $67,700.[2]

Dr. Hawkins was 36 years of age when the Civil War began. There is no record to show that he saw actual military service, although he was placed in command of a reserve unit, Company G, First Florida Reserves, with the rank of Captain. At the close of the War, Dr. Hawkins moved into Tallahassee and resided in a palatial brick house, known as "The Columns,"[3] located at that time at 105 East Park Avenue.

In his politics Dr. Hawkins was a staunch Democrat and firm believer in States Rights, although he never ran for public office nor accepted a public appointment. He did, however, show remarkable business acumen and accumulated considerable wealth. Charitable by nature, he is known to have served as guardian for several orphans and as trustee for several landed estates, all without personal monetary gain. For five years he was receiver for the Florida Central and Peninsular Railroad and was noted for his honesty, recipient of praise from its auditors. He was also known for his experiment in the cultivation of sweet oranges and grapefruit.

Dr. Hawkins never disposed of his property in Franklin County, North Carolina. About 1884 he began spending his summers in Raleigh where he had purchased a house on North Blount Street where he died on April 21, 1921, at the age of 96.

Dr. Hawkins was not a man to flaunt his wealth or social position, an inbred attitude based on his family background and his own intelligence. He never lacked for the means for comfortable living. In addition to the aforementioned wealth, he is shown to have owned 51 slaves in the early 1860s.[4]

1. The greater part of the detail contained in the present sketch is drawn from the obituary notice which appeared in the Raleigh, N.C., *Times* on the day of his death, which was reprinted in the Tallahassee *Daily Democrat* of April 23, 1921.

2. Due to the loss of his slaves and disruptions following the War, his properties had been reduced to an estimated value of $26,000 in 1870.

3. "The Columns" had been built by Dr. Hawkins' father-in-law, William Bailey. It was later moved farther west on Park Avenue where it stands today.

4. Slave Schedule, Leon County, Florida, 1860.

Hawkins, Hamilton S., U.S. Army Physician, 1802-1847

Dr. Hawkins, a native of Maryland, was born about 1802.[1] In 1822 he was graduated from the University of Maryland Department of Medicine located in Baltimore.[2] Two years later he was commissioned Assistant Surgeon in the United States Army[3] and as his first assignment was stationed as post surgeon at Ft. Moultrie, Charleston Harbor, South Carolina.[4] In 1827 he began his first tour of duty in Florida, serving at the Army cantonment near Pensacola, where Dr. Thomas Lawson, later to become Surgeon General, was the chief medical officer.

In August 1827, an outbreak of yellow fever occurred in Pensacola. W. Hasell Hunt, the reputable editor of the Pensacola *Gazette,* in reporting the epidemic, followed the customary practice of the times by minimizing the seriousness of the disease, lest he set off a panic among the residents and, perhaps equally important, do a disservice to the mercantile interests of the town. Both Drs. Lawson and Hawkins, to some degree the custodians of the health of the community, were incensed and took public issue with Hunt, accusing him of deceiving the local populace by concealing the true conditions. They claimed that the fever was far more prevalent and dangerous than Hunt had been willing to admit. A heated controversy ensued.[5]

Dr. Hawkins' next military post was Ft. King, located on the Oklawaha River east of Ocala, an installation which assumed a special importance with the growing hostilities between the white settlers and the Seminole Indians in the late 1820s. There Dr. Hawkins worked in close association with Gad Humphreys, Indian agent in the Territory. In response to complaints from settlers northward in Alachua County that their lives and property were threatened by Indian predators, Dr. Hawkins was dispatched into the area to survey the situation. In his deposition of March 1829 to George Downs, an Alachua justice of the peace, he stated that he had gone as far north as the Santa Fe River settlement, i.e., to Col. James Dell's place, but could find no Indians. It was his conclusion that the fears were unfounded.[6]

At about the same time Humphreys came under attack from Waters Smith and his associates who accused him of malfeasance and mismanagement of his office. These accusations were thought to have been inspired by Smith's ambition to replace Humphreys as Indian agent. Among the several deponents coming to Humphreys' defense was Dr. Hawkins.[7]

By 1830 Dr. Hawkins had been transferred to Cantonment Brooke (later to be reclassified as Ft. Brooke) off the northeast shore of Tampa Bay.[8] Military records indicate that he remained at the base until about the end of 1833 when his Florida career ended. In 1834 he received his second assignment to Ft. Moultrie[9] and a year later he was assistant surgeon at Ft. Severn in his native state of Maryland where on July 4, 1836,[10,11] he was promoted to the rank of Surgeon. Although the documentation is not at hand, it is almost certain that this promotion was recommended by Dr. Lawson, who on June 20 previously had been appointed medical director of the Army of the South..."with general control over all hospitals, and the distribution of duty among the surgeons, assistant surgeons, and surgeons' mates of this army, as well as the distribution among the medical officers of medicines and hospital stores."[12] On November 30, 1836, Dr. Lawson became Surgeon General.[13]

In 1838 Dr. Hawkins was the medical officer at the Army post in New Orleans.[14] Nothing is known of his subsequent career until the winter of 1846-47 which found him serving with American troops in the Mexican War. He died in Tampico on August 13, 1847,[15] whether from wounds received in military encounter or fever is not known. Evidence suggests that Dr. Hawkins was a physician of exceptional competence who carried out his duties efficiently and responsibly. The single letter over his signature which appeared in the Pensacola *Gazette* indicates a high degree of literacy. His death at the age of 45 was a serious loss to the Army and to his profession.

1. This is an approximation based on the assumption that most medical students of the early 19th century entered medical school at about age 18 usually after a few years of "reading medicine" under the guidance of a local physician and received their medical degrees at about age 20.

2. Eugene Fauntleroy Cordell, *Historical Sketch of the University of Maryland School of Medicine, 1807-1890,* Baltimore, 1981, p. 178.

3. *The Medical Department of the United States Army,* Harvey E. Brown, Comp., Washington, Surgeon General's Office, 1873, p. 291.

4. *American State Papers,* Military Affairs, Vol. V, Washington, 1861, p. 278.

5. Pensacola *Gazette,* issues of August 31 and September 7, 1827. In defense of his statement Editor Hunt sought the opinion of local physician Fernando Moreno whose report on sickness in Pensacola for the month of August is printed in the issue of September 7. Dr. Moreno had treated 29 cases of fever, only one of which he identified as yellow fever.

6. *"Gad Humphrey Papers,"* collected by Edward T. Keenan, p. 69. These papers are now in the collection of the P.K. Yonge Library of Florida History, University of Florida, Gainesville.

7. TP, XXIV, p. 213.

8. U.S. Census, 1830, Alachua County, Florida, p. 13.

9. *American State Papers,* Military Affairs, V, 278.

10. Ibid., p. 608.

11. See. n. 3 supra, p. 288.

12. *American State Papers,* Military Affairs, VII, 344.

13. See note 3 supra, p. 286.

14. *American State Papers,* Military Affairs, VII, 929.

15. See note 3 supra, p. 288.

Hawks, Esther Hill, Northeast Florida, 1833-1906

Dr. Hawks, wife of Dr. John Milton Hawks, spent only a small part of her lengthy career in Florida, never actually as a regular practitioner in the state. She was born in Hooksett, New Hampshire, on August 4, 1833,[1] the daughter of Parmenus and Jane (Kimball) Hill. As a young adult she became a school teacher but soon turned to the study of medicine at an unidentified school, becoming a licensed physician in 1857.[2] She married Dr. John Milton Hawks on October 5, 1854. For their wedding trip they headed for Florida, ultimately arriving in Manatee County, south of Tampa Bay, where they spent the winter of 1854-55. During their sojourn the couple apparently had an opportunity to observe the slavery institution first hand and were moved to devote their energies to the amelioration of the plight of the Negro in the South.

With the enunciation of the Emancipation Proclamation on January 1, 1863, the condition of the Negro in some parts of the South actually worsened. The Freedmen's Bureau did not come into being until March 1865. Meanwhile the Freedman's Aid Society had been formed in New York in 1862. The Drs. Hawks volunteered their services to the organization and were sent to Hilton Head and Edisto Island, South Carolina, where he immediately tried to organize a Negro Regiment. He was only partially successful and soon realized that he could better serve the cause of the Negro by devoting his time to medical practice among them. Both he and his wife henceforth devoted their energies to medical practice among the Negroes and the Confederate prisoners in the Charleston area.

In the years immediately following the War, Dr. Esther devoted her time to volunteer work among the Negro children through the office of the Freedmen's Bureau. She also worked to establish an orphan asylum in Charleston. She was also for a time principal of a school in Charleston. In 1870, however, she decided to return to New England. Whether this move was the result of an estrangement from her husband is not made clear, but it is almost certain that it was not. Anyway she returned to Lynn, Massachusetts, where she established a medical practice at 51 Silsbee Street in partnership with Dr. Mary J. Flanders. They were the first female physicians in Lynn and are said to have been successful.

It is not known whether Dr. Esther ever returned to Florida even for a visit with her husband who had established a well-appointed home on spacious grounds, naming the place Hawks Park. It would eventually be engulfed by the town of Edgewater.

Family documents indicate that after 1870 Dr. John regularly spent his summers in Lynn with his wife and two sisters, returning to Hawks Park for the winters. Mrs. Hawks died at Lynn on May 6, 1906.

1. Biographical information on Dr. Esther Hill Hawks is derived almost totally from a publication issued by descendants of the Hawks family, the masthead of which is *Hawkes Talks*, Genealogical Bulletin of the Adam Hawkes Family Association, Inc. The issue of reference here is that of Volume XVI, April 1984.

2. It is not known whether Dr. Hawks earned her medical license by way of the preceptorate system or by graduation from a medical college. The barrier against women attending medical colleges had been broken when Elizabeth Blackwell was admitted to Geneva Medical College, Geneva, New York, from which she was graduated in 1849, "the first woman to be graduated in medicine in the United States." Frederick Clayton Waite, *The First Medical College in Vermont, Castleton, 1818-1862*, Montpelier, Vermont Historical Society, 1949, p. 160.

Hawks, John Milton, Volusia County, 1826-1910

Dr. Hawks, one of the most colorful figures to practice medicine in Florida in the 19th century, first appeared in the state in 1854 when he included Florida in a lengthy wedding trip which had taken him and his bride, the former Esther Hill, as far south as Manatee County. He was born in Bradford, New Hampshire, on November 26, 1826,[1] son of Colburn Hawks and grandson of Farrington Hawks, a native of Dunstable, Maine. He received his early education in the Bradford schools and at age 15 began a teaching career in a country school near his home. From there he went to Albany County, New York, where he taught in 1843-44.

In late 1844 he moved to Houston County, Georgia, where he taught for three years in a private school before enrolling in the Eclectic Medical College of Cincinnati, Ohio, which had been established in 1832. He received his medical degree in 1847. Apparently not satisfied that he had received the best of medical training, he enrolled at the Vermont Medical College, Woodstock, Vermont, in the fall of 1847, remaining there for a term and, according to the records of the College, left without receiving a degree.[2] He entered into practice in Manchester, New Hampshire, in 1848.

Apparently intrigued by the professional and business possibilities in the two recently-admitted states, California and Florida, Dr. Hawks decided to try his luck in California. As the time of departure approached he decided to go to Florida instead. He was favorably impressed with what he saw and a year later returned with his bride to Manatee County, established in 1855, where they spent the winter of 1854-55.

Dr. Hawks was much concerned with the social injustice regarding the Negro which he observed in the South, especially runaway slaves as well as those who had been liberated. He volunteered his services to the Freedmen's Aid Society, serving as physician on Edisto Island, South Carolina, in 1862. At about the same time he assisted in organizing a Negro Regiment, the first to be incorporated into the Union Army, serving as Assistant Surgeon from October 1862 to October 1863. During this service he was promoted to the rank of Surgeon in which capacity he continued until December 1, 1865, when he returned to Florida. His unit was designated the Twenty-First U.S. Volunteer Regiment.

As a resident of parts of Florida which had suffered least from the war and emancipation of the slaves, Dr. Hawks was amicably received upon his return to civilian status in the later 1860s. In the years of reconstruction after settling in Volusia County, his abilities and intelligence were soon recognized and he was called into public service, filling several important posts. In 1868 he was Secretary of the Board of Voter Registration for Volusia County and served as engrossing clerk in the Florida Legislature in 1868, 1869 and 1870. His progressive stance in political matters was demonstrated by his support of a measure which would have given women the voting privilege. While serving as Internal Revenue Assessor in Pensacola he led the effort to establish a public library and is said to have collected the nucleus of books. His presence in East Florida was apparent when he served as postmaster of an office north of Mosquito Inlet to which he gave the name, Orange Point, which still exists.

As a writer and publisher Dr. Hawks is not to be overlooked. While serving as clerk in the Legislature he wrote periodic reports on its transactions for the Florida *Times-Union* of Jacksonville at the same time contributing articles to the Savannah *Morning News*. He published the first two directories for the city of Jacksonville. As a publicist for the attractions and advantages of living in Florida Dr. Hawks published his *Florida Gazeteer*, printed in New Orleans in 1871. This served as a guidebook for hundreds of visitors and settlers entering the state.

Medicine appears to have been a secondary occupation for Dr. Hawks after settling in Florida. His approach to the profession was one of common sense. He emphasized proper nursing for the sick and proper dieting for the prevention of many ailments. It was his conviction that given sensible care nine-tenths of the sick would recover without any medicine whatsoever. He wrote: "The true mission of the medical fraternity is to prevent disease by the timely teaching of the laws of health."

Having explored much of Florida during his extended visits to the state, Dr. Hawks finally decided to build a home in which he might live out the latter years of his life. He knew the East Coast well and selected a beautiful spot on the west bank of Indian River Lagoon two miles south of the New Smyrna city limits where he built a comfortable but not pretentious house in which he spent his last years. Upon occupying the place in 1872 he named it Hawks Park, the name it continued to bear until the area was engulfed by the municipality of Edgewater. It was said to have been a hospitable place where the doctor enjoyed the visits of numerous acquaintances. He died there on April 2, 1910, and was buried in a cemetery nearby. A modest stone marks the place of his burial.

Although not totally estranged from her husband, Mrs. Hawks spent little time in the South. She had obtained a medical degree prior to the Civil War in 1857 and is said to have assisted her husband in his work with colored children through the Freedmen's Bureau. After the war, however, she returned to the North and established a medical practice in Lynn, Massachusetts, in partnership with another female physician, Dr. Lizzie Breed Welch, and later with Dr. Mary J. Flanders. She died in Lynn on May 6, 1906.

1. This biographical sketch has been drawn almost entirely from two sources: a bulletin *Hawkes Talks*, a Genealogical Bulletin of the Adam Hawkes Family Association, Inc., Vol. XVI, April 1984, 4 pp., and a biographical data sheet in the Collection of the P.K. Yonge Library of Florida History, University of Florida, Gainesville, 2 pp., its authorship is unknown.

2. There is some disagreement as to whether Dr. Hawks actually received a medical degree from the Vermont school. See Frederick Clayton Waite, *The Story of a Country Medical College*, a history of the Clinical School of Medicine and the Vermont Medical College, Vermont Historical Society, Montpelier 1845. In the appendices are two lists of students: those who received degrees and those who did not. Dr. Hawks' name appears in the latter list. The full entry is "John Milton Hawkes, entered 1847, Bradford, New Hampshire, Nov. 26, 1826."

Hayward, Charles, Leon County, 1836

Notwithstanding their prominent roles in the antebellum history of Leon County, the activities of the Hayward family are difficult to document. The Florida Haywards appear to have originated in Dorchester County, Maryland. The first to migrate to Florida was Richard Hayward who arrived in Florida about 1831.[1] He and his wife, Harriet, settled in Tallahassee, although he purchased lands nearby and within a couple of decades had become one of the wealthier planters of the county. Several children were born, Charles, the doctor, and a daughter, Anna, who was the second wife of Dr. William Tradewell.

Charles was born in Tallahassee in 1836[2] and christened at St. John's Episcopal Church on March 20, 1838.[3] Nothing is known of either his early education or medical training, but in the Leon County Census of 1860 he is entered as a resident of the home of his parents with the designation M.D. Dr. Hayward was married to Coralie Adelaide Bond and on April 18, 1864, their daughter, Harriet Fort Hayward, was christened at St. John's.[4]

There is no evidence that Dr. Hayward was ever a member of the Confederate armed forces.[5] It is probable that he practiced in Tallahassee during the war; however, the suspension of publication of local newspapers in 1864 and 1865 makes it impossible to verify his presence there as a medical practitioner. His father, Richard Hayward, died in Tallahassee on January 29, 1867.[6] Since the Leon County Census of 1870 does not include the name of Dr. Charles Hayward, it is assumed that he had departed the state by that date.

1. Richard Hayward is not included in the Florida Census of 1830, but the records of St. John's Episcopal Church, Tallahassee, list him as a parishioner in 1832.
2. U.S. Census, 1860, Leon County, Florida, item 116.
3. Parish Records, St. John's Episcopal Church, Tallahassee, Record of Baptisms, p. 13.
4. Ibid., p. 24.
5. Another Charles Hayward, cousin of the doctor, and son of Dr. William R. Hayward of Tallahassee, enlisted in the Confederate Army in May 1861, was commissioned 2nd Lieutenant in April 1862 but resigned his commission in order to reenlist in a military unit from his native state of Maryland. See NA, Service Records, CSA, M 251, Roll 27.
6. Tallahassee *Sentinel*, February 1, 1867.

Hayward, William R., Tallahassee, 1816

Dr. Hayward, a native of Maryland, migrated to Leon County in the early 1840s, doubtless persuaded by certain relatives, notably Richard Hayward, who had moved into the area in the 1830s.[1] The earliest evidence of his presence is his professional card, published in late 1842, in which he announced a partnership with Dr. James Henry Randolph,[2] already an established practitioner of Tallahassee. At about the same time Dr. Hayward purchased the drug firm of Drs. J.H. Pope and J.S. Robinson, a sale brought about by the dissolution of the partnership. The transaction was announced on November 24, 1842.[3]

Within a year after he purchased the drug store the most destructive fire ever to occur in the town swept through the business section.[4] The store was among the casualties although he had been able to salvage most of its contents. The fire had broken out on the afternoon of May 25, 1843, and on June 6, Dr. Hayward announced that he was again open for business in a house occupied by the Surveyor-General, "2nd door below Brown's Hotel."[5]

Dr. Hayward apparently prospered both as druggist and physician. As the 1850s drew on he made frequent appearances in public roles. An adherent to the Whig persuasion, he became State Treasurer in the administration of Governor Thomas Brown in 1849,[6] and in that capacity he became an ex officio member of the Board of Internal Improvements in 1851.[7] Two years later he was elected Intendant (Mayor) of Tallahassee and as such was instrumental in launching the building program for the recently-created West Florida Seminary (now Florida State University).[8]

Dr. Hayward and his wife Eliza, also a Maryland native, were the parents of several children listed in the Census of 1850 as Charles, Delia and William. Another son, Robert Emmett, was baptized at St. John's Episcopal Church, Tallahassee, on January 12, 1853. Beyond this very little is known of the Hayward family. Unfortunately no death dates for Dr. Hayward and his wife have been located.

1. U.S. Census, 1840, Leon County, Florida, pp. 66, 79.
2. Tallahassee *Star of Florida*, January 5, 1843.
3. Ibid.
4. For full account of the disaster see ibid., June 1, 1843.
5. Tallahassee *Florida Sentinel*, June 6, 1843.
6. The complete list of state officers appeared in several issues of ibid. in the summer and fall of 1850.
7. A.W. Thompson, "Florida Senatorial Election of 1851," FHQ, XXXI, No. 3, January 1953, p. 187.
8. William G. Dodd, "Early Education in Tallahassee and the West Florida Seminary, Now Florida State University," FHQ, XXVII, No. 1, July 1948, pp. 21, 22.

Hazell, Ellen Frances Fitzpatrick McCallum, Putnam County, 1826-1905

Unless midwifery be considered medical practice, women were rarely found among the medical practitioners of 19th century Florida. Although many woman were doubtless acquainted with the common home remedies of the times and indeed are known to have administered to their own families and those of their neighbors, none appears to have been designated physician before the middle of the century. The first woman known to have been engaged in actual practice was Ellen Frances Fitzpatrick McCallum Hazell, a native of Ireland, who with her husband and three small children arrived in Florida in the early 1850s.[1] Her husband, Scottish-born Eugene McCallum, was a civil engineer. The family settled at Orange Mills, Putnam County, on the east side of the St. Johns River, where McCallum found work in the sawmill recently established by the wealthy Rhydon Grigsby Mays, physician and planter, who had settled on a large tract of land along the River northeast of Forrester Point.

Ellen McCallum, neé Fitzpatrick, was said to have studied medicine at a Dublin hospital, and soon after her arrival in Florida had begun to practice medicine up and down the River wherever she was needed. She was of intrepid character, colorful yet compassionate. Her neighbor and contemporary, E. Stuart Hubbard, remembered her as "of medium height, rugged frame, possessed of unbounded spirit, dauntless courage and an Irish brogue." She usually traveled on horseback "through the forest, unafraid. She dominated the scene, even in the eighteen-nineties, when she entertained passengers on the mailboat with her spirited conversation."[2]

Three children were born to Eugene and Ellen McCallum prior to their migration to America.[3] Within three years after their arrival at Orange Springs, however, McCallum died, leaving his widow to fend for herself. About 1860 she remarried, this time to John B. Hazell, who had recently driven a wagon from Edgefield, South Carolina, for his employer, Marshall Siegler of Edgefield. Family tradition holds that Hazell chose to remain in Florida, whereupon Siegler introduced him to Dr. Mays, who immediately offered him employment at Orange Mills. Through his industry and intelligence Hazell had soon earned sufficient resources to enable him to purchase a part of the Sanchez land along the River north of Orange Mills on which he turned to farming and orange growing. There he and Ellen reared their two children, a son, Elzy, and a daughter, Margaret affectionately known as Maggie.[4]

Notwithstanding the outbreak of war in 1861, Dr. Hazell continued her medical practice up and down the River even after Union troops had gained control of the waterway. At one point she aroused the suspicion of the captain of a Union gunboat who accused her of doctoring Confederate soldiers and possibly passing on sensitive information to them. She was arrested and taken aboard a boat for Jacksonville for questioning by Union authorities. On arrival there she proceeded to walk off the boat but was immediately reminded that she was a prisoner-of-war. At this point she assumed her purest Irish brogue and declared herself a subject of Great Britain and therefore not subject to arrest. It is said that the baffled boat captain, not wishing to ignite an international incident, decided to set her free.[5]

It is not known how long Dr. Hazell continued her medical practice, but it appears that as the 19th century drew toward a close she retired to the role of housewife and grandmother, her son, Joseph McCallum having married in the 1880s and fathered four sons. Dr. Hazell died at her Orange Mills home on November 29, 1905, after a brief illness. A devout Catholic throughout her life, she was buried in the Catholic Cemetery at Orange Mills.[6]

1. Much of what is known about the remarkable Ellen Hazell is derived from E. Stuart Hubbard, "Memories of Florida," Poughkeepsie, N.Y., 1951-54, published in five parts, mimeographed. Hubbard was born at Federal Point near Orange Mills and in his youth he had known the Hazell family.

2. Ibid., ii, 18.

3. U.S. Census, 1860, Putnam County, Florida, item 57. The children of this marriage were Joseph, Mary and James, aged 14, 13 and seven respectively.

4. U.S. Census, 1870, Putnam County, Florida, item 14, Orange Mills Precinct. The two children of this marriage were Elzy born 1862 and Margaret born 1866. She married M.J. Murphy of Wappinger's Falls, New York. The Putnam County Census of 1900 cites 1860 as the year of Ellen McCallum's marriage to John B. Hazell.

5. Hubbard, "Memories," iv, pp. 19-20.

6. Jacksonville *Florida Times-Union*, December 1, 1905, p. 10.

Heard, Faulkner (Falkner), Marion and Clay Counties, 1850s

Dr. Heard, who practiced medicine for little more than a decade in Florida, was a native of Georgia.[1] He was born about 1828, entered the Jefferson Medical College of Philadelphia in the fall of 1847 and was graduated as M.D. in the spring of 1849.[2] Immediately after graduation he settled as a novice physician in Ocala, taking up residence at Josiah Paine's boarding house.[3] He first advertised his services to the citizens of Marion and adjacent counties in May 1851,[4] with an office facing the public square, where he remained at least until the summer of 1853.[5]

Nothing further is known of Dr. Heard's activities until 1860 when he was entered in the Census Schedule of Clay County as a resident of Hibernia. In the meantime he was married to Lendorska (patronym unknown), an Alabama native, having become the father of two sons, John F., aged six, and Bryan, aged one.[6] Since neither he nor his family appear in subsequent Florida censuses, it is assumed that they had departed the state in the 1860s.

1. U.S. Census, Marion County, Florida, p. 220.

2. *American Journal of the Medical Sciences*, Philadelphia, April 1849, n.s. XXXIV. The appendix to this issue contain a list of Jefferson graduates of March 28, 1849. Dr. Heard's thesis was titled "Pneumonia."

3. See note 1 above.

4. Ocala *Conservator*, October 22, 1851.

5. Ocala *Florida Mirror*, July 8, 1853.

6. U.S. Census, 1860, Clay County, Florida, p. 141. The spelling of Mrs. Heard's Christian name is uncertain.

Heiskell, Henry Lee, Surgeon, U.S. Army, 1855

Dr. Heiskell, a career service physician in the United States Army, was a native of Virginia. He was commissioned Assistant Surgeon on July 13, 1832.[1] Some three years later the hostility which had developed between the Florida Indians and the white settlers encroaching on their territory flared into open conflict near Bushnell when a group of Indian warriors ambushed a couple of companies of United States Army troops making their way from Ft. Brooke to Ft. King, killing all but three soldiers. This event prompted Washington authorities to dispatch a brigade of regular troops to Tampa to deal with the threat. The brigade was led by General Edmund P. Gaines; Dr. Heiskell was its chief medical officer, subordinate to Surgeon General Thomas Lawson.[2]

Dr. Heiskell was promoted to surgeon's rank on July 7, 1838. He remained in the Army until his death, which occurred in Washington on August 12, 1855.[3]

1. Francis B. Heitman, *Historical Register and Dictionary of the U.S. Army*, Vol. I, Washington, 1903, p. 291.
2. Ibid.
3. Ibid., pp. 288

Henley, Thomas N., Gadsden County, 1831

Dr. Henley was hardly more than a sojourner in Florida. He moved from his native North Carolina to Gadsden County about 1860 and settled in the village of Concord in the northeastern corner of the county. On March 12, 1862, he enlisted in Company B (Captain B. Love, commanding), 6th Florida Infantry, with the rank of 5th Sergeant. In the summer of 1862 the 6th was ordered to Tennessee to become a unit of the army of General Braxton Bragg as he was organizing his Kentucky campaign. Upon their return to Knoxville for the winter Dr. Henley became ill and was hospitalized at Chickamauga. He was promoted to Junior 2nd Lieutenant on February 7, 1863, but within a few weeks became a 2nd Lieutenant.

Dr. Henley was captured by Union forces at Nashville on December 14, 1864, and sent immediately to prison at Louisville. A short time later he was moved to Johnson Island in Lake Erie near Sandusky, Ohio, remaining there until his release, on taking the required oath June 16, 1865.

Confederate Army records describe him as six feet tall, of light complexion, blue eyes and dark hair. His age at the time of discharge was 34.[1]

Upon his release Dr. Henley returned to Concord and resumed medical practice. The Census of 1870 lists him as physician, owning property valued at $3,500. His wife, Elizabeth, a Georgia native and some 14 years his junior, and Mary I. Foster, also from Georgia, completed the household.[2] Dr. Henley, a Master Mason, was a member of Concordia Lodge No. 28.[3] Since the Henleys do not appear in subsequent censuses it is assumed that they departed the state in the 1870s.

1. NA, Service Records, CSA, M251, Roll 71.
2. U.S. Census, 1870, Gadsden County, Florida, p. 709.
3. *Returns of Particular Lodges Order of Mason* (no place; 1865), p. 428.

Henry, Thomas Yuille, Gadsden County, 1821-1867

Born in 1819 to one of Virginia's most illustrious families and related by blood or marriage to numerous Virginia aristocrats, Dr. Henry migrated to Florida in the early 1850s.[1] He was the son of Edward Winston Henry, 15th child of Patrick Henry and Jane Yuille Henry, and was born at Red Hill, the Patrick Henry plantation in western Charlotte County near the Campbell County line. Although Thomas was born 20 years after the demise of his famous grandfather, the imprint of the great patriot was still visible in the life-style of Red Hill's residents. His father was a noted race horse breeder and fancier and young Thomas was well-known as a skillful equestrian.[2]

University of Virginia records list Thomas Y. Henry as a student there in the terms of 1838 and 1839 but indicate that he went elsewhere for his medical education.[3] University of Maryland School of Medicine records, however, show him to have been awarded the M.D. degree in the class of 1841.[4]

The career of Dr. Henry for the years immediately following his graduation is not presently accounted for and it is presumed that he entered practice, probably in Virginia. Evidence suggests that upon arriving in Florida he abandoned medicine and turned instead to the life of a planter.[5] His lands lay outside Quincy and by the standards of the time he was not a wealthy man. He did, however, make his presence known in Gadsden County. By 1857 he had gained sufficient prominence in Masonic circles to be named Grand Master of the Grand Lodge of Florida, a position he held for two years.[6]

As reactions to the slavery issue began to intensify in the late 1850s Dr. Henry remained faithful to the convictions of his class. He was among those rejecting the compromise proposals of the old Democratic party at its Charleston Convention which broke up in discord. He was one of the delegates from Gadsden for the subsequent Convention in Baltimore which met on June 18, 1860.[7] Later he was one of Gadsden's delegates to the Secession Convention meeting in Tallahassee on January 3, 1861[8] and was among those voting for secession.

When the Civil War began Dr. Henry, in spite of his 42 years, offered his services to the Confederate cause. The several companies which would compose the 2nd Florida Infantry Regiment were being organized in the early summer of 1861 and in early July Governor Perry tendered to Dr. Henry the appointment of assistant surgeon to Dr. Thomas M. Palmer. On July 13 he was mustered into service.[9] The Monticello *Family Friend* of July 13 took note of the appointment as follows:

> Dr. Henry is a high-toned, honorable man, but as to his ability we have no knowledge. He has abandoned medical practice for several years past, but it does not follow as a necessity that he has thusly disqualified himself for the practice.

In the light of subsequent events it may perhaps be said that this raising of eyebrows by the Monticello paper was understandable. Dr. Henry accompanied his regiment to Virginia in late July but for reasons not at all clear he returned to Florida a few months later. His army record, though incomplete, indicates that he was on leave for the first 10 days of January 1862 and throughout the month of February. Apparently his military career soon ended for in the fall of 1862 he was elected as one of Gadsden County's three members to Florida's House of Representatives where he served for three consecutive terms—1862,

1863 and 1864. In the House he was a leader. In January 1863 he was sent by Governor Milton to Tennessee for the purpose of determining the advisability of establishing a "Florida Hospital" for Florida units serving in General Braxton Bragg's Army. At Tullahoma he consulted with Bragg's medical director, Dr. E.A. Flewellen, and was advised that no such hospital was needed at the time. Dr. Henry's report was included in Governor Milton's address to the General Assembly in November 1863.[10]

Meanwhile Dr. Henry was not idle on the home front. In 1863 Governor Milton assigned to him the responsibility of establishing military hospital facilities in a number of West Florida localities. In Quincy, which was one of six sites for such units, Dr. Henry converted churches and public buildings into hospitals and with the assistance of the Ladies Aid Society maintained 126 beds.[11]

Information on the immediate family of Dr. Henry is not abundant.[12] Other children of Edward Winston and Jane Yuille Henry were Patrick Lafayette, who left no issue, five daughters, Maria Rosalie, Sarah, Lucy Dorothea, Celina, and Ada, all of whom married and had issue, and the youngest, Edward W., who married Anne Ely and had issue. Dr. Henry himself was married to Mary F. Cunningham and is thought to have had issue.[13] His only appearance in Florida census schedules came in 1860 (Gadsden County) where no children are listed. Mrs. Henry is listed as 30 years of age and a native of Georgia.

Dr. Henry did not long survive the close of the war, dying on May 31, 1869. He was buried in the Quincy cemetery. The inscription on his gravestone reads: Thomas Y. Henry, Grandson of Patrick Henry, Born in Red Hill, Virginia, 1821, died May 31, 1869, Grand Master of Masons of Florida, 1857 & 1858.

1. Dr. Henry's whereabouts during the nine years following his graduation from medical school is unknown. It is probable that he was in practice somewhere in Virginia.
2. George Morgan, *The True Patrick Henry*, Philadelphia, 1907, p. 305. See also William Wirt Henry, *Patrick Henry*, New York, 1891, 3 vols.
3. A baccalaureate degree was not a prerequisite for admission to medical colleges of that era. One wonders why he did not enroll at the University of Virginia's medical college.
4. E.F. Cordell, *Historical Sketch of the University of Maryland School of Medicine, 1807-1890*, Baltimore, 1891, p. 179.
5. U.S. Census, 1860, Gadsden County, Florida. Here Dr. Henry's occupation is listed as farming. His property was valued at $32,000; his slaves numbered 13.
6. *Proceedings, Grand Lodge of Florida, 1860-66*, Tallahassee, 1860-66, Tallahassee, 1866, pp. 408, 450.
7. Tampa *Florida Peninsular*, April 28, 1860.
8. *Florida Historical Quarterly*, V, No. 2, October 1926, p. 118.
9. NA, Service Records, CSA, M 251, Roll 38. Incomplete record.
10. *House Journal, State of Florida*, 12th Session, 1863, Entry for November 16, pp. 22, 54-55.
11. Miles K. Womack, *Gadsden, A Florida County in Word and Picture*, place of publication unknown, 1976, pp. 75-76.
12. William Wirt Henry, *Patrick Henry*, II, 638.
13. No trace of offspring of this union has been discovered.

Hentz, Charles Arnould, Jackson, Gadsden, and Brevard Counties, 1827-1894

Dr. Hentz was born in Chapel Hill, North Carolina, on May 28, 1827, son of Nicholas Marcellus Hentz, a French émigré, who was expelled from France because of his revolutionary activities. With the return of the Bourbon dynasty to the throne in 1814 he eventually sought refuge in America, arriving in New York on March 12, 1816. Nicholas Hentz appears to have been a restless, impatient man, seldom settling in any one place for long. His American peregrinations began in Berwick, Pennsylvania, a town on the Susquehanna River some 25 miles from Wilkes-Barre. By 1824 he had moved to Massachusetts, finding employment as a teacher in the Round Hill School in Northampton. On September 30, 1824, he was married to Caroline Lee Whiting[1] of Lancaster, Massachusetts. Their first child, Marcellus Fabius, was born in Northampton on September 6, 1825.

In the fall of 1826 the Hentz family moved to Chapel Hill, North Carolina, where Marcellus had been appointed Professor of Modern Languages in the state university. Charles Arnould was born in Chapel Hill, where the older son died only two months later. Some 65 years later Charles Arnould noted in his diary that "the College is still flourishing."

From Chapel Hill the Hentzes removed to Covington, Kentucky, where they remained for about two years before moving across the Ohio River to Cincinnati. On reflection it would probably have served their interests best if they had remained there. They had become a part of a stimulating literary group headed by the renowned physician, Dr. Daniel Drake. Marcellus Hentz had a position as teacher of Romance languages in a school for girls. Wanderlust overcame his better judgment, however, and lured him on to Alabama for brief sojourns in Florence and Tuscaloosa where he remained in the teaching profession.

During their residence in Tuscaloosa the Hentzes were favored by a visit from Dr. Drake. While there he was much in the company of young Charles in whom he detected an aptitude for learning. Before his departure he urged the youngster to consider seriously the study of medicine. Heeding Dr. Drake's advice Charles became an apprentice to the eminent Tuscaloosa physician, Reuben Searcy, in 1843. He later recalled that he had found Eberle's Therapeutics "dry and dull," and Bell's Anatomy "equally so."

In the meantime Hentz enrolled in a preparatory school in Tuscaloosa, run by Professors Foster and Teague, where he spent time in the study of Greek and Latin. He then enrolled at the University of Alabama where he remained for two terms.

It was soon time for another move, so after a brief stay in Mobile the family moved on to Montgomery where the elder Hentz bought an interest in a military school on the outskirts of Tuskegee. There young Charles enrolled and began the study of French and history. He soon found this tiresome, however, and made his way back to Montgomery where he was cordially received by Dr. Searcy, under whom he resumed his medical studies.

Hentz was ready for medical school by 1846 and he chose the Medical Department of the University of Louisville, doubtless because Dr. Drake, his "mentor and father figure" was there as Professor of Medical Practice. He began his formal medical study in early November 1846 under the watchful eye of Dr. Drake. He later remembered the other professors as being "pleasant and competent" but the inspiration was without question derived from Dr. Drake.

Hentz found his two terms at Louisville stimulating, even exciting; his progress was not. He was practically penniless and found it necessary to work at various jobs and live in comparative privation. Still there appears to have been time for other activities, social and cultural. His recollections of these were often amusing, sometimes touching.

At the end of term in February 1847, Hentz faced a dilemma. He knew that his father could not help him with college fees. Without some financial support he could not meet the college expenses and pay for room and board. He would, therefore, go to Florida where a medical degree was not a requisite for obtaining a license and begin practice. He was about to leave for Marianna, where his brother-in-law, Dr. John W. Keyes, husband of his sister, Julia, was practicing dentistry, when Dr. Drake intervened and he was offered a position as Curator of the College's Museum and almost simultaneously the office of Librarian. His continuation was assured. He wrote: "I joyfully changed my plans...Father sent me $25." In late February 1848, he was graduated Doctor of Medicine.

In the fall of 1848 Dr. Hentz settled at a village on the west bank of the Chattahoochee River, just north of its confluence with the Flint River. It was a dismal location. He had been warned by Dr. Nicholas Long who was practicing in Greenwood north of Marianna. Dr. Long was of the opinion that "medicine was humbug," intimating that only starvation awaited him in Port Jackson. Dr. Hentz was not dissuaded. He heard that a Dr. Caldwell was leaving his practice in Port Jackson and proceeding to Louisiana he located Dr. Caldwell, bought his medical supplies, and after a brief visit to Marianna returned to Port Jackson, arriving there on December 4, 1848. On December 10 he made his first professional call.

At Port Jackson his clients were predominantly tough, hard-drinking, uncouth types, victims of family feuds and drunken brawls. After a few months Dr. Hentz abandoned the wretched place, sold his horse and stock of medicines and instruments at a ridiculously low price, and returned to Marianna, residing briefly in the home of Dr. Keyes before deciding to return to Cincinnati.

On arriving there after a series of mishaps such as losing all his money, he went directly to Dr. Drake who employed him to assist in editing the manuscript of his "On the Diseases of the Mississippi Valley" and getting it through the press.[2] Dr. Hentz's assistance was duly acknowledged in the preface of the book. His meagre stipend from Dr. Drake was supplemented by teaching afternoon classes at a local school for $2.50 per week.

Discouraged and forlorn, Dr. Hentz joined a young medical graduate, Dr. Caroland, in a partnership in Cincinnati in an office located at No. 87 Broadway. Their practice was fairly good but of short duration. On receiving word of his father's failing health, Dr. Hentz departed Cincinnati in the spring of 1851 and returned by a circuitous route to Marianna.

Once more in Marianna, Dr. Hentz's future seemed brighter. Dr. Keyes was enjoying a successful practice and had inherited a plantation while his brother Thaddeus had joined Dr. Keyes in the practice of dentistry. Dr. Hentz was much in the company of Marianna's aristocracy, one member of which was Miss Elizabeth (Bettie) Booth, daughter of Dr. William Booth, the leading physician of Quincy.

Meanwhile Dr. Hentz, always restless and generally dissatisfied, decided to begin his practice in Ochesee, a village on the Apalachicola River in the southwest corner of Jackson County. It was a favorable location which allowed him to practice on both sides of the river, in Gadsden as well as Jackson County. He soon gained a number of clients among whom was Jason Gregory at whose plantation home he obtained board and lodging for $15 per month, "$8 for me and $7 for my horse." He had been able to buy the horse for $25.

On April 5, 1854, Dr. Hentz was married to Bettie Booth in an elegant wedding at the Booth home in Quincy. This marriage brought Dr. Hentz into kinship with the wealthy Coe family, Mrs. Booth having been the daughter of the Reverend Jesse Coe, one of antebellum Florida's wealthiest men.

Although his medical career was on solid footing and his social position secure, Dr. Hentz moved to Quincy in 1858. There he enjoyed the good life. Even the rigors of the Civil War did not seem to have depressed him. His brother Thaddeus, a practicing dentist in Marianna, wrote: "He is a happy fellow, always full of life, imparting gladness wherever he goes; whether he is really so much delighted with everything, I don't know."

Dr. Hentz was 34 years of age at the outbreak of the Civil War but he was never actually inducted into military service. It is assumed that he was considered useful on the home front. The existence of five small children was possibly the explanation for his having avoided actual military service. He was, however, a member of the Gadsden County Board of Military Examiners, sharing its responsibility with Drs. David S. Telfair and Charles A. Gee,[3] the latter of whom saw service on the battlefront. At the end of the War, Dr. Hentz included in a letter to his cousin, Paul Willard, the following statement:[4]

> The War ended without my having been compelled to enter military service—being over thirty-five years old and having been in the practice of my profession over fifteen years, the conscription never touched me. I have fortunately been allowed to stay with my family and continue my business. I had to enter the militia service of the State, obtained a surgeon's situation, and was present at the Battle of Natural Bridge[5] of which I have a trophy in the shape of a large fragment of shell which fell within a few inches of my feet.

The rigors of Reconstruction thrust Dr. Hentz into reduced circumstances. He was barely able to provide for his ever-increasing family. In 1870 the estimated value of his property was only $4,000. In his household at that time were his wife and four children, his sister-in-law, Sarah Booth, and two orphaned grandchildren.

Notwithstanding Dr. Hentz's superior medical education and better than average intellect there is no indication that he ever took more than a passive interest in improving the quality of medical practice and the standards for certification of physicians practicing in Florida. At its third annual meeting, held in Tallahassee in January 1876, he was elected to membership in the Florida Medical Association and was chosen to give the oration at the meeting in Jacksonville in April 1877. Although his signature appeared on the report of the Committee on Fees which was presented at the 1877 meeting, he was not present having resigned from the organization prior to its meeting. The oration was delivered by Dr. Thomas M. Palmer of Monticello instead. No reason for his withdrawal from the group has been discovered.

By 1880 Dr. Hentz was once more exhibiting signs of restlessness. Upon learning that land areas along the Manatee River were open for purchase he explored the possibility of leaving Quincy and taking a chance in a new region. He was able, however, to resist the lure of the Manatee, but on March 7, 1880, his father-in-law, in this instance, Thomas Munroe, of Quincy, joined him on a tour of inspection of the Indian River area of Florida's east coast. Dr. Hentz was favorably taken with the prospects of making a good living there and proceeded to purchase a hundred acres or more on the west bank of the river in the vicinity of

City Point. On returning to Quincy in preparation for the move he advertised his practice and equipment for sale. No doctor was willing to meet his price, which prompted him to remark: "I came to the conclusion that the doctors are a poor lot."

In spite of the difficulties of leaving Quincy (he retained possession of his home there), he made the move, chartering a box car to take his belongings to Jacksonville and thence by boat to Rockledge. He also purchased in Jacksonville the materials for constructing a house in his new location. He had the foresight to purchase a mule in Quincy. To further complicate matters, on January 25, 1881, a daughter, Jessie, was born. On September 22, 1881, Dr. Hentz wrote: "We left our dear old Quincy House...took the afternoon train to Jacksonville...thence to Indian River."

On arrival at their new home site the Hentz family camped out for several weeks while their house was being built. When the carpentry was finally finished Dr. Hentz and his wife painted the interior themselves.

At last, good fortune had smiled on the Hentz endeavors. Their land proved to be fertile and well-drained, well suited to citrus culture as well as truck-farming. Henceforth until the end of his life Dr. Hentz lived in comfort and comparative affluence at City Point. At some juncture, the exact time unknown, Dr. and Mrs. Hentz returned to their Quincy home. The Titusville *Florida Star*, the principal newspaper in the Indian River area, in its issue of February 10, 1893, announced: Dr. and Mrs. C.A. Hentz, of Quincy, Fla., and their son, Dr. W.B. (Willie) Hentz, of Rio de Janeiro, reached this place Thursday night. They have about 2000 boxes of oranges in their grove and will be here until the shipping season is over. Mrs. W.B. Hentz is shopping a few weeks in New York City before joining them.

Finally, on April 14, 1893, the Titusville paper published the following: "Dr. and Mrs. C.A. Hentz returned to their home in Quincy, Wednesday, April 12th." Dr. Hentz died in Quincy on June 30, 1894, and was buried in Quincy's Eastern Cemetery. His wife, Cornelia, had died less than two months earlier, on May 14th.

It is a perplexing task to account for the numerous children born to Dr. Hentz and his two wives. In the case of the first Mrs. Hentz, who died September 20, 1871, after giving birth prematurely to a child who died within a matter of hours (she had been delivered of a stillborn baby within the previous year, an ordeal which had nearly cost her life) she was survived by three daughters, Sallie, Julia and Rebecca, and a son, William who became a physician and emigrated to Rio de Janeiro, Brazil. By the second, Cornelia Fitzgerald Munroe, there were Charles, Alice, Cornelia, Robina, Jessie (daughter), Harry, and finally, John Whiting, born July 21, 1885.[5]

1. Caroline Whiting Hentz, far better known than her husband, gained national recognition as the author of numerous romantic novels and short stories. A native of Lancaster, Massachusetts, she had met her husband when he was a teacher at the Round Hill School in Northampton, Mass. For her play, *De Lara or the Moorish Bride* she won a $500 prize offered by William Pelby, the Boston actor. For further information see *Dictionary of National Biography*, Vol. VIII, pp. 565-66.

2. The book, which was published in 1850, bore the title, *A Systemic Treatise, Historical, Etiological, and Practical, on the Principal Diseases of the Interior Valley of North America, as they Appear in the Caucasian, Indian, and Esquimaux Varieties of Its Population*, Cincinnati, Winthrop B. Smith and Co., 1850, 878 pp.

3. Dr. Gee had been a zealous secessionist, volunteering for military service in 1861. He resigned his military

commission for reasons of failing health in April 1862. NA, Service Records, CSA, M 251, Roll 54.

4. An excerpt from Dr. Hentz's letter dated June 17, 1865. P.K. Yonge Library of Florida History, University of Florida. MSS. Box 51.

5. In his "Autobiography" Dr. Hentz made random entries of dates of births, deaths, and other events relating to his family. For the present purposes these have been verified and augmented by reference to the census schedules of 1860, 1870, 1880 and the Special Florida Census of 1885. In the last of these (1885) compiled only about three years after Dr. Hentz settled in Brevard County, his land was assessed at $10,000. He owned 100 acres, of which 20 acres had been planted in orange groves with only an acre devoted to vegetable crops. It is a matter of interest that the county mortality schedule for that year indicates that Dr. Hentz had attended only one of the deceased persons. See Special Census, Brevard County, Florida, 1885, p. 320, item 11.

Note: This sketch is a mere condensation of Dr. Hentz's voluminous autobiography. The original manuscript exists in the Southern Historical Collection, University of North Carolina, Chapel Hill, Library. It has been laboriously transcribed—Dr. Hentz's hand posed some problems for the transcriber—and a typescript has been used in the preparation of the present sketch. The typescript exists in the collection of the P.K. Yonge Library of Florida History, University of Florida, Gainesville. Annotations have been added only in instances in which a clarification of the original text seems necessary, or when data not included in the original are deemed important. The transcript, it would be added, is divided into two parts; the total pages number 807.

Herndon, John R., Columbia County, 1860

Dr. Herndon, a native of North Carolina, was living in the home of his son, Charles S. Herndon, in Columbia County in 1860. The census that year indicates that the family had only recently arrived in Florida. Dr. Herndon was 60 years of age. It is doubtful that he was ever an active practitioner in Florida.[1]

1. U.S. Census, 1860, Columbia County, Florida, p. 219.

Herron, James Solar, Pensacola, 1834-1915

Dr. Herron, military surgeon and for almost half a century a practitioner in Escambia County, was representative of the most enlightened element of 19th century Florida physicians. Well-educated, intelligent and compassionate, he enjoyed the love and respect of hundreds of patients whom he served during his lengthy professional career. He was born in Chambersburg, Pennsylvania, on November 30, 1834, son of James and Irish-born Fannie Marie (nee Byrne) Herron.[1] Both his grandfather, James Herron, and his father, also named James, were civil engineers, the latter having been assigned to supervise construction work at the Pensacola naval base when his son, James Solar, was still a youth.

After receiving basic education in Pensacola schools, young Herron attended Spring Hill College in Alabama from which he received a baccalaureate degree. In the fall of 1859 he entered the University of Pennsylvania School of Medicine and received the medical degree in the spring of 1861.[2] Immediately thereafter he returned to Pensacola and began medical practice. His services were apparently much in demand at the nearby Navy Yard.[3]

Dr. Herron entered the Medical Department of the Confederate Army on November 25, 1861, with the rank of Assistant Surgeon and was immediately assigned to the headquarters hospital near the Navy Yard. In early 1862 he was transferred to the General Hospital in Pensacola where he remained for about a year before being assigned to the General Hospital in Montgomery, Alabama.[4] He was still in service there at the time of promotion to the rank of Surgeon in August 1864. In a matter of days on August 29, 1864,[5] however, he was ordered to field duty with the army of General Braxton Bragg in Tennessee,[6] where he remained until surrender of the Confederate troops the following April. His detainment as a prisoner-of-war was of brief duration, parole being granted on June 10, 1865. His parole papers described him as: "Surgeon, CSA, five feet, eight inches tall; light hair; blue eyes; and light complexion."[7]

Following parole Dr. Herron chose to remain for a few months in Montgomery where he resumed civilian practice. During this period he received numerous official permits allowing him to move freely in and out of military encampments in carrying on his professional practice. It appears that he remained in Montgomery until some time in 1866 when he moved to Milton,[8] some 20 miles from Pensacola. By mid-1868, however, he was once more established in Escambia County, settling briefly in Warrington[9] before returning to Pensacola where he would live out his life.

Soon after settling in Pensacola Dr. Herron entered into partnership with his brother, Dr. Charles R. Herron, later to practice in Savannah, Georgia. Their professional card indicated their location "on the Bay, at the foot of Herron's Wharf." They made a special appeal for clients among the seamen frequenting Pensacola's harbor as well as ailing military personnel. They offered to treat their patients either at the Marine and General Hospital or at their offices, specifying that Dr. Charles R. would, "if desired, also attend on shipboard."[10]

The partnership was dissolved a few years later when the younger member, Charles, moved to Savannah. In 1873 Dr. Herron purchased the historic site of the old Panton, Leslie & Co. from the heirs of John Inneranity for $7000 and converted what had been the dwelling house into a Marine and General Hospital.[11]

There is abundant evidence that Dr. Herron applied himself unstintingly, even enthusiastically, to his medical practice. Unencumbered by family responsibilities, he was never married, he devoted much of his energy to the care of patients and study of their ailments. A discerning pathologist he developed a deep interest in epidemiology, especially as related to smallpox and yellow fever in which he was generally regarded an expert whose opinions were sought by his fellow physicians. In the local epidemic of 1873 he was appointed acting assistant surgeon at the Pensacola Navy Yard, an appointment which was repeated two years later when he was called to attend Surgeon George M. Sternberg who later became Surgeon-General of the U.S. Army.[12]

Among the growing number of physicians in Pensacola Dr. Herron was a highly-regarded leader.[13] He was twice president of the Pensacola Medical Society and for several terms served as its vice president. In 1891, even though isolated from the mainstream of Florida medicine, he became a member of the Florida Medical Association.

Dr. Herron died at his home, 519 Palafox Street, on February 20, 1915, after an illness of a few weeks. Funeral services were held at St. Michael's Catholic Church after which he was buried in St. Michael's Cemetery.[14] His closest survivors were his only sister, Fannie, unmarried, and his brother, Charles, the Savannah physician.

1. The greater part of these biographical details derive from a lengthy obituary notice in the Pensacola *Journal* of February 21, 1915, and a bundle of Herron papers, uncatalogued, deposited in Manuscripts Section, P.K. Yonge Library of Florida History, University of Florida, Gainesville. References to the former will be cited only as "Obit" and to the latter only as "Herron Papers."

2. Archives, University of Pennsylvania, Lists of Graduates, shows that Dr. Herron's preceptor in medicine had been his cousin, Dr. G.R.B. Horner, U.S. Navy.

3. Herron Papers. Included is a permit, dated March 15, 1861, signed by Acting Inspector General James E. Slaughter, giving Dr. Herron permission to visit the Navy Yard near Pensacola.
4. Obit.
5. Herron Papers. Included is a list of medicines, instruments, and other medical supplies issued to Dr. Herron by Surgeon John F. Young, Medical Purveyor in Atlanta, dated June 1, 1864.
6. Ibid. Special Order of August 29, 1864, ordering Dr. Herron to "report without delay" to Medical Director Foard, Army of Tennessee, for assignment.
7. Ibid.
8. Ibid., Letter, T. Seymour, Savannah, to Dr. Herron, then in Milton.
9. Ibid., Receipt for $174 paid to Dr. Herron of Warrington by Joseph Saurez.
10. Ibid.
11. Elizabeth D. Vickers, "The Golden Gream," *Pensacola Historical Society Quarterly*, Vol. VII, No. 3, Spring 1974, p. 27.
12. Dr. Herron from time to time submitted reports to the Supervising Surgeon, U.S. Marine Hospital Service. Some of these were printed in the Annual Reports of that Agency. One relating to yellow fever was published in 1884. Government Printing Office, Washington, D.C. His report on "Yellow Fever at Barrancas in 1875" was also published. Copy in the P.K. Yonge Library of Florida History.
13. Obit.
14. Obit. Also St. Michael's Cemetery Survey.

Hester, William, Sumter County, 1825-1862

Dr. Hester's Florida career was brief. Born in North Carolina about 1825 he arrived in Florida in the mid-1850s and established a medical practice in or near the village of Adamsville, one of the earliest settlements in Sumter County. With emergence of Sumterville, about five miles southwest of Adamsville, a year or so later he served that community as well. Dr. Hester first appeared in Florida records with the Census of 1860 for Sumter County in which he was listed as physician, aged 35, owning property, all personal, valued at $6,575. He was the sole resident of the household and was assigned the dual addresses, Sumterville and Adamsville.

Dr. Hester enlisted in the Confederate Army on November 9, 1861, joining Company I, First Florida Cavalry Regiment, a unit organized by William D. Clark of Gainesville and composed largely of recruits from Alachua County. He provided his own horse, valued at $150, with saddle and bridle valued at $25. On November 22, the Company assembled at Newnansville; Dr. Hester was 37 years of age.

Soon after joining his unit Dr. Hester was taken ill and for the early part of 1862 granted sick leave. Although able to return to active duty for much of the year, he apparently did not regain good health. Meanwhile, on July 16, 1862, the Confederate Congress passed a conscription act reestablishing the age limit for recruits. Given the condition of his health Dr. Hester was granted a discharge under provisions of the act on February 9, 1863.[2] From that point on nothing is known of Dr. Hester. He was not listed in the Florida Census of 1870 and it is assumed that he had either died or departed the state by that date.

1. U.S. Census, 1860, Sumter County, Florida, p. 822.
2. National Archives, Service Records, CSA, M251, Roll 2.

Hicks, James W., Orlando, 1827-1895

Dr. Hicks[1] was born in Granville County, North Carolina, on January 20, 1827, the only living child of Dr. John R. and Rebecca (Wood) Hicks. His father, born in England, had come to America in 1777 and joined American forces in the

American Revolution. James had the advantage of the best educational opportunities. He attended private preparatory schools, then matriculated at the University of North Carolina from which he was graduated in 1847. He enrolled in the Medical Department of the University of Virginia from which he received his medical degree in 1851.

Dr. Hicks returned to Granville County to begin medical practice. After a year he moved to Rome, Georgia, where he remained, except for time spent in the Confederate Army, until 1875. His military service, which included a stint as surgeon in the 54th North Carolina Regiment engaged in hospital service in Savannah, later took him into Tennessee as surgeon in the Georgia 57th Regiment, a post in which he spent a year.

While practicing in Rome, Dr. Hicks married Minerva Mitchell, daughter of Daniel Mitchell, and their family included 10 children, seven of whom lived to adulthood.[2]

At the annual session of the Florida Medical Association in Sanford in 1885, Dr. Hicks was elected to membership and simultaneously placed on the Committee on Ethics joining Drs. R.A. Lancaster of Gainesville and Columbus Drew of Jacksonville, hold-over members. In 1886 at the meeting of the Association in Palatka, Dr. Hicks as chairman of the Committee had the painful duty to report a fellow physician, Dr. W.P. Lawrence of Orlando, for having violated the Ethics code. At the meeting in St. Augustine in 1887, Dr. Hicks was elected president of the Association, over which he presided at Gainesville in 1888.[3]

In his presidential address, Dr. Hicks dealt at length with the various fevers endemic to the state, setting forth numerous measures, many of them common sense approaches to the problem, e.g., quarantine and sanitation, which he was convinced accounted in large measure for the death toll attributable to the diseases. He also called on the state legislature to enact measures designed to reduce the virulence of the fevers.

There can be no doubt that Dr. Hicks was highly respected in his home town of Orlando. At the time of his death in Orlando on January 14, 1895, the medical faculty of the town, composed of 13 physicians some of whom were from other parts of Orange County, met and drafted a resolution praising his splendid professional skills while offering condolences to the bereaved family. It is an exceptional document, a part of which deserves inclusion here:[4]

> Resolved: That the death of Dr. Hicks is a public calamity; that society has lost an ornament, and humanity a friend; that a wise physician and a philanthropist has been taken from us, a benefactor of the poor, a friend of all suffering humanity has finished his work and gone up higher; and further be it resolved: That his services to his country as surgeon and patriot were distinguished by that lofty bearing, and lofty devotion to duty, so eminently characteristic of his private life.
>
> While we, the medical profession, have lost an esteemed companion and friend, our loss is but slight as compared with the loss to his family, to whom he was indulgent to a fault; a loving husband, an affectionate, tender father. We extend to the family our sincere sympathy in this, their great bereavement.

1. A substantial part of this sketch is derived from *Biographical Souvenir of the States of Georgia and Florida*, Chicago, F.A. Battey & Co., 1899, p. 396. This source indicates that Dr. Hicks also served as a member of the Florida Medical Board of Examiners and the Orange County Board of Health. In addition he was Orlando City Physician for six years, also an Odd Fellow and a Mason.

2. Seven of the ten children living in 1899 were Mrs. Agnes M. Prince, Mrs. Irene R. Harrington, Mrs. Viola M. Hammond, Mrs. Emma V. Church, Olive A., Cora V., and Clarence J.

3. Numerous references to Dr. Hicks' participation in the affairs of the Florida Medical Association are found in the various issues of its *Proceedings* from 1886 until 1895.

4. Orlando *South Florida Sentinel*, January 18, 1895.

Hicks, William Matthew, Suwannee County, 1833-1901

As is so frequently true of the medical practitioners who chose to remain in rural Florida throughout their careers, only meager biographical data have been preserved. This is indeed true of Dr. Hicks, a North Carolina native who moved to Florida after the Civil War, settled in or near the village of Houstoun, and spent the rest of his life practicing among the people of Houstoun and Wellborn. He was born in July 1833[1] and since he does not appear in the lists of students attending any of the major medical schools of the South it is assumed that he obtained medical training through the apprenticeship system so common in antebellum days.

Dr. Hicks is known to have served in the Army of the Confederacy[2] but since he does not appear in the Civil War records of the State of Florida, it is assumed that he served with a North Carolina unit.

Dr. Hicks arrived in Suwannee County about 1869 or 1870 accompanied by his wife Anne, a native of Georgia. Within the year their first child, a daughter named Annie, was born. Their two younger children, a daughter Margaret and a son William M., Jr., were born in 1872 and 1879 respectively.[3]

Scattered evidence suggests that the Hicks family enjoyed a fair degree of prosperity. The 1870 Census shows them owning land valued at $3,500 and other property worth about $1,000 which, considering the depressed years of Reconstruction, would indicated a comfortable living. Besides, his home was free of mortgage.[4]

Cemetery records show that Dr. Hicks died at some unspecified date in 1901.[5] Indications are that he was a highly regarded physician and leading member of the Suwannee County Medical Society. As such in 1897 he joined the other 15 members in signing and publishing a statement that they would not continue to answer calls "from those who do not pay their doctor bills."[6]

1. U.S. Census, 1900, Suwannee County, Florida, Dist. 8, p. 122.
2. WPA, Veterans' Grave Registration Project, Suwannee County, p. 15.
3. Dr. Hicks, providing information for the census enumerator in 1900, indicated that he had been married for 38 years and that of the three children born to him and his wife one was deceased.
4. See note 1, supra.
5. See note 2, supra.
6. Live Oak *Suwannee Democrat*, November 20, 1897. This statement was signed by 16 physicians practicing in Suwannee County. It is indicated that all were members of the medical society.

Hill, B.A., Pensacola, 1871

Dr. Hill, a brief sojourner in Florida, entered medical practice in Pensacola in January 1871. His professional card, first appearing on January 20, announced that he had practiced his profession for 18 years, most recently in Montgomery, Alabama. He offered his services as a specialist in midwifery and diseases of women and children. He solicited "a liberal share of patronage" from the citizens of Pensacola. His office was located at the Drug Store of Henry Cushman while his residence was on Belmont Street.[1]

Since his office was taken over one year later by Dr. W.J. Mitchell it is assumed that Dr. Hill had moved to another locality.[2]

1. Pensacola *Commercial*, February 25, 1871; first printed on January 20 (issue not extant).
2. Pensacola *Mail*, January 30, 1872.

Hill, Henry B., Hamilton and Sumter Counties, 1860s, 1870s

Limited sources provide only fleeting glimpses of Dr. Hill, a native of Georgia, who appears to have moved to Hamilton County in the 1850s. The Census of 1860 identifies him as a physician of Jasper whose household included not only his wife, Louisa, and four-year-old son, Francis, born in Florida, but also four other Georgians, all adults. By the standards of the times he was fairly well off, owning property valued at about $7,000.[1]

Nothing is known of the whereabouts and activities of Dr. Hill during the course of the Civil War but in the 1870s he appears as a resident of Sumter County. In the summer of 1874, as political activity began to mount in preparation for the fall elections, his name was put forth as a candidate for the county's seat in the Florida Legislature. The Ocala newspaper offered its support, recalling the mediocre quality of Sumter's previous representatives and judging Dr. Hill to be an excellent choice.[2] Nothing came of it, however, either he chose not to run for office or local support was not forthcoming. Nothing further is known of him.

1. U.S. Census, 1860, Hamilton County, Florida, p. 2.
2. Ocala *East Florida Banner*, August 8, 1874.

Hill, James H., Lake City, 1820

The medical career of Dr. Hill was brief, spanning less than 20 years. A native of Georgia and a graduate of the Medical Department of the University of Georgia in Augusta in 1845,[1] he practiced in Georgia for a few years prior to moving to Columbia County in the early 1850s. Upon arrival there he appears to have purchased land outside Lake City which he farmed with the labor of his 15 slaves[2] while maintaining a residence in the town and continuing his medical practice. By the year 1860 his household included his wife and six children, the younger three, Joseph, John and Martha, ages eight, six and three, respectively, having been born in Columbia County. The Hills were a family of moderate means, their properties having been valued at $15,000 in 1860.[3]

Soon after outbreak of the Civil War, the 3rd Regiment of Florida Volunteers, Infantry, was organized. It was formally commissioned in July 1861 and included two companies, I and K, made up principally of Columbia County enlistees. On August 10, 1861, Dr. Hill was named Regimental Surgeon and mustered in with other members of the Regiment on Amelia Island. Slightly more than two and a half months later, on October 25, his career took a strange turn when he faced a court-martial. Whatever his offense or indiscretion, it must have been of small consequence in that he was not dismissed from the service, but instead reduced in rank to assistant surgeon. His new contract, negotiated late in 1861, stipulated a monthly pay rate of $80. While awaiting outcome of the court-martial he continued on duty with the Regiment.[4]

In early November Dr. A.H. Mathers, also a Confederate assistant surgeon, visited the headquarters of the 3rd Regiment where he met Dr. Hill. Dr. Mathers was also a graduate of the Augusta school. On November 4 he wrote to his wife in Micanopy: "Nothing worthy of your attention transpired on my trip to Fernandina. I was invited by Dr. Hill to go around with him which I accepted and spent a very pleasant time meating (sic) old friends and class mates."[5]

Having been reinstated and awarded a new contract, Dr. Hill returned to duty sometime in December. On January 24, 1862, he abruptly submitted his resignation claiming pay for only the period January 1 through January 24. His formal statement read, in part: "My residence is Lake City, Florida, and my removal from service was on the 24th of January, 1862. . .I am not indebted to the Confederate States on any account whatsoever."[6]

Beyond this date no information on Dr. Hill has been discovered. He does not appear in the Florida Census of 1870 although his wife and young children are listed. It seems likely that he had died by that date.[7]

1. Medical Department, University of Georgia, *List of Graduates from 1829 to 1891*, Augusta 1891, p. 18.
2. Slave Schedule, Columbia County, Florida, 1860.
3. U.S. Census, 1860, Columbia County, Florida, p. 185.
4. NA, Service Records, CSA, M251, Roll 48. As for the incident of the court-martial, Dr. Hill's service record contains the following notation: "Special Order 63, Dept. of S.C., Ga., and Fla., Col. Dilworth, date Oct 25, 1861," to which is added the following: "This record contains information relative to the above named man upon the subject stated above." Since the charge was of such trivial nature as to result in reinstatement, no further inquiry into the matter has been made.
5. See F.A. Doty, ed., "The Civil War Letters of Augustus Henry Mathers, Assistant Surgeon, Fourth Florida Regiment, CSA," Florida Historical Quarterly, XXXVI, No. 2, October 1957, p. 98.
6. See note 4.
7. It seems probable that Dr. Hill was in poor health at the time of his army service and died soon after his resignation. As for the court-martial affair, it is quite likely that, having left a wife and six children at home in Lake City, he went back to visit them without the formality of a leave. These, however, are only speculations suggested by the context of the sources.

Hines, Whitson J., Madison County, 1812

Dr. Hines, a native of Georgia, probably Lowndes County, moved to Madison County about 1845. His family included his wife, Julia, and four sons, Whitson, Jr., James E., William and Charles.[1] They settled in the village of Clifton some 12 miles northwest of the town of Madison. Dr. Hines purchased a portion of land near the village and henceforth engaged in farming as well as medical practice. He appears to have prospered in both. His slaves numbered 11 in 1850 and increased to 34 by 1860, his real estate was valued at $8,000 while other properties were said to have been worth $24,000.[2]

As a resident of a remote part of the county Dr. Hines' activities were not often noted in the newspapers. One frightening experienced which nearly cost him his life, however, was reported to the Monticello *Family Friend* in a letter from Clifton resident, Thomas F. McCall. The gist was: Dr. Hines was returning to Clifton from Madison after dark on the evening of April 27, 1861, when at some point along the way he was fired upon from ambush by a would-be assassin. He suffered a painful injury which could easily have been fatal. McCall's letter was apparently written to counter the suspicion that he was guilty of the attack. Dr. Hines was said to have had some difficulty with two men of the community, the Hardee brothers. Since McCall had been a close friend of the two the rumor was spread that he had hired a man named Askew to commit the murder. McCall further stated that Dr. Hines had dealt unfairly with the Hardees and that he himself had ceased to use Dr. Hines as his family physician. In closing, he added that "Hines had a very extensive practice and traveled both night and day."[3]

Another event, recorded in the "Plantation Book" of Thomas J. Mays of

Madison County, casts further light upon Dr. Hines although it is by no means an indictment. In 1875-76, Mays was in debt to Dr. Hines in the amount of $350. He discussed the matter with him and concluded that the doctor had acted in a "sort of double-faced manner" to the extent that Mays considered taking the affair to court.[4] One gathers the impression that Dr. Hines did not hesitate to express his opinions, regardless of consequences.

Subsequent to the Mays altercation of 1875-76, nothing further is known of Dr. Hines and his family. Since he did not appear in the Madison County Census of 1880 it is assumed that he had left the county and possibly the state by that date.

In addition to the aforementioned children four others were born in Florida, Harrison, Julia Ann, Elizabeth and Rebecca. The second son, James E., listed as a medical student in the Census of 1860, had matriculated at Oglethorpe Medical College, Savannah, in the fall of 1859 and was the recipient of his medical degree on February 28, 1861.[5] At this commencement his father was awarded the M.D. degree ad eundem.

1. U.S. Census, 1850, Madison County, Florida, p. 188, item 239. Clifton enjoyed the convenience of its own post office in 1846, but soon lost it, only to be eclipsed by the neighboring village of Hamburgh which obtained a post office in 1851 and Cherry Lake where a post office had been established in 1840.
2. U.S. Census, 1860, Madison County, Florida, item 403.
3. Monticello *Family Friend*, May 4, 1861.
4. Terry B. Ziegler, "A Madison County Plantation, 1865-1900." Typed ms. in P.K. Yonge Library of Florida History, University of Florida, 1943-44. See entry of September 24, 1876.
5. Savannah *Daily Morning News*, March 1, 1861.

Hodges, Andrew Elton, Levy County, 1829-1885

That portion of Florida's Gulf Coast between the Suwannee and Withlacoochee Rivers was slow to attract settlers. Only Cedar Key, which had assumed some importance during the Second Seminole War, had emerged as a settlement of consequence. The area, dotted with small islands and cut through with numerous creeks and rivulets, did not invite settlers. In 1854, however, a tough intrepid Georgian of adventurous spirit, Andrew Elton Hodges, explored the Withlacoochee and after some prospecting purchased extensive acreage on the north side of the river, obtaining much of it for as little as 25 cents per acre. His holding extended from the Gulf of Mexico eastward about half way to the town of Dunellon. On a hammock where the present nuclear power plant is situated he built his first Florida home.[1]

Dr. Hodges was born in Dooly County, Georgia, in 1829, the eldest child of Elbert and Selena Hodges, rural people of modest means.[2] After attending local schools and probably reading medicine under a local physician he entered the Medical College of the State of South Carolina, Charleston, where he remained for a term.[3] He returned to Georgia, obtained a license to practice and began his professional career.[4]

A short time later, for reasons not altogether clear, Dr. Hodges went to Waco, Texas, where he met and married Nancy Pinkney Johnson, a young woman 10 years his junior, daughter of a pioneer family of considerable wealth.[5] The Johnsons, who were among the first settlers of Waco, had previously lived in Union Springs (Bullock County), Alabama.

Soon after arriving in Florida Dr. Hodges launched his first business enterprise, operation of a ferry service across the Withlacoochee at a point known as Blanche's Ferry, subsequently known as Hodges' Ferry. On the south side of the river was the plantation of the wealthy and influential David Levy, builder of the railroad linking Cedar Key with Fernandina. Levy and Dr. Hodges became friends,[6] an association which was doubtless mutually advantageous.

Meanwhile Dr. Hodges, with a sharp eye for business opportunity, continued to purchase other properties, especially land containing good growths of cedar and palmetto. From these he harvested lumber and logs for which he found a ready market extending from Florida to the Texas Coast. The cedar slabs were much in demand in Germany and elsewhere for the manufacture of pencils.[7] The principal firms were those of Eberhard, Eagle, and F.A. Wolfe. The palmetto logs were in demand for building wharves and piers along the entire Gulf Coast. From this venture Dr. Hodges reaped a fortune.

Realizing that his remote and modest home on the Withlacoochee was not conveniently situated for the supervision of his developing business interests, Dr. Hodges built a new residence on Hickory Island a short distance north of the mouth of the Withlacoochee facing the open waters of the Gulf.[8] From this vantage point he was able to manage the shipments of timber floated down the river and shipped to Cedar Key and other Gulf ports. Tapping some of his newly acquired wealth Dr. Hodges then proceeded to build a new residence, something more in keeping with his social position and suitable for his rapidly growing family. For this he chose a place five miles north of Hickory Island on the mainland and near the Gulf. There he built a "palatial residence, containing fifteen rooms, outhouses, a well of good water, and a large cistern" surrounded by 500 acres of "choice land," of which 100 acres were under cultivation.[9]

Meanwhile nearby Cedar Key was becoming a boom town. With prosperity and the newly completed railway, the final link having been completed on March 1, 1861, it assumed strategic military importance becoming a prime target as the Civil War began. Dr. Hodges was immediately involved.[10] He was instrumental in organizing a company of militia, becoming its commanding officer.[11] His role in the defense of Cedar Key was a minor one, however, for with seizure of the port city by a Union naval force in January 1862 and subsequent destruction of the railroad, there was little a small militia company could do. Nevertheless Dr. Hodges remained a nuisance to the occupying Union officers and was eventually arrested and jailed after being deprived of his shoes. At the conclusion of the war he was taken to the mouth of the Withlacoochee and released, still without shoes, left to walk the 12 miles through marshes and palmetto thickets to his home.[12]

Although Dr. Hodges retained possession of his Hickory Island and Magnolia property until his death, he appears to have spent the greater part of his postwar years in Cedar Key, the shipping base of his commercial enterprises. As for the practice of medicine, there is little evidence that, subsequent to his settlement in Florida, it was more than a secondary occupation. His medical services were certainly sought from time to time but they were not basis for a livelihood.

Eleven children were born to Dr. and Mrs. Hodges.[13] The eldest, Leo Antonio de Lopez, named for a Texas business partner of Dr. Hodges, Romulus, who died at the age of eight from eating poisonous fruit,[14] and a daughter, Alpine Scott, were born at the Hodges Ferry home. Hickory Island was the birthplace of Yulee, namesake of David Levy Yulee; twin daughters, Leona and Florence; Culpepper Johnson,[15] William Randolph,[16] Jules Comear, Texas Ruff,[17] and May Hortense. Dr. Hodges placed a high value on education, employing private tutors to teach the children until they were of an age to enter an academy or college. Of these children the best known were William Randolph, who ran a successful seafood business in Cedar Key for several years, and Texas Ruff, who edited a newspaper, the *Cedar Key Gulf-Coaster*[18] around the turn of the century and later became the Florida Shell Fish Commissioner. The eldest son, Leo, was a successful steamboat captain, serving for several years aboard the famous Belle of Suwannee.

Dr. Hodges died in early 1885 and was buried in the family cemetery on Hickory Island, beside his son Romulus (1858-66) and daughter, Florence (1864-1880).

1. A few decades ago D.B. McKay, Tampa journalist, published a lengthy biographical sketch of Dr. Hodges written by his youngest son, Texas Ruff. This sketch, somewhat romanticized, is a valuable source not only for the life of Dr. Hodges but also for the early history of Cedar Key and its vicinity. See Tampa *Tribune*, February 21, 1954.
2. U.S. Census, 1850, Dooly County, Georgia, p. 242, item 203.
3. Rowland H. Rerick, *Memoirs of Florida*, Atlanta, Southern Historical Association, 1902, II, 566.
4. In many states, including Florida, licenses to practice medicine could be obtained from a county judge upon the recommendation of a practicing physician.
5. The chronology of Dr. Hodges' early years remains vague. He had probably made trips to Texas prior to attending medical school. Miss Johnson was identified as his "boyhood sweetheart."
6. The brilliant career of David Levy Yulee is well documented. After the rift with his father brought about by his marriage to a non-Jewish woman, David Levy changed his surname to Yulee. The lands of Hodges were separated from those of Yulee by the Withlacoochee River.
7. The early prosperity of Cedar Key relates in large measure to the pencil industry.
8. The Hickory Island house, owned by Mr. and Mrs. Dewey D. Allen of Inglis, Florida, has been restored with care so as to preserve its original character. The larger and more pretentious home, Magnolia, was burned several years ago.
9. *Levy Enterprise*, February 23, 1883.
10. Dr. Hodges enlisted as a private in the Coast Guard Company of Capt. James L. Miller of Crystal River. The unit was organized on May 27, 1861, and disbanded on August 21, 1861. See *Soldiers of Florida*, Tallahassee, 1903, p. 57.
11. See note 1, supra.
12. Ibid.
13. Ibid.
14. Hampton Dunn, *A History of Citrus County, Florida*, Clearwater, p. 31.
15. Following the death of his father Culpepper bought the shares of his brothers and sisters in the Hickory Island property and lived there until his death in 1940. He was buried in the family cemetery on the Island. See Tampa *Tribune*, October 10, 1966, for feature article by Claire Slean.
16. William Randolph Hodges became a successful seafood merchant in Cedar Key.
17. Texas Ruff Hodges was an honorable Florida Shell Fish Commissioner who sought to curb destructive and illegal practices of some of Florida's coastal fishermen, thus incurring their wrath. In his 1917 campaign for the governorship of Florida, Sidney Catts exploited this situation to the limit, vowing that, if elected, he would "rid the State of this man." It was a scurrilous campaign with Catts capitalizing on the ignorances and prejudices of many Florida voters. He won the election and soon carried out his threat to oust Hodges from office. See Wayne Flynt, *Cracker Messiah: Governor Sidney J. Catts*, Baton Rouge, Louisiana State University Press, 1977, pp. 45, 58, 110.
18. A few issues of this paper are extant.

Hodges, Matthew W., Hamilton County, 1837-post 1900

Dr. Hodges was born in Georgia in November 1837.[1] He attended the Medical Department, University of Georgia, Augusta, from which he was graduated Doctor of Medicine in 1860.[2] Soon after graduation he settled in Jasper, Hamilton County, residing for a while in the home of his brother, a young Jasper merchant.[3] In 1862 he enlisted in the Army of the Confederacy as a private in Company B, Fifth Florida Infantry Regiment, reporting for duty at Lake City.[4]

Very soon after enlistment the Regiment was ordered to the Virginia war zone, setting up its headquarters near Petersburg. On July 23, 1862, Dr. Hodges was detailed to the regimental hospital as steward and there he remained until the end of the War. His name continued to appear on the roster of Company B with the repeated explanation that he was to be paid at the rate prescribed for his assignment. There is no explanation, however, for the fact that he was never raised to the rank of assistant surgeon.

On the eve of General Lee's surrender at Appomattox the main contingent of the Fifth Florida Regiment was captured at Farmville, Virginia, the actual date being April 6, 1865. Dr. Hodges soon found himself a prisoner of war at Newport News but his imprisonment was of brief duration. His army file contains this description of the man: light-complexioned, light-haired, blue-eyed, and five feet nine inches tall.

Upon his release Dr. Hodges returned to Florida and resumed medical practice. Soon thereafter he took as his wife Georgia-born Florida,[5] five years his junior and settled down to practice in White Springs on the Suwannee River, a place destined to become a popular resort during the latter part of the 19th century. He appears to have been a successful practitioner. The date of his death has not been discovered but he was practicing medicine in White Springs in 1900. The census of that year lists him as homeowner, aged 63.

Children born to Dr. and Mrs. Hodges were a daughter, Annie,[6] and two sons, Bryant and Pliny. The daughter was married in 1890 to B.F. Bullock of Georgia. Their two children, Bryant and Thelma, were born in Georgia but were members of the Hodges household in 1900.

1. The Census for Hamilton County, 1900, gives the date of Dr. Hodges' birth as November 1837 and that of Mrs. Hodges as April 1842. See Census, sheet 19, item 39. The Census of 1880, Hamilton County, Florida, lists Mrs. Elizabeth Sheffield, aged 76, as a member of the Hodges household. She is identified as "mother-in-law."

2. *Medical Department, University of Georgia, Lists of Graduates, 1829-91,* August 1891, p. 19.

3. Details of Dr. Hodges' military service may be found in National Archives, M251, Reel 63.

4. A recruitment center had been established at Lake City. The main strength of the Fifth Regiment was recruited from that area of the state.

5. U.S. Census, 1880, Hamilton County, Florida, p. 11.

6. The name of the Hodges daughter is not clear. She is designated as Annie and Emma, depending upon the year of the census.

Holbrook, Moses, St. Lucie County, 1783-1844

Dr. Holbrook, a physician of distinction although somewhat eccentric, spent only the last 18 months of his life in Florida, but he made a vivid impression on those who were privileged to have made his acquaintance. Born in Sherborn, Massachusetts,[1] on September 6, 1783, he was one of 10 children of James and Milla Holbrook, his father having been a blacksmith. His remarkable intellect, however, lifted him far above his commonplace background.

Dr. Holbrook matriculated at Harvard University in the fall of 1804 and was graduated Bachelor of Arts in 1808. Some three years later he was graduated Doctor of Medicine after which he practiced for a few years in Sherborn. Harvard records show that he returned to earn a Master of Arts degree in 1829.

In 1819 and 1820 fate dealt Dr. Holbrook a series of dreadful blows when, within a few months, death claimed his wife, sister-in-law and two infant sons, all victims of fevers. Left with two small daughters who required constant care he remarried before the end of 1820. To compound his sorrow the first child of this marriage also died, her death coming in August 1821.

Following these misfortunes Dr. Holbrook turned more avidly than ever to medical practice. Perhaps of more importance to his general well-being was the fellowship provided by membership in Freemasonry in which he rose to the position of Grand Secretary of the Grand Lodge, rising eventually to the elevated rank of Sovereign Grand Commander. He held this position in the period when the "Anti-Masonic Excitement" was gaining substantial support through the country. Apparently the antagonism was less severe in South Carolina than in other parts of the country.

In early 1843, after having practiced medicine in Charleston for more than 20 years, Dr. Holbrook, at age 59, left Charleston for Florida. He took advantage of the United States Armed Occupation Act of August 4, 1842, to obtain a tract of land on the west side of St. Lucie Sound, near the present town of Ankona, some seven miles south of Ft. Pierce.

Robert Ranson of St. Augustine, in a slender pamphlet setting forth some of his recollections of Captain Miles Olcott Burnham, a Florida pioneer, recalled:

> Next to Captain Burnham, on the South, lived Dr. Holbrook, a very talented physician from Charleston, South Carolina, an aged man of powerful build, very bald, and always hatless, who brought down his valuable library and acted as physician for the colony for two years, when he too died and filled an unmarked grave close to George Walker's on the beautiful Ankona bluff overlooking the Indian River.

Ranson continued:

> Below Captain Burnham lived, like a hermit of olden times, Dr. Holbrook, a learned physician of great skill and prominence in his profession while he lived in Charleston, S.C. He was in 1844 a very old man—actually he was only just past 60—but still tall, erect and powerful.

1. This biographical data is derived from two sources: Ray Baker Harris, "Dr. Moses Holbrook, M.D., 1783-1844," *The New Age*, Vol. 68, No. 2, pp. 15-18, and Robert Ranson, *A Memoir of Captain Mills Olcott Burnham, A Florida Pioneer*, St. Augustine, June 1926.

Holden, Julius Thomas, Marianna, 1834-1922

Dr. Holden, for many years an esteemed physician and diligent civic and religious leader in Marianna, was born in Wilmington, North Carolina, on February 23, 1834.[1] After gaining a basic and collegiate education in the schools of North Carolina and Maryland, he was enrolled at the Medical University of the City of New York (later to merge with Bellevue Hospital Medical College to become the University and Bellevue Hospital Medical College) from which he received his medical degree in 1855.[2]

A year or two after graduation Dr. Holden settled in Marianna where two of his uncles had settled earlier.[3] There he met Clara W. Roulhac, daughter of Jackson County Probate Judge Joseph B. Roulhac. They were married in 1860.[4] The census of that year shows that the young couple were living in the home of William E. Anderson whose wife, a sister of Mrs. Holden, had previously died leaving her husband with three small children.[5]

In April 1862, Dr. Holden entered the service of the Confederate Army as surgeon of the Sixth Regiment, Florida Infantry, commanded by Brigadier General Jesse J. Finley. Some years later his military career was succinctly summarized by Col. J.J. Dickison:[6]

> In August 1862, he was promoted to brigade surgeon with the rank of major, and he continued to serve in this capacity until the surrender of the army at Greensboro, N.C. (in April, 1865). In the course of his service he participated in all the campaigns of his regiment and brigade and was often under fire. At Resaca (Ga. Battle of, 13-16 May, 1864) he was five times shelled out of his hospital, and at Jonesboro (Ga. 31 Aug. 1-Sept. 1864) also he found himself in a perilous situation. Major Holden is gratefully remembered by the Florida soldiers of the Western Army as a warm friend and comrade as well as a skillful surgeon and physician.

It should be added that he had been present at the fierce encounter at Missionary Ridge and when the battle was finished he was sent behind enemy lines to treat the wounded soldiers.[7] On May 1, 1865, some three weeks after the Appomattox surrender, he was discharged at Greensboro.

Upon his return to Marianna Dr. Holden settled into the life of a small town doctor, endearing himself to the people of the community and participating in civic and religious affairs. From 1878 until his death on August 1, 1922, he was a warden of St. Luke's Episcopal Church.[8]

According to the Census of 1900, six children were born to Dr. and Mrs. Holden. Of these two did not survive infancy. The eldest, Clara R., 1867-1920, was married to George Farley, a Marianna merchant, in 1894 and a daughter, also named Clara, was born to that union. The second daughter, Eliza H., died prior to 1900; she is listed in the Census of 1880 as nine years of age. The third daughter, Louise, born in 1873, was still a member of the Holden household in 1900 while the youngest, Patty, born in 1877, was a school teacher in Marianna and living with her parents.

1. U.S. Census, 1900, Jackson County, Florida, p. 245, item 175.
2. J.J. Dickison, *Military History of Florida*, Atlanta, 1899, p. 278.
3. J. Randall Stanley, *History of Jackson County*, Marianna, 1950, p. 22.
4. See note 1, supra.
5. U.S. Census, 1860, Jackson County, Florida, item 932.
6. J.J. Dickison, loc. cit.
7. National Archives, Service Records, CSA, M251, Roll 71.
8. *Annual Journal, Diocese of Florida*, 1923, p. 38.

Holden, Thomas Leonard, Jackson County, 1830

Only a single reference establishes Dr. Holden as a resident of Jackson County about 1830. J. Randall Stanley identifies him as brother of Benjamin Holden, native of North Carolina, who settled in the Upper Chipola part of the county in the late 1820s. Benjamin, a farmer, was justice of the peace in the county in the 1830s. He played an important role in the early development of the area. Since Dr. Holden's name never appears in any Florida Census, it may be concluded that he was a brief sojourner in the Territory.[1]

1. J. Randall Stanley, *History of Jackson County*, Marianna, 1950, p. 22.

Holland, Griffin W., Leon County, 1806-1873

Dr. Holland was born in the Borough of Norfolk, Virginia, in 1806.[1] Nothing is known of his early education but it may be surmised that it was both proper and adequate. In 1825 he matriculated at the Medical College of the University of Maryland in Baltimore from which he received his degree in 1827.[2] Having been born into a family of considerable means he was able soon after graduation to move to Leon County and purchase a large tract of land north of Tallahassee which he developed into a well-organized plantation, operated and maintained with the help of 170 slaves.[3] His total wealth in 1860 was estimated at about $105,000, which certainly established him as one of the wealthiest men in Florida. Notwithstanding his medical education it is doubtful that he ever practiced beyond the borders of his own plantation. The censuses of 1850 and 1860 designated him only as "Planter."[4] At his plantation home, which he named "Minerva Hall," he established a school run by three governesses he had brought down from the North.[5]

The emancipation of slaves in combination with the disruptions of the Civil War dealt a disastrous blow to Dr. Holland and his family. Prior to 1870 he had given up his plantation and left Florida. No member of his family was listed in the Census of that year. He had apparently returned to Norfolk. In its issue of September 16, 1873, the Tallahassee *Weekly Floridian* printed the following notice: "Died at Norfolk, Virginia, Sept. 9, 1873, Dr. G.W. Holland, late of Florida, aged sixty-seven."

As for the Holland family, census data show that Mrs. Holland, whose Christian name was Margery, was a native of North Carolina. Their children numbered seven. The eldest, a son, N.L., was 17 years old in 1850. It is indicated that Mrs. Holland had married at age 15. In addition to the son there were six daughters in order of their birth: Laura, Margaret, Mary, Florence, Juliet and Nora.[6]

1. This date of birth from the date of his death in 1873 at age 67.
2. Archives, University of Maryland College of Medicine, List of Graduates.
3. Leon County, Florida, Slave Schedule, 1860.
4. Leon County, Florida, Census, 1850, p. 199; ibid., 1860, p. 70.
5. The plantation of Dr. Edward Bradford, known as Pine Hill, located a few miles north of Tallahassee, lay fairly close to the plantation of Dr. Holland. In her memoirs, Susan Bradford, daughter of Dr. Bradford and wife of Nicholas Ware Eppes, made frequent mention of the Holland family. She had attended the school at the Holland plantation and wondered "why all our teachers came from the North. They are all very pleasant and so are the three governesses Dr. Holland has had to teach at Minerva Hall since I have been going to school." Susan Bradford Eppes, *Through Some Eventful Years*, Facsimile Edition, Introduction and Index by Joseph D. Cushman Jr., Gainesville, 1968, p. 52. Later she mentions having spent Christmas Eve at Dr. Holland's, Ibid., p. 122. December 26, 1859. Later she mentioned that Dr. Holland, being a Methodist, did not permit dancing in his house..."But," she added, "we played games and had music, both vocal and instrumental, and everything good you could think of to eat." Ibid., p. 122. And finally, Mrs. Eppes mentioned the Holland Plantation, "Greenwood, where Dr. Holland lives with a house full of daughters."
6. No attempt has been made here to trace the lives of the Holland children. It is known, however, that on May 19, 1859, at the Holland home, their daughter, Margaret, was married to Dr. George W. Betton of Tallahassee. The Holland son, known only as N.L. was, according to Mrs. Eppes, "among the first to volunteer for military service."

Holland, Henry D., Duval County, 1805-1860

Dr. Holland, a native of Charleston, South Carolina, spent the greater part of his professional life in Duval County. Very little is known of his early life and education. Although the records of the Medical College of South Carolina do not include the date of his matriculation at that institution, they do show that he was graduated in the spring of 1830 after submitting a thesis entitled "Melancholia and Hypochondria."[1] Soon after receiving his degree Dr. Holland settled in Camden County, Georgia, and began practice. In 1831 he was married to Esther Ann Berrie, daughter of a well-to-do South Georgia farming family.[2] In 1833 their first child, a son named Marshall, was born,[3] and by 1837-38 the family had moved to Duval County.

The Hollands arrived in Florida with sufficient funds to purchase a tract of land up-river from Jacksonville at about the location of the present-day Naval Air Station. This they developed into a plantation which they called Mulberry Grove and with the help of more than 60 slaves began a farming operation.[4] For reasons not revealed Mulberry Grove did not prosper. It may have been from poor management, over-extended credit, or lack of productiveness. Whatever the reason the Hollands had abandoned the plantation by the latter 1840s and Dr. Holland had entered into full-time practice in Jacksonville.

In order to supplement his income and provide for a large family Dr. Holland was able to obtain appointment as medical examiner for the New York Life Insurance Company whose Jacksonville agent was J. McRobert Baker.[5] In 1853 he was appointed Port Physician defeating the other candidate, Dr. William J. L'Engle.[6]

By his very nature Dr. Holland could not avoid becoming involved in the civic affairs of Jacksonville and the state of Florida. He ran successfully for the office of Intendant (i.e., Mayor) of the city in 1852, defeating J.D. Hemming by a vote of 54 to 19.[7] He assisted in planning the Fourth of July celebration in June 1853.[8] As the slavery question became a burning issue in the 1850s Dr. Holland came out in strong support of "the institution of slavery against those who would try to encourage the slaves to abscond."[9]

Dr. Holland had fallen into poor health by 1857. In February he retired from active practice, making a public announcement in which he thanked his many friends for their patronage and at the same time urging those in his debt "by note or open account" to come forth and make a settlement by the first Monday in March "or suit will be commenced indiscriminately." Subsequent to that date his books would be placed in the hands of his attorney.[10] Many of his debtors, of course, did not respond and on May 9, 1857, he reminded those who had ignored his request and notified all "who still owed him that Philip Fraser, attorney-at-law, has been employed to prosecute."

By late 1857 Dr. Holland had left Jacksonville and returned to Bethel, Georgia, the former home of his wife,[11] but by late 1859 or early 1860 had returned to Jacksonville. He is known to have been there on June 10, 1860, when the census-taker came his way, and he was also there on June 27, 1860, when he attended a political rally at the Duval County Court House, where he declared his support for John C. Breckenridge as the presidential nominee of Southern Democrats. The reporter for the Jacksonville paper wrote, "He did so in a few earnest and well-timed remarks."[12]

Dr. Webster Merritt of Jacksonville stated with apparent authority that Dr. Holland died in 1860.[13] He did not, however, cite a source for that date. Cemetery records of Duval County list a gravestone for Henry D. Holland in Jacksonville's Evergreen Cemetery and the date of death inscribed thereon is October 25, 1889. Obviously this is not Dr. Holland's grave. The Duval County Census of 1870, page 537, shows Mrs. Holland, then 60 years old, living in the home of her daughter, Jane, wife of Charles C. Barnard, a railroad agent. The residence was located in LaVilla, a Jacksonville suburb. Incidentally, the Christian name of one of the Barnard children, a son, was Holland, aged nine in 1870. The Holland's daughter, Selma, became the wife of William E. Livingstone. She was buried in Evergreen Cemetery.[14]

1. Records of the Medical College of South Carolina, Waring Medical Historical Library, Charleston, list Dr. Holland among the graduates of 1830. The date of his matriculation is not given but is assumed to have been the fall of 1828.
2. The Berrie family of Bethel community, Glynn County, Georgia, was well above average means.
3. U.S. Census, Duval County, Florida, p. 147.
4. Webster Merritt, *A Century of Medicine in Jacksonville and Duval County*, Gainesville, 1949, pp. 17-18.
5. Jacksonville *Florida News*, April 24, 1850.
6. Jacksonville *Florida Republican*, May 12, 1853. The regulations relating to the duties of the Port Physician were explicit. He was to board all vessels and report to the Intendant all diseases or symptoms thereof. He was to receive $3 for each ship boarded, to be collected from the master of the vessel. He was not permitted to board any vessel unless its captain signaled that there was sickness aboard; on the other hand should he fail to board a vessel on which there was sickness, he would be subject to dismissal by the Intendant.
7. Ibid., June 3, 1852.
8. Ibid., June 30, 1853.
9. Ibid., June 3, 1852.
10. Jacksonville *Florida News*, February 7, 1857.
11. Ibid., February 7, 1857.
12. Fernandina *East Floridian*, August 10, 1860.
13. It is unfortunate that Dr. Merritt neglected to cite his source for the date of Dr. Holland's death. The survey for Evergreen Cemetery in Jacksonville, which gives the date 1889, is presumably the gravestone of Dr. Holland's son, Henry D., Jr., who was born in 1850.
14. Notice of daughter Jane Ann's marriage to Charles C. Barnard appeared in ibid., August 4, 1859.

Holland, Mark D., Tallahassee, 1839

Dr. Holland, a resident of Franklin County, Virginia, was a brief sojourner in the vicinity of Tallahassee for the winter seasons of 1837-1839 having gone there for the benefit of his health. He was suffering from tuberculosis. He died on January 9, 1839. His obituary included praise for his "fine qualities" and a lament for his untimely death. His relationship with the other Holland families in Leon County has not been established.[1]

1. Tallahassee *Floridian*, January 12, 1839.

Hollingsworth, William, Bradford County, 1862

Dr. Hollingsworth, a Starke physician for only about 10 years, was born in Cherokee County, Georgia, and moved to Starke about 1851. Of his five children four were born in Georgia, while the youngest, William, Jr., aged nine in 1860, was born in Florida.[1] By inference from the sparse information available he appears to have been a typical country doctor, beloved but hard-pressed to make a living in New River (Bradford) County, then one of the more backward areas of the state.

A single but well-documented incident suggests that Dr. Hollingsworth was a man of exceptional courage.[2] Just prior to the Civil War a group of rough characters from Starke and the surrounding country organized a vigilante group operating in a manner later adopted by the Ku Klux Klan. They claimed to be an agency dedicated to the preservation of "law and order." Under cover of night they resorted to abducting and brutally beating or intimidating persons whom they considered undesirable or whose ideas did not coincide with their own. They thus terrorized the community and gradually became an instrument for private vengeance. Dr. Hollingsworth openly condemned their practices and consequently became the object of their wrath.

He began receiving threatening letters in July 1860 from the group who called themselves "Regulators." These were sufficiently serious to render it hazardous for him to make professional rounds. On July 27, 1860, a Friday, he received a note saying that he was a doomed man and would be dead ere Sunday came. On Saturday night, as the family was preparing for bed, one of the doctor's sons spied a band of "regulators" approaching the house. They were armed and as they came into close range began firing through windows and doors. Meanwhile Dr. Hollingsworth had seized his shotgun and returned their fire, killing their leader, a fellow named Dowling. The exchange continued and the doctor himself received a minor wound and fell to the floor, whereupon his 13-year-old son continued the fight. But the attackers, apparently thinking that they had accomplished their purpose, gathered their dead and wounded and made their departure. It was reported that the Starke community generally applauded the heroic deeds of the doctor and his young son, Franklin.

In September 1861, Dr. Hollingsworth and his eldest son, Gilbert, enlisted for service in the Army of the Confederacy.[3] The doctor was then 38 years old and the son 19. With a wife and four other children his exemption from military service would have been assured. It would appear, therefore, that he was driven by either patriotism or the expectation of a medical appointment. The appointment never came. While on duty at Ft. Clinch near Fernandina early in the following year, he became ill with pneumonia and died on March 6. The efforts of Dr. Hollingsworth's wife, Nancy Ann, to collect her husband's pay for his five months and seven days of service, for which he had at his death received no compensation, produced an exchange of communications and depositions from which a few meagre biographical details have been gleaned. His eyes were blue, his hair and complexion dark, his height was five feet 10 inches and his age at death was 39. He never rose above the rank of private and his total pay for more than five months of military service was $58.30, which was paid to his widow on March 10, 1864.

1. U.S. Census, 1860, New River County (now Bradford), Item 14. NA, Service Records, CSA, M251, Roll 95, gives the place of his birth as the north Georgia county of Cherokee.

2. A preliminary report of the incident appeared in Fernandina *East Floridian*, August 2, 1860. A week later a full-column account of the entire incident and circumstances relating to it, prepared by a resident of Starke, was published in ibid., August 9, 1860. A brief report was published in the Monticello *Family Friend* of August 11, 1860.

3. All details of Dr. Hollingsworth's military service as well as Mrs. Hollingsworth's exchanges with the Confederate agencies are found in the National Archives material mentioned in note 1 supra.

Hollomon, James M., Calhoun County, 1860

Dr. Hollomon, a native of Mississippi, practiced medicine in or near the village of Ocheesee,[1] Calhoun County, about the year 1860. He and his wife, Ailsey, were the parents of two daughters, Sarah J. and Ailsey Ann, both born in Florida, age three years and nine months respectfully in 1860. The doctor and his wife appear to have arrived in Florida about 1856;[2] however, they may have been in the state earlier. The Census of 1850 lists a Dr. Hollaman, the spelling could have been an error, as 37 years of age, possessing property valued at only $300. His wife was a native of Mississippi and his junior by 16 years. They are presumed to have left the state when the Civil War became imminent.

1. Ocheesee (Ochesee), located in the northeastern corner of Calhoun County, had a post office from 1831, except for brief intervals, until 1911.

2. This is an extrapolation based on the age of the elder child who was three years of age in 1860. See U.S. Census, 1860, Calhoun County, Florida, p. 113, item 50.

Holmes, Henry McCall, Marion County, 1834-1899

Born into a family of cultivation and high social position in Charleston, South Carolina, in 1834—a family whose kindred included the Gibbeses and DeSaussures—Dr. Holmes spent about 12 years of his professional life in Marion County.[1]

The third child and eldest son of Dr. Henry McCall and Eliza Ford Holmes,[2] young Henry received his early education in private schools in Charleston. He appears to have shown an early interest in the biological sciences[3] and in his early youth served an apprenticeship under the preceptorate of his kinsman, Dr. Henry W. DeSaussure, one of Charleston's most eminent physicians.[4] In the fall of 1854 he matriculated at the Medical College of the State of South Carolina, Charleston, from which he was graduated on March 6, 1856, after having submitted a doctoral thesis entitled "Aneurism."[5]

In his quest for further training in a specialized field Dr. Holmes left almost immediately for Philadelphia and enrolled at the Philadelphia Institute of Obstetrics from which he received a certificate of graduation in January 1857.[6]

A few months later Dr. Holmes followed the lead of several other South Carolina families who had settled in Marion County. He chose the community of Silver Springs, probably for two reasons: it was near the waterway connecting the community with Palatka and the St. Johns River, and Ocala, the county seat, was well-staffed with physicians. He found lodging in the home of Thomas J. Pasteur, a well-to-do farmer.[7] On October 21, 1858, he was married to the Pasteurs' daughter, Sidney, a union which appears to have been blissful. Their first child christened Henry McCall Jr., was born in late 1859.[8]

Dr. Holmes had scarcely established his professional practice when the clouds of war appeared. Two months after inauguration of President Lincoln and three weeks after the firing on Ft. Sumter in Charleston harbor, the Marion Light Artillery Company was formed. Soon after organization it established quarters on Amelia Island near Fernandina. Dr. Holmes joined the company there on December 12, 1861, with the rank of sergeant,[9] providing his own horse for which he was to receive $12 monthly for "use and risk."

The Marion unit moved northward into Georgia in June 1862, encamping for a few weeks at Dalton before proceeding to Knoxville, Tennessee, where it came under the command of General Kirby-Smith. The outfit moved into Kentucky and saw action at the Battle of Richmond, after which it was cited for bravery. Dr. Holmes' son, Alester, recalled years later having heard his father speak of "sighting the guns that broke up a Yankee band."

On December 17, 1862, Dr. Holmes found his proper niche in the Confederate effort. He was discharged from the Marion Artillery and assigned to the headquarters of the First Florida Cavalry with the rank of Assistant Surgeon, the transfer having been signed by Colonel George Troup Maxwell, eminent surgeon of Jacksonville and other places, and probably a civilian acquaintance of Dr. Holmes.[10]

Henceforth Dr. Holmes' Army career was by no means tranquil, although he was a Field and Staff officer. In September 1863, the First Florida Cavalry was assigned to the Army of General Braxton Bragg, campaigning in north Georgia and eastern Tennessee and participating in the Battles of Chickamauga and Missionary Ridge. In the following year Dr. Holmes participated in the campaign around Atlanta and Nashville. Subsequently, during the latter months of the War, he was with General Johnston's Army and present at the action around Goldsboro and Bentonville (North Carolina). At the close of the War, he was with Johnston's Army in the vicinity of Greensboro, North Carolina, whence he made his weary way home "—by foot and on a broken-down horse."[11] Meanwhile, he had received his proper recognition by promotion to Surgeon (exact date not ascertained).[12]

On returning to Silver Springs in the summer of 1865, Dr. Holmes found a dismal situation. Marion County, predominantly an area of plantations worked by slave labor, was especially depressed. Medical fees were impossible to collect and fevers were rampant. In 1873 he finally decided to return to South Carolina, arriving in Charleston on June 26 and living with his mother while trying to find a suitable location for practice. He considered Spartanburg but was dissuaded on the grounds that the area was particularly depressed. He chose instead Limestone Springs at that time in Spartanburg County but later after its formation in Cherokee County where a college had recently been established.[13] He practiced there for about four years before moving into nearby Gaffney, the county seat of the new county, where he remained until sometime in the late 1880s when his failing health forced him into retirement.

In the meantime Dr. Holmes' son, Wilmot Stuart Holmes, had become a clergyman and was serving a pastorate in Florence, South Carolina, and Dr. Holmes joined him there. When his son moved to Laurens, South Carolina, in 1897, Dr. Holmes accompanied him. He died there on August 6, 1899, and was buried in the City Cemetery. Mrs. Holmes survived her husband by seven years, dying in Laurens in 1906.

Of the several children born to Dr. and Mrs. Holmes, the eldest, Henry M., Jr., died in childhood. The second son, Wilmot Stuart, became an ordained minister. A third son, Alester Garden, became a Professor of History, spending much of his career on the faculty of Clemson College, now Clemson University. A daughter, Caroline Pasteur, married into the Bivens family of South Carolina.

Although there were certainly segments of happiness in the life of Dr. Holmes, there appears to have been a thread of sadness. His career was certainly blighted by the misfortunes of the Civil War and Reconstruction. This is borne out by the number of changes of location dictated by the adversities of the times. He appears to have been a devoted husband and father, certainly revered by his children and grandchildren.

1. The author is much in the debt of Mrs. Alester G. Holmes II, whose husband, now deceased, was Professor of Mechanical Engineering at Mississippi State University, Starkville. He was the grandson of Dr. Holmes and had collected an abundance of information about his grandfather. In 1968 he edited and published *The Diary of Henry McCall Holmes, Army of Tennessee, Assistant Surgeon, Florida Troops*, (Starkville, Miss., 1968). Mrs. Holmes has generously provided vital information about her husband's grandfather. A granddaughter of Dr. Holmes, Mrs. Caroline Pasteur Holmes Bivins, has also supplied useful data.

2. The Holmes family was a prolific one. Dr. Holmes' grandfather and grandmother, John B. and Elizabeth Edwards Holmes, were the parents of 12 children. See *South Carolina Historical Magazine*, LV(1954), p. 25; Dr. Holmes was one of 10 children. Their descendants were numerous. Mrs. Holmes was one of 12 children of William Stuart and Frances deSaussure Gibbes. See ibid., XII (1911), pp. 91-92.

3. Still preserved in the Holmes family is a book on anatomy and physiology bearing the inscription, "To H.M. Holmes, from his friend and teacher, Mr. James Reeves."

4. Lists of matriculants and graduates, Medical College of the State of South Carolina, preserved in the Waring Historical Medical Library, Charleston, South Carolina. See also Charleston *Mercury*, March 11, 1856.

5. Information, courtesy of Mrs. Anne K. Donato, Waring Historical Library.

6. From biographical notes on Dr. Holmes prepared by his son, the Reverend Wilmot Stuart Holmes.

7. U.S. Census, 1860, Marion County, Florida, p. 76. The Pasteurs were a North Carolina family of more than average means, owning property valued in excess of $16,000. Their slaves numbered 47. Dr. Holmes' holdings in 1860 were modest, being valued at less than $2,000.

8. Dr. Holmes' first child, born in 1859, died in early childhood.

9. Information relating to Dr. Holmes' Confederate service derives chiefly from National Archives, Service Records, CSA, items relating to the Marion Light Artillery and the First Florida Cavalry, which are incomplete, and from his Civil War Diary, note 1, supra. The original manuscript of the "Diary" and other Holmes family papers are now in the Southern Historical Collection, University of North Carolina Library, Chapel Hill.

10. Dr. Maxwell, a native of Georgia, had a distinguished military career, rising from private to lieutenant colonel in a matter of four months, ultimately the commanding officer of the first Florida Cavalry.

11. Miss Emma Holmes, sister of Dr. Holmes, presented a heart-rending account of his last weeks in the Confederate Army, and his return to a dismal situation in Florida. See *The Diary of Miss Emma Holmes, 1861-1865*, ed., with Introduction and Notes by John F. Marszalek, Baton Rouge, Louisiana State University Press, 1979.

12. Ibid. p. 415. Miss Holmes states only that he had received his promotion to surgeon, no date is given.

13. Limestone exists today as a thriving four-year private college.

Holt, Pleasant A., Lake City, 1870-71

Little information has been preserved concerning the career of Dr. Holt. A native of North Carolina, he appears to have arrived in Columbia County in the summer of 1868 at which time he announced his services in medicine and surgery to the citizens of the community.[1] His name is entered in the Census of 1870 with the designation "physician." He was then 42 and the owner of property valued at $4,000. Others in his household were his wife, Meta, and his one-year-old son, Pleasant, Jr., the former born in Georgia, the latter in Florida. There were also two others, Annie Scarlett and Dawson Johnson, both 18 and probably close relatives of the Holts.[2]

Dr. Holt was nominated in 1871 by the voters of Columbia for a seat in the lower house of the Florida Legislature but for "professional reasons" he declined to run for the office.[3] In the following year the list of military appointments announced by the Adjutant General of Florida included Colonel P.A. Holt, Lake City, for Surgeon General.[4] Meanwhile he had accepted a local civic responsibility when he became a member of the Board of Public Instruction for the county.[5] Nothing is known of the latter years of Dr. Holt's life.

1. Lake City *Press*, December 17, 1870 (only extant issue), the notice having been first printed in the issue of August 14, 1868. Both his office and his residence were located on the north side of the Public Square.

2. U.S. Census, 1870, Columbia County, Florida, p. 426.

3. Tallahassee *Sentinel*, December 9 and 16, 1871.

4. Ibid., January 30, 1872.

5. J.M. Hawks, M.D., comp., *The Florida Gazetteer*, New Orleans, 1871, p. 22. Serving as Chairman of the Board at this time was a more renowned physician-politician, Dr. Samuel T. Day, sometime lieutenant governor and acting governor of the State.

Homer, Gustavus, Escambia County, Warrington Navy Yard, 1860

Of Dr. Homer it is only known that he was stationed at the Warrington Navy Yard near Pensacola in 1860 and was a native of Virginia, aged 56, with a wife, Maria, aged 26, and an infant daughter, Emma. Mrs. Homer was born in Indiana; the daughter in Florida.[1]

1. U.S. Census, 1860, Escambia County, Florida, p. 89.

Horsey, Charles W., Fernandina, 1844-1878

The year 1877 was a particularly tragic one in the history of Florida medicine. Yellow fever epidemics of extreme virulence prevailed in Jacksonville and Fernandina and the mortality rate in both cities was shockingly high. Among the fatalities in Fernandina was Dr. F. Preston Wellford of Jacksonville who had volunteered his services to the afflicted city. From the standpoint of epidemiology it was significant in that two eminent physicians, Dr. Charles W. Horsey of Fernandina and Dr. R.P. Daniel of Jacksonville, recorded in detail their observations on the origin, characteristics and treatment of the disease. As for the origins, Dr. Daniel concluded that in Jacksonville it was local, arising from accumulations of garbage left at various points in the city. Dr. Horsey, on the other hand, was equally convinced that it had been introduced into Fernandina by the crews and passengers of vessels putting in at the port from various Caribbean areas.

Dr. Horsey was born in Charleston, South Carolina, in 1844.[1] Nothing is known of his childhood and youth but it is assumed that he received his early education in local schools and served an apprenticeship in the office of a local physician. By the time he was prepared to enter medical school the Medical College of the State of South Carolina in Charleston was still closed because of war, but when it reopened in the fall of 1865 he enrolled and on March 2, 1867, was graduated as Doctor of Medicine.[2]

The precise date of Dr. Horsey's move to Florida is not known. The Census of 1870 lists him as a resident of Fernandina, living alone and owning property valued at only $500.[3] It is probable that he arrived in Fernandina within a year or two after receiving his medical degree.[4] His earliest known professional card, published in late 1872, states that he resided at "4th Street, between Centre and Ash" and that his office was "on 3rd Street, near Virginia House."[5]

As was the case with many 19th century Florida physicians, nearly all of whom were born elsewhere, Dr. Horsey was moved to record his impressions of various features of the Florida scene, in his case the climate. His paper, "Remarks on the Climate of Florida," was published in the *American Journal of Medical Sciences*, April 1874.[6]

Yellow fever appeared in Fernandina in August 1877, claiming as its first victim a member of the crew of the Norwegian bark, *The Bjorn*, his death occurring on August 21. In addition there were reports of many deaths at sea by some of the ships in port at Fernandina. Dr. Horsey found himself in the midst of the onslaught which followed. By the second week in November the fever had run its course and Dr. Horsey had survived. The casualties, however, numbered more than 100.

The Florida Medical Association met for the fifth annual session on April 16, 1878. Discussions centered on the recent epidemics of fevers. Though not a member Dr. Horsey was asked to report on the Fernandina experience. His paper was followed by that of Jacksonville physician, Dr. R.P. Daniel. Both were scholarly in method and content, although their conclusions were at odds. After delivering his paper Dr. Horsey was immediately nominated for membership in the Association and elected by unanimous vote, bringing the total membership to 24. Simultaneously he was elected Second Vice President.[7] Both papers were printed in the *Proceedings* of the Association later that year.

As the meeting closed Dr. Horsey appeared destined for a long and distinguished career. It was not to be, however. He died suddenly in Starke on November 2, 1878, at the age of 34.[8]

It is not known whether Dr. Horsey was ever married. His mother, Louisa, had moved from Charleston to Fernandina at some time in the 1870s, accompanied by another son, John Louis, a druggist, and a daughter, Julia. In 1880 she was keeping a boarding house in Fernandina.[9] In the mid-1880s John Louis returned to Charleston and enrolled in the Medical College of the State of South Carolina from which he received his medical degree in 1886.[10]

1. This date of birth is an extrapolation from the Nassau County, Florida Census of 1880, p. 3, which gives his age as 26.
2. Charleston *Courier*, March 4, 1867.
3. U.S. Census, 1870, Nassau County, Florida, item 436.
4. The absence of Fernandina newspapers is frustrating for much of the period under consideration.
5. The earliest known professional card of Dr. Horsey is that of *The Fernandina Observer* of January 18, 1873, first printed in ibid. of November 2, 1872 (not extant).
6. This fairly prestigious journal enjoyed a lengthy circulation extending from 1827 until near the end of the 19th century.
7. Much of the information concerning Dr. Horsey's relationship with the Florida Medical Association is found in its *Proceedings*, 1878, in which his "Report of the Epidemic of Yellow Fever at Fernandina, Florida, in August, September and October, 1877" is printed in toto, pp. 51-88. This is an excellent paper in which is revealed not only Dr. Horsey's professional acumen and meticulous record-keeping but his acquaintance with the literature pertinent to the subject.
8. *Proceedings, Florida Medical Association*, Jacksonville, 1879, p. 9. No explanation of Dr. Horsey's presence in Starke nor of the nature of his fatal illness has been located.
9. U.S. Census, 1880, Nassau County, Florida, p. 3. Six boarders are mentioned.
10. *Centennial Memorial of the Medical College of the State of South Carolina, 1824-1924*, Charleston, 1924, p. 130.

Hort, William P., Jackson County, 1824

Among the earliest settlers of Jackson County none was more active in public affairs than Dr. Hort, who appears to have arrived in early 1824.[1] Of his origins and professional training nothing is presently known but it is inferred that he possessed superior intelligence and qualities of leadership.

When the location of the county seat became an emotional issue in 1825, he was one of three citizens, the others were James Patterson and Owen Williams, selected to choose the site. Although his holdings were in the vicinity of Webbville, a contender for the seat, he acquiesced in the choice of Marianna, which was more centrally located.[2] He was the first among 140 signers of a petition to Congress, dated December 11, 1827, requesting that Marianna be chosen as the seat.

In the further distribution of public lands in 1826 Dr. Hort received an additional three quarters of a section, lying in township No. 5, Range 10, located some five miles northwest of Marianna,[3] establishing him as one of the larger landowners of the county.

As a citizen of substance he assumed public responsibility accordingly. He was a member of the Board of Trustees of Webbville Academy which opened on February 27, 1827; it was the first school in the county to be chartered by the Florida Legislative Council.[4] He also exhibited interest in internal improvement by joining the efforts to gain congressional aid in establishing a satisfactory harbor to serve the settlers in the St. Andrew's Bay area.[5] He also supported the ill-fated project to build a canal linking the Chipola and Apalachicola Rivers.[6]

In spite of these activities Dr. Hort did not abandon medical practice. As a physician he was sufficiently well regarded to receive legislative appointment to the Medical Board of the Territory of Florida, which was created as a regulatory body by the Legislative Council on December 31, 1827, and approved by Governor Duval a week later.[7] In a revision of the Act a year later, Dr. Hort remained a member of the Board.

It need hardly be added that Dr. Hart was an agrarian Democrat who found the administration of President John Quincy Adams repugnant. In a toast delivered at a Fourth of July celebration at Chipola in 1826 he expressed this sentiment: "To the opposition in the Senate and the House of Representatives, may their course prosper and finally prevail."[8] He was doubtless delighted with the Andrew Jackson victory in 1828.

It is unfortunate that nothing further is known of Dr. Hort. It is odd that a man of his local importance should have disappeared without a trace.

1. Clarence Edwin Carter, ed., *The Territorial Papers of the United States*, Washington, Government Printing Office, Vol. XXIII (1824-28), p. 100.
2. Ibid., p. 948. See also J. Randall Stanley, *History of Jackson County*, Marianna, 1950, p. 43.
3. WPA, Writers Project, "Jackson County," Land grants, p. 62.
4. Stanley, *History*, p. 88.
5. *Territorial Papers* (note 1 supra), p. 398.
6. Stanley, *History*, p. 101.
7. Acts, *Florida Legislative Council*, 6th Session, 1827-28, pp. 46-49.
8. Tallahassee *Intelligencer*, September 1, 1826.

Houseal, Henry, Marion County, 1833-1862

The medical career of Dr. Houseal was brief. A native of Newberry District, South Carolina,[1] he received his early education in the common schools of the District. As a young man he served a professional apprenticeship in the office of Dr. O.B. Mayer of Newberry. In the fall of 1854 he matriculated at the Medical College of the State of South Carolina from which he was graduated as Doctor of Medicine on March 6, 1856, after submitting a doctoral thesis entitled "Dysentery."[2]

Soon after receiving his degree Dr. Houseal was married to Nancy Lucius, daughter of Frederick and Nancy Lucius of Newberry District, the wedding having occurred on March 19, 1857. Their only child, a daughter christened Ida, was born in late 1857 or early 1858. At some time in 1858 the Houseals made their way to Marion County which had already become the home of several former South Carolinians.[3]

In early 1862, with the Civil War under way, Madison Starke Perry, later to become the governor of Florida, organized a regiment of troops from various counties of central Florida. To Wade S. Eichelberger, Marion County resident and, like Dr. Houseal, native of Newberry District, was assigned the task of conscripting a company from Marion County. Among those mustered into the company at Gainesville on April 12, 1862, was Dr. Houseal, who committed himself for three year's service. He was assigned the rank of First Lieutenant. When Eichelberger, because of illness resigned his captain's commission, Dr. Houseal was promoted to that rank. His unit was Company "B," 7th Florida Infrantry Regiment.

Within a month after its organization the Seventh Regiment was ordered to eastern Tennessee to become a part of the Army of General Braxton Bragg. Its actual combat service had hardly begun when Dr. Houseal fell ill and died at Chattanooga on July 14.[4]

Mrs. Houseal, left to fend for herself and a five-year-old daughter, apparently elected to remain in Marion County. A few years later she married William McAteer, also a former South Carolinian who, incidentally, had been a private in Dr. Houseal's military unit. He was captured at Missionary Ridge and released at the war's end.[5]

1. The Houseals had been among the early settlers in St. Helen's Parish, Beaufort District, South Carolina. Some members of the family had migrated to Newberry District in the early 19th century.

2. *Catalogue, Medical College of the State of South Carolina,* Session of 1854-55. For a list of graduates in the class of 1856 see Charleston *Mercury,* March 11, 1856.

3. U.S. Census, 1860, Marion County, Florida, item 505. The Houseals were a family of modest means, their property having been valued at $1,500.

4. Some confusion exists concerning the actual place of Dr. Houseal's death. A compilation of data, *Soldiers of Florida,* Live Oak, Florida, 1903, p. 182, cites the place as Chattanooga. National Archives records, however, give the place as Adamsville, Fulton County, Ga.

5. U.S Census, 1880, Marion County, Florida, p. 134. Here the McAteers are shown to have been living in Marion County.

Houston, J.M.J., Apalachicola, 1860

As far as is known Dr. Houston made only one appearance in the historical records of Florida. The year 1860 found him in medical practice in Apalachicola, Franklin County. He was a native of Virginia,[1] aged 55, owning property valued at $6,000. He is believed to have departed the state prior to 1870.[1]

1. U.S. Census, 1860, Franklin County, Florida, p. 423.

Houstoun, George M., Jefferson County, 1860

Very little is known of the Florida career of Dr. Houstoun, who is listed in the Jefferson County Census of 1860 as a Doctor of Medicine practicing in the Waukeenah community. He appears to have been a widower. Two small children, Thomas J. and Henry C., aged three and one respectively, and Dr. Houstoun's mother, Eliza, were the only residents of the household.[1] Both the doctor and his mother were natives of North Carolina; the two children were born in Florida. Since the Houstouns do not appear in the Florida Census of 1870, it is assumed they had left the state by that date.[2]

1. U.S. Census, 1860, item 152.

2. The Jefferson County Census of 1870 shows Eliza Houstoun, age 63, a resident in the home of Robert Kuichen (Kitchen?) of Waukeenah. The editorial note accompanying her name reads: "Living with friends."

Howard, James C., Levy County, 1860-1885

Dr. Howard was a medical practitioner in Levy County during the latter half of the 19th century. A native of Georgia, he is known to have been a resident of the community of Levyville, some 12 miles east of the county seat of Bronson, as early as 1860.[1] He is said to have been among a small group of citizens captured at Fanning Springs by a Union gunboat crew shortly after the fall of Cedar Key to the enemy in 1862. Although a noncombatant, his services were so much needed by Union troops in the area that his release could not be negotiated. Only through the feminine wiles of a local woman who spirited him away under the cover of darkness was he able to escape and rejoin his family.[2]

Censuses of 1870 and 1885 show Dr. Howard still living and practicing in Levy County but no further details of his career have been located.

1. U.S. Census, 1860, Levy County, Florida, p. 19, item 113. He is listed as 30 years of age, a physician, owning property valued at $1,000. His residence was in or near the Levyville Settlement, some eight miles due east of the town of Bronson.

2. William Samuel Yearty, "Yearty Family History," unpublished manuscript, photocopy P.K. Yonge Library of Florida History, University of Florida, Gainesville, pp. 23-24. In this intimate and chatty account of his family Mr. Yearty recalled numerous incidents from his earlier years. The woman mentioned in this connection was his father's sister, Meriah, who by using her charm on the commanding officer of the Union troops at Cedar Key, obtained the release of her father but not of Dr. Howard. She was able later, however, to obtain a boat and by night rowed him from Way Key to the mainland, whence he made his way home.

Howard, John G., Quincy, 1860

Beyond the fact that he was living and presumably practicing medicine in Quincy about 1860, nothing is known of Dr. Howard. A native of Virginia, he was 55 years old in 1860. His wife, Emily, was Kentucky-born while his two children, Emily and John, were born in Louisiana. He was a man of modest means, his property being valued at $7,000 in 1860.[1]

1. U.S. Census, 1860, Gadsden County, Florida, p. 65, item 475.

Howell, David D., Liberty County, 1826

Dr. Howell, a native of South Carolina, spent the greater part of his professional career in the comparative obscurity of rural Liberty County. It appears that he arrived in the state about 1857 accompanied by his wife, Zanetta, and their two small daughters, Americus and Lillie,[1] establishing their home in the Aspalaga community.[2] It is unlikely that he was a graduate of a medical college, but he had doubtless read medicine in the office of a regular practitioner which would have qualified him for practice in Florida at the time.[3]

For reasons unknown no member of the Howell family is listed in the Florida Census of 1870. The year 1880, however, found Dr. Howell sharing his home with two sons, Hayne and Robert, and three daughters, Etta, Leila and Cora.[4] Mrs. Howell is presumed to have died prior to that date. The last reference to Dr. Howell's residence in Florida appeared in the Special Florida Census of 1885 which lists him as a resident in the household of J.N. Howell, thought to have been his brother.[5] All members of the family appear to have been persons of very modest means, earning their living on small farms in northwest Liberty County. No date for Dr. Howell's death has been discovered.

1. U.S. Census, 1860, Liberty County, Florida, p. 10, item 70.

2. Although Aspalaga was situated on the east side of the Apalachicola River, it shared its post office with residents of Liberty County living across the river. As a populated community it virtually disappeared from more recent maps. After October 1898 the Rock Bluff post office served Aspalaga.

3. Prior to organization of the Florida Medical Association in 1874 the issuance of licenses to practice medicine in the state was left to the discretion of county judges who usually required endorsement of a practicing physician.

4. U.S. Census, 1880, Liberty County, Florida, p. 12, item 110.

5. Well into the 20th century Liberty County was still an area of small farmers, timber cutters and turpentine dippers, with here and there a small mercantile operation.

Hoyt, Charles, Jacksonville, 1804-1835

Dr. Hoyt's tragically brief Florida career began in Jacksonville in the winter of 1834-35. His professional card first appeared in the local newspaper on January 29, 1835, when he offered his services to "inhabitants of Jacksonville and this section of Florida as surgeon and physician."[1] His death came "very suddenly" on October 18 of the same year.[2] He had been born in Deerfield, Massachusetts, on August 20, 1804, son of Elihu Hoyt of Deerfield.[3] He had received his medical degree from Vermont Medical College at Woodstock in 1834.[4]

1. Jacksonville *Courier*, February 26, 1835; first printing, January 29, 1835.
2. Ibid., November 19, 1835.
3. Ibid. The only record of Dr. Hoyt's extra professional activities is that of July 4, 1835, when he attended an Independence Day celebration in Jacksonville and offered a toast "To the St. Johns River—may her flood be emigration (sic) and her ebb the exportation of our products." Ibid., July 9, 1835.
4. Waite, F.C., *The Story of a Country Medical College*, Montpelier, Vermont Historical Society, 1945, p. 165.

Huchingson, Marcellus, Lake City, 1839

Dr. Huchingson, son of Abel and Jane Huchingson, was born in Georgia in 1839.[1] He received his medical degree in 1859 from the Medical College of Georgia, Augusta,[2] and soon after joined his family near Lake City and began professional practice. He was barely established in practice when the Civil War began. Two of his brothers, both younger than he, were among early enlistees[3] but more than a year elapsed before Dr. Hutchingson, then 23, was mustered in at Lake City on August 2, 1862.[4] He was assigned to Company C, 2nd Florida Infantry Battalion, but in recognition of his professional training he was "detailed to the General Hospital" in Lake City. He was promoted to assistant surgeon on October 5, 1862, and detailed to assist the surgeon at the hospital. Near the end of the year he was designated "hospital steward." Although his service record is incomplete he appears to have remained at the hospital for the duration of the War.

After his release from military service in 1865, Dr. Huchingson resumed civilian practice in Lake City. At some juncture in the late 1860s he took a wife about whom it is only known that her Christian name was Origan, a native of Florida, and two years younger than her husband.[5]

As a physician Dr. Huchingson soon achieved prominence within the ranks of his profession. He displayed interest in the Florida Medical Association, organized in Jacksonville in January 1874,[6] and was one of 10 doctors present at that meeting. At the second annual meeting, also held in Jacksonville in February 1875,[7] Dr. Huchingson was admitted to full membership and simultaneously elected treasurer. Ironically he never attended another session.

Meanwhile Dr. Huchingson had entered the world of business. In the early 1870s he had joined three other local men, J.V. Brown, Duval Selph and F.M. Weeks, in a mercantile venture operating under the firm name, J.V. Brown & Company. This partnership was dissolved on November 10, 1875, by mutual consent with Brown and Dr. Huchingson authorized to collect all debts due.[8] Simultaneously Dr. Huchingson published the following announcement.[9]

> Dr. M.M. Huchingson, having retired from his professional practice, will in the future devote his entire time to the promotion of the mercantile business.
>
> (Signed) John V. Brown
> M.M. Huchingson

This was apparently an irrevocable decision. Although still treasurer of the Medical Association he did not appear at the 1876 meeting in Tallahassee and in the roster of members in 1885 his name does not appear. In the comprehensive list of 1893 it is stated that he had been dropped from membership for non-payment of dues.[10]

Little more is known of Dr. Huchingson.

1. This date is an extrapolation from the military record of Dr. Huchingson in which his age at the time of enlistment on August 2, 1862, was 23.

2. Medical College of the University of Georgia, *List of Graduates*, 1829-1891, Augusta 1891, p. 19.

3. These brothers were Theodosius and Valerius. The parents were apparently fascinated by Roman names; two daughters were named Hortensia and Octavia.

4. NA, Service Records, CSA, M251, Roll 48.

5. U.S. Census, 1870, Columbia County, Florida, p. 421, item 92.

6. *Proceedings, Florida Medical Association*, 1874-1875, Jacksonville, 1875, pp. 4, 7, 11.

7. Ibid., p. 11.

8. Lake City *Weekly Reporter*, November 10, 1875.

9. Ibid.

10. *Proceedings, Florida Medical Asociation*, Jacksonville, 1893, p. 44.

Hughes, Ellis, Ft. Heilman and Ft. Lauderdale, 1813-1866

Dr. Hughes,[1] native of Annapolis, Maryland, was born in 1813, son of Jeremiah Hughes, sometime editor of *Niles National Register*. He was graduated from the University of Maryland School of Medicine in 1834 at the top of his class. For this achievement he was awarded the gold medal, a prize given annually by the school.[2] Soon after graduation he moved to Tallahassee where for a year or so he was employed as a teacher in the Leon Academy. With a change in the administration of the Academy in 1836 Dr. Hughes returned to Baltimore and for a term (1836-37) served as Demonstrator in Anatomy in the medical school.

Following the Dade Massacre in late December 1835, the War Department began serious preparations for dealing with the Indian problem in Florida. Dr. Hughes was among the considerable number of physicians gaining employment in the Medical Department of the Army, his commission as assistant surgeon bearing the date August 21, 1838.[3] Before the end of that year he was assigned to Ft. Heilman, an outpost on Black Creek near the present site of Middleburg in Clay County. In January 1839, he was ordered to report for duty at Ft. Lauderdale, then a garrison on New River. After a series of misadventures and some loitering on Key Biscayne he arrived on February 15 at the Fort then garrisoned by Co. K, 3rd Artillery, U.S. Army.

Garrison life at remote Ft. Lauderdale, while providing an excessive amount of leisure time, proved to be both debilitating and demoralizing for the gifted young doctor. During his stay he was frequently afflicted with fevers and dysentery, ailments responsible for more casualties than Indian arrows. Equally bad was the boredom which enveloped posts such as Ft. Lauderdale. To beguile the tedium Dr. Hughes, among others, turned to strong drink and his indiscretions while intoxicated led eventually to a confrontation with the Fort commander, Capt. William B. Davidson, and the doctor's arrest on March 25, 1840. Within the week Dr. Hughes was ordered to return to Ft. Heilman. His resignation from the Army, effective as of July 31, 1840,[4] concluded his military career, an inglorious one at best.

From that point on through the next 25 years Dr. Hughes was unable to settle down in any position of permanence. He returned to Maryland where for a brief time he assisted his father in editing the *Niles Register*. Subsequent efforts to reenter a military establishment proved futile, possibly because of his earlier record. He moved to Georgetown, D.C., in 1849 where he published the *Georgetown Advocate*, but by that time his health had deteriorated to the point that any resumption of medical practice was impossible. He died in Georgetown on October 5, 1866.

A casual reflection on the career of Dr. Hughes leads only to the sad conclusion that a life of enormous promise in the medical profession was dissipated and ultimately destroyed by circumstances over which he had lost control.

1. The career of Dr. Hughes has been thoroughly explored and documented by Paul Eugen Camp, Assistant Special Collections Librarian, University of South Florida, Tampa. See "Boredom, Brandy and Bickering," *Broward Legacy*, II, March 1978, 7-12; 31-38. This splended article is based on the "Journal of Ellis Hughes," a manuscript in the Ms. Collection of the Library of the University of South Florida. The present sketch consists largely of information found in Mr. Camp's article. No specific page citations will be appended except in a few instances in which the present writer used sources not cited by Mr. Camp.

2. Eugene F. Cordell, Historical Sketch of the University of Maryland School of Medicine, 1807-1890, Baltimore, 1891, p. 213. It may be noted that Dr. Hughes' date of birth is at variance with that cited by Mr. Camp. The place of birth cited by him was Baltimore. My source is Cordell, op. cit., p. 93, where the following statement may be found: "Ellis Hughes was from Annapolis. He held the demonstratorship for a brief period (1837)."

3. *Medical Department of the Army, 1775 to 1873*, comp. by Harvey E. Brown, Washington, Surgeon General's Office, 1873, p. 292.

4. Ibid.

Hughes, William H., Marianna, 1860

Dr. Hughes is one of many natives of eastern North Carolina who settled in Jackson County in the mid-19th century. He was a practicing physician in Marianna just prior to the Civil War. The Census of Jackson County, 1860, lists him as a resident in the home of Francis Ely, a wealthy merchant-planter, who was also a North Carolina native. Accompanying Dr. Hughes in the move to Florida was his daughter, six-year-old Lenora,[1] which suggests that Dr. Hughes was probably a widower. Lacking evidence to the contrary it is conjectured that Dr. Hughes was a relative of Ely. Whatever the relationship it appears that Dr. Hughes immediately found his place in the top rank of Marianna society. On the invitations to a Dancing Party to take place at the Marianna Seminary on December 24, 1860, Dr. Hughes was listed a one of four Senior Managers in charge of the affair.

As the inevitability of war became increasingly apparent in the winter of 1860-61, Dr. Hughes must have returned to his native North Carolina so that his young daughter could find a home with relatives in case his services should be required by a Confederate Army unit from that state.[2]

1. Charlotte Corley Farley, *Florida's Alamo: The Battle of Marianna*, mimeographed copy, 1981, p. 4. The 1860 Census, Jackson County, Florida, lists Dr. Hughes and his daughter as residents in the home of L.A.C. Ely, a wealthy farmer, owner of property valued at nearly $100,000.

2. Confederate Records, Military Units of Florida, list a William Hughes as a private in Company K, 2nd Florida Cavalry Regiment. He cannot be identified as the subject of the present sketch.

Hull, Oliver P., Waldo, Alachua County, 1832-1862

Very little information on the brief career of Dr. Hull has survived. He was born in Georgia in 1832 but nothing is known of the actual place of birth, his family, early education, nor has the medical school which he attended been identified.[1] In 1859 he was a practicing physician in Waldo, Alachua County, when he attended Stephen Driggers who was mortally wounded by an outraged husband, William Dominick, whose wife had been seduced by, and subsequently eloped with, Driggers.[2]

As secession became the burning issue in the South in 1860 Dr. Hull became an ardent and outspoken proponent of the movement. On November 8, 1860, the probability of Lincoln's election having been generally accepted throughout the country, a group of Waldo citizens met and with Dr. Hull as their leader declared themselves "ready for any emergency, and in favor of immediate disolution of the Union, should Lincoln be elected President."[3]

Dr. Hull was mustered into the Confederate Army on April 19, 1861, as a second lieutenant and assigned to Company C, First Florida Infantry Regiment, the unit being assembled at Camp Magnolia, near Pensacola, but on Janury 26, 1862, he resigned his commission. Shortly thereafter, however, he reenlisted as a private but in the following March was recommissioned with the rank of first lieutenant.[4]

During build-up of the Confederate forces prior to the Battle of Shiloh (Tennessee) General Braxton Bragg's Army which included the Florida First Regiment was ordered to Corinth, Mississippi, to await further orders. These were not long in coming and when the battle was joined at Shiloh on April 6, 1862, Lt. Hull, at that time commander of Company D, was among the early casualties, dying soon after receiving mortal wounds.[5]

Dr. Hull was unmarried at the time of his death. There is some evidence that he had intended to return to Alachua County at the end of the War.[6] Instead he was buried in the Shiloh Military Cemetery among the more than 3,000 other victims of one of the bloodiest battles of the War.[7]

1. None of the four contemporary medical colleges of Georgia, Oglethorpe, Atlanta, University of Georgia at Augusta, Savannah, lists Dr. Hull among its matriculants and graduates.

2. Dr. Hull was moved to report the incident to Dr. William H. Babcock, editor of the Fernandina *East Floridian*, who published the account in the issue of July 14, 1859. Prior to April 1859, Dr. Babcock had been a practicing physician in Gainesville and was doubtless a personal acquaintance of Dr. Hull.

3. Ibid., November 14, 1860.

4. NA, Service Records, CSA, M251, Roll 27.

5. *The War of the Rebellion*, House of Representatives, 48th Congress, 1st Session, Misc. Docs. No. 26, Washington, 1884, Ser. I, Vol. 10, Pt. I, p. 504.

6. In a transaction of February 10, 1860, Dr. Hull had purchased a lot in Gainesville from John C. Richard and wife for $300. Alachua County, Deed Book, E. P. 150.

7. U.S. Census, 1860, Alachua County, Florida, item 73. Here Dr. Hull's age is shown as 28, his birthplace, Georgia, and his property valued at $1,000.

Hulse Gilbert White, Army Physician, 1807-1883

Dr. Hulse was an army physician who served at Tampa Bay and other Florida posts in the 1830s. The following biographical sketch was written by John Hendley Barnhart (1871-1949), for many years bibliographer of the New York Botanical Garden. It appeared as an annotation in John Kunkel Small, "Seminole

Bread—the Conti," *Journal of the New York Botanical Garden,* XXII, p. 132. It is reproduced here in its entirety without alteration or additional notation.

> Gilbert White Hulse was born 12 March 1807, in Blooming Grove Township, near Washingtonville, Orange County, New York. He studied medicine at the College of Physicians and Surgeons in New York City, receiving his degree in 1835. He immediately entered the medical service of the United States Army, being stationed at Tampa Bay from February to April, 1836, in Arkansas during the summer and fall of the same year, returning to Fort Brooke, Florida. In 1837 he went again to Ft. Gibson, Arkansas, returning to Ft. Brooke in January 1838. He was at Tallahassee in March, and before the middle of the year 1838 had settled as a medical practitioner at Rodney, Mississippi. Later he was a planter in Louisiana, and about 1850 he visited northern California, where he collected plants for (John) Torrey as he had done in Florida and Mississippi. Throughout the Civil War he was a surgeon in the Confederate Army, and at its close, his property gone, he returned north, making his home at first with his sister, Mrs. Moffatt, at Rockford, Illinois, and later with her daughter, Mrs. Knapp, at Auburn, New York, where he died 13 November 1883.

In Small's article are found several quotations from various letters written by Dr. Hulse.

Hulse, Isaac, Pensacola, 1797-1856

Dr. Hulse, probably the most eminent physician to practice in West Florida during the Territorial Period, was the subject of a biography written by Charles T. Werner which was published in a limited edition in New York in 1922. It is a well-documented work which includes numerous letters from Dr. Hulse addressed to his close friend, Benjamin F. Thompson. Thompson, like Dr. Hulse, a Long Island native, is known chiefly for his *History of Long Island,* first edition published by E. French in New York in 1833. Data for the present sketch is drawn chiefly from the Werner biography unless otherwise indicated.[1]

Dr. Hulse, a highly esteemed physician who spent the greater part of his professional life in the vicinity of Pensacola, was born near Coram, Suffolk County, Long Island, New York, on August 31, 1797. He was the youngest of the five sons of Major Caleb M. Hulse and Jerusha Petty Hulse. At an early age he exhibited an aversion to the farm labor to which his brothers were assigned and, encouraged by his mother to apply himself diligently to his school work, he soon demonstrated a propensity for scholarship. He completed his basic education at Union Hall Academy in nearby Jamaica, Long Island, where he is said to have become proficient in foreign languages.

About 1840 Hulse made his way to Baltimore where he taught for a brief period in a classical school. In 1821 he enrolled in the Medical Department of the University of Maryland in Baltimore from which he received his medical degree in the spring of 1823. His splendid record placed him at the top of his class and earned for him the gold medal for scholastic excellence.

Meanwhile, while still a medical student, he met and married a Baltimore girl, Amelia Roberts. Notwithstanding his marriage and the birth of his first two children, Dr. Hulse, doubtless in quest of financial security, joined the United States Navy on May 12, 1823. His first assignment was that of Surgeon's Mate aboard the U.S.S. Congress based in Norfolk, Virginia. His voyages aboard the Congress in the following year took him to Gibraltar, Cadiz, Rio de Janeiro, the West Indies and the west coast of Africa.

Back in the United States for land duty in 1824 Dr. Hulse was assigned to the Naval Hospital at Norfolk, Virginia, where he remained for two years during which he was promoted to Surgeon. In 1826 he began his Florida service at the Naval Hospital in Pensacola. For the years 1826-35 his letters to his friend Thompson, if indeed they were written, have been lost. When the correspondence was resumed on January 13, 1835, the letter of that date recounted an altercation which had developed between the doctor and his commanding officer, Captain Wolcott Chauncey, an affair relating to a horse. The gist of the matter was that without authorization of Chauncey the doctor had hired a horse for the purpose of transporting himself from his quarters at the Navy Yard to the Naval Hospital, a distance of perhaps a couple of miles. He justified his action on the grounds that the hospital required some transportation in case of emergency. As he stated it, his sole object was "to prevent the Hospital ever being in want of a horse."

When Dr. Hulse submitted his quarterly expense account, which included the hire of the horse, to Chauncey, it was forwarded to the Navy Department with the recommendation that the expense for the horse be disallowed. Other fuels were in time added to the fire with the result that Dr. Hulse's tour of duty was for a time an unpleasant one. (Werner, pp. 13-14). Dr. Hulse's action was later vindicated, however, when Secretary of the Navy, Mahlon Dickerson, sided with him in the affair (Werner, p. 17).

There is evidence to show that Dr. Hulse was more than a mere practitioner of medicine. The various fevers endemic to the area interested him immensely. He is known to have made careful observations on the numerous cases which came under his scrutiny, taking pains to describe the symptoms and note the results of his various efforts at treatment.[2]

On December 11, 1837, Dr. Hulse's service was rewarded by his appointment as Fleet Surgeon, attached to the West India Squadron. He served in this capacity until September 1840 when he returned to Pensacola as the chief surgeon of the Naval Hospital. This brought him under the direct command of Commander Alexander J. Dallas, who had interceded for him with Secretary Dickerson in the "affair of the horse."

Dr. Hulse's interests appear to have extended well beyond the bounds of the Pensacola Navy Yard. His leadership brought about organization of the Board of Medical Officers, which included those from both Army and Navy in the Pensacola area. It was designed to meet periodically for discussion of health problems common to the two services. He occasionally took time to record his observations on unusual cases which he treated. One of the these reports was published in the St. Augustine *Florida Herald* on November 14, 1833. His monograph on "Yellow Fever" was published in the *Maryland Medical and Surgical Journal,* April 1842. There were doubtless many others. As for his religious persuasion, Dr. Hulse was a Methodist.[3] Records of his contributions to the Methodist Church have survived.

Dr. Hulse was twice married. His first wife was Amelia Roberts of Baltimore. To this marriage were born a son who died in early childhood; another son, Isaac, born January 15, 1824, and a daughter, Georgiana, who was married to Alexander W. McLeon, a clergyman. She became a writer of minor importance, under the nom de plume, Mary A. Holmes. She died in Baltimore on July 2, 1890. Mrs. Hulse died on August 2, 1827, while on a voyage from Pensacola to New York. She was buried at sea.

On January 10, 1833, Dr. Hulse married Melania, daughter of John Innerarity, Scottish-born, who had served as British consul in Pensacola. To this marriage were born John, who became a physician; Albert, about whom nothing is presently known, and Emma, who became the wife of Lewis Boyer Taylor. Her death occurred on April 5, 1924. Mrs. Hulse (Melania) died in Pensacola on January 13, 1875, at the age of 64.[4]

Dr. Hulse's life ended at the U.S. Naval Hospital at Warrington on August 29, 1856, after a painful and protracted illness. His close friend and editor of the Pensacola *Gazette* wrote:

> Dr. Hulse was at his death fifty-nine years of age, having seen thirty-three years of honorable, faithful and efficient service as surgeon of the U.S. Navy. He has spent many years on the station and by his courteous and gentlemanly deportment he had drawn around him a large circle of devoted friends by whom his loss will be long and deeply felt. By his disinterested benevolence and constant readiness to minister to the wants of suffering humanity for which an acknowledged eminence in his profession so well qualified him, he has endeared himself to the hearts of the poor and afflicted by ties which death itself cannot sever.[5]

1. Only 100 copies of Charles J. Werner, *Dr. Isaac Hulse: His Life and Letters*, New York, Charles J. Werner, 44 Whitehall Street, 1922, were published. Dr. Hulse's earliest extant letters date from his stay in Baltimore about 1821.
2. In addition to his published articles much information relating to his practice in Florida is contained in his letters to Thompson. His broad range of intellectual interests is suggested by the following occurrence: In late December 1850, a noted Catholic Divine, Father Mathew (probably an archbishop) visited Pensacola. As a part of formal function he was given a tour of the Naval Station, pausing for an inspection of the Marine Hospital. It was reported that "He observed with pleasure the marked attention paid to the suffering of invalids in the different wards, and was highly gratified to find a valuable Library of nearly 2000 volumes collected through the zeal of Dr. Hulse, and specially intended for the use of the convalescent patients." Pensacola *Florida Democrat*, January 9, 1851.
3. F.W. Haskins, *The History of Methodism in Pensacola, Florida*, Nashville, 1928, pp. 112, 114.
4. Information from gravestones, St. Michael's Cemetery.
5. Pensacola *Gazette*, September 2, 1856.

Hunter, George Baxter, Marion County, 1830-1865

Dr. Hunter, whose professional career was spent almost entirely in the Wacahoota community of Marion County, was born in Harrisonburg, Virginia, on August 12, 1830.[1] After attending local schools he entered the University of Virginia where he completed what was then known as a "classical education."[2] Hunter then enrolled at Jefferson Medical College in Philadephia from which he received his medical degree in the spring of 1851.[3] He had scarcely launched himself into medical practice when failing health, brought on by tuberculosis, forced him to seek a more benign climate. For reasons which are not clear he chose to settle in the village of Wacahoota, located on the northwestern border of Marion County, arriving there in 1853. He soon began practice and before many months had elapsed he had gained the confidence and respect of the community.

About 1859 Dr. Hunter was married to Sallie Fleming, daughter of John Fleming, a plantation owner near Wacahoota. To this marriage was born a son, George Baxter Jr., who died on August 16, 1867, at the age of three years and 10 months.[4]

Owing to the delicate state of his health Dr. Hunter was not conscripted into Confederate military service. There is evidence, however, that he was active in the civic affairs of the community. He was much involved in the efforts of the local citizens to obtain railroad transportation for Marion County.[5]

Upon reaching what should have been the best years of his life Dr. Hunter was struck down by the disease that had plagued him throughout his career, his death coming on October 12, 1865, a mere two months after his 35th birthday. His death evoked a wave of sorrow throughout the community. The Gainesville *New Era* noted his demise in two issues,[6] the second included the following estimate of the man: "He practiced up to the time of his death with benefit to the people and credit to himself...The community lost an excellent physician and a good citizen...The Doctor was a gentleman of superior education, good talents, and amiable disposition."[7]

In November following Dr. Hunter's death his widow, administratrix of his estate published the following notice:[8]

> To be sold at the residence of John Fleming, near Wacahoota, December 20th, house and lot of Dr. George B. Hunter, horse, cattle, hogs, household and kitchen furniture, Medical Library, Surgical Instruments—sold on credit. S.W. Hunter, Admx. Wacahoota.

But the times being difficult, the sale was delayed. In May 1867 the following notice appeared:[9]

> Important to physicians in search of a Location. The house and lot at Wacahoota where the late Dr. Hunter lived...is for sale. There is no better location for a physician or merchant in Florida.

1. Gainesville *New Era*, November 4, 1865.
2. Archives, University of Virginia, Lists of Students.
3. Jefferson Medical College, Philadelphia, Pa., "List of Dead or Lost Graduates in Classes from 1826 to 1879," p. 77.
4. Gainesville *New Era*, September 7, 1867.
5. Fernandina *East Floridian*, June 23, 1859.
6. Gainesville *New Era*, October 21, 1865; ibid., November 4, 1865.
7. Ibid., November 4, 1865.
8. Ibid., December 9, 1865.
9. Ibid., May 12, 1867.

Hunter, Green H., Lake City, 1860

Dr. Hunter, a Georgia native, received his medical degree from the Georgia Medical College, Augusta, in 1851,[1] whereupon he appears to have entered practice in Georgia where he remained for some nine years.[2] He arrived in Lake City too late to have been included in the census count of 1860 but in time to enlist in the newly organized 3rd Florida Infantry Regiment on July 3, 1861.[3] He joined his regiment at Ft. Clinch, Fernandina, the following month with the rank of 3rd lieutenant, remaining with this regiment until the following May, although spending much of his time on detached service in Tallahassee with the Commissary Department. He had enlisted for a 12-month period and although he had been promoted to the rank of brevet 2nd lieutenant on May 8, 1862, he declined any extension of his term of service.

On September 2, 1862, the following item appeared in the *Florida Sentinel*, Tallahassee:

> The citizens of Lake City have raised a thousand dollars and Mrs. Governor Reid, General M. Whit Smith and Dr. Green H. Hunter have volunteered their services to go and attend the sick in Virginia. They have been there for some time ministering to the wants of the soldiers, and are exerting themselves to establish a hospital in Richmond for the Florida Regiments.

Further information indicates that the hospital was successfully established. Subsequent to his participation in this civilian effort, Dr. Hunter joined the 9th Florida Infantry Regiment on February 11, 1863, for the duration of the war.

His rank was that of 1st Lieutenant. Later in the year he accompanied his unit northward into the combat zone near Petersburg and on June 3, 1864, was seriously wounded in a minor skirmish known as the Battle of Gaines Farm. A bullet penetrated the back of his right shoulder joint coming out in front above the right clavicle, disabling his right arm. A Medical Examining Board composed of Drs. Abel S. Baldwin (surgeon), John L'Engle (assistant surgeon), and Malcolm (assistant surgeon) on October 7, 1864, recommended his discharge. On December 17, 1863, he had been promoted to captain.

Prior to his discharge Dr. Hunter's name had been placed on the ballot as a candidate for the House of Representatives from Columbia and Suwannee Counties. He was elected on October 3, 1864, and served for the session of 1864.

With the war behind him but still carrying the damaged right arm, Dr. Hunter settled down to the practice of medicine in Lake City. From his marriage about 1860 a son had been born.[4] The boy, an only child named Joseph Howell, grew up to join his father in operating a drug store,[5] an establishment which lasted well into the 20th century. Dr. Hunter continued to live in Lake City until his death, the date of which has not been determined.

1. *Medical Department, University of Georgia, List of Graduates,* Augusta, 1890, p. 19.
2. No record has been uncovered which might place him in Florida before 1860.
3. U.S., AGO., CSR., M251, Roll 59. All information relating to Dr. Hunter's military service has been gleaned from documents contained in this collection.
4. U.S. Census, Columbia County, schedules for 1870 and 1880.
5. Lake City *Reporter,* May 8, 1885. This issue advertised "Triple Extracts at Dr. Hunter and Son's."

Hunter, James, Leon County, 1810

Dr. Hunter, a native of eastern North Carolina, migrated to Leon County about 1835. He had previously married Sarah Branch, second daughter of Governor John Branch.[1] Their eldest child, Eliza, had been born in North Carolina. The Hunters purchased a plantation some six miles northeast of Tallahassee on the Meridian Road to which they gave the name "Hickory Hill." Dr. Hunter's professional notice first appeared in the summer of 1835,[2] but there is little evidence that medicine ever became his full-time occupation. Instead he turned to farming at which he was apparently successful. His slaves numbered 45 in 1850. The census of 1850 lists him only as "planter."[3]

After they had settled in Florida five additional children were born to the Hunters, viz., Martha, Rebecca, Josephine, James B. and Mary.[4]

1. Susan Bradford Eppes, *Through Some Eventful Years,* Facs. Ed., Gainesville, 1868, genealogical table facing p. xxviii.
2. Tallahassee *Floridian,* June 27, 1835.
3. U.S. Census, 1850, Leon County, Florida, p. 137.
4. Ibid.

Hunter, John M.G., Quincy and Apalachicola, 1805-1880

Dr. Hunter, a native of Virginia, moved to Quincy about 1829 soon after the town had been incorporated. The Census of 1830 indicates that he was married but without children. His slaves numbered five.[1] Ten years later, however, his household included five children among whom were twins.[2] Very little is known of Dr. Hunter's activities during the first decade of his Florida residence, although it is apparent that he was a respected member of the community. In 1829 he was among the group of practitioners requesting President Andrew Jackson to take measures to safeguard land titles held by purchasers of tracts within the Forbes Grant.[3] More significant, however, was his election as one of four Gadsden County representatives at the historic St. Joseph Constitutional Convention in December 1838.[4] Two years later he was a member of the Gadsden Committee organized to press for statehood for Florida.[5] In 1842 he was elected colonel in the Gadsden militia regiment.[6] He joined a group of Middle Florida physicians meeting in Quincy in 1848 to organize a state medical society.[7]

In an unexplained move Dr. Hunter left Quincy about 1849 for a brief sojourn in Calhoun County. The census of the following year lists him as "phisition," a native of Georgia (an obvious error) with a wife, Elizabeth, and seven children.[8] By 1856 he had established his practice in Apalachicola and announced his location "over H.F. Abell's Drug Store, Corner of Commerce and Chestnut."[9] Two years later he was still at that address.[10]

Dr. Hunter was too advanced in years to become directly involved in military service during the Civil War. He continued to practice in Apalachicola where his services were much needed. In early 1863 the State Treasurer was authorized to disburse to him $60 for assistance in postmortem examinations.[11] The Census of 1870 lists Dr. Hunter sharing his house with his eldest daughter, Anna.[12] Since he does not appear in the Census of 1880, it is assumed that he had died prior to that date.[13]

1. U.S. Census, 1830, Gadsden County, Florida, p. 148.
2. Ibid., 1840, p. 97.
3. TP, XXIV, 159.
4. Apalachicola *Gazette*, December 8, 1838. The Gadsden delegation of four included three physicians: Banks Meacham, John W. Malone, and Hunter. The fourth was Samuel B. Stephens.
5. Quincy *Sentinel*, December 4, 1840.
6. Tallahassee *Florida Sentinel*, July 22, 1842.
7. Quincy *Times*, May 20, 1848.
8. U.S. Census, 1850, Calhoun County, Florida, p. 63. In all other censuses Dr. Hunter is listed as a native of Virginia. His children and their ages were: Anna, 18; Nathaniel, 17; Adam, 15; Marthey (Martha), 15; Elizabeth, 5; Marianna, 3; Jane, 3.
9. Apalachicola *Commercial Advertiser*, December 3, 1856.
10. Ibid., March 10, 1858.
11. Tallahassee *Florida Sentinel*, February 24, 1863.
12. U.S. Census, 1870, Franklin County, Florida, item 114. It appears that Anna was never married. In the 1880 census she appears as the head of the household, sharing the residence with her sister Elizabeth and brother-in-law F.E. Harrison, and their son William, aged 12.
13. Both Hunter sons, Nathaniel and Adam, were among the earlier volunteers for military service, both receiving commissions as officers in infantry regiments.

Hutchins, Joseph, Pensacola, 1834

Dr. Hutchins is thought to have arrived in Pensacola in late 1832. Although a native of Philadelphia he does appear to have been a graduate of either Jefferson Medical College or the University of Pennsylvania School of Medicine. Soon after settling in Pensacola he formed a partnership with George F. Baltzell for the operation of a drug store, an arrangement which was terminated by mutual consent in April 1833.[1] On April 8 Dr. Hutchins married Margaret McPherson.[2]

Dr. Hutchins' brief career ended with his death on September 15, 1834.[3] His erstwhile partner, George Baltzell,[4] was named executor of his estate and on November 1, he called upon all Dr. Hutchins' creditors and debtors to respond so that the settlement of the estate could be concluded.[5] Simultaneously it was announced that "The Drug Store formerly occupied by Dr. Joseph Hutchins is again open and under the superintendence of a person well acquainted with business."[6]

1. The store was located on Palafox Street. Pensacola *Gazette*, April 11, 1833.
2. Ibid.
3. Ibid., September 20, 1834.
4. Ibid., November 1, 1834. Baltzell was at the time Clerk of Escambia County Superior Court. He later studied medicine and in 1850 was a medical practitioner in Washington County. See Washington County Census, 1850.
5. Ibid.
6. Ibid.

Hyams, Moses S., Duval County, 1814

Dr. Hyams, member of a prominent Jewish family of Charleston, South Carolina, and an 1834 graduate of the Medical College of South Carolina,[1] established his medical practice in Jacksonville prior to 1840. Soon after his arrival he became the proprietor of a drug store from which he carried on his practice. In April 1840 he advertised that he had added a "soda water fountain...and now offers...that cool and pleasant beverage, pure from the fountain, with all kinds of syrups."[2]

A year or so later Dr. Hyams settled in the Black Creek community in what is now Clay County. There he presided at a meeting on July 11, 1843, called for the purpose of nominating a candidate to represent Duval County in the Florida Legislative Council. Benjamin Frisbee was the nominee.[3]

Nothing further has been learned of this physician.[4]

1. Charleston *Courier*, March 10, 1834. His doctoral thesis was entitled "Inflammation."
2. Jacksonville *East Florida Advocate*, June 16, 1840.
3. St. Augustine *Florida Herald and Southern Democrat*, July 24, 1843.
4. Some confusion exists as to the precise identity of Dr. Moses Hyams. The 1850 Census of Duval County lists a Mordecai Heims, druggist, as a resident of Black Creek District. Ten years later he appears in the census of Clay County (into which a portion of Duval was incorporated) as M.E. Hymes, druggist, aged 40. By this date he and his wife, German-born Caroline, were the parents of three sons and a daughter. With the advent of war in 1861, Mordecai enlisted for service in the Confederate Army as a private in the 2nd Florida Infantry Regiment. He served for about nine months in the Regiment's medical department before being discharged for reasons of health at Yorktown, Virginia, on April 15, 1862. The question remains, Were Mordecai and Moses the same person? If not what was their relationship?

Ingle, James, Jacksonville, 1870

Dr. Ingle,[1] a native of South Carolina, was a brief sojourner in Jacksonville about 1870. The Duval Census of that year gives his age as 31. His property was valued at a mere $300. He was apparently the only person living in his household. No further information on this doctor has been located.

1. U.S. Census, 1870, Duval County, Florida, item 388.

Irvine, Osmund B., Marion County, 1805-1860

Dr. Irvine, who spent the latter years of his professional life in the northern part of Marion County, was born in North Carolina in 1805.[1] Nothing is presently known of his childhood and youth nor has any information concerning his education, either general or professional, emerged. Since his name does not appear in the student rosters of any of the major medical colleges of the South during the mid-19th century, it is suspected that he was trained for his profession through the apprenticeship system.

Dr. Irvine appears in the 1850 Census of Greenville County, South Carolina, as "physician," aged 45, and owner of property valued at $10,000. His wife, Frances McMahan, whom he appears to have married when she was only 15, was a native of South Carolina, presumably born in Greenville County. By 1850 four children had been born, Pinckney, nine; daughter Frances, six; son Dixon, five; and a daughter Maryanna, one. All were natives of South Carolina. Ten years later the census of Marion County included the names of three additional children, daughter Adelia, and sons W.H. and F.H., born in Florida.[2]

By 1860 Dr. Irvine could look with satisfaction, even pride, upon his career. He was a planter, owning property, real and personal, valued at more than $65,000. His slaves numbered 37. His plantation, located on the west side of Orange Lake, in one of the most picturesque parts of Marion County, indicated a successful career. As for his medical practice, nothing is known, although it was doubtless confined to his plantation and the neighborhood. The management of the plantation was left to an employed overseer, Irish-born James Stewart.[3]

The woes of the Civil War doubtless dealt a devastating blow to Dr. Irvine. The date of his death, notwithstanding his prominence in the community and in Marion County generally, has not been discovered. One would assume that he would have been buried in Millwood Cemetery near the Irvine plantation where his two eldest sons, Dixon Hill and Daniel Pinckney, were buried but no gravestone has been discovered. Perhaps his death occurred during the Civil War or Reconstruction at a time when there may have been insufficient funds for such extravagance and in the years following the War the family never "got around to" erecting a gravestone.

As for the surviving children, Dickson Hill remained on the Irvine plantation where he died on January 19, 1929, at the age of 82.[4] He is said to have owned a beautiful home which, after his death, was converted into a home for retired railroad employees. His funeral services were held in Grace Episcopal Church, Ocala. Daniel Pinckney was never married and is presumed to have remained on the plantation where he died on October 19, 1871. He was also buried in Millwood Cemetery. As for the other Irvine children, no effort has been made to determine their dates of death nor their places of burial.

It should be added that the Irvine name has been perpetuated by the establishment of a post office near the plantation house on December 12, 1871. It was discontinued on February 4, 1872, reestablished on February 10, 1875, and discontinued on March 22, 1876. It was reestablished on June 23, 1896, and is still in existence.

1. U.S. Census, 1850, Greenville County, S.C., p. 478.
2. Ibid, p. 206.
3. Ibid.
4. Ocala *Banner*, January 25, 1929.

Irwin, Henry, Jackson County, mid-19th century

Dr. Irwin remains a somewhat obscure member of the medical profession. Born in Ireland about 1795, he arrived in America in the mid-1820s, settling first in North Carolina where he met and married his wife, Mary, and where his first three children, Arabella, William H., and Robert, were born.[1] About 1840 he moved to Georgia, where three additional children, Lorenzo, C.C., and John, were born.[2] Although the censuses of 1850 and 1860 designate him Doctor of Medicine, there is no reliable evidence that he was a regular practitioner.

No gravestone for Dr. Irwin is listed in the Jackson County Cemetery Survey.[3]

1. U.S. Census, 1850, Jackson County, Florida, p. 577.
2. Ibid., 1860, item 838.
3. Doris E. Pamphilon, compiler, *Cemeteries of Jackson County, Florida*, Vol. I (1984).

Jackson, James Maxwell, Levy, Orange and Hamilton Counties, 1828-1911

The role of the beloved and trusted country doctor, noble in bearing, gentle and compassionate in manner, is exemplified in the career of Dr. Jackson who for the greater part of his professional life served the people of Levy County. Born in Chester District, South Carolina, in 1828[1] into a family of moderate means, he received his basic education in the local schools. He subsequently enrolled at the Medical College of New Orleans, later to become a part of Tulane University, from which he received his medical degree in 1856.

Leaving his younger brother to take care of their aging mother and her farming interests,[2] he settled at White Springs, Florida, a popular spa in the latter part of the 19th century.[3] There he was married in 1858 to Mary Glenn Shands, a native of Spartanburg, South Carolina.[4] Soon thereafter they moved to the Mellonville community of Orange County where the census enumerator found them in 1860. At that time Dr. Jackson was the only qualified physician in the county.

By 1861 the Jacksons were again living at White Springs. With the outbreak of war in 1861 Dr. Jackson responded to the call by enlisting as a private in Company E, First Florida Cavalry, and was mustered in on November 14, 1861, committing himself to 12 months of service while providing his own horse and saddle valued at $190. In March 1862 he was placed on detached service at Camp Mary David, as assembly area six miles south of Tallahassee. A few weeks later he was with his regiment near Chattanooga, Tennessee, where he was discharged "by substitution" to return to Florida and private practice.[5]

In the critical year 1864, Dr. Jackson reentered the military service and was commissioned an assistant surgeon in the independent company of Capt. E.J. Lutterloh who commanded a small cavalry unit at Clay Landing.[6] He remained there until the end of the war after which he returned to White Springs where his only son, James M., Jr., was born on March 10, 1868.[7] Two daughters had died in early childhood. Two years later Dr. Jackson moved to Levy County, settling in the village of Bronson, where he remained for the remainder of his professional career.

Dr. Jackson's routine daily practice remains only scantly documented. In the occasional issues of Levy County papers which have survived there are occasional professional notices of Dr. Jackson. More frequently are advertisements of the numerous patent medicine in his well-stocked drug store. As was customary these advertisements were often interspersed with social items and other news of the community.[8] When the Levy County *Times* of April 1, 1886, published a lengthy account of Bronson and its attractions and advantages, Dr. Jackson was portrayed as "the big-hearted Mayor of the Town." In addition to his stint as mayor, Dr. Jackson was postmaster from March 11, 1873, until July 16, 1874.[9] For several years he was superintendent of the Bronson Methodist Sunday School.[10] Even though he resided in a rural area, remote from the main centers of medical professionalism, Dr. Jackson was ever interested in improving the quality of medical education and medical practice. In 1881 he attended the meeting of the Florida Medical Association in Tallahassee and subsequently was accepted for membership and elected second vice president.[11] He attended only one other meeting, that of 1897 in Palatka, when he joined his son, James M. Jackson Jr., who had recently entered practice in Miami. Nevertheless, he continued to pay his annual dues to the Association almost to the time of his death.

Soon after the death of his wife on March 30, 1907, Dr. Jackson went to Miami to live with his son. He died there before dawn on May 11, 1911, at the age of 83. His body was returned to Bronson for burial.[12]

1. George M. Chapin, *Florida, Past, Present and Future*, 2 vols., Chicago 1914, II, 48. Of the several dates for the birth of Dr. Jackson, the year 1828 seems the correct one since it was provided by his son for an obituary notice.
2. U.S. Census, 1850, Chester District, S.C., p.19. Here Dr. Jackson at age 24, a farmer, is living with his widowed mother, Esther, whose property was valued at $33,000.
3. Chapin, op. cit. These springs, known also as White Sulphur Springs, continued to attract visitors well into the 20th century.
4. William M. Straight, "James M. Jackson, Jr., Miami's First Physician," Journal Florida Medical Asociation, August 1972, pp. 54-62.
5. NA, Service Records, CSA, M251, Roll 2.
6. *Soldiers of Florida*, Live Oak, 1903, p. 320. Clay Landing, situated on the east bank of the Suwannee River, some 12 miles from its mouth, was a minor military post, later achieving some commercial importance as a shipping point for pine products.
7. Straight, op. cit. This son was destined to become one of Florida's most eminent physicians and civic leaders. After practicing briefly in Bronson he removed to Miami where he remained for the remainder of his life. Miami's Jackson Memorial Hospital was named in his honor.
8. See e.g., Bronson *Weekly Artery*, October 24, 1874, and the Bronson *Levy County Times*, April 20, 1893.
9. Ruth Verrill, *Romantic and Historic Levy County*, Gainesville, 1976, p. 71.
10. Levy County *Times-Democrat*, October 3, 1895. Dr. Jackson also served as a county commissioner for Levy County, 1879-81.
11. *Proceedings, Florida Medical Association*, 1881, p. 4.
12. Miami *Daily Metropolis*, May 11, 1911, Miami *Herald*, May 12, 1911.

Jackson, Robert, Tampa Bay, 1802-1865

Dr. Jackson, one of the first American born physicians to settle in the Tampa Bay area, was born in Philadelphia, Pennsylvania, on May 2, 1802. He was the son of Robert and Euphemia (nee Parker) Jackson, the former a civil engineer said to have assisted in construction of Ft. Moultrie, Charleston, S.C.[1] Little is known of his early childhood and youth. Family tradition maintained that he had been a cadet at the United States Military Academy, West Point, but no confirmation of this claim has been discovered. Although nothing is known of his medical training it is very probable that he had served as an apothecary's apprentice. At any rate, when he appeared at Ft. Brooke (Tampa) in 1834, he was employed as hospital steward and intern.[2] Another source identifies him as a "compounder of medicines and surgeon's chief steward."[3] In this capacity he served as an associate of Dr. Robert Crooke Wood, assistant surgeon at Ft. Brooke.[4]

Meanwhile the Coller family, whose head was Levi Coller, moved into Florida. The family had lived on the north side of the St. Mary's River in Camden County, Georgia, but to escape marauding Indians had moved across the river into Florida. Discouraged with the quality of land they moved farther south, homesteading for a while in Alachua County before moving to Tampa Bay about 1822. There they laid claim to a tract on the east bank of the Hillsborough River near its entrance into the Bay. This land was a choice property and soon appropriated by the United States Government as the site for Ft. Brooke. This forced the Collers to move up-river a short distance where they resumed farming operation, selling fruit and vegetables to the Fort's quartermaster.

A deadly fever struck the area in 1834 and among its victims were four of the Coller children. Mrs. Coller, also desperately ill, was said to have been attended by the recently-arrived Dr. Robert Jackson, in the course of which he made the acquaintance of Nancy Coller whom he married in September 1836. The wedding was performed in the office of Judge Augustus Steele, one of Florida's most prominent citizens, who would later play an important role in the development of Cedar Keys.

In 1838 Dr. Jackson resigned his position at the Fort and moved across the Hillsborough River to its west bank where he homesteaded on a tract of 160 acres, a portion of which came to be known as Jackson's Point and more recently Hyde Park. He appears to have prospered as a grower of farm produce for which he found a ready market. He became a popular and trusted citizen of the area soon to be elected to the judgeship of Hillsborough Probate Court, a position he held for many years. The family's comfort and happiness suffered a severe shock when in September 1848 a hurricane swept the area and the accompanying tidal wave completely destroyed the Jackson home, nearly claiming the lives of Mrs. Jackson and her small baby.[5] From that time until the start of the Civil War the Jacksons were busy reorganizing their lives and replacing their home. During these years Dr. Jackson was often called into consultation with other physicians facing difficult cases.

When war came in 1861 two of the Jackson sons enlisted in the Confederate Army. Oscar, the eldest son, living in Georgia, joined a Georgia unit, while John Brown, eight years younger, enlisted in Company K, 7th Florida Infantry Regiment. Dr. Jackson himself, although already in failing health, joined the Tampa Home Guard. On March 2, 1865, he succumbed to the illness and was buried in Oaklawn Cemetery. A younger son, Parker, died in late 1865.

The union of Robert and Nancy Jackson was blessed with 11 children, four of whom died of fever at an early age. The other seven survived their father, Parker by only eight or nine months. Four sons lived out their lives in the Tampa area; all were prominent in business and public service in the community. Mrs. Jackson, the highly respected matriarch of the family, died on March 24, 1907, at the age of 92. The Jackson daughters married into prominent Florida families and like their brothers were the ancestors of many present-day Floridians.[6]

1. The principal sources of biographic data on the Jackson family are two interviews granted by Mrs. Jackson in her later years. The first, "Pioneer Women in Tampa Lived Dangerous Lives," recorded by the Honorable B.D. McKay, well-known Tampa journalist, was published in the Tampa *Tribune* of February 16, 1947. The other, "Nancy Jackson, 1815-1907," based on an interview with Mrs. Jackson recorded in 1900 by Cynthia K. Farr and presented in an article prepared by Martha Lester Nelson, a direct descendant of Dr. Jackson, and published in *The Sunland Tribune*, Tampa Historical Society, Vol. IX, December 1983, pp. 22-25. For further information see Charles E. Harrison, et al, *Genealogical Records of the Pioneers of Tampa*, Tampa, 1915, pp. 62-66.

2. Harrison, *Gen. Recs.*, p. 62.

3. Nelson, "Nancy Jackson," pp. 22-23.

4. Some confusion exists regarding the association of Dr. Jackson with Dr. Wood. There is no doubt that they were acquaintances, probably close friends. The question arises as to the date at which they became acquainted. Mrs. Jackson remembered Dr. Wood as present at her wedding in 1836 but he, son-in-law of General Zachary Taylor and medical officer at Ft. Brooke under Taylor's command, does not appear in Florida until 1837. Mrs. Jackson also recalled that both the Taylors and the Woods had sent wedding gifts. Of course these could have been presented to the recently-wedded couple at a later date. This question is left unanswered for who is to say that Mrs. Jackson did not recall the date and other details of her own wedding.

5. This baby was William Parker Jackson, an infant at the time of the storm.

6. The Jackson home still stands today at 205 Platt Street in the Hyde Park area.

Jackson, Samuel, Newnansville, 1870

Dr. Jackson, born in South Carolina, was a resident of the Newnansville community in 1870.[1] His property, real and personal, was valued at $1,000. Residing in his household were Jane Bashaw, born in Georgia, and two Bashaw children, Sallie, aged three, and Julia, aged 17, who were probably relatives of Dr. Jackson. Nothing more is known of this physician.

1. U.S. Census, 1870, Alachua County, Florida, p. 326, item 2969.

Jackson, S.H., Hamilton and Madison Counties, 1860s

The Hamilton County Census of 1860 lists Dr. Jackson as a medical practitioner, native of South Carolina, aged 24, and resident in the home of F.T. Wilson, a merchant, also born in South Carolina.[1] Six years later he joined Dr. R.H. Shaffer in a professional partnership in the town of Madison. Their notice first appeared in the local newspaper on March 6, 1866.[2] No further information on Dr. Jackson has been discovered.[3]

1. U.S. Census, 1860, Hamilton County, Florida p. 35, item 240.
2. Madison *Southern Messenger*, April 20, 1866. The issue of March 6th no longer exists.
3. Records of Floridians serving in the Army of the Confederacy do not include S.H. Jackson nor does the Florida Census of 1870.

Jackson, Theophilus Hardee, Liberty County, 1836-1917

Dr. Jackson, a native of Georgia, was born in October 1836.[1] By 1859 he was living in Liberty County, a resident in the home of John McCray, a farmer whose homestead was located in the Aspalaga community, although the post office was on the north side of the county line in Gadsden County. In the fall of 1859 he entered Oglethorpe Medical College, Savannah, from which he was graduated on January 28, 1861.[2] Although his Confederate Service Record is incomplete, he appears to have enlisted almost immediately after receiving his medical degree, joining Company A, Fourth Florida Infantry Regiment, without military rank. He subsequently served also in Company H, Fifth Florida Infantry, and later in Company A, Second Florida Cavalry, from which he was mustered out on April 26, 1865.[3]

At some unknown date in 1862, Dr. Jackson was married to a native of South Carolina known only as Nancy, 10 years his junior. The year 1870 found them living in the village of Rock Bluff, some 10 miles north of Bristol, the seat of Liberty County. They had 13 children but by 1900 only seven survived.[4]

At some time after the Civil War Dr. Jackson had acquired a tract of land in Liberty County shown in the Special Census of 1885[5] to have been 1,500 acres, of which only about 40 were under cultivation with an additional portion devoted to grazing. In this instance his occupation is listed only as farming although in the Mortality Schedule for the County that year he was the attending physician of two person who had died, so it is assumed that he attended others who had not died. The Census of 1900, however, lists him as "physician and farmer."[6] Apparently his sons were the farm laborers of the family. The list of Florida physicians practicing in 1893 indicates that he was Liberty County's only practitioner at that date although a Dr. Carson had practiced there earlier.[7]

Dr. Jackson died at his farm home near the village of Rock Bluff in 1917 and was buried in the Rock Bluff cemetery, situated "one half mile west of the post office."[8]

1. U.S. Census, 1900, Liberty County, Florida, p. 11, item 223. Ibid., 1860, item 71.
2. Savannah *Daily Morning News*, March 1, 1861.
3. *Soldiers of Florida in the Seminole Indian, Civil, and Spanish-American Wars*, Live Oak, 1903, pp. 121, 149 and 262.
4. The surviving children: Sarah, Frank, Theophilus Jr., Saphronia, Clara, Clark, and Ross.
5. See Special Florida Census, 1885, Liberty County, Agriculture and Mortality Schedules, and Schedule of Inhabitants, p. 21.
6. See note 1, supra.
7. Dr. L.D. Carson, a native of South Carolina.
8. *Liberty County Veterans' Graves Registration Project*, St. Augustine, 1940-41, p. 15.

James, Thomas E., Liberty and Gadsden Counties, 1835-1892

Dr. James, a native of Norfolk, Virginia, was born about 1835. As a recent graduate of medical school he migrated to Florida in 1857 and settled in the village of Bristol in Liberty County. The circumstances relating to his decision to make this move as well as those which greeted him upon his arrival were recalled with amusement by Dr. Charles A. Hentz who had recently moved to Quincy from Ochesee, a short distance upriver from Bristol. It appears that the community was without a physician. A local cotton grower and warehouse owner, Matthew McAliley, placed advertisements in several newspapers inviting any physician interested in settling in the area to contact him. Several responded to the advertisement which had described Bristol in glowing terms. It lay "at the head of sloop navigation" and among its many attractions were "a courthouse, stores, a blacksmith, etc." Of the several who answered the call McAliley chose Dr. James, a young graduate "whose penmanship and style were the most promising."[1]

Dr. James' arrival in Bristol was most inauspicious. The steamer on which he had come up the Apalachicola River docked on the bluff in the middle of a dark and dismal night. McAliley, whose house was some distance away, was asleep and did not hear the boat whistle. Dr. James, yelling as loudly as he could, failed to arouse anyone so he sat on his trunk the balance of the night, as Dr. Hentz told it, "listening to the raccoons and the owls, and straining his eyes for the sight of the stores, sloops, courthouse, offices, etc., of the flourishing city." With dawn came total disillusionment. But, says Dr. Hentz, "James was full of grit, and staid, and did well."

In 1858, Dr. James married Emma Hudnall, daughter of Willis Hudnall, a farmer of some substance. They had three sons and two daughters.[2]

Due to remoteness of the area and the absence of newspapers, there are only occasional glimpses of Dr. James as a local practitioner. Early on the morning of April 29, 1860, the steamer, *John C. Calhoun*, making its way upriver from Apalachicola to Chattahoochee, "while rounding out from Ridleysville (Bristol Landing)...exploded and burned." Several of the crew were killed. "In attendance, rendering aid, was Dr. T.E. James, of Bristol, using every exertion to save and relieve the sufferers that he possibly could."[3]

On another occasion he was called to the home of James Evans, son-in-law of Dr. William Booth of Quincy and, therefore, Dr. Hentz's brother-in-law, to attend the illness of Evans' little daughter, Eva. Meanwhile Dr. Hentz, not noted for modesty when it was a matter of his medical skills, arrived on the scene. He reported: "It was well that I came...for Dr. James did not know how to treat the disease," pneumonia.[4]

By 1870 the James family had moved to Midway in the southeastern part of Gadsden County where the doctor and his wife lived out their days although Mrs. James in the meantime had inherited her father's plantation. Of his extra professional activities it is known only that in 1880 he was a trustee of the local Midway common, i.e., public, school.[5] Since Dr. James is not listed in the directory of Florida practitioners of medicine in 1892, it is assumed that he had died by that date.

1. Charles A. Hentz, "Autobiography," typed copy of a transcription, original in Southern Historical Collection, University of North Carolina, Chapel Hill, I, 229.

2. The James children were Virginius eldest son, who is listed in the 1860 Census as Virginia, a daughter. This is corrected, however, in the census of 1870; the others were Stephen, Sue, Emma, and Thomas E., Jr.

3. Monticello *Family Friend,* May 12, 1860.

4. Hentz, "Autobiography," I, 342. Dr. Hentz was generally unrestrained in recording estimates of his medical colleagues.

5. Miles Kenan Womack Jr., *Gadsden: A Florida County in Word and Picture,* Quincy, 1870, p. 90.

Jane, R., Newnansville, 1856

Dr. Jane scarcely merits inclusion in a roster of active physicians who practiced in Florida in the mid-19th century. He is recognized only because he was a delegate at the Newnansville Court House for a meeting of Democrats on May 13, 1856, assembled for the purpose of ratifying the action taken at the State Democratic Convention, held in Madison, Florida, in April 1856. The Committee readily endorsed the action taken at the Convention.[1]

1. Jacksonville *Florida News,* May 24, 1856. Dr. George B. Payne was also in attendance at the meeting. The others, all prominent in public affairs of the county, were Colonel J.C. Pelot, John B. Stanley, W.F. Perry, E.N. Adkins, V.R. Prescott, and Colonel E. Earle.

Jarrott, Richard, Gadsden County, 1810

Dr. Jarrott, a brief sojourner in Florida but one of its most eminent antebellum practitioners, was born in Fayetteville, North Carolina, in 1810.[1] About 1830 his sister, Elizabeth, and her husband, Carter T. Baughn, moved from Fayetteville to Williamsburg District, South Carolina, settling in the little town of Kingstree.[2] They were joined by Richard who began the study of medicine under the preceptorate of local physician, W.S. Burgess.[3] In the fall of 1832 he matriculated at the Medical College of South Carolina from which he was graduated in March 1834 after submitting a thesis entitled "Incubus," a subject which suggests that he may have had an interest in psychiatry.[4] So excellent was his academic record that he was chosen by the students and faculty to deliver the valedictory address. As reported in the Charleston *Southern Patriot,* "the oration of this gentleman, as had been anticipated, was pleasingly and touchingly written, and amply confirmed the propriety of his selection."[5]

Following graduation Dr. Jarrott returned to Kingstree and entered the practice of his profession. Like many physicians of the 19th century he supplemented his income by running a drug store, an enterprise in which he was joined by his brother-in-law, Carter T. Baughn. Their business was soon expanded into a general merchandise store, occupying the ground floor of the old Williamsburg courthouse, with the Baughn family residing in the upper story. At about the same time these Fayetteville natives were joined by Dr. Jarrott's brother, John M., who opened a shop in what had earlier been the county jail.[6]

Dr. Jarrott's business and professional enterprises apparently prospered. Dr.Samuel D. McGill, historian of Williamsburg County, wrote: "Dr. Richard Jarrott, a most remarkable man for his intelligence and dignity, was for many years the most prominent among our physicians."[7] At the full tide of his success Dr. Jarrott married Louisa E. Shaw, a Kingstree girl, some 10 years his junior. As Dr. McGill recalled, she was endowed with "ample property," being the daughter of Henry D. Shaw, one of the country's wealthiest planters and owner of 65 slaves in 1840.[8] The young couple proceeded to build "a handsome residence on Vinegar Hill," presumably Kingstree's most desirable location. Meanwhile Dr. Jarrott had acquired additional properties in the town.[9]

In addition to his business and professional responsibilities Dr. Jarrott found time to supervise the medical apprenticeships of Kingstree youths bent on becoming physicians. At least one of his protégés, Samuel Singletary, was an 1841 graduate of the Medical College of South Carolina.[10] He was also an active member of the Williamsburg Presbyterian Church, his last appearance in church records bears the date December 31, 1844.[11]

In the 1840s, with Indian hostilities in abeyance, the 2nd Seminole War had been concluded in 1842, and vast tracts of fairly cheap land available, many South Carolinians were induced to uproot themselves and venture to Florida. Middle Florida, as it was designated, that is, the area between the Suwannee and Apalachicola Rivers, was especially attractive. About 1846 Dr. Jarrott's brother, John M. Jarrott, whose wife was Georgianna Witherspoon of Kingstree, moved to Quincy, the seat of Gadsden County, and established a cotton-ginning business. Before the end of 1846 Dr. Jarrott, his wife and three small children had moved to Quincy.[12]

Dr. Jarrott announced his services to the people of the Quincy community on May 18, 1847, with the reassuring statement that he had been "constantly engaged during the last twelve years in the practice of his profession in South Carolina...and flatters himself that he is familiar with the characteristics and modes of treatment of the prevailing diseases of the South." His office was located "at the New Drug Store of Dr. W.L. Davis & Co., next door to the Marshall House."[13] He could also be reached at his residence, "the place belonging to the estate of Stephens (Godfrey)" a half mile from Quincy.[14] The estate was soon to pass into the hands of Samuel Stephens, a prominent Quincy attorney.

Dr. Jarrott's commitment to his profession was total. He appears to have been appalled at the low quality of the medical service he observed on his arrival in Florida. Procedures were slipshod for licensing physicians; practitioners of dubious qualifications were not uncommon. Worst of all there was no statewide professional organization which might have improved the situation. In mid-May 1848, a small but determined group of physicians from Gadsden, Leon, Jefferson, Calhoun and Jackson Counties, all in Middle Florida, met in Quincy for the purpose of organizing a state medical society. Although physicians throughout the state had been notified in advance and urged to be present, only 12 appeared. Five were from Gadsden County. At the first session Dr. Jarrott presided. He also participated in writing a charter for the proposed society. All was for nought, however, for the Legislature, meeting the following January, rejected the proposal by a single vote in the House, the negative vote being cast by a physician, the Senate having given its approval.[15] Florida must wait until 1874 for a state medical society.

Except for his professional activities little is known of the doctor's Quincy years. He is said to have been an active member of the Quincy Presbyterian Church.[16] Although a comparative newcomer he was present at a Fourth of July celebration in Quincy in 1847 where he offered a toast to the Orator of the Day, the distinguished Dr. John M.W. Davidson.[17] Being of the Whig persuasion he was present at a gathering of Gadsden Whigs in August 1850 at which the actions of the recent Nashville Convention were discussed. The tone of the meeting was nonconciliatory as far as the slave question was concerned. Dr. Jarrott ended the proceedings with a resolution that "The Southern Press newspaper at Washington is entitled to the support of the Southern Public."[18] Two years later he was among the Gadsden citizens offering tributes to Henry Clay, recently deceased.[19]

By 1854, for reasons unknown, the Jarrotts had moved to Baker County, Georgia, settling in the village of Milford.[20] For the family it appears to have been a time of comparative happiness and prosperity. Their four youngest children were born there, while their properties, personal for the greater part, were valued at nearly $20,000.

On the eve of the Civil War the Jarrotts moved once more, to adjoining Miller County, settling in the town of Colquitt, were the doctor resumed his medical practice. Henceforth their lives took an unfortunate turn. They did not escape the common hardships brought on by the War and the following Reconstruction. Shattering indeed were the deaths of five of their nine children during the decade of 1860s. These tragedies, combined with the collapse of his own health, left Dr. Jarrott a broken and desolate man. By 1870 his holdings were valued at a mere $400.[21]

The unhappiness of Dr. Jarrott's last years is reflected in a letter which he wrote on August 12, 1869, to his niece, Mrs. Charles Edward Jarrott of Florence County, South Carolina.[22] It was a reply, long overdue because of his illness, "a debilitating affection of haemophilia" which had kept him confined to bed and quite unable to write. He urged his niece and nephew to abandon the struggle against the lawlessness and general civil disorder attending Reconstruction in South Carolina and seek a better life in Texas whither his (Dr. Jarrott's) brother, Edward, had settled some years earlier. The sad letter ended with the lament for the loss of five of his children, "gone to the spirit world."

The Miller County Census of 1870 lists the Jarrott family reduced to four. Besides Dr. Jarrott, aged 60, and Mrs. Jarrott, aged 48, there were Arthur, aged 14, a farm laborer, and Roddy, aged nine, "at school."[23]

As a man of medicine Dr. Jarrott earned the respect of patients and colleagues alike. As a citizen he concerned himself with public issues and, although not known to have run for public office, participated in numerous discussions. As a Southerner of the land-owning class he held fast to the principles so eloquently enunciated by John C. Calhoun. It is likely, on the basis of two articles he contributed to the *Charleston Medical Journal and Review* in 1849,[24] that had he chosen to remain in South Carolina in close proximity to the medical faculty of Charleston he would have become a medical scholar of national importance.[25]

1. Dr. Richard Jarrott was the son of John Jarrott of Fayetteville, N.C., whose name appears in the Cumberland County, N.C., Censuses of 1810 and 1820.
2. Samuel D. McGill, M.D., *Narrative of Reminiscences in Williamsburg County*, Columbia, S.C., 1897, p. 243.
3. Lists of Graduates and Matriculants, Medical College of South Carolina, Waring Medical History Library, Charleston.
4. Report of Commencement of May 7, 1834, Charleston *Mercury*, May 8, 1834.
5. Charleston *Southern Patriot*, March 8, 1834.
6. McGill, *Narrative*, loc. cit.
7. Ibid., p. 245.
8. U.S. Census, 1840, Williamsburg County, S.C.
9. Deed Book E, Office of Clerk of Court, Williamsburg County, S.C., pp. 348, 542. When Dr. Jarrott left Kingstree in 1846, he appears to have mortgaged his Kingstree lots and never bothered to redeem them. Letter, William J. Cooper, Kingstree, S.C., to Emory J. Jarrott, March 14, 1983.
10. See note 3, supra.
11. See reference Cooper Letter, note 9, supra.
12. U.S. Census, 1850, Gadsden County, Florida, p. 356. Here three of the Jarrott children, Elizabeth, Richard and Miranda, are shown as South Carolina natives while the fourth, Clara, was born in Florida.
13. Tallahassee *Southern Journal*, May 18, 1847.
14. The Stephens family was one of prominence in Gadsden County. The elder Stephens, whose name was Godfrey, had settled there in the 1820s, obtaining large acreage in and around Quincy, and was an important figure in the early development of the area. His son, Samuel B., a man of great influence, was a successful attorney in Quincy and a member of the Florida House of Representatives in 1841, 1842 and 1848. The Stephens family moved to Florida from Cumberland County, N.C., and possibly account for the decision of the Jarrotts to move to Quincy. The fact that Dr. Jarrott resided on Stephens property seems to confirm this assumption. See Miles Kenan Womack, *Gadsden, A Florida County in Word and Picture*, 1948, no place, p. 13.
15. This effort to organize is well documented in the Quincy *Times*, May 29, 1848. The subsequent failure of the effort has been explored in detail in E. Ashby Hammond, "Medical Regulation and Organization in Florida, 1821-74," *Journal of the Florida Medical Association*, January 1974, pp. 62-70.
16. This assertion is not documentable due to destruction of Church records.
17. Tallahassee *Floridian*, July 17, 1847.
18. Jacksonville *Florida Republican*, August 15, 1850.
19. Quincy *Sentinel*, July 20, 1852.
20. U.S. Census, 1860, Baker County, Georgia. This date, possibly inaccurate, is an extrapolation based on the age of the sixth Jarrott child, J.E., who was six years old in 1860 and a native of Georgia.
21. U.S. Census, 1870, Miller County, Georgia, p. 6.
22. Mrs. Jarrott, nee Emma Engle Brown, was the wife of Charles Edward Jarrott, son of Dr. James Howard Jarrott.
23. This leaves two of the Jarrotts' nine children unaccounted for. It is assumed that they had married or for some other reason had left the household.
24. The two articles were: "Amputation for Gangrene of the Foot Successfully Performed on a Negro at the Advanced Age of One Hundred and Two Years," *Charleston Medical Journal and Review*, Vol. IV, No. 3, 1849, pp. 301-303, and "On the Sulphate of Iron in Chlorosis," ibid., pp. 553-559.
25. No date of death for either Dr. or Mrs. Jarrott has been discovered. It appears probable that they lived out their lives in Colquitt, Ga.

I am indebted to Emory L. Jarrott of Savannah for substantial data. He is a great-great-grandson of Dr. James Howard Jarrott, brother of Dr. Richard Jarrott. Dr. James Jarrott spent the greater part of his professional career in Florence and Darlington Counties, South Carolina.

Jelks, Edward A., Hamilton County, 1830

Although Dr. Jelks spent part of his youthful years in Hamilton County, Florida, it is doubtful that he ever practiced medicine in the state. Born in Georgia about 1830, son of Oliver and Margaret P. Jelks, he was brought to Bellville, Hamilton County, in the late 1840s or early 1850s.[1] As for his early education records of the Medical College of the State of South Carolina indicate that it was of a classical nature, meaning that he had exposure to some Latin and possibly a little Greek. He began his medical study under the guidance of local physician, Dr. Lewis E. Folsom, and in 1858 was enrolled at the College. He was graduated Doctor of Medicine on March 10, 1860, after submitting a thesis entitled "Tetanus."[2]

Nothing is known of Dr. Jelks' practice after 1860 except that he had chosen to live in Georgia. It has been discovered, however, that he invested in land in Orange County near Oviedo in Seminole County which he planted in citrus and that until the great freeze of the winter of 1894-95 had been a profitable venture. The date of his death has not been ascertained.[3]

1. Cora Hinton, comp., *Early History of Hamilton County, Florida*, 2nd ed., Jasper, 1983, pp. 93, 132.

2. "Catalogue, Medical College of the State of South Carolina," 1859-60, p. 417. See also Charleston *Daily Courier*, March 14, 1860.

3. Two members of the Department of History, University of Central Florida, Orlando, have discovered that Dr. Jelks, "a physician from Georgia," was one of several who invested in land in the Oviedo community of Orange County which they planted in citrus. Oviedo is now located in Seminole County. It was a profitable investment until the freeze of 1894-95. Dr. Jelks owned nearly 60 acres of orange groves which were producing "1700 boxes worth $2500." See Richard Adicks and Donna M. Neely, *Oviedo, Biography of a Town*, Oviedo, 1979, p. 21.

Jenkins, Charles J., Hamilton County, 1833

Except for vital data in the census schedule of 1860 very little is known of the life and career of Dr. Jenkins. A native of Georgia, he had settled in Jasper about 1857, married, was the father of a son and daughter, and owned property valued at almost $11,000.[1] His age was 27. He had barely established his medical practice when the War between the States began. In spite of domestic obligations, he enlisted in the Confederate cause and was mustered into service on December 3, 1861, with the rank of captain. He was assigned to command Company B, 10th Florida Infantry Regiment.[2]

The service record of Dr. Jenkins is garbled and incomplete, therefore, a valid resume of his military career is impossible. It is known that he was in Virginia with his regiment in 1863, became ill, overstayed his sick leave, was placed under arrest and exculpated, and probably participated in the Battle of Cold Harbor[3] in June 1864. A short time later he became ill again and was hospitalized in October at Howard's Grove Confederate Hospital near Richmond, and on November 11, 1864, submitted his resignation which was supported by Hospital medical officers who affirmed that Dr. Jenkins was suffering from tuberculosis and unfit for further service.

Since no further evidence linking Dr. Jenkins to Jasper and Hamilton County has been discovered it is presumed that upon his discharge from the Army he terminated his Florida practice and moved to another state.

1. U.S. Census, 1860, Hamilton County, Florida, p. 2, item 12. Mrs. Jenkins is shown to have had property valued at $2,800.

2. NA, Serv. Recs. M251, Roll 95.

3. It is stated in *Soldiers of Florida*, Board of State Institutions, Live Oak, 1903, p. 222, that Dr. Jenkins was killed at Cold Harbor. This is not in agreement with information in his service record.

Jenkins, Joseph G., Levy County, 1860

Except for the information contained in the Levy County Census of 1860 nothing is known of Dr. Jenkins. That year he is shown to have been a resident of Atsena Otie Key with his wife, Mary and their nine children who ranged in age from one to 14. Both the doctor and his wife were natives of South Carolina as were seven of the nine children. The second child, Joseph Jr., was born in Alabama, indicating the family's brief residence there, while the youngest, Benjamin, aged one, was born in Florida. In addition to the family there were 11 residents of the household. They were of assorted trades—mariners, blacksmiths, printers and mechanics—apparently renting from the householder, a man named John Gomez, a native of Madeira Island, himself a "coaster."

Since Dr. Jenkins does not appear in later censuses it is assumed that his stay in Levy County was short.[1]

1. U.S. Census, 1860, Levy County, Florida, item 51. Confederate Service Records, 7th Florida Infantry Regiment, include an entry for Nicholas A. Jenkins, eldest child of Dr. Jenkins, showing that he enlisted at Gainesville in May 1862 at age 16 and was assigned to Company D. He was captured at the Battle of Missionary Ridge, Tennessee, on November 25, 1863, and spent the last years of the War at Rock Island Barracks, Illinois, as a prisoner of war.

Jennings, George, Madison and Hamilton Counties, 1790

There is no certainty that Dr. Jennings was actually a practicing physician although contemporary documents refer to him as such.[1] He was born in England in 1790, emigrated to America at age 12 and settled in North Carolina. He moved to South Georgia in 1820 but at some time prior to 1830 moved to Old Town, also known as Suwannee Old Town, in what was then Madison County. In spite of the misfortune of losing all his personal belongings when his boat capsized on the Suwannee while making his way to Florida,he was able to obtain a portion of land on the River some three miles south of the village of Old Town which he developed into a plantation.

In the earlier stages of the 2nd Seminole War the scattered settlements became targets of Indian depredations. Dr. Jennings' place was among the first casualties. The Jacksonville *Courier* of December 31,1835, contained the following item:

> Mr. Isaac Watson passed through place last evening from his plantation on the Suwannee. He says that Dr. Jennings' house at Suwannee Old Town has been burned, one negro is missing, killed or carried away...and that Ft. Jennings at Old Town has been evacuated.[2]

Soon thereafter Dr. Jennings abandoned the Suwannee settlement, relocated on the east side of the Alapaha River in Hamilton County and began once more the life of a planter. There he was to remain until his death.[3]

Before coming to Florida Dr. Jennings had married a North Carolina native whose Christian name was Elizabeth. At least two children, George S. and William T., both natives of North Carolina, were born to this union. Dr. Jennings' name was perpetuated in Hamilton County when the town of Jennings was named for him.[4]

1. Some biographical data on Dr. Jennings appear incidentally in Rowland H. Rerick, *Memoirs of Florida*, Francis P. Fleming, ed., Atlanta, Southern Historical Association, 1902, I, 385-86, in the biographical sketch of his grandson, James R. Jennings, son of George S. Jennings.

2. Dr. Jennings was apparently well-known and highly-respected.

3. The date of Dr. Jennings' death has not been determined. The Census of 1850, Hamilton County, p. 433, lists him as "planter," aged 60; his wife, Elizabeth, was 53. Ten years later, he was a widower, aged 69, listed as "farmer," whose property was valued at $17,000.

4. He is said to have been a county commissioner who built Hamilton County's first courthouse and jail. See note 1, supra.

Johns, Edward W., Key West and Miami, 1829-1892

Dr. Johns, a native of South Carolina, was born about 1829 and is thought to have received his education in that state. He matriculated at the University of Maryland School of Medicine in 1847 from which he was graduated in the spring of 1849.[1] Within months after graduation he offered his services to the Medical Department of the United States Army, his appointment as assistant surgeon having been approved on June 29, 1849.[2]

Dr. Johns' posts of duty for the next few years are not known. His name, however, appears in a list of officers serving at Ft. Dallas, Miami, in 1856.[3] A short time later he was transferred to Key West as surgeon to the army post located there.

In March 1858, Dr. Johns prepared to leave Key West. His reasons are unknown but given the political turmoil of the times, it is conjectured that he may have been considering his choices in case of war. The Key West newspaper, *Key of the Gulf,* published two notices on March 6, 1858, relating to his imminent departure. In the first he invited all persons whom he owed to present their demands, adding that all who owed him for medical services should make immediate payment. In the second he offered for sale "small bay mare." George D. Allen, Key West druggist, was named as his collection agent.[3]

On his return to Maryland Dr. Johns apparently resumed his duties as Army Surgeon, continuing to serve for the next three years. The bombardment of Ft. Sumter began on the morning of April 12, 1861. On April 22 Dr. Johns resigned his army commission and immediately offered his services to the Confederacy. His offer was accepted and he was inducted into the service with the rank of Surgeon. He served throughout the War[4] in this capacity.

At the conclusion of the war Dr. Johns returned to civilian practice in Maryland and continued in his profession until near the time of his death which occurred on June 13, 1892.[5]

1. Eugene F. Cordell, *Historical Sketch of the University of Maryland School of Medicine*, 1807-1890, Baltimore 1891, p. 182.
2. Francis B. Heitman, *Historical Register and Dictionary of the United States Army*, Washington 1903, I, 574.
3. Key West *Key of the Gulf*, March 6, 1858.
4. Heitman, loc. cit.

Johns, Samuel W., Tampa, 1857

Dr. Johns, or John, thought to have been a native of New Hampshire and a graduate of the Berkshire Medical College, Pittsfield, Massachusetts,[1] settled in Tampa in early 1855. Shortly thereafter he entered into a professional partnership with Dr. Franklin Branch, already a well-established physician and druggist.[2] Dr. Johns also became a partner in the drug store which appeares to have been a well-stocked and prosperous enterprise dispensing not only medicines but also a variety of household commodities such as perfume, tobacco, soap, and oils.[3]

The partnership continued more than two years and was terminated by the illness and eventually the death of Dr. Johns. Perhaps he had been suffering from some lingering illness prior to settling in Florida and probably had made the move in the hope that the more benign climate might prove beneficial to his health. He died in the fall of 1857.[4] Soon after Dr. Johns' death, Dr. Branch was joined in partnership by his son, Dr. Darwin A. Branch.

1. The similarity of his name and certain coincidences of dates as well as his partnership with Dr. Franklin Branch invite the speculation that Dr. Johns, or John, may be identified as Samuel W. Jones, a native of Bradford, New Hampshire, who matriculated at the Vermont Medical College, Woodstock, in 1848 and who later was graduated from Berkshire Medical College, Pittsfield, Massachusetts. If this is true, then he is known to have been born in Bradford in December 1821. The fact that Dr. Branch, a native Vermonter, was a graduate of the Medical College at Castleton, Vermont, seems further to support this speculation.

2. Tampa *Florida Peninsular*, February 10, 1855.

3. Ibid, August 11, 1855.

4. Although no obituary for Dr. Johns has been located, the executor of his estate, Tampa lawyer James Gettis announced the settlement of his estate on November 7, 1857. Ibid., Dr. Johns' estate included a land purchase he had made through the Land Office in Newnansville. Ibid., January 11, 1856.

Johnson, Alexander, Leon County, mid-19th century

Very little is known of the medical career of Dr. Johnson.[1] He was the eldest of eight children born to George C.S. and Mariah Johnson of rural Leon County. The elder Johnson, a farmer of fairly substantial means, was a native of Maryland who had apparently settled in Leon County about 1830. In the Leon County Census of 1850 Alexander is listed as "student," aged 18 and born in Florida. Ten years later, at 28, he is designated "physician," still a resident in his father's home, and owning personal property (doubtless professional equipment) valued at $300. No further information relating to him has been located.

1. Confederate Records of the First Florida Infantry Regiment include the Civil War Record of an Alexander Johnson of Company D who enlisted for service April 5, 1861, who was wounded at Shiloh, Tenn., in April 1862, at New Hope Chapel, Dallas, Georgia, in March 1863, and at Missionary Ridge near Chattanooga in December 1863. It has not been verified, however, that he was the Dr. Johnson.

Johnson, Benjamin, Jefferson County, 1798-1856

Dr. Johnson, native of Virginia and 1818 graduate of the University of Maryland School of Medicine,[1] was born in 1798.[2] In 1836, with his wife, Sarah, their three children, slaves and household goods, he arrived in Jefferson County,[3] obtaining a portion of the lands previously belonging to Abram Cabell but at the time in the possession of Edward Carrington Cabell. The elder Cabell had named the place Dulce Domum (Sweet Home) which Dr. Johnson changed to Jumper Run.[4]

For a brief but undetermined period after moving to Florida Dr. Johnson practiced medicine in the Monticello vicinity but appears to have later abandoned it for the more lucrative business of planting at which he is said to have been very successful. By Jefferson County standards the Johnsons were not wealthy, owning only 33 slaves in 1850, such families as the Gambles, Gadsdens, Baileys owned several times as many,[5] but they were educated folk and property-wise would have been considered well-to-do. Mrs. Johnson was regarded as a fine lady, model wife and mother.

Five children were born to the Johnsons, the eldest was Julia, the only daughter. The four sons were George, Benjamin W., Robert S., and William. Only Robert was not educated in the Monticello schools. Because of a congenital affliction he was taught at home. The other boys were sent to Davidson College in North Carolina for further education.

Dr. Johnson died in 1856. The conduct of the plantation was henceforth the responsibility of Mrs. Johnson and her sons, George and William. Benjamin W., having studied pharmacy, became a practicing druggist in Monticello. The Civil War, however, brought untold sorrow to the family. The three able-bodied sons enlisted in the Confederate Army, and George was killed in action near Tullahoma, Tennessee, on March 23, 1863,[6] and William in Georgia in 1864. Benjamin W. returned home to face the responsibility of caring for his mother and invalid brother. Mrs. Johnson died in 1879. Benjamin W. continued to operate a drug store in Monticello until his death in 1906 when the business passed to his son, J. Robert Johnson.

1. Eugene F. Cordell, *Historical Sketch of the University of Maryland* School of Medicine, Baltimore, 1891, p. 182.
2. U.S. Census, 1850, Jefferson County, Florida, p. 61. Here Dr. Johnson is shown as aged 52 with dual occupations of farmer and physician.
3. Ibid., Slave Schedule, Jefferson County, Florida.
4. Much of the data included here derives from "Plantations, Jefferson County," WPA, Writers Project, Florida. Typescript, P.K. Yonge Library of Florida History, University of Florida. No further references from this work will be specifically cited. The name, Jumper Run, is derived from a creek which ran through the plantation. The Seminole Indian Chief, Jumper, is said to have established his headquarters on this creek.
5. The rolling hills and fertile lands of Jefferson County had attracted many wealthy Virginians and Carolinians whose slaves in some instances numbered in the hundreds.
6. NA, Service Records, CSA, M251, Roll 49, 3rd Florida Infantry Regiment, Company H.

Johnson, E.C., Gadsden County, 1860

Dr. Johnson, son of Randall Johnson, a prominent farmer of Gadsden County, was born in Florida about 1832.[1] He was graduated from the Medical College of the State of South Carolina in March 1859 after submitting a thesis entitled "Pneumonia."[2] He appears to have returned soon thereafter to Gadsden County where he entered medical practice. In June 1860 he was a delegate from his county at the State Democratic Convention in Quincy.[3] Nothing further is known of him.[4]

1. U.S. Census, Gadsden County, Florida, 1860, p. 71. Here Dr. Johnson's age is shown to have been 28. Both his parents were natives of North Carolina. They had settled in the Sycamore community in the western part of the county.
2. Charleston *Mercury*, March 16, 1859.
3. Fernandina *East Floridian*, June 21, 1860.
4. Dr. Johnson's name does not appear in the Service Records of the Confederacy nor is he listed in the Gadsden Census of 1870.

Johnson, Elisha G., Lake City, 1839-1875

Dr. Johnson, native of North Carolina, settled in Lake City soon after the Civil War.[1] A short time after his arrival he entered into a professional partnership with a local physician, Marcellus M.T. Huchingson; they also operated a drug store.[2] Arriving as he did just as the winds of bitterness began to swirl in Florida's northern precincts, Dr. Johnson soon found himself caught up in the maelstrom of Reconstruction politics. Although he was of southern origin he could not in good conscience join the forces of the predominantly southern Conservative-Democratic Party, aligning himself instead with the Republicans, the party largely under the control of "carpetbaggers" who held most of the federal offices in the state.

At considerable risk of life Dr. Johnson was persuaded in the fall of 1870 to become a candidate for the Florida Senate, representing Columbia County, the 14th senatorial district. His opponent on the Conservative-Democratic ticket was Charles B. Ross. As election day, November 8, approached the Democrats were determined that the recently enfranchised Negroes would not be permitted to vote and by rowdy intimidation virtually succeeded. At the polls the Democrats prevailed, though only by a small majority, but the Republicans, no strangers to fraud, were not finished. They controlled the State's Canvassing Board and proceeded to name the Republicans winners, among them Dr. Johnson.[3]

When Dr. Johnson arrived in Tallahassee for the opening session of the Legislature on January 3, 1871, he was confronted by opposition from members of the body bent on seating Ross. After a review of the November election and considering the argument that Dr. Johnson, had the Negroes been permitted to vote, should have been the winner, he was duly seated on January 12.[4]

But Dr. Johnson's troubles were not over. In the spring of 1871 his life was threatened in a letter obviously prepared by the Ku Klux Klan.[5] He was undaunted and in the elections of 1872, 1873, 1874, and 1875 was reelected.

It is said, however, that for about three years he dared not sleep in his own home for fear of murder. Finally, on the night of July 21, 1875, as he was returning home, lighting his way with a lantern, an assassin laying in wait called his name. Upon facing the direction whence the voice came he was twice shot in blasts from a double-barreled gun. His death was instantaneous.[6]

The aftermath of Dr. Johnson's death included some of the most disgraceful behavior on the part of public officials known to the Reconstruction period. The basic civil rights of more than one individual[7] were blatantly ignored in the zeal to apprehend a culprit. Eventually an Alachua County farmer, Harney Richard, was arrested and charged with the crime. After his arrest Richard was taken to Palatka and then by steamer to Jacksonville where a Federal marshal presided over a preliminary hearing. Stated the Jacksonville Union:[8] "The evidence against him (Richard) was almost conclusive;" yet when a battery of witnesses came forward to establish an alibi for the accused Richard, he was set free. The trial ended on September 20 and the following day the Union reported, "The entire community finds it (the verdict) an outrage, and strong indignation is expressed everywhere."[9] It was assumed that perjury, not justice, had prevailed.

1. U.S. Census, 1870, Columbia County, Florida, item 123.

2. J.W. Hawks, ed., *The Florida Gazetteer*, New Orleans, 1871, p. 21. Dr. Johnson's identity as a partner of Dr. Huchingson is mentioned in *Senate Journal*, Florida, 1871, p. 50.

3. An account of this critical election is found in several publications, notably Edward F. Keuchel, *A History of Columbia County, Florida*, Tallahassee, 1981, pp. 129-30; William Watson Davis, *The Civil War and Reconstruction in Florida*, Columbia University Studies in History, Economics and Public Law, New York, 1813, pp. 355 et passim and John Wallace, *Carpet-Bag Rule in Florida*, Jacksonville 1888, pp. 127 et passim.

4. *Senate Journal*, Florida, 1871, p. 67.

5. Davis, *Civil War*, loc. cit. It is a matter of interest at this point that another Florida physician, John N. Krimminger, member of the Florida Senate from the 12th District, had also died from an assassin's bullet as he sat on his porch in New Troy, Lafayette County, on the morning of October 5, 1871. He too was a native of North Carolina.

6. This shocking event was widely publicized. The Tallahassee *Floridian*, a Republican newspaper, was particularly diligent in reporting the details as they emerged. Unfortunately only an occasional issue of other Florida papers has been preserved.

7. The case of the unfortunate Lewis L. Lutes of Appling County, Georgia, is a good example of the general hysteria of the period. He happened to have been in the area at about the time of the murder, was sought and eventually found in Key West. He was arrested, put in chains and held briefly in the Key West jail, then still in irons was brought by

ship to Tampa thence to Cedar Keys and eventually to Columbia County, only at last to establish his innocence.

8. Tallahassee *Floridian*, September 14, 1875, quoting from the Palatka *Herald* of September 11, 1875.

9. Ibid., September 21, 1875.

Johnson, William W., Alachua County, 1834-1900

Dr. Johnson, native of South Carolina, was born on September 17, 1834.[1] He received his medical degree from the Medical Department, University of Georgia, in 1859[2] and shortly thereafter moved to Florida settling in what was then a remote rural locality known as Morrison's Mills, site of a sawmill and gristmill built in 1848 by Daniel Morrison,[3] located near the Putnam County line some two miles east of present-day Hawthorne.[4] The census enumerator who canvassed the area in 1860 found Dr. Johnson residing in the home of John W. Peacock, owner of a country store. He was 25 years of age and unmarried[5] but shortly thereafter he married an Alabama girl named Evalina. They had seven children, four sons and three daughters.[6]

Dr. Johnson apparently shunned political activity and other involvements which might have gained for him the usual publicity. Instead, besides his medical practice, he devoted much of his time and energy to orange groves and other agricultural interests. With onset of the general economic collapse of 1873 and its disastrous impact on farmers, the Grange movement, which had begun in 1867, suddenly flourished. Dr. Johnson was among the organizers of a Grange in eastern Alachua County,[7] holding the office of assistant steward.

Dr. Johnson continued medical practice and farming until his death on February 13, 1900. He occasionally served as preceptor for local young men, e.g., W.J. Jolly,[8] entering the study of medicine. Dr. Johnson, his wife, and other members of his family were buried in the family lot in the Hawthorne Cemetery. There is no record of his ever having affiliated with the Florida Medical Association.

1. Dates of Dr. Johnson's birth and death are from his gravestone in the Hawthorne Cemetery.

2. *Medical Department, University of Georgia*, List of Graduates, 1829-91, Augusta 1891, p. 19.

3. Morrison's Mills, situated near the crossing of two much traveled roads, had its own post office except for two brief intervals from 1859 till 1874.

4. By 1881 the two railroads serving the area had been completed; the first running from Waldo to Ocala in 1879 and the second from Palatka to Gainesville in 1881. Both by-passed Morrison's Mills but crossed about two miles to the west giving rise to the town of Hawthorne and blighting any urban potential for Morrison's Mills.

5. U.S. Census, 1860, Alachua County, Florida, item 171.

6. Ibid., 1880, p. 120.

7. Gainesville *New Era*, August 30, 1873. The following item appeared in ibid., July 6, 1866: Letter, George Arnow, Solicitor, to Editor. Reference to a controversy between Dr. William W. Johnson, "a justice of the peace for the District of Fernandina who, I know personally, is a gentleman, and a Paul Crippen, of whom I have heard much and know a little professionally." No further information concerning this altercation or the possibility that Dr. Johnson may have resided for a time in Fernandina has been located.

8. Archives, Medical College of South Carolina, show Dr. Jolly as a resident of Waldo, student at the College, 1880-82, and M.D., 1882.

Jones, F.E., Liberty County, 1856

A single reference establishes the presence of Dr. Jones as a resident in Liberty County in 1856. At a meeting of the county's Democrats at Ridleysville on July 5, 1856, he was among the delegates elected to attend the convention of the party to be held in Quincy a short time later.[1]

1. Tallahassee *Floridian and Journal*, July 19, 1856. Ridleysville, originally in Gadsden County, received its name from John Clark Ridley, its first postmaster. When Liberty County was formed from a portion of Gadsden County in December 1855, it became the seat of the new county. Its name was changed to Bristol in April 1859. Mrs. Harold Major Pickett, Kenneth L. Rice, and Henry M. Spelman, III, *Florida Postal History and Postal Markings During the Stampless Period*, Florida Federation of Stamp Clubs, Handbook No. 1, Palm Beach, 1957, mimeographed, p. 40.

Jones, Hilton S., Ocala, 1858

Dr. Jones was one of several physicians whose medical careers in Ocala were of short duration. Nothing is known of his place of birth and educational background. He apparently came to Florida in the mid-1850s soon after receiving his medical degree in 1853[1] and began practice in an unidentified Florida locality.[2] In the summer of 1857, Ocala lawyer Samuel St. George Rogers was authorized by Florida Governor James E. Broome to organize a volunteer regiment to assist in the major effort to put an end to the Indian threat in south Florida.[3] By August 10 the main cadre had been assembled and on the 13th moved on to Ft. Brooke at Tampa. Seven days later they arrived at Ft. Myers. Dr. Jones joined the unit known as the First Regiment, Florida Mounted Volunteers, on September 15 as regimental assistant surgeon and saw service at Ft. Myers, Ft. Deynaud and other places along the Caloosahatchee River. When the six month period, for which the regiment was committed, ended on February 10, 1858, Dr. Jones was among those mustered out.[4]

Upon release Dr. Jones went immediately to Ocala and began civilian practice, perhaps prompted to do so by Colonel Rogers. On February 23 the Ocala newspaper stated in an editorial item: "It affords us pleasure to inform our citizens that Dr. Hilton S. Jones has yielded to the persuasions of his friends, and will locate in Ocala. He has long been known as a practitioner in the State, and during the recent campaign served as Assistant Surgeon in Col. Rogers' Regiment...."[5] Shortly after arrival in Ocala Dr. Jones joined Dr. George Wilson in professional partnership, an affiliation which was terminated by mutual consent on January 1, 1860.[6]

Dr. Jones' whereabouts for the next three years are unknown but in 1863 he reappeared as surgeon in the 8th Regiment of Tennessee Volunteers and by mid-1863 had been promoted to the rank of brigade surgeon under the command of Brigadier Marcus J. Wright. In this capacity he was present at the battle of Chickamauga in September 1863 and two months later at the encounter at Missionary Ridge, November 24-25. Some months later General Wright, in his report to Confederate Army Headquarters in Atlanta, singled out Surgeon Jones for special commendation for his service in the Chattanooga Campaign.[7] Nothing more has been discovered on the career of Dr. Jones.

1. An extrapolation from a statement that he was 25 years of age in 1858. See note 4, infra.
2. See note 5 infra. If Dr. Jones was indeed 25 in 1858 he could hardly have "long been known as a practitioner in the State."
3. This move was a part of the final stage of the so-called Third Seminole War which had begun on December 20, 1855, and would end in March 1858 when the last major resistance of the Indians was crushed.
4. Records, Adjutant General's Office, Group 94; Compiled Service Records, Volunteers Soldiers, Florida Indian Wars, 1835-1858, M. 1086, Roll 51.
5. Ocala *Florida Home Companion*, February 23, 1858. Dr. Jones' professional card appeared in the same issue.
6. Ibid., January 10, 1860.
7. *War of the Rebellion, Official Records*, I, xxxi, Part 2, p. 709.

Jones, James S., Alligator, 1850s, 1860s

Except for his title there is no evidence that Dr. Jones ever practiced medicine in Florida. A native of Virginia, he appears in sources relating to Alligator (Lake City), Columbia County, as early as May 1848, at which time he was about 31 years of age.[1] He was present at a meeting of Columbia County Democrats at Alligator on May 9, 1848, serving as secretary of the gathering and becoming a member of the County Democratic Committee.[2] In July of the same year he presided over the County Democratic Convention.[3] His popularity with fellow Democrats won him a seat in the Florida House of Representatives in the fall of 1850, but when in 1854 he was the nominee by acclamation for a seat in the Florida Senate which he could easily have won, he declined the honor and was replaced by William H. Cone, who won handily over his Whig opponent.

In November 1854 the editors of the recently founded Tampa *Herald*, M. Whit Smith and C.S. Reynolds, both former residents of Columbia County, chose to dissolve their partnership, whereupon the former sold his interest in the newspaper to Dr. Jones who moved to Tampa about the end of the year. A few months later the name of the paper was changed to the *Florida Peninsular*. Dr. Jones sold his interest to Simon Turman in August 1855, explaining that it provided insufficient income to support his family.[4] Within a matter of weeks he had purchased another newspaper, the Tallahassee *Floridian and Journal*, previously owned and edited by Charles E. Dyke whose failing health had prompted the sale. In the first issue following the sale, November 17, 1855, Dyke sought to bless the transition with an editorial praising his successor. He wrote:

> Dr. Jones is a Virginian by birth, a Democrat of the Jeffersonian strict construction, State rights school, and consequently the opponent of all modern isms that have sprung up like noxious weeds to infect the moral atmosphere and introduce the seeds of decay and death into the body politic...

Two years later Dyke returned to obtain half interest in the paper. His name appeared on the masthead along with that of Dr. Jones in the issue of November 21, 1857. The editorial partnership lasted until November 1859 when Dr. Jones sold his interest to J.B. Carlisle and moved to Pensacola where he eventually became a partner of A. Marzoni in the publication of the Pensacola *Observer*.[5] It is not known how long he remained in this position. The last extant issue of the *Observer* bearing the names Marzoni and Jones was that of June 9, 1861, Vol. II, No. 19.

Only a few references remain concerning Dr. Jones' sojourn in Pensacola. He continued to be a loyal Democrat as evidenced by attendance at the Florida Democratic Convention in Quincy during the week of June 4, 1860, as a delegate from Escambia County.[6] He was named a member of the State Democratic Committee. He was in Pensacola as late as December 1861 when his stepdaughter, Louisa A. Summerlin, was married to John Frink, Esq., on December 23.[7]

Dr. Jones was twice married, first to Mrs. Mary A. Summerlin, widow and native of Georgia who had two daughters by a previous husband. She was quite possibly the mother of the three Jones children, Minor S., Anna and William J.[8] His second wife, Elizabeth (no patronym known), was also Georgia-born.

Beyond the year 1861 no information on the Jones family has emerged. He was not listed in the Escambia County Census of 1870; quite possibly they had left Florida by that date.

1. The U.S. Census, 1850, Columbia County, Florida, item 5, gives his age as 33 and that of his wife, Mary, as 31. Their son, Minor S., was six months old.
2. Tallahassee *Floridian*, May 9, 1848.
3. Ibid., July 27, 1848.
4. Karl H. Grismer, *Tampa*, St. Petersburg, 1950, p. 122.
5. Since Dr. Jones and family are listed in the Pensacola Census of 1860, it may be assumed that he had moved to Pensacola immediately after sale of the Tallahassee paper. Only a few issues of the Pensacola *Observer* of the early 1860s have survived. The only one bearing the name of Dr. Jones as coeditor is that of June 9, 1861. When publication of the paper was resumed after the Civil War neither Marzoni nor Dr. Jones were connected with it.
6. Monticello *Family Friend*, June 16, 1860; Fernandina *East Floridian*, June 21, 1860.
7. Tallahassee *Floridian and Journal*, January 19, 1861.
8. In the Census of 1850, Dr. Jones is designated "farmer" with real estate valued at $1,400; in that of 1860, he is listed as "editor" with real property valued at $5,000.

Jones, S.F., St. Augustine and Key West, 1840s, 1850s

Dr. Jones, native of Virginia, is thought to have arrived in Florida in 1840. In mid-May of that year the shipping news of the St. Augustine newspaper listed among the arrivals on board the schooner, Stephen and Frances, from Charleston "Dr. S.F. Jones, lady, and five children."[1] Two weeks later he announced his services to the citizens of St. Augustine from his office on Carlota Street. His residence on St. George Street was the house formerly occupied by a Mr. Dupont.[2] His presence in the city was verified a few weeks later by the census enumerator who listed the doctor and his wife as between 30 and 40 years old while their five children, three sons and two dughters, were under 10.[3]

About a year later on July 20, 1841, Dr. Jones was appointed[4] Port Physician replacing Dr. Charles Byrne. In his report to the City Council on October 1 he noted the general cleanliness of the city, praising the Mayor and Aldermen for their diligence in enforcing sanitary regulations. His main concern was the Sebastian River an arm of which was not adequately drained, resulting in a hazard to the city's health.[5]

Before the summer of 1841 was over, however, by sheer inadvertence he incurred the wrath of Dr. Byrne, his predecessor, when he reported to the Council that he had discovered two cases of fever aboard a steamer in St. Augustine harbor, neither of which he regarded as contagious but which, he stated, had been "grossly exaggerated and perverted" presumably by his predecessor. Dr. Byrne was outraged. He inferred that Dr. Jones was referring to him since he had attended an ailing man aboard the ship. In a blistering attack, published in the newspaper, he denounced Dr. Jones' slipshod diagnosis. When Dr. Jones read Dr. Byrnes' letter (apparently it was only then that he discovered Dr. Byrne was attending the man) he was stunned into a public response in which he defended his actions regarding the ailing mariner. The incident, though apparently patched up, was never quite forgotten by either physician.[6]

There can be no doubt that the altercation with Dr. Byrne, a highly respected citizen, was damaging to the reputation of Dr. Jones as far as the people of St. Augustine were concerned. And yet he continued to practice there until the summer of 1844 when he moved to Key West. A few weeks earlier Dr. Edward S. Aldrich had settled in St. Augustine. Mrs. Aldrich, in a letter to her brother in Utica, New York, wrote: "The Dr. who led the van here has removed to Key West. He was a very unpopular man and Edward (Mrs. Aldrich's husband) was urged to come here before he left, and I think his coming was an added inducement for the other to quit." She continued, "However, since his removal to Key West he has been urging Edward to join him in practice there, assuring him that he can make more in one year than in five here."[7]

After a year or two in Key West Dr. Jones moved once more, in this instance to Gadsden County where as a staunch Whig he was active in the 1848 campaign to elect fellow-Virginian, Zachary Taylor, to the presidency.[8] In 1849, however, he returned to Key West and in August of that year was appointed surgeon to the Marine Hospital.[9] This appointment, doubtless made in payment of a political debt, was a severe blow to the ambitions of Dr. Aldrich who had vigorously sought the position. Wrote Mrs. Aldrich, "Dr. Jones is appointed...a man scarcely capable of spelling his own name...Key West people have gotten a petition to have Dr. Jones removed and Ed appointed in his place...the charge is incompetency." Such was the sting felt by the Aldriches.[9]

The Monroe County Census of 1850 shows Dr. Jones as a resident of Key West at the age of 48.[10] Four years later he was relieved of his duties at the Hospital and replaced by Dr. William J. L'Engle, a native Floridian and a Democrat.[11] It was sheer misfortune for Dr. Jones that within the three months prior to his dismissal Key West suffered the worst yellow fever epidemic in more than a decade. Twenty-five cases were recorded of which nine were fatal. The majority of the cases had been admitted to the Marine Hospital.

On learning of Dr. Jones' dismissal, obviously for political reasons, a number of Key West friends subscribed a sum of money for a piece of silver plate, presented to him "for his unremitting attention to the sick during the late epidemic." This was a well-earned tribute, "for no person could do more in attention and services to those requiring it than did Dr. Jones...To the poor and penniless he was particularly kind...no small quantity of medicines were given to those whom he knew had not the means for paying..."[12]

Beyond this point nothing is known of Dr. Jones. Very probably he departed the state never to return. It seems a fair assumption that he was a far better physician and citizen than the Byrne rebuke and the Aldrich letters would indicate.

1. St. Augustine *Florida Herald*, May 15, 1840.
2. Ibid., June 5, 1840.
3. U.S. Census, 1850, St. Johns County, Florida, p. 119.
4. St. Augustine *Florida Herald*, July 30, 1841. This appointment was made by the City Council. It entailed responsibilities which were not to be taken lightly in that it demanded the detection of infectious diseases on all incoming ships and, if necessary, imposition of quarantine. With the pervading fear of yellow fever a great responsibility rested with the port physician.
5. Ibid., October 1, 1841.
6. See Dr. Byrne's letter in ibid., July 30, 1841, and Dr. Jones' reply in ibid., August 6, 1841.
7. Corine Aldrich to her brother, Mandeville Aldrich, July 15, 1844. Letter #219 now in the possession of Mrs. Louis Goolsby of Gainesville.
8. Tallahassee *Floridian*, March 4, 1848; Marianna *Florida Whig*, May 17, 1848.
9. Corine Aldrich to Mandeville Aldrich, August 17, 1849.
10. U.S. Census, 1850, Monroe County, Florida, item 5.
11. Jacksonville *Florida Republican*, July 27, 1854. With Franklin Pierce, a Democrat in office (1852-56), this change is presumed to have been politically dictated.
12. Ibid., August 10, 1854.

Jones, William L., Gadsden County, 1834-1900

Dr. Jones, native of North Carolina, began his medical training under the preceptorates of Drs. W.A. Culbertson and William H. Byrd, both graduates of the Atlanta Medical College, Atlanta, in the classes of 1855 and 1856 respectively.[1] Jones himself matriculated at the same institution in the fall of 1857, remaining for only one term.[2] There is no evidence that he ever returned to Atlanta for his degree.[3]

On May 7, 1859, Dr. Jones and Dr. Richard L. Byrd, a native of Georgia, announced the formation of a professional partnership which they expected to locate at the twin villages of River Junction and Chattahoochee in the northwest corner of Gadsden County.[4] It may be significant that in the announcement the designation followed each name. The announced plan did not materialize, however, for in the census of the following year Dr. Jones is listed as unmarried and a resident in the home of William Banks Meacham, a prominent Quincy merchant.[5] Dr. Jones announced in the Quincy *Republic* the opening of his office at the Chattahoochee Hotel in Chattahoochee on June 2, 1860, offering his services to its citizens and those of the surrounding country at "moderate charges."

In late 1860 or early 1861 Dr. Jones married a Georgia native, known only by her Christian name, Lovie Ann. In the following year, with mobilization for war already well under way, he enlisted for military service as a private in the Second Florida Cavalry.[6] Unfortunately his military record is incomplete. It appears, however, that soon after enlisting he was given the rank of Third Lieutenant and a short time later promoted to Second Lieutenant. In reorganization of the Regiment in May 1862, Dr. Jones' commission was not renewed which prompted him to resign from the service later in the year.

With his undistinguished military service behind him, Dr. Jones returned to Quincy and resumed medical practice. The Census of 1870 lists him as "physician" living in Quincy with his wife and three children, daughter, Carrie, aged eight, and sons, William and Walter, aged three and two, respectively.[7]

At some unknown date, probably the early 1870s, Dr. Jones moved to River Junction-Chattahoochee where he spent the remaining years of his life. By 1880 five additional children had been born and the eldest, Carrie, was 17; the youngest, Julia, was one.[8] Twenty years later in 1900 at age 66, Dr. Jones was still practicing medicine at River Junction-Chattahoochee. The household included Mrs. Jones, daughter, Stella, aged 21, and their youngest child, a son, Carlton, who had been born in March 1881.[9] No date of death for Dr. Jones has been discovered.

1. *Annual Announcement of the Medical College of Atlanta*, Atlanta, 1872, p. 11. This bulletin lists all graduates of the College from 1855 through 1871.

2. Ibid., 1858, p. 13.

3. It is reasonable to assume that the B.L. Jones, who was graduated from the College in 1858, was indeed W.L. Jones. Typographical errors were by no means uncommon. He could have been familiarly known as Bill Jones.

4. In their public announcement, first appearing in the Quincy *Republic* on May 7, 1859 (this issue not extant) and continuing to appear as late as October 7, 1859, it was stated that their office was located "on the street leading from the Arsenal to the River." See ibid. of the latter date.

5. U.S. Census, 1860, Gadsden County, Florida, p. 473. Town of Quincy.

6. The information found in the Confederate Service Records relating to Dr. Jones is both incomplete and confusing. It is shown that he enlisted at Lake City on October 12, 1861. He apparently remained in service until early summer, 1862.

7. U.S. Census, 1870, Gadsden County, Florida, p. 788, item 1129.

8. Ibid., 1880, p. 271.

9. Ibid., 1900, p. 271, item 302. The information in this schedule is valuable in that it includes the month and year of birth of all family members and number of years married also.

Jordan, James Arthur, Hamilton County, mid-19th century

Dr. Jordan was apparently a brief sojourner in Hamilton County about the middle of the 19th century. Records of Transylvania University, Lexington, Kentucky, indicate that he was enrolled there for the 1829-30 term. His name does not appear in the Florida census schedules of either 1840 or 1850. From the following obituary it is apparent that he was a medical practitioner there about 1847.[1]

> Died, on the 22nd ult. (i.e. December 22, 1846) of typhus fever, at the residence of Dr. James A. Jordan, Hamilton County, Major Henry P. Heath, in the 24th year of his age.

Dr. Jordan is known to have been a native of Autauga, Alabama, where he had begun his medical studies under the guidance of a Dr. Andrew.[2] Since he does not appear in the Florida Census of 1850, it is assumed that he had departed the state.

1. The Tallahassee *Floridian*, January 23, 1847.
2. Transylvania University Alumni Records.

Jordan, M.G.W., Monticello, 1850s and 1860s

Information on the medical career of Dr. Jordan is by no means abundant. This is true in some measure because of the garbled and incomplete record of his military service in the Army of the Confederacy. A native of Thomasville, Georgia, he matriculated at the Medical College of the State of South Carolina in the fall of 1852 and was graduated in March 1854 with the degree Doctor of Medicine. The subject of his doctoral thesis was "Acute Bronchitis."[1]

After practicing medicine in a place presently unknown, he appeared in Monticello in the summer of 1860. His professional card, first published on August 18, announced his practice from an office at Bless' Hotel.[2] The census that year shows him to have been a man of modest means, sharing his house with his brother, John W. Jordan, whose occupation was farming.[3]

With the outbreak of war in 1861 Dr. Jordan enlisted in the military unit known as the Jefferson Rifles being locally organized which became Company H, 3rd Florida Infantry Regiment. He apparently enlisted for a term of one year and was given no rank, then after a year resigned and returned to his practice in Monticello. A short time later he returned to the Regiment as Assistant Surgeon on the regimental staff.[4] During the interim an outbreak of smallpox occurred in Monticello and Dr. Jordan was prevailed upon to cope with the threat of epidemic. With the assistance of a nurse and by a rigid quarantine he was able to contain the disease. A board of physicians recommended that he be paid $200 for his heroic services. The Jefferson County Commission readily authorized the payment.[5]

There is evidence that after serving with his regiment in Tennessee, Mississippi and Georgia throughout the war, Dr. Jordan was mustered out on April 26, 1865, at Greensboro, North Carolina,[6] and returned to Monticello and his practice. Apparently it was only for a brief period since he does not appear in the Jefferson County Census of 1870. Possibly he had left the county and state.

1. Charleston *Mercury*, March 15, 1854.

2. Monticello *Family Friend*, August 18, 1860.
3. U.S. Census, 1860, Jefferson County, Florida, item 448. Dr. Jordan's property was valued at $1,000.
4. Dr. Jordan's war record is garbled, generally illegible and incomplete. National Archives, Service Records, CSA, M251, Roll 49.
5. Jerrell H. Shofner, *History of Jefferson County*, Tallahassee, 1976, p. 261.
6. See note 4, supra.

Judge, William H., Santa Rosa County, 1819-1893

Dr. Judge was born in Alabama on February 5, 1819.[1] By extrapolation from the Florida Census of 1860 it is reckoned that he moved to Florida in the mid-1840s, settling on the outskirts of the village of Milton, Santa Rosa County, where his three children were born. Nothing is known of his early life and education or his medical training. At the time of his arrival Santa Rosa County, except for portions contiguous to Pensacola Bay, was a virtual wilderness. Dr. Judge contributed in substantial measure to the development of the area. He was a man of above average means, owning property valued at about $20,000 in 1860.[2]

Ten years after arrival in the county Dr. Judge became involved in politics, running for a seat in the Florida House of Representatives in 1856 against James R. Mims. He was unsuccessful but 20 years later in 1875 returned to politics and ran successfully for the House seat. Four years later he was a candidate for the Florida Senate from the Second District winning handily. He was returned to the Senate in the sessions of 1881 and 1887. A scrutiny of his Senate record indicates that he was progressive in his outlook, notably in the area of improving the quality of medical practice and in raising the standards for the licensing of physicians, surgeons and obstetricians.[3]

Meanwhile Dr. Judge carried on an extensive medical practice in Santa Rosa and adjoining counties. The Special Florida Census of 1885, Mortality Schedule, shows him to have been the attending physician for several persons who died during the year beginning June 1, 1884.

Dr. Judge was twice married. His first wife, known only by her initials, E.C., was a native of South Carolina. She was the mother of three children, a son, Thomas J., aged 13 in 1860, and two daughters, Mary and Margaret, 11 and nine respectively. After the death of his first wife Dr. Judge married Martha, a native of Georgia, listed in the Census of 1880 as a school teacher. They were residents of a hotel managed by Mrs. Maria Laffen.[4] Dr. Judge died on July 3, 1897.[5] He was buried in the Milton Cemetery.

1. Thanks to the diligence and perseverence of Richard Earl Jernegan in compiling and editing the gravestone inscriptions in the cemeteries of Santa Rosa County and the West Florida Genealogical Society for supporting the publication of same in 1987, this treasure of information is now readily available.
2. U.S. Census, Santa Rosa County, Florida, 1860, p. 711.
3. For his candidacy, see *Tallahassee and Journal*, August 30, 1856. For the dates of his service in the Florida Legislature, see Allen Morris, *The People of Lawmaking in Florida*, Tallahassee, 1977, unpaginated, but alphabetically arranged. *The Florida Senate Journal*, 1881. Act of March 7, 1881. Here is evidence of his professional concern.
4. U.S. Census, 1880, Santa Rosa County, Florida, p. 54, item 507.
5. See note 1 above.

Judson, W.H., Pensacola, 1834

Notwithstanding the effusiveness of his professional announcement in the Pensacola newspaper of November 15, 1834, Dr. Judson does not appear to have impressed the people of Pensacola very favorably. Having established himself "permanently" on Palafox Street with an office in the Collins Hotel, he hoped that "by his undivided attention and punctial attendance to gain a liberal share of public patronage." Furthermore, he had been educated "in both Europe and America, in different colleges and hospitals" and had had "eighteen months of intensive internship in City Hospital in New York City." More recently he had spent his "last four years in practice during which his treatment of cholera, yellow fever, and congestive fevers," he was happy to say, "had been very successful."[1]

There followed immediately Dr. Judson's professional card which stated that as Professor of Surgery, Medicine and Midwifery he was especially qualified. But with a hint of quackery he added that "his treatments were peculiar to himself." He assured his potential patients that his charges were reasonable.

Nothing further is known of this unusual man. He had left Pensacola by the year 1840.

1. The Pensacola *Gazette*, November 13, 1834.

June, Daniel R., Alachua County, 1802-post 1870

A degree of mystery or uncertainty beclouds the Florida career of Dr. June, an Alachua County resident for more than two decades. A native of New York State he had studied medicine and possibly received a medical degree prior to moving to Charleston, South Carolina, probably in the late 1830s. Better known for business acumen than medical practice, he arrived in Alachua County in the early 1850s bringing with him a number of slaves and soon thereafter purchasing a large tract of land in what is now southwest Gainesville. Accompanying him or following soon afterward were his son, William E., and another young Charlestonian, James Doig, both members of the June household in 1860.[1] Census data show that Dr. June was a man of far more than average means, owning property valued at more than $76,000 in 1860. His slaves numbered 30.

An amusing insight into Dr. June's affairs derives from a series of recollections written by Doig and published in the Gainesville *Sun* in 1917. About 1857 Doig had contracted to supervise the building of a part of the Florida Transit and Peninsular Railroad, later to become a part of the Seaboard Railroad System, extending from Gainesville to Archer. As Doig recalled the affair:[2]

> We had to go through some land owned by Dr. June, now the University farm. As we started to clear the way through Dr. June with his overseers came out and drove us away, telling us not to go through without paying. Therefore we had to fall back and remain where we were. Finally Dr. June went to South Carolina and we "jumped" him and went through. We continued right on through until we reached Archer, known then as "Deer Hammock"....That was in 1859.

The Civil War brought disaster to Dr. June as it did to most Southern planters dependent on slave labor for the cultivation of their lands. In the 1870 Census his total properties were valued at $10,000.[3] More devastating, however, was the death of his son, William, killed in battle at Missionary Ridge, near Chattanooga, on November 25, 1863.[4] The Census of 1870 shows Dr. June living alone at the age of 68.

The date of Dr. June's death has not been discovered although an earlier obituary notice was published in a Jacksonville newspaper. The inadvertence bears inclusion here:

> Item, The Gainesville *New Era*, September 20, 1867...Obit, Dr. Daniel R. June, an old and highly esteemed citizen of Alachua County, died near Gainesville on Thursday last (Sept. 11, 1867). Item in Jacksonville *Times*, September 19, 1867. The Gainesville *New Era* Sept. 20, 1867, responded: "This will doubtless surprise the venerable doctor, and when he reads this item of news he will, we think, laugh heartily over it. The *Times* has been misinformed. Dr. June has been quite ill but is now better and we hope he may live for many years to come.
>
> On the same page of the *New Era* there appeared the following notice: A horse stolen from Dr. D.R. June, near this place a few weeks since, together with the alleged thief, was captured in Madison a few days ago.

1. U.S. Census, 1860, Alachua County, Florida, p. 75. Another resident of the June household in 1860 was Charlestonian, Dr. Thomas Jefferson Myers, a veteran of the Mexican War who had been wounded at the Battle of Churubusco. Dr. Myers was an ardent secessionist, eager to return to South Carolina and join his old regiment, the Palmettoes. Doig had been brought from Scotland at the age of three by his parents. His father had been an engineer and the son James, a bright youngster, turned to the study of engines practicing his trade throughout his life in Gainesville. In 1917 he was persuaded to write an account of his early years in Gainesville. Three installments were published in the Gainesville *Sun* on July 15, 22 and 29, 1917, under the title: "Reminiscent Sketches of Gainesville's Early Days."

2. The affair apparently did not damage the friendly relationship of Dr. June and Doig. The latter was still a resident in the June home in 1860.

3. U.S. Census, 1870, Alachua County, Florida, p. 21.

4. NA, Serv. Recs., CSA. Young June had been mustered in as a Third Lieutenant at Gainesville on March 20, 1862. At the time of his death he held the rank of captain.

Kearney, John H., Navy Surgeon, mid-19th century

Dr. Kearney,[1] surgeon to the Marine Corps group stationed at Ft. Brooke, Tampa Bay, was the chief medical officer for the Marine Hospital at the Fort. He was relieved of his duties on May 22, 1837, and replaced by Assistant Surgeon Charles S. Tripler. For Dr. Kearney this was a promotion in that he assumed direction of all medical units south of the Withlacoochee River. He was, however, only one of several medical officers to serve in Florida during the Seminole Wars.

Some 10 years later with the Mexican War going on, Dr. Kearney was once more on the scene of battle, having been promoted to the rank of Captain with a company of the First Dragoons under his command. It was reported that his unit "exhibited activity and zeal in the pursuit of the enemy" in one of the skirmishes in the environs of Mexico City.

Dr. Kearney's activities after the Mexican War are presently unknown.

1. The information included in this sketch is derived almost entirely from two sources: Rodenbough, Theo F., compiler, *From Everglade to Canon*, New York, Van Nostrand, 1875, and McLellan, Major Edwin North, *Indian Campaigns, 1835-1852*, An Account, prepared as Chapter VI, Vol. 2, Part I, History of the United States Marine Corps.

Keddie, John W., Jackson County, 1823

Among the earliest settlers in Jackson County was Dr. Keddie who practiced medicine briefly at Chipola (Webville). On the night of July 1, 1823, he was murdered in his bed. His unknown assassin fired a gun through an aperture in the chimney of Dr. Keddie's house, killing him instantly.[1] Nothing further is known of this unfortunate man.

1. Pensacola *Floridian*, August 30, 1823.

Keep, Lester, Key West, 1858

Dr. Keep was a brief sojourner in Key West in the 1850s. Nothing is known of his origin, education, or medical training. His professional card, which appeared in the *Key of the Gulf* of March 6, 1858,[1] indicates that he was indeed a Doctor of Medicine. He was a resident in the home of O.T. Braman, where his office was also located, but his stay was apparently of brief duration since he does not appear in the Florida Census of 1860.

1. Key West *Key of the Gulf*, March 6, 1858.

Keitt, William J., Marion County, 1820-1860

Dr. Keitt, one of several prominent South Carolinians to settle in Marion County in the antebellum period, was born on August 30, 1820, on his father's plantation in St. Matthew's Parish, Orangeburg District. His parents were George and Mary M. Wannamaker Keitt.[1] He received his early education in Parish schools; his medical preceptor was a Dr. Glover. In the fall of 1839 he matriculated at the Medical College of the State of South Carolina, Charleston, from which he was graduated on March 16, 1841.[2] He was awarded a silver cup for having submitted a thesis on "Caloric," judged to have been the best of the class.[3]

With his degree he returned to his father's plantation and began the practice of medicine among the people in the surrounding community. He also had a brief fling at local politics, running successfully for the lower house of the South Carolina General Assembly in 1850. He was said to have "acquitted himself well in all the duties of his legislative position."[4] It was an eventful session, following as it did the adoption by Congress of the controversial Compromise of 1850, and for Dr. Keitt it was an important learning experience.

Early in 1854 Dr. Keitt purchased a plantation in Marion County and moved there from South Carolina. The land was located some three miles west of Ocala and he combined the roles of physician and farmer but was not long in emerging as a leader among the pioneers of the area. In 1856, having fulfilled the residency requirements, he was elected to the Florida Senate, an office to which he was returned for the sessions of 1858 and 1859.[5]

Shortly after his return home, subsequent to adjournment of the Legislature in January 1860, tragedy overtook Dr. Keitt. Living alone and suffering from a minor illness he was lying in bed on the night of February 17, 1860, when two of his slaves broke into his house and murdered him. When his house servant arrived early the next morning to build the fires he found his master lying dead on the floor. An inquest revealed that he had been brutally beaten, "his throat cut from ear to ear."[6]

The murder of Dr. Keitt was widely publicized and, together with similar incidents, sent shock waves throughout the South. Even the Key West newspaper published the horrible details. Dr. Keitt's sister-in-law, writing from Marlborough County, South Carolina, to a friend in the North, concluded: "No longer can we open the door to the waferer (sic) and offer a Southern cheerful hospitality. The midnight dagger and the poisoned bowl may, many days after, come to us. Thus it was that my noble brother-in-law, the kind master and true gentleman..."[7] There can be no doubt that Dr. Keitt was held in high esteem as physician and public servant.

1. U.S. Census, 1850, Orangeburg District, S.C., p. 581. The George Keitt property was valued at $25,000. Several biographical details relating to Dr. Keitt are found in his obituary. Charleston *Mercury*, March 10, 1860.

2. Archives, Waring Historical Library, Medical University of South Carolina, Charleston, S.C., "Lists of Matriculants and Graduates."

3. Charleston *Courier*, March 19, 1841. The word "Caloric" used in Old Chemistry is now obsolete.

4. Charleston *Mercury*, March 10, 1860. Obit.

5. Allen Morris, *The People of Lawmaking in Florida*, Tallahassee, 1977.

6. Fernandina *East Floridian*, March 3, 1860.

7. Elmer Don Herd Jr., "Sue Sparks Keitt to a Northern Friend," March 4, 1861, *South Carolina Historical Magazine*, LXII, 1961, p. 86. Susan Sparks Keitt was the wife of Laurence M. Keitt, brother of Dr. Keitt. He was a distinguished South Carolina politician and leader in the secessionist movement. He is the subject of a Master of Arts thesis, unpublished, University of South Carolina, 1956, by Elmer Don Herd Jr.

Kellum, James, Caloosahatchee Settlement, post-1870

Dr. Kellum, perhaps the earliest physican to practice medicine in that portion of Monroe County which encompassed the Caloosahatchee River, was born in Ohio about 1832.[1] Of his childhood and professional education nothing is known. He is thought to have arrived in South Florida about 1870 and staked out a claim to land on the north side of the Caloosahatchee River some 20 miles upstream from its mouth. Much of what is presently known of his activities is derived from an account by an explorer-writer who made an exploratory journey through the interior of central and south Florida and under the pseudonym James published an account of the trip serially in the Ocala *East Florida Banner* in 1875-76.[2]

Upon his arrival at the Kellum homestead James was received most hospitably. He marveled at the lush tropical growth along the river and the variety of fruits and vegetables under cultivation. He referred to the locality as the "Caloosahatchee Settlement, up the river from Ft. Myers, where Dr. Kellum is the practicing physician." He added, "He also served the citizens of Ft. Myers...But the area is so healthy that Dr. Kellum is free to devote most of his time to the cultivation of his plants."[3]

Due possibly to the remoteness of his homestead and the remissness of the census enumerator Dr. Kellum does not appear in the Monroe County census of 1880. Five years later, however, he was included in the Special Florida Census of 1885. A Monroe County entry includes some vital data on the family: the doctor was 53 years of age; his wife, Sallie, a native of Mississippi, was 26 years his junior. Two children, Sallie, four, and James, two, were born in Florida. A nephew, Medford Kellum, aged 10, was also a member of the family.

Dr. Kellum appears to have been a typical rural practitioner, unstinting in his attention to patients, willing to travel considerable distances by boat or horseback to attend to the ailing. A neighboring homesteader, in an interview of January 20, 1939, recalled Dr. Kellum as a man of compassion, never declining to respond to calls for his services and, as often as not, never sending a bill. This homesteader, John C. English, told of an illness of his sister for whom Dr. Kellum was summoned. English remembered: "Dr. Kellum homesteaded down there and he came and treated her. He didn't make a charge for his services but he had a little chopping for me to do in return for his services...I did it for him." English, a native of Bainbridge, Georgia, added, gratuitously, "Dr. Kellum was a Catholic...lots of people hates Catholics."[4]

The date of Dr. Kellum's death has not been determined, nor has the actual location of his homestead been pinpointed. It is believed to have been on the river near the village of Alva between Ft. Denaud and Olga. As for the surviving members of the Kellum family, it is only known that in 1900 son James F., aged 17, was a schoolboy, boarding in the home of Mrs. Margaret English, who kept a boarding house in Alva.[5]

1. An extrapolation from the Monroe County, Caloosahatchee Settlement, 1885, p. 22, item 206, where Dr. Kellum's age is given as 53. It is to be remembered that until 1887 Dade County had extended northward to Charlotte Harbor and Lake Okeechobee.

2. This informative article, one of several written by Mr. James, was published in the Ocala *East Florida Banner* of February 19, 1876.

3. Ibid. The James description sets forth an idyllic picture of the Caloosahatchee. Even the Indians settled in the area are depicted as friendly and cooperative.

4. This interview, recorded by A. Brenner, is one of a number of items relating to the history of Lee County, prepared under auspices of the the Federal Writers' Project. Typescript copy in the P.K. Yonge Library of Florida History, University of Florida, Gainesville.

5. Mrs. English, aged 74 in 1900, is presumed to have been the mother of John C. English.

Kelly, James, Alachua and St. Johns Counties, 1822-1843

About all that is presently known about Dr. Kelly is derived from a deposition taken on November 27, 1832, in which his knowledge of certain land claims put forth by Moses Elias Levy was solicited.[1] He made known that he had arrived in St. Augustine in 1822 and remained there for three months before moving to Palatka and shortly thereafter into the Alachua country where he was employed to replace Dr. Samuel R. Ayers as medical practitioner for the settlement being established by a group of New York and New Jersey speculators known as the Florida Association.[2] Dr. Kelly is identified as a Charleston physician.

Dr. Kelly probably remained in the employ of the land company until 1824, when he returned to St. Augustine and established a practice. His professional card first appeared in the local newspaper on June 26 of that year giving his place of residence as "the shipyard."[3] There is evidence, however, that he was once more in Alachua County. The census schedule of that county in 1830 lists him as a resident with a wife and two children both under five years old. His post office was Spring Grove.[4] He was among the Alachua inhabitants who in December 1831 signed a memorial to President Jackson endorsing Judge Joseph L. Smith for reappointment.[5]

Dr. Kelly had returned to St. Augustine by 1837. Late that year he was one of the citizens of the city petitioning Congress for federal assistance in improving and maintaining the harbor.[6] In the following year he lent his support to a similar request.[7] Although he disappeared from public documents after 1838, it is probable that he was still living in St. Augustine in 1843 when the local newspaper announced the death of John C. Kelly, "youngest son of Dr. James Kelly," which occurred on August 8, 1843.[8]

1. HRS, "Spanish Land Grants," II, 78-79.
2. Ibid., II, 106.
3. St. Augustine *East Florida Herald*, June 26, 1824.
4. U.S. Census, 1830, Alachua County, Florida. The precise location of Spring Grove is unknown. Inhabitants listed in the Spring Grove portion of the Census who can be identified as those who had received land grants in identifiable sections of the county suggest that it was in the northwest quadrant of the county probably a few miles from Gainesville and between the roads leading from Gainesville to Newberry and Archer. See Jess G. Davis *History of Alachua County*, Gainesville, Florida, 1969, Mimeographed, Sect. IV, Chap. II, 13, Norman LaCoe, contributor.
5. TP., XXIV, 599.
6. Ibid., XXV, 451.
7. Ibid., 548.
8. St. Augustine *Florida Herald and Southern Democrat*, August 14, 1843.

Kendrick, Robert James, Hillsborough County, 1829

Dr. Kendrick moved from his native Georgia about 1849 and settled in the vicinity of Ft. Brooke in Hillsborough County. He was accompanied by his brother, Hardy D. Kendrick, a fledgling lawyer. The two men found lodging at a boardinghouse operated by another Georgian, Elizabeth Mattair.[1] Dr. Kendrick remained in Tampa for about four or five years before deciding to risk a move to the northeastern part of the county. On February 10, 1855, the following professional card appeared in the Tampa *Herald*:

> Dr. R. Kendrick—Respectfully informs the citizens of Ichepucksassa, Pease Creek and Alafia Settlements that he has located in their midst for the purpose of practicing his profession, and believing himself thoroughly qualified and prepared, if perfect satisfaction is not given, NO PAY WHATEVER will be demanded. He can be found at the residence of Joseph Howell, Esq., when not professionally engaged.

Dr. Kendrick had scarcely established himself in the new location when remnants of the Seminole Indian nation, aware of the growing threat of the white man's encroachments into what they believed was their rightful territory, began to strike back. Ft. Brooke became a recruiting headquarters for assembling volunteer companies of both mounted and foot soldiers to eliminate the threat. Edward T. Kendrick, probably a brother of Dr. Kendrick, with the rank of captain, hurriedly raised a company of mounted soldiers which were joined on September 26, 1856, by Dr. Kendrick as assistant surgeon with the rank of First Lieutenant. They moved forthwith "to the frontier," which probably meant Pease Creek near its entrance into Charlotte Harbor.[2] Dr. Kendrick presumably remained with the Company until its term of service was over in early January 1857 and throughout its second term (it was reorganized in July 1857 for six months' service) ending on January 12, 1858.[3]

Nothing is known of Dr. Kendrick subsequent to his military service in the 3rd Seminole War. He does not appear in the Florida Census of 1860 nor was he a member of any Florida unit in the Confederate Army.[4]

1. U.S. Census, 1850, Hillsborough County, Florida, p. 48.

2. Throughout the brief conflict the frontier was constantly changing but only in the latter stages was it established along the Caloosahatchee River.

3. Records of the Adjutant General's Office, Record Group 94; Compiled Service Records, Volunteer Soldiers, Florida Indian Wars, 1835-1858, 112-B, Microcopy 1086, Roll 63.

4. For his services in the war Dr. Kendrick was paid $417.25. Years later the state of Florida, which had borne the expense of the 3rd Seminole War to some degree, sought reimbursement from the Treasury of the United States. On February 26, 1887, the U.S. Senate authorized the Secretary of the Treasury to settle and pay the claims. The measure had passed the House of Representatives on January 27, 1887. Only a few claims were actually paid, no vouchers having been preserved as evidence. The payment to Dr. Kendrick was among those disallowed, no voucher or receipt having been found.

Kelly, J.W., New River County (Bradford), 1860

Dr. Kelly,[1] native of South Carolina, was a resident of rural New River County in 1860. His wife, Margaret, was a native of Georgia, while their eight-month-old daughter, Julia, was born in Florida. Since he does not appear in the Census of 1870 he is presumed to have been only a brief sojourner in the state.

1. U.S. Census, 1860, New River County (name changed to Bradford County in 1861), p. 478.

Key, Gilbert L., Hillsborough and Polk Counties, 1830

Dr. Key, a native of Georgia, settled in rural Hillsborough County about 1859 offering his medical services to the citizens of his community. He was of modest means, owning property valued at $1,250 in 1860.[1] After a brief period of unremunerative practice he moved with his family to Ft. Meade in Polk County where he turned to farming.[2] In the latter part of the Civil War he tendered his professional service to the Confederacy and his offer was accepted. He was assigned the rank of assistant surgeon and permitted to remain at Ft. Meade as physician to a company which had been recruited by Captain F.A. Henry. His commission was dated 1864.[3]

Dr. Key remained in Polk County after the close of the war. The Census of 1870 lists him as "farmer" owning property valued at a mere $200. Members of the family included his wife, Rachel, also a native of Georgia, and six daughters, Fannie, Sallie, Rachel, Mary, Nancy and Susan, all Florida-born, except Fannie who was born in Georgia.[4] Beyond this date nothing is known of the Key family. They do not appear in the Polk County Census of 1880.

1. U.S. Census, 1860, Hillsborough County, p. 645.
2. Ibid., Polk County, Florida, p. 476.
3. *Soldiers of Florida in the Seminole Indian, Civil and Spanish-American Wars*, Live Oak, p. 320.
4. Another daughter, Martha, aged eight in 1860 does not appear in the Florida Census of 1870.

Kilmer, Washington, Orange County, 1838-1919

Dr. Kilmer, a man of great courage, intelligence and high moral principle, was born in New York State in 1838. Nothing is known of his early education but in 1858 he matriculated at the Albany Medical College, Albany, New York, and was graduated in 1860. He apparently began practice in Albany. In the following year, however, with mobilization of troops under way, he offered his services to the Union Army in which he served, probably as medical officer, until conclusion of the war in 1865. He then settled in Ironton, Ohio, a town known for its iron and steel production as well as Portland cement. There he remained in practice from 1865 until 1872.[1]

For reasons not known Dr. Kilmer decided at that juncture to move to Florida and lacking funds for transportation decided to walk the entire distance from Ironton to central Florida, some 1,400 miles. Making his way through central Florida he eventually arrived at Altamonte Springs. He was impressed with the natural beauty of the place and decided to settle there. Citriculture had already begun in the area. Dr. Kilmer joined in the enterprise and for the next three years conducted a medical practice and observed the growth of his orange grove.

Dr. Kilmer moved into nearby Orlando in 1875 where he established a good reputation as both physician and public servant. Two years later he was elected Chairman of the Orange County Board of Public Instruction, a post he held until 1885.

The city of Tampa suffered one of its most deadly yellow fever epidemics in 1887 and with some of its own physicians falling victim to the disease a call for help went out to other towns. Dr. Kilmer was one of the first to respond, making his way immediately to the city. He too soon came down with the disease but survived. On the basis of observations he theorized that yellow fever was spread by germs (the mosquito theory had not yet been proven) and that the disease could not thrive in pine lands but required marsh lands and fresh water lakes for propagation. Following his recovery he took his family north for an extended visit and afterwards settled again in Orlando where he would spend the rest of his life. The citizens of Orlando, touched by his courage in the Tampa epidemic, awarded him a gold medal on which the following words were engraved:

> Presented to Dr. Washington Kilmer by the citizens of Orlando in appreciation of his service in the yellow fever epidemic at Tampa, Florida, November 25, 1887.

The greater part of Dr. Kilmer's service in the Union Army was spent in Alexandria, Virginia, where he was in charge of the Grace Church Hospital which cared for wounded Union soldiers. He was there for approximately three years and in 1864 he met and married Florience (patronym unknown).[2] She was a Virginia native whose father was English-born. Census records give the date of her birth as August 1844. To that marriage were born two daughters, Alice, born in Maryland in 1866, and May, born in Ironton, Ohio, in 1872, just prior to the removal of the family to Florida.

Dr. Kilmer lived in Orlando until 1919, dying at the age of 81. He was buried in Greenwood Cemetery in Orlando.

1. No complete biographical sketch of Dr. Kilmer has been located. The most useful of the brief treatments is that of William R. O'Neal, *Memoir of a Pioneer*, Orlando, privately printed, no date. Another useful source is E.H. Gore, *From Florida Sand to the City Beautiful*, Orlando 1951, pp. 160 and 205. Not to be overlooked is William Fremont Blackman, *History of Orange County*, Mickler House, Publ., Chuluota, Fla., 1973, pp. 50, 55, and 90.

2. Very useful, although not totally reliable, are the Censuses of Orange County, Florida, 1880 and 1900, as well as the Special Florida Census of 1885.

King, Benjamin, St. Marks, 1821

Dr. King, who was commissioned surgeon's mate and assigned to the 7th Infantry Regiment on October 14, 1818, served only briefly in Florida. Soon after being promoted to assistant surgeon on June 1, 1821,[1] he was assigned to the St. Marks post from which he made the following report for the third quarter of that year:[2]

> At St. Marks there were 7 deaths. The prevailing diseases were remittent and intermittent fever, diarrhoea (sic), and dysentery....My hospital is very bad, and more or less wet at every rain; on the 16th September, the tide rose uncommonly high, which nearly inundated this place and the adjacent country; the water was a foot deep in the hospital; in fact, I visited my sick and went through it in a canoe. The bunks were sufficiently high to keep the sick out of the water; but this occurrence, as well as the dampness from the rains, had a very injurious effect on my patients, more particularly those laboring under dysentery and diarrhoea.

By 1823 Dr. King had been transferred to a post in Augusta, Georgia,[3] and in 1825 was stationed at Ft. McHenry, Md.[4] Since he was a native of Maryland he probably was pleased to remain in that area. He appears to have spent the greater part of his lengthy service in Washington, D.C.; at least, he was there at the time of retirement from the Army on November 9, 1863.[5]

1. MDUSA., p. 291. The 7th Infantry Regiment was assigned to Louisiana with headquarters in Baton Rouge.
2. Lawson, *Statistical Report*, p. 29.
3. ASP., II, 516.
4. Ibid., p. 838.
5. MDUSA., p. 291. See also ASP., V, 278, 608; VI, 35, 1006; VII, 929.

Kneeland, Lucius, Ft. McCoy, Marion County, 1822-1852

Dr. Kneeland was born in Waterbury, Vermont, on March 20, 1822. He was graduated from the University of Vermont at Burlington with the Bachelor of Arts degree in 1846 and two years later enrolled at the Clinical Medical School at Woodstock, Vermont,[1] from which he received his medical degree in 1850. Soon thereafter he was commissioned as a medical officer in the United States Army and assigned to service at Ft. McCoy,[2] located in the northeastern part of Marion County, a few miles west of the Oklawaha River, an assignment which was far from desirable. He died there on August 11, 1852, probably from one of the fevers endemic to the area.

1. The brief biographical data presented here is derived from F.C. Waite, *A History of the Clinical School of Medicine, Woodstock, Vermont, 1827-1856*, Montpelier, Vermont Historical Society, 1945, p. 166.

2. Ft. McCoy as it existed in the mid-19th century was an isolated post around which the village of Ft. McCoy later grew. It exists today as the hub of a thriving farming community.

Knight, Albion W., Jacksonville, 1823-1889

Much of the biographical data relating to Dr. Knight are well documented by Wanton S. Webb and Dr. Webster Merritt.[1] He was born in Brunswick, Maine, on January 5, 1823, and in 1841 was graduated from Bowdoin College in Brunswick with a Bachelor of Arts degree. He remained in Brunswick and attended the Medical School of Maine from which he was graduated Doctor of Medicine.[2]

Following medical school he joined his brother in Brunswick, Georgia, doubtless fascinated by the name, and practiced for a year or more. He met and married Carolina Demere and prior to 1850 moved to White Sulphur Springs, now White Springs, on the Suwannee River in Hamilton County where he practiced until 1871.[3] It was there that six of his children were born. In 1850 the Knight household included in addition to the immediate family two of Mrs. Knight's sisters, Mary and Martha Demere.

On August 26, 1871, the following announcement appeared in the Live Oak *Times*:[4]

> Dr. Knight, having recently removed from the White Springs and located in Jacksonville, respectfully solicits a share of the patronage from all those unfortunate enough to need a physician.

Soon after settling in Jacksonville Mrs. Knight died.[5] Dr. Knight did not long remain without a wife for after a "decent" interval he married Miss Anna Bishop to whom three children were born.

It appears that Dr. Knight did not want for patronage. Once in Jacksonville he adjusted quickly to urban surroundings by associating himself with professional colleagues and assuming a position of influence and leadership in the medical societies of both Duval County and the state. For seven years he was secretary of the state organization and a member of numerous committees.[6] Beyond this he served for several years as health officer for the city of Jacksonville and found himself in the irksome situation of defending his report on the outbreak of yellow fever in Jacksonville in 1877 against the probing skepticism of Dr. R.P. Daniel.[7] He faced other occasions which called for patience and perseverance as, for example, when the Florida Times-Union refused to publish his report on the yellow fever epidemic in the city in 1883 fearing damaging publicity. He was also incensed by the general disregard for quarantine precautions on the part of the citizens.[8]

Dr. Knight carried on his professional duties vigorously and efficiently almost until the time of his death on September 6, 1889. In January he had attended the annual meeting of the Florida Medical Association in St. Augustine and had assisted in preparation of a report.[9] At the Association's annual meeting in 1890 in Ocala, Dr. R.A. Lancaster, presiding, offered a fitting tribute to the memory of his departed colleague.[10]

1. Wanton S. Webb, *Historical, Industrial and Biographical Florida*, New York, 1885, I. 155. Webster Merritt,

A Century of Medicine in Jacksonville and Duval County, Gainesville, 1949, pp. 95-96.
2. These dates were verified by Dr. Knight's family for Dr. Merritt.
3. White Sulphur Springs on the north bank of the Suwannee River in the southeast corner of Hamilton County enjoyed considerable popularity as a spa in the mid-19th century.
4. The issues for 1871 are not extant. The issue of March 22, 1873, however, indicates that the notice was first printed on August 26, 1871.
5. Mrs. Knight's death occurred on February 24, 1873. She was buried in the Old City Cemetery.
6. *Proceedings, Florida Medical Association*, 1874-1890, passim. Various issues include references to Dr. Knight's activities within the Association.
7. Ibid., 1878, pp. 22-49. It should be stated that Dr. Daniel's queries were in no sense malicious, but rather in the nature of scientific inquiry.
8. Merritt, *Century*, pp. 131-132.
9. *Proceedings, FMA*, 1889, pp. 6, 24.
10. Ibid.

Kock, Karl, Fernandina, 1870

Dr. Koch practiced medicine for a brief period in Fernandina about 1870. The Census of that year lists him as a native of Saxony, aged 50, and owner of property valued at $1,800. He was a resident of a rooming house owned by Mrs. Carolina Clark. Nothing further is known of this physician.[1]

1. U.S. Census, 1870, Nassau County, Florida, p. 398, item 355.

Kovaleski, Kayeton, Pensacola, early 1840s

As far as can be determined Dr. Kovaleski was only a brief sojourner in Florida. He appears in the Escambia County Census of 1840 as a resident of Pensacola, between 30 and 40 years of age, and unmarried.[1] It appears, however, that he had earlier in the year been a practitioner in St. Joseph, Florida,[2] but on June 6, 1840, he announced he was moving his office "to the house adjoining the residence of Joseph Ballada on Church Street near the Episcopal Church."[3] Two years later, however, the following notice appeared in the local newspaper: "Dr. K. Kovaleski, having returned to Pensacola, tenders medical services, etc. Residence opposite that of Captain Baker's."[4] No further reference to his Florida practice has been discovered.

1. U.S. Census, 1840, Escambia County, Florida, p. 17.
2. St. Joseph *Times*, March 11, 1840.
3. Pensacola *Gazette*, August 10, 1840, 1st printing, June 6, 1840.
4. Ibid., June 11, 1842, 1st printing May 14, 1842.

Krimminger, John Newton, New Troy, Lafayette County, 1871

Although he is designated physician in the U.S. Census of 1870, there remains some doubt that John Newton Krimminger was ever a legitimate member of the medical profession. Born in North Carolina he had migrated to Darlington, South Carolina, probably in the 1840s, married a Darlington girl, and settled down there as a farmer. The Census of South Carolina for 1860 shows him and his wife, Rebecca, to be the parents of six daughters, the eldest aged 13 and all born in South Carolina.[1]

With the coming of the Civil War Dr. Krimminger had been drafted into the Confederate Army but had managed to escape through the enemy lines and join the Union cause.[2] When the conflict was over he moved with his family to Lafayette County, one of the less populated areas of North Florida, and settled in the village of New Troy which had a population of less than 100. If indeed he had been seeking a locality in which his past would remain concealed he had found it in New Troy. The Census of 1870 for Lafayette County lists him as physician and includes, in addition to his wife, three daughters, all South Carolina-born, and a son, Franklin, aged four, and born in Florida.[3]

All might have gone well but Dr. Krimminger's moral convictions were deep and fervent. He was quick to ally himself with the radical Republicanism designed to benefit the emancipated blacks and prevent the return to power of the southern white conservatives. It was in this role that he became a member of the Constitutional Convention of 1868 which met in Tallahassee on January 20th. It is well documented that Dr. Krimminger's voting record in the Convention established him as a radical Republican in spite of his southern origin.[4] With the implementation of the newly-devised constitution later in the year, Dr. Krimminger found himself the representative of Lafayette and Taylor Counties (10th District) in the Florida Senate, an office which he was to hold again in 1869 and 1870.

Failing to win his senate seat for the fourth time, Dr. Krimminger appears to have settled down to the profession of country doctor in New Troy while his wife Rebecca became the postmistress of the town. His political activities understandably had incurred for him the hatred of some of his neighbors and rendered him a target for local Klansmen. One of these, a man named Ponchier, harboring a grievance said to have grown out of the election campaign of 1870, decided to rid the county of this traitor to the southern cause. Concealing himself in the county courthouse, which stood near the Krimminger home, he waited throughout the night of October 4, 1871, and at dawn next morning the doctor came out the door and took a seat on the porch. Ponchier took aim with his rifle and shot Dr. Krimminger through the heart, killing him instantly. Mrs. Krimminger emerged from the house in time to see the assassin leaving the courthouse rifle in hand. It was her verdict that her husband was the victim of the Klan.[5]

There is no reason to assume that Dr. Krimminger was not an honorable man and a conscientious medical practitioner. He was simply unfortunate to have lived in a time and place where the violence triggered by reconstruction was especially rampant.[6] At the time of his death he was a county judge of Lafayette County.

1. U.S. Census, 1860, South Carolina, Darlington District, p. 58.

2. Ralph L. Peek, "Lawlessness in Florida, 1868-71," *Florida Historical Quarterly*, XL, 167. New Troy, a settlement on the Suwannee River about five miles north of Branford and 20 miles south of Live Oak, no longer exists. It enjoyed briefly the distinction of being the county seat of Lafayette, an honor later transferred to Mayo.

3. U.S. Census, 1870, Florida, Lafayette County, p. 33. The age of the son, Franklin, suggests that the Krimmingers arrived in Florida about 1866.

4. Richard L. Hume, "Membership of the Florida Constitutional Convention of 1868," *Florida Historical Quarterly*, LI, July, 1972, 1-21. This is a carefully documented treatment of the voting behavior of the members of the Convention.

5. A complete report of the assassination is found in the Tallahassee *Sentinel*, October 21, 1871.

6. Peek, "Lawlessness." The U.S. Census, 1880, Lafayette County, p. 48, shows Mrs. Krimminger, daughter Caroline, aged 16, and son Franklin, aged 12, still living in New Troy.

Lacy, Robert A., Key West, 1820

The actual date of Dr. Lacy's arrival in Key West remains undetermined but it appears that he was there by the late summer of 1827. Among appointments to public office announced by Acting Governor and Secretary William M. McCarty in the summer of 1827 was that of "Doctor Lacy, Auctioneer for the County of Monroe."[1] Such appointments were subject to approval by the Legislative Council, however, and in action by that body on August 8, 1827, Dr. Lacy was rejected for the auctioneer's post but simultaneously approved for a notary public office.[2] He was later reconsidered and approved for the position of auctioneer, however, and was still serving in that capacity when he left Key West after some two and a half years.

Dr. Lacy was born about 1804. He was awarded his medical degree by the University of Pennsylvania with the class of 1824, having written a thesis on "Gonorrhea."[3] Upon settling in Key West he had established medical practice and in spite of his public offices appears to have been a busy practitioner. Because of the frequent recurrence of yellow fever on the island its reputation as a place of disease and death or as one writer put it, "a Perfect Graveyard," had been widely publicized not only through northern newspapers but also in those of Pensacola and St. Augustine. Consequently it became an obligation of Key West physicians to counterbalance such unfavorable reports. Both Dr. Lacy and his colleague, Dr. Henry S. Waterhouse, used the columns of the Key West newspaper to reassure potential settlers, investors and persons in failing health that Key West was healthful and safe. In a letter to Dr. Edward Macomb, an Army surgeon at Tampa Bay, Dr. Lacy wrote: "I have resided on this Island near twelve months, and during that whole period but two cases of disease of any importance has occurred. The one yellow fever, the other bilious remittent."[4]

The problems of medical regulation and public health were from the very beginning serious ones for Florida's territorial government. In its session of 1827-28 the Legislative Council finally created a medical regulatory body, giving it the power to control the licensing of physicians. The act designated the physicians, nine all told, who would constitute the Medical Board. Dr. Lacy was among them.[5]

The year 1829 was an eventful one for Dr. Lacy. On February 9 one of the most sensational and widely-publicized duels ever fought in Florida took place on Key West's south beach. Involved were Capt. Charles E. Hawkins, an American serving in the Mexican Navy, and William Allison McRea, U.S. Attorney for the Southern Judicial District of Florida. The challenge was issued by Hawkins whose winsome wife had lured McRea into her bedroom. Although four shots were fired by each man, only one bullet found its mark and that one lodged in McRea's thigh. Within a few weeks he had recovered.[6]

In the meantime, Dr. Lacy and McRea took a brief sojourn in Havana returning to Key West on March 29.[7] Hawkins also left Key West on February 20 for Vera Cruz to return within a few weeks. In the late afternoon of May 24 he concealed himself in a house on Whitehead Street near its intersection with Carolina Street and as McRea walked past he rushed out with his shotgun and unloaded two rounds of buckshot in the back of the attorney. This time the wounds were fatal.[8]

In March 1829 Dr. Lacy announced his candidacy for a seat in the Legislative

Assembly but in the June elections he was unsuccessful, losing to Theodore Owens largely because of the vote in Indian Key.[9]

As the very devastating yellow fever epidemic of 1829 began to engulf Key West in September the local newspaper suspended its publication thus making it impossible to follow the professional activities of Dr. Lacy. We must assume that he remained on the island ministering to the needs of the sick as best he could. It is known that he survived the epidemic. On December 7 he announced his intention to be absent from the city for an unspecified period of time, appointing Fielding A. Browne his agent during his absence and empowering Browne to act as auctioneer in his stead.[10] It appears that Dr. Lacy never returned to Key West except possibly for the purpose of settling his affairs there. In February 1830 he joined a group of Leon County citizens in protesting to President Jackson against what they deemed to be high-handed misuse of judicial power by a judge of the Middle District of Florida in a matter relating to the use of public lands.[11] It seems certain that Dr. Lacy was at that time a citizen of Leon County.

Beyond this nothing is known of Dr. Lacy. An item of shipping news in the Key West *Inquirer* of January 9, 1836, announced the arrival at Sand Key[12] of the brig Chieftain from Apalachicola. Aboard was "Robert Lacy of Tuscaloosa (Ala.)." It is purely conjectural to identify this man as Dr. Lacy.

1. T.P., XXIII 927.
2. Ibid., p. 1007.
3. Archives, University of Pennsylvania, List of Medical Graduates.
4. Key West *Register*, March 26, 1829.
5. *Acts, Legislative Council, Territory of Florida*, 6th Session, 1827-28, Tallahassee 1828, pp. 46-49. This bill was printed in toto in the Key West *Register*, April 30, 1829.
6. Ibid., February 12, 1829. This is a brief account. Additional details may be found in Thelma Peters, ed., "William Adee Whitehead's Reminiscences of Key West," *Tequesta*, XXV, 1965, pp. 24-25.
7. Key West *Register*, April 2, 1829.
8. Ibid., May 28, 1829. See also Peters, n. 6, supra.
9. Key West *Register*, March 19, 1829, June 4, 1829, June 11, 1829.
10. Ibid., December 31, 1829.
11. T.P., XXIX, 365.
12. Sand Key lies 8½ miles south, southeast of Key West.

LaFitte, David Montague, Leon County, 1829-1864

Dr. LaFitte, descendant of a prominent South Carolina Huguenot family, was born in Barnwell District, South Carolina, in 1829. His father, of the same name, had been born in Savannah, Georgia, in 1791, but prior to 1818 had moved to South Carolina, where he married Mary, daughter of James and Elizabeth Garvin.[1] Dr. LaFitte received his medical degree from the Medical Department, University of Georgia, Augusta, in 1852[2] and soon thereafter settled in Leon County near Lake Miccosukee where he practiced until the beginning of the Civil War.

Dr. LaFitte's sole excursion into politics occurred in the summer of 1860 when he was a Leon County delegate to the State Democratic Convention which met in Quincy on June 4 in what became a notoriously boisterous session.[3] In August of the following year, he was commissioned by Governor Madison S. Perry to organize a company of volunteers for service with the 5th Florida Infantry Regiment, "to be formed into a camp of instruction."[4] Wrote the Monticello newspaper of this undertaking: "Dr. LaFitte is a high-toned, intelligent gentleman, and there exists not a doubt that he will make a popular and useful commander."[5] On September 7 he announced: "I have concluded to go into camp on the 10th of September at Miccosukie Lake. All members are requested to appear there on that day, come prepared for camp life. Bring your blankets, clothing, a cup, a knife, a tin plate, etc..."[6]

For reasons not clear but doubtless dictated by the urgent need for medical personnel, Dr. LaFitte was not permitted to remain for very long with his Leon County company before being called into medical service with the Confederate Army in Alabama. While on duty in Mobile in 1864 he was taken ill and sent home to Florida where he died within a few weeks. He was buried near his Miccosukee home.[7]

Dr. LaFitte was twice married. His first wife was Mary Jane, daughter of Alexander and Elizabeth Brisbane Lawton of Barnwell District, S.C. She died without issue. After moving to Florida he married Sarah Ann Miller in 1857 and they had two children, Charles, who died in infancy, and Rondeau Boyd who, on reaching manhood, settled in Lloyd, Jefferson County, where he operated a mercantile business.[8]

1. For more genealogical information on the LaFitte family see W.T. Cash, *The Story of Florida*, New York, American Historical Society, 1938, IV, 619.
2. Medical Department, University of Georgia, *List of Graduates from 1829 to 1891*, Augusta, 1891, p. 20.
3. Fernandina *East Floridian*, June 21, 1860.
4. Monticello *Family Friend*, August 24, 1861.
5. Ibid.
6. Ibid., September 7, 1861.
7. See note 1, supra.
8. Rondeau Boyd LaFitte was married to Ida Lee Sydnor. They became the parents of Dr. Lincoln Sydnor LaFitte, 1892-1963, alumnus of the University of Florida, Rhodes Scholar at Oxford University, and medical graduate of the University of Pennsylvania. He had a distinguished career as a physician in Jacksonville and served a term as the president of the Duval County Medical Society, 1947.

Lamar, Thompson Bird, Leon and Jefferson Counties, 1828-1864

Scion of a distinguished Southern family, Dr. Lamar was born in Oxford, Georgia, in 1828. His father, Lucius Quintus Cincinnatus Lamar,[1] a lawyer and superior court judge, had died at the age of 37. After attending the local school young Lamar attended Emory College at Oxford from which he was graduated in 1848.[2] In the fall of that year he matriculated at Jefferson Medical College in Philadelphia and in the spring of 1850 was graduated as Doctor of Medicine.[3] The following year he moved to Leon County where he met and married Sarah Bellamy Bailey, daughter of William Bailey, wealthy banker and planter of neighboring Jefferson County.[4]

Dr. Lamar announced his medical services in January 1864 to the people of Leon and adjoining counties available from his home on the Thomasville Road, eight miles north of Tallahassee. It had formerly been the home of Dr. James Hunter.

With proper family connections[5] and endowed with extraordinary charm and intelligence, Dr. Lamar quickly achieved recognition in public life. He was sufficiently well known by 1856 to become the Democratic candidate for a seat in the Florida Senate which he won in a close race with the "Know Nothing" candidate. He was returned to the Legislature for the session of 1858 and was also present for the adjourned session of 1859.[6]

Near the end of 1859 or early 1860 Dr. Lamar moved with his family which included four children to the Bailey plantation northeast of Monticello.[7] His father-in-law was 70 years of age and it was doubtless his need for care that prompted the Lamars to make the move. By this juncture the slavery issue had become all-engrossing and Dr. Lamar had become an effective spokesman for the Southern cause. At a meeting of the Jefferson County Democrats on March 31, 1860, he gave a speech "lengthy and eloquent" directing attention to the "inroads the Black Republicans are endeavoring to make upon the Constitution, and the rights of the States under it, and the course of action to be pursued by the South in the present emergency."[8] In Quincy on June 4 he addressed an inebriated and boisterous crowd exhorting them to support secession.[9] Similarly in Monticello on August 4 he responded to a request to speak extemporaneously and it was reported that he "talked an hour and a quarter, eloquently...to much applause."[10] As soon as the November election returns had assured a Lincoln victory, Dr. Lamar spoke at a mass meeting convened to discuss what was to be done "following the shocking election."[11] At the special convention assembled in Tallahassee on January 3, 1861, to consider the secession matter, Dr. Lamar was one of four delegates from Jefferson County. Not surprisingly he was among those voting for the secession proposal, which carried 62 to seven.[12]

With war looming little time was lost, especially on the plantation counties of middle Florida, in augmenting the militia. In the earlier stages it was a volunteer effort, somewhat haphazard. Before the end of March Dr. Lamar had made his service available. He was mustered in on April 19 with the rank of captain and assigned to command Company I, First Florida Infantry.[13] From this post he was honorably discharged by special order on January 30, 1862, however, less than three months later he was mustered in with the rank of lieutenant colonel and assigned to Headquarters, 5th Florida Infantry. He was promoted to the rank of colonel on July 6, 1863, and saw service under the command of General Joseph E. Johnston.

Fate was brutal, however, to this brave man. In early May 1864 he was wounded in one of the early skirmishes of the Battle of the Wilderness near Fredericksburg, Virginia. Having lost the index finger of his left hand and suffering a gunshot wound in his left leg, he was admitted to the General Hospital of the Confederacy at Richmond on May 8. A recuperation furlough permitted him to return to his Jefferson County home from which he wrote his commanding general, Patton Anderson:[14] "I look upon my wound as a blessing...I am at present in that pleasant state where I get sympathy without any occasion for it..." His respite was brief. By early August he had returned to his unit in Virginia and on August 30, 1864, he was killed on the field of battle at Petersburg.[15]

1. Better known was his brother, Lucius Quintus Cincinnatues Lamar, II, U.S. Senator from Mississippi, Secretary of the Interior under President Cleveland and later Justice of the U.S. Supreme Court. The younger brother, Jefferson Mirabeau Lamar, commanded a Georgia Regiment under General T.R.R. Cobb in the Civil War and was killed during a skirmish at Crampton Gap, Md., in September 1862.

2. Some biographical data concerning Dr. Lamar are found in *Makers of America*, Florida Edition, Atlanta 1911, IV, 503-509, which also includes a sketch of Dr. Lamar's son, William Bailey Lamar.

3. Jefferson Medical College, Philadelphia, *List of Dead and Lost Graduates in Classes from 1826 to 1879*, Philadelphia, 1879, p. 79.

4. William Bailey was one of the wealthiest men in antebellum Florida having owned 330 slaves in 1850. In 1860 his properties were valued at more than $600,000.

5. Tallahassee *Floridian and Journal*, January 28, 1854.

6. Allen Morris, *The People of Lawmaking in Florida, 1822-1977*, Tallahassee, 1977, unpaginated.

7. U.S. Census, 1860, Jefferson County, Florida, p. 45.

8. Monticello *Family Friend*, April 7, 1860.

9. Ibid., January 9, 1860.

10. Ibid., August 11, 1860.

11. Ibid., November 17, 1860.

12. *Florida Historical Quarterly*, v(2), 118.

13. NA, Service Records, CSA, M251, Rolls 28 and 65.

14. T.B. Lamar to J. Patton Anderson, June 3, 1864. J. Patton Anderson Papers, P.K. Yonge Library of Florida History, University of Florida, Gainesville.

15. See note 13 supra.

Lang, Thomas, Leon County, 1798-1850

Dr. Lang was one of many physicians who migrated to Florida during its Territorial Period only to find life rigorous and remuneration not only inadequate but difficult to collect. He arrived in Florida early in 1841 lingering briefly in Tallahassee before moving into the area northeast of the city on the west side of Lake Miccosukee. On April 23, 1841,[1] he informed the public that he was locating at a residence until recently occupied by Colonel Augustus Aalston.[2] About a year later he announced he was moving to a "place recently owned by Mr. Levi Massey, within 14 miles of Tallahassee on the Monticello Road and within one mile of Major Edward Mills, Post Office address still Tallahassee."[3] On June 24, 1842, he offered for sale 1,500 bushels of corn "on credit until Jan. 1, next."[4] He was still advertising his services in January 1843.[5]

At some subsequent date Dr. Lang gave up the struggle in Florida and moved to Bibb County, Georgia, where he died in East Macon on May 19, 1850. His obituary notice gave Charleston, S.C., as the place of birth and his age as "about fifty-three."[6]

1. Tallahassee *Sentinel*, September 24, 1841. First printing, April 23, 1841.
2. Col. Augustus Aalston was killed in a duel with General Leigh Reid in 1839. His plantation was later bought by Colonel Joel Blake. See Joy Smith Paisley, *The Cemeteries of Leon County, Florida*, Tallahassee, 1978, p. 11.
3. Tallahassee *Sentinel*, March 18, 1842.
4. Ibid., June 24, 1842.
5. Ibid., January 6, 1843.
6. Tallahassee *Floridian and Journal*, May 25, 1850.

Langford, Thomas E., Madison and Lee Counties, 1847-1900

Dr. Langford, whose medical career spanned only a few years, was born in Madison County in 1847.[1] He was the first son and third child of Thomas Langford, planter,[2] and his wife Lucinda neé Overstreet. Both the Langford and Overstreet families were fairly prominent in the public affairs of early Madison County. Nothing is known of Dr. Langford's education at either the elementary or professional level but he is thought to have served a medical apprenticeship[3] in the office of Dr. Silas T. Overstreet, a native of Madison County, who later practiced in Live Oak, Suwannee County.

Dr. Langford appears in the Madison County census of 1870 as a resident of Ellaville, a village on the west bank of the Suwannee River near its junction with the Withlacoochee. In 1869, at age 22, he married Annie Jane Galloway of Live Oak[4] and soon thereafter decided to abandon the practice of medicine and turn to cattle raising, a pursuit in which he appears to have been moderately successful. About 1878 he moved to Ft. Myers where he joined James E. Hendry Sr. in the cattle business, apparently becoming affluent largely by supplying beef for the Cuban market.

Dr. Langford died in Bartow on January 21, 1900[5] whence he had gone for treatment under Dr. Frank Wilson. He had suffered from Bright's disease for some time and Dr. Wilson had recognized his condition as incurable. A day or so prior to his death he experienced a brief period of remission but death came suddenly. Even allowing for the mannered style of his obituary, there can be no doubt that he was held in high regard. His eulogist wrote: "Dr. Langford was a gentleman of fine character, who stood high in the esteem of those who knew him...He came to Lee County comparatively poor, but by thrift and industry he had accumulated quite a handsome fortune."

Dr. Langford was survived by his widow and five children.[6] His body was returned to Ft. Myers for burial.

1. Some data have been derived from Karl H. Grismer, *The Story of Ft. Myers*, St. Petersburg, St. Petersburg Printing Co., 1949, p. 282.
2. See Censuses of Madison County, Florida, 1850, 1860 and 1870.
3. It was not until founding of the Florida Medical Association in 1874 that completion of the Doctor of Medicine

degree was generally held to be an absolute requisite for obtaining a license to practice in Florida.

4. Annie J. Galloway was the eldest daughter of John T. Galloway, who brought his wife and three daughters, all South Carolina-born, to Columbia County about 1859. He began his Florida residence as a farmer. Later he "read law" and by 1870 was a practicing lawyer in Houstoun, Suwannee County.

5. Bartow *Courier-Informant*, January 24, 1900.

6. The children were Walter G., Stella, James, Homie and Eunice. Walter G. became a successful businessman in Ft. Myers. He was instrumental in the early development of the town, having been in large measure responsible for persuading the Atlantic Coast Line Railroad to extend its services to Ft. Myers. See note 1, supra.

Langley, Samuel, Monticello, 1830

Dr. Langley apparently arrived in Monticello about 1831 for the Tallahassee newspaper published a notice on January 3, 1832, announcing the dissolution of the partnership previously existing between him and Dr. Albert J. Dozier.[1] In the same issue Dr. Langley announced that he would continue to reside in Monticello and offer his services to the people of Jefferson and adjoining counties, however, a short time later he is believed to have moved to the Waukeenah community where he owned land and engaged in planting.[2] In September 1835, as abolitionist sentiment in the North intensified, Dr. Langley presided over a gathering of concerned planters of Jefferson County called for the purpose of meeting the threat of northern "fanatics" to southern "property rights."[3] No further information on Dr. Langley has been discovered.

1. Tallahassee *Floridian*, January 10, 1832.

2. Jerrell Shofner, *History of Jefferson County, Florida*, Tallahassee, 1976, p. 61.

3. Tallahassee *Floridian*, September 19, 1835. This meeting occurred on August 7 at the Cross Roads south of Monticello.

Langner, Henry G., Volusia County, 1835

Dr. Langner, a native of Maryland, settled in or near the village of Volusia[1] just prior to the beginning of the Civil War, too late to have been listed in the Census of 1860. The 1870 Census of Volusia County lists him as 35 years of age, owning property valued at $550. Included in his family were his wife, Annie,[2] aged 36, and three children, Henry, aged 10, Charles, four, and Kate, five months old. All three were Florida-born, indicating that the Langners arrived in Florida about 1859-60. Since they do not appear in subsequent censuses, they are presumed to have left the state by 1880.

1. The village of Volusia was located on the east bank of the St. Johns River between Lake George and Lake Monroe across the river from present-day Astor.

2. Mrs. Langner was born in New Jersey about 1834.

Lassiter, Craven, Alachua, Suwannee and Madison Counties, 1829

Dr. Lassiter was a native of North Carolina[1] but while still a child his family moved to Darlington County, South Carolina, settling on a farm located on Swift Creek.[2] As a young man he began the study of medicine under the preceptorate of Dr. Christopher Flinn, a physician of the town of Darlington who was a graduate of the Medical College of the State of South Carolina, class of 1849.[3] Lassiter enrolled at the college in 1851, and in March 1853[4] received his medical degree. His thesis topic was "Tetanus."

Within a year after graduation Dr. Lassiter had settled in Newnansville where he joined Dr. E.R. Power in a partnership which included operation of a drug store.[5] They announced their intention in February 1854 to "Keep constantly on hand and for sale a complete assortment of the Best Drugs & Medicines, Fancy Articles, Fine Cigars, etc;" however, in 1854 Newnansville lost its bid for the county seat of Alachua to Gainesville and began a decline which eventually led to its extinction. The year 1860 found Dr. Power practicing in Lafayette County while Dr. Lassiter had settled in the village of Houstoun in Suwannee County.[6] Meanwhile the post office had been established at Houstoun on December 22, 1859, with Dr. Lassiter as its first postmaster.[7]

The decision to take Florida out of the Union having been made at the Secession Convention in Tallahassee on January 7, 1861, mobilization for possible conflict was soon under way. Among the first to offer his services to the Confederacy was Dr. Lassiter who enlisted as a private on April 2, two weeks before the firing on Ft. Sumter.[8] He was assigned to Co. C, 8th Florida Infantry Regiment, a unit to which he belonged for the first 12 months of his service. He was mustered out on April 19, 1862.[9]

Dr. Lassiter was quick to reenlist and in May was mustered once more into the 8th Florida Regiment, this time as Second Lieutenant, having signed for "three years, or the duration." Soon thereafter his Regiment was ordered to Virginia and in August participated in the 2nd Battle of Manassa. Although Dr. Lassiter's official war record is garbled, it appears that he was with the 8th on its Maryland campaign in the autumn of 1862 returning to Fredericksburg in December.

Dr. Lassiter was promoted to a first lieutenancy on April 23, 1863. He had actually been recommended for a captaincy but before his promotion papers could be processed he fell wounded at the Battle of Chancellorsville on May 3 and thereafter was shortly taken prisoner and sent to the dreaded Union prison at Johnson's Island on Lake Erie. His first lieutenant's commission was approved, however, and in April 1864 he was transferred to Point Lookout, Maryland,[10] but the damage to his health was done. Later in the summer of 1864 he was returned to the Confederate Army, presumably in a prisoner exchange, whereupon he was listed as "sick at hospital" in Petersburg. On September 19, 1864, he was granted a leave of absence for 50 days. A hospital report issued at the General Hospital in Richmond on August 9, 1864, diagnosed his illness as "Debilitas" resulting from chronic diarrhea contracted while a prisoner of war. His age was 35. He was paroled on April 9, 1865.

On his return to Suwannee County Dr. Lassiter resumed medical practice, and in October 1865 he was persuaded to offer himself as a candidate for a seat in the Florida House of Representatives. He was elected. The House *Journals* do not suggest that he was a legislative leader although he appears to have been regular in attendance at its sessions; finding himself frequently on the winning side when votes were tallied. When the House came to vote on a Senate Bill designed to establish a Medical Board for the state, a bill which had passed the Senate by a vote of 20 to 3, Dr. Lassiter was among those voting "Nay,"[11] this notwithstanding the fact that two physicians who were members of the Senate, Holmes Steele and Daniel W. Whitehurst, both displaying leadership qualities, had achieved the passage of the bill in their branch.[12]

Soon after adjournment of the Legislative Assembly in December 1866, Dr. Lassiter moved to Madison County and settled near the village of Hamburg some 10 miles northwest of Madison. He resumed medical practice while operating a small farm. Meanwhile, probably in 1868, he married a Florida woman, known only by her given name, Alice, who was about 19 years younger than he, and in 1869 their first child, a son Jacob, was born.[13] Three other children followed: Robert, Gertrude and Lauren, aged eight, five and three, respectively in 1880.[14]

No other information on the Lassiter family has been discovered. They were not included in the Special Census of Florida in 1885, and it is not known what became of any members of the family.

1. U.S. Census, 1860, Suwannee County, Florida, p. 772.
2. Swift Creek, originated northwest of the Town of Darlington, flowed in a southeasterly direction into Black Creek which in turn joined the Great Pee Dee River. In earlier times there was a post office on Swift Creek.
3. Dr. Flinn, a Darlington practitioner, was a graduate of the Medical College of the State of South Carolina in March 1849, Charleston *Courier*, February 24, 1849.
4. Ibid., March 15, 1853.
5. The professional notice of Drs. Power and Lassiter appeared in the Tampa *Herald* for the first time in the issue of February 22, 1854, not extant. Extant, however, is the issue of January 20, 1855, in which the notice is found.
6. See note 1, supra.
7. Suwannee Centennial Program, Souvenir, 1958, p. 13. Copy in P.K. Yonge Library of Florida History.
8. NA, Service Records, CSA, M251, Roll 84. The 8th Florida Infantry at this stage was apparently a militia unit, not to become a part of the Army of the Confederacy until the following year.
9. Ibid.
10. Pt. Lookout, Maryland, situated on the spit of land where the Potomac River enters Chesapeake Bay, though more benign than Johnson's Island, was nevertheless bitterly cold and damp in winter. Besides it was generally overcrowded with prisoners.
11. Florida *House Journal*, 1866, p. 192.
12. Florida, *Senate Journal*, 1866, pp. 38, 41, 43, 57.
13. U.S. Census, 1870, Madison County, Florida, p. 12, item 6.
14. U.S. Census, 1880, Madison County, Florida, p. 515, item 29.

Laub, Charles Henry, Ft. Mellon, Lake Munroe, 1816-1876

Dr. Laub, army surgeon, was born in Washington, D.C., about 1816. Nothing is known of his early life and education. He was appointed Assistant Surgeon in the United States Army[1] on November 30, 1836, and soon thereafter was assigned to Florida where the Second Seminole War was reaching a critical stage.

He received orders to report to Captain Charles Mellon whose Company, a unit of the Second Artillery Regiment, was positioned on the south side of Lake Munroe in present-day Seminole County. He was present at the battle which occurred there on February 8, 1837, an encounter in which Captain Mellon lost his life, "having received a ball in the chest, and fell dead at his post" and was replaced by Captain David H. Vinton.[2]

In his report of the battle, prepared by Vinton and submitted by Brevet Lieutenant Colonel A.C.W. Fanning to General Thomas S. Jesup, Fanning singled out Dr. Laub for special commendation. He wrote:[3]

> Assistant surgeon Laub dressed the wounded under the fire of the enemy. In fact, I have never seen the sick soldier more promptly and faithfully attended to....His duties have been very arduous and he has discharged them with vigor, zeal and ability.

Having survived the perils of the Second Seminole War, Dr. Laub spent the next 10 years in routine medical practice on various army posts but as an experienced military surgeon and veteran of the war he was sent to Mexico as a medical purveyor with the beginning of the war there in 1846. After the fall of Vera Cruz to the army of General Winfield Scott in March 1847, Dr. Laub set up a medical purveyance depot in that city and remained there until the end of the conflict.

Notwithstanding his meritorious service it was not until October 17, 1854, that Dr. Laub was rewarded with promotion to surgeon or "major surgeon," according to the official record. With onset of the Civil War he was confronted with wartime responsibility and as a lieutenant colonel became assistant medical purveyor for the Union Army, a service for which he was rewarded with the permanent rank of colonel "for faithful and meritorious service during the War."

Dr. Laub died in Washington on December 2, 1876. No information about his family, if indeed he had a family, has been discovered. Dr. Ellis Hughes, who kept a journal of his service in the Second Seminole War, quite unnecessarily included the recollection of Dr. Laub as "a remarkably ugly man."[4]

1. Unless otherwise indicated the biographical information concerning Dr. Laub is derived from two sources: *Medical Department of the Army, from 1775 to 1873*. Harvey E. Brown, compiler, Washington, D.C., Surgeon General's

Office, 1873, and Francis B. Heitman, *Historical Register and Dictionary*, Vol. I, Washington 1903, p. 617.

2. John T. Sprague, *The Origin, Progress and Conclusion of the Florida War*, Facsimile Edition, with Introduction by John K. Mahon, Gainesville, University Press, 1964, p. 168.

3. Ibid., p. 169.

4. Ellis Hughes, Manuscript Journals, pp. 56, 57. These Journals are in the Manuscript Collection of the University of South Florida Library, Tampa.

Law, Charles R., Micanopy, 1836

Very little is known of the career of Dr. Law. He was born about 1836 in South Carolina and moved with his widowed mother, Mary Law, and six brothers and sisters to Alachua County in the late 1850s,[1] settling in the town of Micanopy. Records of the Oglethorpe Medical College, Savannah, show him as a matriculant in 1855 and a graduate in the spring of 1857.[2] His professional card offering his services in surgery, medicine and obstetrics at his residence on the "west side of town" first appeared on August 24, 1860.[3] When the Civil War began in 1861 he would have been of proper age to enlist in the Army of the Confederacy but the service records of Florida military units make no mention of him. It is probable that he returned to either South Carolina or Georgia for enlistment.

The Census schedules of 1870 list Dr. Law's mother, two brothers and two sisters,[4] among the residents of Micanopy, but the name Law does not appear in the Census a decade later. No further information on Dr. Law has emerged.

1. U.S. Census, 1860, Alachua County, Florida, item 234.

2. Lists of Graduates and Matriculants, Oglethorpe Medical College, Savannah. Records, Georgia Historical Society, Savannah. His doctoral thesis bore the title "Phthisis Pulmonalia."

3. Micanopy *Cotton States*, September 28, 1861, 1st printing, August 24, 1860. It appears likely that Dr. Law began practice in Micanopy prior to appearance of the first issue of the newspaper.

4. U.S. Census, 1870, Alachua County, Florida, p. 165. The entry includes Robert Y.H. Law, the younger brother, who enlisted in the Confederate Army as a 2nd lieutenant and was assigned to Co. C, 1st Florida Infantry Regiment. He resigned his commission in November 1861, then reenlisted in 1862, was assigned to the Florida 7th Infantry and was captured at Missionary Ridge. In 1870 he was employed as a clerk in a general merchandise store in Micanopy.

Lawson, Thomas, Surgeon-General, United States Army, 1780-1861

Considering the stature and eminence of Thomas Lawson it is astonishing that so little is known of his early life. The date and place of his birth are unknown as are the nature and extent of his education. Even his medical education remains a mystery; it is possible that he was trained as a physician's apprentice and after achieving promise as a military surgeon was accorded the title Doctor of Medicine *honoris causa*. His military career, however, is well documented.[1]

A Virginian by birth, Thomas Lawson began his military career on March 1, 1809, as a surgeon's mate in the United States Navy. Two years later, on January 12, 1811, he resigned this appointment and a short time later became garrison surgeon's mate in the United States Army. He was named surgeon on May 21, 1813, in the Sixth Infantry from which he was transferred on May 17, 1815, to the Seventh Infantry where he became staff surgeon on June 1, 1821. For the next 15 years he served in a number of military posts including one or possibly two in Florida. He reached the pinnacle of his career on November 30, 1836, when he was appointed surgeon-general following the death of Surgeon-General Joseph Lovell on October 17.[2]

Dr. Lawson's Florida service began in February 1827 when he was assigned to the Fourth Infantry as staff surgeon. This unit under the command of Colonel Duncan L. Clinch was located at Cantonment Clinch (later Ft. Clinch) near Pensacola. Returns from the post indicate that he had been expected to report for duty in February but actually arrived a few days late. He is known to have been present for duty from March 1827 until January 1828 when he joined General Winfield Scott on a two-month inspection trip to various points in Florida. On his return in March he remained at Ft. Clinch until January 1830. Indications are that Dr. Lawson did not actually live on the post but instead maintained a house in Pensacola[3] during much of his three years at Ft. Clinch.

Some seven and a half years later, Dr. Lawson was among the troops hurriedly assembled, volunteers for the most part, following the Dade Massacre of late December 1835. A part of this preparation was reported as follows:[4]

> A regiment of Volunteers was raised in Louisiana by Colonel P.F. Smith, of which Surgeon Thomas Lawson was offered a Colonelcy. He accepted...did major service as he had done previously in his more accustomed work. In May, 1836, the troops from the North destined for service in Florida and Alabama were concentrated at Ft. Mitchell, Alabama, and Dr. Lawson (whose term as a volunteer had expired) was assigned to duty as Medical Director.

Dr. Lawson had been in Pensacola in early February and met with General Edmund Pendleton Gaines on February 6, discussing with him the intelligence that General Winfield Scott had recently been placed in command of the Florida campaign. They spoke of the advisability of Gaines' proceeding with his own campaign plans until such time as Scott should actually appear on the scene, a course of action which Dr. Lawson approved. On their arrival in Tampa a few days later General Gaines prepared for a march to Ft. King with the troops he had assembled in Pensacola. Dr. Lawson was second in command under Col. Persifor Smith of one of the columns. They followed the main military route which led them past the site of the Dade Massacre arriving in Ft. King on February 22.[5]

As a result of his participation in the march he became a major witness at a senatorial inquiry into the failure of the Indian war at which he testified that he had been among those officers who had advised General Gaines to proceed.[6] Just how long Dr. Lawson remained in Florida is not known but it is apparent that his support of General Gaines in no way jeopardized his career. Before the end of the year he was named Surgeon General.

Two years later Dr. Lawson's considerable knowledge of Florida and the Indian problem was solicited by Senator Thomas Hart Benton of Missouri, a firebrand expanionist with a no-nonsense, no-temporizing attitude regarding the Indians. He wrote in strong support of Benton's policy on December 30, 1838. Small scale skirmishes, he concluded, were useless and a waste of manpower. The United States should launch a forceful campaign in substantial numbers, then establish block houses from which to defend the gains. With no consideration for the inherent rights of Indians to exist in the Florida Territory, he proposed their quick removal westward, dismissing them as savages.[7]

Dr. Lawson during his Florida residence had gained abundant knowledge of the geography and topography of the Territory. More important for his later career, however, he had ample opportunity to observe at first hand the various diseases, especially the fevers, endemic to the area. He is reputed to have been an exceptionally fine diagnostician although his treatments would in more recent times be looked upon with horror. He resorted to calomel followed by enemas for a variety of ailments. After becoming surgeon-general in 1836 he kept voluminous records of sickness and death not only in far-flung military posts but also in adjacent civilian communities. *The Statistical Report on the Sickness and Mortality in the Army of the United States, 1819-1839*, compiled and prepared under his direction and printed in Washington in 1840, is an invaluable document on the subject, a useful source on contemporary medical practice in America.

For his meritorious service in the Mexican War, Dr. Lawson was breveted Brigadier General. He died in Norfolk, Virginia on May 15, 1861. He was never married.

1. *Medical Department of the Army, from 1775 to 1873*, compiled by Harvey E. Brown, Washington, Surgeon General's Office, 1873, pp. 269, 286, 287.
2. Ibid.
3. An incident in which a young white man "of a prominent Pensacola family" shot and killed a Negro girl who was the property of Dr. Lawson. The magistrate making the inquiry judged it to have occurred "more the result of an accident than design." The man was nevertheless bound over to the next term of court on $1000 bond. Pensacola *Gazette*, November 27, 1830.
4. *Medical Department*, see n. 1, supra, p. 154.
5. U.S. Congress, Senate Document, 224, May 1836, p. 384.
6. Ibid., p. 686.
7. TP, XXV, 554-7.

Leavenworth, Melines Conklin, Micanopy, 1796-1862

Dr. Leavenworth[1] was born in Waterbury, Connecticut, on January 15, 1796. At a fairly early age he matriculated at Yale University from which he received his medical degree in 1817. While a student at Yale he developed an interest in botany which he maintained as an avocation throughout his life. Soon after graduation he began medical practice at Augusta, Georgia, but perhaps motivated by a desire for a steady income he accepted a commission as Assistant Surgeon in the United States Army on September 1, 1833. He retained this position for seven years, resigning on September 30, 1840.

Dr. Leavenworth's army service included tours of duty at Ft. Towson, Arkansas (at that time in eastern Oklahoma), and eastern Texas. In the late 1830s he was stationed briefly at a post near Micanopy and later at Ft. Frank Brooke near present-day Steinhatchee. Wherever he was stationed he spent his spare hours collecting plant specimens which he is said to have sent to two of America's most famous botanists, John Torrey of Princeton University and Charles Wilkins Short who spent his latter years in Louisville, Kentucky.

With the War Between the States already well under way, Dr. Leavenworth, at age 66, offered his services as surgeon to the Union Army. He was assigned to the 12th Connecticut Militia, serving with this unit in Louisiana but spending the greater part of his time collecting plants. He died near New Orleans on November 16, 1862.

1. The more important data included in this sketch are derived from John K. Small, "Seminole Bread—The Conti," *Journal of the New York Botanical Garden*, XXII, 1921, p. 131. The details relating to Dr. Leavenworth's military career are found in Francis B. Heitman, *Historical Register and Dictionary of the United States Army*, Vol. I, 1903, p. 622, and *Medical Department of the Army, 1775-1873*, Harvey E. Brown, comp., Washington, D.C., Surgeon General's Office, 1873, p. 292.

Leavitt, J.E., Tallahassee and Key West, 1850

Dr. Leavitt established his professional practice in Tallahassee in May 1858 in an office located in "Nash's New Building" near the post office.[1] Before the end of the year, however, he had moved to Key West where his professional card first appeared in the local newspaper on October 23.[2] He could be found at Russell's, presumed to have been the residence of William D. Russell, a local watchmaker. Later in the year he announced that he had moved to "the Parsonage," the residence of the Methodist minister. His professional notice continued to appear in the paper until October 15, 1859. Since he is not listed in the Monroe County Census of 1860, it is assumed that he had left the state prior to the enumeration of that year.

1. Tallahassee *Floridian and Journal*, May 22, 1858.
2. Key West *Key of the Gulf*, October 23, 1858, and subsequent issues.

Lee, J.C., Monticello, 1855

Dr. Lee, native of Georgia and graduate of the Medical College of Georgia in 1854,[1] made his appearance in Monticello in January 1855 offering his services "in the various branches of his profession" to the people of the town and surrounding country. His professional card first appeared on January 13, 1855, with the announcement that he could be found at Monticello. It continued to appear for several months thereafter.[2] He is thought to have departed Monticello before the end of the year. Nothing further is known of him.

1. Medical Department, University of Georgia, *List of Graduates, 1829-1891*, Augusta, 1890, p. 20.
2. Tallahassee *Floridian and Journal*, January 13, 1855; July 28, 1855.

Lee, William States, Penscacola, 1828

Dr. Lee was born in South Carolina about 1829.[1] When he was a small child his family moved to Alabama settling in a rural locality called Carlowville. When he enrolled at the Medical College of the State of South Carolina in the fall of 1848 he gave Carlowville as his home address.[2] In March 1850 he received his medical degree, having presented a thesis entitled "Peritonitis."[3]

Dr. Lee's whereabouts for the next few years is not presently known. On February 28, 1856, the following notice appeared in the Pensacola *Florida Democrat*: "Dr. W.S. Lee, having permanently located in Pensacola, offers his services in medicine and surgery..." His office was that which had previously been occupied by Dr. George Maxwell.[4] It was located on Intendencia Street.

About 1865 Dr. Lee married an Alabama native known only by her Christian name, Susan. Two children, Susan and Frank, had been born to Dr. and Mrs. Lee by 1870. Other members of the household that year included two of the doctor's brothers, Joseph and D.M., both civil engineers, and two sisters, Julia and Mary, both teachers in Pensacola schools. In the same census Dr. Lee was also identified as "Civil Engineer." His property was valued at $4,000.[5] A list of physicians compiled by the Medical College of the University of Pennsylvania in 1870, however, includes Dr. Lee as a Pensacola physician.

Dr. Lee apparently had given up his medical practice by 1876. On February 14 that year he was named to replace Elijah Zebulon as Postmaster of Pensacola, a position he held until June 18, 1880, when he was replaced by George E. Wentworth.[6] It is doubtful that he ever resumed medical practice. The date of his death has not been discovered.

1. This date is an extrapolation from census data.
2. Records, Medical College of the State of South Carolina, preserved in the Waring Historical Medical Library, Medical University of South Carolina, Charleston.
3. Ibid. This thesis has been preserved.
4. Tallahassee *Florida Democrat*, April 3, 1856.
5. U.S. Census, 1870, Escambia County, Florida, p. 630.
6. U.S. Post Office Department, List of Appointments.

Leitner, Edward Frederick, Jupiter Inlet, 1812-1838

Dr. Leitner,[1] whose brief but brilliant career was terminated by an Indian scalping party in 1838, was far better known as a botanist than as a physician. Born in Stuttgart, Germany, on February 4, 1812, son of Johann Frederick and Karoline Friedericke (Bühler) Leitner, he was destined by birth to pursue dual professions, his father having been Royal Court Gardner in Stuttgart's Botanical Garden and his grandfather a barber-surgeon of Eckersdorf. After the early death of his father, Edward Frederick's mother returned with her children to her birthplace, Schönfort, a small town near Tübingen. Leitner is said to have attended lectures of Professor Gustav Schubler at the University of Tübingen. A list of his students includes the name Friedrich Leitner, Gartner-Student, indicating that he was part-time gardner and student. His record at Tübingen indicates that he attended lectures in Medical Botany, Economic Botany and Plant Physiology in 1828-30.

Leitner arrived in the United States in 1831. After a few months in New York and Pennsylvania he made his way to Charleston, South Carolina, where he found a friendly German community whose dominant father-figure was the Reverend Dr. John Bachman, founder and pastor of St. John's Lutheran Church. Dr. Bachman was also a naturalist and, equally important, a close friend of John J. Audubon.[2] The bright and engaging young Leitner had immediate access to the company of Charleston's intellectual circle which included Dr. John Edwards Holbrook, eminent physician, who is thought to have influenced him to consider a career in medicine.

Leitner began an apprenticeship under Dr. Holbrook and simultaneously advertised his services as instructor in botany and German. Doubtless through the influence of Dr. Bachman he was able to obtain recommendations as to his competence from several Charleston physicians in addition to Dr. Holbrook: Andrew Hasell, Eli Geddings, Henry R. Frost and Elias Horlbeck. Other than botany and German, Leitner stated that, if need be, he was prepared to offer instruction in Latin and Greek. On his behalf Dr. Bachman wrote: "Mr. Leitner has been regularly educated at the University of Tübingen. He is a good classical scholar and is particularly qualified to give instruction in German, it being his native language."

Leitner's knowledge and enthusiasm as a teacher of botany soon aroused the interest of a large number of Charlestonians, many of them women. On July 1, 1832, he wrote: "My efforts were so blessed that as of now 15 gentlemen and 17 ladies are my students in Botany, 5 in German, 1 lady in Latin, and 1 gentleman in Latin and Greek."

Meanwhile, having completed his apprenticeship under Drs. Holbrook and Thomas L. Ogier, Leitner matriculated at the Medical College of the State of South Carolina, Charleston, in the fall of 1832.

It was natural science, however, and not medicine which claimed Leitner's primary attention. He had heard much of the marvelous variety of plant and animal life in Florida, very little of which had been the subject of close examination and classification. He longed to go there but without subsidy it was impossible. He advertised his projected research trip, outlining his proposed itinerary, and offering to collect specimens of plants unknown to the Carolinas which he would distribute to local botanists, ornithologists, et al, in exchange for cash contributions to support his trip. He was successful in obtaining adequate funds and in January 1833 left for Florida on a journey much publicized by the Charleston *Courier* and supported by many prominent Charlestonians.

Leitner's Florida expedition was fraught with danger as well as fascination. The territory through which he roamed was unchartered for the most part. He traversed the Everglades alone and is thought to have been the first white man to undertake such a journey. It was not without incident. He came near death after being bitten by a moccasin and suffered the mishap of losing his entire collection, botanical, ornithological et cetera and faced the necessity of repeating the arduous task.

On September 3, 1833, the Charleston *Courier* reported that Dr. Leitner was "safe in Key West and will leave for Charleston...aboard the Schooner John Dennison." He arrived in Charleston on September 11.[3] He resumed medical study in early November and on March 7, 1834, was graduated as Doctor of Medicine.[4] His thesis was awarded the prize for the best one written in Latin.

For the next two years Dr. Leitner remained in Charleston living at 137 Meeting Street continuing his studies and occasionally lecturing on botanical subjects, and probably doing some writing. In the summer of 1836 he returned to the Florida Keys. On September 14, 1836, Dr. Bachman wrote to Audubon: "Dr. Leitner is among the Keys. I gave him my own gin and whiskey for his specimens." In October Dr. Leitner joined Lt. Levin M. Powell, a Navy officer on an exploratory expedition along the east coast of Florida and into the Everglades. The surgeon for the expedition was Dr. Jacob Rhett Motte of Charleston who like Leitner was a graduate of the medical college in Charleston. Dr. Leitner was accorded the temporary rank of Assistant Surgeon. Since he had previous knowledge of the area to be explored his role was obviously more guide than physician. His personal mission was more that of naturalist than physician.

In mid-January 1838 the main complement of the expedition had established its headquarters inside Jupiter Inlet. Upon information provided by an Indian that several parties of Indians were encamped nearby, a detachment under Lt. Powell's command had moved out in search of them. Suddenly they were beset by Indians in a far larger force than anticipated. The detachment began its retreat in disarray but not before several members of the party, including Dr. Leitner, had suffered mortal wounds.[5]

Dr. Motte was grief-stricken. In his diary he recorded the tragic incident: "Poor Leitner! He was my friend and fellow student, (we) having pursued our professional studies together in the same office in Charleston, under the auspices of Dr. J.E. Holbrook... ."[6]

Dr. Motte continued to praise his fallen friend for his ability, diligence, scholarship and zeal in acquiring knowledge pertaining to natural science. Thus ended the brief but brilliant career of Edward Frederick Leitner.

1. Some years ago the late George E. Gifford Jr., a distinguished physician of Cambridge, Massachusetts, published a splendid paper on the career of Dr. Leitner. This sketch has been drawn extensively from Dr. Gifford's work, "Edward Frederick Leitner, (1812-1838), Physician-Botanist." *Bulletin of the History of Medicine*, XLVI, No. 6, November, December, 1972, pp. 568-590.

2. Dr. Bachman's spiritual and intellectual influence upon the young people of Charleston, especially those of German-Lutheran extraction, was beyond measure. He was a close friend of John James Audubon, the great ornithologist. Two of Dr. Bachman's daughters were married to the two Audubon sons.

3. Charleston *Courier*, September 12, 1833.

4. Ibid., March 8, 1834. See also Charleston *Mercury* of the same date.

5. Several accounts of the skirmish in which Dr. Leitner lost his life have been published. The most complete and perhaps the most accurate is that of Dr. Motte, *Journey Into Wilderness*, edited by James F. Sunderman, Gainesville, University of Florida Press, 1953, pp. 182-185.

6. The two physicians, Leitner and Motte, were obviously close friends, both having begun their medical studies under the preceptorate of Dr. Holbrook. Leitner, one year ahead of Motte, was graduated in 1834. Since he was basically a botanist it is not surprising that his doctoral thesis, *De Hippomano Mancinello*, dealt with a plant which exudes a milky, poisonous sap, contact with which causes blistering of the skin.

L'Engle, Edwin Walter, Jacksonville, 1847-1893

Dr. L'Engle, sixth son and ninth child of Capt. John Claudius and Susan Fatio L'Engle, was born in Jacksonville in 1847.[1] He was the third member of the L'Engle family to enter the medical profession, two of his older brothers, William Johnson and John Claudius Jr., having followed the same calling. From his early childhood Edwin appears to have had problems. When he was two his brother William, writing to their aunt, Miss Leonis L'Engle, remarked, "Edwin, I think, has improved lately in his behavior."[2] When he was barely 15 he managed to enlist in the Confederate cause and shortly thereafter suffered a bullet wound in his leg, a mishap which plagued him for many years.[3]

In spite of poor health L'Engle entered the Medical Department of the University of Georgia at Augusta in 1868 and was graduated in the spring of 1870.[4] Soon afterwards he married Eliza Hart Elliott and began his professional practice in Savannah. A short time later, however, he returned to Florida and resumed practice in Gainesville as a partner of the highly-regarded physician, Newton

D. Phillips. Very little is known of his Gainesville experience due largely to the nonexistence of newspapers of the period. Miss L'Engle wrote only "Dr. L'Engle had a home in Gainesville and other properties, including a farm, but he lived in town on account of his medical practice."[5]

During the decade of the 1870s Dr. L'Engle's health began to fail. Although no description or diagnosis of his ailment has survived one must suspect that he himself knew it was tuberculosis. When a complete breakdown occurred about 1880,[6] his doctors advised a complete change of climate, suggesting Denver, Colorado, as a healthful place. Almost two years later on April 13, 1882, he and his family began the long trek to Colorado. The entourage consisted of a surrey drawn by two mules and a small covered wagon, laden with trunks, tents and household things, driven by a black servant. Mrs. L'Engle and their three children completed the group.[7]

After many adventures and much hardship the family arrived in Denver in mid-August 1882. The Doctor immediately consulted a physician who examined him and discovered that his ailment, tuberculosis, was already in an advanced stage. He urged the L'Engles to move on to New Mexico for a more favorable climate. He recommended that they settle in a small town where Dr. L'Engle's practice would keep him much out of doors exposed to the fresh dry air. They chose Santa Fe and the Doctor once more began his medical practice. The move had been a fortunate one; Dr. L'Engle lived and practiced for 11 more years, dying in Santa Fe in 1893. The Denver physician had indicated five years at the most.[8]

Dr. L'Engle, like other members of his family, was a staunch Democrat. Even though he was far from well he was active in the presidential campaign of 1876. In the summer prior to the election he made an extensive journey into South Florida for the cause of Samuel J. Tilden. He apparently foretold the closeness of the election, reporting to his brother, Henry, the critical importance of a few extra votes for the Democratic ticket.[9]

Dr. L'Engle, due to his long struggle with sickness and the needs of his family, never enjoyed the financial ease achieved by several of his brothers and sisters. In late 1876 after visiting him in Gainesville his brother Edward wrote:[10]

> I have seen Edward today...He had been very sick and is still weak and has a troublesome cough...He has recently had a hemmorhage (sic) which may have been from the lungs...If he were to die his wife and children would be without a stiver...Fortunately the Lord has given me the means of helping him if it should be wanted.

There is no indication that such help was "wanted."

Four children were born to the L'Engle's. The eldest, Jennie Elizabeth, was born in Gainesville in 1872. She was married to a Mexican citizen, Mauro Santos Ortega, and died in Guadalajara, Mexico, in 1898. The second child, Elliott Fleming, was born in 1874, became a mining engineer, and died in 1927. The third child, Edward McCrady, was born in Gainesville in 1876, also became a mining engineer, and died in Bridgeport, Connecticut, in 1942. A fourth child, John Claudius, named for his grandfather, was born in Santa Fe, N.M., in 1888 and died in Tallahassee, Florida, in 1905. Mrs. L'Engle, born in 1855, died in London, England, in 1913.[11]

1. Nearly all the information contained in this sketch is derived from Gertrude Nelson L'Engle, "A Collection of Letters, Information and Data on Our Family," Jacksonville, 1951. This exists as a typed manuscript, a photocopy of which is in the P.K. Yonge Library of Florida History. In one instance another work of Miss L'Engle, a compilation of letters of William Johnson L'Engle and his wife, Madeline Saunders L'Engle, existing in typed copy in the P.K. Yonge Library has been cited. The former work is cited as "Our Family."
2. Letter, William J. L'Engle to Miss Leonis L'Engle, December 29, 1849. See "Letters," p. 23.
3. L'Engle, "Our Family," p. 167. No service record for Edwin Walter L'Engle has been located in CSA files.
4. Medical Department, University of Georgia, *List of Graduates from 1829 to 1891*, Augusta, 1891, p. 20.
5. L'Engle, "Our Family," pp. 167, 168.

6. Ibid., p. 168.
7. Ibid., pp. 168-170.
8. Ibid., p. 170.
9. Ibid., p. 167. Edward L'Engle to his wife, Frances Wirt L'Engle, Jacksonville, September 22, 1876.
10. Ibid., p. 168. Edward L'Engle to his wife, Frances Wirt L'Engle, Jacksonville, June 1878.
11. Ibid., p. 170. During the last decade of his life Miss L'Engle states that L'Engle and his daughter, Jennie, "made rather frequent trips back to Jacksonville." She adds, however, that his son, Edward, did not return for 65 years. It was from Edward (the son) that much of the detail relating to the first trip to New Mexico was obtained by Miss Gertrude L'Engle who was his first cousin.

L'Engle Jr., John Claudius, Jacksonville, 1840-1914

John Claudius Jr.,[1] fourth son and fifth child of John Claudius L'Engle, was born in Jacksonville on October 22, 1840, and soon after the family moved to Hamilton County where the elder L'Engle had purchased a farm in the vicinity of the mineral springs, present day White Springs, where for a brief time he was a cotton planter. The family soon returned to Jacksonville, however, when the father found employment in railroad building, in which the son also worked for a while.[2]

The early education of the L'Engle children was entrusted to private tutors who were no doubt under the constant scrutiny of Mrs. L'Engle, said to have been a well educated woman. At the age of 16 or 17 John Claudius Jr. chose to prepare for a career in medicine. Under the preceptorate of the eminent Dr. Richard P. Daniel of Jacksonville he read medicine and observed the practice of his preceptor. In the fall of 1859 he matriculated at the Medical College of South Carolina, Charleston, from which he was graduated in March 1861.[3]

Two months after receiving his degree on May 9, 1861, Dr. L'Engle enlisted for service in the Confederate Army, committing himself for a period of 12 months. He was mustered in on July 13 as a private in Company G, 3rd Florida Infantry Regiment. Before the end of summer he was promoted to a lieutenancy and assigned to a hospital unit. He continued to serve in the Medical Department as surgeon throughout the war, remaining with his unit in several Virginia campaigns. At the conclusion of the war he was mustered out with the rank of major.[4]

On his return to Jacksonville Dr. L'Engle does not appear to have resumed medical practice but instead opened a drug store which he continued to manage until near the end of the century. The Duval County Census of 1870 lists him only as "druggist," owning property valued at $15,000.[5] When Jacksonville's most devastating epidemic of yellow fever struck in August 1888, Dr. L'Engle brought his medical skills back into service working, it is said, around the clock with the sick and dying. When death came to his brother, Henry Augustus, and brother-in-law, J.J. Daniel, he stepped into the breach performing noble service on both the Executive Committee of the Jacksonville Auxiliary Sanitary Association and the Jacksonville Board of Health.[6]

Besides his drug store located at 23 West Bay Street, Dr. L'Engle turned his attention to other enterprises including coal supply and a towing service on the St. Johns River, his boat being located at the foot of Washington Street.[7] Upon the death of his brother, Henry, he joined the banking firm which had been established by him and another brother, Edwin. The bank, known as the State Bank of Florida, was located at 24 West Bay Street; Dr. L'Engle eventually became its president.[8]

Dr. L'Engle's home was among those destroyed by the great Jacksonville fire of 1901. He was elected chairman of the Board of Public Works and in this capacity aided significantly in the relief of the homeless and reconstruction of the burned out homes. He rebuilt his own house as a replica of the former one.

At the age of 59 (1899), Dr. L'Engle became active in politics running successfully for the Florida House of Representatives in 1899 and again in 1901. Ten years later he represented Duval County, the 18th Senatorial District, in the Florida Senate in the sessions of 1911 and 1913.[9]

Dr. L'Engle was twice married; first, in 1861 to Sarah Cornelia Daniel, daughter of James M. Daniel and sister of Col. J.J. Daniel. They had five children, Claudia, Rosa, Edward Jaquelin, John Claudius, and Mary Evelyn. John Claudius died on Christmas Day in 1889; only Edward and Mary Evelyn enjoyed long lives. Mrs. L'Engle died on October 13, 1901, and two years later the Doctor married Florence Miller of Virginia. He died on September 9, 1914.

Known as a quiet, introspective and gentle man, abstemious in both food and drink, Dr. L'Engle was highly esteemed by his fellowmen. In later years he is said to have become more urbane and cheerful. The untimely death of his son was a blow from which he was slow to recover; Christmas was not celebrated in the household for many years thereafter. Still so well was he regarded in the Jacksonville community that on the day of his death all city offices were closed from ten o'clock till noon as a tribute to his memory.

1. This sketch has been drawn extensively from Gertrude Nelson L'Engle's "Collection of Letters, Information and Data on Our Family," Jacksonville, 1951, Vol. I. A photocopy of the original tyewritten work has been used. It is in the collection of the P.K. Yonge Library of Florida History. Unless otherwise indicated the information derives from this source.
2. Ibid., p. 156.
3. Archives, Waring Historical Library, Medical University of South Carolina, Charleston.
4. L'Engle, "Collection...", loc. cit. See also NA, Service Recs., CSA, M. 251, Roll 39.
5. U.S. Census, 1870, Duval County, Florida, item 32.
6. *Report of the Jacksonville Auxiliary Sanitary Association*, Chas. S. Adams, ed., Jacksonville, 1889, p. 35, et passim.
7. Jacksonville City Directories for several years beginning in 1880 are the principal sources for Dr. L'Engle's career.
8. Dr. L'Engle apparently became president of the bank shortly after the death of his brother, Henry, in 1888.
9. Allen Morris, comp., *The People of Lawmaking in Florida, 1822-1977*, Tallahassee, 1977.

L'Engle, William Johnson, Jacksonville, 1832-1861

Dr. L'Engle,[1] scion of one of Florida's most distinguished families, was born in St. Augustine on July 25, 1832, the second son of Captain John Claudius and Susan Fatio L'Engle. Soon after birth he was taken to Hamilton County where his father owned and operated a cotton plantation near Mineral Springs, now White Springs. The family had moved to Jacksonville by 1848 and settled in a house located at the corner of Bay and Laura Streets on the St. Johns River. At that time the L'Engle children numbered eight, one christened Henry Trescot having died in early childhood in 1847.

In his youth William made several visits to Charleston and Raleigh where relatives of his father's foster parents resided.[2] In Raleigh he became acquainted with the family of Judge Romulus Saunders whose daughter, Margaret Madelline, became his wife on April 3, 1854.[3]

Meanwhile young L'Engle had entered the Medical Department of the University of Pennsylvania in the fall of 1851, graduating in March 1853, four months prior to his 21st birthday.[4] Returning to Jacksonville he announced the opening of his practice on April 21.[5] Some four weeks later several Jacksonville physicians met in his office and organized the Duval County Medical Society, choosing Dr. L'Engle as secretary.[6] For reasons not clear but possibly because of his failure to obtain the port physician's post, he abandoned his practice in the summer of 1853 and settled in St. Mary's, Georgia, where he had expected to become a partner of a well-established physician, identified only as "Dr. C."[7] When that did not materialize he made his way to New York where on December 15 he took the qualifying examination for appointment to the Medical Department, United States Army. This accomplished, he returned to Raleigh where he waited anxiously for the result. Word of his success came on February 20, 1854.[8]

Although his actual commission as assistant surgeon was not forthcoming for more than two years Dr. L'Engle was ordered into government service and assigned to the Marine Hospital in Key West. Leaving his bride of a few weeks with his family in Jacksonville, Dr. L'Engle made his way to Key West in early summer and in July arranged for her to join him there. In spite of some hardships living there, judging from their letters, appears to have been almost idyllic. They made agreeable friends, including the Mallorys, and managed to survive the "sickly season" without harm. Mrs. L'Engle became pregnant.[9]

Dr. L'Engle received his commission as Assistant Army Surgeon on August 28, 1856, the papers having been signed by President Franklin Pierce and Jefferson Davis, Secretary of War. From that point on life became difficult. Dr. L'Engle was ordered to California and assigned to Ft. Miller, a remote post in the San Joaquin Valley. Their first child, a son William Johnson, was born there on February 11, 1857. The doctor wrote of observing the practice of medicine by the medical men of the local Indian tribe (Yokuts) and of being called on one occasion to assist in a difficult case.[10]

Other assignments followed in rapid succession in Oregon, Washington Territory, Fort Moultrie, S.C., and Texas. His last post was Fort Jefferson on the Dry Tortugas (Florida) from which in April 1861 he submitted his resignation from the Army of the United States.[11] No sooner had he returned to Jacksonville than he left his wife and children (then three) with his family at their country place, Palermo, and went to Montgomery, Alabama, to offer his services to the Army of the Confederacy. While awaiting the processing of his commission he decided to return to Florida, going by way of Pensacola. He arrived there "with some fever and quite sick." The hotel at which he had stopped being overcrowded he contacted the brother-in-law of Stephen R. Mallory who moved him to the Mallory home and summoned a physician. Due to an error on the part of the druggist Dr. L'Engle was administered a massive dose of morphine, 20 grains, it is said, which was quickly fatal, his death occurring on May 11, 1861.[12] It is a bitter irony that Dr. L'Engle's commission as Surgeon in the Medical Department, Army of the Confederacy, with the rank of major, arrived on May 13, two days after his death. Funeral arrangements were handled by Mr. Moreno, Stephen Mallory's brother-in-law, who arranged for burial in Pensacola. Years later, his son, William J., located his grave and had his remains reinterred in Evergreen Cemetery, Jacksonville, by the side of his beloved wife.

Mrs. L'Engle and her three children lived on into the 20th century, her death coming in 1917. William Johnson L'Engle Jr. died in New York City in 1924. The second son, Camille (Camillus) was born in late 1857 and died in 1907, while the daughter, Carolina (Lina) Hallowes, who was born in 1859, died in 1935.

1. Thanks to the untiring effort and perseverance of Gerturde Nelson L'Engle of Jacksonville, daughter of Dr. William Johnson L'Engle's youngest brother, Henry Augustus L'Engle, the genealogical material on the entire L'Engle family is abundant. The information contained in this sketch is drawn principally from her work: Gertrude N. L'Engle, "A Collection of Letters, Information and Data on Our Family," Jacksonville, 1949. Photocopy of a typed manuscript, P.K. Yonge Library of Florida History, Gainesville. Also extremely valuable is the collection of the Letters of William Johnson L'Engle, M.D., and his wife, Madelline Saunders L'Engle, compiled and edited by Gertrude N. L'Engle and Katherine Tracy L'Engle. Typed and bound in looseleaf notebook in the P.K. Yonge Library. See also Webster Merritt, *A Century of Medicine in Jacksonville and Duval County*, Gainesville, 1949, pp. 43-44. The letters are particularly valuable in that they reveal the high level of cultivation and gentility enjoyed by the entire L'Engle family.

2. Jean L'Engle, father of John Claudius, was of French birth. He and his wife had immigrated to Charleston. Upon his premature death Mrs. L'Engle turned over the upbringing of her small son to Judge William Johnson, in whose home he lived until he entered the United States Military Academy. In due time John Claudius honored his foster father by naming his second son, William Johnson L'Engle.

3. See "Letters," pp. 32-33. William Johnson L'Engle to Col. Miller Hallowes, dated at Smithfield, N.C., March 29, 1854, for account of wedding arrangements.

4. Archives, University of Pennsylvania Department of Medicine.

5. Jacksonville *Florida Republican*, April 21, 1953; Jacksonville *Florida News*, April 23, 1853.

6. Merritt, *Century of Medicine*, p. 44.
7. Dr. "C" was doubtless Dr. G.P. Cohen. See U.S. Census, 1850, Camden County, Georgia.
8. This proved to be an agonizing interval for Dr. L'Engle in that he had delayed proposing marriage to Miss Saunders until he had received the results of his examination.
9. Miss L'Engle has assumed that Dr. L'Engle's commission was conferred immediately upon passing the examination, i.e., in early 1854. This seems to be in error, however. Records of the Medical Department, U.S. Army, show that his commission was issued on August 28, 1856. His prior medical service had been in the role of Contract Surgeon.
10. Gertrude N. L'Engle, *Our Family*, p. 131.
11. Dr. L'Engle's resignation was submitted on April 30, 1861, 18 days after the firing on Ft. Sumter. By this date nearly all the states which would form the Confederacy had already seceded from the Union. *MDUSA*, p. 294.
12. An obituary for Dr. L'Engle appeared in the Jacksonville *St. John's Mirror* of July 17, 1861. This was subjoined by a touching letter of condolence to Dr. L'Engle's father, John Claudius, written at Pensacola on May 27, 1861, by Stephen R. Mallory, describing in some detail the sad event of his son's death.

Leonard, Theobald M., Pensacola, 1851-1885

Dr. Leonard, whose successful medical career spanned a mere 12 years, was born in Pensacola, on January 6, 1851, the eldest child of Samuel A. and Virginia (Sierra) Leonard.[1] His father, an Alabama native, had come to Pensacola as a school teacher[2] and obtained lodging in the home of Joseph Sierra, a prosperous merchant. On April 11, 1850 he married the Sierra daughter, Virginia, the Bishop of Mobile having performed the ceremony at St. Michael's Church.[3]

Very little information relating to Dr. Leonard's early education has emerged. Mrs. Elizabeth Dwyer Vickers, medical historian of Pensacola, has discovered that he was a graduate of Spring Hill College in Mobile[4] but the medical college he may have attended has not been identified.[5] He is known to have served his apprenticeship under the preceptorate of Dr. Robert B.S. Hargis of Pensacola.

Dr. Leonard practiced in Pensacola from 1873 until 1876. His entry into the ranks of practitioners was no doubt sponsored and encouraged by Dr. Hargis and Dr. John Cary Whiting in whose drug store he found office space. Incidentally his residence was located on Romana Street next door to Dr. Hargis.[6]

Dr. Leonard gave up his civilian practice on September 7, 1876, to accept appointment as quarantine physician in Pensacola harbor replacing Dr. William A.W. Spotswood, a move which brought him into close association with the Port Inspector, William Henry Davison, a Harvard-educated New Englander with whom he developed a cordial friendship. From the daily log dutifully kept by Davison it is possible to follow the activities of both men; for Dr. Leonard it was a difficult and often frustrating assignment. On September 7, 1876, Davison wrote: "Dr. Leonard brings verbal instructions (as he thinks) to compel all vessels, even from healthy ports, to discharge all their ballast in quarantine...I don't think even the stupidity, or the rascality of the officials of Pensacola could go to such lengths."

In his earnest effort to perform his assigned duties Dr. Leonard was frequently confronted by outright refusals on the part of some ships' captains to obey the orders, and what was more discouraging he found on occasion that his orders were countermanded by the mayor himself, or by other members of the Board of Health, sometimes after the ship's captain had favored a member of the Board with a keg of rum or some other bribe or token appropriated from the ship's cargo.

In spite of such unpleasant encounters Dr. Leonard retained the post of quarantine officer until May 1882 when he was relieved by a Dr. Carrington of New Orleans thought to have been a medical graduate from Tulane University. As the fever season approached in late August 1882, Dr. Leonard was instructed by the Board of Health to return to the quarantine station to assist Dr. Carrington. His sole duty was to attend to the fumigation of all vessels entering the harbor. This action on the part of the Board provoked criticism from certain citizens of the town who addressed a series of questions to the Board, one of which was:

"Why are (both) Dr. Leonard and Dr. Carrington on salaries by order of the Board of Health?" The implication was that with the yellow fever raging in the town one of the doctors could have been spared to attend fever victims.[7]

Dr. Leonard himself appeared to regard his presence at the quarantine station as unnecessary. As the epidemic reached its peak in late September and early October his communication to the editor of the Pensacola *Commercial* expressed his wish to be relieved of his assignment, feeling "that he can do more good in Pensacola than where he was at present."[8] He was permitted to return to Pensacola on October 15 and resume his practice there.[9]

It is clear that Dr. Leonard was a physician of excellent reputation. More to the point is the fact that he enjoyed the confidence and support of Pensacola's most eminent physicians, Drs. Hargis and Whiting. His good standing within the profession was indicated when, at the meeting of the Florida Medical Association in Pensacola in mid-April 1882, he was chosen Secretary pro tem for the meeting, and subsequently Secretary for the coming year. His dear friend, Dr. Hargis, was elected President. The annual meeting for 1883 was to be held in Jacksonville.[10]

In December 1882, Dr. Leonard wrote an impassioned letter urging the support of all Pensacola physicians in the affairs of the Florida Medical Association, calling for a good representation at its meeting in April following. The two important issues to be discussed were regulation of the medical profession and establishment of a Florida State Board of Health. He thought it was time to end the isolation of Pensacola and its doctors from the mainstream of medical matters in the state. He countered the common excuse of the high cost of transportation for the failure of Pensacola's physicians to join their professional organization by promising to persuade the railroads to reduce the fares for those attending meetings in distant towns. Since both he and Dr. Hargis were expected to be present at the Jacksonville meeting he would campaign immediately for reduced fares.[11]

His hopes and promises remained unfulfilled. By April 1883, ill health had overtaken Dr. Leonard; Dr. Hargis, for reasons not known, was unable to attend but honored his obligation in part by sending his presidential address entitled "The Natural History of Plagues" which was read by Dr. C.J. Kenworthy of Jacksonville.[12]

Dr. Leonard died at his home in Pensacola on June 30, 1885, at age 34. Both Pensacola newspapers, the *Pensacolian* and the *Commerical*, took proper notice of his death.

1. The dates of Dr. Leonard's birth and death are found on his gravestone in St. Michael's Cemetery, Pensacola.
2. U.S. Census, 1850, Escambia County, Florida, p. 242.
3. Escambia County, Marriage Book C, p. 10.
4. Elizabeth Dwyer Vickers and F. Norman Vickers, M.D., "Notations on Pensacola's Medical History," *Journal of the Florida Medical Association*, January 1974, p. 91.
5. It appears probable that he attended the Medical College of Alabama, Mobile, at least for one term. The College's list of graduates, however, does not include his name.
6. Pensacola *Gazette*, April 20, 1875.
7. Pensacola *Commerical*, October 3, 1882.
8. Ibid., October 10, 1882.
9. Ibid., October 13, 1882. He returned from quarantine on the 12th and resumed his practice a day or so later.
10. *Proceedings, Florida Medical Association*, 1882, Jacksonville, 1882.
11. Although attendance at the meeting of the Florida Medical Association in 1882 was small, it was significant. Four Pensacola physicians joined the organization at that session. In addition to Dr. Leonard, Drs. E. Bouvier, W.T. Fordham, and J.C. Whiting became members. Previously only Dr. Hargis, who joined in 1878, had been a member. For Dr. Leonard's letter, see the Pensacola *Commercial*, December 29, 1882.
12. *Proceedings, Florida Medical Association*, 1883, Jacksonville, 1883.

Leonard, Thomas K., Leon County, 1820-1865

Dr. Leonard, a Leon County practitioner, was born in North Carolina about 1820. His mother, Margaret Ann Leonard, widowed when Thomas was still a small boy, migrated to Florida in the 1820s[1] and settled in the Miccosukie community near the Georgia line. She married Jacob Carr, a widower with one son by a previous marriage on October 26, 1830.[2] To this marriage three daughters were born.[3] Since Carr does not appear as a member of the household in 1850 it is assumed that he had died by that date.

Meanwhile Dr. Leonard had attended medical school (unidentified) and returned to Leon County where he appears to have practiced for a brief period in Tallahassee.[4] With the death of his stepfather,[5] however, he returned to Miccosukie and the home of his mother, becoming a member of the household. For the next 15 years he appears to have practiced in the Miccosukie community.

In the summer of 1846 Dr. Leonard won a seat in the Florida House of Representatives in the Whig landslide of that year.[6] In the years immediately following he continued to be active in the public life of northern Leon County. As a captain in the local militia, known as the Miccosukie Cavaliers, he participated in local gatherings and military funerals.[7] He was, for example, an eloquent speaker at Monticello's Fourth of July celebration in 1847, an affair attended by many notables,[8] including Governor William D. Moseley. In subsequent years, however, he failed to reach such eminence again.

Very little information has survived regarding Dr. Leonard's activities in the 1850s. In 1860, at age 40, he appeared in the census as the head of a household which included a young wife, Mary, and his mother, 68. His property was valued at $22,000. In the following year, however, his career took a weird turn. In October the Monticello *Family Friend* printed the following professional announcement:[9]

> As much as I detest the notoriety which this notice will give me, I am induced to do so from feelings prompted by no personal ambition or desire for gain, but I do affirm that I can, and do warrant to cure Spermatorrhea, or Seminal Weakness; also Ulcerated Os Uteri. Patients must apply to me in person. My fee for the first is one hundred dollars—for the latter, fifty. I ask my brother physicians not to judge me too harshly, but wait the issue of a fair trial—even the worse case that can be sent or brought to my office.
> Thomas K. Leonard, M.D., Oct. 12, 1861.

In its issue of November 2, 1861, the same newspaper printed the following:[10]

> To the Medical Public: Under the notice styled "Special Medical Notice," I have published that I could cure Spermatorrhea or Seminal Weakness and Ulcerated Os Uteri. I withdraw that notice, being under the delusion of an evile spirit. God in his mercy has convinced me of it, and I take this method to request every paper which published that notice to publish this one only, the influence which induced its publication having been withdrawn from me.
> Thomas K. Leonard, Miccosukie, Fla.

One week later the same *Family Friend* carried the following item:[11]

> NOTICE. The subscriber is desirous of collecting enough money to pay his DEBTS. He knows of no other method so effectual as to let his friends know by this notice that he is in want, and humiliating as it is, justice to those he is indebted to requires that he should make it known.—Thomas K. Leonard.

If Dr. Leonard served in the army of the Confederacy no record of such service has survived. He continued to reside in Miccosukie, at least until late 1865, when the following advertisement appeared:[12]

> I offer for sale a small tract of land, most pleasantly situated, about the centre of Miccosukie neighborhood. If you want a good home, apply soon to T.K. Leonard, Miccosukie, Nov. 10, 1865.

Nothing further is known of this unusual physician.

1. U.S. Census, 1830, Leon County, Florida, p. 126. She is listed as a householder, owning four slaves.
2. Marriage Records, Leon County, Florida.
3. U.S. Census, 1850, Leon County, Florida, p. 70.
4. Henry E. Palmer, M.D., "Physicians of Early Tallahassee and Vicinity," *Apalachee*, Tallahassee Historical Society, p. 41.
5. Date of death unknown; probably in early 1840s.
6. Tallahassee *Southern Journal*, September 1, 1846, and subsequent issues.
7. Ibid., June 7, 1847.
8. Ibid., July 19, 1847.
9. Monticello *Family Friend*, October 26, 1861.
10. Ibid., November 2, 1861.
11. Ibid., November 9, 1861.
12. Tallahassee *Semi-Weekly Floridian*, November 10, 1865.

Lesesne, C.W., Marion County, 1810-1880

Dr. Lesesne was one of several medically-educated South Carolinians who migrated to Marion County in the antebellum period, bringing with them sufficient funds to purchase land and settle down to the planter's style of living. He was an 1831 graduate of the Medical College of South Carolina, Charleston, having written a doctoral thesis, "General and Local Bloodletting."[1] The Lesesne family to which he belonged was of French Huguenot origin; its members were considered to be of the gentry.

The South Carolina roots of the Lesesne family date from the 18th century. They were prominent in both the Charleston and Georgetown Districts. It has not been determined to which branch Dr. Lesesne belonged, although a single reference points to the Charleston branch. The "Journal of Carson and Sons, Charleston cotton factors and commission" for 1854-55 includes the mention of the account of C.W. Lesesne *(South Carolina Historical Magazine*, Vol. LXXXI, p. 277.) This possibly suggests the disposal of property or goods prior to his departure for Florida.

Dr. Lesesne probably arrived in Florida in the mid-1860s. The earliest known reference to his presence is found in the list of arrivals at *Ocala House* in early March 1858, where he is identified as "Dr. Lesesne of Belvue."[2] His properties were estimated to have been worth $17,000 in 1860. His slaves numbered 14. Apparently unmarried at the time, he shared his abode with his overseer, a South Carolinian named Perry.[3]

In the early months of reconstruction Dr. Lesesne is known to have had an encounter with the military authority of Marion County. On October 24, 1865, he was ordered by Lt. Charles A. Northrop, military commander at Ocala, to "sell no cotton...until claims and charges preferred against him by Dr. R.H.Y. Thomas, administrator of the estate of Kitchen W. Syms, deceased...are investigated and settled."[4]

As late as 1880 he was still living on his farm near Ocala. He is listed in the Marion County Census of 1880 as "doctor," aged 70, widower.[5] There appears to be no evidence that Dr. Lesesne ever practiced medicine beyond the bounds of his own estate although the census of 1860 styled him "planter and doctor."

1. Charleston *Courier*, March 19, 1831.
2. Ocala *Florida Home Companion*, March 6, 1858. Belvue was a variant spelling of Belleview, a village 11 miles south of Ocala. The fact that Dr. Lesesne was of French ancestry accounts for the fact that the village was given the French spelling, Bellevue, later to be anglicized to Bellview.
3. U.S. Census, 1860, Marion County, Florida, item 126.
4. Letter, Lt. Chas. A. Northrop to Dr. C.W. Lesesne, October 24, 1865. MS., Box 20, MSS, P.K. Yonge Library of Florida History, item 126. Dr. Thomas, also a native of South Carolina, practiced at various times in Marion, Alachua and Levy Counties.
5. U.S. Census, 1880, Marion County, Florida, p. 30.

Lesesne, John Frederick, Fernandina, 1817

Dr. Lesesne, who for a few years was a practicing physician in Fernandina, was born in Georgetown, South Carolina, on January 12, 1817.[1] The Lesesne family was one of note in the early history of the state, having arrived in the early 18th century along with others of the French Huguenot persuasion. His parents, Joseph and Anne Lesesne, were natives of the Georgetown District. Though not wealthy, they were moderately well-off, having owned 19 slaves in 1830.[2]

He began the study of medicine in the Georgetown office of Dr. S. Gasque and at age 20 matriculated at the Medical College of the State of South Carolina, Charleston, from which he was graduated Doctor of Medicine on March 13, 1839.[3] Soon thereafter he returned to Georgetown and began practice in which he was apparently popular and successful. For two terms, 1841 and 1842, he served as mayor of the town. On June 13, 1844,[4] he married Hannah E. Porter, member of a prominent Georgetown family. They had two daughters, Hannah and Josephine, the former born in Alabama about 1845, which invites the speculation that Dr. Lesesne practiced briefly in that state. The second child was born in Fernandina in 1856.[5]

The Lesesnes arrived in Fernandina in 1855. He immediately set up practice there and appears soon to have gained the confidence and respect of the people of the town. He changed his church affiliation from Methodist to Episcopalian, Mrs. Lesesne having been an Episcopalian, and became one of the organizers of St. Peter's Church, which began services in 1858 in temporary quarters, with Dr. Lesesne as a member of its first vestry.[6] In the following year the church was ready for occupancy, and Mrs. Lesesne was among those contributing substantially to its support.[7]

Meanwhile Dr. Lesesne came into possession of a building in the town, using a portion of it for his own purposes while renting space to others among them Dr. L.M. Butler. In May 1858, Dr. Lesesne entered into a professional partnership with Dr. D.P. Beatty, a North Carolinian, recently arrived in Fernandina.[8]

With the onset of war in 1861 Fernandina became a prime target for Union occupation. Its harbor would be a convenient gateway for further advances into Florida. In early March 1862, the town fell into Federal hands, the majority of its white inhabitants having fled prior to the landing of enemy troops. Only a few had been able to remove their household belongings. The Lesesnes were among those who could not so their property fell into enemy hands as did that of other prominent citizens, including some of the wealthiest such as David L. Yulee and Joseph Finegan.[9] Subsequent to this misfortune nothing further is known of the Lesesne family. Presumably they fled into the interior of the state and doubtless made their way eventually to South Carolina.

1. "Records of the Georgetown Methodist Church," *South Carolina Historical Magazine*, LXI, 101.
2. U.S. Census, 1830, Georgetown District, S.C.
3. Charleston *Courier*, March 21, 1839.
4. *South Carolina Historical Magazine*, LXXIV, 172. This marriage apparently enhanced Dr. Lesesne's financial standing. In 1850 his property was valued at $5,000 in 1860 at $46,000.
5. U.S. Census, 1860, Nassau County, Florida, item 130.
6. WPA Writers Project, "Fernandina," a potpourri of documentary materials. Typed copy in P.K. Yonge Library of Florida History, Gainesville, p. 318.
7. Ibid., p. 319. During the Federal occupation of Fernandina the silver utensils of the Church, "originally a gift through the cooperation of Mrs. Dr. Lesesne, wife of the vestryman, and the Rev. Toomer Porter, of Charleston, S.C. had been placed in charge of the U.S. Customs House..." These items were returned to the Church in 1866.
8. Fernandina *East Floridian*, June 2, 1859. 1st printing, May 26, 1859. In ibid., August 9, 1860, is a report on fine grapes grown by Dr. Lesesne. These were of the "herbemont Madeira" variety from plants set in the spring of 1859.
9. Mary Elizabeth Dickison, *Dickison and His Men*, Facsimile edition, Gainesville, 1962, p. 169. The property of two other Fernandina physicians, D.P. Beatty and Jacob Cohen, was also confiscated.

Lespeyre, Bernard, Washington County, 1832-1863

The professional career of Dr. Bernard Lespeyre (Laspier) was brief. A native of North Carolina, he migrated to Florida prior to 1860, settling in what was then one of the more remote and undeveloped parts of the state. Vernon, although the county seat, was little more than a village. There Dr. Lespeyre found room and board in the home of A.M. Skipper, a local merchant, and began his practice as the only physician in the county.[1]

With the outbreak of war in 1861 Dr. Lespeyre was one of the first local men to offer his services to the Confederacy. He was mustered into Company H, 4th Florida Infantry Regiment, a unit commanded by Captain William F. Lane, who at the time of his enlistment was 57 years of age.[2] The company was organized on September 13, 1861, at Ft. William.[3] Dr. Lespeyre, with the rank of First Lieutenant, was second in command.[4] The official record does not indicate that he was ever considered a medical officer.

For much of the first year of its service the Fourth Regiment was assigned to duty on the Gulf Coast of Florida. Dr. Lespeyre's Company was assigned to the section in and around St. Marks where it remained until mid-1862 when it was ordered to proceed to Chattanooga, Tennessee. Dr. Lespeyre's service record indicates that he was at Chattanooga in July 1862 when he was issued equipment by Quartermaster A.L. Pope. Before the end of the year his unit had moved into the vicinity of Murfreesboro, Tennessee, where it became a part of the Brigade of General William Preston and participated in the Battle "in front of Murfreesboro," in which encounter Dr. Lespeyre was wounded on January 2, 1863. Although the records are not completely clear, it appears that he remained in service, although never completely recovering from his wounds. He died on October 29, 1963, at Uniontown, Alabama, his death, according to the Confederate record, the result of "disease."[5]

1. U.S. Census, 1860, Washington County, Florida, p. 288.
2. Captain Lane at the age of 57 was doubtless quite unfit for military service. He had joined the Regiment and was mustered in at Ft. William on September 18, 1861, dying at Lake City on May 22, 1862, "of disease." National Archives, Service Records, CSA, Co. H., 4th Florida Regiment.
3. Ft. William (Williams?) has not been accurately identified. Even Francis B. Heitman, Historical Register and Directory, 2 vols., Washington, D.C., 1903, was unable to give its precise location.
4. After the death of Captain Lane in May 1862, Dr. Lespeyre was promoted to the rank of captain in his stead.
5. In most instances of death, the records do not specify the disease.

Letherman, Jonathan, Physician, U.S. Army, 1825-1872

Dr. Letherman (Letterman) was born in Pennsylvania in 1825.[1] His name suggests a German origin. There is no record of his having attended a medical college, which probably indicates that he prepared for a medical career as a physician's apprentice. He was commissioned Assistant Surgeon in the United States Army on June 29, 1849.[2] The following year found him on duty in the Alifia Settlement of Hillsborough County, Florida.[3] He was apparently successful in his military career in that on April 16, 1862, he was promoted to the rank of major surgeon. For unknown reasons, but probably because of health problems, he resigned his commission on December 22, 1864, although the War Between the States was far from over. He died in Pennsylvania March 15, 1872.[3]

1. This date is an extrapolation from the Census of 1850 which shows age as 25.
2. Francis B. Heitman, *Historical Register and Directory of the United States Army*, Vol. I, Washington, U.S. Government Printing Office, 1903, p. 629.
3. Ibid.

Levitz, William A., Tampa, 1860

Dr. Levitz practiced medicine for a short time in Tampa. The Census of 1860 lists his age as 27, birth place as Kentucky, and his property valued at about $1,800. He and his young wife, Fanny, a native of Mississippi, were residents in the home of the Reverend J.J. Wells, a Methodist clergyman.[1] In the Wells household there was also E.M. Wells, aged 21, a medical student. Dr. Levitz is presumed to have left Florida prior to the outbreak of war in 1861.

1. U.S. Census, 1860, Hillsborough County, Florida, item 440.

Lewis, C.W., Alachua County, mid-19th century

About all presently known of Dr. Lewis, native of South Carolina, is derived from the records of the Medical College of the State of South Carolina, Charleston, where he matriculated in the fall of 1858.[1] He had prepared for admission by serving an apprenticeship under the guidance of Dr. Gabriel P. Thomas who had settled in Gainesville in 1855. Dr. Lewis was graduated with a medical degree in the spring of 1860, having submitted a doctoral thesis entitled "Malaria." Dr. Lewis was actually a resident of the Waldo community north of Gainesville near which his family had settled in the early 1850s. He is thought to have been the son of Edward and Martha Lewis, natives of South Carolina.[2]

1. Catalog, Medical College of the State of South Carolina, Sessions of 1858-59 and 1859-60. In the first of these his residence is shown to have been Gainesville, in the second, Waldo.
2. Several members of the South Carolina family of Lewises settled in the Waldo area in the 1850s. Edward Lewis was a man of considerable means having owned property valued at more than $60,000 in 1860. His slaves numbered 41.

Lewis, George H., Tallahassee, 1804-1834

Dr. Lewis, whose brief career was terminated by death on October 17, 1834,[1] was a native of Connecticut. He was graduated from the Jefferson Medical College of Philadelphia in the spring of 1830,[2] after which he began practice in Hartford, Connecticut. Plagued by poor health, probably tuberculosis, he moved to Tallahassee in the winter of 1832-33 in search of a more benign climate. In February 1833 he announced his professional services to the people of the town and county. He would treat all branches of his profession from his residence "the first house south of Major R. Lewis,"[3] where he died after a protracted illness. He was buried in the Old City Cemetery on October 18.[4]

1. Tallahassee *Floridian*, October 25, 1834.
2. Jefferson Medical College, Philadelphia, List of Dead or Lost Graduates in Classes from 1826 to 1879 (date?), p. 79.
3. Tallahassee *Floridian*, February 16, 1833.
4. Tallahassee Cemetery Records.

Lewis, H.T., Jackson County, 1850

Dr. Lewis, a native of Georgia, was practicing medicine in rural Jackson County in 1850. He was 27 years of age and a boarder in the home of farmer, William B. Dickson, a North Carolina native. His name does not appear in lists of graduates of any Southern medical colleges. It is therefore assumed that he entered the profession by way of the apprenticeship procedure.[1]

1. U.S. Census, 1850, Jackson County, Florida, p. 586.

Lewis, James S., Marion County, 1812-post 1876

Dr. Lewis, a South Carolina native, and one of many well-to-do citizens from that state to settle in rural Marion County in the antebellum period, arrived in Florida with his wife, Mary, and a young overseer, W.D. McAteer, in the 1850s. The Census of 1860 lists him as the owner of property valued at about $50,000.[1] His slaves numbered 59. His land was located in the northern part of the county in the community of Flemington.

Dr. Lewis, whose marriage was childless, was among the first to respond to the call to arms as the Civil War got under way. He enlisted at Ocala on March 8, 1862, without military rank but three months later was commissioned Assistant Surgeon and assigned to the Seventh Florida Regiment. A short time later he became staff surgeon under regimental commander, Madison Stark Perry, soon to become Governor of Florida. By the spring of 1863 Dr. Lewis was with his regiment in Tennessee, stationed at various posts including Knoxville, Chickamauga and Jonesboro. Throughout much of 1864 he was with his outfit at Dalton, Georgia. He was on duty "in the field" when the war ended and was among those paroled at Greensboro, N.C., on May 1, 1865.[2]

After the war Dr. Lewis returned to his farm in Marion County and resumed the dual operations of farming and practicing medicine. Although he was omitted from the Marion County Census of 1870, there is evidence that he continued to live beyond that date.[3]

1. U.S. Census, 1860, Marion County, Florida, p. 317.
2. NA, Service Records, CSA, Roll No. 78.
3. A University of Pennsylvania document listing the physicians practicing in Florida in 1870 includes "Dr. Lewis, of Flemington." University of Pennsylvania Archives, MSS. 2.3 #16. The Ocala *East Florida Banner* July 11, 1874, included an item about an unusual cucumber, called the "serpentine cucumber," grown on the plantation of Dr. J.S. Lewis. It was said to have been five feet, two inches long. This, of course, does not constitute proof that Dr. Lewis was still living at that date. There is also the information in Dr. Lewis' army record indicating that he was in poor health during a part of his army career, so poor, in fact, that he was granted two lengthy leaves of absence for recovery.

Lewis, J.O.A., Jackson County, 1850

The Register of Students of the Medical College of Georgia, Augusta, lists J.O.A. Lewis of Greenwood in Jackson County as an M.D. graduate in 1854. For an earlier term, 1851-52, however, he is shown to have been a resident of Sand Fort, Russell County, Alabama. No evidence has been located which would establish him as a Florida practitioner.[1]

1. Register of Students, 1832-1861. Registrar's Office, Medical College of Georgia. W.P. Lewis, probably his physician-father or kinsman, is named as his preceptor.

Ligon, Thomas H., Gainesville, 1826

The name of Dr. Ligon,[1] a Gainesville resident in 1865, has survived in Florida records chiefly because of his political activities during the difficult times following the Civil War. He was a native of Laurens District, South Carolina, and a graduate of the Medical College of the State of South Carolina in 1846.[2] His doctoral thesis bore the title "Congestive Fever." His preceptor had been Dr. W. Anderson of Laurens.

Following graduation Dr. Ligon practiced medicine in Atlanta for a few years, moving to Gainesville in 1865.[3] In the late summer of 1865 Florida's Provisional Governor William Marvin, in order to return Florida to its viable place in the Union, ordered that a constitutional convention be held in Tallahassee, beginning on October 25. October 10 was the date set for election of delegates, two of which were to represent Alachua County. Dr. Ligon was one of six whose names were placed in nomination. His political convictions, shared by many Alachua County citizens, were summarized in the Gainesville *New Era*: "Dr. T.H. Ligon, formerly of Atlanta, Georgia, is a gentleman of good ability and strict integrity. He advocates the colonization of the Negro to South Florida and opposes Negro suffrage and the receiving of Negro testimony in Court."[4] The election results show him to have placed fourth in the race, the two winners being Col. W.W. Scott of Newnansville and Col. S. Spencer of Gainesville.[5]

The new constitution having been completed, general elections were set for November 29, 1865. Col. Scott's name was placed in nomination for a seat in the Florida Senate but he declined to run for the office. Dr. Ligon was persuaded to allow his name to be placed on the ballot. Shortly before the election, however, Prof. J.H. Roper, Principal of the Gainesville Academy, became a candidate, whereupon Dr. Ligon withdrew from the contest. His decision came too late for the removal of his name from the ballot, and of the 335 votes cast he received 23.[6]

These political skirmishes apparently ended Dr. Ligon's Florida career. In late 1866 when his brother-in-law, John Leak, was killed in an altercation in Levy County, the Gainesville paper in its report of the incident referred to Dr. Ligon as "formerly of this place."[7] Presumably he had left the state by that date. His name has not been found in subsequent records.

1. The 1850 Census for Fairfield District, South Carolina, includes an entry for Thomas Ligon, a Virginia-born carpenter, aged 40. Among his seven children ranging in ages from two months to 15 years is a son, Thomas, aged 12, who is thought to be Dr. Ligon.

2. Charleston *Mercury*, March 23, 1846. Here are listed the names of those receiving degrees on March 7, 1846, together with their home districts and thesis titles.

3. Gainesville *New Era*, October 7, 1865.

4. Ibid., September 23, 1865. Here Dr. Ligon sets forth his proposals for dealing with the Negro problem. These included laying off 18,000 square miles (11,200,000 acres) of land in South Florida, using latitude 27 degrees 30 minutes as the northern boundary, extending to the headwaters of the Peace River and down the river to Charlotte Harbor. He calculated that since there were about 60,000 Negroes in Florida his proposal would provide 100 acres for each Negro. The area was to be colonized only by blacks.

5. Ibid., October 14, 1865.

6. Ibid., December 2, 1865. In reporting the results the editor was careful to point out that Dr. Ligon's meagre vote was attributable to the fact that he was not actually a candidate.

7. Ibid., October 19, 1867. The date of Dr. Ligon's departure from Gainesville is unknown as are his reasons for leaving.

Lindsey, W.K.D., St. Augustine, 1833

On January 10, 1833, Dr. Lindsey advertised his professional services to the citizens of St. Augustine and vicinity. He was both physician and surgeon, as were most medical practitioners of the times. Since no other information relating to his practice or even his residence in the Territory has been discovered, it is assumed that he was only a sojourner in Florida.[1]

1. St. Augustine *East Florida Herald*, January 10, 1833. Dr. Lindsey also claimed to have on hand an adequate supply of medicine.

Lipford, Albert T., Gadsden and Jefferson Counties, 1837

Dr. Lipford was born in South Carolina in 1837. Nothing is known of his education nor does his name appear on any of the available lists of graduates and matriculants of any of the better known medical colleges of the South. He is presumed to have been either the son or the nephew of Henry M. Lipford, a planter of considerable wealth, who arrived in Gadsden County in the mid-1850s.[1] Both men settled in this vicinity. The Census of 1860 lists Dr. Lipford as unmarried, aged 23, owning property valued at $20,000, and the sole resident of his house.[2]

With the Civil War already well under way Dr. Lipford enlisted as a private in the Second Florida Cavalry Regiment on May 8, 1862, at Camp Gladden,[3] bringing with him his horse and equipment, the combined value of which was $410. Soon after enlistment he was placed on detached service, probably as a medical aide. On at least two subsequent occasions his company commander, unaware of his whereabouts, listed him in reports as "absent without leave" although he was actually serving as medical officer with another unit. He was "discharged by promotion to Assistant Surgeon" on April 9, 1864, and in February 1865 was stationed at Baldwin, Florida, having recently been assigned to relieve Assistant Surgeon A.P. Smith. He was taken prisoner at Tallahassee and paroled on May 13, 1865. His parole papers give his height as five feet nine inches, his age as 25, his hair dark, his eyes dark, his complexion fair.

With his war experience behind him Dr. Lipford returned to the Quincy community and resumed medical practice. Census data indicate that Dr. Lipford had actually been married just prior to enlisting in the Confederate Army. His wife, Sally, was 30 years old in 1870 while their first child, Albert Jr., was eight years old that year.[4] By 1870, however, the family had moved to Jefferson County and settled in the village of Waukeenah. Meanwhile a daughter, Willie, five years old in 1870,[5] had been born. As far as is presently known Dr. Lipford lived out his life as a practitioner in Jefferson County. The date of his death has not been discovered.

1. Henry M. Lipford, probably the father of Dr. Lipford, was a wealthy planter, owning property valued in excess of $100,000 in 1860. His slaves numbered 60. Dr. Lipford's professional card first appeared in the Quincy *Republic* of March 15, 1859 (not extant). See ibid. of October 15, 1859.

2. U.S. Census, 1860, Gadsden County, Florida, p. 509.

3. NA, Service Records, CSA, M251, Roll 10.

4. U.S. Census, 1870, Jefferson County, Florida, p. 417.

5. In the Benjamin Chaires Cemetery, Verdura, located in the southeastern part of Leon County there is a gravestone with the inscription, "Willie Lipford Farmer, daughter of Dr. Albert Thaddeus Lipford, (dates unknown)." There is this added note: "Her unnamed daughter is also buried here."

Little, Robert Edmonds, Quincy, 1840

There is little information relating to Dr. Little. He arrived in Quincy in the early part of 1844, rented an office just north of the county courthouse and offered his services to the citizens of Gadsden County.[1] Obviously a scholarly young man, a rare quality among practitioners of the frontier, he found time for observation and reflection on the relationship of health to climate in Gadsden County. His paper on the subject was published in 1845.[2] Within two years two additional medical treatises found their way into print.[3]

Dr. Little was among those physicians employed by the state to provide medical attention for prisoners. Near the end of the session of 1846-47, the Comptroller of Public Accounts was authorized by the Legislature to issue a warrant for payment of an account which had been submitted by Dr. Little. It received final approval on January 6, 1847.[4]

Only one other reference to Dr. Little has been located, that being his endorsement of a patent medicine published in a local paper.[5] It appears that he had died prior to 1850.[6]

1. Tallahassee *Florida Sentinel*, April 9, 1844. In this notice he identified himself as R.E. Little, M.D., "late of Kentucky."

2. Robert Edmonds Little, M.D., "Remarks on Climate, Disease, etc., of Middle Florida, Particularly in Gadsden County," *Southern Medical and Surgical Journal*, September 1845, pp. 526-535.

3. Ibid., November, 1845, pp. 618-625, "Thoughts of Syphilitic Ulcers, Their Treatment, etc." And in ibid., March, 1847, pp. 141-147, "Observations on Various Diseases."

4. Acts and Resolutions, General Assembly, State of Florida, 2nd Session, p. 95; 3rd Session, p. 57.

5. Tallahassee *Florida Sentinel*, April 2, 1848.

6. Information from the Census of 1850 strongly suggests the demise of Dr. Little prior to 1850. Note the following entry:

Edmonds, Robert L.	aged 60	b. Ireland
Edmonds, Julia	aged 44	b. Virginia
Edmonds, Jeanette	aged 25	b. Virginia
Little, Susan	aged 23	b. S.C.
Little, Robert	aged 3	b. Florida

Robert Edmonds Little was almost certainly a nephew of Robert L. Edmonds. The surmise here is that after Dr. Little's death his widow and young son became members of the Edmonds household.

Lively, William A., Tampa, 1833

Dr. Lively, a native of Kentucky,[1] moved to Tampa in the mid-1850s. He is thought to have already attended lectures in a medical school for a term or possibly served an apprenticeship under a practicing physician. Anyway, he had been able to find some type of employment by which he earned a living and made a favorable impression upon the citizens of the town. At the annual convention of the Hillsborough County Democrats on August 2, 1857, he was chosen as candidate for Clerk of the Circuit Court, the office which he won handily in the following October.[2]

After serving as Clerk of the Court for about a year[3] he decided to resign and resume his medical education. He returned to Kentucky for the 1858-59 term (thought to have been at the University of Louisville, Department of Medicine) and in March 1859 he returned to Tampa to begin his new career. His return was noted in the following item:[4]

> Dr. Lively, our Worthy Clerk of the Circuit Court, has been attending Medical Lectures in Louisville, Kentucky, for the past few months...and now returns to his home "with a sheepskin" to begin practice as an M.D.

During his earlier stay in Tampa Dr. Lively had found lodging and board in the home of Methodist minister, Jesse J. Wells. On January 10, 1860,[5] he married the elder Wells daughter, Fanny, and a son was born a year later. Meanwhile Dr. Lively had formed a professional partnership with one of Tampa's best known physicians and public figures, Dr. Franklin Branch,[6] a fortunate alliance for him in that Dr. Branch was not only a well-regarded physician but also owner of the best drug store in town.

When the Civil War was well under way and with the sick and wounded from the Florida regiments being returned to the state from the combat zones, several hospitals were established for their care. One was located on the west side of Tampa Bay on a key shown on early maps as Hospital Key which lay a short distance from Mullet Key. In early 1864 Dr. Lively was commissioned Acting Assistant Surgeon and assigned to hospital duty at the temporary encampment named Camp Cook.[7] He was officially assigned to Major John T. Leslie's Company (Company K, 4th Florida Infantry) composed for the greater part of men from Tampa. He was thus able to enjoy occasional visits to his wife and little son.

In the summer of 1860 the partnership of Drs. Branch and Lively had been dissolved, it is thought, because of a conflict of opinion regarding the proper role of the Democratic Party of the South on the slavery issue. The public notice of the breakup first appeared in the Tampa *Florida Peninsular* of June 2, 1860. It bore only the name of Dr. Branch. Since the notice continued weekly for seven months at Dr. Branch's expense, it appears that he had harbored a grudge against his former friend and professional partner.

Nothing further is known of Dr. Lively until 1866. He ceased to appear at the meetings of Tampa Democrats after 1859 but reappeared at a meeting in Tampa on March 15, 1866, called for the purpose of "organizing a Union Party." It was the hope of the group to enlist the support of all men who "have taken the oath of allegiance, i.e., President Johnson's Amnesty Oath, to support in elections candidates who during the rebellion have been known to sympathize with the Government of the United States." The central committee for the Party included Dr. Lively.[8]

This courageous stand did not terminate Dr. Lively's political life in Tampa. In elections of August 28, 1866, he won a seat on the Tampa City Commission,[9] but if we may trust a statement by Dr. Branch in June 1867 he did not immediately resume medical practice at the end of the War. In mid-June, 1867, Dr. Branch wrote a letter to the *Peninsular* which began: "As no physician has desired to practice here until very recently except myself, I have had charge of all the sick in the town and vicinity." He then proceeded to dismiss as false the rumors that Tampa was not a healthful place.[10]

The summer of 1867 brought devastating sorrow to Dr. Lively when the death of his wife, Fanny, was followed a few weeks later by the death of his son, John Laurens Lively. His eulogist wrote:[11]

> The noble, manly sweet-tempered, truthful, obedient boy...a few weeks ago we saw him stand by the grave of his departed mother, while her friends were laying her away in her last resting place....

Apparently shattered by this double tragedy, Dr. Lively did not long remain in Tampa. Within weeks he had departed, presumably to return to his native Kentucky. His father-in-law, Jesse Wells, soon followed his daughter in death. The medical tradition of the family was carried on, however, by Mrs. Lively's brother, Richard M. Wells, who became a physician and practiced medicine in the Crawford Mill community outside Tampa.[12] Nothing is known of the later years of Dr. Lively.

1. U.S. Census, 1860, Hillsborough County, Florida, p. 681, item 440.
2. Tampa *Florida Peninsular*, October 10, 1857.
3. Dr. Lively was still Clerk of the Circuit Court as late as April 1858. See ibid., April 3, 1858.
4. Ibid., March 19, 1859.
5. Ibid., June 14, 1860.
6. Ibid., June 18, 1859.
7. Positive identification of the Key and encampment has not been made. A Geodetic Survey map of 1875 identifies it as Hospital Key but the name does not appear on later maps. For Dr. Lively's military assignment see *Soldiers of Florida*, Live Oak, Florida, Board of State Institutions, 1903, p. 320.
8. Jacksonville *Florida Union*, May 5, 1866.
9. Tampa *Florida Peninsular*, September 1, 1866.
10. Ibid., June 29, 1867.
11. Ibid., September 7, 1867.
12. U.S. Census, 1870, Hillsborough County, Florida, p. 122; also ibid., 1880, p. 431, item 139.

Lockhart, John Porter, Jackson County, 1830

Dr. Lockhart was among the earlier settlers in Jackson County. He was already there at the time of the founding of the town of Marianna in 1827 and in the controversy over the selection of a county seat he was among those favoring Marianna over Webbville.[1] Although J. Randall Stanley, the Jackson County historian, identifies him only as "lawyer," the evidence indicates that he was more concerned with the medical profession.[2]

The list of matriculants in the medical department of Transylvania University of Lexington, Kentucky, for the year 1824-25, includes the name, John Porter Lockhart from Franklin County, Alabama, as a first-year student.[3] When, in the sixth session of the Legislative Council of the Territory of Florida, an act for establishment of a Medical Board for the Territory was passed on December 31, 1827, the Gadsden County member was Dr. William P. Hort.[4] In a revision of the Act in November the following year, Dr. Lockhart was added to the Board.[5] The 15-member Board included most of the eminent physicians practicing in the Territory at the time.

Dr. Lockhart also accepted important civic responsibilities. In 1829 he was a member of a commission charged with letting the contract for the building of the Jackson County courthouse and jail.[6] He was active in expansion of the Bank of West Florida in 1831, serving on the committee to receive monies for the newly authorized issues of capital.[7] In 1832 he was one of three commissioners appointed to select a permanent site for the capital of the Territory.[8]

Very little is known of Dr. Lockhart's personal life. The Jackson County Census of 1830 gives his age as between 20 and 30 but lists one male slave as the only other member of this household.[9] He ceases to appear in the records after 1832. One may assume that he left the Territory for permanent residence elsewhere.

1. J. Randall Stanley, *History of Jackson County*, Marianna, 1950, p. 24.
2. Ibid., pp. 24, 63.
3. Archives, Transylvania University, Medical Department (Microfilm, courtesy of Prof. Eric Christiansen, University of Kentucky).
4. Acts, Legislative Council, Territory of Florida, Sixth Session 1827-28, pp. 46-49.
5. Ibid., Seventh Session, 1828, pp. 258-60.
6. Stanley, op. cit., p. 48.
7. Ibid., p. 114.
8. St. Augustine *East Florida Herald*, January 5, 1832. The other commissioners were Dr. Malcolm Nicholson of Gadsden County and E.B. Gould, Esq., editor of the St. Augustine newspaper.
9. U.S. Census, 1830, Jackson County, Florida, Sheet 81.

Long, Nicholas A., Jackson County, 1815-1869

Dr. Long, son of a distinguished Georgian, Richard H. Long, and grandson of the even more distinguished Col. Nicholas Long, who had made a fortune in land dealing just after the American Revolution, was born in Wilkes County, Georgia, on December 10, 1815. When he was still a youth he was brought to Florida by his father who purchased property in Jackson County some eight miles north of Marianna in the Greenwood community. Other members of the Long family were brothers, Richard H., Jr.; Felix Gilbert Hay, and Thomas T., and their sister, Rebecca, later to become the wife of George F. Baltzell, a judge of note in the county.[1] From their base at Greenwood, the father and his four sons participated actively and constructively in the early development of Jackson County.

Although Dr. Long was a graduate of the Medical College of the State of South Carolina, Charleston, in the class of March 1838,[2] his medical career was overshadowed by involvement in politics. He was elected for six terms in the Florida Legislature, serving in the Territorial House of Representatives in 1842, and as a senator from the Western District in the sessions of 1843 and 1844. After statehood was achieved in 1845, he was returned to the House in the sessions of 1848, 1850 and 1852.[3] From the beginning of his public career he embraced the principles of the Whig Party to which he remained faithful until its dissolution in the 1850s.

The actual extent and nature of Dr. Long's medical practice cannot be determined but it is clear that except for his absences in Tallahassee he was a regular practitioner. He was not, however, among the small group of physicians from central Florida who met in Quincy on May 15-16, 1848, to discuss the condition and quality of medical practice in the state and draft a charter for a state board or society which was to be presented to the Legislature at its session the following November. But it was Dr. Long who assumed sponsorship of the bill and undertook to guide it through the House.[4] His toleration of professional deviation of more orthodox practice is apparent in his support in the session of 1850 of a bill which would allow a Thompsonian doctor to practice in Benton, later Hernando County.[5]

No record of marriage for Dr. Long has been located; it is assumed that he remained single throughout his life. In the Census of 1850 he was shown to have been a householder, owning property valued at $17,000. He shared his residence with his brother, Felix, a farmer, and an overseer, Wilton P. Whatley, also a native Georgian.[6] Ten years later his real estate was valued at $25,000; he was living with his father, aged 70. He died on August 28, 1869, and was buried in the Long Cemetery.[7]

1. For additional data on the Long family, see Eliza A. Bowen, *The Story of Wilkes County, Georgia*, Marietta, Georgia, 1950, pp. 105-108.
2. Charleston (S.C.) *Mercury*, March 19, 1838. His doctoral thesis bore the title, "On Hepatitis."
3. Allen Morris, *The People of Lawmaking in Florida*, Tallahassee, unpaginated but alphabetically arranged.
4. The bill met strong opposition in the House and was defeated by a vote of 18 to 14 on December 28, 1848. The Journals of the House for the session, 1848-49, do not include the text of the bill as first presented, although the legislative processes involved are recorded. A similar bill was passed by the Senate on January 9, 1849, and subsequently by the House. For the Act of early January 1849, see *Acts and Resolutions, General Assembly of the State of Florida*, Tallahassee, 1849, pp. 74-75.
5. This bill, supported by a petition from Benton County citizens, related to the Thompsonian, George W. Andrews. It passed the House handily but met opposition in the Senate led by Dr. John L. Crawford of Wakulla. The Senate eventually passed it by a vote of 11 to seven.
6. U.S. Census, 1850, Jackson County, Florida, p. 588, item 285.
7. U.S. Census, 1860, Jackson County, Florida, item 63.

Lorimer, John, British West Florida, 1732 or 1733-1795

Dr. Lorimer's reputation as a military surgeon was established several years prior to his appearance on the American scene.[1] Born in England about 1732, he had apparently entered the medical profession by way of the apprenticeship system. Entering the British Army as a Surgeon's Mate, he was promoted to the rank of Regimental Surgeon and in 1762 was involved in the British-French hostilities which had resulted in the capture of Belle Isle, a French possession off the south coast of Brittany.

The British occupation of Florida in 1763, a fairly peaceful affair, was followed by a division of the territory into an East and West Florida. The British presence was supported by establishment of military bases or garrisons in each part. In 1765 Dr. Lorimer was dispatched to Pensacola as surgeon to its garrison, arriving there in August of that year. His duties allowed him sufficient time to pursue his interests in hydrography and cartography.[2]

Authors Rea and Holmes,[3] who have studied the career of Dr. Lorimer, discovered that he gained prominence in the affairs of the Territory, having been elected in 1766 to the first session of the West Florida Assembly, becoming speaker *pro tempore* on two occasions. He was also surveyor as well as auditor of the royal revenues of the colony. As for his professional duties he found the summer fevers endemic to the area a challenge; however, he was unable to impose successfully sanitary regulations and avoid a discouraging death rate among the soldiers of the garrison.

As expected, Dr. Lorimer took advantage of his situation to pursue interests in local flora, especially plants of medicinal value. As the months passed he was joined by other medical personnel. These included Dr. Michael Grant, John Ramsey and Park Maxwell, and even the renowned William Bartram. Bernard Romans, in his *Concise and Natural History of East and West Florida*, referred to Dr. Lorimer as "My very worthy friend, Doctor J. Lorimer, at Pensacola."[4] Not to be overlooked, of course, was his interest in cartography. He joined George Gault in exploring the Gulf Coast and the Mississippi. Dr. Lorimer remained in West Florida until Spanish rule was reestablished in 1782.

From Pensacola Dr. Lorimer went to New York where he accepted the post of Inspector of Military. Soon thereafter he returned to England where he died in July 1795.

1. Dr. Lorimer was born about 1732 in England. He is thought to have been a relative to two distinguished Scots, James Lorimer, 1818-1890, a native of Perthshire, who was a professor at the University of Edinburgh, and Peter Lorimer, 1812-1879, a prominent Presbyterian clergyman, also of Edinburgh.
2. Much of the biographical data is from Robert R. Ray and Jack D.L. Holmes, "Dr. John Lorimer and the Natural Sciences in British West Florida," *South Humanities Review*, IV, No. 4, Fall 1970, pp. 363-372.
3. Ibid.
4. See Notes on the Life and Works of Bernard Romans, by P. Lee Phillips. A facsimile reproduction of the 1924 edition with an Introduction and Index by John D. Ware, Gainesville, University of Florida Press, 1975. See especially pp. 27-28 in which Romans expresses his high esteem of Dr. Lorimer.

Loring, John McC., St. Augustine, 1812-1839

Dr. Loring, graduate of the South Carolina Medical College in the class of 1834,[1] practiced briefly in St. Augustine where he died on April 18, 1839, at the age of 27.[2] He was the eldest son of Reuben Loring, native of North Carolina, who died in St. Augustine in late 1837.[3] Certain civic concerns of Dr. Loring are reflected in his signature to petitions of St. Augustine citizens requesting congressional aid to the city for road and bridge building and for harbor improvements.[4] He was very probably the brother of William W. Loring, who represented St. Johns County in the Florida Legislative Council in the sessions of 1844 and 1845 and who went on to a distinguished military career following resignation from the legislative body in 1845.[5]

1. Medical University of South Carolina, Archives, List of Graduates.
2. St. Augustine *News*, April 20, 1839; St. Augustine *Florida Herald and Southern Democrat*, April 18, 1839.
3. Reuben Loring appears in the St. Johns County Census of 1830 as head of a large family. His widow, Hannah, is listed in the 1850 Census as a native of North Carolina, rendering it fairly certain that Dr. Loring was also born in that state.
4. TP., XXV, 451, 548.
5. St. Augustine *Florida Herald and Southern Democrat*, November 13, 1843. Allen Morris, *The People of Lawmaking in Florida*, Tallahassee, 1977.

Lykes, Howell Tyson, Hernando and Hillsborough Counties, 1846-1906

Dr. Lykes' career in medicine was brief and totally overshadowed by his tremendous success in the world of business. He was born in Columbia, South Carolina, on August 25, 1846, the son of Frederick and Margaret Howell Tyson Lykes. In 1851 the Lykes family moved to Florida, settling in Spring Hill, a village in Hernando County some four miles west of Brooksville. Concerning his early education nothing is known. In due time he enrolled at the Medical College of the State of South Carolina, where he remained for one term, leaving without his degree. Returning to Florida he practiced medicine for a brief period but soon abandoned it for the more lucrative world of business.

His first business success came by way of the cattle industry. Acquiring large acreage in Hernando County he turned to production of beef cattle, soon taking advantage of the Cuban market. This led into the shipping business and in cooperation with his brothers the Lykes Steamship Company was soon sending its ships to ports around the world. In due time the Lykes enterprises had offices in New York, Galveston, Houston, as well as Havana, Tampa, Rotterdam, Hamburg and Bremen. Medicine was no longer one of his concerns.

On July 8, 1874, Dr. Lykes was married to Miss Almeria Bell McKay and they had eight children. Seven were sons, Frederick, Lipscomb, Thomas, John, Joseph, Howell and James. The daughter, Tillie, became the wife of Solon H. Turner. Needless to add, the Lykes family has played important roles in the business, cultural and social life of Tampa.[1]

1. Several biographical sketches of various members of the Lykes family have appeared. Much of this data is derived from *The Book of Florida*, compiled by The James O. Jones Company, 1925. Also useful for the early years of Dr. Lykes was Richard J. Stanaback, *A History of Hernando County*, 1840-1976, Brooksville, Florida, 1976.

Lyons, J.M., Wakulla County, 1832

A single but significant reference establishes Dr. Lyons as a medical practitioner in St. Marks in the early 1830s. On November 15, 1832, he wrote a letter to the editor of the Tallahassee *Floridian* protesting publication of exaggerated reports about the spread of cholera in St. Marks. Such reports were, in his opinion, false and irresponsible. He claimed that there was no case of cholera in the town nor had there been, assuring the editor that should a case of cholera appear the public would be promptly informed. The letter was signed by 14 citizens of St. Marks.[1] Since Dr. Lyons was not listed in the censuses of 1830 and 1840, he is presumed to have been a brief sojourner in the Territory.

1. Tallahassee *Floridian*, November 20, 1832.

Lytle, James H., Alachua County, 1843

Dr. Lytle, presently known only because of his participation in a Fourth of July celebration at Newnansville in 1843, was apparently a person of some local importance. He not only gave the main address of the day but offered two toasts: the first to Nicholl Turnbull, a land speculator who had laid claim to 58,300 acres of land in the vicinity of New Smyrna, a claim which was later challenged in the Federal Court,[1] and the second, which perhaps reflected some impatience with the Territorial government in Tallahassee, "To East Florida: May she yet be rid of her collateral kin, Middle and West Florida, and go on her own hook." In addition to these functions Dr. Lytle also presented the flag[2] to the Alachua County Troop commanded by Capt. R.G. Livingstone, followed by an address to which Livingstone responded.

1. *Florida Territorial Papers*, 1828-34, XXIV, 708; ibid., 1839-45, p. 200, et passim.
2. The account of the celebration appeared in the St. Augustine *Florida Herald and Southern Democrat*, July 24, 1843. The flag was presented "on behalf of a Lady."

MacKay, Stephen, Putnam County, 1860

Dr. MacKay, a native of Canada, was a practicing physician in Palatka for a brief period just prior to the Civil War. His wife, Susan, was a native of Florida. These two facts argue for the probability that Dr. MacKay had been a resident of Palatka for several months, or at least for sufficient time to have made the acquaintance of his wife-to-be and propose marriage. His age in 1860 was 38; hers 25. His properties were valued at $2,500.[1]

Dr. MacKay does not appear in subsequent censuses and is presumed to have left Florida with the outbreak of war in 1861.

1. U.S. Census, 1860, Putnam County, Florida, Item 74.

Macomb, Edward, Surgeon, U.S. Army, 1844

Dr. Macomb, a native of New York and citizen of that state when he was commissioned Assistant Surgeon on January 20, 1824, saw military service in Florida from 1824 until about 1830.[1] His first assignment appears to have been with the Fourth Infantry Regiment, nine companies of which were stationed in Florida.[2] Dr. Macomb's station was Ft. Brooke on Tampa Bay where he remained throughout his Florida career except for brief intervals of detached service at other cantonments.

The evidence strongly suggests that he was a highly-respected member of the Medical Department. On two occasions he was dispatched to Key West on special assignments. On the second in 1829 he accompanied his commanding officer, Col. George M. Brooke, "to examine the harbor and select a suitable site for the erection of barracks and a military station."[3] In 1829 he was granted a leave of absence for four months "because of ill health and private business;"[4] probably because of health he was transferred out of Florida in 1830.

In 1833 Dr. Macomb was at Ft. Wood in New York.[5] The following year he was promoted to the rank of surgeon and assigned to Ft. Leavenworth.[6] His last years were spent at Ft. Monroe in Virginia where he died on March 26, 1844.[7]

1. MDUSA, p. 288.
2. ASP, Military Affairs, II, p. 838. At this juncture the Fourth Regiment was divided, with nine companies assigned to Florida at Ft. Brooke, St. Marks, Ft. Barrancas, and Cantonment Clinch and seven companies to various posts in Louisiana.
3. Ibid., IV, p. 411. See also Key West *Register*, March 12, 1829. On one of these visits Dr. Macomb became acquainted with Dr. Robert Lacy, a prominent Key West physician who wrote a lengthy letter to Dr. Macomb on March 16, 1829, giving his observations on the health of the island city during his residence there. See ibid., March 26, 1829. At about the same time the two doctors were in Havana, presumably together, returning to Key West on the Revenue Cutter Pulaski which arrived on March 29. Ibid., April 2, 1829.
4. ASP, Military Affairs, IV, 441.
5. Ibid., V, p. 278.
6. Ibid., VII, p. 929. See ibid., VI, pp. 35, 205 for information relating to pay and allowances received by Dr. Macomb.
7. MDUSA., p. 288. If we assume that Dr. Macomb was in his early 20s at the time of commissioning in 1824, he would not have been more than 45 at the time of his death. A thorough search has not revealed that he was a kinsman of Major General Alexander, Commanding General of the Army.

Macomb, John L., Walton and Escambia Counties, 1820

Dr. Macomb arrived in West Florida as early as 1822 and probably settled first in Pensacola. Later, however, he acquired land on the southeast side of Pensacola Bay in what was then, or was soon to become, Walton County.[1] In 1827 he and a colleague, Dr. Randolph, are known to have attended Captain W. Armstrong, an officer stationed at Cantonment Clinch, in his last illness. It was reported that in spite of "the assiduous care" of the two physicians, the illness, diagnosed as consumption, was fatal.[2]

A random social note provided additional identification of Dr. Macomb when the marriage of Mr. John Brown to Mrs. Eliza Simmons was held "at the plantation of Dr. Macomb, on the Yellow Water." The date was September 24, 1829.[3]

Dr. Macomb was listed in the Census of 1830, Walton County, as a householder, aged between 40 and 50. Also in the house were four male children under 20, and five females besides 14 slaves, all female.[4] His name does not appear in the Florida Census of 1840.

1. The earliest reference to Dr. Macomb is found in the Pensacola *Floridian*, July 27, 1822, in the list of persons for whom letters were being held in the Pensacola post office.

2. Pensacola *Gazette*, February 16, 1827. Cantonment Clinch, established by Col. Duncan U. Clinch some four miles west of Pensacola as a healthier site than the Pensacola waterfront. This move was prompted by the outbreak of yellow fever in 1822. The identity of "Dr. Randolph" remains uncertain although he was possibly Dr. Arthur W. Randolph, later a Leon County practitioner.

3. Ibid., September 29, 1829. This item established Dr. Macomb as more than a casual sojourner in the area. John Lee Williams *A View of West Florida*, facsimile edition, Herbert J. Doherty Jr., ed., Gainesville, 1976, contains a map citing the Macomb plantation on Pensacola Bay near the effluence of the Yellow Water River.

4. U.S. Census, 1830, Walton County, p. 74. The Census of 1840 does not include his name.

Magill, William G., Lake City, 1803-1865

Dr. Magill spent only a brief part of his career in Florida. He was born in Georgetown, South Carolina, in 1803.[1] He graduated from the South Carolina College in Columbia, after which he attended Jefferson Medical College in Philadelphia, then enrolled at the Medical College of South Carolina and was graduated in 1826, having submitted a doctoral thesis entitled "Febris Intermittens" (Intermittent Fever).[2] He served as surgeon in Major Harlee's South Carolina Regiment in the Florida Seminole War. He later entered the Civil War as surgeon assigned to the Chatham Artillery in Savannah. In February 1864 he was transferred to hospital service in Lake City, Florida, and subsequently assigned to the Army of Tennessee, in which he served during the campaign around Dalton and Atlanta. After his capture he served at the infamous Andersonville Prison in Georgia and finally in Florence, Alabama, where he became ill. In his debilitated condition he was finally sent to Athens, Georgia, where he died on Febrary 24, 1865.[3]

1. Some of the data included in this sketch is derived from J.J. Dickison, *Military History of Florida*, p. 314, the accuracy of which is not to be totally trusted.

2. Charleston *Mercury*, April 5, 1826.

3. Dickison, op. cit.

Magill, William Joseph, Jacksonville, 1827-1890

Although he was well-qualified in the field of medicine, there is no evidence that Dr. Magill ever practiced medicine in Florida. He arrived in the state in 1876, settling in Jacksonville where he lived until his death years later. Soon after arriving he began growing oranges but soon abandoned this to become a justice of the peace and an inspector of fertilizers. Throughout the 1880s he resided at 69 West Union Street, which was also the residence of his son, Frederick J., and daughter, Mrs. Edward B. King. Both the son and son-in-law held positions with the railroad. Although he was married to Mary E. Percival, of Albany, New York, her name did not appear in local records until Dr. Magill's obituary in the Jacksonville *Times-Union* of September 18, 1890 (he had died the previous day), in which it is stated that Mrs. Magill was in New York but would arrive in Jacksonville in time for the funeral.

James D. Moody, of Charleston, has provided detailed biographical information on Dr. Magill from his birth up to the time he settled in Florida in 1876. This information is gratefully acknowledged and is appended here verbatim.

William Joseph Magill born at Richmond Hill Plantation, Georgetown District, S.C., March 10, 1827, son of Dr. John Daniel Magill and Mary Eliza Vereen of Waccamaw Island.

Graduated from the Citadel in Nov., 1846.

Mexican War-commissioned Second Lieutenant, 3rd Regiment U.S. Dragoons, April 1847; Unit disbanded at the end of the War.

Merchant, Savannah, Georgia, 1848-1850; M.D. Medical College of S.C., 1852.

Capt. of Police, Charleston, 1856; employed at Custom House, Charleston, 1857. Professor, Kentucky Military Institute, Marietta, 1859-61.

C.S.A. 1st Lieutenant Kennesaw Dragoons (local defense company of Georgia State Troops) 1861; Captain, Co. A. 1st Regt. Georgia Regulars, Feb. 1, 1861; promoted to Lt. Colonel, 1st Ga. Regulars, June 8, 1861; promoted to Colonel, Feb. 6, 1862; lost an arm at Sharpsburg; Retired to Invalid Corps, Aug. 3, 1864; commanded the post at Columbia, S.C., Aug.-Oct. 1864; commanded post at Athens, Ga., thereafter.

Post-War: Superintendent of Agencies, Cotton States Life Insurance Company, 18? to 1876; moved to Florida in 1876 to become orange grower; moved to Jacksonville, 1885, where he was justice of the peace and Inspector of Fertilizers.

Married Mary Percival of Albany, N.Y.

Died at Jacksonville Sept. 19, 1890.

Note that the date of death does not agree with that stated in Dr. Magill's obituary. See info supra.

Mallory, W. Clay, Suwannee County, 1870

Very little information on the career of Dr. Mallory, a medical practitioner in Suwannee County during the last part of the 19th century, has been located. He and his wife, Betty, aged 34 and 35 respectively in 1870,[1] were natives of North Carolina. They are thought to have arrived in Florida about 1869, settling first in the Wellborn community, but later moving to Branford. He was still a practicing physician in Branford as late as 1897 when, as a member of the Suwannee County Medical Society, he attached his name to a public notice signed by 16 members of the Society stating that they would not continue to answer calls from those who had not paid their doctor bills.[2] The date of Dr. Mallory's death has not been determined.

1. U.S. Census, 1870, Suwannee County, Florida, p. 692.
2. Live Oak *Suwannee Democrat*, November 29, 1897.

Malone, John, Madison County, 1850

Dr. John Malone,[1] thought to have been a native of Jasper County, Georgia, practiced medicine for a brief time in Madison County. The only reference to his presence in the state is the entry in the Census of 1850 which shows him to have been a physician, 23 years of age, living with his wife, Lucy, and one-year-old daughter, Rosa. In the household also was Dr. Lucius Malone, aged 21, presumably a brother. Neither physician appears in the later censuses. A search through lists of graduates of the more important medical schools of the South in the antebellum period did not reveal their names.

1. U.S. Census, 1850, Madison County, Florida, p. 148. Another Dr. Malone, John Wood, also a native of Georgia, was a prominent medical practitioner in Quincy during the 1830s and early 1840s. No kinship with the Madison County Malones has been established.

Malone, John Wood, Quincy, 1810-1844

Dr. Malone, a native of Georgia, moved to Quincy about 1833[1] and quickly established himself as a reputable physician and civic leader. There is no present information concerning Dr. Malone's medical education. He was regarded as a skilled, compassionate practitioner. His success was probably aided by his marriage to Louisa Booth, one of the charming daughters of William Fitzgerald Booth.[2] To this union were born three sons, William B., Alfred and John W., and one daughter, Florida.[3]

Dr. Malone, a conservative (Whig) in politics, was from the time of his arrival in Quincy a public figure. As early as May 1834 he participated in a Fourth of July celebration,[4] having been chosen to deliver the oration. His speech was reported as "classic, chaste, eloquent and a patriotic oration;"[5] the full text was later published.[6] It is a fine example of the grandiloquent style of oratory in vogue at the time and its numerous classical allusions suggest the basic soundness of Dr. Malone's early education.

In 1838 Dr. Malone was a Gadsden County representative at the famous St. Joseph Constitutional Convention[7] and four years later represented the county in the Territorial Legislative Council as a member of the House.[8] He was among the conservative leaders of Middle Florida who fought valiantly to preserve the Union Bank of Tallahassee which had virtually collapsed because of mismanagement and the Panic of 1837.[9]

Dr. Malone died at his home in Quincy on January 18, 1844, at age 33, after an illness of 11 days. He was said to have been a highly endowed physician and a distinguished public servant.

1. An obituary notice appeared in the Tallahassee *Florida Sentinel* of January 22, 1844. A full account and eulogy appeared on January 30, 1844.

2. William F. Booth's daughters numbered seven. Their respective husbands included, in addition to Dr. Malone, other socially prominent men of Quincy such as Samuel Stephens, Jesse Coe, David L. White, Arthur J. Foreman and Hudson Muse. See J. Randall Stanley, *History of Gadsden County*, Quincy, 1948, p. 139.

3. The three Malone sons served in the Army of the Confederacy. William, the eldest, was commissioned as First Lieutenant and later promoted to Captain. As commander of Company C, 6th Florida Infantry, he was wounded in combat and spent the last months of the War in Way Hospital, Meridian, Mississippi. Alfred F., the second son, was Second Lieutenant, also in the 6th Florida Infantry. He was captured by Sherman's forces near Atlanta and spent the last months of the War in various Union prisons. The youngest, John W., Jr., entered the service as a Sergeant, later became Second Lieutenant. He was wounded, taken prisoner at Gettysburg and hospitalized. He was paroled on May 16 following. NA, Serv. Recs., CSA, M251, Rolls 72, 28, and 84.

4. Tallahassee *Floridian*, June 7, 1834.

5. Ibid., July 12, 1834.

6. Ibid., July 19, 1834.

7. See note 1, supra.

8. Allen Morris, *The People of Lawmaking in Florida*, Tallahassee, 1977.

9. Some details of Dr. Malone's role in the banking controversy appeared in the Quincy *Sentinel*, issues of October 9 and 16, 1840.

Malone, Lucius, Madison County, 1850

Dr. Malone[1] appears in the Madison County Census of 1850 as a resident in the home of his brother, Dr. John Malone. He was also a native of Georgia. As was true of his brother, he appears to have been a brief sojourner in Florida.

1. U.S. Census, 1850, Madison County, Florida, p. 148. Dr. Lucius Malone was 21 years old in 1850.

Manes, Ellis, Wakulla County, post-1865

Little is presently known of the career of Dr. Manes. It appears that he moved from his native Georgia soon after the Civil War and settled in Crawfordville, where he was for several years the town's only physician.[1] The Census of 1870 shows him to have been 49 years old, while his wife, Ann Eliza, also a native of Georgia, was 31.[2] Ten years later the couple were still living in Crawfordville. Meanwhile a daughter, Mattie B., had been born in 1873.[3] Since they do not appear in the special census of 1885, it is assumed that the doctor had either died or left the state.

1. Dr. Manes is listed in J.M. Hawks, *Florida Gazetteer*, New Orleans, 1871, as Crawfordville's only doctor.
3. U.S. Census, 1870, Wakulla County, Florida, p. 12.
2. U.S. Census, 1880, Wakulla County, Florida, p. 22.

Manning, Andrew May, Leon and Jefferson Counties, 1831-1907

Dr. Manning was born in Alabama in March 1830.[1] His father, Benjamin Manning Jr., and mother, Silvia Little Manning, were natives of Edgecomb County, North Carolina, who had moved to Alabama in the 1820s. They were a family of considerable means who, upon moving to Florida about 1832, purchased a tract of land situated on the west side of Foshalee Slough and extending northward to the Georgia border. A portion of this Leon County property was developed into farm land. The homestead, on which a village developed, was known as Mannington, later Iamonia. It enjoyed the convenience of a post office from 1833 to 1853.

Nothing is known of Dr. Manning's early education. It may be conjectured that he was taught at home by his mother or possibly a tutor. As for basic medical training he probably served an apprenticeship under a nearby practitioner. By whatever means he was qualified to matriculate at the Medical Department of Tulane University in the fall of 1851. He was graduated Doctor of Medicine in the spring of 1853.[2]

Dr. Manning began medical practice in south Georgia, presumably in Thomas County, where he remained for a few years and where he married Emily Blackshear. Prior to 1860, however, he elected to return to Florida, settling in Jefferson County, but by this time medical practice appears to have become a secondary occupation. In 1860 the census enumerator designated him as "farmer and miller" owning property valued at $25,000. His slaves numbered 17.[3]

Soon after arriving in Jefferson County Dr. Manning was drawn into the arena of local politics. As a farmer of well above average means, relying on slave labor for cultivation of his crops, he could not escape the conflict which was developing by the mid-1850s. He quite naturally embraced the Democratic cause and in the election of 1858 won a seat in the Florida House of Representatives, remaining in that body for the adjourned session of 1859. Again, in the critical election of 1865, he was elected to a seat in the House.[4]

By 1870 Dr. Manning, like most plantation owners of the South, had experienced the pain of Reconstruction and the economic depression leading to the Panic of 1873. His slaves had been freed and his properties reduced in value to a mere $5,000. In desperation, and possibly out of true conviction, he turned to preaching as a primary vocation. The Census of 1885 designates him only as Minister of the Gospel.[5] Having abandoned medical practice almost entirely and having apparently inherited the family land in Leon County, he devoted himself to farming. In 1885 he is shown to have owned 640 acres of "improved land" and 100 acres of woodsland, altogether valued at $7,000. The annual farm produce was estimated to have been worth $3,650.

Dr. Manning lived until 1907. He was buried in the family cemetery located 16 miles north of Tallahassee on what is presently known as Cherokee Plantation. He was twice-married, first to Emily Blackshear, who bore three children, Edward Blackshear, Lucien, and daughter, Ann, who died in early childhood. Mrs. Manning died in the mid-1870s and within a year or so Dr. Manning remarried. The second Mrs. Manning, known only as Martha R., was Florida-born, as was her father. To this marriage were born four daughters, Silvia, 1878; Benula or Eula, 1879; Martha J., 1881; and Helen or Nellie, 1882, and two sons, Andrew M., Jr., 1889, and Charles W., 1892.[6]

It is apparent from census schedules that Dr. Manning was engaged in medical practice hardly at all during the last 25 years of his life. He died at his rural home near Foshalee Slough in 1907 and was buried in the family cemetery. Numerous descendants still live in Leon and Jefferson Counties.[7]

1. The Leon County Census, 1900, p. 46, item 122, states that he was born March 1830 and was 70 years old. His gravestone gives his date of birth as 1831.

2. *Alumni Catalogue of the Medical Department, Tulane University of Louisiana*, New Orleans, 1901, p. 25. His state of residence was Georgia.

3. U.S. Census, Jefferson County, Florida, Monticello, p. 874.

4. Allen Morris, compiler, *The People of Lawmaking in Florida*, Tallahassee, 1971. Verified by checking House Journals.

5. Special Census, Florida, 1885, Leon County, p. 152, item 1436. See ibid. "Agricultural Production," p. 11.

6. See note 1, supra.

7. Additional genealogical information on the Manning Family is found in Joy Smith Paisley, *The Cemeteries of Leon County, Florida*, a compilation, sponsored by the Colonial Dames, Dominie Everardus Bogardus Chapter, Tallahassee, 1978. The information on the Manning Family was compiled by Miss Ethel Manning, a descendant of Dr. A.M. Manning. Attention should also be directed to a lengthy article by Mrs. Paisley on the old family cemeteries of Leon County published in the *Tallahassee Democrat*, March 28, 1874, Special Edition, Section 15, p. 2 B.

Mapp, John L., Army Surgeon, 1863

Dr. Mapp, a native of Georgia or more certainly a resident there at the time of his matriculation at Jefferson Medical College in Philadelphia in 1860, resided only briefly in Florida. With the Civil War having reached its most intense phase in the spring of 1863, he was commissioned assistant surgeon and assigned to the Fifth Florida Battalion. Although no information relating to his subsquent career has been disovered, it is assumed that he survived the conflict and eventually returned to civilian practice. Since his name does not appear in the Florida Census of 1870, it is assumed that he did not return to practice in this state.

1. This brief data is derived from the *General Alumni Catalogue of Jefferson Medical College*, 1917, p. 81, and also *Soldiers of Florida*, Board of State Institutions, Publishers, Macclenny, 1983, p. 320.

Marion, Nathaniel Peter, Hamilton County, 1820-1909

Dr. Marion,[1] grandnephew of Francis Marion ("Swamp Fox"), famous South Carolina patriot, was born in the village of Cokesbury, Abbeville District, South Carolina, on February 19, 1820. In 1839 he matriculated at the Medical College of the State of South Carolina from which he was graduated in the spring of 1841.[2] Two years later accompanied by several family slaves and endowed with adequate funds, he migrated to Hamilton County and purchased a large tract of land on the Suwannee River six miles south of Jasper. This was some of the most fertile land of the county and although it was a wilderness through which Indians still wandered he soon converted it into a prosperous plantation. The small community of Marion which had the distinction of its own post office from 1877 to 1916 as well as a railway station on the Savannah, Florida and Western Line, memorializes the presence of the Marion family there.

The Marion property was valued at $40,000 in 1860 while his slaves numbered 50.[3] By 1870, however, the ravages of war and the loss of his slaves had reduced the value of his holdings to $5,760.[4] A large measure of Dr. Marion's success in farming was owed perhaps to the skill and good judgment of his neighbor and overseer, a Scotsman named Angus McLeod.

For the first few years of his Florida residence Dr. Marion practiced medicine but there is no evidence that his practice was extensive, nor that he wished it so. Like many medically-trained sons of wealthy Southern families in the antebellum period, he apparently invested his inheritance in land and led the life of a well-to-do planter, a more honorable and prestigious calling in that era. Doubtless he looked after the medical needs of his family and his slaves, as was the custom.

Dr. Marion appears to have preferred the quiet and reclusive existence which his plantation home provided, and since he could afford to indulge his preferences he was seldom seen away from his rural home. Especially was this true after the death of his wife in 1879. Yet it is said of him that "in his home no more social, genial, companionable gentleman ever lived."[5] Only once did he emerge into public life, in 1856 when he served as County Commissioner. He was never affiliated with a church, although his wife was a founding member of the non-denominational Nunn Church which later became the Mount Pleasant Methodist Church.[6]

Dr. Marion returned to Abbeville in 1845 to marry Eugenia Ann Hayne, the wedding ceremony occurring on November 27. They had several children although only two lived to adulthood. The older, daughter Martella Jane, became the wife of John C. Reynolds; the younger, Nathaniel Wolfe, married Alice L. Frink, member of a prominent Hamilton County family.[7]

In his later years Dr. Marion suffered a mental decline. He died at his home on March 20, 1909, at the age of 89.[8] He was buried in the family cemetery on the plantation by the side of his wife who had died 30 years earlier.

1. Some of the biographical data included in this sketch is derived form Cora Hinton, comp., *Early History of Hamilton County, Florida*, Jasper, 1976, pp. 45, 81.

2. Archives, Medical College of the State of South Carolina, Waring Memorial Library, Charleston, S.C. See also Charleston *Courier*, March 19, 1841, in which is printed a list of medical graduates of March 16. Here Dr. Marion's home is identified as the village of Cokesbury, Abbeville District.

3. U.S. Census, 1870, Hamilton County, Florida, p. 17. See also Slave Schedule of same year.

4. U.S. Census, 1870, Hamilton County, Florida, p. 61.

5. Jasper (Fla.) *News*, March 26, 1909.

6. Hinton, *Early History*, p. 81.

7. Ibid., p. 45.

8. Jasper *News*, *loc. cit.*

Marshall, S. Joseph, Micanopy, mid-19th century

Dr. Marshall was among the early settlers in the Micanopy community. A native of Abbeville, South Carolina, and a graduate of the Medical College of the State of South Carolina, Charleston in 1846,[1] he settled shortly thereafter on the shores of Lake Tuscawilla, on the fringe of the town where he became better known as a citrus grower than as physician. Since his name does not appear in the Florida Census of 1860, he is presumed to have left the state by that date.

1. Charleston, S.C., *Courier*, March 21, 1846. Dr. Marshall's doctoral thesis was titled "Hepatitis."

Martin, Edward R., Jackson County, 1839-1911

Very little is known of the life of Dr. Martin who spent his later years near the village of Kynesville, Jackson County. He appears to have been born in Alabama; at least he served in an Alabama Infantry Regiment during the Civil War. He was born in December 1839 and died on April 15, 1911. He was buried in the Martin Family Cemetery, located about two miles southeast of Kynesville.[1]

1. This information comes from Dr. Martin's gravestone and is entered in the survey of cemeteries in Jackson County.

Martin, Martin H., Quincy, 1840

Among the numerous members of the Martin clan of Georgia who moved to Middle Florida in the 1830s and 1840s was Dr. Martin, an 1838 graduate of the Medical College of Georgia in Augusta.[1] Although he does not appear in the Gadsden County Census of 1840, he is thought to have arrived in Quincy[2] later that year after the enumeration had been completed. In December 1840 he was present at a public meeting in Quincy assembled for the purpose of pressing for statehood for the Florida Territory.[3]

A month later he joined five other physicians of Gadsden County in drafting a schedule of charges which would be made for their professional services.[4] Dr. Martin married a widow, Mrs. Caroline, also of Quincy,[5] on July 22, 1841. Since no further trace of him has been found in Florida sources, he is presumed to have left the state prior to 1850, possibly to return to Georgia.

1. Medical Department, University of Georgia, "List of Graduates, 1829-1891," Augusta, 1890, p. 21.
2. The Gadsden Census of 1840 includes a Martin but he cannot be identified as the physician under consideration.
3. Quincy *Sentinel*, December 4, 1840.
4. Miles Kenan Womack, Jr., *Gadsden: A Florida County in Word and Picture*, Quincy, 1976, p. 61.
5. Tallahassee *Sentinel*, August 6, 1841.

Mason, Zelotes H., Orange County, 1814-1893

Dr. Mason,[1] a native of Pennsylvania, was one of the pioneer white settlers of Orange County, having arrived there in the early 1850s from his native state of Pennsylvania. Nothing is presently known of his early life and education, either general or professional. Since his name does not appear in the lists of graduates of the two major medical colleges in Pennsylvania, Jefferson and the University of Pennsylvania, both in Philadelphia, it appears probable that he entered practice by way of the apprenticeship system or abandoned medical college without a degree.

Regardless of education, general and professional, he was "one of the most respected and intelligent citizens in Orange County," so stated one of his neighbors to members of the Florida Legislature. His business acumen was sufficiently keen that he recognized the bright future awaiting those who were bold enough to purchase real estate and plant orange trees. He was one of the founders of the Town of Apopka, in which he built his home and on whose Board of Aldermen he served. He was a member of the town's first school board, which was formed in 1869. He was also one of the organizers of the Apopka Presbyterian Church, which was established in 1873. With investments in real estate and orange groves, his medical practice was limited to very occasional or emergency calls.

Prior to moving to Florida Dr. Mason was married to an Ohio-born lady, known only by her Christian name, Christianna, nine years her husband's junior.[2] The marriage was apparently childless.

Dr. Mason died in 1893 and was buried in the Edgewood Cemetery near Apopka.[3] He is remembered not for medical practice but for his important role in the development of the citrus industry in central Florida, and his influence on the early growth of Apopka.

1. The biographical data are drawn in large measure from Jerrell H. Shofner, *History of Apopka and Northwest Orange County*, copyrighted in 1982 by the Apopka Historical Society, which contains numerous references to Dr. Mason.
2. U.S. Census, 1870, Orange County, Item 320.
3. *The Cemetery Survey*, a part of the Veteran's Grave Registration Project, St. Augustine, 1940-41, p. 21, lists Dr. Mason's service in the Civil War as membership in the Florida Home Guard.

Mathers, Augustus Henry, Alachua County, 1825-1914

Dr. Mathers was born in Monticello, Florida, on April 22, 1825,[1] son of William Henry and Elizabeth Clarke Mathers who had settled in Jefferson County in the 1820s. After spending his youth in Jefferson County he moved to Madison, Florida, and opened a tailor shop.[2] On October 28, 1848,[3] he married Mary Ann Cooper, daughter of Dr. James A. Cooper, who had moved to Madison from Farmington, Oconee County, Georgia. In 1856, at the age of 31, and probably at the urging of his father-in-law, he entered the Medical College of the University of Georgia, Augusta, from which he was graduated in the spring of 1858.[4]

Meanwhile Dr. Cooper and his son, James L. Cooper, had opened a drug store in Micanopy and, instead of returning to Madison, Dr. Mathers joined the Coopers in Micanopy and on April 6, six weeks after obtaining his degree, announced the opening of his medical practice.[5] His office was located in the Cooper Drug Store.

A little more than two years later Dr. Mathers announced the formation of a professional partnership with Dr. James G. Cameron, who had recently arrived in Micanopy. They designated themselves "physicians and surgeons," stating that they could be found at their office "one door south of the Post Office."[6] The same paper carried a conspicuous notice calling attention to the drug store of "Drs. Mathers and Cameron, Druggist and Apothecaries."

With the onset of war in 1861 Dr. Mathers, in spite of age (he was 36) and family obligations (wife and nine-year-old son, James Cooper Mathers), was one of the first to enlist for military duty.[7] The record of his service is incomplete but it is known that he joined the Fourth Florida Infantry, was assigned to the medical staff, spending at least the first year of the War at Ft. Hopkins on Sea Horse Key near Cedar Key and later at Fernandina. His letters to his wife, dated September 12, 1861 to February 27, 1862, reveal much concerning the scarcity of supplies and equipment, presence of dysentery and fevers among the troops as well as the tender devotion of the doctor for his wife and son. Although no records have been located which might supply the details of his service from 1862 until 1865, family tradition holds that he served honorably until discharged on April 17, 1865. Throughout the conflict he bore the rank of Assistant Surgeon.

Dr. Mathers' partner, Dr. Cameron, died in the fall of 1865;[8] henceforth he appears to have devoted the greater part of his time to the drug store, which had come into his possession with the retirement of his father-in-law, Dr. Cooper.[9] At some time in the 1870s the business was passed on to Dr. Mathers' son, James Cooper, who continued to operate it until his death in 1904.[10] For reasons which have not been discerned Dr. Mathers moved to Tampa in 1900 and established a drug store known as the Nebraska Pharmacy.[11] A short time before his death on April 12, 1914, he returned to Micanopy. He was buried in the Micanopy Cemetery in a lot containing the graves of several other members of the family.

Of the nonprofessional aspects of Dr. Mathers' life very little information has emerged. As one of six physicians practicing in the little town about 1860, he, like others of his profession, turned to additional pursuits to supplement his income. His orange and tangerine groves attracted much attention and were said to have yielded about $1,500 a year profit.[12] His drug store was apparently another profitable venture. As early as 1858 when the proposed incorporation of the town of Micanopy was presented to the voters, Dr. Mathers was one of five who opposed incorporation,[13] presumably on the grounds that such a measure would result in increased taxes. Nevertheless the measure was approved.

In the postwar years Dr. Mathers was occasionally involved in civic matters. In 1876, for example, he was secretary at a meeting of Micanopy citizens gathered to promote the construction of a railroad from Gainesville to Orange Lake via Micanopy.[14]

Dr. Mathers outlived the other members of his immediate family; his wife died in 1892, son James in 1904, and father-in-law in 1883. Only his daughter-in-law, Modes Hunter Mathers, survived him.

1. Gravestone, Micanopy Cemetery, Micanopy.
2. U.S. Census, 1850, Madison County, Florida, p. 160.
3. Some important biographical information relating to Dr. Mathers is found in Franklin A. Doty, "The Civil War Letters of Augustus Henry Mathers, Assistant Surgeon, 4th Florida Regiment, CSA," *Florida Historical Quarterly*, XXXVI, No. 2, October 1957, pp. 94-124. The introduction includes data provided by Mrs. Catherine Mathers Simpson of High Springs, granddaughter of Dr. Mathers.
4. *Medical Department, University of Georgia, List of Graduates, 1829-91*, Augusta, 1891, p. 21. Here it is stated

that Dr. Mathers read medicine under the guidance of Dr. J.A. Williams, physician of Sand Town, Ga., a suburb of Marietta.

5. Ocala *Florida Home Companion*, April 6, 1858.

6. Micanopy *Cotton States*, September 28, 1860.

7. Information relating to Dr. Mathews' military career is confusing. The letters referred to in note 3 confirm his service as Assistant Surgeon in 1861-62. Papers preserved by the Mathers Family indicate that he served until the end of the War in 1865. This information is not found in Service Records, CSA, National Archives.

8. Gainesville *New Era*, November 4, 1865. Legal notice announcing that Mrs. Cameron would administer her husband's estate.

9. Dr. Cooper, a Georgian, would have been 68 in 1865. The drug store was burned in September 1867 but later rebuilt.

10. Although the younger Mathers was referred to as Dr. Mathers, he was actually a pharmacist. See U.S. Census, 1880, Alachua County, Florida, p. 147.

11. See note 3 supra. Several Florida Gazeteers of the period list him as physician.

12. Charles H. Webber, *The Eden of the South*, New York, 1883, p. 98.

13. Voting against the proposal, in addition to Dr. Mathers, were Drs. Payne, Montgomery, Cooper and Stewart; voting for it was Dr. Carn. See Manuscript in Glunt Collection, P.K. Yonge Library of Florida History, Box II.

14. Ocala *East Florida Banner*, April 1, 1876. Another obituary for Dr. Mathers appeared in the Gainesville *Daily Sun* of April 17, 1914; its states that Dr. Mathers "recently realized he could not live long and just ten days previous to his death he moved back to Micanopy...Had he lived a few days longer he would have been eighty-nine years old."

Mattox, Thomas Jefferson, Bartow and Wauchula, mid-19th century

Dr. Mattox, a native of Georgia, spent the latter years of his life in southern Florida. He is said to have been a graduate of the "Medical College of New York" in the class of 1823.[1] He saw military service in both the Seminole and Civil Wars and in 1867 settled in Bartow where he resumed civilian practice. Three years later he moved to the settlement later to become Wauchula, seat of Hardee County. The date of his death has not been determined.

The name of Dr. Mattox has been preserved in connection with a feud between the Lucas and Crews families of Polk County which culminated in a gunfight between John Lucas and Dempsey Crews, resulting in the death of Crews. Dr. Mattox, who was called to the scene, was unable to save his life but he did prepare the body for burial. Meanwhile, he had removed a bullet from the body of Lucas who recovered. A short time later a reward of $500 was offered for capture of the murderer of Bud Sauls of Zolfo Springs. Lucas ambushed and killed the murder suspect, Jim North, and collected the reward but subsequently met his death in the same manner.[2] So much for frontier justice.

1. Since there was only one medical college in New York at the time, Medical College of New York, it is assumed that Dr. Mattox received his medical education at that school.

2. The brief information set forth here is derived from a handwritten note by one of Dr. Mattox's descendants, a copy of which is preserved in the Albert DeVane Papers, P.K. Yonge Library of Florida History, University of Florida, Gainesville.

Maurice, R.F., Marion County, 1833

Dr. Maurice was born at Indian Town, Williamsburg District, South Carolina, in 1833 and is presumed to have begun the study of medicine in the office of a local physician, probably in nearby Williamsburg.[1] He matriculated at the Medical College of the State of South Carolina, Charleston, in the fall of 1855 and was graduated in March 1857, having submitted a thesis bearing the title "Intermittent Fever."[2] Soon thereafter he was persuaded to begin practice in Marion County, a section of Florida which had attracted many settlers from South Carolina. Dr. Maurice advertised his professional services to the citizens of Ocala and surrounding areas on June 4, 1860, stating that his office was located in the rear of Joseph Bell's Store[3] in Ocala.

With the outbreak of the Civil War in 1861 Dr. Maurice is thought to have returned to South Carolina, presumably to join a South Carolina regiment as medical officer. His fate beyond this point has not been determined. There is no evidence that he ever returned to Florida.

1. Indian Town, not to be found on modern maps, is shown on the Mills Map of 1825. It was located about 15 miles southeast of Kingstree, Williamsburg District, South Carolina. The Charleston *Mercury*, March 21, 1857, in its list of recent graduates from the Medical College of the State of South Carolina, simply gives his home address as Williamsburg District.

2. Ibid.

3. Ocala *Florida Home Companion*, June 5, 1860.

Maxwell, George Troup, Leon County, 1827-1897

Dr. Maxwell, a man of superior intelligence and numerous interests but of restless spirit, was born in Savannah, Georgia, on August 6, 1827.[1] He was the son of William M. and Rebecca Elwell Maxwell of the prominent Maxwell family of Bryan County, Georgia. After completing basic education at Savannah's prestigious Chatham Academy he enrolled at New York University where he is said to have completed the arts course at the age of 16. After an interval of a year or two he entered the Medical Department of the same institution and received his degree in 1848, a few months prior to his 21st birthday.

Meanwhile several members of his family had moved to Florida and purchased valuable land a short distance south of Tallahassee in what came to be known as Bel Air. The area, enjoying a higher elevation than surrounding territory, became a popular summer retreat for well-to-do families. Dr. Maxwell, after an interlude of perhaps a year, joined the clan there in 1851. His professional card, appearing in a Tallahassee newspaper on June 24, 1851, stated that he was living in the home of Col. John J. Maxwell in Bel Air.[2] By December, however, he had moved into Tallahassee and rented an office "over C.C. Byrd's Store."[3]

Dr. Maxwell married Augusta Jones of Tallahassee in 1850. They continued to live in Leon County until 1857, with the doctor dividing his time between medical practice and farming. His interest in farming was not merely avocational as he was instrumental in formation of the Leon County Association, serving on its executive committee.[4] He was also actively involved in the State Agricultural Association which was responsible for organization of the Florida State Fair.[5]

In early 1857 Dr. Maxwell received a presidential appointment as surgeon and health officer at the Marine Hospital in Key West. His experience and observations at this post were to have a profound effect on his professional career, developing in him a zealous concern for protective public health measures.[6] His move to the island was ill-timed and ill-fated, however, for in September 1857 a severe yellow fever epidemic claimed the lives of Mrs. Maxwell, their young son, and the wife of Dr. Maxwell's brother, Dr. Jackson Maxwell, a Key West physician.[7] Before the end of the year Dr. Maxwell had abandoned Key West and returned to practice in Tallahassee. The Key West paper lamented his departure as "a loss to Key West."[8]

With the secession of Florida from the Union on January 7, 1861, military preparations followed quickly. The 1st Florida Cavalry Regiment, composed of volunteers from several north Florida counties, was mustered into service in July. Dr. Maxwell, an ardent secessionist, entered the service as a private but within four months he was elevated to the rank of lieutenant colonel, second in command of the Regiment.[9] In the following year, when the commanding officer, Col. William G.M. Davis, was promoted to general, Dr. Maxwell assumed command with the rank of colonel. The Regiment remained in Florida for more than a year before being ordered into combat in the summer of 1863. It moved into eastern Tennessee where it saw action in the fighting around Chattanooga. At the Battle of Missionary Ridge Dr. Maxwell led his regiment in a defensive action designed to allow the retreat of General Braxton Bragg's army but which resulted in the capture of all surviving members of the unit including Col. Maxwell himself. He spent the remainder of the war as a prisoner on Johnson's Island in Lake Erie.[10] On the very day of his capture a special order for his promotion to the rank of general had been issued at Confederate headquarters.[11]

Dr. Maxwell returned to practice in Tallahassee in the summer of 1865, apparently with the aura of war hero. Shortly he married a cousin, Martha Ella Maxwell.[12] On the order of the provisional governor, William Marvin, elections were held for a state constitutional convention and Dr. Maxwell was one of four delegates chosen to represent Leon County.[13] The new constitution was completed in mid-November and in the general election on November 27, Dr. Maxwell won a seat in the Florida House of Representatives.[14]

Having discharged his political responsibilities, Dr. Maxwell elected to leave Tallahassee and settle in Fernandina. On March 13, 1866, the Tallahassee *Semi-Weekly Floridian* reprinted an item from a Jacksonville newspaper announcing his decision to resume practice and congratulating Fernandina on acquiring the services of a physician of such splendid abilities. It reported: "He has sheathed the sword and again draws the lancet." He lived in Fernandina briefly, however, soon moving on to Jacksonville where he obtained the post of city physician.

Dr. Mitchell did not long remain in his new position before the wanderlust of his nature prevailed. In this instance he left the state and for the next 20 years resided in the state of Delaware. He practiced first in Middletown, then in New Castle, and finally in Wilmington, where he stayed for several years and edited a newspaper espousing the Democratic cause. While in Wilmington he became an active member of the Masonic Order, rising to the honored post of "Most Worshipful Grand Master of the State of Delaware." The death of his second wife in Wilmington appears to have prompted his return to the South. After a brief sojourn in Atlanta where he joined a Dr. Johnson in a medical partnership he returned to Florida, stopping first in Fernandina, then to Ocala and later (1888) to Lake City where he received appointment to the Veterinary and Physiological Section of the Experiment Station, Florida State Agricultural College.[15]

Dr. Maxwell's last move came in the fall of 1888, once more to Jacksonville, and he arrived when the yellow fever outbreak which was terrorizing the city was at its peak. He is said to have endeared himself to the people of the city by his diligent and tireless attention to many of those stricken with the disease. He remained in Jacksonville for the rest of his life, not only practicing his profession but also writing articles on a variety of subjects, and assisting in the work of the Florida Medical Association.[16] He does not appear to have become a member of the Association, however, until 1895.

In 1896 Dr. Maxwell was present at the meeting of the Association in Sanford, which he attended as the official delegate of the Duval County Medical Society. He gave a lengthy paper on "Hygiene in Florida," an intriguing potpourri based on his personal experiences and the medical theory of the time. He also tendered the invitation to the Association to hold its next meeting in Jacksonville, issued, it was reported, "in his customary hearty and forceful manner."[17] In the following year, at the age of 69, he attended the annual meeting of the Association in Palatka. Again he read a paper, in this instance "So-called Typho-Malarial Fever," which provoked animated discussion and was referred to the Committee on Publication of which he was a member.[18] At this meeting he was elected chairman of the Committee on Hygiene.[19] In his obituary it is stated that Dr. Maxwell had published an article concerning his invention of the laryngoscope for which he claimed full credit.[20]

Dr. Maxwell remained in vigorous health until the summer of 1896 when he suffered a paralytic stroke while listening to a speech in Jacksonville delivered by William Jennings Bryan, Democratic candidate for the presidency of the United States. From this he recovered sufficiently to attend the Florida Medical Association meeting at Palatka the following April. A few weeks later he suffered another stroke and in late August another which was fatal. He died on September 2, 1897, in the home of his daughter, Ann (Mrs. C.W. Maxwell), in the Riverside section of Jacksonville. His body was sent to Tallahassee for burial.

There can be no doubt that Dr. Maxwell was generally admired and respected by his colleagues and acquaintances. He was described as an impressive figure of a man, "splendid and erect in stature, possessing a fine physique and a commanding appearance."[21] Elsewhere, after laudatory remarks about his military career, one writer described him as "a man of great breadth of character, generous to a fault, enthusiastic in all things he undertook, and a serious, indefatigable worker."

1. The two principal sources of biographical data on Dr. Maxwell are the Jacksonville *Florida Times-Union*, September 3, 1897, and Appleton's *Cyclopaedia of American Biography*, Vol. IV. Since the factual information was probably provided by members of the Maxwell family, it is assumed to be reliable. Unless otherwise indicated the material here presented is from these two sources which differ as to the place of Dr. Maxwell's birth. The Appleton version identifies it as Bryan County, Georgia, while the other indicates Savannah.

2. Col. John J. Maxwell was a brother of Dr. Maxwell's father. The Leon County Census of 1850 lists him as a resident, aged 66, and a planter. See Tallahassee *Sentinel*, August 12, 1851, 1st printing, June 24, 1851, not extant.

3. Ibid., December 2, 1851.

4. Ibid., December 30, 1851.

5. Ibid., December 14, 1852. See also Jacksonville *Republican*, January 6, 1853.

6. Jacksonville *Florida News*, March 28, 1857. In his later years Dr. Maxwell showed deep concern about hygiene and public health in the state. He worked closely with Dr. J.Y. Porter, who became Florida's first public health officer in 1889.

7. Tallahassee *Floridian and Journal*, issues of September 19, October 3, and 24, 1857. Another victim of the fever was Dr. Maxwell's son, Elliott, one of his three children, the others being a son, George, and a daughter, Anna.

8. Ibid., December 12, 1857.

9. *Soldiers of Florida*, Live Oak, Board of State Institutions, 1903, p. 247. Dr. Maxwell had been appointed Professor of Obstetrics and Diseases of Women and Children at Oglethorpe Medical College, Savannah, for the term beginning November 4, 1861. See Annual Circular of the Oglethorpe Medical College, Savannah, 1861, original in collection of the Georgia Historical Society, Savannah. It is probable, however, in view of his early involvement with the 1st Florida Cavalry Regiment that he never actually filled the Oglethorpe position.

10. The 1st Cavalry remained in Florida until the early summer of 1863; as late as January 1863 he is known to have

engaged in civilian practice (part-time). In February he received $23 from the State Treasurer for performing postmortem examinations. Tallahassee *Sentinel*, February 24, 1863.

11. Florida *Times-Union*, cited in note 1, supra. Dr. Maxwell was lauded for his modesty in refusing always to use the designation, General.

12. Ibid. To this second marriage was born a son, John Stevens Maxwell, who was destined to become a noted military figure as well as a judge.

13. Tallahassee *Weekly Floridian*, October 27, 1865.

14. Allen Morris, *The People of Lawmaking in Florida*, Tallahassee, 1977.

15. Dr. Maxwell's brief tenure at the Experiment Station was a period of meager salary ($50 per month) and constant altercations with the Director, Dr. John Kost. These led to charges of mismanagement and incompetence which resulted in Dr. Kost's dismissal. For details of this episode see Samuel Proctor, "The University of Florida, Its Early Years," doctoral dissertation (unpublished) MS, P.K. Yonge Library of Florida History, University of Florida, Gainesville, pp. 353, 356-357.

16. Although Dr. Maxwell became president of the Duval County Medical Society, he did not appear in the *Florida Medical Association Proceedings* until 1895, when he was credited with having paid his annual dues. *Proceedings Florida Medical Association*, 1896, p. 50.

17. Ibid., p. 23.

18. Ibid., 1897, pp. 17, 18. The paper was never published.

19. Ibid., p. 32.

20. Dr. Maxwell's paper, "Hygiene in Florida," was published in ibid., 1896, pp. 60-84. There is no indication of the work on the laryngoscope already done by the Bohemian, Johann Czermak (1873), and the Viennese, Ludwig Turck (1868).

21. See note 1, supra.

Maxwell, R.T., Pensacola, 1850

Dr. Maxwell, a native of Pennsylvania, is listed in the Census of 1850, Escambia County, Florida, as a Doctor of Medicine practicing in Pensacola. His wife, Mary W., and daughter, Ellen M., aged 25 and five respectively, were natives of Pennsylvania. No further information on this family has been discovered.[1]

1. U.S. Census, 1850, Escambia County, Florida, p. 241.

Mays, Rhydon Grigsby, Madison, St. Johns, and Putnam Counties, 1802

The vicissitudes of fortune in 19th-century Florida are nowhere more poignantly demonstrated than in the career of Dr. Mays, pioneer citrus grower, cotton planter and sometime physician in Madison, St. Johns and Putnam Counties. He was born in Edgefield District, South Carolina, about 1802,[1] the third son of Samuel and Nancy (Grigsby) Mays, who had settled on the Saluda River just prior to the American Revolution.[2] After receiving a medical degree from the University of Maryland School of Medicine in 1823,[3] he is thought to have begun practice in Edgefield County, but he is known to have emigrated to Florida in the early 1830s, settling on the right bank of the St. Johns River at a place known as Buena Vista[4] after acquiring the orange groves planted by the fabulous Zephaniah Kingsley. For the first year or so the venture was successful but on February 8, 1835, the temperature dropped to seven above zero, remaining well below the freezing point for more than 24 hours, destroying not only the current fruit crop but killing the trees as well.[5]

Following this disaster Dr. Mays returned to Edgefield. The 1840 Census lists him as a practicing physician in the town of Edgefield[6] and shows him to have been the owner of 57 slaves which suggests that he was also a planter of means. Meanwhile he married a cousin, Sarah Butler Smith, a union to which six or seven children were born.[7]

At some date in the 1840s Dr. Mays returned to Florida, settling in Madison

County as a planter, having purchased land in the southern part of the county west of Sampala Lake.[8] He remained here for a few years but by the mid-1850s was once again on the St. Johns River where, in partnership with his son, Sumter, and son-in-law, E.C. Simkins (husband of daughter Elizabeth), he built a couple of sawmills about a mile east of the river at a site to be known as Orange Mills. With a vast acreage of virgin pine and an abundance of cypress trees ready for cutting, the enterprise was very successful.[9] In addition, Dr. Mays bought a plantation in west Putnam County in the vicinity of Ethoniah, situated north of present-day Grandin and Florahome. This venture was also successful.[10] In the meantime he had replanted his groves at Buena Vista and these also proved to be profitable. It is no surprise that the census enumerator of St. Johns County in 1860 appraised his real estate at $20,000 and his other properties at $100,000,[11] while his slaves, listed in the Putnam County Census of that year, numbered 88.[12] So important was his cotton production that a Charleston cotton broker, Lawton and Co., used Mays' endorsement as a testimonial to its integrity.[13]

With the coming of the War in 1861 calamity once more befell the aristocrats along the St. Johns. Several, Dr. Mays, Francis L. Dancy, E.C. Cole and A.H. Cole, had built imposing homes along the River north of Palatka. Jacksonville, by virtue of its commercial importance, was an early target of Union military attack and by March 1862 was controlled by Federal troops. A Federal gunboat, accompanied by detachments of Negro troops recruited for the most part from South Carolina, made their way up the river as far as Palatka, pillaging and burning as they advanced.[14] Some homes were destroyed, others simply ransacked, including the Mays home. In most instances the inhabitants had fled to the interior of the state as the Federal troops continued to patrol the river. Many, such as the Mayses, had relatives in Middle Florida where they found refuge. Only at the end of the conflict did most venture to return. For some it was a sorrowful homecoming, as this touching recollection of John Francis Tenney indicates:[15]

> It was while residing at Orange Mills that one of the most pathetic scenes that came to our notice was enacted. One cold, dark, rainy night a steamer blew for the landing, and as we were living not far away we lit our lantern and went to take her lines as she tied up. She landed Dr. R.G. Mays and wife, an aged couple, who were coming home for the first time after the close of the war. Their house stood about one-half mile from the landing, and to reach it they had to cross a foot bridge through a small swamp. Their house had been shelled by a Union gunboat during the war and robbed of nearly all of its furniture. They were formerly wealthy people, owning many slaves and a large cotton plantation, besides an interest in the big saw-mill which lay in ashes. The night was very dark, cold and stormy, as I have written. We gave them our lantern and saw them start off through the gloom unattended, with feelings too deep to be written in cold type.

As for the fate of Dr. Mays and his family after his return, Tenney provides some clues. Although his mills had been destroyed, slaves freed and fortune vanished, his groves, though neglected, had survived. With the help of sons and a black laborer or two who had chosen to work for hire, and with oranges soon bringing a good price once more, Dr. Mays was able to live comfortably.[16]

It becomes apparent that as the years passed Dr. Mays virtually abandoned his medical practice for the more lucrative occupations of farming and lumbering. In fact, no census after that of 1840 designates him as "physician," only as "planter" or "farmer." But this was the course of many antebellum Florida physicians, especially those who came from families of means.

Throughout his years in Florida Dr. Mays played an active and influential role in the politics of the state. During his sojourn in Madison County he was among the leaders of the planter aristocracy who spoke out emphatically against what they regarded as the erosion of states' rights. When a band of Madison planters gathered at the court house in 1847 to express formally and collectively their anger at the passage of the Wilmot Proviso by the U.S. House of Representatives—a bill which would have prohibited the introduction of slavery into any territory acquired in the Mexican War — it was, in fact, Dr. Mays who presided over the meeting and assisted in preparing a stinging rebuke to the House.[17] In 1851, as a member of the "Friends of Cuban Independence," he addressed a meeting in St. Augustine,[18] and in 1852 represented his precinct at a Democratic convention in Picolata.[19] When E.J. Dummett, St. Johns County representative in the Florida House, resigned after the 1854 session, Dr. Mays ran unopposed for the adjourned session of the following year.[20] In late 1860 he was elected to represent the 17th Senatorial District (St. Johns and Putnam Counties) at the "Secession Convention" which met in Tallahassee in early January 1861. Needless to add, he voted for secession.[21]

Dr. Mays' last years were marked with sorrow. In the early 1870s his beloved wife, Sarah, died. She was buried in a plot on the homestead designated by her husband as a family burial ground. Soon thereafter his two surviving daughters, Elizabeth (Simkins) and Sallie Stark (Call) also died. Facing the imminence of death in June 1878, he was persuaded to write his last will and testament in which he set forth with remarkable clarity the disposition of his estate. The document, in his own hand and signed on June 19, 1878, is preserved in the Archives of Putnam County. He bequeathed the major portion of his property to his younger son, Thomas Sumter, stipulating, however, that a trust be established for the support and education of his two granddaughters, Lucy and Annie, Thomas Sumter's daughters. He was especially mindful of the possible needs of his grandson and favorite, Rhydon Mays Call, until such time as he "gets into some business to support himself."[22] Nor did he overlook his two black household servants, Sarah and Lavinia Roberts.

No trace of the Mays family residence remains, only a highway marker, a half mile from the St. Johns River, pointing to Mays Landing, where the river boats used to stop. The vista from the pier kept in good repair is still beautiful. The house and even the cemetery have long since given way to the encroaching cabbage fields.

1. The date of Dr. Mays' birth is an extrapolation from census data for the years 1860 and 1870.

2. The locations of Mays family lands are shown on the map of Edgefield District in Robert Mills, *Atlas of South Carolina*, edition of 1825, and republished in Columbia, S.C., in 1865. For valuable information on the Mays family in the 19th century see Patty Mays, "Richard Johnson Mays, Pioneer, Preacher, Patriot," Madison County Historical Society Publication, 1941, pp. 19-28.

3. E.F. Cordell, *Historical Sketch of the University of Maryland School of Medicine, 1807-1890*, Baltimore, 1891, p. 187.

4. Buena Vista was situated on the right bank of the St. Johns River a short distance north of present-day Orange Mills. Kingsley is said to have planted the original grove with budded stock brought from Spain. See Edwin Stuart Hubbard, *Memories of Florida*, Mimeographed, Poughkeepsie, New York, 1951-54, 5 parts, bound as 1, IV, 16.

5. The freeze is thought to have been the most severe ever to occur in northeast Florida. Ibid., pp. 18-20.

6. U.S. Census, 1840, Edgefield District, S.C., p. 52.

7. See Mays, "Richard Johnson Mays," cited in note 2.

8. U.S. Census, 1850, Madison County, Florida, item 473.
9. Hubbard, *"Memories,"* p. 17.
10. W.S. Webb, *Webb's Florida*, New York, 1885, p. 93. Here Webb stated that in one year Mays had produced 100 bales of cotton on 100 acres of unfertilized land which would have been a phenomenal yield.
11. U.S. Census, 1860, St. Johns County, Florida, item 424. It is to be recalled that until 1868 that portion of Putnam County lying east of the St. Johns River had been a part of St. Johns County.
12. Only William D. Moseley, sometime governor of Florida, a resident of Putnam County in 1860, owned more slaves, 114.
13. Fernandina *East Floridian*, December 12, 1858.
14. For an account of these raids see William W. Davis, *The Civil War and Reconstruction in Florida*, Facsimile edition, Gainesville, 1964, p. 232.
15. John Francis Tenney, *Slavery, Secession and Success: Memoirs of Florida*, San Antonio, Texas, 1934, p. 23. See also Hubbard, Memories, p. 12.
16. Tenney, *Slavery*, etc. p. 32.
17. Tallahassee *Floridian*, August 7, 1847.
18. Jacksonville *Florida Republican*, September 11, 1851.
19. St. Augustine, *Ancient City*, August 14, 1852.
20. *House Journal, Florida Legislature*, 7th Session, adj., Tallahassee, 1855, p. 5.
21. Mays was chairman of a meeting of Putnam County citizens held at Etoniah, near which his plantation lay, on November 29, 1860, for the purpose of discussing the secession issue. Fernandina *East Floridian*, December 12, 1860. For his acceptance as the representative at the Convention see St. Augustine *Examiner*, December 22, 1860.
22. Rhydon Mays Call was the only son of George W. Call Jr., and grandson of Dr. George W. Call, who practiced medicine in Fernandina. The senior George W. Call was a brother of Richard Keith Call, Territorial Governor of Florida. George W. Call Jr., a Confederate major, was among the early casualties of the War, having been killed at the Battle of Seven Pines on May 31, 1861. Henceforth, for several years, his widow and little son, Rhydon Mays, lived with her father, Dr. Mays. This explains the special affection of Dr. Mays for his grandson. Rhydon Mays Call studied law, practiced in Jacksonville, and later became a highly successful judge, dying without issue in 1924.

Mays Jr., Richard Johnson, Madison County, 1836—post 1900

Although he was a student at the Medical College of the State of South Carolina for the session of 1857-58, there is no evidence that Dr. Mays ever practiced medicine.[1] Born in South Carolina, Edgefield District, in 1836, the eldest of eight sons of Richard Johnson Mays Sr. and his wife, Eliza Ann, he came to Florida about 1845 when his father purchased a tract of land in the Clifton community northwest of Madison Court House.[2] The Mays family was one of considerable means, having owned 80 slaves in 1850, with total property valued at $15,000.[3] The Florida venture was prosperous. Ten years later, their slaves numbered 125; their total property was valued at $102,000.

Nothing is known of young Richard's early education but it appears probable that he attended the well-regarded St. John's Seminary of Learning in the town of Madison. It is a matter of record, however, that he began his medical education under the preceptorate of Madison's foremost physician, Dr. John H. Pope.[4]

With the Civil War already under way Dr. Mays enlisted for Confederate service in March 1862 and was mustered in at Camp Jolo located at Station No. 5, later to become Greenville, on May 15. Without military rank he was assigned to Company I, Second Florida Cavalry, his promotion to sergeant following shortly. Four months later, however, he was discharged after providing a substitute, young John Poppell. One year later, with the War taking an unfavorable turn for the South, Dr. Mays reenlisted with the rank of Second Lieutenant, soon advancing to First Lieutenant. He remained with his outfit until its surrender to Union General E.M. McCook at Tallahassee on May 10, 1865. He was paroled two days later.[5]

The remaining years of Dr. Mays' life were spent in comparative obscurity. He was married soon after discharge from military service and settled as a farmer on land, doubtless his portion of his father's estate, in Jefferson County.[6] His career was quite overshadowed by that of his younger brother, Dannittee H. Mays, who settled in Jefferson County, represented the county in the Florida Legislature for several terms and for two terms his district in the Congress of the United States.

1. Lists of Students, Medical College of the State of South Carolina, Waring Historical Medical Library, Charleston, South Carolina.

2. Madison County, Florida, WPA, Writers' Project, Typed Copy, p. 71. In 1846 Clifton acquired a post office with Richard J. Mays becoming its first postmaster. He was a man of exceptional energy and ability. Having become an ordained minister in the Missionary Baptist Church prior to leaving South Carolina, he continued his active role in the church, affiliating with the Concord Baptist near Greenville. He is said to have assisted in the organization of other churches in both Madison and Jefferson Counties, and preaching "wherever needed." Mary Oakley McRory and Edith Clarke Barrows, *History of Jefferson County, Florida*, Monticello, 1935, p. 58.

3. U.S. Census, 1850, Madison County, Florida, p. 234. See also Slave Schedule of the same year, Madison County. U.S. Census, 1860, Madison County, Florida, p. 205, and Slave Schedule, same year.

4. See note 1, supra.

5. Service Records, CSA, 2nd Florida Cavalry, National Archives, RG-109, Roll 10.

6. U.S. Census, 1870, Madison County, Florida, p. 358. The person under consideration is not to be confused with a cousin of the same name, Richard J. Mays, of Monticello, a retail merchant and partner of his father-in-law, Shirley C. Bott.

McBride, Milton J., Gadsden, Leon and Wakulla Counties, 1818-1859

Dr. McBride, a native of Green County, Georgia,[1] came to Florida with his family in the late 1820s. His father, the Reverend David S. McBride, a clergyman and planter, settled in Gadsden County outside the town of Quincy but by 1840 had moved into the town. He appears to have been a man of moderate means, his property being valued at $8,300 in 1850, while his slaves numbered less than 20.

Nothing is known of Dr. McBride's education but he is presumed to have attended Quincy's Male Academy. No record of his medical training has been located but on July 29, 1845, however, he announced that he and Dr. Thomas K. Leonard, two years his junior, had formed a professional partnership and were prepared to offer their services, their offices being located "at the residence of the late Capt. J.D. Parish, one-half mile northwest of J.B. Beard's Store on Lake Miccosukie," in north Leon County.[2] Within a short time Dr. Leonard withdrew from the association but Dr. McBride continued the practice for about three or four years.

From the beginning of his professional career Dr. McBride took an active interest in Florida politics. He was a dedicated member of the Whig Party, supporting it until its demise, and afterwards preferring the Know-Nothings to the reinvigorated Democrats. In the summer of 1847 he was persuaded to become a candidate for a seat in the Florida Legislative Assembly.[3] His wife, Mary Ann, had died on May 28, 1847, at the age of 22[4] and rumors were planted that "the force of private and personal considerations would compel him to decline." These were dispelled, however, by a letter from Dr. McBride to Editor Joseph Clisby of the Tallahassee *Sentinel*, an ardent Whig, who responded with a strong endorsement of Dr. McBride's candidacy. The chief drawback, said Clisby, was that the doctor was not well-known outside his own community. He further stated that Dr. McBride was "a most unassuming and gentlemanly man, whose quiet and earnest devotion to the duties of his profession had hitherto prevented that extensive acquaintance with the people which is ordinarily so serviceable to the candidate."[5] In the subsequent election Dr. McBride handily carried his own precinct but lost in the county by the mere margin of four votes. The *Sentinel* lamented the loss.

A year or so later Dr. McBride moved to New Port, Wakulla County, where the census enumerator found him in 1850 as a resident in the home of his 62-year-old father. His brother, Albert C. McBride, and wife and child were also New Port residents which probably accounts for the doctor's decision to settle there.[6] Dr. McBride once more entered the political arena in 1856, this time as a Know-Nothing candidate for the Florida Senate from the Ninth Senatorial District, Wakulla County. He easily won, notwithstanding the fact that statewide the Democratic Party won a major victory.[7]

Subsequent to his service in the Senate Dr. McBride appears to have devoted full time to his medical practice. Evidence points to the probability that by 1858 he was in failing health. Twice within the last two years of his life he publicly assured the citizens of the community that he would continue his professional practice.[8] In October 1859 he came down with a fatal illness, his death occurring on October 24 at the age of 41.[9] He was mourned by citizens of the county. The Masonic Lodge of New Port, of which he had been a member, buried him with the solemn rites of the Order, then met and drafted a tribute to his memory. It read, in part:[10]

> [He was] cut down in the prime of life and in the midst of his usefulness, we mourn not only a broken link in our circle, but we deplore the loss of one so richly qualified and eminently useful and devoted to his profession...We have lost an upright and worthy brother, the community a tried and good physician.

1. The obituary for Dr. McBride appeared in the Tallahassee *Floridian and Journal* of December 31, 1859, although a death notice had appeared on November 1.
2. Tallahassee *Florida Sentinel*, January 27, 1846, 1st printing, July 29, 1845.
3. Ibid., September 21, 1847.
4. Tallahassee *Floridian*, June 5, 1847.
5. Tallahassee *Sentinel*, October 5, 1847.
6. U.S. Census, 1850, Wakulla County, Florida, p. 504.
7. Tallahassee *Floridian and Journal*, November 5, 1856.
8. Wakulla *Times*, June 23, 1858; February 9, 1859.
9. See note 1, supra. See Charles A. Hentz, "Autobiography," MS, in Southern Collection, Library, University of North Carolina, Chapel Hill, vol. 1, p. 324. Microfilm of transcription in P.K. Yonge Library of Florida History, University of Florida. Dr. Hentz, seldom one to excuse human frailties, even among his medical colleagues, was called to New Port from Quincy by the wife of Dr. David Telfair, who was Dr. McBride's sister. When he arrived he found Dr. McBride desperately ill, and Dr. Telfair, who was supposed to be treating him "on one of his sprees." As Dr. Hentz recalled it, Dr. McBride "was critically sick...out of his mind...had sniffed chloroform. Dr. Telfair had given him large doses of Calomel...in vain. He became maniacal before he died."
10. Tallahassee *Floridian and Journal*, November 26, 1859. Dr. McBride was survived by his aged mother, three sisters, Frances, Louisa (Mrs. Telfair), and Sophia; his wife and two small sons.

McCaa, Thomas Whitaker, Gainesville, 1828-1871

Dr. McCaa, eldest child of Dr. John and Amelia Whitaker McCaa, was born in Kershaw County, South Carolina, on April 20, 1828. The elder McCaa, also a physician, was a farmer of modest means who owned property on the west side of the Wateree River only a few miles west of Camden, the county seat. Thomas was the eldest of the seven McCaa children.[1] He began his medical study under the preceptorate of the Camden physician, Dr. Edward M. Boykin, who had received his medical degree from the Medical College of the State of

South Carolina in 1841.[2] In the fall of 1848 young McCaa matriculated at the same institution and in early April 1850 he was graduated as Doctor of Medicine, having submitted a thesis bearing the title, "Pneumonia."[3]

Soon after receiving his degree Dr. McCaa returned to Camden to begin practice. In the summer of 1850 he married Mary Matheson, daughter of Scottish-born Christopher Matheson, a prominent Camden merchant. The Census of 1850 lists the newlywed couple as residents in the Matheson household.[4]

When Dr. McCaa moved to Gainesville has not been determined; however, the evidence suggests late 1855 or early 1856.[4] It is known that in the spring of 1857 he purchased a plot of land in a transaction handled by Andrew Robb, trustee for James B. Bailey.[5] As near as can be determined it lay just east of Sweetwater Branch in the vicinity of the Christopher Matheson house on N.E. First Avenue, formerly East Union Street.[6] Alachua County Deed Books for subsequent years indicate that the McCaa family was one of above average means, the most important item being purchase of 1,920 acres from John Mathews for $15,000 on April 9, 1864.[7]

Dr. McCaa appears to have entered fully into the public life of the small Gainesville community, only recently designated as the seat of Alachua County. He presided over a meeting of Gainesville citizens on July 22, 1857, called for the purpose of choosing delegates to the Southern Commercial Convention in Knoxville, Tennessee, in August.[8] He was an active member of the Gainesville Presbyterian congregation and also found time to serve as preceptor for several young men, instructing them in the fundamentals of medical practice and thus preparing them for matriculation at medical schools.[9] Meanwhile his practice was extensive. Included among his patients were some of the town's most prominent families, among them the James B. Bailey family.[10]

With the onset of war Dr. McCaa volunteered for service with the Seventh Florida Infantry Regiment, was assigned to the post of Regimental surgeon in April 1862, and served with his unit in the Army of Tennessee under the command of General Braxton Bragg.[11] He is presumed to have been with General Bragg in the unsuccessful Kentucky campaign in the summer of 1862.

Dr. McCaa remained in Confederate service until April 26, 1865. Upon his release he returned to Gainesville and resumed medical practice. Very little information concerning his day-to-day practice has been preserved; however, years later a citizen of Fernandina, recollecting his experiences in Gainesville while a refugee from his coastal home, remembered "pleasantly Dr. McCaa and the ever-jovial J.H. Roper, Principal of the Gainesville Academy."[12] In September 1866 when yellow fever appeared in several North Florida communities, the Gainesville Town Council ordained "that no person shall be permitted to stop in the Town of Gainesville, from the cars (i.e., the trains) unless permitted to do so by a physician to be appointed by the Council to examine the trains on their arrival at the depot."[13] Drs. McCaa and Gabriel P. Thomas were appointed to enforce the ordinance.[14]

Death came to Dr. McCaa as the result of his devotion to professional duty. In the late summer of 1871 a deadly epidemic of yellow fever befell the town of Cedar Key, causing a majority of its citizens to flee.[15] The fugitives included the two or three physicians who resided there. Upon learning of the plight of the town and hearing of the desperate need for medical assistance, Dr. McCaa hurried to the Island to offer his services. He soon became ill and returned to Gainesville where he died on September 22 "despite the efforts of his physician-friends" to save him.[16] He was 43 years of age. He was buried in Gainesville's Evergreen Cemetery.

Six children were born to Dr. and Mrs. McCaa, the two eldest natives of Camden, South Carolina. They were, in order of date of birth: Kate, who married Gainesville businessman, Harry C. Denton, and lived at 309 East Main Street, North; Amelia (Lillie), Mrs. Dozier, of Tampa; Julia (unmarried) a resident of Portsmouth, Virginia; Mary (Mrs. Ichabod M. Cox) of Jacksonville; Mrs. Elizabeth Joiner, a resident of South Dakota; and son Boykin, also a resident of Portsmouth, Virginia.[17]

Mrs. McCaa, born on December 29, 1829, in Camden, South Carolina, died in her 80th year at the home of her daughter, Mrs. Kate M. Denton, in Gainesville. She was a member of Holy Trinity Episcopal Church and was buried by the side of her husband in Evergreen Cemetery.

1. U.S. Census, 1850, Kershaw Dist., S.C., p. 75, item 59. Dr. McCaa and his wife were residents in the home of her father, Christopher Mathewson. See ibid., p. 127, item 887, entry for John McCaa, which lists the names and ages of Dr. McCaa's brothers and sister.

2. Archives, Medical University of the State of South Carolina, Catalogue of 1840-41.

3. Ibid., Catalogue of 1849-50.

4. This conjecture is based on the ages of the McCaa children as shown in the Alachua County Census of 1860, which lists the second McCaa daughter, Amelia, aged six, as South Carolina-born, while the third child, Julia, aged three, was born in Florida.

5. Alachua County, Florida, Deed Book, E, p. 580.

6. The Matheson House is occupied (1987) by Mrs. Sarah Hamilton Mathewson, widow of Christopher Mathewson. It is the second oldest house in Gainesville, being antedated only by the Bailey House, N.E. 6th Street. The McCaa House is thought to have stood just east of Sweetwater Branch and north of the Mathewson House.

7. Alachua County, Deed Book, C, p. 15.

8. Jacksonville *Florida News*, August 1, 1857.

9. See note 2, supra. J.P. Richardson, medical graduate of Medical College of the State of South Carolina, Charleston, in 1861, was a protege of Dr. McCaa.

10. The Bailey MSS, P.K. Yonge Library of Florida History, MS Box 27, include Dr. McCaa's itemized bill for services to the Bailey family in 1860-61.

11. National Archives, Service Records, CSA, M251, Roll 78. Dr. McCaa's Military Record is incomplete.

12. Sanchez Papers, "Civil War Gainesville," P.K. Yonge Library of Florida History, MSS, Letter, Samuel A. Swann to E.F. C. Sanchez, Sept. 26, 1908.

13. Gainesville *New Era*, September 14, 1866.

14. Ibid.

15. Tallahassee *Sentinel*, September 23, 1871. This paper reported: "The fever is raging but on the wane...because so many people have fled...there has been a general stampede to get out."

16. Tampa *Peninsular*, October 7, 1871. See "State News." This date of death is possibly questionable. The Tallahassee *Sentinel* assigns his death to September 24. No date of birth or death appears on his gravestone in Evergreen Cemetery, Gainesville.

17. A lengthy obituary for Mrs. McCaa appeared in the Gainesville *Daily Sun* of November 4, 1908. In this are listed her children, their places of residence, surnames of their spouses as well as the names of her brothers and sisters. The brothers were J.D. and W.C. Mathewson, both of Gainesville; sisters, Mrs. E.P. McCuen of Santa Fe, N. Mexico, and Mrs. B.M. Adamson, of Gainesville. A curious error occurred in the published obituary, the contents of which were doubtless conveyed by word of mouth to the *Sun's* reporter. The family name appears throughout as *McCall*, which leaves no doubt that the proper pronunciation was *McCaw*, not McKay.

McCall, Stephen, Gainesville, 1802-1876

Dr. McCall, one of the first physicians to practice in Gainesville, was a native of Savannah, Georgia, where he was born on November 22, 1802.[1] No information relating to his education, either general or professional, has been discovered. Since his name does not appear in the lists of graduates of any of the medical schools of the United States which existed prior to 1830, it is assumed that he entered the profession by way of the apprenticeship system. He was one of two physicians who settled in Gainesville soon after it became the county seat in mid-1850s. The other was Gabriel P. Thomas.

Soon after his arrival in Gainesville Dr. McCall established a drug store at the northeast corner of East University Avenue and North East First Street, a location later to be occupied by pharmacist A.J. Vidal.[2] Soon after establishing his Gainesville practice Dr. McCall purchased a spacious lot on the east side of Sweetwater Branch, the site on which the Kirby-Smith School was later built. He is also said to have built a fine house, sufficiently large to accommodate himself, his wife Priscilla, and his seven daughters and four sons, all said to have been charming and intelligent. Either by inheritance, industry, or perhaps by marriage, Dr. McCall had become a man of substantial means by 1860. In that year his real property was valued at $47,250, and his personal property at $34,575.[3] It was said of the McCall family that by settling in Gainesville, "They have provided not only medicine for the citizens, but also brought seven daughters, possibly of more interest to the swains of the town than all his herbs and compounds."[4]

When J.H. Roper arrived in Gainesville in 1856 to establish its first school, the Gainesville Academy, he was able to obtain lodging, at least temporarily, in the McCall Drug Store.[5] The two men, both intellectuals, became steadfast friends.

Dr. McCall was married in 1842 to a Savannah native, whose Christian name was Priscilla, eight years younger than her husband. She survived him by 25 years, dying in Gainesville on December 18, 1901. In the post-Civil War period Dr. McCall served as Clerk of Gainesville's Town Council.[6]

1. The dates cited here are from gravestones in Gainesville's Evergreen Cemetery.
2. Charles Halsey Hildreth, *A History of Gainesville, Florida*, Gainesville; University of Florida Press, p. 18.
3. U.S. Census, 1860, Florida, pp. 78-79.
4. Hildreth, op. cit., p. 18. Hildreth quotes Dr. McCall's contemporary, W.L. Finger, a statement appearing in the Sanchez Papers preserved in the Manuscript Collection, P.K. Yonge Library of Florida History, University of Florida.
5. Ibid.
6. Gainesville *The New Era*, September 14, 1866.

McCants, Archibald Campbell, Jefferson and Duval Counties, 1832-post 1880

Dr. McCants was born in Jefferson County shortly after his South Carolina-born parents, Joseph and Elizabeth McCants, had migrated to Florida from the Abbeville District. The family settled on land some two miles south of Monticello where three of their four children were born.[1] Soon after arrival in Florida Joseph McCants entered vigorously into the political and social life of his community. By profession he was a lawyer.[2] There was scarcely a public issue that did not evoke his interest and participation. As early as 1832 he was vocal in his support of the effort to open the Aucilla River for navigation. In 1834 he was appointed justice of the peace and in 1839 President Van Buren appointed him Secretary of the Territory of Florida.[3] Meanwhile he had become a county judge. He was also among the subscribers for stock in the ill-fated Union Bank of Tallahassee. He represented his county in the Territorial Legislative Council in 1836 and two years later was a delegate at the St. Joseph Constitutional Convention.[4] He was equally active in community matters.[5]

Young Archibald McCants received his early education in the schools of Monticello, including the highly-regarded Monticello Academy, and for his early medical instruction was sent to Quincy to "read medicine" under the guidance of Dr. E.S. Byron.[6] The fall of 1854 found him at the Medical College of the State of South Carolina, Charleston, but after one term he decided to pursue instead the somewhat questionable study of homeopathy,[7] presumably under one of the Charleston practitioners. Anyway, in April 1855, he opened an office at the home of his father offering his services as homeopathic physician.[8]

In March 1859 Dr. McCants moved his office to Monticello, "five squares directly north of the Court House."[9] Three months later he announced that he had joined Dr. G.T. Waggoner in a partnership and that they would practice from two offices—in the home of Dr. McCants in Monticello and the City Hotel in Tallahassee.[10]

Meanwhile Dr. McCants had married Julia Clark, daughter of William G. Clark, well-to-do farmer of Monticello,[11] who did not live long. Soon after her untimely death he remarried, in this instance, Sarah Scruggs, a union to which four children were born.[12]

With the coming of the Civil War Dr. McCants, although 29 and the father of a year-old son, enlisted for Confederate service on August 10, 1861. He was assigned to the company of Capt. W.O. Girardeau with the rank of first sergeant. He was soon promoted to a first lieutenancy but in reorganization of the unit in May 1862 he was deprived of his commission and immediately sought a discharge. His plea went unheeded.[13] In 1863 a group of Monticello citizens, concerned by the lack of a physician in the town, petitioned President Jefferson Davis for the release of Dr. McCants, "as his services as a resident physician are much needed." The request was denied.[14] Instead he was assigned to the Miter Bureau.[15] It is not known how long he remained in this organization but by early 1864 he was serving without officer rank in the light artillery company of Capt. Robert H. Gamble. When this unit participated in the Battle of Olustee, Dr. McCants suffered a slight wound from a shell fragment.[16] After this encounter Capt. Gamble reporting his casualties declared him still fit for duty.

When the war was over Dr. McCants returned to practice in Monticello but for unknown reasons moved to Jacksonville. The Duval County Census of 1870 designated him M.D. and valued his property at a mere $500. Within a few years he returned to Monticello, probably for financial reasons. For the remainder of his life association with the medical profession was tenuous, if indeed he practiced at all. He turned instead to religious service and was for at least 10 years pastor of the Monticello Baptist Church which his mother had helped to establish in 1845.[18] The date of his death has not been determined but he is known to have been living as late as December 1882 when he was mentioned as pastor of the Monticello Baptist Church.[19]

1. U.S. Census, 1850, Jefferson County, Florida, p. 19. The McCants children were Ann, Caroline, A.C., Jr. and Joseph E., the latter three having been born in Florida.

2. The McCants law partners were Barton V. Pope and Richard R. Stone. Jerrell H. Shofner, *History of Jefferson County*, Tallahassee, 1976, p. 59.

3. *Territorial Papers*, XXIV, 640-650, 699, 967.

4. Allen Morris, *The People of Lawmaking in Florida*, Tallahassee, 1977; Shofner, *History of Jefferson County*, p. 173.

5. For example, he helped in the establishment of the Presbyterian Church of Monticello.

6. Medical College of the State of South Carolina, Lists of Matriculants and Graduates, Waring Medical Historical Library, Charleston, S.C.

7. By this date homeopathy and other medically related professions such as Thompsonianism, hydropathy, isopathy, etc., were falling into disrepute among most regular physicians. In 1856, a Jefferson County physician, Dr. E.S. Gaillard, published a denunciation of the Thompsonians, homeopaths and certain empiricists, *Charleston Medical Journal and Review*. This may be why in later life Dr. McCants abandoned medicine and became a Baptist minister.

8. Tallahassee *Floridian and Journal*, April 28, 1855.

9. Monticello *Family Friend*, March 22, 1859.

10. Ibid., May 10, 1859. Each styled himself M.D. and Homeopath.

11. Tallahassee *Floridian and Journal*, May 24, 1856.

12. The children are listed in the Duval County Census, 1870, City of Jacksonville, item 109 as Archibald C., Sarah, Margaret, and Charles G.

13. N.A.M. Service Recs., CSA, M251, Roll 49.

14. Shofner, *History of Jefferson County*, p. 263.

15. *War of the Rebellion, Official Record*, "Report of Capt. Robert H. Gamble, Leon Light Artillery," Ser. IV, 1, p. 1115.

16. Ibid., Ser. I, Vol. 35, p. 346, Report of February 22, 1864.

17. See note 12, supra.

18. Shofner, *History of Jefferson County*, pp. 54, 412, 422.

19. Tallahassee *Floridian*, December 5, 1882.

McCoskry, Charles N., St. Augustine, 1821

Dr. McCoskry (McCrosky), native of Carlisle, Pennsylvania, was commissioned post surgeon in the United States Army on April 12, 1820.[1] About a year later he was assigned to service with a detachment of two companies of troops under the command of Capt. John R. Bell ready to leave Boston for Amelia Island and St. Augustine.[2] Shortly after his arrival in Fernandina on May 15, 1821, Bell reported to John C. Calhoun, Secretary of War: "At Charleston, we took on board Dr. McCrosky who is to be stationed at this post."[3] A few days later Bell and one company proceeded to St. Augustine where they were expected to establish a semblance of military control during the final negotiations for the cession and until civil authority could assume control. Dr. McCoskry was army surgeon for the post.

In the meantime a civil government for East Florida was taking shape. By August 20 the various positions had been filled, though not without some difficulty, and a Board of Health for St. Augustine had been set up with Dr. Micah Stone as its president.[4] When this Board, acting in cooperation with the City's Board of Aldermen who were ex officio members, resolved to order the army detachment to abandon the hospital, located on the central plaza, and as a public health precaution transfer patients to the Flour Magazine south of the City, Capt. Bell called upon Dr. McCoskry to support him in his refusal to comply. It was Dr. McCoskry who also declared Ft. St. Marks uninhabitable, a decision which necessitated the appropriation of the most desirable public buildings for army use. This move sparked a bitter controversy with Drs. Stone and McCoskry the medical adversaries.[5] The civil authorities won the struggle, but by that time the City was ravaged by a yellow fever epidemic which ultimately claimed both physicians as its victims.

Meanwhile, Dr. McCoskry, presumably with time on his hands, or perhaps responding to citizens' demand for his professional service, advertised on July 21, 1821, that he was offering his services to the public and could be found "at the Old Government, in the Square."[6] He was still there as late as the beginning of November when Col. Eustis ordered both him and Capt. Bell to vacate the building.[7]

Dr. McCoskry died in St. Augustine on November 16 before he had reached the age of 30. He was succeeded as post surgeon by Dr. J.C.P. McMahon.[8]

1. MDUSA, p. 283.
2. TP, XXII, 20.
3. Ibid., p. 46. Letter, Capt. Bell to John Calhoun, May 18, 1821.
4. Ibid., p. 359.
5. See infra, item on Dr. Micah Stone. Regarding the removal of soldiers from Ft. St. Marks, Col. Abraham Eustis wrote to the Acting Governor on September 27, 1821, "Candour obliges me to state to your Exy. that on the representation of Dr. McCrosky, army surgeon on this station, I did advise Capt. Bell immediately to withdraw the troops from Ft. St. Marks, & place them in any suitable building within his control." Ibid., p. 218.
6. St. Augustine *Florida Gazette*, July 28, 1821.
7. TP, XXII, 273
8. MDUSA, p. 290. In his medical report for the year 1821 Surgeon General Thomas Lawson identified Dr. McCoskry's fatal illness as yellow fever. SRSMAUS., p. 31.

McCoskry, William, St. Augustine, 1823

It is a reasonable conjecture that Dr. McCoskry, a native of Carlisle, Pennsylvania, arrived in St. Augustine even before the death of his brother, Dr. Charles N. McCoskry, on November 16, 1821. He is known to have been active in the public affairs of the city in early 1822, first appearing in the public records as a signer of a petition to Congress requesting improvement in the postal service.[1] A month later, on March 3, 1822, he joined other citizens in an expression of support of Judge William P. Duval, a candidate for the governorship of Florida.[2] A short time later he subscribed to a letter recommending George Murray as a replacement for Bernardo Sequi in the Legislative Council of the Territory.[3] On June 26, 1822, he sponsored the baptism of Maria, infant daughter of John Johnson of St. Augustine, at Trinity Episcopal Church.

Upon transfer of Dr. J.P.C. McMahon, President of the Board of Health and Resident Physician of St. Augustine, to Pensacola in the summer of 1822, Dr. McCoskry was appointed to replace him. While serving in this dual capacity he also offered his services to the people of the city, his professional card appearing for the first time on November 14, 1822. At that time he occupied the office formerly used by his brother in the old Government House.[4] Henceforth until the time of his death only a single reference to his work as public health officer has been found. On May 7, 1823, he presided over a meeting of the Board of Health called to discuss the preservation of the health of the city, where it was resolved that the quarantine law should become effective immediately, weeks before the "sickly season" was expected to begin.[5] The resolution bore the signature of Dr. McCoskry.

As was the fate of many physicians during that era, Dr. McCoskry fell victim to the fever on September 14, 1823. His obituary bears inclusion at this point. "Died, in this City on Sunday morning last of bilious fever, Dr. William McCoskry, aged 25 years. Dr. McCoskry was a native of Carlisle, Pennsylvania. As a physician he had acquired reputation, was amiable in his manners, and had drawn around him a large circle of friends, some of whom, in his sickness, by their kind ministrations of comfort, did much to 'smooth the pathway to the tomb.'"

He was buried at his request on the glacis of St. Marks by the side of his brother who "had gone before him about two years ago."[6]

A measure of Dr. McCoskry's intellect is suggested by a list of books he had loaned to various persons which the administrator of his estate was attempting to recover. It included: Nicholas Gouin DuFief, *Nature Displayed in Her Mode of Teaching Language to Men.* This was a popular work on the learning of languages, originally published in French but translated into several languages; Johann Friedrich Blumenbachm, *Elements of Physiology;* Nathan Chapman, *Elements of Therapeutics and Materia Medica;* John Locke, *Essay Concerning Human Understanding,* and *The Poems of Ossian,* ancient Gaelic verses popularized by the 18th century Scottish poet, James MacPherson.

The list of medical officers of the United States Army for the years 1789-1818 includes Dr. William McCoskry, commissioned surgeon's mate from Pennsylvania in 1791 and assigned to the 2nd Infantry Regiment in March 1792. He was promoted to the rank of surgeon April 30, 1798, resigning his commission on February 1, 1802. It is very probable that he was the father of the two Drs. McCoskry, Charles and William.

1. TP., XXII, 367.
2. Ibid., p. 372.
3. Ibid., p. 450.
4. St. Augustine *East Florida Herald,* January 4, 1823. It is indicated that the initial notice first appeared in the issue of November 13, 1822 (missing).
5. Ibid., May 10, 1823. Glacis: a slope leading up to the wall of the fort.
6. Ibid., September 20, 1823. The following entry was found in the diary of an itinerant missionary, J.N. Glenn, who arrived at St. Augustine on April 8, 1823, and was still there at the time of Dr. McCoskry's death. Perhaps it should not be taken at its face value. "Sunday the 14th (Sept.). This morning we had Two Deaths in Town, Dr. Wm. McCroskey and Mr. Cashen, both in about two hours and it is said both of them by intemperance ... what a pity .. what a pity ... as young a man as Dr. McC. should so far forget humanity (he was 22). I precht twice and attended his funeral."

McCranie, Daniel W., Santa Rosa and Walton Counties, 1823-1857

Information on Dr. McCranie is not abundant. He was born in Decatur County, Georgia, on December 17, 1823.[1] No record has been located of his early education, apprenticeship or formal medical training, but in 1850 he was included in the Santa Rosa County Census as physician, aged 26.[2] Two years later he moved to neighboring Walton County, settling in the town of Euchee Anna (Eucheeanna) which was the county seat.[3] His professional card, published initially on June 19, 1852, advertised his services to the citizens of Walton and Holmes Counties, with the additional commitment to "obey calls in Washington County as far as possible."[4] He claimed competence "to perform operations connected with minor surgery." He died in Decatur County on March 14, 1857, and was brought to the Euchee Valley Cemetery for burial. His grave marker bears the inscription: "Gravestone erected by his friend, Dr. Angus Douglas McKinnon."

1. Lola Lee Daniell Bruington, "Walton County, Florida," Pensacola Chapter, Daughters of the American Revolution, Pensacola, 1951, p. 20. Typescript copy, P.K. Yonge Library of Florida History.
2. U.S. Census, 1850, Santa Rosa County, Florida, p. 229. The name McCranie was of frequent occurrence among the multitude of Scotch Highlander settlers of Walton County.
3. Euchee Anna was Walton County's second seat, the first having been the village of Alaqua. The seat was later relocated at DeFuniak Springs.
4. Marianna *Florida Whig,* June 19, 1852.

McDonald, Norman G., Jefferson County, 1831-1860

The Florida career of Dr. McDonald was brief, spanning only six or seven years. Nothing is known of his early life and education. He was born in 1831,[1] arrived in Jefferson County in late 1855, and his earliest professional card bears the date, March 22, 1856. In it he announced his services to the people of Jefferson County, promising to "attend with assiduous care, all cases entrusted to him."[2] His office could be readily located since it adjoined the office of Col. William S. Dilworth, Jefferson County's most eminent lawyer.

Soon after settling in Monticello Dr. McDonald expressed his concern about the poor quality of medical practice and the incompetence of some of the practitioners. At a meeting of a small group of doctors in Monticello on February 11, 1856, presided over by Dr. John G. Pettus with himself as secretary, he assisted in the organization of the Jefferson County Medical Society, one of the first in the state.[3] In the early weeks of his residence Dr. McDonald had shown his political colors by attending a meeting of County Democrats held at the Court House in Monticello on March 22, 1856.[4]

After little more than a year of practice in Monticello, Dr. McDonald moved his residence and practice to Waukeenah, a village 12 miles south of the county seat. As for his motives for the move it seems certain that he found Monticello over-staffed with physicians, there being six others in practice in the little town at the time of his arrival. After the move, his altered professional card, first appearing on May 9, 1857, advertised "a well-selected stock of Drugs and Medicines" to be sold "on liberal terms." "Physicians' prescriptions and Planters' Orders" would be filled "with care...each article warranted."[5]

For the next four years Dr. McDonald practiced his profession and ran his drug store in Waukeenah. Meanwhile he had married into one of the county's most illustrious families, having taken as his wife Harriet Giroude Palmer, youngest of the nine children of Martin and Amelia (Miles) Palmer, the wedding having taken place at the Palmer home in Monticello on October 6, 1858. During their residence in Waukeenah two children were born, Norman J. and Jane, the former dying at an early age, the latter living on to the age of 93.[6]

In the summer of 1861 the McDonalds returned to Monticello and again the doctor offered his professional services to the people of the town and vicinity. They resided with Mrs. McDonald's mother, then a widow, her husband having died in 1857. It appears that Dr. McDonald was by that date already in failing health and that he did not live for more than a few months. The historians of the Palmer family only tell us that "Dr. McDonald did not live long."[7] The precise date of his death has not been ascertained. Mrs. McDonald later married the Reverend J. Hamilton Quinby, a union to which no children were born.

1. Theresa Yaeger Palmer, *The Palmer Physicians*, Hugh Archer Palmer, ed., 1966.
2. Tallahassee *Floridian and Journal*, March 22, 1856.
3. Ibid., February 16, 1856.
4. Ibid., April 5, 1856.
5. Ibid., May 9, 1857. Waukeenah had been the site of a 17th century Spanish mission but soon after Spanish cession of Florida the land in the area had come into the hands of John Gamble, who called his plantation Waukeenah. It was a prosperous area in antebellum days.
6. See note 1, supra. Jane McDonald became the wife of Thomas Hopkins in 1889. To this union were born two children, Norman and Helen Gignilliat, who married John Felder Charlton. Children of this line still live.
7. Ibid., p. 53. After her marriage to Mr Quinby the couple went to Japan as missionaries. On their return home in 1876 she died aboard ship and was buried at sea.

McDougall, Charles E., Milton, 1830-1916

Dr. McDougall, a native of Pennsylvania, whose parents had been born in Maine,[1] spent the greater part of his lengthy career as a citizen of Milton, Florida, serving in the dual roles of physician and clergyman. For more than 50 years he practiced medicine in the town and surrounding area before accepting the call to become rector of St. Mary's Episcopal Church. Nothing is presently known of his early education and medical training, but it is evident that he was a well-educated man and competent physician. Besides, he was a trusted civic leader in Milton and Santa Rosa County.

About 1854 Dr. McDougall married an Alabama native, Sarah (patronym unknown).[2] Theirs was a long and happy union to which were born two sons, William, who became a druggist in Milton, and Charles, and three daughters, Ethel, who became the wife of Lewis P. Golson; Mabel and Bessi, the former two living well into the the 20th century.

The esteem in which Dr. McDougall was generally held is indicated by the account of his funeral which was conducted by the eminent clergyman, the Right Reverend Edwin G. Weed, Bishop of the Diocese of Florida, assisted by the Reverend John H. Brown, Rector of Christ Church, Pensacola.

1. U.S. Census, 1880, Santa Rosa County, Florida, p. 54.

2. The essential biographical data relating to Dr. McDougall is derived from his obituary published in the Milton *Gazette* of May 26, 1916. His death had occurred on May 24.

McGehee, W. Scott, Leon County, 1817-1854

Very little can be told of the professional career of Dr. McGehee[1] which was of brief duration and melancholy conclusion. A native of South Carolina, he settled in Leon County in the 1840s, doubtless following the path of his older brother, John C. McGehee, who had settled in Madison County as a substantial planter and who later became a county judge. Judge McGehee, an ardent secessionist, is best remembered as the presiding member of the Florida Secession Convention which met in Tallahassee in January 1861. On February 6, 1849, Dr. McGehee married Evelyn M. Byrd of Wakulla County,[2] member of a Lenoir County, North Carolina, family which had migrated to Middle Florida some years earlier.[3]

What had promised to be a happy and lasting union was cut tragically short in 1854 when Dr. McGehee, apparently in robust health, died suddenly at the age of 37. His grieving widow and their two small daughters were taken into the household of Judge McGehee in Madison County. Only a few months later while on a visit with her brother, Waitstell Byrd, in Wakulla County, Mrs. McGehee, a frail woman, was stricken with erysipelas, dying on March 6, 1855.

1. U.S. Census, 1850, Leon County, Florida, p. 117. Here Dr. McGehee's age is recorded as 33; his property is valued at $3,000. The older child was one year old.

2. Tallahassee *Florida*, February 10, 1849. Several Byrd families settled in Leon and adjoining counties. No effort has been made in the present study to determine their interrelationships.

3. A doleful account of this tragic family is found in Tallahassee *Floridian and Journal*, April 14, 1855. The actual date of Dr. McGehee's death is not stated, although the writer of the notice states that it had occurred "a few months since," i.e., a few months prior to Mrs. McGehee's death.

McHan, Mark, Chattahoochee, 1832

Dr. McHan, one of the earliest settlers in Gadsden County, lived in the vicinity of Chattahoochee near the Georgia state line. He appears in the Census of 1830 as aged between 30 and 40. His household included his wife, Mary B., aged between 20 and 30, and two daughters, both under five.[1] His death occurred in the early fall of 1832.[2] His slaves numbered 15, which suggests that he was engaged in farming as well as medical practice. Dr. McHan's widow continued to live in Gadsden County until at least late 1834 when her seven-year-old daughter, Catherine, died on September 21,[3] but no McHan entry appears in the 1840 Census.

1. U.S. Census, 1830, Gadsden County, Florida, p. 142.
2. An extrapolation from the public notice announcing the administration "of the estate of Dr. Mark M'Han, late of Gadsden County, now deceased," which appeared in the Tallahassee *Floridian*, October 30, 1832.
3. Ibid., October 4, 1834.

McHenry, Thomas P., Alachua County, 1826-1875

Dr. McHenry was born in Alabama on February 21, 1826, and died in Newnansville on February 6, 1875.[1] Nothing is known of his early education and professional training. The earliest notices of his Florida practice show him to have been a resident of Adamsville, Sumter County, now Okahumpka, Lake County, in 1854. He advertised himself as druggist and practicing physician, who "keeps on hand and for sale a complete assortment of drugs, medicines, etc."[2] By early 1860 Dr. McHenry had moved to Alachua County, settling in the town of Newnansville, where on February 15 he announced his professional services to the citizens of the community, stating that he could be found at his office "between Gunnel's Store and his hotel."[3] Unlike so many of his medical colleagues he was by no means an impoverished practitioner. The census schedule of 1860 shows him owning property valued at $5,000, while that of 1870 indicates real estate worth $10,000 and personal property valued at $13,000.[4]

Dr. McHenry seems to have been keenly aware of the importance of establishing a viable professional society for the physicians of Florida. This concern he demonstrated by affiliating with the Medical Society of Marion County, his own county of Alachua having no such organization at the time. He was one of 11 physicians who met in Jacksonville on January 14, 1874, and organized the Florida Medical Association.[5] Unfortunately, he did not live to attend the second meeting of the Association which convened in Jacksonville on February 17, 1875; his death occurred on February 6, just two weeks prior to his 49th birthday. It was the sad duty of his Newnansville colleague, Dr. J.A. Williams, to announce his death to the Association.[6]

Nothing more is known of Dr. McHenry. He was survived by his wife, Harriet, native of Georgia, and a young man, Calvin J. McHenry, born in South Carolina, probably a son.[7]

1. Information from gravestone in Newnansville Cemetery.
2. Tampa *Herald*, February, 22, 1854.
3. Newnansville *Florida Dispatch*, May 11, 1860. First printed in the issue of February 15.
4. U.S. Census, 1860, Alachua County, item 716, and ibid., 1870, item 3730.
5. *Proceedings, Florida Medical Association*, 1874, Jacksonville, 1875, p. 4.

6. Ibid., 1875, p. 12.

7. The census schedule of 1860 does not include Calvin J. McHenry as a member of the household, while that of 1870 gives his age as 17.

McIlvaine, Robert H., Cedar Key, 1820-1889

Notwithstanding his relative prominence in the public affairs of Cedar Keys and north Florida generally, the biographical data on Dr. McIlvaine are fraught with annoying hiatuses. A Delaware native, born on April 23, 1820,[1] he followed a circuitous course before arriving in Florida about 1855. Upon completion of medical studies at Jefferson Medical College in 1848, he married a Kentuckian, Mary Jane Bledsoe, and began professional practice in Tennessee where the three eldest of his nine children were born.[2] About 1849 he moved to North Carolina where he remained for some six years and where three more children were added to the family.

Prior to 1855 the Cedar Keys had little attraction for settlers. Way Key (now Cedar Key), Depot Key (now Atsena Otie), and Sea Horse Key had emerged from obscurity during the Second Seminole War (1835-42) when they became a base of supply for troops engaged in the effort to subdue the Indians. In 1855 they assumed importance when the value of the cedar forests of the area was recognized and two German pencil manufacturing firms bought or leased the forested land and began the rash harvesting of the timber. Five years later David Levy Yulee, a major investor in property in Levy and adjoining counties, completed his railroad linking Cedar Keys with the interior of the state.

Dr. McIlvaine first established his practice on Atsena Otie where a post office had been located in 1852. The Levy County Census of 1860 designated him "physician, Presbyterian," owning land valued at $600 and personal property valued at $300. With the coming of the Civil War and the seizure of the Keys by Union troops in 1862 the McIlvaines seem to have left, not to reappear until well after the end of the War.[3]

Dr. McIlvaine had returned to Levy County by 1876, settling this time in Cedar Keys, so-called until well into the 20th century when it came to be known as Cedar Key. In addition to the practice of medicine, however, he turned to business, acquiring a hotel known as Island House, later to be called the Suwannee Hotel. The Gainesville *Times* noted that he was "improving his hotel at Cedar Keys" and called attention to his bath house, "a great institution in this warm weather."[4] Later in 1876 the Commissioners of Levy County appointed him Tax Collector,[5] and soon thereafter Col. J. Ira Gore, owner and editor of the Cedar Keys *Florida State Journal*, sold his newspaper "to Dr. McIlvaine, proprietor of the Island House."[6]

When the *Florida State Journal* a short time later published a list of deliquent taxes (probably a lengthy list, given the economic depression of the times), L.B. Lewis, Chairman of the Levy County Board of Commissioners, was sufficiently outraged to condemn "the dishonest practices of Dr. McIlvaine." He accused the doctor of having purchased the paper primarily for the purpose of advertising delinquent taxes and charging the taxpayers "outrageous rates to have their delinquencies exposed to the public." Commissioner Lewis also leveled charges of collusion to defraud between David Levy Yulee and the Doctor.[7]

In 1880 Dr. McIlvaine was again in medical practice, the Census of that year designating him only as "doctor" while Mrs. McIlvaine was identified as "hotel keeper." The three younger McIlvaine children were still members of the household while three of the older sons, Frank, William and Edmund, with homes and children of their own, were engaged in maritime occupations.[8]

Dr. McIlvaine's newspaper venture was apparently of brief duration, the sole ownership being resumed by Colonel Gore. In 1886, however, he turned to journalism once more launching his own paper, the Cedar Key *Gulf View* in July of that year. The masthead of the two surviving issues proclaim him editor and proprietor. In the issue of March 12, 1887, the following notice appeared: "McIlvaine, R.H., M.D., physician and surgeon, will resume the practice of his profession. Office opposite the Suwanee Hotel."[9]

Dr. McIlvaine's remaining days were few. Death came for him on February 28, 1889. The following notice seems to be an adequate summation of his Florida career:[10]

> Dr. R.H. McIlvaine, editor of the Cedar Key Gulf View, died on Thursday last after a very short sickness. Dr. McIlvaine intended starting a newspaper in Micanopy soon, and the *Times-Union* says of him: He was a man of great energy of character and more than ordinary ability. He had been a citizen of Florida for more than a quarter of a century, having accumulated a very handsome property during a very busy and successful life. Of pronounced views, and firm in expressing them, he made enemies as well as friends. As a writer he ranked among the ablest in Southern journalism, and we join the press of the State in deploring the loss of one whose counsels will be missed in the discussion of grave public issues.

1. A few biographical notes on Dr. McIlvaine including dates of his birth and death as well as the name of his wife are included in the biographical sketch of his grandson, Eugene Thomas McIlvaine, appearing in Harry G. Cutler, *History of Florida, Past and Present,* 3 vols., New York, 1923, II, 89. Eugene Thomas McIlvaine, a successful Tampa attorney, was the son of Victor B. McIlvaine, Dr. McIlvaine's youngest son.
2. U.S. Census, 1860, Levy County, Florida, Item 62.
3. Ibid.
4. Gainesville *Times,* August 10, 1876.
5. Ibid., February 27, 1878.
6. Only a single issue of the *Florida State Journal* (that of August 5, 1882, Vol. VIII, No. 31) has survived. By that date the sole ownership and editorship had been resumed by Col. Gore.
7. The implication is clear. Yulee expected to profit immeasurably by having the distressed properties identified and the amount of taxes due made public. On the basis of the scant evidence it is hardly possible to substantiate the Lewis charges. His letter is a fine piece of satire couched in Biblical language. Yulee appears as King David and McIlvaine as his *hakim* (judge) and *satrap* (petty prince).
8. U.S. Census, 1880, Levy County, Florida, p. 10.
9. The two extant issues of the *Gulf View* are those of March 12, 1887, Vol. I, No. 35, and April 14, 1888, Vol. II, No. 40.
10. Madison *Recorder,* March 8, 1889.

McKay, John P., St. Augustine, 1832

Dr. McKay was one of three physicians practicing medicine (the others were Drs. G.H. Simmons and William F. Shine) in St. Augustine in 1870. He was a native of France, born of American parents in 1832. Except for the fact that he was married to Mary F., a native of Vermont, nothing further is known of this physician. It seems probable that he was only a brief sojourner in Florida.[1]

1. Dr. McKay was identified as one of three physicians in a manuscript, University of Pennsylvania Collection, UPC 2.3, No. 16, p. 1.

McKinnon, Angus D., Walton County, 1827-1870

Dr. McKinnon, eldest son of Col. John L. McKinnon, pioneer settler of Walton County, was born in Richmond County, North Carolina, on September, 23, 1827.[1] Col. McKinnon, a native of the Isle of Skye, Scotland, was one of many Scottish Highlanders who made their way to America in the last decades of the 18th century, settling in large numbers in North and South Carolina. Even prior to the cession of Florida to the United States, Col. McKinnon had made a trip to Pensacola in the expectation of finding a suitable site for settling.[2] In 1826 he married Catherine Campbell, also of Richmond County, and in 1828 with his wife and small son migrated to Florida, laying claims to land in the fertile Euchee Valley of Walton County.[3]

The numerous children of Col. McKinnon were brought up in the strict religious atmosphere of Scotch Presbyterianism. They were exposed also to the best educational opportunity available in the area. The best, however, was probably quite mediocre until the arrival in the valley in 1848 of John Newton,[4] a well-educated Pennsylvania clergyman who came in search of a favorable professional situation. He arrived by way of Pensacola where he had met Dr. John Brosnaham, from whom he learned of the Euchee Valley Settlement. He determined to go there. By chance, the small schooner on which he found passage was run by none other than Angus D. McKinnon and his brother C.L. McKinnon[5] who gave him a warm welcome and took him to the home of their father. Within a short time Newton was not only preaching but also teaching in what came to be an academy of some renown.

Soon thereafter, under the encouragement of Newton, Augus McKinnon began the study of medicine in South Alabama under the preceptorate of a relative, Dr. D.D. McKinnon.[6] In 1853 he was enrolled in the Medical College of the State of South Carolina in Charleston where he remained for one term,[7] returning in the next year to begin practice in Euchee Valley at Mossy Bend near the eastern end of the Valley. At about the same time he married Catherine Douglass, member of another Scottish pioneer family from North Carolina.

When the sounds of the firing on Ft. Sumter were heard in Euchee Valley it was a virtual call to arms to the young men of Walton County. A unit of militia, the Walton Guards, was hurriedly assembled. In a reorganization of February 1862, these troops were incorporated into Company D., 1st Florida Infantry Regiment, Captain C.L. McKinnon, commanding. Although by this time three children had been born to Dr. McKinnon and his wife, he entered his brother's unit as 3rd Sergeant, committing himself for three years of service, his enlistment dating from February 28. The Company assembled at Camp Walton, now the site of Ft. Walton Beach, where it remained until August 1862 when it was moved to Tennessee, first to Camp Moccasin on the Tennessee River and later into Kentucky, where it was engaged in the Battle of Perryville. Although his war record is fragmented it appears that he was wounded at the Battle of Chickamauga in September 1863 and subsequently discharged to return to his home in Florida. He ended his military career as a 1st sergeant.[8]

For the next four or five years Dr. McKinnon carried on a medical practice in the Euchee Valley. As the war came to an end there was general breakdown of law and order as bands of deserters organized themselves into terrorists groups, directing their pillaging and plundering upon the rural families of Walton County and South Alabama. Dr. McKinnon narrowly escaped death at their hands. A small band of ruffians had secreted themselves near the home of the doctor one night and shot him down as he emerged from his house. The order to kill him was given by their leader, a man named Clark. Assuming that he was dead they left him lying in his blood. Mrs. McKinnon sent for a doctor and his life was saved. Some time later this band was apprehended near Elba, Alabama; Clark was taken into custody, and just before he was hanged he confessed that it was indeed he who had ordered the shooting of Dr. McKinnon.[9]

At some date prior to 1870 Dr. McKinnon and his family moved to Geneva, Alabama, about eight miles across the state line from Walton County. He died there on June 1, 1870, leaving his widow with four children, Augustus, Arabella, Wallace and Angus M., aged 14, 10, nine and four, respectively.[10] His body was returned to Florida for burial in the Euchee Valley Cemetery. Mrs. McKinnon died on April 8, 1890, and was also buried there.

1. The dates of birth and death of Dr. McKinnon are found in the pamphlet, "Walton County," prepared by the Pensacola Chapter, Daughters of the American Revolution, Pensacola, 1951. Typed copy, P.K. Yonge Library of Florida History, gift of Lola Lee Daniell Bruington. This pamphlet includes a brief history of the county, a survey of three of its cemeteries, and a useful index.

2. John L. McKinnon, *History of Walton County*, Introduction by A.G. Campbell, Gainesville, Kallman Publishing Co., 1968. This is a fascimile edition of the original, published in Atlanta in 1911. This work, authored in his latter years by John L. McKinnon, was written largely from his own memories. Its chronology is sometimes difficult to follow. It includes a useful map and a superb index. It is an intimate and often romantic treatment. See pp. 22-27.

3. Ibid., map, p. 8.

4. Ibid., p. 181.

5. Ibid., p. 182.

6. Archives, Waring Historical Library, Medical University of South Carolina, Charleston. Lists of Matriculants.

7. Ibid.

8. NA, Service Records, CSA, M251, Roll 28. There is some confusion here. His wound may have occurred at Murphreesboro, Tennessee, earlier in the year.

9. McKinnon, *History*, p. 323.

10. U.S. Census, 1870, Geneva County, Alabama, p. 533, item 198.

McKinnon, Charles, Walton County, 1834

Dr. McKinnon was born in Kershaw District, South Carolina, in 1834. He is presumed to have been the son of Scottish-born Charles McKinnon, who emigrated to North Carolina where he married Mary Johnson. He later moved to Kershaw District, South Carolina, where his two sons Charles and Neill J. were born.[1] Dr. McKinnon began his medical education in the office of Dr. B.S. Lucas of Kershaw. He matriculated at the Medical College of the State of South Carolina, Charleston,[2] in 1852 and was graduated with the M.D. degree in the spring of 1854.[3] By that date his brother and several other McKinnon relatives had settled in Walton County, so Dr. McKinnon joined them in the Eucheeanna community where he entered the practice of his profession. The Walton County Census of 1860 lists him as a resident of Eucheeanna, living alone, and owning property valued at $8,500.

With the outbreak of war in 1861, Dr. McKinnon was among the early enlistees, joining Company E, 1st Florida Infantry Regiment, on July 20, 1861, for a three-year stint. He entered as a private. In the following year he was with his outfit in Tennessee. His military service was terminated at Chattanooga on November 21, 1862, by a disability discharge. His discharge papers, signed by two surgeons, give the following diagnosis of his ailment: "Chronic

Rheumatism of a severe character which totally unfits him for duty in any department of the government." His papers also include the following personal data. He is "28 years of age; was born in Kershaw Dist., S.C., is 5 ft. 10 inches tall, of fair complexion, blue eyes and light hair, and by occupation a physician. During the last two months he was unfit for duty for 50 days."[5]

Following his discharge Dr. McKinnon returned to Walton County, setting up practice in Mossy Bend, east of Eucheeanna. It is possible that at some juncture he returned to military service, although it has not been confirmed. John L. McKinnon, in his *History*, described the dramatic moment when the people of Walton County first learned of the end of the War. Postal service into the County had been almost completely disrupted during the last stages of the War. Private arrangements were made for a special courier to bring such mail as was addressed to Walton citizens from Marianna to Know Hill in the eastern part of the County, near the Choctawhatchee River. There representatives of the important families would gather at appointed times to await the arrival of the special postman to appear with the mail pouch. They met under a large oak. As McKinnon recalled the particular occasion many years later,[6]

> One evening as these McLeans, McPhersons, McKenzies, McDonalds, Campbells...among whom was Dr. Charles McKinnon, a surgeon of the Confederate army at home in Mossy Bend on furlough...the postman rode up, handed over the mail pouch, and while they sat around examining this mail matter, he dismounted, took his knife from his pocket, ripped open a small sack that was neatly and securely placed between two of his saddle cloths, took a newspaper from it and passed it on to these gentlemen, saying, "This paper Judge Bush in Marianna placed here and charged me 'that I see that you get it!' " The paper was handed over to Dr. McKinnon who was requested to read it aloud. He read in a full distinct voice as follows: "General Lee Has Surrendered...Our Cause Lost."...When through, the paper fell from his hands to the ground and they all sat, with heads downward for several moments as silent as Job's comforters. Dr. McKinnon lifts his head, the silence is broken by his exclaiming: "Gentlemen, we as a Southern people are politically irredeemably damned."

Thus did Walton County get the news that the War was at last over.

Nothing further is known of Dr. McKinnon. If he indeed did continue the practice of medicine, it was probably in another state. He does not appear in the 1870 Walton County Census.

1. See Sketch of Charles B. McKinnon in H.G. Cutler, *History of Florida, Past and Present*, Chicago & New York, 1923, pp. 137-138.
2. Archives, Waring Historical Library, Medical University of South Carolina, Charleston, Lists of Matriculants and Graduates.
3. Charleston *Mercury*, March 15, 1854. Charles McKinnon's doctoral thesis bore the title, "Digestion."
4. U.S. Census, 1860, Walton County, Florida, p. 14, item 87.
5. NA, Service Records, CSA, M251, Roll 28.
6. John L. McKinnon, *History of Walton County*, Atlanta, 1911, pp. 321-322.

McKinnon, John Wesley, Walton County, 1827-1871

Dr. McKinnon, physician and surgeon, practiced medicine in Walton County for only a brief period following the Civil War. Born in North Carolina on February 6, 1827, he was one of a multitude of Scottish Highlanders who made their way into Florida and southern Alabama seeking a better life. Nothing is known of his early education and medical training. He appears to have begun his professional career in Alabama about 1855. Soon thereafter he married Sarah, by whom he became the father of two children, Robert and Edward, both born in Alabama.[1] About 1865 the family moved to Walton County, settling in the village of Freeport,[2] only a few miles inland from Choctawhatchee Bay, where two additional children, Mary E. and John Francis, were born.[3]

Dr. McKinnon was the only physician known to have practiced in the Freeport community during the early postbellum period. John L. McKinnon, the historian of Walton County, recounted an incident which indicated either the courage or the foolhardiness of the doctor. Jesse Evans, then living in Aliqua, a few miles distant, rode to Freeport to summon the doctor to Aliqua to see some member of the Infinger family who was very ill. As they rode toward Aliqua Evans' dog discovered a large rattlesnake lying close to the road. As the snake's attention was engaged by the dog, Dr. McKinnon lassoed the snake with his bridle rein, held him up full length, opened his pocket knife with his teeth and severed the creature's head. The historian claimed to have verified the story.[4]

Dr. McKinnon's Florida career was of short duration, however. He died on April 20, 1871, at the age of 44 and was buried in the Euchee Valley Cemetery. Of his survivors it is known only that his daughter, Mary E., became the wife of Stuart Knox Gillis and died on December 28, 1830, while his son, John Francis, died on May 9, 1841.[5] As for Mrs. McKinnon and the two older children no information has emerged.

1. U.S. Census, 1870, Walton County, Florida, p. 26. It was by no means uncommon for errors to occur as census enumerators transcribed their data to the prescribed forms. In the item cited here Dr. McKinnon's name appears as Joseph. The error was rectified, however on the gravestone in the Euchee Valley Cemetery, on which it appears as J.W. But John L. McKinnon, his kinsman, cites the full name, John Wesley McKinnon. See John L. McKinnon, *History of Walton County*, Gainesville, Kallman Publishing Co., 1868, p. 157.

2. Ibid.

3. See n. 1, supra.

4. McKinnon, *History*, p. 157.

5. "Walton County, Florida." Information on Walton County, Florida including a survey of a few of its cemeteries, collected under supervision of the Pensacola Chapter, DAR, 1951. Typed copy in P.K. Yonge Library of Florida History, pp. 8, 28.

McKinstry Sr., James Fletcher, Gainesville, 1842-1926

Dr. McKinstry Sr., son of John W. and Margaret E. McKinstry, was born near Winnsboro, Fairfield County, South Carolina, on December 17, 1842. When he was four years old his family moved to Florida and bought a tract of land in the northern part of Marion County.[1] A few years later they moved across the county line settling near Newnan's Lake in Alachua County. John McKinstry appears to have been a farmer of more than average means, having owned property valued at nearly $20,000 in 1860. His slaves numbered 12.[2] The McKinstry household included Georgia-born Henry Gainey, overseer of the McKinstry farming operation.

Very little information concerning Dr. McKinstry's youth has been preserved. It is surmised that he attended such schools as were available in Gainesville. He likely was a student at the academy founded by J.H. Roper in 1856, which was Gainesville's most prestigious school for several years. It was located on East Main Street, North, the present location of the First United Methodist Church.[3]

McKinstry was barely 18 years of age when the Civil War began, a circumstance which doubtless interrupted his plans for further education. By early

1862 it had become apparent that the conflict would not be quickly finished and in the spring the Seventh Florida Infantry Regiment was organized with recruits from Alachua and Marion Counties. On March 20 Company C was organized with Philip B.H. Dudley as its commanding officer. McKinstry was among those mustered in, committing his services for "three years or the duration." Two months later he was transferred from the Company to Regimental Headquarters with the designation "musician" to become a member of the band.[4]

Official Confederate records provide very little information about Dr. McKinstry's military career. Presumably he was with his Regiment in Tennesseee under the command of General Braxton Bragg. Near the end of the war he was taken prisoner, then paroled on May 26, 1865.

In the fall of 1865, when most of the medical schools of the South had not yet resumed operation, James McKinstry enrolled at the Long Island Hospital Medical School and in the following summer was awarded a diploma.[5]

By early September 1866, Dr. McKinstry was once more in Gainesville where, on September 12, he married Miss Isabelle McCall, the wedding ceremony taking place at the home of her father, Stephen McCall, a well-to-do planter.[6] Slightly more than a week later Dr. McKinstry announced his professional services to the citizens of Gainesville and vicinity. His office was "for the present at the residence of S. McCall, Esquire."[7] Two months later the following item appeared in the local newspaper: "We understand that Dr. J.F. McKinstry has purchased the residence of Colonel J.M. Richardson, with the land attached, for the sum of $2300."[8]

A few months after launching his medical practice Dr. McKinstry joined the highly-regarded Dr. Gabriel P. Thomas in a professional partnership which endured for nearly two decades, only to be terminated when Dr. Thomas' son, Thomas F. Thomas, returned to Gainesville as a recently graduated physician to become his father's partner.

Throughout many years of practice in Gainesville and the surrounding area Dr. McKinstry maintained a splendid reputation as physician and concerned citizen. He was active in negotiating for establishment of the East Florida Seminary (later to become the University of Florida) in Gainesville. In 1915 he was appointed postmaster, a position he held for six years. He occupied offices at several different locations in the town, the last one having been 204 West Main Street, North (now simply North Main Street), directly across from the Atlantic First National Bank. His residence was for many years at 108 S. Pleasant Street (presently SW Second Street).

Dr. McKinstry was active as physician and citizen almost to the time of his death, which occurred on September 7, 1926. His survivors included, in addition to his son, Dr. James F., Jr., his widow, Belle (Isabelle), two daughters, Jane and Isabelle, and several grandchildren.

1. U.S. Census, 1850, Marion County, Florida, p. 249.
2. U.S. Census, 1860, Alachua County, Florida, p. 83.
3. Additional biographical data on Dr. McKinstry may be found in Webster Merritt, "Physicians and Medicine in Early Alachua County and Gainesville, Florida," *Journal of the Florida Medical Association*, October 1955, p. 306. Dr. Merritt, now deceased, was a native of Gainesville. He combined his medical practice in Ponte Vedra and Jacksonville, Florida, with diligent research in the medical history of Florida.
4. National Archives, Confederate Service Records, Company C, Seventh Florida Infantry Regiment.
5. Most Southern medical schools suspended their operations from 1861 until the fall of 1865 or later.
6. Gainesville *New Era*, August 21, 1866.

7. Ibid., September 21, 1866.
8. Ibid., November 9, 1866.

McKnight, George B., Ft. Barrancas, 1823

Dr. McKnight, born in Pennsylvania and resident of that state when he was commissioned surgeon's mate in 1817,[1] was only a brief sojourner in Florida. Having resigned his commission in 1818, he reentered military service with the rank of post surgeon on October 13, 1820.[2] On the first of June the following year he was promoted to assistant surgeon.[3]

The precise date of Dr. McKnight's transfer to Florida is uncertain. It is probable, however, that he was sent to Ft. Barrancas in late 1822 or early 1823. Records show him as medical officer there in 1823.[4] By the end of that year he had been transferred to nearby Dauphin Island at the entrance to Mobile Bay.[5] He resigned his commission and presumbably returned to civilian practice on June 1, 1824.[6]

Uncertainties in identification of early military assignments result from occasional inconsistencies in official records. In some cases, for example, a place of assignment is recorded as simply Pensacola, although for much of the 1820s at least two military posts, Ft. Barrancas and Cantonment Clinch, existed in the Pensacola area. To add to the confusion, Cantonment Clinch was for a brief period known as Ft. Hope.

1. MDUSA., p. 290.
2. Ibid.
3. Ibid.
4. ASP. II, 614.
5. Ibid., p. 516.
6. MDUSA., p. 290.

McLemore, John, Leon, Jefferson and Suwannee Counties, 1810-1836

Dr. McLemore, physician and soldier, was born in Richland District, South Carolina, about 1810.[1] He matriculated at the Medical Department of Transylvania University, Lexington, Kentucky, in the fall of 1828 but the following year transferred to the Medical College of South Carolina where he received a medical degree in the spring of 1830.[2] In 1831 he moved to Tallahassee and in December announced the launching of his professional career to the citizens of the community. His office was located in town but his residence was a few hundred yards out on the Quincy road.[3] Within a few weeks he had obtained an office "next door to Drs. Perkins (Elisha) and Bradford (Edward)" and a residence at the corner and Adams and Call Streets.[4]

Indications are that Dr. McLemore was well received by the Tallahassee community and that his patients were numerous. In March 1833, as was true of many physicians, he opened a drug store stating in his announcement that Dr. William Tradewell (Treadwell), "a gentleman of fine talents and first-rate medical reading had been engaged for a few months, until the practicing season, to superintend the establishment." The store was located "at Mr. Blake's large Building, corner of Clinton and Adams Streets."[5] When it became necessary for him to return to South Carolina for four or five weeks later in the year, he left his affairs in the hands of attorney Richard Hackley, while his accounts were turned over to Leigh Read for collection with instructions that no further indulgence would be granted to those owing since 1832.[6] In the meantime he had formalized his association with Dr. Tradewell as a practicing colleague.[7]

Dr. McLemore announced that he was moving to Monticello in November 1834 where he would offer his services to the people of Jefferson County. His accounts were left for Attorney Hackley to collect.[8] Nothing is known of his Monticello practice, although his appointment as an appraiser for the Union Bank of Florida, as one of five Jefferson County appointees, suggests that he was a person of good reputation in the County.[9]

At some undetermined date in 1835 Dr. McLemore purchased a spa, known as Suwannee Sulphur Springs,[10] located about 11 miles down the Suwannee River from the more famous White Sulphur Springs. He apparently moved to the Springs with the intention of developing the resort. This venture, however, coincided with the outbreak of Indian hostilities, particularly along the Suwannee and Withlacoochee rivers, actions characterized by raids on isolated homes and small settlements, which reached a climax with the Dade Massacre of December 27, 1835. Responding to Governor Eaton's call for an augmented militia to meet the situation, Dr. McLemore raised a volunteer unit of some 50 men recruited from Columbia and Hamilton Counties, which became a part of the Sixth Regiment of the Florida Militia. Dr. McLemore assumed command of his company with the rank of captain.[11]

Dr. McLemore and his company saw immediate action around the Alachua Savannah (Payne's Prairie) in mid-December 1835. A short while later they escorted about 250 persons who had fled the Wacasassa area around present-day Otter Creek and taken refuge at Suwannee Old Town to a camp at Newnansville in Alachua County.[12] Dr. McLemore's most notable exploit, however, was carried out in early April 1836 when, bearing his newly-acquired rank of major, he led a group of 50 men to the mouth of the Withlacoochee, then upriver for nine miles in the face of Indian ambush and within a matter of four or five days built a block house on the south bank of the River. This feat was carried out on the orders of General Winfield Scott, who had expected the structure to be used as a supply depot,[13] and was accomplished between March 30 and April 4.[14]

Having accomplished his mission, Dr. McLemore left 40 men behind at the block house under the command of Capt. E. Holloman, killed by Indians on May 3.[15] But the doctor's days were few. He was apparently not a man of strong constitution and the rigors of wilderness warfare and constant exposure to the elements had destroyed his health. Nevertheless he was able to make his way from the Withlacoochee station, which was named Camp McLemore,[16] to the Suwannee, thence up the river as far as Charles Ferry,[17] where on April 16 he wrote a pathetic letter to Governor R.K. Call asking to be relieved of his command. After recounting briefly his experiences on the Withlacoochee, which he had departed on April 4, he added:[18]

> My health for the last month has been gradually declining. I am now but a walking skeleton, with a chronic cough and chill and fever. My prayer to your excellency is, to permit me to resign my command. Mine is really a case of life and death. If I remain in service I shall certainly lose my life. By retiring to some healthier climate, with good nursing, I may regain my health...

Within three weeks he was dead at the age of 26.[19]

1. Archives, Transylvania University, Lists of Matriculants.
2. Archives, Medical College of South Carolina, Joseph I. Waring Medical Historical Library, MUSC, Lists of Students.
3. Tallahassee *Floridian*, December 27, 1831.
4. Ibid., February 16, 1832.
5. Ibid., March 9, 1833.
6. He was away in South Carolina and New York for the greater part of November and December 1833. Ibid., November 2, 1833; November 9, 1833; December 21, 1833.
7. Ibid., April 27, 1833.
8. Ibid., November 22, 1834.
9. TP. XXV, 102. List for Jefferson County signed by Gov. Eaton.
10. Also known as Suwannee Medical Springs, Jacksonville *Courier*, December 17, 1835.
11. Ibid., December 24, 1835. Dr. McLemore's company was known as "Columbia Volunteers." See ibid. for brief account of his campaign activities. See also John K. Mahon, *History of the Second Seminole War*, Gainesville, 1864, pp. 150-153.
12. Jacksonville *Courier*, December 31, 1835.
13. Numerous accounts of this exploit exist and the most reliable is that of Dr. McLemore himself in *Senate Documents*, 19th Congress, 1st Session, pp. 38-39.
14. Ibid.
15. The failure of General Scott to rescue the beleaguered soldiers left at the block house touched off a furious attack on him. It was led by the *Tallahassee Floridian*. In veering off the main route from Tampa to St. Augustine, Scott led his troops straightway to St. Augustine, leaving the abandoned men to face repeated Indian attacks and starvation. The death of Capt. Holloman left Lt. L.B. Walker in command of the block house. Unaware of Dr. McLemore's death, Walker addressed a letter to him, dated May 10 at Camp McLemore, setting forth the desperate situation. Ibid., p. 48. A few days after Walker's letter was written a rescue party under the command of Major Leigh Read removed the men from the block house. See Norristown, Pa., *Register and Montgomery Democrat*, July 13, 1836.
16. Apparently the block house was designated "Camp McLemore" by the party which had been abandoned there.
17. Charles Ferry, located on the Suwannee River just west of present day Dowling Park, was at that time headquarters of the 12th Florida Regiment.
18. See note 13, supra.
19. Dr. McLemore is presumed to have died at Charles Ferry. It is odd that, notwithstanding the widespread publicity relating to the block house, the precise date of Dr. McLemore's death is still unknown. It occurred between April 16, the date of his letter of resignation, and May 21, the date of the *Floridian* in which Dr. McLemore is first referred to as "the late Major McLemore." Strange it is that the paper never printed an obituary.

Dr. McLemore's friend and companion-in-arms, Joseph McCants, a Monticello attorney, was named administrator of his estate. Tallahassee *Floridian*, September 10, 1836.

Addendum: Senate Document, 24th Congress, 2nd Session, No. 224, pp. 163-165. This document sets forth the proceeding of the Court of Inquiry in the case of Major General Winfield Scott regarding failure of the Florida Campaign in 1836. It contains a review of the circumstances of the construction of the block house on the Withlacoochee and includes the General's attempts to exculpate himself from the disaster which befell the garrison. Major McLemore is praised as "a highly meritorious Floridian." Scott added that he had "further penetrated the River, established a block house, and left it garrisoned...with a promise to return and relieve it in 8 or 10 days. Unfortunately, however, as he entered the Suwannee, he was assailed with a fever, and fell victim of its effects," p. 185.

McLeod, Leddy, Madison County, mid-19th century

Notwithstanding the diligent searches for positive identification of Dr. Leddy (Lodry) McLeod by Madison County's historian, Edwin B. Browning,[1] he remains a somewhat shadowy figure, although an important one in antebellum Madison County. The Census of 1850 indicates that he was a native of Georgia, aged 22, and a resident in the home of Dr. Theodore Hartridge, later to gain eminence as a physician and businessman in Jacksonville. In the Hartridge home in Madison was also another young physician, Dr. Samuel A. Bradford, of South Carolina.[2] It is possible, even probable, that the two young physicians had been apprentices under the preceptorate of Dr. Hartridge. Dr. McLeod's name does not appear in subsequent censuses of Florida.

1. Edwin B. Browning, *History of the Greenville Missionary Baptist Church, 1849-1979*, Monticello, Florida, Monticello Printers, 1980, p. 14. Browning suggests the reasonable assumption that Dr. McLeod was the owner of a

number of slaves received into the Concord Baptist Church, Madison County, on October 17, 1858, following closing of the nearby Shilo Church. He also suggests the possibility that Dr. McLeod may be identified as the I.D. McLeod named in a Madison County document of 1854 as the owner of 65 slaves and more than a thousand acres of land in the county.

2. U.S. Census, 1850, Madison County, Florida, Item 9.

McLeod, Moses D., Madison County, 1829

Dr. McLeod (McCloud) was a mid-19th century practitioner in Madison. Born in Sumter District, South Carolina,[1] son of Moses B. McLeod, he read medicine under the guidance of Sumter physician Dr. J.A. Mayes, and in 1850 was graduated from the Medical College of the State of South Carolina.[2] The title of his doctoral thesis was "Hints on the Medical Treatment of Negroes."

Upon receiving his medical degree Dr. McLeod returned to Sumter where he practiced for several years. In the winter of 1857-58 he and his newly-acquired wife, Mary, migrated to Madison where he established a practice in March 1858.[3] His professional card, first appearing on March 20, 1858, gave his address as Madison Court House, "two doors south of the Hotel." The census enumerator in 1860 assigned a value of $10,000 to his property. It also listed as members of his household two infant daughters, May and Lenora, as well as two of his sisters, Margaret and Martha, who upon the death of their father, had come to live with the doctor.[4]

So far as is known Dr. McLeod continued to practice in Madison through the Civil War years. When the Madison newspaper resumed publication in March 1866, Dr. McLeod's professional notice reappeared.[5] The absence of his name from the Madison County Census of 1870 seems to suggest that he had left the state by the date.

1. U.S. Census, 1850, Sumter District, S.C., p. 114, it. 924.
2. Archives, Waring Historical Library, MUSC, Charleston, S.C., Catalogue, 1849-50.
3. Madison *Southern Messenger*, December 25, 1858.
4. Their father was 72 years of age in 1850.
5. Madison *Southern Messenger*, April 20, 1866; 1st printing, March 29, 1866.

McLoring, John, St. Augustine, mid-19th century

Except for the fact that he entered the Medical College of the State of South Carolina in the fall of 1832 giving his place of residence as St. Augustine, nothing is known of the early years of Dr. McLoring. The 1830 Census for St. Johns County has no McLoring entry. He did, however, receive a medical degree from the Charleston institution on March 7, 1834, having submitted a thesis entitled "Dysentery."[1] He subsequently returned to St. Augustine, began practice and was still there in 1837 when he signed a petition to Congress requesting an appropriation for the completion of the seawall protecting the city.[2]

It is assumed that Dr. McLoring did not long remain in St. Augustine. In 1838 he was married in New York to Elizabeth A. Clark, daughter of William Clark of that city.[3] Since the Florida sources such as censuses of 1840 and 1850 do not list him, it is assumed that he had departed the state, perhaps as early as 1837.

1. Charleston *Courier*, March 14, 1834. The graduates in this class numbered 39, an indication of the prestige achieved by the College which had graduated its first class (only five in number) in March 1825. One other Floridian, Theodore Turnbull of Jefferson County, was among the graduates in 1834.
2. *Florida Territorial Papers*, XXV, 451.
3. St. Augustine *Florida Herald*, September 29, 1838.

McMahon, J. Ponte Coulant, St. Augustine and Pensacola, 1837

Nothing is known of the early years of Dr. McMahon prior to his receiving a commission as surgeon's mate on November 21, 1817, soon after which he was assigned to serve with the 3rd Infantry Regiment.[1] His place of birth was not indicated although he is shown to have been a resident of Washington, D.C. On August 5, 1826, he was promoted to the rank of surgeon.[2]

Dr. McMahon arrived in St. Augustine in the late summer of 1821, just in time to observe the ravages of yellow fever which had made its appearance in the city in August.[3] His notes on the epidemic followed by specific details of his mode of treatment form one of the most informative and valuable accounts of the disease to have been preserved from that era.[4]

Following the death of Dr. Micah Stone, first president of the Board of Health of St. Augustine under the recently organized government, Dr. McMahon was appointed to replace him as Resident Physician and President of the Board.[5] Dr. McMahon remained in the dual capacity of military surgeon and civilian health officer for about six months after which he was ordered to accompany Colonel Duncan L. Clinch and his regiment to the new post at Pensacola.[6]

The "sickly season" of 1822 in Pensacola was one of the deadliest on record. This epidemic prompted Florida's first legislative assembly to discontinue its session in Pensacola and move deliberations to the comparative safety of the Gonzales Plantation some 14 miles northwest of the town. Also this epidemic took the lives of two prominent Pensacola physicians, Dr. James C. Bronaugh who had been Andrew Jackson's personal physician, and Dr. M.H. Elliott, post physician at Ft. Barrancas. Dr. McMahon was brought down by the fever but managed to survive.[7]

In a letter addressed to the Adjutant General on October 5, 1822, Colonel Clinch reported on the dismal situation at Barrancas where the only surviving physician, Dr. Ayers P. Merrill, lay desperately ill. He explained that he was moving his troops to a more healthful location some three miles west of the city to a site which he called Camp Hope, later to be known as Clinch Cantonment. Parenthetically he mentioned that he was sending Dr. McMahon to relieve Dr. Merrill whose condition appeared to be hopeless. Enclosed with this dispatch was Dr. McMahon's full report on the Pensacola military, prefaced by Colonel Clinch's remark: "The following report is from Assistant Surgeon McMahon, whose opinions derive additional importance from the fact that he had witnessed the disease the previous year in St. Augustine."[8] This report, like his previous one, is a carefully prepared and intelligent assessment of the public and military health problem.

Further evidence, although scarce, indicates that Dr. McMahon remained as military surgeon in Pensacola. Mystery surrounds his participation in a duel with Colonel (George?) Walton, erstwhile acting Governor of Florida, an affair of honor which elicited a one-page special edition of the Pensacola *Gazette* on June 2, 1818. The Key West *Register* of July 2, 1828, explained that the altercation was the upshot of bitterness growing out of a recent political election. Walton had been the challenger; both men received wounds and both were recovering. Dr. McMahon was identified as an "army physician."

The passenger list of the U.S. Transport *Florida*, published in the Pensacola *Gazette* of August 21, 1830, included the name of Dr. McMahon, indicating that he had just come from Tampa on August 16. Except for resignation from the army in 1834 and mention of his death in New Orleans on April 14, 1837, no further information on Dr. McMahon has been discovered.

1. MDUSA, p. 287. *American State Papers, Military Affairs*, III, 570, lists Dr. McMahon as Surgeon, rank attained August 5, 1826, assigned to 5th Infantry. Ibid., III, 665, lists him as still with the Fifth as of January 12, 1838.
2. Heitman, HRDUSA, I, 676.
3. House Documents, Nos. 28-53, 17th Congress, 2nd Session, Vol. III, Item 38, p. 10. This includes payment to Dr. McMahon for travel expenses, Charleston to St. Augustine, latter part of 1821, $43.20.
4. NA, Record Gp. 94, Adj. Gen. Office (1780s-1917). Letter, J.C.P. McMahon, Asst. Surg. USA, to Surg. Gen. Joseph Lovell, December 31, 1821, St. Augustine.
5. TP, XXII, 359. Dr. Stone died on December 5, 1821.
6. The date of Col. Clinch's arrival in Pensacola has not been determined. A letter, Clinch to President Monroe, dated at Pensacola, June 24, 1822, seems to establish his presence there during early June.
7. Thomas Lawson, SRSM, p. 35. Here Surgeon General Lawson states: "Three medical officers, Drs. Elliott, McMahon and Merrill, were seriously attacked, the first of whom fell a victim of the disease."
8. Ibid.
9. For an account of this duel see Leora M. Sutton, *The Walton House*, Pensacola, 1968, p. 31.

McMannin, Charles T., Hamilton and Suwannee Counties, 1832-1900

Dr. McMannin (McManan), a native of North Carolina, migrated with his family to Hamilton County sometime between 1865 and 1870, settling outside the town of Jasper, the county seat.[1] Nothing is presently known of his early education and medical training, although he probably qualified for practice through the apprenticeship system. His various properties were valued at $1,200 in 1870. A few years later, and for reasons quite unknown, he elected to move to adjoining Suwannee County, settling at the village of Houstoun a few miles southeast of Live Oak.[2]

By 1890, however, Dr. McMannin had returned to Hamilton County,[3] locating at White Springs on the Suwannee River which had become a popular resort and health spa. In November he joined eight other physicians in the county in the formulation of a policy regarding the failure of so many patients to pay their bills. Their statement was as follows:[4]

> (The Hamilton Physicians) having lost patience with people who do not try to pay their doctors for services rendered, so henceforth, they will not answer summons for anyone who has wilfully refused to settle his medical bills, except in cases where it is known that they cannot afford to pay without depriving their families of the necessities. They will provide each other with lists of delinquents. Neither prejudice nor personal differences will determine the lists. The policy will become effective on January 1, 1891.

Dr. McMannin's wife, Mary, was also a native of North Carolina, having been born there in 1832, which was also the year of Dr. McMannin's birth. Their three eldest children, Walter, Fannie and Elizabeth, were also natives of that state. Their other children, daughters Malinda and Alice, were born in Florida.[5]

The last available information on the McMannin family, which is found in the Hamilton County Census of 1900,[6] lists the doctor at the age of 68 living at White Springs with his daughter, Alice, 24, and a granddaughter, Ella Matiell, 20. The date of Dr. McMannin's death has not been ascertained.

1. U.S. Census, 1870, Hamilton County, Florida, p. 71.
2. Ibid., 1880, p. 342. Dr. McMannin is also listed in the Special Florida Census of 1885, Mortality Schedule, as one of the physicians attending patients who died in that year.
3. Jasper *News*, November 14, 1890. His post office was Houstoun.

4. Ibid.
5. U.S. Census, 1900, Hamilton County, Florida, p. 286.
6. Many discrepancies in ages as well as spellings exist in the census schedules for the two counties cited here. The Census of 1880 appears to be fairly reliable. The schedule of 1900 is useful in that it gives both month and year of birth as well as actual age at the time the census data was obtained.

McMeekin, Francis M., Putnam County, 1830-1889

Dr. McMeekin was born of Irish parents in Union County, South Carolina, on January 14, 1830.[1] He received a basic education in the schools of his home community. Upon reaching adolescence he decided upon a career in medicine and moved to adjoining Fairfield County where he apprenticed himself to a local physician preparatory to entering a medical school.[2] In 1853 he was admitted to the Medical College of the State of South Carolina, Charleston, and in March 1855 was graduated as Doctor of Medicine, the Faculty having approved his doctoral thesis which bore the title "Intermittent Fever."[3]

Following graduation Dr. McMeekin appears to have returned to his home in Union District to begin practice. A short time later he married a South Carolina girl known only by her Christian name, Harriet. The McMeekins moved to Florida in 1857, purchasing a fairly large tract of land on the western boundary of Putnam County some four miles east of the town of Hawthorne.[4] In 1860 the census enumerator designated him as "M.D. and Farmer." His property was valued at more than $12,000 while his slaves numbered 14.[5]

Notwithstanding family responsibilities — wife, two small children, and a farm to be cultivated — Dr. McMeekin enlisted for service at Camp McCarthy near Orange Springs on May 14, 1862. He was given the rank of second lieutenant and assigned to the Sixth Florida Battalion, Company B, commanded by Capt. J.W. Pearson. His first two years in service were uneventful, limited for the most part to garrison duty. In early 1864, however, he became involved in the actual fighting, having been present at the Battle of Olustee on February 20. A short time later, as the struggle in Virginia became more critical, the Sixth Florida Battalion became a part of the Ninth Florida Infantry Regiment, which became a part of General Joseph Finegan's Brigade in the Virginia war zone.[6]

Meanwhile Dr. McMeekin had been assigned to the Quartermaster Department and in July 1863 was ordered to "proceed to Sanderson or Lake City to arrange your business connected with the Quartermaster and Commissary Departments and report" (to Ft. Brooke) as soon as practicable. Subsequently, at an unknown date, Dr. McMeekin returned to his Regiment which became a unit in General Joseph Finegan's Brigade. He was with the Regiment as it moved to Virginia in early 1864 and participated in the bloody battle at Cold Harbor in early June. He was wounded in this encounter but apparently not sufficiently serious to be retired; he was encamped near Petersburg in December 1864.[7]

Although the war record of Dr. McMeekin does not indicate his whereabouts during the latter months of the war, stating only that he was mustered out on April 9, 1865, with the rank of first lieutenant,[8] it is assumed that he was required to take the customary oath of allegiance to the United States.

With his military career finished Dr. McMeekin returned to his Putnam County home, resuming his dual role of physician and farmer. Living as he did in a remote part of the county, his day-to-day activities did not often come to the attention of newspaper editors in either Palatka or Ocala. Not until 1876, when he was persuaded to run for the Florida Senate, did he emerge as a public figure. A staunch Democrat in a county which was fairly equally divided between the two parties, he won the seat. The Senate *Journal* makes it clear that he was an influential member. As chairman of two committees, Agriculture and Corporations,[9] his responsibilities were considerable. He was elected once more in 1878,[10] and in 1880 to the Assembly (House) with another Putnam physician, Dr. L.L. Newsom, winning the other seat.[11] The voting results were very close with the Republican candidates, losing by margins of less than 50 votes in each instance.[12]

Henceforth Dr. McMeekin's career was apparently not out of the ordinary for a country doctor engaged in the routines of attending the local sick, running a farm, and rearing a family. Six children were born to Dr. and Mrs. McMeekin, all natives of Florida. The two oldest, Mary (called Molly) and Jefferson, were born prior to the Civil War. Jefferson appears to have come into possession of the major part of the family lands. The Census of 1900 lists him as farmer, aged 39. Others in the household were his wife, Louise, and their two-year-old son.[13] Dr. McMeekin's descendants are numerous and widely scattered. Biennial family reunions have been established by members of the clan, the gathering at Lake City in 1984 was typical.

Dr. McMeekin died at his plantation home on August 8, 1889, in his 60th year. He was buried in Ochwilla Cemetery some three miles north of the family home on State Road 21. The McMeekin house, a spacious three-story structure, equipped with eight fireplaces, still stands today. Its present owners (1984) are Mr. and Mrs. Steven Brown.

1. Dates of Dr. McMeekin's birth and death are from his gravestone, Ochwilla Cemetery, six miles south of Melrose.
2. Charleston *Courier*, March 16, 1855. Although born in Union County, there is evidence that he was a resident of Fairfield District at the time of his matriculation at the Medical College. See U.S. Census, Fairfield District, S.C., 1850, p. 232, where he is shown as a student, aged 19, resident in what appears to have been a boarding house. The Medical College records also indicate that he was a resident of Fairfield District at the time of his graduation.
3. See Frank Rathbun, "Reunion at Olustee," *North Florida Living*, April 1984, pp. 16, 17; also Frank Rathbun, "Star Cooks," *North Florida Living*, August 1984, pp. 16, 17.
4. The site of the McMeekin property is indicated on the Florida State Road Department General Highway Map, Putnam County.
5. U.S. Census, 1860, Putnam County, Florida, p. 585. Dr. McMeekin's post office was Orange Springs, Marion County, Hawthorne not being assigned a post office till 1879.
6. *Soldiers of Florida*, Live Oak, 1903, pp. 206-209.
7. National Archives, Service Records, CSA, M251, Roll 90. In this instance Dr. McMeekin's service record is somewhat garbled, lacking chronological order, and in certain parts open to question.
8. *Soldiers of Florida*, loc. cit.
9. *Florida Senate Journal*, 1877, et passim.
10. Ibid., 1879, et passim.
11. *Florida Assembly Journal*, 1881.
12. The final count was McMeekin, Democrat, 759; Newsom, Democrat, 754; C.A. Cowgill, Republican, 739; and Sawyer, Republican, 713. Tallahassee *Weekly Floridian*, November 16, 1880.
13. U.S. Census, 1900, Putnam County, Florida, 18th Precinct, item 116.

McMillan, Benjamin, Quincy, 1814

Only meager biographical information on Dr. McMillan has survived. He was born in North Carolina, the son of John McMillan[1] who was among the earliest white settlers in Gadsden County. His lands were located in the western part of the county just east of the Apalachicola River near the village of Aspalaca.

The McMillans belonged to the considerable number of Scottish people who migrated to Florida from the Cape Fear settlement of eastern North Carolina in the 1820s.

Dr. McMillan enrolled at the Medical College of the State of South Carolina in the fall of 1832 and was graduated as Doctor of Medicine in March 1834.[2] Immediately thereafter he returned to Quincy and began practice. He appears to have found a secure place in the medical faculty of the town. In 1841 he joined the four other physician of the community in setting forth a schedule of charges which would be assessed on all medical services.[3]

It is not known how long Dr. McMillan continued to practice, nor has the date of his death been ascertained. He is presumed to have been the medical preceptor for Robert McMillan, probably his brother, also of Quincy, who matriculated at the Medical College of the State of South Carolina in 1841 and was a member of the class of 1843.[4]

1. The date of Dr. McMillan's arrival in Florida is unknown. He was, however, included in the Gadsden Census of 1830.

2. Lists of Marticulants and Graduates, Medical College of the State of South Carolina, Waring Historical Library, Medical University of South Carolina, Charleston.

3. The group met "in Dr. McMillan's room" on January 6, 1841. Present, in addition to Dr. McMillan, were Drs. John M.W. Davidson, John W. Malone, William Booth and M.H. Martin, all men of prominence in the early history of Gadsden County.

4. See note 2, supra.

McMillan, James Templeton, Gainesville, 1837-1913

Dr. McMillan,[1] one of Gainesville's most beloved physicians and respected civic leaders, was born in Beaufort, South Carolina, on June 13, 1837. His parents, Thomas Moncur and Agnes Urquhart McMillan, were natives of Scotland, the former having been born in Glasgow, the latter in Edinburgh. Soon after their marriage Thomas Moncur's grandfather, a Glasgow shipbuilder, gave the young couple a sailing ship in which they crossed the Atlantic, arriving in Charleston, South Carolina, where they lived for a few years before removing to Beaufort. Young James Templeton received his early education in Beaufort where he also "read medicine" and observed medical practice and procedures as an apprentice to a local physician.

In the fall of 1859 Dr. McMillan enrolled at the Medical College of the State of South Carolina, Charleston. According to his own account:[2]

> In the year 1859 (I) returned to South Carolina, entering the South Carolina Medical College at Charleston, ...for the term 1859 and 1860, and also for 1860 and 1861 two years.

He did not, however, receive his degree, having withdrawn as the war clouds gathered in 1861, although classes at the College were not suspended until March of that year. Immediately following this interruption he went to Jacksonville where he began medical practice. This was interrupted by bombardment of Ft. Sumter in Charleston Harbor and soon after Dr. McMillan returned to the place of his birth to join the Beaufort Artillery. In a matter of days he was placed in charge of the hurriedly-constructed army hospital at nearby Hardeeville.

Dr. McMillan was scarcely settled in his new post when he received notice that his father, who had established a drug store in Starke, had fallen seriously ill. He hurried to Starke only to be greeted with the sad news that his father had died and that burial had already taken place. He was faced with a dilemma: what to do about the stock of drugs in his father's store? For reasons now unknown he decided to gather up his father's belongings, including the drugs, and open a drug store in the village of Wellborn near the eastern boundary of Suwannee County. His stay there ended in 1866 when he moved to Gainesville and, in partnership with his brother-in-law, Fitch Miller, opened a drug store on the north side of the Court House Square, an enterprise which enjoyed a long and successful existence.[3] Becoming afflicted with failing eyesight, Dr. McMillan retired from the business in 1893 after selling his interest to pharmacist-physician, Dr. J.S. Bodiford.

Notwithstanding his success as physician and pharmacist Dr. McMillan maintained an active interest in the general economic development of Alachua County. One of his major concerns was the plight of numerous families living around Alachua Lake (now known as Payne's Prairie), especially those of the Micanopy area, who had no means of transporting their produce to market, their closest railway being the Fernandina-Cedar Key line built by David Levy Yulee. Gainesville was their nearest station. But how were the people on the south side of the lake going to transport their produce to Gainesville? To solve the problem Dr. McMillan was the prime mover in establishing the Alachua Navigation and Canal Company which provided regular steamboat service across Alachua Lake.[4]

Dr. McMillan was married in 1863 to Mary Amelia,[5] a South Carolinian, whose parents, like his own, were born in Scotland. She was a woman of cultivation and good sense. Ten children were born to the couple but only four were living in 1900.[6] They were Augusta, affectionately known as Gussie, who was married to Charles F. Smith; Myra Avery, who never married; Nellie, who became the wife of Lewis C. Smith; and a son, James Harry McMillan.

Dr. McMillan was a devout Baptist, having been one of the organizers of the first church of that denomination to be built in Gainesville; this is spite of the fact that Mrs. McMillan remained a staunch Presbyterian throughout her life. She died at her Gainesville home, located at 201 North Virginia Avenue (now N.E. Second Street), on December 13, 1917. Dr. McMillan had preceded her in death, having died on September 4, 1913. He had patiently endured almost total blindness throughout his last years.[7]

1. For two important sources of biographical information on Dr. McMillan, see: Obituary notice, Gainesville *Daily Sun*, September 6, 1913; and Barbara Foster, a biographical sketch, "Civil War Caused Doctor to Move to this Area," Gainesville *Sun*, Sunday, August 23, 1887.

2. It was not uncommon in those years and later, especially in the South, for a person to obtain a license to practice medicine after only a year in medical school or even after having served an apprenticeship in the office of a practicing physician who would recommend him to the State Legislature or their authorized licensing board. After the establishment of the Florida Medical Association in 1874, licensing procedures were more rigidly controlled.

3. Long after the death of Dr. McMillan the drug store on the north side of the Square was known as the McMillan Drug Store.

4. Gainesville *Weekly Bee*, March 9, 1883. Vital information relating to this utility and its establishment is found in Caroline B. Watkins, *The Story of Historic Micanopy*, Gainesville, Alachua County Historical Commission, 1976, p. 41, et passim.

5. See note 1, supra.

6. U.S. Census, 1900, Alachua County, Florida, p. 207. See also Alachua County Cemetery Records. A copy may be found in the Gainesville Public Library. Several members of the McMillan family were buried in Evergreen Cemetery, Gainesville.

7. An obituary notice for Dr. McMillan appeared in the Gainesville *Sun*, September 6, 1913. Mrs. McMillan's obituary appeared in ibid., December 14, 1917.

McMillan, R., Quincy, 1840

Almost nothing is known of Dr. McMillan's career. He was a resident of Quincy at the time of matriculation at the Medical College of the State of South Carolina in the fall of 1842. The following spring he was graduated as Doctor of Medicine after submitting a thesis bearing the title "Prophylaxis." His preceptor prior to entering medical college had been Dr. Benjamin McMillan, thought to have been his older brother, also a graduate of the Charleston institution.[1]

1. Lists of Matriculants and Graduates, Medical College of the State of South Carolina, Waring Historical Library, Charleston.

McRae, A.L., Santa Rosa County, 1860

A.L. McRae, occupation: Doctor of Medicine, appears in the Santa Rosa Census of 1860.[1] His age was 26 and his birthplace Mississippi. He was married, his wife was 18 years old. She was also a native of Mississippi. It appears that his Milton career was brief.

1. U.S. Census, 1860, Santa Rosa County, Florida, p. 138.

McRae, Duncan J., Putnam and Orange Counties, 1827-1893

Available sources permit only a loose genealogical framework for the life of Dr. McRae. The Putnam County Census of 1870 presents several problems, one being the listing of two sons named John, ages 21 and 14. It is obvious that Dr. McRae was twice married; his second wife, a South Carolina native, is identified only as M.C., aged 34 in 1870. The children ranged in age from 21, the elder of the Johns, to Lerian, a son of four months. Of the children, four were born in Florida, four in South Carolina.

Dr. McRae settled in Florida in the late 1840s after purchasing a tract of land in the southwest corner of Putnam County in what was known as the Timmons District.[1] His post office was Waldo in Alachua County some 10 miles distant. After a few years, however, he moved to South Carolina, where four of his children were born. On his return to Florida, he settled in Sanford, at that time located in Orange County. There he lived out the last years of his life.

At the Gainesville meeting of the Florida Medical Association in 1888 Dr. McRae was proposed for membership in the organization.[2] The fact that he was readily accepted speaks well for his qualifications. He was not present at the meeting of 1889 in St. Augustine but the following year was present at the meeting in Ocala. It is understandable why, given his age, he was not present at the gathering of 1891 in Pensacola, nor that of 1892 in Key West. Death came in 1893, an event which was brought to the attention of the members of the Association at its Tampa meeting in 1894.

Dr. McRae served briefly as a sergeant in Company I, First Florida Infantry, during the Civil War. He was buried in Lakeview Cemetery, located on the south side of Sanford.[3]

1. Notwithstanding his active public life, biographical information on Dr. McRae is surprisingly scarce. The Timmons District in which he settled was totally rural. Apparently Palatka took little note of him. See Putnam County Census 1870, p. 541, item 53.

2. Dr. McRae's affiliation with the Florida Medical Association is fairly well documented in the Proceedings of

the organization in spite of his rare appearances at its annual meetings.

3. The identification of the McRae burial site is derived from the Veterans' Graves Survey, Seminole County, which provides explicit directions for locating the cemetery as well as the grave.

McRae, George W.A., Putnam County, 1829-1900

Dr. McRae was born in South Carolina in September 1829.[1] After graduating from the Medical Department, University of Georgia, Augusta, in 1853,[2] he migrated to Florida and settled in the northwestern corner of Putnam County about one mile south of the town of Melrose.[3] He apparently arrived with sufficient funds to purchase a tract of land which in 1860 was valued at $12,000.[4] The Slave Schedule of the same year numbered his slaves at 19.

With the Civil War well under way Dr. McRae enlisted for service on April 14, 1862, for a period of three years or the duration. He was given the rank of first lieutenant and assigned to Company I, Seventh Florida Infantry Regiment, commanded by ex-Governor Madison Stark Perry. There is no evidence that his duties were in any way medical. He accompanied his regiment into Tennessee where it became a part of the army of General Braxton Bragg. In the winter of 1862-63, Dr. McRae became ill with a serious lung ailment and was returned to Florida for a 60-day furlough. Failing to recover, however, he wrote to Col. Perry on March 20 that he had suffered two lung hemorrhages and upon the advice of his physician was requesting permission to resign from the service. The physician, Dr. Thomas W. McCaa of Gainesville, endorsed the request, declaring Dr. McRae "totally unfit for service" because of hemoptysis and recommending his discharge which was approved and became effective on April 22, 1863.[5]

Very little is known of Dr. McRae's activities subsequent to his discharge. Presumably he returned to his farm at McRae's Mills[6] and settled down to the life of a country doctor, while running a grist mill and cotton gin on Etonia Creek a short distance from his home. With his recovery complete by 1866 he entered into a medical partnership with Dr. J.M. Perry of Waldo. Their professional card, interestingly, was addressed to the citizens of Alachua and Marion Counties while their respective residences were some 12 miles apart.[7]

Henceforth the extent of Dr. McRae's medical practice is not clear. The Putnam County censuses of 1870 and 1880 designate him only as physician, while the special census of 1885 in its mortality schedule shows him to have been the physician of a few patients who did not recover, while designating him as M.D. and fruit grower. In the Census of 1900 he is listed as "Retired Physician." In the Florida *Gazetteer* of 1884 there appears the following entry: "McRae, G.W.A., gen'l mdse, grist mill and physician."[8]

Dr. McRae's wife, Frances, was also a native of South Carolina. They had no children of their own. The 1870 census lists younger members of the family but their ages suggest that they were younger brothers or nephews and not sons of Dr. McRae. The Census of 1880 makes it clear that the children of the household, Ellen aged seven, Archibald five, and Mattie four, were adopted, all natives of South Carolina.

Dr. McRae died at his home near Melrose on August 17, 1900, a month short of his 71st birthday. His wife, Frances, or Fannie as she was known, died on

October 18, 1902, at the age of 66. Both were buried in the Elam Cemetery just south of Melrose.

1. McRae gravestone, Elam Cemetery, Melrose.
2. *Medical Department, University of Georgia, Augusta, List of Graduates, 1829-91,* Augusta, 1891, p. 21.
3. The site of McRae's homestead was known as McRae's Mills. It is not to be confused with McRae, a few miles distant in Clay County.
4. U.S. Census, 1860, Putnam County, Florida, p. 29.
5. NA, Service Records, CSA, M251, Roll 78.
6. Dr. McRae's little community later became known as Banana. In 1875 it was assigned a post office, which was discontinued in 1894.
7. Gainesville *The New Era,* September 14, 1866.
8. Ross A. Smith, comp., The Florida State Gazetteer and Business Directory, Charleston, S.C., 1884, p. 139.

McSherry, Richard, Army Physician, 1807-1890

Florida can make only a slight claim to the services of Dr. McSherry,[1] army physician and in his later life private practitioner of distinction. Born in Martinsburg, Virginia, on November 21, 1817, he received his medical degree from the University of Pennsylvania in 1841. Previously he had served as medical officer in what Professor Charlton Tebeau has called "the Wars of Indian Removal" in Florida under the command of Colonel Zachary Taylor and later in the Mexican War under General Winfield Scott. In 1850 he published a book "embodying his Mexican experiences" entitled *Il Puchero*, or *A Mixed Dish From Mexico*, Philadelphia, 1850.

Dr. McSherry was appointed to the chair of Materia Medica at the University of Maryland in 1862 and a year later was raised in rank to a full professorship. He also found time to publish two books: *Essays and Lectures on Various Subjects*, Baltimore, 1869, and *Health, and How to Promote It*, New York, 1879. A reviewer of his writings included the following estimate of Dr. McSherry's various qualities and skills:

> He wrote good English, but was fond of apt classical quotations. His knowledge and reading were extensive and encyclopaedic. His articles were practical in character and exhibit close observation and judicious thinking. As a teacher he was safe and inclined strongly to conservatism. ....His mind was one ever open for the reception of new truths... His manners were quiet, unostentatious and grave....He was particularly polite and condescending to the young graduates. He was a strict Catholic, but his religion was never obtrusive. His professional honors included... those of first president of the Baltimore Academy of Medicine, 1877-79, and president of the Medical and Chirurgical Faculty, 1883-84.

It is obvious that Dr. McSherry possessed the finest qualities which could accrue to a member of his profession. Florida could claim, however, only an all-too-brief glimpse of this exceptional physician.

1. The information presented here is drawn almost entirely from Eugene F. Cordell, *Historical Sketch of the University of Maryland School of Medicine*, 1870-1890, Baltimore, 1991, p. 145.

Meacham, Banks, Gadsden and Liberty Counties, 1800-1895

Dr. Meacham, whose role in the early development of Gadsden County was significant, was born in North Carolina about 1800.[1] Of his early life and medical training nothing is known. As a sojourner in South Carolina during his early manhood he met and married Sarah, and there their eldest son, Byrd, was born.[2] The Meachams arrived in Gadsden County about 1827, the Doctor making his first known appearance in the Florida public records in February 1829 as a signer of a petition addressed to President Andrew Jackson requesting executive action to validate titles to land held by settlers within the area of the Forbes Purchase.[3]

The extent and nature of Dr. Meacham's medical practice cannot be estimated, nor can it be stated with certainty that he ever actually practiced in Florida in spite of the title "Doctor" invariably accorded him in Territorial records. In 1840, for example, as a leader of Gadsden County's political conservatives, "Dr. Meacham" presided at a meeting in Quincy on April 15.[4] On the other hand it is quite clear that by 1840 he had acquired land near Quincy and settled down to the life of a planter. His slaves that year numbered 40, which would have established him as a man of moderate means. Censuses of subsequent years, which include occupational designations, list him only as "farmer."

From the beginning of his Florida residence Dr. Meacham was active in the public affairs of Gadsden County. In February 1833 he was appointed justice of the peace by Governor Duval.[5] He was reappointed to that office in 1838[6] and again in 1841.[7] In the mid-1830s he was among the elite of the county who purchased shares (20) in the Central Bank of Florida and a short time later in the ill-fated Union Bank (57 shares, each at a par value of $100).[8]

Given his social and economic status he could not escape involvement in state politics. He was a successful candidate in 1833 for a seat in Florida's Legislative Council;[9] Gadsden County's other member was Joseph McBride. Seven years later, Florida in the meantime having established a bicameral legislature, he was elected to the House of Representatives[10] for the session of 1840.

Meanwhile Dr. Meacham had served his county as a delegate to the St. Joseph Convention, brought into session in 1838 to draft a constitution for the Territory in anticipation of statehood.[11] Beyond such distinctions he had shown deep concern for general civic improvement. As a trustee for both the male and female academies of Quincy, he joined other trustees in 1841 in petitioning Congress for a gift of public land adequate for establishment of other academies in the county.[12] As the effort of Floridians to obtain statehood intensified, Dr. Meacham was among the leaders, having presided over a meeting called for the purpose in Quincy on April 30, 1842.[13]

Beyond this point it is impossible to follow Dr. Meacham's career. Only a few scattered issues of Quincy newspapers of the 1850s and 1860s have survived. One of the rare extant issues is that of the Quincy *Times* of May 20, 1848, which carried a full account of a meeting of physicians of Gadsden and adjoining counties in Quincy for the purpose of establishing a Florida Medical Society. Dr. Meacham's name is conspicuously absent from the list of 12 doctors in attendance. This would appear to confirm the conclusion that by this date he was not a member of the medical fraternity.

There is sufficient evidence to suggest that by the late 1840s things had gone badly for Dr. Meacham. In 1850 his slaves had been reduced in number from 40 to 20. His seven children were still members of his household, although they ranged in age from 29 to 13.[14] In 1855 Liberty County was established out of a portion of Gadsden and Dr. Meacham was henceforth a resident of Liberty.

The Census of 1860 shows him owning only four slaves, his total properties being valued at less than $6,000.

Of the Meacham sons only Joseph was in Confederate service. He had enlisted in the Infantry Company of Capt. William T. Gregory (Co. H, 5th Fla. Inf.) on April 19, 1862, at Rickoe's Bluff of the Apalachicola River. He was killed on May 3, 1863, in the fighting at Chancellorsville. Months later Dr. Meacham appeared before a justice of the peace to make a claim for such pay as was owed his son ($109.89). In his sworn affidavit he included the statement that his deceased son "leaves neither wife, child or mother." It is thus apparent that Mrs. Meacham had died prior to July 14, 1864, the date of the claim.[15] Nothing further is known of Dr. Meacham, except that a cemetery survey of Gadsden County includes a gravestone in Quincy's Eastern Cemetery bearing the inscription: Banks Meacham Died January 25, 1895.

1. An extrapolation from the Liberty County Census of 1850, p. 15, item 137.
2. Ibid. Although the evidence is not conclusive it is probable that B.B. Meacham, an 1843 graduate of the Medical College of the State of South Carolina, Charleston (Charleston *Courier*, March 18, 1843), and listed as a resident of Colleton District of South Carolina, was Byrd Meacham, eldest son of Dr. Banks Meacham.
3. T.P., XXIV, p. 159.
4. Quincy *Sentinel*, August 21, 1840.
5. T.P., XXIV, 815.
6. Ibid., XXV, 476.
7. Ibid., XXVI, 257.
8. Ibid., XXV, pp. 47, 111. He was also an appraiser of the latter bank in 1835. Ibid., p. 135.
9. J. Randall Stanley, *History of Gadsden County*, Quincy, 1948, p. 39.
10. Ibid., p. 40.
11. For an account of the Convention see *Florida Historical Quarterly*, XVII, No. 2, 1938. The entire issue is devoted to the St. Joseph Convention in recognition of the 100th Anniversary of the event. Gadsden's other delegates were Dr. John W. Malone, Dr. John M.G. Hunter and Samuel B. Stephens. See F.W. Hoskins, "The St. Joseph Convention," Ibid., XVI, p. 41.
12. T.P., XXVI, 241.
13. Miles Kenan Womack, *Gadsden*, Quincy, 1976, pp. 30-31.
14. U.S. Census, 1850, Gadsden County, Florida, p. 367, item 195.
15. NA, Service Records, CSA, M251, Roll 65.

Meals, Henry H., Apalachicola, 1845

Dr. Meals was among a large number of physicians who settled in Florida in the mid-19th century only to discover it was not quite the paradise they had envisioned. Dr. Meals, whose origin and ultimate fate remain unknown, arrived in Apalachicola in January 1845, established himself in the Mansion House, the leading hostelry, and advertised his professional services to the citizens of the community.[1] In the following month he joined a man named Crawford in establishing a drug store on the southwest corner of Chestnut and Commerce Streets.[2] Typical of such enterprises of the times, it offered, in addition to medicines, a variety of merchandise including oils, paints and horehound candy. Dr. Meals informed his patients on May 17, 1845, that requests for his services might be left at the "Drug Store of Meals and Crawford, or at his residence opposite the New Methodist Church."[3]

For unknown reasons neither the drug store nor Dr. Meals' practice lasted the year out. The only subsequent mention of either man is found in the post office notice of October 1, 1846, to the effect that a letter was being held for Meals and Crawford.[4]

1. Apalachicola *Commercial Advertiser*, January 11, 1845. Only a few scattered issues of the Apalachicola paper have survived (none subsequent to May 17, 1845).

2. Ibid., May 17, 1845 (1st printed in issue of February 1, not extant).

3. Ibid.

4. Apalachicola, after a brief but bitter rivalry with neighboring St. Joseph for commercial advantage, gained the upper hand about 1838 while St. Joseph suffered a decline. With its location near the mouth of the Apalachicola River it became a boomtown about mid-century, serving as the entry point for vessels going up river to Columbus, Georgia, and other towns. But Dr. Meals no doubt found the competition keen since three very competent physicians, John Gorrie, Alvan W. Chapman and Samuel W. Spencer, were already there.

Means, Daniel, Alachua County, 1880

Dr. Means, a native of South Carolina, moved to Florida shortly after the Civil War and settled in the Newnansville community of Alachua County where he practiced medicine for several years. He was one of the few Negro physicians practicing in Florida in the 19th century. The Census of 1880 lists him and his wife, Easter, also a native of South Carolina, to have been the parents of four children: Lemon, 14; William, 11; Annie, nine; and Manuel, four, all born in Florida.[1] Nothing further is known of this physician and his family.[2]

1. U.S. Census, 1880, Alachua County, Florida.

2. Although it is clear, as shown in the Census of 1880, that Dr. Means had been a resident of Florida as early as 1866 (his eldest child, aged 14 in 1880, having been born in Florida), he is not listed in the Florida Census of 1870. This omission cannot be accounted for.

Means, T. Sumter, Alachua County, 1833-1900

The Florida career of Dr. Means had scarcely begun when it was terminated by the outbreak of the Civil War. He was born in Union County, South Carolina, on April 1, 1833, son of James K. and Margaret (Clowney) Means. After receiving his early education in local schools and presumably reading medicine under the direction of a local physician, he entered the University of Pennsylvania School of Medicine from which he was graduated in the spring of 1859.[1] He then spent a year or more as resident physician at Blockley Hospital in Philadelphia, resigning in the early summer of 1860.[2]

For reasons not known Dr. Means decided to go to Florida immediately, where he settled in the thriving little town of Micanopy in Alachua County adding his services to those of five other physicians already in practice there. In the initial issue of the Micanopy newspaper, which appeared on August 24, 1860, he announced his services from an office located opposite the St. Nicholas Hotel where he had taken a room.[3]

Dr. Means terminated his Micanopy practice in April 1861 and responded to the call for volunteers for military service, enlisting in a unit which a short time later would become Company C, 1st Florida Infantry Regiment, Army of the Confederacy. He entered as a private, committing himself for a period of 12 months. Within a matter of weeks the commanding officer of the outfit, 1st Lt. J.D. Turner, was promoted to a captaincy with Dr. Means becoming 1st lieutenant in his stead. Meanwhile the several Florida volunteer companies had been assembled at the Chattahoochee Arsenal in Gadsden County and on April 5 had been mustered into the Confederate Army. The regiment was then ordered to Pensacola, arriving there on April 12 to become a part of the Army of General Braxton Bragg.[4]

Dr. Means' company remained in Pensacola for several months in what was known as Camp Magnolia. On October 8, 1861, General Bragg ordered part of his troops to attack an installation held by federal troops on Santa Rosa Island across the bay from Pensacola. Dr. Means participated in the action which took place the next day. He was said to have distinguished himself by his bravery under fire.[5]

Dr. Means moved with his unit to Corinth, Mississippi, near the Tennessee border in March 1862. In a reorganization of the regiment he was promoted to the rank of captain and given command of Company B, one of four companies composing the battalion of Major T.A. McDonnell.[6] In this capacity he entered the Battle of Shiloh where he was wounded and taken prisoner. In an exchange of prisoners he was released to Confederate authority. Soon thereafter he resigned from military service; however, before the end of 1862 he reentered, spending several months in Eufaula, Alabama, in conscription service. By order of the Secretary of War, dated February 20, 1864, he was placed on detached service as Surgeon in the Confederate Hospital in Newnan, Georgia. The last months of his military career were spent as Brigade Surgeon in the Carolinas Campaign under General Joseph E. Johnston who surrendered to General Sherman on April 26, 1865, following the Confederate loss at the Battle of Bentonville, N.C.[7]

Following the War Dr. Means resumed medical practice, this time at Glenn Springs, Spartanburg County, S.C., near the place of his birth. In 1872 he moved to Spartanburg where he remained in practice until his death on June 19, 1900. He was an active member of the medical societies of Spartanburg and the State of South Carolina. In 1863 he was married to Celina E. Moore, only daughter of Dr. Maurice Moore of Glenn Springs. No children were born to the union.[8]

1. A brief biographical sketch of Dr. Means is found in J.B.O. Landrum, *History of Spartanburg County*, Atlanta, Franklin Publishing Co., 1900, pp. 464-465. The date of Dr. Means[1] graduation from medical school as cited by Landrum, 1858, seems to be in error. In its issue of March 21, 1859, the Charleston *Mercury* published a list of South Carolinians recently (March 1859) graduated from the University of Pennsylvania Department of Medicine. T. Sumter Means name is included.

2. Landrum *History*, states that he spent two years at Blockley. This appears unlikely.

3. Micanopy *Cotton States*. It is probable that Dr. Means was persuaded to settle in Micanopy by a relative, G.W. Means, a South Carolinian, lawyer and wealthy landowner, who had settled there a few years earlier. The initial issue of the *Cotton States* is not extant but the notice continued to appear in later issues.

4. Several sources for the military career of Dr. Means, each incomplete, have been consulted. See *Soldiers of Florida*, Board of State Institutions, Tallahassee, 1903, pp. 38-39. See also NA, Service Records, CSA, M251, Roll 28; Landrum, *History*, p. 464.

5. Landrum, *History*, loc. cit.

6. *Soldiers of Florida*, p. 39.

7. Landrum, *History*, loc. cit.

8. Ibid.

Mellichamp, Benjamin, Leon, Jefferson and Washington Counties, 1807

Due chiefly to his peregrinations the career of Dr. Mellichamp remains obscure. A native of South Carolina[1] and 1827 graduate of the Medical College of South Carolina, Charleston,[2] he made his initial appearance in Florida in early 1832 when he announced to "his friends and the public" that he was beginning medical practice in Leon County and could be found at "General I.W. Searcy's farm...a few miles from Tallahassee." He promised punctual attention to the various duties of his profession.[3]

Dr. Mellichamp's stay in Leon County was a mere sojourn, however, for late in 1833 he joined Dr. William F. Taylor in a medical partnership in Monticello, the county seat of Jefferson.[4] The two had apparently become acquainted earlier in the year when Dr. Taylor had practiced briefly in Leon County.[5] It is not known how long their association lasted but it is known that by 1840 Dr. Mellichamp had moved to Washington County and settled in or near the village of Econfina. There he was counted by the census enumerator along with his wife, three children and five slaves.[6] Elba Wilson Carswell, historian of Washington County, discovered that Dr. Mellichamp was one of the earliest members of Ebenezer Baptist Church, founded in 1846 on the site where the Moss Hill Church now stands. This would indicate that he had moved from Econfina into the vicinity of Vernon prior to 1846.[7]

After Florida achieved statehood in 1845 a Board of County Commissioners was established in Washington County. Dr. Mellichamp was one of four members of the first Board which took office on October 31, 1845. He was reelected the following year.[8] He was appointed as the county's first Commissioner of Fisheries in 1845, an office which he declined to accept.

Nothing further is known of Dr. Mellichamp. His name does not appear in the Florida Census of 1850 which would indicate that he had either died or left the state. He remains something of an enigma in that, with a Charleston background and prominent connections in the Charleston area, he should have chosen to lose himself in what was in the 1830s and 1840s one of the least developed areas of north Florida.

1. The Mellichamps, a family of French Huguenot origin, immigrated to the Charleston District of South Carolina in the 18th century. Abundant references to various members of the family may be found in the *South Carolina Historical and Genealogical Magazine*, redesignated *South Carolina Historical Magazine*, beginning with issue LIII, No. 1, January 1952.

2. *Centennial Memorial of the Medical College of the State of South Carolina, 1824-1924*, Charleston, 1924, p. 116.

3. Tallahassee *Floridian*, March 20, 1832, 1st printed March 13, 1832.

4. Ibid., December 21, 1833.

5. Ibid., March 30, 1833.

6. U.S. Census, 1840, Washington County, Florida, p. 179.

7. Elba W. Carswell, *Holmes Valley, a West Florida Cradle of Christianity*, Bonifay, Central Press, 1969, pp. 72, 75. The Moss Hill Church is located three miles southwest of the town of Vernon.

8. Elba W. Carswell, *Tempestuous Triangle, Historical Notes on Washington County, Florida*, Chipley, 1974, pp. 279, 298. Here the name is erroneously spelled Millichamp. See also the Jacksonville *News*, January 9, 1846.

Meredith, William E., Duval County, 1863

Only meagre biographical data concerning Dr. Meredith have survived. A resident of Jacksonville in mid-19th century, he enlisted for military service in Company A, 1st Florida Infantry Regiment, on April 5, 1861.[1] He was mustered in on April 21 at Camp Magruder, Virginia, committing his services for 12 months. His actual term of service was tragically brief, however; he was killed while walking along the plank road between Jacksonville and Lake City.

1. The brief data presented here are derived from a letter, Winston Stephens to his wife, Octavia, dated March 16, 1863. It is worthy of mentioning that Stephens did not long survive Meredith's death. He died at Cedar Creek near Jacksonville on March 4, 1864. See Stephens Papers, "Diary of Mrs. J.W. Bryant," early 1863. Mention is made of the death of Dr. Meredith, surgeon in her husband's company.

Merrill, Ayers P., Pensacola, 1822

Dr. Merrill, a native of Massachusetts, entered the Medical Department of the U.S. Army as surgeon's mate on March 19, 1819.[1] He was assigned immediately to the 8th Infantry Regiment whose headquarters at that time were near New Orleans.[2] Dr. Merrill's actual post was probably Bay St. Louis, Mississippi, some 30 miles east of New Orleans. His medical report to the Surgeon General for the third quarter of 1820 originated there.[3]

This report, judged by modern standards of practice, is something of a horror. As the "sickly season" came on Dr. Merrill faced a raging epidemic of yellow fever and as the medical officer of the post, the decisions relating to treatment were his alone. He claimed to have initiated his regimen by bleeding the patient, "extracting from 30 to 36 ounces of blood." This was followed by massive doses of calomel — 15 to 20 grains per dose—"with an equal quantity of jalap (another purgative)—with cooling mucilagenous and acidulated drink." Shortly thereafter the calomel was resumed, two or three grains every hour, "combined with a sufficient quantity of opium to prevent a cathartic effect..."[4] It was his claim, however, that no death occurred after he had begun this treatment, although 10 deaths had occurred previously.

Dr. Merrill was promoted to the rank of assistant surgeon on June 1, 1821, and his whereabouts for the next few months cannot be documented beyond the fact that early in 1822 he received $38 in remuneration for travel expenses[5] incurred in late 1821. By June 1822 he was at Ft. Barrancas as medical officer. At a meeting of the Pensacola Board of Health, of which he already was a member, held on June 10 he was unanimously nominated for the post of Health Officer for the city.[6]

In September Dr. Merrill again faced a major epidemic of yellow fever, one of the deadliest ever to attack Pensacola. Ft. Barrancas was especially hard hit—to the extent that Col. Duncan L. Clinch, commanding officer of the area, ordered an evacuation of the base, transferring the sick to a makeshift hospital near his own headquarters at Camp Hope outside Pensacola. In the meantime, however, Dr. Merrill had come down with the disease which had prompted Col. Clinch to send his own post surgeon, Dr. M.M. McMahon, to cope with the situation at Ft. Barrancas. Although Dr. McMahon's report on the situation has been lost, a fragment has been preserved in a Clinch letter, "The Doctor reports very little hope of Dr. Merrill."[7]

Perhaps miraculously, Dr. Merrill recovered. How long he remained in Florida is not known. On September 21, 1823, he resigned his commission and entered private practice.[8]

Twenty years later the name, Ayres P. Merrill, appeared on the faculty roster of the newly organized Memphis Medical College as Professor of Materia Medica and Therapeutics.[9]

1. MDUSA., p. 291.
2. Ibid. By a Congressional Act of March 2, 1821, a general reorganization of the army was ordered. As a result the number of regiments was reduced from eight to seven, with the 8th Regiment of Infantry the casualty of the order. Its personnel were reassigned.
3. Lawson, SRSMAUS, p. 20.
4. Ibid. It is recorded that General Lawson himself had advised similar treatment for "bilious remitting fever," prescribing as a preliminary measure the drawing of "12-20 ounces of blood." He also prescribed calomel in similarly large doses. See P.M. Ashburn, *History of the Medical Department of the United States Army*, Boston, 1929, pp. 45-46.
5. House Documents, Nos. 28-53, 17th Cong., 2nd Session, 1822-23, Vol. III, No. 38, p. 8. This was compensation for two trips, one in east Tennessee (Ocoee to Madisonville) and one from his base in Mississippi to the Per River (possibly Perdido) and return.

6. Pensacola *Floridian*, June 15, 1822. Dr. Merrill was actually not present at this session.
7. TP, XXII, 538-39, Col. Clinch to Acting Adj. Gen. Maj. C.J. Nourse. Camp Hope later became Cantonment Clinch.
8. MDUSA, p. 291.
9. Advertisement inside back cover of *The Charleston Medical Journal and Review*, Vol. VII, No. 4, July 1852. Although this announcement promised an opening of the College in November 1852 it did not begin operating until 1854.

Mettauer, E.M., Wakulla County, 1865

Dr. Mettauer, a native of Virginia, is listed in the Wakulla County Census of 1860 as a medical practitioner in Newport, Wakulla County, owning property valued at almost $30,000.[1] He was the sole member of his household. He died in late October or early November 1865 and on November 21 Daniel Ladd, administrator of his estate, announced the upcoming settlement.[2] His age, 33 in 1860, as well as the absence of any military record, suggest that he may have removed to Florida because of poor health and, hence, was not qualified for military service.

1. U.S. Census, 1860, Wakulla County, Florida, p. 2.
2. Tallahassee *Semi-Weekly Floridian*, November 21, 1865.

Miller, John William, Orange County, latter 19th century

Very little is known of the career of Dr. Miller who homesteaded on Lake Apopka in 1874 and soon thereafter purchased lots in Orlando on Jackson Street across from what is in more recent times Beardall Park. His property ran from Boone Street through to Orange Avenue. Dr. Miller owned a drug store at the corner of Orange Avenue and East Church Street.[1]

E.H. Gore, historian of Orange County, places the date of Dr. Miller's move to Orlando in 1881. No account of his death and burial has been located. He is known, however, to have died prior to 1898.[2]

1. E.H. Gore, *From Florida Sand to the City Beautiful*, Orlando, 1951, p. 212.
2. This assumption is inferred from the fact that the complete list of Florida physicians published by the Florida Medical Association in 1898 does not included Dr. Miller. This list was not limited to Association members.

Mills, O.P., Key West, 1831

In the early days following the purchase of Key West from Spain, a significant event of January 19, 1822, the island's importance was essentially its function as a military outpost guarding to some degree the shipping lanes in and out of the Gulf of Mexico. As a consequence the physicians who practiced there were usually attached to military units. This was true of Dr. Mills who arrived on January 2, 1831, as surgeon to the detachment from the Fourth Infantry Division.[1] His arrival in the town was also noted by William R. Hackley who on January 3, 1831, recorded the arrival of troops at the army post, "among them Lieutenant Newcomb and his Lady, Lieut. Manning and Dr. Mills."[2] Nothing more is known of him.

1. Key West Gazette, March 28, 1831.
2. "The Diary of William R. Hackley, 1830-1857," P.K. Yonge Library of Florida History, Gainesville.

Mims, James M., Gadsden and Suwannee Counties, 1833

The career of Dr. Mims appears to have been brief. Born in Orangeburg District, South Carolina, he had moved into Gadsden County prior to 1850. In that year the census enumerator located him as a resident in the household of Jacob Bradcock, also born in South Carolina, a fairly prominent farmer living near Quincy. The Bradcock household was exceptional in that it included, in addition to Bradcock, his wife and five children, Samuel Love, sheriff of Gadsden County; Edward Byron, a 35-year-old physician; William K. Johnson, an English-born watchmaker, and two other South Carolinians, Clark Matthews and Joseph Dunn.[1]

Young Mims began medical study under the guidance of Dr. Byron. Prior to entering medical school, however, he returned to Orangeburg to complete an apprenticeship under Dr. J.F. Rumph,[2] who graduated from the Medical College of South Carolina in 1836. Mims enrolled at that institution in the fall of 1853 and was graduated in March 1854.[3]

Henceforth the career of Dr. Mims becomes obscure. In the Suwannee County Census of 1860, there is listed "James Mims, aged twenty-six, South Carolina-born, a farmer." This entry is followed by "James Mims, Sr., South Carolina-born, farmer, aged sixty-nine," owning property valued at only $1300.[4] Was the younger James Mims the physician?

The Civil War record of a James Mims sheds little light. Information on the 8th Florida Infantry Regiment, Company H, lists a James Mims, private, who enlisted in Columbia County in the 8th Florida Infantry Regiment on January 27, 1862. His record, if indeed he was the person being considered here, was dismal. He is shown to have deserted on July 11, 1862.[5]

No further information on Dr. Mims has been discovered.

1. U.S. Census, Gadsden County, Florida, p. 342, item 23.
2. *List of Graduates of the Medical College of the State of South Carolina*, Charleston, 1924, p. 118.
3. Ibid., p. 124. He gave his home address as Quincy. His doctoral thesis bore the title, "Hygiene."
4. U.S. Census, 1860, Suwannee County, Florida, p. 783.
5. National Archives, Civil War Records, 3rd Florida Infantry Regiment, Co. H.

Mims, Thomas S., Gadsden County, 1850

Dr. Mims, a native of Barnwell, South Carolina, and graduate of the Medical College of the State of South Carolina, Charleston, practiced medicine in Gadsden County during the 1850s. His doctoral thesis bore the title, "Acute Gastritis."[1] His presence in Florida is verified somewhat indirectly in records of the Medical College of Georgia which show that he had been the preceptor of Thomas Tabb of Sandy Ford (later to be known as Greenville) in Gadsden County.[2] Dr. Mims' residence in Florida was brief. As the War Between the States became imminent he apparently returned to his native state.

1. Charleston *Mercury*, March 27, 1840. Report of the commencement of the College and list of graduates receiving degrees on March 19.
2. Records of the Medical College of Georgia, Augusta. Lists of Graduates.

Minding, (Christian name unknown), Hernando County, 1850

Dr. Minding, whose given names are unknown, was a native of Mississippi.

For a brief period in the mid-19th century he practiced medicine in the Buddy's Lake Settlement of Hernando County.[1] He shared a house with a laboring man named Augustus Mizell, also a Mississippi native. Since his name does not appear in the Census of 1860, it is presumed that he did not linger long in Florida.[2]

1. The name of Hernando County was changed to Benton on March 6, 1844, to honor U.S. Senator Thomas Hart Benton of Missouri. Benton had endeared himself to many for his support of measures reducing the price of public lands, suppression of land speculation and other legislation calculated to make land more available to settlers. His antislavery stand led to failure to regain his Senate seat in 1850. It also brought the change of the county name back to Hernando.

2. See U.S. Census, 1850, Benton County, Florida, item 25.

Mitchell, Benjamin J.J., Madison County, mid-19th century

Dr. Mitchell's Florida medical career appears to have been brief. The meager biographical data relates more to his political activity than medical practice. A native of Georgia, he attended the Medical College of Georgia, Augusta, from which he was graduated in 1843.[1] A year or so later he moved to Madison where he soon became a leader in the Democratic Party. In the summer of 1847 he was persuaded to enter the race for the Florida House of Representatives and although there were numerous candidates for the county's two seats he won by a fairly comfortable margin while another Democrat, Thomas A. Hall, won the other seat.[2] B.G. Liddon, an ardent Whig, had only a short time earlier begun publication of the *Florida Whig* in Marianna, and in a doleful editorial in the second issue, October 6, 1847, he blamed the defeat of his party on its lackadaisical attitude and failure to organize.

There is no reason to label Dr. Mitchell an exceptional member of the Florida House; he was, however, competent and conscientious. His standing committee assignments were Finance and Public Accounts (a very demanding assignment) and Propositions and Grievances. Toward the end of the session he exhibited a praiseworthy stance when the legislative body received a communication from the National Medical Convention, which had met in Philadelphia in May 1847, announcing the formation in Pennsylvania of a state agency responsible for the Registration of Births, Marriages and Deaths occurring therein and urging the Florida Legislature to organize a similar agency.[3] A committee of five was appointed to consider the matter and report to the full body. The committee consisted of three physicians, Drs. Mitchell, John L. Crawford and James L. Shields, and two others, Daniel Bradwell and the chairman, W.O. Forward. This very worthwhile proposal failed to gain the support of a majority of the House, however, and Florida waited until 1899 when its Central Bureau of Vital Statistics was established.

A second argument employed by proponents of a Bureau of Vital Statistics brought under consideration the excessively high life insurance rates prevailing in Florida—twice as high as those in other states—which might well be lowered by revealing the causes of death and giving a true estimate of the relative duration of life in Florida as compared with that of other states. It was also brought to the attention of the House that clerks of county courts were already required to register all marriages; adding a record of births and deaths would not place an unreasonable burden upon them. This argument, too, was unavailing.[4]

Apparently disappointed, possibly disgusted, with the refusal of the House to give serious consideration to their proposal, the committee drew up a bill, "which they respectfully submit for the consideration of the House, and ask to be discharged from further consideration of the subject."[5]

With the triumph of the Whig Party in national politics, Zachary Taylor followed James K. Polk, a Democrat, into the White House. In local politics even in remote Florida the Whig Party took control. In the Jackson County elections of the first of October 1848, Whigs handily captured the two seats in the House with Dr. Mitchell coming in fifth out of a field of six. Editor Liddon had cause to gloat.[6]

No further information on Dr. Mitchell has been located. His name does not appear in the Census of 1850. It is, therefore, concluded that he had either died or left Florida by that date.[7]

1. Medical Department, University of Georgia, *List of Graduates from 1829 to 1891*, Augusta, 1890, p. 22.
2. Marianna *Florida Whig*, October 6, 1847.
3. Florida House of Representatives, *Journal of Proceedings*, Tallahassee, 1847, p. 5, et passim.
4. Ibid., p. 167.
5. Ibid.
6. This defeat was a devastating blow to Dr. Mitchell. It had come about largely as a result of the enormous popularity of Zachary Taylor, hero of the Mexican War and a Whig adherent, who was elected president.
7. Although the survey of Jackson County cemeteries includes the names of dozens of Mitchells, Dr. Mitchell's name is not among them. It is conjectured that he returned to his native Georgia to spend his last years.

Mitchell, Charles L., Polk County, 1848-1900

Dr. Mitchell, an eminent citizen and beloved physician of Polk County, was born in the Alifia Settlement of eastern Hillsborough County in 1848. He was the son of Thomas and Elizabeth (nee Stearns) Mitchell, who had moved to Florida from Alabama in the mid-1820s.[1] When Charles Mitchell was still a small boy his family settled on a farm in the vicinity of Tampa and it was there that he received his education. The name of his medical preceptor is not known. In the fall of 1868 he matriculated at the Medical College of the State of South Carolina, Charleston, from which he was graduated on March 1, 1870.[2]

Soon after receiving a degree Dr. Mitchell returned to Hillsborough County, launching his career in Tampa where his brother, Henry Laurens Mitchell, later to become Governor of Florida (1893-97), had established a law practice. For at least a brief period Dr. Mitchell was a member of his brother's household.[3]

After two years of practice in Tampa Dr. Mitchell moved to Ft. Meade, at that time a mere village in Polk County located 10 miles south of Bartow, the county seat. He became Ft. Meade's first resident physician.[4] Although the people of the little community were no doubt pleased to have a physician, the reasons for his departure from Tampa, then a rapidly growing city, to live and practice in a somewhat remote rural area, remain unknown. Of course Polk County had a bright future.

Meanwhile Dr. Mitchell had married. His wife known to us only by her Christian name, Ellen, was a native of Florida, some eight years junior to her husband. Several children were born to this marriage.[5]

Surprisingly Dr. Mitchell gave up medical practice in 1882,[6] leaving patients in the hand of Dr. M.O. Arnold. He continued to live in Ft. Meade, however, until 1899 when he moved to Bartow where he died on March 15, 1900,[7] a victim of la grippe. His brother, ex-Governor Mitchell, and other members of his family were at his bedside when death came.

1. Thomas Mitchell was a native of South Carolina; his wife, Elizabeth, was born in Tennessee. They had begun their married life in Georgia, later moving to Alabama before moving to Florida.
2. Charleston, S.C., *Daily Courier*, March 2, 1870.
3. U.S. Census, 1870, Hillsborough County, Florida, p, 44.
4. M.F. Hetherington, *History of Polk County, Florida*, St. Augustine, 1928, p. 79.
5. U.S. Census, 1880, Polk County, Florida, p. 24, item 299; ibid., 1900, Town of Bartow, p. 47.
6. Hetherington, *History*, p. 76.
7. Bartow *Courier-Informant*, March 21, 1900. The notice here printed is a lengthy eulogy containing no biographical data.

Mitchell, Henry N., Quincy, 1836

Dr. Mitchell, a Georgia native and 1856 graduate of the Medical College of Georgia, Augusta, practiced for a short time just prior to the outbreak of the Civil War. The Census of 1860 shows him unmarried and living alone in or near Quincy. His property was valued at $800. Since nothing more is known of him it is presumed that he left Florida for his native state, possibly for military service.[1]

1. U.S. Census, 1860, Gadsden County, Florida, p. 91, item 684. For reference to Dr. Mitchell's medical degree see *Medical Department, University of Georgia*. "List of Graduates, 1829-1891," Augusta, 1891, p. 22.

Mitchell, Isaac W., Leon County, 1830

Nothing is known of Dr. Mitchell's early years whose Florida residence began in the late 1820s and career in Leon County spanned more than a decade. His place of origin, youth, as well as medical education are still undiscovered despite the fact that his role in political and medical affairs in Leon County was significant. He appeared in Tallahassee, probably in 1828, and on January 31, 1829, purchased a house on North Calhoun Street from Turbott R. Betton, later known as the Bowen House.[1]

Although a newcomer (most Tallahasseans were newcomers) he announced his candidacy for a seat in the Legislative Council in February.[2] By election time the candidates for the county's two seats numbered eight, but Dr. Mitchell was a winner, along with Thomas Brown.[3] Dr. Mitchell's performance as a legislator, however, was undistinguished and when in the following year he sought the office again he ran third in a field of five.[4] As a legislator on one occasion he cast the deciding vote which defeated a bill to suppress dueling.[5]

Among the physicians practicing in Tallahassee Dr. Mitchell appears to have been a maverick. He was not among the five who on February 2, 1833, published a list (31 items) of fees which they had agreed to charge for their various medical and surgical services.[6] Some four weeks later, however, possibly responding to public pressure, he published his own list, preceded by an introductory statement laden with sarcasm.

> Now the very intelligent brethren of the faculty of the City of Tallahassee, who possess so eminently too, so much of the learning and science of the profession, are assured that their own peculiar elysium is not about to be invaded, that their fee bill of happy memory is not either about being attacked, nor a new version given...If there be any who feel any indisposition to pay the price set forth below, he [i.e. Mitchell] would most respectfully request them not to honor him with their calls...

There follows his list of 26 items which in several instances are slightly less dear than the charges published by his colleagues.[7]

Such petulance does not appear to have affected Dr. Mitchell's status in the community; however, he remained an active participant in civic matters. In February 1833, he was a gubernatorial appointee as appraiser to the much-troubled Union Bank of Tallahassee.[8] In 1836 he was vice president of a Leon County group organizing a public dinner honoring Major Leigh Read for his gallantry against the Indian raiders along the Withlacoochee River.[9] The affair featured castigations and denunciations aimed at General Winfield Scott, then in very bad odor among Floridians for having abandoned the beleaguered Florida volunteers in their struggle to protect their homes against the Creeks. Dr. Mitchell set the tone with an imprecatory toast.[10] In 1838 he was among those lauding Governor Call for his defense efforts "in spite of the fact that the Federal Government has not done its share."[11]

Information concerning the Mitchell family is meager and some details defy verification. The 1830 census lists him as residing outside Tallahassee; two males under five are included, presumably his two sons, Thomas and William. His own age appears as between 30 and 40. The two females are doubtless his wife, between 30 and 40, and mother-in-law, between 60 and 70.[12] St. John's Episcopal Church, Tallahassee, records indicate that he was a parishioner in 1832, while both he and his two sons, Thomas and William, were baptized in 1837.[13]

Dr. Mitchell is said to have owned land a few miles north of Tallahassee in the area known today as Killearn Lakes Properties. His other property was on the south shore of Lake Iamonia where his name has survived as Mitchell Point and Mitchell Island within the lake. On this land is located the cemetery, much neglected, where Mrs. Mitchell was buried. Her gravestone bears the inscription: "To the Memory of Ann Mitchell, who Departed this Life on April 6, 1837. Age 38. Wife of Dr. Isaac Mitchell." The only other gravestone presumably marks the burial place of Mrs. Mitchell's mother. It bears the inscription:

"Prussia Cole, who departed this life, Mar. 19, 1837. Aged 68 Years."[14]

Nothing is known of the later years of Dr. Mitchell, nor of the time and place of his death. Conceivably he lived out his life quietly on Lake Iamonia. If he were indeed buried in the Mitchell Cemetery, there was none to place a marker at his grave.

1. Evelyn W. Henry, "Old Houses of Tallahassee," Tallahassee Historical Society Annual, I, 26.
2. Tallahassee *Florida Advocate*, February 28, 1829.
3. Ibid., June 13, 1829.
4. Tallahassee *Floridian and Advocate*, January 5, 1830; August 17, 1830.
5. Tallahassee *Florida Advocate*, October 27, 1829, and subsequent issues.
6. Tallahassee *Floridian*, February 2, 1833.
7. Ibid., March 9, 1833; April 6, 1833.
8. TP., XXIV, 815.
9. Tallahassee *Floridian*, June 18, 1836.
10. Ibid.
11. Ibid., February 3, 1838.
12. U.S. Census, Leon County, Florida, p. 235.
13. "Parish Records, St. John's Episcopal Church, Tallahassee." Copied under auspices, Tallahassee Chapter, DAR, Tallahassee, 1936, pp. 9, 13.
14. Joy Smith Paisley, comp. & ed., "The Cemeteries of Leon County, Florida." Mimeographed, Tallahassee, 1978, p. 83.

Mitchell, Joseph Davis, Jacksonville, 1823-1893

Dr. Mitchell,[1] who from 1852 till 1893 (with the exception of the years of the Civil War) was an eminent practitioner in Jacksonville, was born on a farm near West Newfield, Maine, on March 10, 1823. Life on a New England farm in the early 19th century was rigorous but it developed in young Mitchell a toughness of character and mind which lingered with him throughout his long and useful life. As for his early education, he is said to have been largely self-taught. In his teens he attended a local seminary, working to pay the expenses of tuition and board. He was graduated in 1845 and the following year gained admission to the Harvard Medical School from which he received a medical degree in 1850.[2]

Dr. Mitchell began practice in St. Stephens, New Brunswick, where he remained for two years before moving to the more benign climate of Jacksonville. There he practiced for 10 years, building for himself a splendid reputation as physician and surgeon. A major event of the decade was his marriage in 1858 to Myra H. Chase, like himself, a native of West Newfield, Maine.

With the War Between the States already under way Dr. Mitchell in 1862 followed the dictates of his conscience and conviction by offering his services to the Union Army, feeling that the Union cause was the just cause. His first military assignment took him to Beaufort, South Carolina, already under Union control, where he took over management of the general hospital. Before the end of 1862, however, he was commissioned surgeon and transferred to the Eighth Maine Volunteers. In 1864 he was assigned the post of Surgeon to the Thirty-first Maine Regiment, which was regarded as the finest of the Maine units, having the rare distinction of being composed of soldiers six feet tall or taller.

At the end of the war in 1865 Dr. Mitchell returned to Jacksonville and resumed practice. One would expect hostility from the local people on his return but such was not apparent. Perhaps his honesty and firmness of character brought him general acceptance. If animosity were present it was not openly expressed. The diligent effort put forth by both Dr. Mitchell and Mrs. Mitchell in establishing St. Luke's Hospital, Jacksonville's first, which was opened on March 11, 1873,[3] would have helped dissipate any ill feeling.

The last two decades of Dr. Mitchell's life were, professionally, very successful. He had established himself as a physician of exceptional insight and ability and enjoyed the respect of his professional colleagues. Furthermore he had established a lucrative practice and had no pecuniary worries. In 1878 the Florida Medical Association meeting[4] at the Florida Yacht Club in Jacksonville had elected him to membership, and yet he was plagued with physical problems. In his youth he had suffered a knee injury which had never properly healed, leaving him permanently lame. In his later years in Jacksonville he could be frequently seen making his rounds in a wheelchair and sometimes on pony back. Besides, in early life he was the victim of a severe case of pneumonia, accompanied by lung hemorrhages, leaving his lungs permanently weak and susceptible to frequent pulmonary disorders.

On the advice of his family and probably some of his colleagues he was persuaded to curtail his practice or abandon it completely. In the early 1880s he gradually relinquished his practice to his elder son, Neal, who had begun his medical practice in Jacksonville in 1881. A few years later, the younger son,

Sollace, also a physician, joined Neal in practice in Jacksonville.

Dr. Mitchell died at his home at the corner of Forsyth and Julia Streets in Jacksonville on July 15, 1893, following a recurring attack of fever. He was buried in Jacksonville's Evergreen Cemetery.[5] Mrs. Mitchell lived on until May 19, 1915. Dr. Mitchell's death evoked many expressions of love and respect. The following excerpt from the Florida Times-Union, Jacksonville, of July 16, 1893, is indicative of the esteem in which he was held.

> Dr. Mitchell was one of the most prominent physicians, not only in this city and state, but in the South, and was recognized as an authority on medical matters, especially on consumption. His reputation as a skillful physician was well-known in the North where he had many friends.... He was an honest, upright man, and commanded the utmost respect and confidence of every one in the community. His death is a great loss to this city where he was one of the leading and oldest citizens.

1. The chief sources of information on Dr. Mitchell are: Obituary, Jacksonville *Florida Times-Union*, July 16, 1893; Webster Merritt, *A Century of Medicine in Jacksonville and Duval County*, Gainesville, University of Florida Press, 1949, pp. 56-57, and *Proceedings, Florida Medical Association*, Jacksonville, 1894, pp. 45-50.
2. While a student at Harvard Medical School Dr. Mitchell is said to have assisted in a surgical operation in which the anesthesia used was ether, said to have been its first use. This is open to question, however, in that Dr. Crawford Long of Jefferson, Jackson County, Georgia, had first used it in surgery on March 30, 1842. See Arturo Castiglioni, *A History of Medicine*, trans. by E.B. Krumbhaar, New York, Alfred A. Knopf, 1958, p. 723.
3. Merritt, *A Century of Medicine*, p. 86.
4. *Proceedings, Florida Medical Association*, Jacksonville, 1878, p. 11.
5. *Grave Markers of Duval County, 1808-1916*, Comp. by Lucy Ames Edwards, Jacksonville, 1955, p. 159.

Mitchell, W.J., Pensacola, 1808-1884

The brief Florida career of Dr. Mitchell remains obscure. He was born in Charlottesville, Virginia, in 1808,[1] but there is no proof that he was ever a student at nearby University of Virginia. At an unknown date he married Emily (family name missing), a native of Columbia County, Georgia.[2] Since his two daughters were natives of Alabama (Mary and Kate, aged 17 and 11 respectively in the Census of 1860), perhaps he practiced for some years in Alabama.[3]

Dr. Mitchell appears to have migrated to Florida in 1866 for his professional card first appeared in the Pensacola newspaper in November that year. It bore the information that his office was located on Palafox Street "next to Maloney's Store."[4] In early January 1872 it was announced that he had moved to Henry Cushman's Drug Store and would occupy the office previously belonging to Dr. B.A. Hill.[5] He had ceased to practice quite some time before his death which occurred on April 25, 1884.[6] The cause was stated to have been "General Debility." His survivors included his wife, Emily, who died in 1887,[7] daughter, Mary (Mrs. Grace),[8] and daughter, Kate, who is shown in the 1885-86 *Pensacola Directory* to have been a liquor dealer operating at the wharf at the foot of Palafox Street.

1. Gravestone, St. Michael's Cemetery, Pensacola. Another W.J. Mitchell received a degree from the Medical College of Georgia, Augusta, in 1876 and was a resident of Georgia at the time of matriculation.
2. Ibid., the dates given are 1813-1887.
3. U.S. Census, 1870, Escambia County, Florida, item 250.
4. Pensacola *West Florida Commercial*, November 15, 1867. First printed in issue of November 18, 1866 (not extant).
5. Pensacola *Mail*, January 30, 1872.
6. Pensacola *Commercial*, May 3, 1884. Listed in mortuary report for April 1884.
7. Gravestone, St. Michaels Cemetery.
8. Ibid.

Montgomery, Lucius, Alachua County, 1841-1914

Dr. Montgomery, one of Alachua County's most respected citizens, was born in Missouri in 1841.[1] Nothing is presently known of his early years, professional training, or ancestry. He arrived in Florida soon after the end of the Civil War and after surveying the various possibilities decided to settle in Micanopy, which he considered the loveliest place he had seen. Besides it was the largest town in the whole area and seemed to offer the greatest opportunity. He was soon able to earn a splendid reputation both as physician and enterprising businessman. Except for opposition to incorporation of the town,[2] he was supportive of nearly every civic enterprise calculated to improve the conditions for living.

An innovative and visionary man, Dr. Montgomery was quick to invest in and around Micanopy, notably a tract of land on nearby Lake Levy on which he planted orange trees. These he carefully cultivated thereby producing fruit of excellent quality. The warmth of the lake water was sufficient to preserve the trees through cold winters, even the severe freeze of 1894, with only minimal damage. Besides his groves Dr. Montgomery engaged in other enterprises. Carl Webber, who visited Micanopy about 1881-82, recalled that "adjoining his grove he has a cotton gin and a grist mill, both of which are run by steam power."[3] On October 26, 1879, the Gainesville *Sun* published the following:

> Dr. Lucius Montgomery has his steam machinery now in operation, with a new improved Harrison Mill, which ran last Saturday to the satisfaction and admiration of all. In addition, he is ginning and grinding...He expects this fall to put in machinery for cleaning and polishing rice.

Dr. Montgomery was a civic-minded man, illustrated by his gift of two acres of land for a town cemetery. His concern for the low quality of education led him to organize a private school, begun primarily for the education of his son, Harvey, but available to a few other children. He is said to have consulted with certain colleges in an effort to obtain qualified teachers.[4] In the area of religion he leaned toward Presbyterianism, becoming a trustee of the local church and giving it financial support.

Dr. Montgomery was twice married. His first wife, Madora (called Dora), a native of Laurens, South Carolina, was drowned in Orange Lake on June 16, 1871. No children resulted from this union. He then married another South Carolinian, known only as L.J. She was 11 years his junior. To this marriage was born the aforementioned Harvey on February 26, 1876.[5]

There can be no doubt that Dr. Montgomery enjoyed the good life. He was highly regarded as both citizen and physician. He built a spacious home (unfortunately destroyed by fire in 1930) adequate to accommodate guests as well as boarders. Carl Webber, a writer who traveled extensively in the South, lingered for several weeks in Alachua County, which he described at length in his book *Eden of the South*. He devoted a full page to Dr. Montgomery. A portion bears citing.[6]

> Dr. Lucius Montgomery, of Micanopy, has his residence there, an orange grove containing 600 trees, occupying 21 acres of ground. These trees are planted 35 feet apart, and a number of them, thirteen years from seed, measure 41 inches in circumference....He also has a number of lemon trees, the Cicily (sic) and ever-bearing varieties which, with his house and stable, occupy three acres more....He keeps cattle of the improved breed, and five hundred head of poultry....He feeds his cows largely on wheat bran. They give excellent milk in generous quantities, from which comes the richest milk. At Kirkwood, near Levy's Lake,

the doctor has 800 orange trees planted in verdant hammock land...Two and a half miles northeast of Micanopy he has 220 trees on forty acres.

Elsewhere Webber described the Montgomery residence as "the finest in town. It is two stories high, with a two-story cupola, and is built in the finest style of architecture." Census records indicate that the daily upkeep of the mansion was handled by two live-in black servants.

Dr. Montgomery died on the evening of May 11, 1914, of a heart attack. For the previous few days he had mentioned not feeling well. On the afternoon of the 11th he took a walk to his orange grove, some three miles distant. On returning he decided to rest before supper. An hour or so later Mrs. Montgomery went to the bedroom to summon him only to find him dead. Mrs. Montgomery and son, Harvey, also a physician, survived.

1. Dr. Montgomery's grave marker in the Micanopy Cemetery gives the date of his birth as 1841; the Census of 1900 indicates that he was born in October 1842.

2. Thirty-three Micanopy citizens voted on the issue. Of these 25 favored incorporation, eight opposed. Of the six physicians voting five were opposed, only Dr. F.E. Carn voted for. Ms. James D. Glunt Papers, P.K. Yonge Library of Florida History, Manuscript Collection.

3. Carl Webber, *The Eden of the South*, New York, Leve & Alden, 1883, p. 97.

4. Caroline B. Watkins, *The Story of Historic Micanopy*, Gainesville, Alachua County Historical Commission, 1976, p. 57.

5. Gravestone, Micanopy Cemetery. Harvey died on June 18, 1924.

6. Webber, loc. cit.

Moody, Sloman William, Marion County, 1834-1898

Dr. Moody, for more than 40 years a citizen of Marion County, was a native of Sumter, South Carolina. With the early death of his father the responsibility for bringing up young Sloman rested with his mother, Susan.[1] His earliest employment, entered upon when he was still an adolescent, was an apprenticeship in a print shop, but soon developing an interest in medicine he went to Columbia where he found work as a clerk in a drug store.[2] In his spare time he began reading medicine in the office of the eminent surgeon Dr. Samuel Fair, said to have been the finest surgeon in the state. When Dr. Fair and his associate, Dr. Huot, began offering lectures in anatomy and surgical procedures, Moody was among their students. Moving on to the Medical College of the State of South Carolina in the fall of 1855 he was graduated in the fall of 1857, having submitted a thesis on "Syphilis" and achieving honors.[3]

Soon after graduation Dr. Moody moved to Ocala, doubtless persuaded to settle there by former South Carolinians who were numerous in Marion County. From the beginning he appears to have been a popular and successful practitioner. His eulogist described him as an exceptionally handsome man, endowed with a splendid physique, gentleness of spirit and "Chesterfieldian" manners. In 1860 he married Carrie Howse, second daughter of Capt. Edward D. Howse, well-to-do Marion County planter. This happy union to which two children were born was sadly terminated by Mrs. Moody's death soon after birth of the younger child, a daughter also named Carrie. Two years later Dr. Moody married Annie, younger sister of his first wife. This marriage, blessed by the birth of a son, Edward, ended sadly after only two years with Mrs. Moody's untimely death. Dr. Moody's third wife was Eliza Pierson, daughter of the prominent Col. John

W. Pierson of Orange Springs. This marriage produced nine children, seven sons and two daughters, all of whom outlived their father.

About the time of his third marriage Dr. Moody moved to Orange Springs, a village north of Ocala near the Putnam County line. His sojourn there was brief, however, and within a few months he moved to Palatka where he purchased a drug store, harking back to his early experience in Columbia. He appears to have been successful. An Ocalan visiting in Palatka in August 1874 wrote: "...we had the pleasure of meeting an old citizen of Ocala in the person of Dr. S.W. Moody.... The Doctor is prospering in life and is delighted with his new home." In another dispatch he added: "Dr. Moody has a handsome and well-appointed Drug Store in the business center of the town and is rapidly acquiring a good practice," adding, Dr. Moody "is the most valuable acquisition, both as a citizen, a physician, and a business man Palatka has had since the surrender of the Confederacy."[4]

For reasons not known Dr. Moody returned to Ocala with his family, which then included seven children, in 1879. He resumed medical practice but with a large and increasing family he felt the need for additional sources of income. He purchased a tract of land just east of the town on which he planted orange trees which, with the help of his numerous sons, he was able to develop into a profitable enterprise. On the property he also built a handsome dwelling. Success prompted him to invest in additional acreage also to be planted in oranges but to achieve this he mortgaged his other properties. The promising project was well under way when the great freeze of the winter of 1894-95 destroyed everything. He was left practically penniless.

The disaster virtually destroyed Dr. Moody physically as well as financially. Soon thereafter Bright's disease developed which, in spite of his fine physique and robust health, proved fatal on March 20, 1898. He was 64.[5]

Professionally Dr. Moody was an outstanding physician. He was a strong and good man whose presence instilled trust and hope in his patients. As a citizen he served his community well. Although he never ran for public office he held the appointive post of county treasurer for two terms in the days when no bond was required of the holder. In politics he was a Democrat.

Dr. Moody was elected to membership in the Florida Medical Association in 1890. Although there is no record of his having attended an annual meeting, he is known to have paid his dues for 1890 and 1891. Membership was discontinued in 1896 for nonpayment of dues but by that time his health was seriously impaired.[6]

Dr. Moody's funeral was held in the Ocala Methodist Church which he had attended only irregularly. He was buried in Greenwood Cemetery. His eldest sons were pallbearers. His eulogist described it as a "pathetically sad but beautifully touching sight."

Unless otherwise indicated the information in this sketch is derived from a lengthy obituary-eulogy published in the Ocala *Banner* of March 25, 1898. Some uncertainty exists as to the spelling of Dr. Moody's first name. In several instances it appears as Solomon but more often as Sloman, and occasionally as Slowman.

1. U.S. Census, 1850, Sumter District, S.C., p. 876, item 1872. This entry lists Mrs. Moody's age as 45, her son's as 17 (presumed an error). They were residents of Sumterville, later to be known simply as Sumter.
2. Ocala *Banner*, March 25, 1898.
3. Archives, MCSSC, MUSC, Lists of Matriculants and Graduates. For further information on Drs. Fair and Huot see Joseph I. Waring, *A History of Medicine in South Carolina, 1825-1900*, Charleston, 1967, pp. 89, 228.
4. One of the few extant issues of the Palatka *Eastern Herald*, that of April 13, 1874, contains Dr. Moody's adver-

tisement of "FRESH GARDEN SEED," obtainable at THE PALATKA DRUG STORE. See also the Ocala *East Florida Banner*, September 5, 1874.

5. A brief obituary notice for Dr. Moody appeared in the Jacksonville *Times-Union* of March 22, 1898.

6. *Transactions, Florida Medical Association*, Jacksonville, 1890, et. seq.

Moore, Matthew L., Suwannee and Columbia Counties, 1830-1870

In March 1858 Dr. Moore announced his intention to launch a medical practice in the village of New Boston[1] in Suwannee County. Census data, although not necessarily reliable, indicate that he was born in Georgia about 1830. He is thought to have prepared himself for medical practice by serving as an apprentice to a practicing physician.[2] He was living in the vicinity of New Boston by 1860, a mere village which enjoyed the distinction of having a post office from 1857 to 1867. The 1860 Census, Suwannee County, lists him as "physician," whose wife, Elinor, was 11 years younger. His properties were valued at more than $2,000.

For the war years, 1861-1865, no trace of Dr. Moore's activities or whereabouts has been found but it is probable that he returned to Georgia to serve in a military unit. He had returned to Florida by 1870 and was living in the vicinity of Suwannee Shoals. His property value had diminished to less than $1,000. He was obviously carrying on a small farming enterprise in addition to a medical practice. The census entry shows David L. Moore, farm laborer, aged 24, native of Louisiana, as a member of the Moore household.[3]

The Florida Census of 1880 yields no information relating to Dr. Moore. It is fairly certain, however, that at some time in the early 1880s he had become a resident of Alachua County. Soon thereafter he accepted the invitation to become a member of the Alachua County Medical Society; he was expelled from the organization in 1887. At the annual meeting of the Florida Medical Association in St. Augustine in early May, Dr. R.A. Lancaster in his report of the activities of the Alachua County Medical Society made the following statement: "Things are O.K. except for the painful duty of expelling a member for criminal abortion." When the Chairman asked for the name of the guilty party, Dr. M.L. Moore was named.[4]

In spite of the disgrace which Dr. Moore was presumed to have suffered the incident apparently had little effect on his local reputation. He did not linger long in Gainesville, however. In its issue of May 26, 1887, the Gainsville *Alachua Advocate* published the following item:[5]

> Dr. M.L. Moore left yesterday for Los Angeles, California, where he will take a half interest in the extensive practice of Dr. Bidwell of that city. Dr. Moore has perhaps as many friends in Gainesville as any other man in our City, and his departure will be much lamented. His office here will be taken charge of by Dr. A.L. Wagner, a young man who graduated last year from the London, England, College of Physicians and Surgeons. Dr. Moore left in answer to a telegram telling him to come at once. His family will follow him in a short time.

His departure had none of the aspects of being driven out of town on a rail.

1. Alligator Lake City, *Columbia Democrat*, November 27, 1858.

2. Dr. Moore was born and reared in Georgia but he apparently did not attend any of the three or four medical colleges existing in Georgia in the mid-19th century nor was he a student at the prestigious Medical College of the State of South Carolina, Charleston.

3. U.S. Census, 1870, Columbia County, Florida, Town of Suwannee Shoals, p. 361.

4. *Proceedings, Florida Medical Association*, 1887, p. 17.

5. This issue of the Alachua *Advocate* is quite faded, but still legible.

Moragne, Nathaniel H., Palatka, 1826-1880

Dr. Moragne, physician and druggist of Palatka, was born in 1826 near the town of Willington, Abbeville District, South Carolina, son of Isaac and Margaret (nee Blanton) Moragne, the former a native of Bordeaux, France, born in 1774.[1] The Moragne family were among the earliest settlers along the Savannah River in Abbeville District 2 and in religion were of the Huguenot persuasion.[2] After an early education in the Willington school and an apprenticeship under a local doctor, Dr. Moragne attended medical school and returned to his home community to practice. There is evidence that he was a degree holder.[3] The 1850 Census lists him as physician living in the home of his widowed mother.[4]

Soon after the death of his mother in October 1852,[5] Dr. Moragne moved to Palatka and resumed the practice of medicine. From the beginning of his residence there he appears to have gained the confidence and respect of the community. In 1851, William D. Moseley, first Governor of the State of Florida, moved from his Jefferson County home to Palatka where his daughter, Elizabeth, wife of T.S. Haughton, was living. Moseley's youngest daughter, Alice Hill, became the wife of Dr. Moragne in 1856; they had five daughters. By 1870 the Moragne household numbered 12, two of the doctor's sisters, an elderly Negro servant, and two other relatives having been added.[6]

Dr. Moragne opened a drug store in 1856, said to have been Palatka's first. Judging from expansive advertisements which appeared in the local newspapers for years, it was a profitable business. It become evident that as the years passed he gradually relinquished the practice of medicine, devoting more time to the drug store and a variety of other interests. Still his advertisements never failed to designate him M.D.[7]

From the start Dr. Moragne was involved in the civic, religious and fraternal life of Palatka and Putnam County. He was a member of the Masonic Order. Both he and Mrs. Moragne were among the organizers of St. Mark's Episcopal Church. Its first congregational assembly, numbering only 18, included Mrs. Moragne. George R. Fairbanks, historian of the Florida Diocese, cited Dr. Moragne as a devoted parishioner.[8]

In the realm of politics Dr. Moragne served with distinction. As a secessionist he left little doubt as to his dedication to the preservation of Southern traditions. As the conservative candidate in 1868 he ran successfully for a seat in the Florida Senate, representing the 17th District. During the campaign the St. Augustine *Examiner* said of him: "Our nominee for Senator, Dr. Moragne of Palatka, is an old citizen of that place, a man of sterling qualities, uncompromisingly conservative in all his political views and one of the most popular men of his county."[9]

The legislative session which convened on June 8, 1868, was a stormy one, featuring a struggle between radical Republican elements (some of them Carpetbaggers) and the conservative Democrats. Dr. Moragne's seat was immediately challenged by F.A. Dockery but the Senate Committee on Privileges and Elections could find no flaw in the doctor's election.[10] His colors were immediately displayed when he voted with the majority against ratification of the Fourteenth Amendment of the U.S. Constitution. Later in the year he was appointed to a committee to deal with the proposed annexation by Alabama of that portion of Florida west of the Apalachicola River. The Montgomery (Alabama) *Advertiser* described him as a "State Senator, a gentleman of property, influence and intelligence."[11] He appears to have served his constituents satisfactorily; he was returned to the Senate in 1869, 1870, 1871 and 1872.[12]

Dr. Moragne died before 1880, exact date unknown. Having no sons to continue the business of the drug store, it was disposed of after his death. He was survived by his wife and five daughters. Mrs. Moragne died in 1888. The eldest daughter, Susan Moseley, who never married, died on February 19, 1940; Margaret Blanton, the second daughter, became the wife of W.M. Husson of New York. She died on November 15, 1900. The third daughter, Marie Louise, unmarried, died in Palatka on March 25, 1920; the fourth, Alice Natalie, unmarried, died on March 6, 1944; the youngest, Cecile Elizabeth, who became the wife of Judge Lake Jones of Jacksonville, died in July 1930 and was buried in Jacksonville.[13]

1. U.S. Census, 1850, Abbeville District, S.C., p. 20. See also "Inscriptions from Cemetery, Old Presbyterian Church, Willington, S.C.," *South Carolina Historical and Genealogical Magazine*, XXVIII, January 1927, pp. 249, 254.

2. U.S. Census, 1850, Abbeville District, S.C., p. 20.

3. *Centennial Memorial of the Medical College of the State of South Carolina*, Charleston, 1924. The list of graduates, arranged on a yearly basis, does not include the name of Dr. Moragne. It is possible that he attended the College but did not complete the work for his degree.

4. See notes 1 and 2, supra.

5. Ibid.

6. U.S. Census, 1870, Putnam County, Florida, p. 4, Town of Palatka. In 1860 Dr. Moragne is shown to have owned nine slaves. Since he was interested in citriculture and apparently owned a grove, these slaves were probably employed in that enterprise.

7. As an example see Palatka *Eastern Herald*, April 5, 1873.

8. *A History of St. Mark's Church, Palatka, Florida*, pp. 3, 5. See also George R. Fairbanks, "Early Churches of Florida," *Semi-Centennial, Diocese of Florida*, Jacksonville, 1889, App. D, p. 13.

9. St. Augustine *Examiner*, April 25, 1868; May 2, 1868.

10. *Florida Senate Journal*, 1st Session, 1868, Tallahassee, 1868, pp. 12, 30.

11. Cited in Hugh C. Bailey, "Alabama and West Florida Annexation," *Florida Historical Quarterly*, XXXV, No. 2, p. 223.

12. Allen Morris, *The People of Lawmaking in Florida, 1822-1983*, Tallahassee, Office of the Clerk, House of Representatives, 1982, unpaginated.

13. The author gratefully acknowledges the abundant genealogical information supplied by Mrs. Janice S. Mahaffey, Archivist, Putnam County Archives and History Commission, Palatka.

Moreno, Fernando, Pensacola, 1763-1828

Although Dr. Moreno's residence in Florida spanned only a few years, he merits inclusion here as an influential citizen and practicing physician during the territorial period.[1] Dr. Moreno's father, Fernando Sr., and mother, Lorenza, were natives of Malaga, Spain, where Fernando Jr. was born in 1763. When still a child he was brought to Louisiana where he spent the great part of his youth. In 1781, at the age of 18, he enlisted in the Spanish navy and in the course of his military duty was stationed in Havana. In 1784, while still on naval duty, he visited Pensacola. Apparently pleased with the locality he chose, upon completion of his naval duty, to study medicine (presumably in Havana) with the prospect of serving as a surgeon in the Spanish navy.

Dr. Moreno married Florentina Senae of New Orleans in 1783. To this union were born three sons, Fernando III in 1789; Arthur in 1791, and Francisco in 1792.

In the course of his navy service Dr. Moreno saw duty in Placaminos, Plaquemine, located near Baton Rouge, for a few years prior to September 1809 when he became the surgeon at San Carlos de Barrancas, Pensacola. Just how long Dr. Moreno remained in Pensacola has not been determined. It is known, however, that he returned to New Orleans, where Mrs. Moreno died, Subsequent to her death he returned to Havana where he died in 1828.

1. Data included in the present sketch are drawn entirely from Leora M. Sutton, "The Walton House" (mimeographed), Pensacola, 1968, Chapter IV.

Moseley, John G., Wakulla County, 1812

Only slight evidence establishes Dr. Moseley as an active medical practitioner in Florida. The evidence is fairly clear, however, that he was a close relative, probably a nephew, of William Dunn Moseley, first governor of the state of Florida (1845-49), who, in at least two instances, referred to him in his diary.[1] Evidence points to the probability that he was married to a sister of Dr. Jacob Elliott who died a few years after her marriage to Dr. Moseley leaving him with three young daughters. Apparently for reasons of poor health the doctor was unable to assume total responsibility for rearing the children who became the wards of Dr. Elliott, who at the time was a physician in Centreville in Leon County.[2] On February 13, 1850, the ex-Governor wrote in his diary, "John's children began to go to school at the expense of Dr. Elliott."[3]

Following the death of Dr. Elliott in 1856 the three Moseley daughters were taken into the home of William Newton Taylor, a landowner of substance (property valued at $17,000 in 1860) of Wakulla County. Dr. Moseley was also a member of the Taylor household in 1860. The census of that year lists him as physician but with no indication of wealth.[4] He was 48 years old. Since his name does not appear in any subsequent Florida census it is assumed that he did not long survive the year 1860. No military record for him has been discovered.

1. Only a few pages of the Moseley Diary, all from the year 1850, have survived.Typed transcripts of those pages are in the P.K. Yonge Library of Florida History.

2. U.S. Census, 1850, Leon County, Florida, p. 125, item 369.

3. Moseley Diary, entry of February 12, 1850. The entry for April 22, 1850, includes the following: "Sent John's children to Dr. Eliot."

4. U.S. Census, 1860, Wakulla County, Florida, p. 28, item 196. The three Moseley daughters in the Taylor home were: Virginia, 21; Elizabeth, 18, and Mary A., 16, all born in North Carolina.

Motte, Jacob Rhett, 1811-1868

It would be superfluous to include biographical notes on Dr. Motte. James F. Sunderman, ed., *Journey Into Wilderness*, has an account of Dr. Motte's experiences in the Creek and Seminole Wars in Florida, 1836-1838. In the introduction Professor Sunderman includes an excellent biographical sketch of Dr. Motte.

Mountien, Miles, Washington County, 1830-1894

Miles Mountien,[1] physician and state senator, was born in Ireland on February 16, 1830. His early life was spent on a farm and he attended a local parish school. At 14 he migrated to the United States, settling in Sumter County, Georgia, probably in the town of Americus, where he engaged in brick making for about 10 years. He entered medical school in his mid-20s and in 1858 was graduated Doctor of Medicine. Soon thereafter he began practice at Ft. Gaines, Georgia, the county seat of Clay County, situated on a bluff overlooking the Chattahoochee River. With the outbreak of the Civil War, Dr. Mountien enlisted in Co. D., 9th Georgia Infantry Regiment. He was with his Company in Virginia in late 1861. In the latter stages of the war he was transferred to the navy, serving in the command of Admiral Raphael Semmes. He was paroled in Greensboro, N.C., in May 1865.

The following year Dr. Mountien moved to Florida, settling at the little town of Vernon in Washington County. Not surprisingly, he was soon elected to the Washington County Commission, an office which he held for six years. He married Annie Johnson in 1870 and they had three sons, Loren, Julian and Charles, and one daughter, Birdie.[2]

In the fall of 1882 Dr. Mountien ran successfully for the Florida Senate representing the Fourth Senatorial District. He served in the sessions of 1883 and 1885. In politics he was a Democrat; in religion he was, according to his own statement, orthodox (Catholic).

Dr. Mountien continued to live and practice in Vernon until his death in 1894. He was buried in the local cemetery.[3] Little is known of his survivors. Mrs. Mountien died prior to 1900, by which date her daughter had married. The Census of 1900 indicated that the three sons still lived in Vernon, where the eldest, Loren, had become a merchant and Charles had become a school teacher.[4]

1. The greater part of the biographical data presented here is derived from the sketch written by Dr. Mountien himself for inclusion in the Legislative Directory of 1883. See J.V. Drake, ed.; comp., *The Florida Legislature (12th Session); An Official Directory of the State Government*, Jacksonville, 1883, pp. 28-29.

2. See U.S. Censuses for Washington County, Florida, 1885 and 1900. As was so frequently the case, the ages recorded are not totally reliable.

3. *Veterans' Graves Registration Project, Washington County, Florida*, Mimeograph, St. Augustine, 1940-41.

4. U.S. Census, 1900, Washington County, Florida, p. 157.

Mowe, James Fuller, Hamilton County 1824-1868

The medical career of Dr. Mowe remains only scantily documented. He was born in Andover, New Hampshire, on January 19, 1824.[1] In the fall of 1851 he matriculated at the Vermont Medical College at Woodstock, giving as his home address the neighboring town of Bradford.[2] The records of the College indicate that he attended only one session, leaving without a degree. Soon thereafter he departed for the South and in 1853 was appointed to the faculty of the newly-organized East Florida Seminary at Ocala. He was designated "male assistant" at an annual salary of $700.[3] His appointment doubtless came as a result of an earlier acquaintance with the principal, S.S. Burton, A.M., who was a graduate of the Thetford Academy of Thetford, Vermont, located only a short distance from Woodstock.

Dr. Mowe's tenure at the Seminary was brief, thought to have terminated after one session. It is possible that he was tarred with the brush which had resulted in the dismissal of Burton, who had been found guilty of an indiscretion with Miss Underwood, the Seminary's music teacher.[4]

Soon thereafter (about 1854) Dr. Mowe was married to Sarah (surname unknown), a South Carolina native, two years his senior.[5] It appears to have been a financially advantageous union for in 1860 Dr. Mowe was living in rural Marion County as a "planter-physician" with property valued at almost $20,000. He owned 16 slaves.[6]

At some juncture, probably after leaving the East Florida Seminary, Mowe decided to turn his year's training at the Vermont Medical College to advantage. Given the lax procedures for licensing medical practitioners it was possible for a person of minimal qualifications to obtain a license to practice through the office of the county judge. He apparently availed himself of the opportunity and began practice in Marion County soon after leaving the Seminary; henceforth he was known as Dr. Mowe.

With the coming of war in 1861 Dr. Mowe is thought to have joined the Confederate cause, notwithstanding his family responsibilities, i.e., a wife and four small children. There is no record of his having served in any Florida military unit, however, although a graves registration survey lists him as a veteran.[7] It is fairly certain that the war proved to be an economic disaster for the Mowe family. The postwar years found him living and practicing medicine in Hamilton County, in the town of Bellville. There he died in 1868 and was buried in the Baptist Cemetery of the town. Of his widow and children nothing is presently known.

1. Cora Hinton, *Early History of Hamilton County, Florida*, Jasper, 1976, p. 45.
2. Frederick Clayton Waite, *The Story of a Country Medical College*, The Vermont Medical College, Woodstock, Vermont, Montpelier, 1945, p. 194.
3. *Journal, Florida House of Representatives*, 7th Session, 1854-55, App., p. 17. Besides Mowe, who was designated Master of Arts, there were three other members of the faculty, viz., S.S. Burton, A.M.; Laura Chamberlain, Female Assistant; and Miss P.L.A. Underwood, Teacher of Music.
4. Samuel Proctor, "The University of Florida: Its Early Years, 1853-1906," Ph.D. dissertation, University of Florida, Gainesville, 1958, p. 39.
5. U.S. Census, 1860, Marion County, Florida, p. 321. The names and ages, respectively, are shown as James F., 35; Sarah N., 37; Mary J., 5; Susan, 4; Eliza, 3; Fuller (male), 2. Listed also is their farm overseer, Georgia-born William C. Smith, aged 40.
6. Florida Slave Schedule, Marion County, 1860.
7. Hinton, *Early History*, loc. cit.

Munroe, Thomas, Tallahassee and Quincy, 1803-1880

Dr. Munroe was born in Scotland about 1803,[1] migrating to America in the early 1820s. Soon after arrival he enrolled in the University of Maryland School of Medicine from which he was graduated in the class of 1829.[2] He then made his way to Florida, settling first in Tallahassee where he quickly emerged as a leader in medicine and politics, in addition to becoming a leader in society. With establishment of a medical regulatory board following enactment by the Legislative Council in 1828, the Territory showed some interest in guarding its citizens against the quackery which was likely to flourish in most frontier areas. Dr. Munroe was among the early appointees to the Board.[3] This was soon followed by appointment to the clerkship of the Legislative Council.

Meanwhile Dr. Munroe had opened a drug store in Tallahassee, a venture which he shared with Dr. Lewis Willis, a fellow practitioner and colleague on the Medical Board.[4] The two physicians announced their partnership in medical practice on January 5, 1830, from their office on Adams Street.[5]

For reasons not made clear, the Munroe-Willis partnership was dissolved in 1832 at about the time the Legislative Council rejected Dr. Munroe's candidacy for reappointment to the clerkship. He received only a single vote of the 15 which were cast.[6] Soon after this action by the Council and probably because of it, Dr. Munroe moved to Quincy, joining his brother William, who had arrived in Gadsden County from Scotland in 1828, purchased extensive farming land and became a merchant. Dr. Munroe also purchased land in the county and upon settling in Quincy he, as was true of so many professional men of the times, settled into the dual roles of doctor and farmer.[7] He married Sarah Elizabeth Fitzgerald, member of a prominent Gadsden family, on June 21, 1832.[8]

In politics Dr. Munroe embraced the Democratic cause to which he remained faithful through most of his life. He was a vocal advocate of statehood for the Florida Territory, aiding in the preparation of a petition to Congress demanding favorable action on the issue.[9] In 1847 he was an unsuccessful candidate for a seat in the Florida House of Representatives.[10] Two years later he was elected Intendant (mayor) of Quincy for the 1850-51 term.[11] Finally, in 1860, he was one of Gadsden's delegates to the State Democratic Convention meeting in Monticello at which he was appointed to the party's State Executive Committee.[12]

Both Munroes, Thomas and William, prospered in their respective fields and accumulated substantial estates, the latter leaving at the time of his death property valued at about a quarter of a million dollars. The two families were frequently mentioned in the "Autobiography" of Dr. Charles A. Hentz, a Quincy physician, whose second wife was a daughter of William Munroe, and who was the medical preceptor of her brother, Thomas F., when he began his medical apprenticeship. Dr. Munroe also served as executor of the estate of Dr. William Booth, Quincy physician and father of Dr. Hentz's first wife.[13]

Dr. Munroe died on July 4, 1880 after an extended illness, the details of which were described by Dr. Hentz. His burial took place the following day and on July 6 the family gathered for the reading of the doctor's will by Dr. Hentz, whose wife, as a niece of Dr. Munroe, was one of the beneficiaries.[14]

1. U.S. Census, 1850, Gadsden County, Florida, p. 349. It is an intriguing thought that Dr. Munroe belonged to the family which had produced the three famous Scottish physicians, the Doctors Munroe: Primus, Secundus, and Tertius, of Edinburgh.

2. Eugene F. Cordell, *Historical Sketch of the University of Maryland, 1807-1890*, Baltimore, 1891, p. 190. Munroe is listed as a resident of Maryland.

3. *Acts, Legislative Council of Florida*, 8th Session, 1820, Tallahassee, 1829, p. 258. See. ibid., 8th Session, Tallahassee, 1829, and Tallahassee *Floridian and Advocate*, October 13, 1829.

4. Ibid., November 3, 1829. This announcement was accompanied by a lengthy list of patent medicines in stock, typical of the drug store offerings of the times.

5. Ibid., June 5, 1830.

6. *Journal, Proceedings of the Legislative Council, Territory of Florida*, 10th Session, Tallahassee, 1830.

7. U.S. Census, 1860, Gadsden County, Florida, p. 49. Here his land was valued at $15,000, other properties at $130,000.

8. Tallahassee *Floridian*, June 26, 1832.

9. Tallahassee *Sentinel* December 4, 1840.

10. Tallahassee *Floridian*, September 11, 1847.

11. J. Randall Stanley, *History of Gadsden County*, Quincy, 1948, p. 33.

12. Fernandina *East Floridian*, June 21, 1860; Monticello *Family Friend*, June 16, 1860.

13. Charles A. Hentz, "Autobiography." Typed transcript of the MS in the Southern Historical Collection, University of North Carolina, Chapel Hill, I, 305 et passim.

14. Ibid., II, 180-183.

Munroe, Thomas Freeman, Gadsden County, 1846

Dr. Munroe was born in Quincy in May 1845.[1] He was the son of William Munroe, merchant and planter, and nephew of the well-known Dr. Thomas Munroe. In 1861, or thereabout, he began the study of medicine under the preceptorate of Dr. Charles A. Hentz.[2] Since he was only 15 at the outbreak of war in 1861 he waited for two years before enlisting on August 22, 1863, in the 5th

Florida Cavalry Battalion as a private, a grade in which he was to remain until 1864 when he was promoted to 4th Sergeant.[3] Near the end of the conflict he was captured by Union troops, spending a few weeks as a prisoner of war before being released on May 13, 1865. A Confederate document described him as five feet eight inches tall, dark hair, gray eyes, and light complexion.[4]

Upon his release Munroe returned to Quincy and it may be inferred from an entry in the Dr. Hentz "Autobiography" that he resumed medical studies under the guidance of Dr. Hentz.[5] In the fall of 1866 he entered the Medical School of the University of Maryland from which he was graduated as Doctor of Medicine in the spring of 1868. Soon thereafter he returned to Quincy and began medical practice, shortly after which he married Martha Harriet Jones.[6] He continued to practice in Quincy until the time of his death.[7]

1. U.S. Census, 1900, Gadsden County, Florida, p. 56.
2. C.A. Hentz, "Autobiography," transcription of MS in the Southern Historical Collection, University of North Carolina, Chapel Hill, I, 342. Dr. Hentz wrote: "Tom Munroe began reading medicine with me (1861)...He had to go into service later on...after the surrender, he returned to his books."
3. NA, Service Recs. CSA, Microfilm M251, Roll 17.
4. Ibid.
5. Hentz, "Autobiography."
6. J. Randall Stanley, *History of Gadsden County*, Quincy, 1948, p. 80.
7. The date of Dr. Munroe's death has not been determined. Four daughters and one son were born to Dr. and Mrs. Munroe. These children with the year of birth are Rebecca, 1873; Max, 1875; Alice B., 1877; Mary C., 1882; and Sarah, 1886.

Murdoch, John Smith, Jacksonville, 1818-1860

Among the early physicians of Duval County Dr. Murdoch was one of the most highly regarded. Although his span of service was brief—he died at the age of 42—his professional career was eminently successful. Born in Frederick, Maryland, on November 9, 1818,[1] he moved with his parents to Columbia, South Carolina, at an early age and there he received his early education and prepared for admission to medical school. In the fall of 1837 he matriculated at the Medical College of the State of South Carolina, Charleston, from which he was graduated on March 13, 1839,[2] after submitting a thesis on obstetrics which was not at that time a popular field of practice, most deliveries being attended by midwives who, in the South, were for the most part black.[3]

Following graduation Dr. Murdock returned to Columbia to launch his practice and in 1842 married Emma Wallace there. The young couple continued to live in Columbia until early 1850 when they moved to Jacksonville. Dr. Murdoch's opposition to the slave system of the South was demonstrated prior to his move to Florida when he offered freedom to any of his slaves who desired to be free.[4]

On his arrival in Jacksonvile Dr. Murdoch purchased a house on the south side of Forsyth Street, between Liberty and Washington, from which location he began his practice. In the following year he joined Dr. Richard P. Daniel[5] in a professional partnership which continued until Dr. Murdoch's death nine years later.

Dr. Murdoch did not shun civic responsibilities and on several occasions assisted in Fourth of July celebrations. At more than one event he offered toasts befitting the day, such as that of 1852: "To the Crackers of East Florida and the Tigers of Jacksonville."[6] He was elected to the office of Intendant of Jacksonville in 1858, an office later redesignated mayor.

In spite of professional success and popularity with the citizens of Jacksonville Dr. Murdoch suffered occasional spells of manic depression.[7] In one of these he used a pistol to take his own life on October 10, 1860.[8]

Several children were born to Dr. and Mrs. Murdoch. In order of birth they were: Sarah and Eleanor, aged six and four respectively in 1850. Both were natives of South Carolina. Others were: Emma J., Sally D., Wallace (son), and Alexino, aged 11, seven, three and one in 1860. All were natives of Florida.[9]

1. Some of the biographical data included in the present sketch is derived from Webster Merritt, *A Century of Medicine in Jacksonville and Duval County*, Gainesville, University of Florida Press, 1949, pp. 42-43, et passim.
2. See List of Graduates in Charleston *Courier*, March 21, 1839. The measure of Dr. Murdoch's achievement is indicated by the fact that he wrote his doctoral thesis in Latin, for which he received a special award.
3. Merritt, op cit., p. 42. Here Dr. Merritt discusses prevailing attitudes concerning the practice of obstetrics in the 19th century.
4. Ibid., loc. cit.
5. Jacksonville *News*, December 13, 1851.
6. Jacksonville *Florida Republican*, July 8, 1852.
7. Merritt, op. cit., p. 43.
8. Gravestone, Old City Cemetery, Jacksonville.
9. U.S. Censuses, Duval County, Florida, 1850 and 1860.

Murphy, Miles Jones, Middleburg and Jacksonville, 1819-1882

Dr. Murphy, a native of South Carolina, arrived in Florida about 1857, settling in Middleburg in Clay County. He had apparently begun his career a few years earlier in Georgia where his eldest child was born. Nothing is presently known of his educational background. The earliest indication of his presence in Florida is an advertisement of the new Middleburg Seminary in which prospective students were assured that "Board can be obtained on reasonable terms at Dr. Murphy's or Mrs. Dillon's."[1] The Clay County Census of 1860 lists Dr. Murphy as a resident of Middleburg, 41 years of age. His wife, Maria, a native of Maryland, was 26 and his two children, Henry and Florence, two and four respectively.[2] The Murphy property was valued at a modest $1,000.

With the outbreak of war in 1861 Dr. Murphy enlisted in a reserve unit designated as Company A, Florida Reserves. Although he was a physician at the age of 42, he was inducted without military rank. Soon after organization of the Tenth Florida Infantry Regiment in September 1841, he was commissioned First Lieutenant and placed in command of Company A stationed at Ft. Clinch on the outskirts of Fernandina. He remained there as commanding officer until late 1864 when he was elected to the Florida Assembly (House) by the voters of Clay County. Although the Legislature had convened on November 21, Dr. Murphy was not able to take his seat until December 6, and only after the Confederate Secretary of State, James A. Seddon, accepted his resignation.

At the end of the legislative session in 1865, Dr. Murphy resumed medical practice in Jacksonville. In July 1865, he announced he had established his office and residence at the corner of Hogan and Forsyth Streets where he would be specializing in diseases of women and children.[3] Later that year, with revival of the Duval County Medical Society,[4] he became an active member and on November 4, 1865, was one of eight Jacksonville physicians meeting to formulate a professional manifesto or statement of policy for the Society.[5]

Dr. Murphy continued to live and practice medicine in Jacksonville until his death in 1882.[6] No information concerning the last two decades of his life has emerged. It appears that the depressed economic conditions of the postwar years and the attendant difficulty in the collection of fees resulted in strained circumstances for the Murphy family. After her husband's death in 1882 Mrs. Murphy continued to run her boarding house, located at 335 East Forsyth Street, well into the 20th century. Her death occurred in 1920.

Although Dr. Murphy was never a member of the Florida Medical Association, which had been established in Jacksonville in 1874, he continued membership in the Duval County Medical Society. He was one of the group of physicians who met in November 1865 and declared their intention to withhold their services from any client who showed no inclination to pay his just medical bills, adding that they were willing to do the "work of charity and administer to the truly indigent."[7]

In addition to the two children previously mentioned, Henry and Florence, a son, Robert E. Lee, and two daughters, F.K. and Maria, were born to the Murphys. The eldest child, Florence, was married to a real estate broker, James H. Cooley, the couple having moved away from Jacksonville prior to 1900. She is known to have returned on one occasion to arrange for the placing of a gravestone for her parents in the Old City Cemetery. Incidentally she was also buried in the same plot subsequent to her death on September 27, 1824. The other daughter, Maria, became the society editor of the Jacksonville *Metropolis.* As for the two sons, Henry Ernest and Robert E. Lee, the former was for many years employed as ticket agent for a steamship company and for the railroads operating in and out of Jacksonville. The younger brother, Robert E. Lee, was for several years employed by Armour & Company, meatpackers.[8]

1. Jacksonville *Republican,* March 24, 1858.
2. U.S. Census, 1860, Clay County, Florida, p. 145.
3. Jacksonville *Florida Union,* October 14, 1865.
4. In response to the medical needs of the Confederacy nearly all of Jacksonville's physicians enlisted for service, leaving the home front almost without professional medical care.
5. By July 1865 the Duval County Medical Society had been revived. Its statement, drawn up on November 4, included the following provisions: (1) Payment for services due on completion of services. (2) Charity to be extended where required. (3) Patients delinquent in paying their bills will after notification find their delinquency made known to all members of the Society.
6. Dr. Murphy's gravestone bears the following inscription: "Miles Murphy, M.D. First Lt., Co. A, 1st Fla. Regt. C.S.A. 1819-1882."
7. There were apparently some members of the community who failed to pay for medical services, even when they were judged by the physicians as being quite able to pay.
8. *Jacksonville City Directory,* 1889, 1907, 1908.

Murray, Richard, St. Augustine, 1820s

Historical documents indicate that Dr. Murray, a native of Ireland, was a resident of St. Augustine as early as 1816, although there is no record of his having applied for or received a land grant from the Spanish crown.[1] He was among the first inhabitants of the city to take the oath of naturalization to the United States following the cession of Florida in 1821, an event which is a matter of record for August 30, 1821. At this time he gave his age as 30 and indicated that he was the head of a family.[2] In the "Temporary Organization of St. Augustine" completed in mid-July 1821, he was named the medical member of the Board of Health.[3] In the permanent organization of the East Florida Territory, announced on February 1, 1822, he was confirmed in this position with the title Health Officer.[4]

In the succeeding months Dr. Murray's interest and participation in public matters affecting the Territory are indicated by the frequency with which his signature was attached to petitions and memorials addressed to Washington officials.[5]

Although the evidence is lacking it can be reasonably assumed that prior to the cession of 1821 Dr. Murray had gained the reputation as a reliable physician. His first professional card appeared in the St. Augustine paper of July 28, 1821, announcing his practice from an office in Mrs. Lindsay's Hotel.[6] This was followed by a lengthy notice enumerating the "fresh and genuine supply of medicines" recently received from New York and Charleston.[7] Similar notices continued to appear from time to time throughout the year 1823.

Dr. Murray was an active member of the Catholic Church of St. Augustine. So excellent were his devotion and reputation that upon the resignation of G.W. Perpall from a wardenship of the Church in April 1825, Dr. Murray was elected to succeed him. At about the same time he joined other wardens in expressing gratitude to a departing priest, the Reverend Francis Boland, who was transferring to Savannah.[8] In further support of Dr. Murray's reputation for piety was the fact that he owned a copy of Timothy Dwight's "Theology," a series of sermons which was so much in demand that the volume went through numerous editions in the 18th and early 19th centuries.[9]

Toward the end of the year 1826, Dr. Murray became inadvertently involved in a court action resulting from a duel between his colleague, Dr. Richard Weightman, and Edgar Macon, former United States attorney for East Florida. Dr. Murray had served as Dr. Weightman's second.[10] His death occurred during the month of October 1827, it is thought, of yellow fever.[11]

1. TP., XXII, 702. In this instance Dr. Murray joined a number of St. Augustine citizens in attesting to the integrity of Eusebius Gomez, who was formally protesting the presence of Alexander Hamilton on the three-member Land Grant Commission of Florida and accusing him of abuse of his public office. In this document Dr. Murray stated that he had resided in St. Augustine for seven years. The Gomez letter bears the date, June 12, 1823. Hamilton, incidentally, was the son of the great Federalist statesman.
2. Ibid., 434.
3. Ibid., p. 121. See also St. Augustine *Gazette*, August 4, 1821.
4. TP., XXII, 359.
5. Ibid., pp. 367, 450, 530, 762, 764, 858, 986.
6. St. Augustine *Florida Gazette*.
7. Ibid. This list is a virtual catalogue of drugs and patented compounds in general use at the time.
8. St. Augustine *East Florida Herald*, May 7, 1825.
9. The "Diary of Joshua Nicholas Glenn," a portion of which was written when he was a sojourner in St. Augustine in 1823, includes the following entry: "This morning I got Dr. Dwight's Theology of Dr. Murray and commenced reading them threw (sic)."
10. Office of the Clerk of Circuit Court, Miscellaneous File, Drawer T-3. St. Johns County, Florida. Edgar Macon, a controversial public figure in St. Augustine, engaged for several months in a bitter feud with Judge Joseph L. Smith, during the course of which much invective was exchanged. Ultimately President Adams ordered Macon's dismissal from office (summer 1826), an action probably related to the duel. See TP., XXIII, p. 634.
11. St. Augustine *East Florida Herald*, November 7, 1827.

Murray, Robert Duke, Key West, 1845-1903

Dr. Murray, a highly-regarded physician and man of adventurous spirit, spent several of the latter years of his life in southern Florida.[1] He was without doubt a physician of exceptional competence, an unwavering etiologist ever concerned with the causes of disease. In addition, he was a highly regarded medical administrator. Born on April 21, 1845, at Ohlton, Trumbull County, Ohio, he began the formal study of medicine in 1865 at the Tripler Army Hospital at Columbus, Ohio. He then served an apprenticeship in medicine under Dr. J. Augustus Seitz in Bluffton (Allen County), Ohio. From Bluffton he moved to Cleveland where he continued medical study under Dr. John E. Darby. Having thus qualified for medical college he enrolled at Cleveland Medical College from which he was graduated in 1868. Still not satisfied that he was adequately prepared for medical practice he enrolled at prestigious Jefferson Medical College in Philadelphia from which he received a second medical degree in 1871, having served as resident physician for 15 months.

At this juncture Dr. Murray become interested in the cause and treatment of yellow fever. He made his way to Key West to seriously study the disease and attempt to devise an effective treatment. There he made the acquaintance of Miss Lillie Fulwood, daughter of the Reverend C.A. Fulwood, whom he soon married. To this union were born five children, daughters Reba, Gille and Karlia; and sons Robert Fulwood and Joseph Arbour. Mrs. Murray did not long survive the birth of the fifth child, dying at Ship Island Quarantine in 1887.

There can be no doubt that Dr. Murray was a serious and intelligent medical practitioner, much concerned for advancement of medical knowledge and competence of its practitioners, which he demonstrated by affiliating with the American Medical Association, American Public Health Association, as well as the Florida Medical Association. Although he was not present at the organizational meeting of the Florida Association in the office of Dr. Abel S. Baldwin in Jacksonville in 1874, he was elected to membership and was present at the meeting in Jacksonville in 1875.

For the last 25 or 30 years of his life Dr. Murray devoted the greater part of his time and energy to the study of yellow fever, making significant observations during the epidemics in Key West, Pensacola, New Orleans, Vicksburg and elsewhere. He conducted the first *cordon sanitaire* in the United States, which was imposed on Brownsville, Texas, in 1882. He was the first physician to impose a winter quarantine, this having been ordered for Manatee County.

Notwithstanding his active professional life Dr. Murray was much involved in fraternal organizations, having been a Mason, Knight Templar, member of the American Pomological Society, Medico-Legal Society of New York, and several other organizations. His last known role was that of physician in charge of the quarantine on lonely Dry Tortugas, located in the Gulf of Mexico, some 35 miles due west of Key West.

Dr. Murray's death occurred while on a visit to Laredo. It resulted from injuries received when he and a colleague, Dr. G.M. Guiteras, were thrown from their carriage when their frightened horse ran away.

1. The present sketch has been constructed almost entirely from the biography of Dr. Murray which is found in Rowland H. Rerick, *Memories of Florida*, Vol. 11, Atlanta, 1902, pp. 633-634. Accompanying the sketch of Dr. Murray is a splendid portrait which portrays him as a man of dignity and distinction.

Myers, Thomas Jefferson, Gainesville, 1828

The chief biographical data relating to Dr. Myers are found in a letter which he addressed to Governor William Gist on December 2, 1860.[1] Dr. Myers had apparently arrived in Gainesville about 1858 and found lodging in the rural residence of D.R. June, a planter of substantial means and also a native of South Carolina.[2] The letter to Governor Gist reveals that Dr. Myers had been a member of the South Carolina Volunteer Regiment known as the "Palmettos" which had been assembled for service in the Mexican War. He had been wounded at the Battle of Churubusco sometime between August 18-20, 1847, seriously enough to qualify him for a federal pension but which had apparently not dampened his belligerent spirit.

With secession of South Carolina from the Union already imminent, though not officially declared until December 20, Dr. Myers wrote a passionate letter to Governor Gist predicting that Florida would follow South Carolina. Nevertheless, he wrote: "I would prefer to stick to the 'Palmetto'. If Florida does not go, my Company will immediately move for South Carolina..." With "Victory or Death" as his motto, he could scarcely wait to join the battle for "Southern Rights against our common enemy."

Although he was, as he expressed it, an "Invalid Pensioner," he looked forward with enthusiasm "to joining the little remnants of that Glorious Regiment" in the righteous cause. He asked only for the opportunity "of fighting under the dear Old Palmetto," hoping to be placed "near the flashing of the guns."

If Governor Gist ever acknowledged Dr. Myers letter, no record of a response has survived. He enlisted for Confederate service on March 24, 1861,[3] at Gainesville and was assigned to the "Gainesville Minute Men," Company H, 1st Florida Infantry, as commanding officer with the rank of captain. Just how long he remained with this unit is unknown. His military record ends with a pay voucher in the amount of $520 for the period April to July 31, 1862.

It is not known how long Dr. Myers remained in Confederate service. He is known to have returned to his plantation near Gainesville in the mid-1860s where the census enumerator found him in 1870. He is listed as "Dr. Thomas Jefferson Myers, Planter, aged forty-two."[4] Nothing further is known of him.

1. This letter reveals Dr. Myers as a firebrand filled with indignation at the threat to his properties and eager for a fight. The Myers family of Charleston was one of wealth and social position. Letter found in Myers' Confederate Service Record.

2. U.S. Census, 1860, Alachua County, Florida, p. 76, item 578. June's properties were valued at more than $81,000, those of Dr. Myers at $8,200. Other members of the household were William E. June, aged 21, and James Doig, a Scottish-born engineer, who became one of Gainesville's most prominent citizens. Near the end of his life Doig wrote a series of reminiscences, biographical in nature, in which mention is made of many of Gainesville's early settlers. It is strange that he made no reference to Dr. Myers, since both had resided in the home of D.R. June. See Gainesville *Sun*, July 15, 22, 29, 1917.

3. National Archives, Confederate Service Records, 1st Florida Infantry Regiment.

4. U.S. Census, 1870, Alachua County, Florida, p. 57.

Nash, Miles, Leon County, 1797-1873

As physician, druggist, clergyman and postmaster, Dr. Nash was much involved in the antebellum development of Tallahassee. He was born in Norfolk County, Virginia, in 1797,[1] and after his marriage in North Carolina to Martha, daughter of General Ely Whitaker, he migrated to Florida in 1836, settling in Leon County. He moved to Tallahassee in 1843 where, according to local historians, a house was built for him at 131 North Calhoun Street.[2] He soon acquired a large and lucrative practice and within a year or so was able to construct a building at 509 North Monroe Street which housed his professional offices as well as drug store.[3] During the administration of President John Tyler he was appointed postmaster, an office he held for several years.[4] A portion of his building was used as the post office.

References to his medical practice are not abundant, but it is evident that Dr. Nash was a popular and highly respected physician. His obituary abounds with praise for his godlike character, generosity, and humanitarian concerns. So successful was he that his properties were valued at $25,000 in 1850. Only a few Leon County physicians, principally those from wealthy planter families, could boast of more material possessions.[5]

Dr. Nash was closely associated with the propagation of Methodism in Middle Florida. As an ordained minister he made frequent appearances in Leon County pulpits and was without doubt an effective speaker. Leon County marriage records identify him as the officiating clergyman at numerous weddings, especially between the years 1837 and 1857. The account of the marriage of Sarah Whitaker to Lewis H. Branch on October 17, 1843, states that the ceremony was performed by "the Reverend Miles Nash, M.D."[6] An ecumenical element entered his ministry when he officiated at the funeral service for the wife of General George W. Whitfield at St. John's Episcopal Church[7] "in the absence of the rector." Of his dual capacities a Tallahassee historian wrote: "Dr. Nash was a Methodist minister as well as physician. We are told that 'there were times when his duties as a physician interfered with his duties as pastor; sometimes he was called from the pulpit to usher a new soul into the world.' "[8] Subsequent to his election as a delegate from Tallahassee's Trinity Methodist Church on June 6, 1867, to the forthcoming District Conference, however, nothing is known of his religious activities.[9]

Six children are known to have been born to Dr. and Mrs. Nash. In the order of birth they were Miles H., who also practiced medicine in Tallahassee; Francina; John W., a lawyer, who served with distinction in the Army of the Confederacy and died in Tallahassee in 1903;[10] Emma, who became the wife of Judge D.W. Gwynn of Leon County,[11] and Fletcher W. Another son, Joseph Branch, died on October 16, 1840, at the age of five.[12]

Dr. Nash died at the home of his son-in-law, Judge Gwynn, near Tallahassee, on January 15, 1873, in his 75th year.[13]

1. Obituary notice of Dr. Nash, Tallahassee *Weekly Floridian*, January 21, 1873.
2. Evelyn Whitfield Henry, "Old Houses in Tallahassee", *Tallahassee Historical Society Annual*, I, 1934, p. 43.
3. Ibid.
4. See note 1, supra.
5. U.S. Census, 1860, Leon County, Florida, p. 21.
6. Tallahassee *Sentinel*, October 17, 1843.
7. "Parochial Records," St. John's Episcopal Church, Tallahassee, 1832-1880, Tallahassee Chapter, DAR, typed copy, p. 39.

8. Whitfield, "Old Houses," p. 43.
9. Theo Frances Rowe Delp, *History of the Tallahassee District of the Methodist Church*, Tallahassee, 1965, p. 25.
10. Tallahassee *Weekly Tallahassean*, December 4, 1903. Obit.
11. Ibid, March 17, 1874. Obit.
12. Tallahassee *Floridian*, October 24, 1840. Obit.
13. See note 1, supra.

Nash Jr., Miles Henry, Leon County, 1833

Dr. Nash, son of Dr. Miles Nash Sr. and Martha Whitaker Nash, was born in Virginia in 1833. Soon after his birth the family moved to Tallahassee and occupied a house at 131 North Calhoun Street.[1] He presumably received his basic education in the common schools of the town. At adolescence he began the study of medicine under the preceptorate of his father and in 1833 at the age of 20 matriculated at the Medical College of the State of South Carolina, Charleston.[2] In the following year, however, he transferred to the Jefferson Medical College in Philadelphia from which he received his medical digree in the spring of 1855.[3]

Soon after graduation Dr. Miles returned to Tallahassee and on May 2, 1855, announce the launching of his professional career to the people of Leon County. He had entered into a partnership with his father in both medicine and the operation of a drug store, his office and the store being located at 509 North Monroe Street.[4] Over the next four or five years his professional card appeared with regularity in the local newspapers. He was still residing in the home of his father in 1860 and his assets at the time were valued at $2,000.[5]

For the activities of Dr. Nash for the next six years there is no information. Since he was 28 years of age in 1861 and still unmarried he would have been a likely conscript for Confederate service, and particularly so in view of his professional skills, but the service records for Floridians serving in the Army of the Confederacy do not include him, although his younger brother, John W., had a distinguished war record. We can only conclude that he either served in a civilian capacity or that he enlisted in another state. At any rate, he does not reappear in the sources until June 1866 when he resumed practice in Tallahassee, with his "office in the rear of the Post Office, and his Residence with Dr. M. Nash."[6]

As late as 1870, Dr. Nash, still unmarried, was residing in the home of his father, as were his sisters, Emma and Francina. Within the next year or so he married a Miss Randolph of Washington, Wilkes County, Georgia. Soon after the death of his father, which occurred on January 15, 1873, Dr. Nash left Tallahassee to enter medical practice in Georgia. The following item appeared in the Tallahassee *Weekly Floridian* of March 4, 1873:

> Dr. Miles H. Nash left us last week for his new home in Washington, Wilkes County, Georgia, his excellent lady having preceded him some weeks since. In the Doctor's departure our County has lost a good physician, the community a substantial citizen, and his personal associates a warm, trusty friend.

The date of Dr. Nash's death has not been ascertained.

1. Mary W. Keen, "Some Phases of Life in Leon County During the Civil War," *Tallahassee Historical Society Annual*, IV, 1939, p. 21.
2. *Lists of Matriculants and Graduates*, Medical College of the State of South Carolina, Waring Historical Library, MUSC, Charleston.

3. Jefferson Medical College, "List of Dead or Lost Graduates in Classes from 1826 to 1879," p. 82.
4. Tallahassee *Florida Sentinel*, March 2, 1858. Here it is indicated that his professional notice first appeared on May 29, 1855.
5. U.S. Census, 1860, Leon County, Florida, item 180.
6. Tallahassee *Semi-Weekly Floridian*, June 5, 1866.
7. Henry E. Palmer, M.D., "Physicians of Early Tallahassee and Vicinity," *Apalachee*, 1944, p. 31.

Newsom, Lewis L., Jackson and Putnam Counties, 1828

Dr. Newsom, a native of Georgia, moved to Jackson County in the late 1850s accompanied by his wife, Mary, and their two sons, Edward and Charles, aged seven and five respectively. The Census of 1860 gives the doctor's age as 33; his property was estimated to have been worth $11,365.[1]

With the coming of the Civil War in 1861 Dr. Newsom did not become immediately involved but on March 14 of the following year he enlisted for military service and was mustered into the 15th Florida Cavalry, Company B, with the rank of sergeant.[2] Although no further data concerning his military service has been located it is likely that he served in some medical capacity. Meanwhile Mrs. Newsom gave her services to the Ladies Hospital Aid Society of Marianna.[3]

At the conclusion of the war Dr. Newsom moved with his family to Putnam County, settling in the village of Welaka on the St. Johns River south of Palatka where he resumed medical practice and where the census enumerator located him in 1870. By that date three other childrne, Louis, Mary and Lavinia, had been born to the Newsoms.[4]

After a few years in Welaka the Newsoms moved once more, to Crescent City on Crescent Lake in the southeast corner of Putnam County where Dr. Newsom spent the last years of his life.[5] He was still practicing medicine as late as 1885, having been the attending physician of a patient who died that year.[6] Meanwhile his sons, Edward and Charles, had become orange grove owners in the vicinity.

By the year 1900 Dr. Newsom was deceased, although the exact date of his death has not been determined. The census of that year lists Mrs. Newsom, then a widow, living in the proximity of her daughter, Mary (Mrs. Benham) also a widow. Of the seven children born to the Newsoms only four were still living in 1900.[7]

No record of Dr. Newsom's civic or religious activities has survived. Neither is there any record of his having ever been affiliated with a state or county medical society.

1. U.S. Census, 1860, Jackson County, Florida, item 629.
2. *Soldiers of Florida*, Live Oak, 1903, p. 280.
3. J. Randall Stanley, *History of Jackson County, Florida*, Marianna, 1950, p. 182. Dr. Newsom was a Marianna practitioner.
4. U.S. Census, 1870, Putnam County, Florida, Welaka Precinct, p. 97, item 117.
5. U.S. Census, 1880, Putnam County, Florida, Crescent City Precinct, p. 38.
6. Florida Special Census, 1885, Mortality Schedule, 1884-85, p. 38.
7. U.S. Census, 1900, Putnam County, Florida, p. 150.

Newsome, Solomon, Bradford and Baker Counties, 1836-post 1900

The professional career of Dr. Newsome was similar to that of many Florida physicians of the mid-19th century. He settled in Florida with the apparent intention of practicing medicine, but upon becoming aware of the availability of cheap land, he gradually abandoned medical practice, purchased land, and turned increasingly to farming. Born in Georgia in January, 1836,[1] he matriculated at the Medical College of Georgia in Augusta in 1856 and in March 1858 he was graduated as Doctor of Medicine.[2] Soon thereafter he made his way to Bradford County (then known as New River County), Florida, settling in the Lake Butler precinct.[3]

Dr. Newsome found lodging in the home of prominent citizen, William J.C. Prevatt, who was the Bradford County Judge. He could not have chosen a better lodging for the Prevatt home was apparently spacious. In addition to the Judge his wife and their five children, other lodgers included two lawyers, James P. Hunt and Reubin Fitzgerald, both natives of South Carolina; three carpenters, all North Carolina-born, and Elizabeth Clements, probably a relative of Mrs. Newsome.[4]

Within a few months after outbreak of the Civil War in April 1861 and doubtless at the urging of the two South Carolina tenants, Hunt and Fitzgerald, Dr. Newsome enlisted for military service on May 21, 1862. The month of July 1862 found him on duty at Camp Ward, Escambia County, with the rank of Assistant Surgeon.[5] His subsequent military record has not been found but it is known that he was mustered out of the Army on April 26, 1865.

Although no information relating to the death of Mrs. Newsome has been located, it is apparent that she died in the early 1860s. At any rate, about 1866, Dr. Newsome married a South Carolina native known only as Susan L., some 14 years his junior. To this union were born several children: daughters Lucy, Mary, and Frances; and sons William and Lemuel.[6]

The Special Florida Census of 1885 (Bradford County) indicates that Dr. Newsome was dividing his time and energy between medical practice and farming. He then owned about 40 acres of land of which 25 acres were "improved," i.e., under cultivation. Its value was $2,500. He continued to practice medicine, however, the mortality schedule of 1885 lists only a single death among his patients, that one due to "brain fever."[7]

Dr. Newsome continued to live beyond the scope of the present biographical register. He was still living in 1900 at the age of 64. His home was located in the Providence Precinct of West Bradford County. Obviously several of the children had departed his household. His wife, Susan, was 51. His daughter, "Lizzie", Elizabeth, was 34. The date of Dr. Newsome's death has not been determined. It is perhaps of significance that in the Census of 1900 he is designated "farmer" and not "physician."

1. The Bradford County Census of 1900 definitely states that he was born in Georgia in January 1836.
2. Medical College of Georgia, "List of Graduates, 1829-1891," Augusta, June 1890, p.22.
3. *Webb's Florida*, New York, W.S. Webb & Co., 1885, p. 31.
4. U.S Census, 1860, New River County, p. 482.
5. Soldiers of Florida, Board of State Institutions, Macclenny, 1983, p. 128.
6. U.S. Census, 1880, Bradford County, p. 251.
7. Special Census, Florida, 1885. Agricultural Schedule, Bradford County, p. 243. See ibid., Mortality Schedule.

Newton, Isaac D., Leon County, 1806-1848

Dr. Newton, a native of Jefferson County, Georgia, settled in rural Leon County about 1842, apparently hoping that the more benign climate would be beneficial to his health. His health problem was said to have been manifested by inflammation of both lungs and bowel, which resulted in a long and painful illness. His death came on May 19, 1848. It is doubtful that he was ever a medical practitioner in Florida. He was survived by his widow. The obituary notice mentioned that he was a member of the Methodist Church.[1]

1. Tallahassee *Florida Sentinel*, May 23, 1848.

Nicholson Sr., Malcolm, Gadsden County, 1790-1840

Dr. Nicholson, one of Gadsden County's earliest white settlers, was born in Cumberland County, North Carolina, about 1790. His ancestors were Scottish Highlanders, belonging to that massive migration to America in the 18th century, substantial numbers of which settled along the Cape Fear River from Wilmington to Fayetteville and beyond.[1] When he was still a child his family moved to "one of the Northern Districts of South Carolina" and there "with very limited advantages he prosecuted the study of that profession in which he afterward became so distinguished."[2]

Having qualified for the practice of medicine by whatever means, Dr. Nicholson moved into Burke County, Georgia, where "surrounded by a wealthy and intelligent population, a most extended practice afforded him an opportunity of bringing the energies of a powerful intellect, and the sympathies of a feeling heart to bear on the malignant fevers of the Southern country."[3]

Dr. Nicholson's patients were presumably numerous and he apparently prospered. He was able to migrate to Florida about 1823 and purchase extensive acreage in northeast Gadsden County, his properties lying some three miles west of present-day Havana, north of the fire tower. There he built his home which still stands today as the oldest house in the county.[4]

Being a man of intelligence, integrity and material substance Dr. Nicholson was soon drawn into public life. In 1825 he was one of three commissioners chosen to select a county seat and is thought to have helped in laying out the plan for the Town of Quincy.[5] In the following year Governor Duval appointed him election judge for Florida's Sixth District which comprised all of Gadsden County.[6] On December 31, 1827, the Florida Legislative Council established a Territorial Medical Board charging it with the regulation and licensing of all practicing physicians in the Territory. Dr. Nicholson was one of nine physicians named to carry out its functions.[7] Finally, in 1833, he was appointed appraiser for the newly-organized Florida Union Bank, his second gubernatorial appointment.[8]

Nothing is known of Dr. Nicholson's wife beyond the fact that she was still living when the Census of 1830 was taken. Two adults and six children belonged to the household. The absence of Christian names makes further identification impossible. Ten years later the census enumerator omitted all mention of the Nicholson family. The Census of 1850, however, lists three sons, Donald, Archibald and Angus, the two elder ones married (each with one child) while Angus, 17 at the time, would later marry Sarah Wyatt, sister of his brother Archibald's wife, Adelia. The marriage occurred on February 9, 1854. A fourth son of Dr. Nicholson, also named Malcolm, and also destined to become a physician, is not listed in the Census of 1850.[9]

Dr. Nicholson died at his plantation home on April 19, 1840. His numerous descendants, some of whom still live today, were destined to exert considerable influence on the subsequent economic and social development of Gadsden County.

1. Information on Dr. Nicholson's early years is derived solely from his obituary, signed "W.W.W.," which appeared in the Tallahassee *Floridian*, of April 20, 1840. The eulogy, although effusive, appears to have expressed the true feelings of those who knew him well. The obituary is thought to have been written by Dr. William Woodson Waddel, a distinguished Tallahassee physician.

2. Ibid. It is probable that Dr. Nicholson had prepared for his profession through the apprenticeship system which prevailed in many parts of America throughout much of the 19th century. Neither the Medical College of South Carolina nor the Medical Department of the University of Georgia was in existence until 1824 and 1828 respectively.

3. Ibid.

4. Miles Kenan Womack Jr., *Gadsden, A Florida County in Word and Picture*, 1976. See page 15 for photograph of the Nicholson House. Womack has included useful maps showing lands acquired by Gadsden's early settlers.

5. Ibid., p. 15.

6. TP., XXIII, 625.

7. Florida Legislative Council, Acts, 6th Session, 1827-28, pp. 46-49. This act superseded a less restrictive act of December 30, 1824.

8. TP., XXIV, 815.

9. Additional information of value may be found in J. Randall Stanley, *History of Gadsden County*, Quincy, 1948, p. 31, et passim.

Nicholson Jr., Malcolm, Gadsden County, 1837-1899

Malcolm Nicholson Jr., youngest of the four sons of Dr. Malcolm Nicholson Sr., was born at the home of his father a few miles northeast of Quincy about 1837.[1] Upon the death of his father in 1840 he appears to have become for the remainder of his childhood a ward of relatives. In 1850 he was living in the home of James M. Gilchrist whose wife, Mary, was young Malcolm's sister.[2] Ten years later with his medical study completed, he resided with his brother, Angus, at the Nicholson plantation near Quincy.[3] Their father having been one of the wealthiest of the county's pioneer settlers, the sons became through inheritance well endowed.[4] Malcolm himself is shown to have owned property valued at $20,000 in 1860 while his slaves numbered 12. In the values of the times this would have established him within the ranks of the well-to-do.[5]

As for Malcolm's early education no information has emerged, but given the proximity of the Nicholson lands to Quincy, it is almost certain that he attended the Quincy Academy, the most reputable school in the county. For his early medical study, however, he appears to have gone to South Carolina to read medicine under the preceptorate of Dr. Joseph Rice of Barnwell District, an 1849 graduate of the Medical College of the State of South Carolina. After serving his apprenticeship young Nicholson matriculated at the same institution in the fall of 1855 and two years later, in the spring of 1857, he was graduated as an M.D.[6] His doctoral thesis bore the title, "Inflammation."

Dr. Nicholson's professional career was scarcely launched when it was interrupted by the outbreak of war. He enlisted in the Confederate cause in March 1862, committing himself for a term of three years. He was assigned to the Sixth Florida Infantry Regiment with the rank of 3rd sergeant. On August 11 following he was promoted to the rank of 2nd lieutenant by election in Company "B." His service record permits only a bare outline of his military career, but it appears certain that his medical training was never officially utilized by the Army authorities.

Dr. Nicholson was with his unit for the Kentucky campaign in the summer of 1862, subsequently returning to Knoxville for the following winter. On February 19, 1863, he was promoted to the rank of captain, replacing Captain Samuel B. Love as commander of Company "B." Soon thereafter he was beset by a series of misfortunes. In August 1863 he was hospitalized for an extended period and toward the end of that year a Medical Examining Board at Dalton, Georgia, recommended for him a leave of absence to begin on December 6, his ailment: chronic dysentery, emaciation and general debility. A year later when his company was encamped near Atlanta the company roster of August 11 listed him "sick." It is not known whether he was still with the Sixth Regiment when it was transferred to North Carolina in the spring of 1865 but it is probable that he was at Bentonville where he became a prisoner of war. His official record concludes with the information that as a prisoner of war he was paroled at Greensboro, North Carolina, on May 1, 1865, according to the terms of a "military convention of April 26th."[7]

With the war finished Dr. Nicholson returned to Gadsden, settling down on his farm and engaging in the dual occupations of farming and practicing medicine. There is no record that he was ever married, nor is there any indication that he was ever drawn into politics or public life generally. He was still living on January 25, 1899, when some 38 or more members of the Nicholson family gathered at the home of his brother and sister-in-law, Mr. and Mrs. Archibald Nicholson, to celebrate the 50th anniversary of their marriage. In a photograph of the family Dr. Nicholson is shown standing near the center of the group adorned in snow-white walrus moustache and flowing chin whiskers, bearing a striking resemblance to his brother.[8]

1. The Nicholson lands lay some four to six miles northeast of Quincy and southwest of present-day Havana. See Miles Kenan Womack, *Gadsden: A Florida County in Word and Picture*, Quincy, Gadsden County Bicentennial Committee, 1976, for a useful map on which are designated owners of Gadsden County lands during the years 1835-70. The original of this map is in the Strozier Library, Florida State University, Tallahassee. The date of Dr. Nicholson's birth is an extrapolation from Censuses of 1850 and 1860.
2. U.S. Census, 1850, Gadsden County, Florida, p. 180.
3. U.S. Census, 1860, Gadsden County, Florida, p. 83.
4. Both Angus and Archibald Nicholson owned property valued at $20,000 in 1860. Each owned 17 slaves.
5. A decade later, with the emancipation of slaves and the general disruptions following the war, the Nicholsons found themselves in greatly reduced circumstances.
6. Charleston *Daily Courier*, March 20, 1857. Records of the Medical College of the State of South Carolina now preserved in the Wing Historical Library, Medical University of South Carolina, identify Dr. Rice as Dr. Nicholson's preceptor.
7. NA, Service Records, CSA, M251, Roll 73.
8. Womack, *Gadsden*, p. 16.

Nixon, James M., Gadsden County, 1835

Among the early white settlers of Gadsden County were the Nixon family who had migrated from Duplin County, North Carolina, in early territorial days settling in or near Quincy. The senior member of the family, Dr. Nixon, was one of the first to practice medicine in the county. He appears to have arrived about 1830, purchased property, and settled down to the dual occupations of practicing medicine and farming.[1] Apparently a man of above average education and certainly one of intelligence, he soon entered into the public life of the county. In 1834 he was a member of the committee to make plans for the celebration of the upcoming Fourth of July. When the occasion arrived he was among those offering toasts.[2] He announced his candidacy for a seat in the Florida Legislative Council in December 1834, only to lose to the other candidate, John C. Love.[3] As late as March 1835, he was still looking toward the future when he announced the purchase of the Quincy Hotel, stating that he intended to operate it as Nixon's Hotel.[4]

Death intervened, however. On August 1, 1835, the Tallahassee *Floridian* announced the death of "Mrs. Temperance Nixon, consort of Dr. J.M. Nixon, and daughter of the late Thomas James, Esquire, of Duplin County, North Carolina, of consumption, after many months of illness." She was buried in Quincy. Only a few weeks later Dr. Nixon was also dead.[5]

Apparently in anticipation of an early death Dr. Nixon had made a will which bore the date April 1835. Among other provisions he requested that three tracts of land be sold to pay any expenses accruing to his estate. One of the parcels was described as the "Track or parcel of land near the Town of Quincy and commonly known as The Race Track."[6]

Survivors included two sons, Thomas and James, both natives of North Carolina, and both engaged in farming, and one daughter, Mary, who became the wife of Alexander Gregory. She too was born in North Carolina.[7]

1. Dr. Dixon owned land outside the town of Quincy and is assumed to have farmed it although he is not referred to as farmer.
2. Tallahassee *Floridian*, June 7, 1834. Ibid., July 12, 1834. His toast: "Gadsden County—May all her fellow crafts be entitled to receive better wages."
3. Ibid., December 27, 1834.
4. Ibid., April 4, 1835.
5. Ibid., September 17, 1841.
6. Miles Kenan Womack Jr., *Gadsden, A Florida County in Word and Pictures*, Quincy, 1976, p. 56.
7. Children were born to the two sons of Dr. Nixon, thus perpetuating the Nixon name in Gadsden County.

Noland, James T., Gainesville, 1870

Dr. Noland, a native of South Carolina and graduate of the Medical College of South Carolina in the class of 1861,[1] was a Gainesville practitioner for a brief period about 1870. The census that year lists him as 31 years of age, with a wife named Jane and a three-year-old daughter, Annie, both born in South Carolina.[2] No further information has been discovered.

1. Archives, Medical College of South Carolina, List of Graduates, p. 127. Here he is listed as J.F. Noland.
2. U.S. Census, 1870, Alachua County, Florida, item 1398.

Noyes, Charles, St. Augustine, 1841

Dr. Noyes, a physician in the United States Army, was a native of Massachusetts. He was commissioned Assistant Surgeon in Washington, D.C., on August 21, 1830.[1] After several years of hospital duty he was assigned to the Florida theater of war during the latter months of the Second Seminole War, serving in the army hospital in St. Augustine. He died there on July 26, 1841.[2]

1. Francis B. Heitman, *Historical Register of the United States Army*, Vol. I, Washington, D.C., Government Printing Office, 1903, p. 763.
2. St. Augustine, *Florida Herald and Southern Democrat*, July 30, 1841.

Oates, David Dunlap, Marion County, 1834

Dr. Oates was a sojourner in Florida. A native of North Carolina,[1] he spent his youth there where he presumably received his early education as well as basic medical training. He enrolled in the University of Virginia's Medical Department in 1857[2] and completed only one year of the regular two-year program. That institution's records state only that he went elsewhere for his degree.

By late 1859 Dr. Oates had made his way to Florida, probably because a relative had become the wife of Dr. Washington Agnew and was living in the northwestern corner of Marion County in what was known as the Wacahootie settlement.[3] The 1860 Census lists him as a resident of the Agnew household and since he was designated "physician," it is assumed that he had begun the practice of medicine in the community.[4]

With the outbreak of war in 1861 Dr. Oates enlisted for Confederate service, committing himself for a period of 12 months. He was mustered in at Fernandina on December 12, 1861, without rank in spite of his medical training and assigned to the Marion Light Artillery commanded by Captain John M. Martin. Only in the summer of 1862 were his medical skills recognized, whereupon he was placed on detached service with the rank of hospital steward to report to the Confederate Hospital at Knoxville, Tennessee. He also served in a similar capacity at the Lookout Mountain Hospital near Chattanooga. Gaps in his military record do not permit a precise account of his Tennessee service.[5]

As far as is known Dr. Oates remained in military service for the duration of the war, however with cessation of hostilities his immediate whereabouts are not known. Later information compiled by the University of Virginia Medical College about 1878 indicates that by the 1870s he had settled down to practice in Leeds, Alabama, an industrial town a few miles east of Brimingham, where he is thought to have lived out his life.

1. U.S. Census, 1860, Marion County, Florida, item 345.
2. University of Virginia, Charlottesville, Archives, "Lists of Students."
3. The 1850s saw numerous removals, amounting almost to a mass migration, out of South Carolina into Florida, doubtless attracted by the abundance of cheap land and final disposal of the Indian threat. Several members of the Agnew family had made the move from their native Abbeville District to the western part of Marion County.
4. The 1860 Census, note 1, supra, shows Dr. Washington Agnew as owning property valued at nearly $30,000.
5. NA, Service Records, CSA, M251, Roll 24. The record is incomplete.

Oates, John, Duval County, 1830

Dr. Oates arrived in Florida in early 1833, settling in Mandarin, Duval County. In April 1833 he offered his professional services to "the inhabitants of Mandarin and on the St. Johns River."[1] No record of the length of his practice in Florida has been located.

1. St. Augustine *Florida Herald*, April 25, 1833, and subsequent issues.

Oates, Philip, Marion County, 1870

Dr. Oates is known only through the Marion County Census of 1870 where he is listed as physician, aged 51, native of South Carolina, and owner of property valued at only $400. Other members of his household were his wife, Carrie, aged 50, daughter, Sophia, aged 27, and two sons, Wade and Samuel, aged

16 and 13 respectively. All the children are shown to have been natives of Florida.[1] The family appears to have lived on a farm outside Ocala.

1. U.S. Census, 1870, Marion County, Florida, p. 233. There seems to be no explanation why the family was not listed in earlier censuses.

Oliver, William J., Wakulla County, 1835

Little is known of the career of Dr. Oliver who practiced medicine briefly in Wakulla County immediately prior to the Civil War. He was the second son and third child of Berrien and Mary Oliver, the former a South Carolina native, the latter a North Carolinian,[1] whose three eldest children, Mary who married a Lawrence and was widowed by 1860, Peter and William J., were born in Georgia, and the youngest, James L., in Alabama.[2] The Oliver family apparently moved to Florida in the 1850s, settling in the Shell Point community[3] where the elder Oliver purchased a tract of land and built a cotton gin.[4] His properties were valued at $18,000 in 1860, which would establish him as one of the wealthiest men in the county.

Dr. Oliver announced the opening of his practice at Shell Point on January 26, 1859, adding that for the first couple of months his office would be located in the home of his father but beginning on March 1 he could be found at the residence of R.B. Forbes.[5] Apparently his plan did not materialize for in the summer of 1860 the census-taker found him still residing in the home of his father. He married Lucy L. Fisher, daughter of A.A. Fisher, Sheriff of Leon County and hotelkeeper in Tallahassee, on May 15, 1860.[6] Subsequent to June 16, 1860, when the census-taker called at the Oliver home and listed the newlyweds as residents there, nothing is known of either Dr. Oliver or his father.

Mrs. Elizabeth F. Smith published a genealogy of the Oliver Family of Wakulla County in 1964. She was able to account for James L., brother of the doctor, who married and continued to live in Wakulla County until his death in 1908. She also discovered that a second brother, Peter, moved to Gainesville where he reared a family, but of the other members of the family she found no trace.[7]

1. U.S. Census, 1860, Wakulla County, Florida, p. 24.
2. Mrs. Lawrence and her two sons, Lund and Oliver, were members of the Oliver household in 1860. Family tradition holds that the family had moved to Florida from a plantation near Phoenix City, Alabama, in the 1860s. See *The Magnolia Monthly*, Elizabeth F. Smith, Editor, II, No. 12, December 1964.
3. Shell Point later came to be known as Crawfordville, honoring Dr. John L. Crawford, perennial Florida legislator and Secretary of State, 1881-1902, who resided there. The name Shell Point at present applies to the area along the Gulf Coast of Wakulla County, lying between Live Oak Point and Spring Creek.
4. This cotton gin and other valuable property housed in it were burned in February 1859. Wakulla *Times* February 9, 1859. Berrien Oliver's losses were estimated at $2,000.
5. Ibid, January 26, 1859. Richard B. Forbes, also a Georgia native, was a farmer in the Medart community some 10 miles south of Crawfordville. See *Magnolia Monthly*, October 1964.
6. Tallahassee *Floridian and Journal*, June 2, 1860.
7. Descendants of Berrien Oliver may still be found in Wakulla County but his fate and that of his son, William J., are unknown.

Overstreet, Silas T., Suwannee County, 1830-1905

Among the earlier settlers to arrive in Middle Florida were several members of the Overstreet family who migrated from South Carolina in the 1820s. One of those was George E. Overstreet who settled in Madison County. When the wrath of the Seminole Indians was vented upon the white encroachers in the mid-1830s, the George Overstreet family was among the victims. Two of his children were slain while his wife suffered wounds from which she later died. Among the survivors was Silas T. Overstreet, a boy of five or six at the time of the Indian raids.

Silas Overstreet was born in Madison County on April 3, 1830. The circumstances of his childhood were such as to deprive him of any formal education, although the hardships of rural life in Madison County, and later in Hamilton County to which his family moved, toughened his fibre and bred into him the determination to make something worthwhile of his life. At the age of 17 he was hired by a party of surveyors commissioned to explore the swamplands of southwest Florida where he spent several months. In the meantime his family had returned to Madison County, and the Census of 1850 shows him living in the home of his father along with his brother Kayton and sister Phoebe.

At some unknown date in the 1850s, Overstreet decided to undertake the study of medicine. He apprenticed himself to Dr. Charles Hardee and began "reading" medicine and observing practice. In 1857 he was accepted as a matriculant at the Philadelphia College of Medicine and Surgery, where he was graduated as M.D. in the spring of 1859. Returning soon thereafter to Florida he began his medical practice in the village of Columbus, located on the west bank of the Suwannee River and later to be known as Ellaville.[1]

With the outbreak of war in 1861, Dr. Overstreet, aged 31 and unmarried, enlisted in the Madison County militia, soon to be mustered into the Second Florida Infantry Regiment of the Army of the Confederacy.[2] He was assigned to Company I, known as the Hamilton Blues, with the rank of private. He spent the first few months of service at Camp Stockton near Jacksonville.

The Second Regiment left Jacksonville for Richmond on July 15, 1861. It was the first Florida unit to be sent into the combat zone. After two months it was ordered to Yorktown where it would encamp for the winter. In the following spring it would see action in the defense of Yorktown and subsequently would participate in some of the bloodiest campaigns of the war. It is not clear from the war records, however, that Dr. Overstreet was with the Regiment after it entered combat. It appears that he was sent on detached service to one of the Confederate hospitals in Richmond and that he was himself a patient, having suffered an inguinal hernia and varicocele.[3] He received a discharge from the service on October 25, 1862, his papers having been signed by surgeon Emil T. Sabal of Jacksonville. The following year he returned to active duty and was assigned to the Medical Department with the rank of Assistant Surgeon, in which capacity he served until the end of the war. He was paroled in April 1865.[4] His military papers describe him as "six feet tall, of light complexion, light hair and blue eyes."

On his return to Florida Dr. Overstreet settled in Live Oak, Suwannee County, where he would remain for the rest of his life except for the years 1879-81 when he was at Chattahoochee as Superintendent of the Florida Hospital for the Insane.[5] Dr. Overstreet's public life was noteworthy. He was elected on October 10, 1865, to the State Constitutional Convention which met in Tallahassee on October 25. He represented his county in the Florida House of Representatives for two terms, where he was instrumental in the passage of a civil service pension bill. He was an active member of the Live Oak Methodist Church and a strong advocate of temperance, being himself a total abstainer.

In addition to his extensive medical practice, Dr. Overstreet was deeply interested in the improvement of the medical profession. In 1881 he was elected to membership in the Florida Medical Association.[6] Although he did not retain his membership he became the moving force behind the Suwannee County Medical Society, serving as its president for several terms and helping to make it one of the most vigorous in Florida. For 12 years he presided over the Board of Medical Examiners of the 3rd District of Florida.

In 1877 Dr. Overstreet was persuaded to set forth for publication his outlook for the future of Florida.[7] His first sentence bears quoting here:

> I am a native of Florida; forty-seven years of age; have followed close in the wake of the Seminoles from Madison to the Everglades; have lived in and visited nearly every portion of the State; have practiced medicine for twenty years in different localities, therefore have had an opportunity of observing Florida at her varied stages, from her infancy to her present state on the broad road to prospective prosperity.

Dr. Overstreet was twice married. On April 5, 1864, he married Elizabeth Hardee Goodbred; they had three children, George Pierce, Julia and Texas Langford. His second wife, whom he married on November 6, 1877, was Adeline Lang. Their daughter became the wife of Samuel C. Humphries. At his death, which occurred in Live Oak on October 3, 1905, he was survived by his widow and two children.[8]

1. Columbus was situated just south of the confluence of the Withlacoochee and Suwannee Rivers. It was at one time an important lumbering town.
2. Unfortunately the Civil War record of Dr. Overstreet has been only partially preserved and is found only in garbled form in NA, Service Records, CSA, M251, Roll 40.
3. An entry in Dr. Overstreet's war record under the date October 21, 1862, from Chimborazo Hospital, Richmond, Va., states: "Returned from furlough; transferred to Florida Hospital." This entry was made four days prior to his discharge.
4. Board of State Institutions, *Soldiers of Florida*, Tallahassee, 1903, p. 94.
5. R.B. Chardkoff, "The Development of State Responsibility for the Care of the Insane in Florida, 1830-1950," unpublished. M.A. thesis, Florida State University, 1964.
6. Florida Medical Association, *Proceedings*, 1881, Jacksonville, 1884, p. 4.
7. *Florida Dispatch*, October 17, 1877. This paper, published in Live Oak, was devoted primarily to promoting travel and the sale of real estate in Florida. It was sponsored by the railroads serving the state. At that time the southernmost terminals were Cedar Key in the west and Mellonville in the east.
8. Biographical sketches of Dr. Overstreet are found in Rowland W. Rerick, *Memoirs of Florida*, Atlanta, 1902, I, 642-43, and *Florida Medical Transactions*, Jacksonville, 1906, pp. 40-41. Dr. Overstreet was graduated with the final class of the Philadelphia College of Medicine and Surgery which opened in 1846 and closed in 1859.

Orr, Thomas, Tallahassee, 1827

Dr. Orr, one of the first professionally trained physicians to practice in Leon County, was a native of Scotland. On June 24, 1826, he respectfully informed his friends and general public that he had located in Tallahassee and was offering his services as a practitioner of medicine and surgery "having studied his profession in the Universities of Glasgow, Dublin and Edinburgh."[1] He further stated that "having practiced in Europe, North and South America, he hoped to merit a share of public patronage." He could be found at the tavern of Colonel Pendarvis. Some three weeks later he attended a Fourth of July celebration at which he offered a toast "to the memory of Emmet and Orr, to Irish patriots, glorious martyrs in the cause of Irish freedom."[2]

Dr. Orr had scarcely established himself in Tallahassee when his death occurred on January 15, 1827.[3] He was not among the doctors who subscribed to the posted list of fees.[4]

1. Tallahassee *Florida Intelligencer,* July 22, 1826.
2. Ibid., September 8, 1826.
3. Pensacola *Gazette,* February 9, 1827.
4. Bertram H. Groene, *Antebellum Tallahassee,* Tallahassee, 1971, p. 56.

Owens, James Byeram, Marion County, 1816-1889

Dr. Owens, a native of Fairfield County, South Carolina, was born about 1816. He was educated for the Baptist ministry at Edgefield Academy, later Furman University, at Greenville, South Carolina, and subsequently preached for a year or so in Alabama, then for a number of years in Mississippi.[1] He appears to have arrived in Marion County about 1858, having followed his two brothers, S.H. and W.A., who had moved to Florida a year or so earlier. As was true of his brothers,[2] the Reverend Mr. Owens arrived well-endowed, owning 89 slaves and total property valued at $118,000 in 1860. His Florida lands were said to have totaled 1,800 acres located in the vicinity of present-day Sparr. In addition to the usual farming pursuits—cattle, corn and cotton—he is said to have turned his attention to citrus and to have originated what is known as the "pineapple orange."

Family tradition holds that at some juncture Owens studied medicine which he proceeded to practice in the postbellum period in Marion County. At any rate the title "Doctor" was attached to him.

Census records indicate that Dr. Owens was the father of nine children and that he was twice married. Of the nine children, seven were daughters. The two eldest were born in Alabama, the next six in Mississippi, and the youngest, Ida, aged one in 1860, in Florida.[3]

Dr. Owens continued to live on his plantation until his death on August 1, 1889. He was buried in Evergreen Cemetery in Ocala. Among his many descendants was John W. Martin, grandson, who was governor of Florida, 1925-29.

1. Unless otherwise indicated, the substance of this brief sketch is derived from Ezra J. Warner and W. Buck Yearns, *Biographical Register of the Confederate Congress,* Baton Rouge, Louisiana State University Press, 1975, pp. 191-2.
2. Dr. Owens' brothers, Col. S.A. and W.A., had arrived in Marion County in the middle 1850s. They were among the most affluent settlers in the state. The eldest, Col. Owens, owned 156 slaves in 1860; his properties were valued at $230,000, while W.A., the youngest, owned 120 slaves and had property valued at $118,000.
3. U.S. Census, 1860, Marion County, Florida, pp. 16, 81.

Owen, J.J., St. Augustine, 1821

Dr. Owen is identified only through his obituary notice. He died in St. Augustine on December 5, 1821, at the age of 50, and was said to have lived previously in Baltimore, Maryland.[1]

1. St. Augustine *Florida Gazette,* December 10, 1821. Dr. Owen was one of several St. Augustine physicians who died within the first year of American occupation.

Pacetti, Joseph Anthony, St. Augustine and Jacksonville, 1837-1894

Dr. Pacetti, for several years a physician of prominence in northeast Florida, was born in St. Augustine on April 7, 1837,[1] the son of Joseph R. and Mary B. Pacetti. After receiving his basic education in the schools of St. Augustine he matriculated at the Medical College of the University of Maryland, Baltimore, in the fall of 1856 and was graduated Doctor of Medicine on March 10, 1858.[2] A few weeks later he began practice in St. Augustine. For reasons unknown, but probably because of the proportionately large number of physicians practicing in Jacksonville, or possibly because he had been urged by some of its citizens to settle among them, he chose to practice in the village of King's Ferry, located on the St. Mary's River[3] in Nassau County some 30 miles west of Fernandina. He remained there for only a few months before returning to St. Augustine, where he opened a drug store and for a brief period engaged in the dual occupations of pharmacist and physician.

Dr. Pacetti had scarcely begun his professional career when the Civil War began. He was not among the first to volunteer but as the war quickly assumed greater proportions he offered his services and was mustered into Company D, 8th Florida Infantry Regiment, in August 1861. A few weeks later he was raised to the rank of 1st lieutenant and on February 17, 1863, became a captain, a rank he retained until the end of the war.[4]

With his military career behind him, Dr. Pacetti returned to civilian practice, not in Florida but in Cardenas, Cuba, the land of his ancestors, where he is said to have practiced for about 20 years. There he met Amelia Morales whom he married on December 19, 1879. Because of unsettled conditions in Cuba Dr. Pacetti returned to Florida in 1885 and settled in Jacksonville, having purchased a house at 63 Julia Street where he was destined to live out his life.

Dr. Pacetti appears to have been much concerned for the quality of medical practice in Florida. This prompted him in 1888 at age 51 to become a member of the Florida Medical Association.[5] He paid his annual dues through the year 1892.

Dr. Pacetti died at his Jacksonville home at nine o'clock Friday morning, January 12, 1894. He was buried in Evergreen Cemetery there. As late as 1887 he was still practicing in his office on West Monroe Street at the southwest corner of Julia near his home.[6] He was survived by his wife of many years, sons Joseph A., who was employed as clerk for the Florida East Coast Railroad, and Richard, who held several clerical positions with Jacksonville business firms, and a daughter, Amelia.[7]

1. Vital statistics were provided by J.H. Higbee, of Jacksonville, whose wife, Amelia, was Dr. Pacetti's daughter. Material relating to Dr. Pacetti's military career and ancestry was made available by Professor Naaman J. Woodland Jr., of Lamar University, Beaumont, Texas. Mrs. Woodland is a lineal descendant of Gumercindo Pacetti of St. Augustine and Cardenas, Cuba.

2. Eugene F. Cordell, *Historical Sketch of the University of Maryland College of Medicine, 1807-1890*, Baltimore, 1891, p. 191.

3. See note 1, supra.

4. In Florida's general elections held in early October 1864, Dr. Pacetti's name was placed on the ballot as a candidate for a seat in the lower house of Florida's Legislature. This occurred at a time when he was on military duty in the fighting around Richmond, Virginia. On learning that he had been elected he immediately wrote to Florida's Secretary of State, Benjamin F. Allen, explaining his dilemma and resigning the legislative post. His letter is preserved in the National Archives (Civil War Records).

5. *Proceedings, Florida Medical Association*, 1888, and subsequent issues.

6. In the later years of his life Dr. Pacetti's address was changed to 228 Julia Street. See Jacksonville City Directories.

7. Ibid.

Palmer, James Lawrence, Jefferson County, 1831-1901

Dr. Palmer,[1] seventh son of Martin and Amelia Miles Palmer, was born in Monticello in 1831. Family tradition maintains that after a preparatory education in the schools there he entered the Medical Department of the University of Louisville from which he received the M.D. degree about 1853. He is said to have practiced for some three or four years in Logan County, Kentucky.[2] In 1857, however, he returned to Jefferson County and about midyear joined young Dr. Robert Gorman, also a Jefferson County native, in a medical partnership in Waukeenah, a village some 10 miles southwest of Monticello.[3] This arrangement was terminated in 1862 when Dr. Gorman enlisted in the Fifth Florida Infantry Regiment[4] and, so far as records indicate, was never resumed.

Dr. Palmer married Calidonia Rhodes in 1859, daughter of the Rev. J.W. Rhodes, pastor of the Monticello Methodist Church, recently deceased.[5] The couple continued to live in Waukeenah for several years before resettling in the northeastern part of Jefferson County in the village of Ashville. Three children were born, a daughter who died in childhood, a son, Frank, who died when still a youth, and Lawrence, Jr. The latter son settled in Tampa where his father joined him for the last years of his life. Dr. Palmer died in Tampa in July 1901 and was buried in the family cemetery in Monticello.

Unlike his brother, Dr. Thomas M. Palmer, and other Palmer physicians, Dr. Palmer spent his professional life in comparative obscurity, content to serve the medical needs of rural people of Jefferson and adjoining counties. A Jefferson County historian has portrayed him in the following passage:

> He belonged to that much beloved class known as the Country Family Physician. He was kind, affable, considerate and charitable. None but a Recording Angel will know of the many kind deeds and comfort rendered to suffering humanity by this good man.[6]

1. Theresa Yaeger Palmer, comp., and Hugh Archer Palmer, ed., *The Palmer Physicians*, 1966, p. 12.
2. This statement is based on inference. Samuel W. Butler, *The Medical Register and Directory of the United States*, Philadelphia, Office of Medical and Surgical Reporter, 1877, contains an entry, "J.L. Palmer, M.D., Keysburg, Kentucky," who is presumed to have been Dr. Palmer of Jefferson County.
3. Tallahassee *Floridian and Journal*, August 15, 1857.
4. NA, Service Records, CSA, M251, Roll 62. The record indicates that Dr. Gorman enlisted on March 1, 1862, for a period of three years.
5. Monticello *Family Friend*, December 17, 1859.
6. Mary Oakley McRory and Edith Clarke Barrows, *History of Jefferson County, Florida*, Monticello, 1935, p. 29.

Palmer, John Dabney, Monticello, 1841-1909

Dr. Palmer,[1] son of John Miles and Margaret Fletcher Palmer, was born in Monticello on June 27, 1841. After receiving a basic education in the schools of Monticello he entered the Medical Department of the University of Louisville from which he was graduated M.D. in 1866. He returned to Monticello to begin practice but soon turned his primary attention to pharmacy, an area in which his father was already well established. He was no mere drug store operator, however. Much of his energy was devoted to pharmacology and to the general improvement of pharmaceutical practice in Florida. He was elected president of the Florida State Pharmaceutical Association in 1888 (its second president) for a one year term. In 1889 Governor Francis Fleming appointed him to the first Board of Pharmacy in the state.

While still a part-time practicing physician in 1877, Dr. Palmer was elected to honorary membership in the Florida Medical Association on the recommendation of his uncle, Thomas M. Palmer, then president of the organization.[2] Even though he had ceased to practice medicine he enjoyed this honorary status for the rest of his life.

Dr. Palmer married Laura Josephine Willie in 1867 and from 1891 until 1896 they resided in Tampa, returning to Monticello in the latter year. He died there of pneumonia on February 21, 1909.

1. Theresa Yaeger Palmer, comp., and Hugh Archer Palmer, ed., *The Palmer Physicians*, 1966, pp. 13-14. Except for the note concerning Dr. Palmer's membership in the Florida Medical Association, the material used here is drawn from the work cited. Since he was primarily a pharmacist, much of the information has been omitted.

2. *Florida Medical Association Proceedings*, Jacksonville, 1877, p. 12; ibid., 1893, p. 48.

Palmer, John Denham, Monticello, Fernandina and Jacksonville, 1850-1912

Dr. Palmer, second son of Dr. Thomas M. and Jane Denham Palmer, was born in Monticello on July 14, 1850.[1] After attending the local schools of Monticello, during which he began to show an interest in medicine, he entered the University of Virginia where he spent the academic year, 1869-70.[2] In the fall of 1870 he transferred to the University of Maryland Medical College in Baltimore from which he received the medical degree in the spring of 1872.[3] Returning to Florida he established a practice in Fernandina where he was to spend the greater part of his professional life. In 1906 he moved to Jacksonville.[4]

Although he enjoyed the admiration and respect of his medical colleagues, Dr. Palmer was never an "organizational man." At the initial meeting of the Florida Medical Association in Jacksonville in January 1874, Dr. Palmer, though not present, was elected to membership.[5] There is no indication, however, that he was ever involved in the affairs of the Association. It was only in 1878 that he got around to paying his dues; in this instance $20 for the first four years of membership.[6] The *Proceedings* of the Association for the year 1893 list him as having been dropped from membership for "non-payment of dues."[7]

In Fernandina, however, Dr. Palmer was a dedicated practitioner. After surviving an attack of yellow fever during the deadly epidemic of 1877 he devoted much time and effort to the study and treatment of the disease. A few years later when the city of Memphis, Tennessee, experienced a particularly virulent epidemic of the disease, Dr. Palmer hastened to offer his knowledge and assistance to the afflicted people of the city. Through such humanitarian service he so endeared himself to the citizens of Memphis that they expressed their gratitude by awarding him an elaborately designed gold medal.[8]

Dr. Palmer married Sarah Rogers Walker, daughter of James Walker and granddaughter of the famous Dr. Henry Perrine who was murdered on Indian Key. Six children, three sons and three daughters, were born to the union. The second son was christened Perrine after his great-grandfather.

Dr. Palmer died as the result of a bizarre accident occurring in his office in the Doty Building in Jacksonville on November 3, 1912. He had just finished an examination and minor treatment of a patient, a young man whose pistol had been laid upon a table while the examination was in progress. As he was retrieving his coat preparatory to departure the pistol was accidently knocked to the floor whereupon it discharged, sending the bullet into the thigh and upward into the body of Dr. Palmer. Although he was rushed to St. Luke's Hospital his fellow physicians were unable to save his life. He died at 7:30 that evening, five hours after the accident.[9] He was buried in the family cemetery in Monticello.

At its annual meeting in Miami in the following spring the Florida Medical Association took formal notice of Dr. Palmer's death with fitting resolutions of affection and respect.[10]

1. Some material derives from Theresa Yaeger Palmer, comp., and Hugh Archer Palmer, ed., *The Palmer Physicians*, 1966.
2. "Students of the University of Virginia, 1825-75," a manuscript in MSS Department, University of Virginia Library, Charlottesville.
3. Eugene F. Cordell, *Historical Sketch of the University of Maryland School of Medicine, 1807-90*, Baltimore, 1891, p. 192.
4. Obituary notice in Jacksonville *Florida Times-Union*, November 4, 1912. The date of Dr. Palmer's death stated in note 1 appears to be incorrect.
5. *FMA, Proceedings, 1874*, Jacksonville, 1874, p. 6.
6. Ibid., 1879, p. 26.
7. Ibid., 1893, p. 46.
8. Palmer and Palmer, *Palmer Physicians*, pp. 6-7.
9. Jacksonville *Florida Times-Union*, November 4, 1912. The young patient, whose name is not revealed in the obituary notice, explained that he was carrying the weapon because of the present unrest about the city and that he would be returning home, some distance away, after dark. Apparently the angle and direction of the bullet upon entering Dr. Palmer's body removed all doubt that the shooting was anything but accidental.
10. *Transactions*, FMA, 1913, p. 29. There can be no doubt that Dr. Palmer was held in high esteem by his medical colleagues and that their tribute to his memory was a heartfelt expression of their sorrow.

Palmer, Thomas Martin, Monticello, 1821-1895

No Florida practitioner better exemplifies the ideal country doctor of the 19th century than Thomas Martin Palmer of Monticello. An imposing figure of a man at six feet four, of serious demeanor and superior mentality, he was for half a century one of Jefferson County's most beloved and respected citizens. He was the first of a long line of physicians in the Palmer family extending over five generations. At least 14 medical practitioners are numbered among the descendants of Martin Palmer, the first of the clan to settle in Florida.[1]

Dr. Palmer, second son and fifth child of Martin and Amelia Miles Palmer, was born in Pendleton District, South Carolina, on January 6, 1821. When he was eight his father sold off his considerable holdings in South Carolina, packed his movables into a number of wagons and carriages and with his wife and nine children, slaves and livestock, made the long trek to Florida, a journey requiring several days. He had chosen Monticello as his destination and on arrival purchased spacious lots within the recently platted village as well as large acreage just east of the settlement. Martin Palmer was both shrewd and industrious; he prospered. Although he achieved financial security, his children, 12 all told (three were born in Florida), were reared with a wholesome respect for work and a keen awareness of their expected roles as citizens.

Dr. Palmer received his early education in the school at Monticello. Although there is no supporting documentation, it is likely that he began medical study under the direction of Dr. James G. Pettus, Monticello's leading practitioner in the 1830s. He is said to have pursued his education further in Mobile and

New Orleans.[2] In the fall of 1842 he entered the Medical School of the University of Maryland from which he was graduated as M.D. in the spring of 1844. Returning to Monticello Dr. Palmer set up his practice and, except for the interruption imposed by the Civil War, remained there for the rest of his life.[3] He died on June 3, 1895. As was frequently true of physicians of the times he purchased a drug store whose wares were regularly advertised in the local newspaper.[4]

Dr. Palmer married Jane Denham, Scottish-born daughter of William Denham on December 9, 1847, a union which produced four children, three sons and a daughter. The eldest son, John Denham Palmer, became a physician and for several years practiced in Fernandina. After the death of Mrs. Palmer in October 1860, Dr. Palmer remained unmarried for more than two years, but on September 2, 1862, took as his second wife, Jessie Denham, sister of his deceased wife, Jane.

From the time of his graduation from medical school until the outbreak of war, Dr. Palmer carried on a routine medical practice in Jefferson County, treating fevers, healing wounds, delivering babies and, on occasion, employing his surgical skills. His success in amputating the leg of an injured railroad worker in February 1860 was noted in the Monticello newspaper as well as the *East Floridian* of Fernandina.[5] Now and then his services were required by state agencies. In 1850, for example, the Legislature authorized payment of $30 to "Dr. Thomas M. Palmer of Jefferson County" for postmortem examination of the body of one John Stafford, while in the following year, Dr. Palmer and his partner, Dr. B. Waller Taylor, received from the state $100 "for medical and surgical services rendered to Redding Evans, a prisoner in the Jefferson County jail."[6]

Dr. Palmer's community interests were numerous and varied. They ranged from representing the Jefferson Hussars, a local militia unit, at the Fourth of July celebration in Tallahassee[7] to judging mules at the Leon County Agricultural Fair.[8] More important were his political concerns. Shock waves touched off by the election of Lincoln in November 1860 were keenly felt in Florida. Dr. Palmer made a hurried trip to East Florida, stopping briefly at Newnansville, Gainesville, Micanopy, Jacksonville, Lake City and Fernandina. He reported strong secession sentiment all along his route, especially in Fernandina.[9] Upon returning to Monticello, he headed the local secessionist movement, representing his county at the State Convention meeting in Tallahassee on January 3, 1861. He was among the substantial majority voting for secession.

Having already been a member of the Jefferson Hussars, Dr. Palmer was among the first to become involved in military preparations for war. He received an appointment from Governor Madison S. Perry on July 13, 1861, as surgeon of the Second Florida Infantry Regiment about to leave for duty in Virginia.[10] In reporting the event the Monticello *Family Friend* added:

> In accepting same, Dr. Palmer makes a great sacrifice; but he was one of the first to boldly advocate the right and policy of secession, and he deems that he would be recreant to duty if he failed, now in our day of trial, to make sacrifices and aid in the struggle for maintenance of our rights, which the act of secession entails.

The item further cited Dr. Palmer as "a worthy gentleman, a competent and experienced physician." Within the month the dissolution of the partnership between Drs. Palmer and Taylor was announced.[11]

Dr. Palmer wrote to his friends in Monticello a lengthy letter filled with details on August 29, 1861. He had left Monticello on July 16, marched for nine hours and then had taken the train for Savannah where he and his unit were joyously received. Proceeding northward they arrived in Richmond on July 22, or as he put it, "on the day after the Battle of Manassas."[12] On September 20 he wrote from "Camp Bragg" near Yorktown to report on the sick and to outline for folks back home the more pressing needs of his medical unit.[13]

On becoming incapacitated by illness in the summer of 1862, Dr. Palmer was granted a leave of absence for recuperation. His return to Monticello was reported by the Monticello paper on August 9: "We have not had the pleasure of seeing him (Dr. Palmer) but understand that his health is very much shattered. He will doubtless, by a few weeks rest, sufficiently recuperate to permit him again to assume his position in the army, which, we are informed, is his intention."[14] It was during this furlough, on September 2, that Dr. Palmer married his second wife, Jessie.

In the meantime, a hospital for the care of Florida soldiers was established in Richmond and Dr. Palmer became its chief surgeon. Its doors had opened on September 20, 1862.[15] His frequent reports on the operation of the hospital, especially that of September 20, 1863, are valuable for their medical statistics.[16] In February 1864, the Florida Hospital as a separate facility was discontinued and Dr. Palmer was transferred to the General Confederate Hospital at Howard's Grove near Richmond[17] and here he served until the end of the war. On April 17, 1865, just eight days after General Lee's surrender. Dr. Palmer was paroled and permitted to return to Monticello.

Once more in Monticello Dr. Palmer resumed full-scale medical practice. At about this juncture, his father and mother having died (in 1857 and 1862 respectively), Dr. Palmer moved into the fine old family home, a magnificent place still occupied at the present time.

The Florida Medical Association was founded by a group of physicians meeting at the office of Dr. Abel Seymour Baldwin in Jacksonville on January 14, 1874, but Dr. Palmer was not among those present. He did, however, attend the meeting in Jacksonville the following year and was elected to membership. The Association met in Tallahassee in 1876 and Dr. Palmer was there. He was chosen president of the organization for the coming year, a testimonial to his splendid reputation and the esteem in which he was held.[18] At the meeting of the group in Jacksonville, convening on April 18, 1877, Dr. Palmer presided and in the evening delivered his presidential address. It was not a particularly distinguished speech, medically speaking, but a somewhat rambling and informal discourse entitled "Medical History of Florida," based on his recollections and observations during his 48 years of residence in Florida.[19] He dealt extensively with the various fevers endemic to Florida, their causes, symptoms and treatments, repeating at one point the not-yet-exploded theory of miasmatica, on which he offered the following: "It is not strange that malarial diseases should have prevailed as long as this new soil and luxuriant vegetation came into cultivation. The cotton plant was cultivated to a large extent, and this always causes malarial exhalations under a hot and rainy season."[20] It is recorded that a discussion followed on the subject of haematuria miasmatica in which Drs. Baldwin, Palmer and Daniel participated.

Dr. Palmer was present at the meeting of the Association in Jacksonville the following year (1878) where he found the president's chair draped in mourning for Dr. Francis Preston Wellford,[21] president-elect who had died in 1877. Since neither of the vice presidents[22] were present Dr. Palmer found himself once more in the chair, until later relieved by the election of a new president, Dr. R.D. Murray of Key West. In addition to his presidency Dr. Palmer served on several committees, most notably one charged with obtaining from the Legislature an "Act of Incorporation for the Association." Although he was not in attendance at the session of 1879 he was selected as one of four delegates to represent the Association at the next meeting of the American Medical Association. As far as the records show he did not attend any subsequent meetings but continued to pay his annual dues and remained in good standing until near the end of his life. He had been appointed in absentia orator for the session of 1884 but declined the honor.

1. Biographical material on Dr. Palmer is found in two published works, viz, (1) Theresa Yaeger Palmer, comp., and Hugh Archer Palmer, ed., *The Palmer Physicians*, 1966, place of publication not given, and (2) Mary Oakley McRory and Edith Clarke Barrows, *History of Jefferson County Florida*, Monticello, 1935, pp. 26-31; 42-45. Much of the genealogical information included here has been gleaned from these items. The sketch included in Col. J.J. Dickison, *Military History of Florida*, Atlanta, 1899, pp. 326-27, contains information on Dr. Palmer's military career.
2. Ibid. Only in Dickison's sketch have I found references to Dr. Palmer's sojourns in Mobile and New Orleans.
3. Family tradition maintains that Dr. Palmer also served in the Mexican War. While this appears probable no official documentation for such a claim has been located.
4. The Monticello *Family Friend*, March 22, 1859, contains a typical advertisement, listing medicines in general use at the time.
5. Fernandina *East Floridian*, February 23, 1860, copied from the Monticello *Family Friend* (not extant).
6. Laws of Florida, Tallahassee, 1851, Ch. 458, No. 147.
7. Tallahassee *Floridian*, July 10, 1846.
8. Tallahassee *Sentinel*, October 26, 1862.
9. Monticello *Family Friend*, November 17, 1860.
10. Ibid., July 13, 1861.
11. Ibid., August 24, 1861.
12. Ibid., September 7, 1861. Included is interesting information of treatment of wounded.
13. Ibid., October 5, 1861.
14. Ibid., August 9, 1862.
15. Tallahassee *Sentinel*, October 13, 1863. Here is printed a report submitted by Dr. Palmer on September 20, 1863, "on the first anniversary of the opening" of the Florida Hospital. For additional information see James C. Craig, "Cedar Point, Sawpit Bluff, Once Thriving Plantations," Jacksonville *Florida Times-Union*, April 22, 1951, p. 17.
16. Tallahassee *Sentinel*, August 4, 1863, and October 13, 1863. These two reports of Dr. Palmer contain important data on the operation of the hospital and types of injuries and illnesses under treatment.
17. NA, Service Records, CSA, M251, Roll 40.
18. *Proceedings, Florida Medical Association*, Sessions, 1876-77, Jacksonville, 1877, pp. 8-9.
19. Ibid., pp. 29-40.
20. Ibid., p. 33. Here Dr. Palmer was simply reiterating a theory generally held within and without the medical profession until discredited a few years later by the researches of Finlay, Reed, Gorgas, et al.
21. Ibid., Session, 1878, Jacksonville, 1878, p. 5, et passim.
22. The vice presidents-elect were Drs. R.P. Daniel, Jacksonville, and R.D. Murray, Key West.

Pardee, Frank, Alachua County, 1839

Dr. Pardee was one of many South Carolinians who settled in Alachua County in the year immediately following the Civil War.[1] He acquired land in the Micanopy community where he became engaged in farming while carrying on a limited medical practice. The Census of 1870 indicates that he was married to a Georgia native, known as Missouri. They shared their home with Dr. Pardee's mother Martha, who was 60. Nothing further is known of Dr. Pardee.

1. Dr. Pardee's name has been preserved in the little volume, *The Eden of the South* by Carl Webber, New York, 1883, and recently reprinted with an Introduction by Louis C. Goolsby.
2. U.S. Census, 1870, Alachua County, p. 3.

Parker, John H., Tallahassee and Pensacola, 1798-1837

Dr. Parker, a native of Halifax County, North Carolina, matriculated at the University of Maryland School of Medicine in the fall of 1820 and was graduated in the spring of 1822.[1] A few years later he moved to Leon County where he became a professional partner of Dr. Edward Bradford. The two men dissolved their partnership "by mutual consent" on March 17, 1832, and invited their clients to come in and settle their accounts.[2] Simultaneously Dr. Parker announced that he would continue to practice medicine from his office which "fronts the Capitol, just above Brown's Tavern." At the same time Dr. Bradford announced that he would continue his practice, presumably at his plantation a short distance north of Tallahassee.

It is not known how long Dr. Parker remained in Tallahassee. A year later, however, his professional card appeared in the Pensacola *Gazette* announcing the opening of his office in the Cillins Hotel.[3]

For the next four years Dr. Parker practiced medicine in Pensacola, presumably with success. At some unspecified juncture he purchased a tract of land on an island in the Escambia River, some 25 miles north of Pensacola, thought to have been some two or three miles north of the little town of Molino. Suddenly, on November 7, 1837, tragedy befell him. He went by horseback, apparently on the west bank of the river and, arriving alongside the island, hitched his horse, got into a pirugue (canoe) to row himself across to the island to check on the progress some of his slaves were making with their work. He was never heard from again. No evidence of foul play was ever discovered. A search party from Pensacola could find no clue as to his fate. The horse was found hitched to a tree; the pirogue was missing.[4]

Some time later a stone slab was erected to his memory in St. Michael's Cemetery by his Pensacola friends.

1. Eugene Fauntleroy Cordell, *Historical Sketch of the University of Maryland School of Medicine*, Baltimore, 1891, p. 192.
2. Tallahassee *Floridian*, April 10, 1832.
3. Pensacola *Gazette*, April 11, 1833.
4. Ibid., November 11, 1837. A search through subsequent issues of the *Gazette* revealed no further information as to his fate.

Parkhill, George Washington, Leon County, 1824-1862

Dr. Parkhill was born near Richmond, Virginia, in 1824. His father was John Parkhill, a native of Ireland who, with his brother, Samuel, had settled in Virginia in the early years of the 19th century. Both appear to have possessed exceptional business acumen for by the time they migrated to Leon County in 1828 they had accumulated sufficient means for the purchase of land and slaves and to become members of Leon County aristocracy. George Parkhill's mother, a Copeland of Virginia, died sometime in the 1830s and in 1838, his father married Lucy B. Randolph, also a Virginian.[1]

John Parkhill's lands lay in and around the village of Tuscawilla, a short distance northeast of Tallahassee on the Monticello post road. Soon after his arrival he obtained a post office for Tuscawilla and had himself appointed its postmaster.[2] He appears to have been instrumental in establishment of the Tuscawilla Academy at which his son, George, received an early education. In due time George entered the College of Physicians and Surgeons in New York City from which he was graduated as M.D. in the spring of 1845.[3]

Immediately following graduation Dr. Parkhill returned to Florida and on May 6, 1845, announced the launching of his medical career from an office at the home of his father at Tuscawilla.[4] From this point onward references to his medical practice are few but it may safely be assumed that he was a competent and well-respected practitioner. One wonders, however, why he was never involved in the numerous efforts of his colleagues to establish the much-needed professional organizations which might have improved the quality and standards of general practice in the state.[5]

Early in his career Dr. Parkhill became a political activist, embracing the convictions of his class regarding the major issues of slavery and states' rights. Quite naturally he was affiliated with the Whig Party whose strength in Florida derived chiefly from the planter aristocracy. Among his closest political associates was Edward C. Cabell, a Florida congressman for two terms.[6] Dr. Parkhill was a key figure at Leon County's Whig Convention in 1864. Observing the rapid disintegration of his party he offered a compromise which he hoped would strengthen its position in the state. He suggested abolishing both party names—Whig and Democrat—and presenting a Union ticket for the principal state offices.[7] He called himself a Constitutional Unionist. Democrats seemed willing to accept the plan but not his fellow Whigs.

Soon thereafter Dr. Parkhill, shunning the makeshift Know Nothing Party in which many Whigs had found a home, assumed a leadership role in the Democratic Party. In 1856 he was nominated for one of the four Leon County seats in the Florida House, winning handily as did the other three Democratic nominees.[8]

In the next four years, though continuing medical practice, Dr. Parkhill was drawn more and more into the vortex of political activity. With the breach between North and South widening Florida took the preliminary step toward war by augmenting its militia. In early 1860 Dr. Parkhill was nominated for the office of major general in the Western Division, Florida State Militia. In the election of May 7, 1860, he defeated two opponents by a vote of 235 to 24 and in the following month won the statewide election by a vote of 1,406 to 1,001.[9] The Apalachicola newspaper's evaluation of the man bears repeating here.

> He is favorably known to the people of the State. As a Democrat and delegate to the last two Democratic Conventions, his name has figured in a modest yet efficient manner. He has also served in our State Legislature, and his record is at once flattering to himself and eminently Southern. Educated in a Southern and Military School, he is fully qualified for the post to which his friends are endeavoring to elect him. A gentleman of the old school; born and raised in the South; generous, whole-souled and zealous advocate of Southern rights and Southern honor, he is peculiarly fitted in the present emergency of political affairs, for the office of Major General.
>
> Of Irish descent, he has all the soul, fire and courage of the sons of the Emerald Isle. We bespeak for him a cordial support.[10]

Dr. Parkhill was a Leon County delegate at the Secession Convention in Tallahassee in January 1861. He was among the huge majority voting for secession.

After the Battle of Bull Run in July 1861, preparations for war became more frantic in the South. Dr. Parkhill responded to the call to arms by enlisting in the Confederate Army on August 20, exchanging his rank of major general in the militia for that of captain in the Confederate Army and recruiting a company of volunteers under his command. His officers included his cousin, Richard Call Parkhill, with the rank of 2nd lieutenant. Early in 1862 the 2nd Florida Infantry Regiment, of which Capt. Parkhill's Company M was a component, was ordered to Virginia to help defend the Confederate capital, Richmond, the prime target of the Union Army. In a bloody battle at Gaines' Mill near Richmond, Dr. Parkhill was killed. The date was June 27, 1862.[11] He was buried in Shockoe Cemetery at Richmond, Va.

Dr. Parkhill was survived by his widow, Elizabeth, to whom he was married in 1858, a young son, Charles Breckenridge, born in 1859, and a daughter, Emmala, who was to become the wife of Dannitte H. Mays.[12]

1. Rowland H. Rerick, *Memoirs of Florida*, I, 644.
2. Mrs. Harold Major Pickett, Kenneth L. Rice, and Henry M. Spelman, *Florida Postal History and Postal Markings*, Palm Beach, 1957, p. 50.
3. Rerick, *Memoirs*, I, 644.
4. Tallahassee *Sentinel*, March 3, 1846, 1st printed in edition of May 6, 1845 (not extant).
5. At least two valiant efforts were made by groups of physicians of Middle Florida to establish a statewide medical association, one in 1848, another in 1856. Both failed because of indifference of physicians or legislative hostility. See Quincy *Times*, May 20, 1848, and Tallahassee *Floridian and Journal*, February 2, 1856.
6. Tallahassee *Sentinel*, July 11, 1854. In a letter Cabell protested strongly that he did not wish to be nominated for a third term in Congress.
7. Jacksonville *Florida Republican*, August 3, 1854.
8. Tallahassee *Floridian and Journal*, June 28, 1856; October 11, 1856.
9. Monticello *Family Friend*, May 12, 1860; June 23, 1860.
10. Ibid., Apalachicola *Times*, April 18, 1860 (not extant) reprinted in the Monticello paper on April 28, 1860.
11. The records of Dr. Parkhill's military service are fairly complete. See NA, Service Records, CSA, M251, Roll 40.
12. Mrs. Parkhill was the eldest daughter of William and Emmala (Simkins) Bellamy and granddaughter of the eminent pioneer, John (Jack) Bellamy. Her younger sister was married to Richard Call Parkhill, son of Samuel Parkhill and first cousin of Dr. Parkhill. Dr. Parkhill's son, Charles Breckinridge, went into law and enjoyed a distinguished career as a lawyer in Pensacola. See Rerick, *Memoirs*, I, 644.

Parramore, Henry J., Madison County, 1832-1901

Dr. Parramore, the eldest of the eight sons of Reddin W. Parramore, was born in Georgia in June 1832.[1] He was brought to Madison County by his parents when he was 13 years old. The family was one of considerable means, having owned 3,260 acres of land and 85 slaves just prior to the Civil War.[2] Their holdings were exceeded by only one other planter of the county, John Lipscomb.

Very little is known of Dr. Parramore's education and medical training. It is assumed that, since their home was situated near the town of Madison, he attended such local schools as the town afforded. He was possibly a student at the St. John's Seminary of Learning in Madison, a school that enjoyed a fine reputation. As for his medical education, since his name does not appear in the lists of students and graduates of the medical colleges of the South during that period it is assumed that he made his way into the medical profession by way of an apprenticeship under a Madison physician, very probably the highly-regarded Dr. John H. Pope. Dr. Parramore began his practice about 1853.

Dr. Parramore was married to Miss Antoinette Brinson in 1857, a native of New York, and the following year joined Dr. Thomas A. Perry in a professional partnership.[3] By 1860 he had established himself as a prosperous and well-regarded citizen of the Madison community, his properties being valued at $5,000, for those times a fair estate although far less than those of some of his brothers who had chosen planting as an occupation. Meanwhile, two daughters, Willie and Korah, had been born to the couple.

With the coming of the War in 1861 the Parramores were beset by troubles. Dr. Perry, who had volunteered for service in the Confederacy, was killed in the Battle of Seven Pines in Virginia in May 1862. Such property as Dr. Parramore had acquired had vanished under the stringencies of war. Meanwhile, his third child, born about 1861, had died. Since the family does not appear in the census of 1870, it is assumed that they had left the state at some time in the late 1860s.

By 1880 Dr. Parramore was once more in Madison. At about this date he became a partner with the popular Dr. Joseph F. Bythewood. For a brief period they practiced in Greenville, a village a few miles west of Madison but were soon reestablished in Madison where they advertised that "in case of necessity the attention of both will be given at no extra charge."[4] After a year or so the partnership was dissolved and Dr. Parramore continued to practice alone almost to the time of his death, which occurred on October 4, 1901.[5]

Dr. Parramore's wife had preceded him in death as had both of his daughters, Willie and Korah, the former having married Henry J. McCall. The two granddaughters of that marriage were his only survivors. They were Antoinette and Susie McCall, aged 17 and 12 respectively at the time of their grandfather's death.

1. U.S. Census, 1900, Madison County, Florida, Item 163.
2. Edwin B. Browning Sr., *History of the Greenville Missionary Baptist Church, 1849-1979*, Monticello, 1980, p. 11.
3. Madison *Southern Messenger*, December 25, 1858; first printed in issue of September 25, 1858, not extant.
4. Madison *Recorder*, November 4, 1882.
5. Record of death, Office of County Judge, Madison County Court House, Madison.

Paschall, Eaton O., Waldo, Ocala, Bronson, 1849

Dr. Paschall, eldest son of Dr. Edwin P. Paschall, was born in Orange County, North Carolina, in 1849.[1] As a lad of eight or nine he was brought to Florida by his parents who settled in the Waldo community, Alachua County. There the father carried on a medical practice, supplementing his meager income by operating a small farm. The war years of the 1860s brought hardships but the crushing blow was the death of Dr. Edwin Paschall about 1866 leaving his widow with the responsibility of rearing six sons. As late as 1870 young Eaton, then about 21 years old, was listed as a farm laborer, as was his younger brother, William B., aged 15.[2]

In spite of hardships Eaton Paschall was accepted for admission to Savannah Medical College, Savannah, in the fall of 1873 and on March 1, 1875, was graduated as Doctor of Medicine.[3] Soon thereafter he returned to Florida and within the year had begun medical practice in Ocala in partnership with Dr. Zephaniah Butt, an aging practitioner.[4] The arrangement was terminated about two years later when, for unknown reasons, Dr. Paschall decided to return to Waldo and begin his practice there. Meanwhile he had taken a wife, known only by her Christian name, Lily. The 1880 census lists the couple and their two children, Mary, aged three, and Louis G., aged three months.[5]

Dr. Paschall had some interest in organized medicine or at least was aware of the Florida Medical Association which was still in the formative years. In a notice in the Gainesville *Times* of April 8, 1878, he addressed the "Physicians of Alachua County," directing their attention to a published Association statement regarding the propriety of physicians in each county forming medical societies and sending delegates to the Association's meeting in Jacksonville on April 16. He emphasized the importance of the proposal, which should have been apparent, and expressed the hope that the older physicians would act on the matter, relying on the hearty cooperation of the medical fraternity.

Dr. Paschall had moved to Levy County by 1881 and settled in the village of Bronson where the drabness of daily life was occasionally broken by acts of violence which called for the attention of a physician. In 1881, for example, he appeared as a witness in the indictment of three Lancaster brothers for the murder of a Cedar Key citizen, Edward L. Drummond.[6] His published advertisement offered his services as "Physician, Surgeon, Accoucheur...promising prompt attention to calls at all hours." Charges were moderate.[7]

Many Florida physicians of the period found the collection of fees slow and difficult. Dr. Paschall was no exception. In 1883, he published this notice:[8]

> All persons indebted to me for past services are cordially invited to come forward and settle as early as possible. Otherwise they need not send for me in the future. Mr. W.J. Jones will collect and receipt for me in my absence. E.O. Paschall, M.D.

This notice apparently signaled his intention to seek a more lucrative situation elsewhere. Beyond this date nothing further is known of Dr. Paschall. He appeared in none of the Florida gazetteers or listing of physicians published after 1883 and it is concluded that he departed the state in late 1883 or soon thereafter.[9]

1. U.S. Census, 1850, Orange County, N.C., item 1566. Here Dr. Paschall is listed as a baby of nine months, having been born in late 1849.
2. Ibid., 1870, Alachua County, Florida, item 2378.
3. Savannah *Morning News*, May 2, 1875.
4. Ocala *East Florida Banner*, May 27, 1876. In directing attention to the professional card which appeared in this issue the editor wrote: "Dr. Paschall is a young physician and has recently moved to our village. He is studious and energetic and bears very high testimonials as to his proficiency in his profession."
5. U.S. Census, 1880, Alachua County, Florida item 148.
6. *Search for Tomorrow*, Levy County Archives Committee, Bronson, no date, Chapter 4, p. 10.
7. Bronson *Levy Enterprise*, February 23, 1883.
8. Ibid.
9. Dr. Paschall apparently returned to Waldo for at least a brief sojourn. The Tallahassee *Weekly Floridian*, December 18, 1883, printed the following notice: "Died at Waldo, Florida, Mrs. Paschall, wife of Dr. E.O. Paschall." No date of her death is given.

Paschall, Edwin P., Alachua County, 1829

Dr. Paschall, a native of Orange County, North Carolina, began his medical practice there about 1849.[1] Ten years later he moved with his wife, Mary C., and their three sons to Waldo where he purchased a farm outside the village and appears to have carried on the dual occupations of farming and practicing medicine. Insofar as records go he remained a somewhat obscure figure.[2]

With the coming of the Civil War Dr. Paschall enlisted and was mustered in on July 13, 1861, receiving an assignment in Company B, 2nd Florida Infantry, without officer rank. In the following year he was mustered out and discharged because of "disabilities."[3] But his army career was not finished. On March 15, 1864, he was commissioned Acting Assistant Surgeon and assigned to a unit of the Corps of Engineers located at Live Oak. The date of his final discharge remains unknown.[4]

An unfortunate circumstance developing in the summer of 1865 brought Dr. Paschall to public notice. M.A. Williams, presumably a citizen of Waldo, brought charges against him having to do with the loss of a quantity of cotton stored at Waldo when the town was under military rule. Responding to the charges authorities arrested Dr. Paschall and placed him in a military prison in Jacksonville "on charges to be preferred later." Weeks passed, however, while he languished in prison awaiting charges which were never preferred. On September 9, 1865, the Jacksonville *Florida Union* published his lengthy letter complaining of false arrest and imprisonment and hoping by this method to bring his plight to public attention. The implication was that Williams had a personal grievance against him. Presumably his plea was heard and he obtained release, although the paper made no further mention of the case.[5]

Dr. Paschall died at some time prior to 1870 but no date of death has been found. Meanwhile three other sons were born to the Paschalls after they moved to Florida, the youngest, christened Lunsford, was four years old in 1870. The two older sons, Eaton O. and William B., appear as farm laborers in the census of that year while the next two, James and Adolphus, were listed as school boys. The two youngest, Edwin, seven, and Lunsford, had no further designation.[6]

1. U.S. Census, 1850, Orange County, North Carolina, item 1566.
2. Ibid., 1860, Alachua County, Florida, item 67. The evaluation of his property at $500 suggests that Dr. Paschall was a man of very modest means.
3. *Soldiers of Florida*, Live Oak, 1903, p. 82.
4. Ibid., p. 320.
5. Since this incident occurred during the military occupation and since Dr. Paschall was held in a military prison, it is probable that Williams held a minor office in the Union Army and in the wholesale confusion after Appomattox the prisoner was simply overlooked.
6. U.S. Census, 1870, Alachua County, Florida, item 2378. *Records of the War of the Rebellion*, U.S. War Department, I, 42, 43, and 46, identify a Lunsford Paschall as a Captain in the 54th N.C. Infantry Regiment, serving in the Army of General Jubal A. Early in the Valley of Virginia, possibly a brother of Dr. Paschall. Eaton O. Paschall, the eldest son, also became a physician, entering practice in 1877 in Ocala as a partner of Dr. Z. Butt. Ocala *East Florida Banner*, May 17, 1877.

Paschall, Zebulon M., Columbia County, 1815

Dr. Paschall, a native of Virginia and for several years a resident of Granville County, North Carolina,[1] moved to Columbia County with his wife, Eliza, and their seven children in 1859. He acquired land in the vicinity of Lake City[2] on which he settled, presumably with the idea that his two older sons, Richard and Robert, would operate the farm while he resumed the practice of medicine. He could hardly have arrived at a less propitious time. His financial resources, estimated at about $25,000 in 1860, he had invested in land and slaves. By early 1861 the prospects for a prosperous future had begun to dim.

Florida joined South Carolina and Mississippi in seceding from the Union on January 10, 1861. In April South Carolina militia fired on Ft. Sumter; it was only a matter of weeks before Florida was committed to the struggle.

Dr. Paschall's second son, Robert, enlisted for service on July 13, 1861. He was assigned to Company I, 3rd Florida Infantry Regiment, and sent to Amelia

Island at Fernandina, the regimental rendezvous area. He was barely 17 years old. After a winter in encampment near Jacksonville, he was with his company at its reorganization at Midway, Gadsden County, in May 1862. In August he went with the Regiment to Chattanooga where he became ill. He was hospitalized at nearby Ringgold, Georgia, where he died on December 5.[3]

Meanwhile the eldest son, Richard, had enlisted in the same regiment on May 8, 1862. He too was with the regiment at Chattanooga, was hospitalized in March and April 1863, was wounded at Chickamauga on September 25 and furloughed back to Florida. He returned to his unit in 1864 only to fall ill with hepatitis and diarrhea, resulting in his discharge.

Following such misfortunes, and deprived of slaves, the Paschall family did not remain long in Florida but returned, it is thought, to North Carolina.

1. U.S. Census, 1850, Granville County, North Carolina, item 66. Besides the sons, Richard and Robert, other children here listed were Mary, eight; Martha, six; and Mildred, two.

2. U.S. Census, 1860, Columbia County, Florida, p. 46. Listed here are three additional children, all born in North Carolina. They were Sallie, nine; Cornelia, seven; and Charles, one. It is the age of the youngest, Charles, which leads to the conclusion that the family did not arrive in Florida until 1859.

3. NA, Service Records, CSA, M251, Roll 50.

Pasley, Elhanan C., Marion County, 1833-1913

Dr. Pasley (Paisley) was a native of Laurens District,[1] South Carolina, born into a family of considerable means. In 1850 he matriculated at the Medical College of the State of South Carolina from which he was graduated on March 18, 1852, after having written a thesis on "Contagion." His preparatory education was said to have been classical.[2] The two decades prior to the Civil War witnessed the migration of numerous young South Carolinians into Marion County where they purchased tracts of land and settled into the life of plantation owners. Most were people of modest wealth, owners of a few slaves. It was among such settlers that Dr. Pasley came to reside in the mid-1850s, staking out his own claim near the village of Flemington.[3] Like his kinsmen, cousins Enoch and Washington Agnew, he was both planter and physician.

With the coming of war in 1861 Dr. Pasley, accompanied by this brother Charles, made his way to Fernandina where on September 12, 1861, he enlisted in the Second Florida Cavalry Regiment, providing his own horse. Notwithstanding his medical degree, he was inducted without rank. As the winter came on, however, the chilling damp of Ft. Clinch, located on the Atlantic Ocean north of Fernandina, proved too rigorous. He was incapacitated by severe rheumatic pains and on February 17, 1862, was given a discharge suggested by the surgeon's certificate of disability. From this document, a few details about Dr. Pasley may be gleaned. He was 27 years old, five feet nine inches tall, of fair complexion, with blue eyes and blonde hair. He was by profession a "physician." He would be returning to Flemington.[4]

Upon his discharge Dr. Pasley returned to Flemington where he recovered his health and spent the rest of his life as a rural physician-planter. Living as he did, on the northern fringe of Marion County, his activities seldom came to the attention of the Ocala newspapers. His caustic wit was well illustrated, however, in one communication which the newspaper chose to publish during the hectic days of Recontruction. With local government under "Carpetbagger" control, a liberated slave, Louis McGee, had been elected to the Marion County Commission. In this role he had sought Commission approval for payment to his wife, Amanda, for attention to her mother in her final illness. Upon hearing of this Dr. Pasley was moved to write to the Commision:[5]

> Sirs, Mrs. Amanda McGee came to me for a certificate (by the advice of a county commissioner) for pay for her diligence and kind attention to her own mother during her last illness. She expects to be remembered by the County, and as the times are very flush...taxes a mere nothing...the country free from debt, and in a prosperous condition...I think she should be handsomely rewarded for her parental love, that others with parents in like circumstances, may be stimulated to do their duty as becomes affectionate children. Therefore I think that the Honorable Board of Commissioners will be derelict of their duty unless they appropriate at least One Million Dollars in County certificates to the applicant. I remain very respectfully, E.C. Pasley, M.D., one of the tax payers, Marion Co.

Dr. Pasley lived on and continued medical practice until the night of July 17, 1913, when he was thrown from a horse, receiving injuries from which he died within a few hours. The editor of the Ocala *Banner* remembered him with affection and respect.[6]

> It is with profound sorrow that we announce the death of Dr. E.C. Pasley, who has been a resident of the County for nearly three score years. His name has been on the subscription list of the *Banner* continuously since it was founded in 1866...He was one of the most popular and widely known men in the County.

Of the doctor's departed wife the editor wrote: "Mrs. Pasley was a woman of superior culture and attainments and was very fond of literature, and had a wide circle of friends. She died many years ago..."

Dr. Pasley was buried in the family cemetery, located between Wacahoota and Flemington, beside his wife, Anne. His gravestone bears the following inscription:

> Dr. E.C. Pasley, b. Dec. 5, 1833, Died July 17, 1913
> Anne A. Williams "wife of Dr. E.C. Pasley," b. Jan. 25, 1842, d. Aug. 12, 1897.[7]

1. Dr. Pasley's place of birth is indicated in his Civil War Record. See: NA, Service Records, CSA, M251, Roll 11. See also U.S. Census, 1850, Laurens District, S.C., p. 211. Here he is listed as the son of Edmund and Caroline Pasley, second of their 10 children.
2. Archives, Medical College of South Carolina, List of Graduates. The account of the annual commencement of the College, in the spring of 1852 (March 18th), shows Dr. Pasley as having a "classical education" prior to entering medical school. Charleston *Courier*, March 18, 1852.
3. Dr. Pasley first appears in the Census records of Florida in 1860, as a resident in the home of Dr. and Mrs. Enoch Agnew.
4. See note 1, supra.
5. Ocala *East Florida Banner*, July 18, 1874.
6. Ocala *Banner*, July 25, 1913.
7. Mrs. Pasley was the daughter of Dr. Jesse Kendrick Williams, a resident of the Wacahoota-Flemington part of Marion County and a sister of Dr. Retis Joseph Williams of the same community.

Patterson, John, Madison County, mid-19th century

Obvious discrepancies in the biographical data relating to Dr. Patterson make it impossible to do more than merely identify him as a resident of Madison County in the middle of the 19th century. He was born in South Carolina, the eldest child of John H. and Sarah Patterson, both natives of South Carolina.[1] The family moved to Madison County in the latter 1840s settling on a farm outside the town of Madison.

As slavery became a more burning issue in the spring of 1861 and the threat of war loomed, citizens of the counties of north Florida, Escambia, Franklin, Jackson, Madison, Gadsden and Jefferson, began the mobilization of troops which resulted in the organization of the First Florida Regiment, which came into formal existence on April 5, 1861, seven days before the firing on Ft. Sumter.

John H. Patterson, not at that time a physician, was among the first to volunteer for service, enlisting on April 5 and joining Company F, of the First Florida Regiment.[2] Richard H. Bradford was the company commander. The company moved immediately to Camp Magnolia, located near Warrington, Escambia County. Although the records are missing, it is thought that Patterson was with the company when it participated in the attack on federal camps on Santa Rosa Island on October 8, 1861, when his company commander was killed.

Soon thereafter he was with the unit of Major John T. Miller which participated in the Battle of Shiloh in Tennessee in April 1862. A reorganization of the Regiment had taken place in January 1862 during which Patterson had been transferred to Company B. No further record of his military service has survived although it is stated that he was mustered out on April 4, 1862.[3]

Nothing is known of Dr. Patterson's medical training, which he probably underwent after release from army duty, and since his name does not appear on the lists of students and graduates of any of the medical schools of the South, it must be assumed that he prepared for medical practice through the apprenticeship system.

Whatever his professional training might have been, Dr. Patterson appears in the Census of 1870 as "Physician," aged 30, living at the rural home of his mother in Madison County. Amazingly, no further information on him has come to light.[4]

1. U.S. Census, 1850, Madison County, Florida, p. 346.
2. NA, Services Records, CSA.
3. This mustering out apparently refers to his leaving Company F and reenlisting in Company B.
4. U.S. Census, 1880, Madison County, Florida. Here is found a listing for Dr. Patterson's brother Franklin, a lawyer practicing in Madison County. Also listed is his mother, Sarah, at the age of 58, p. 522, item 402, his sisters, Catherine and Sarah A., ages 24 and 29, respectively, and two grandsons, Frazier and Robert, ages 16 and 18, respectively.

Payne, George B., Alachua County, 1840s

Dr. Payne, native of Virginia, moved to Florida in the early 1840s and purchased land in and around Micanopy where he engaged in medical practice.[1] Tradition has it that he was the first physician to establish a permanent practice in Alachua County and that his services were available to the citizens of Marion County as well. He is said to have sold his property in Micanopy and moved to Ocala in 1854. One of the purchasers was a fellow physician, Dr. James S. Stewart.[2] It appears, however, that he did not remain long in Ocala for in the spring of 1858 he attended several meetings of the stockholders of the proposed Ocala-Alachua railroad. In each instance the newspapers identify him as physician and resident of Micanopy.[3] Furthermore, as a Micanopy resident in 1858, he was among those voting against incorporation of the town.[4]

The census schedule of 1850 indicates that he and his wife, Catherine, were parents of two children, Ida, aged seven, born in Virginia, and a son Marion born in Florida. These data indicate that he came to Florida between 1843 and 1847.[5] No date of death for Dr. Payne is known, but the absence of his name from the Census of 1860 suggests that he was deceased by that date.[6]

There is some confusion regarding the identity of Dr. Payne due to a George

Morton Payne residing in Marion County seven miles south of Micanopy. The Marion County Census of 1850 lists him as a lawyer and native of Virginia. He was doubtless a close kinsman of Dr. Payne. With his wife, Eliza, and their children, he lived on a plantation overlooking the southwest part of Orange Lake. It was known as "Lochbie" and contained about a thousand acres. An obituary notice of his younger son, Robert, who died on February 9, 1854, mentions that the boy's father was deceased. It also indicates that the family had moved to Florida about 1849. An older son of George M., named John M., was also a Florida physician.

There is a possibility that George Morton Payne was a medical practitioner, although not so designated in the census schedule. This assumption is based on the fact that a George M. Payne of Henry County was a medical student at Transylvania University, Lexington, Kentucky, in 1826-27. Since both Kentucky and Virginia have a Henry County, this student could well have been the later Florida resident.[7]

1. Webster Merritt and others have stated that Dr. Payne arrived in Florida about 1835 after a devastating freeze and began the cultivation of citrus, especially the Chinese "sweet orange," but the documentation for this has not been offered. Webster Merritt, "Physicians and Medicine in early Alachua County and Gainesville, Florida," p. 26. Fritz W. Buchholz, *History of Alachua County, Florida*, p. 168, and Charles L. Norton, *A Handbook of Florida*, p. 291.

2. Caroline B. Watkins, *The Story of Historic Micanopy*, p. 74.

3. *The Florida News*, Fernandina, March 31, 1858; *The Florida Peninsular*, Tampa, May 1, 1858; ibid., June 19, 1858.

4. Glunt MSS., Box II, P.K. Yonge Library of Florida History, "Poll Book, or List of Voters for and against Incorporating Town of Micanopy."

5. 7th U.S. Census, 1850, Alachua County, p. 1.

6. An entry in the Alachua County Census of 1860 appears further to confirm his death prior to 1860. Here the household of E.H. Jordan, Virginia-born probate judge, included not only Jordan, his wife and four children, but also three Payne children, Ida, aged 16, Rosa, aged 10, and Virginia, aged three.

7. Jacksonville *The Florida News*, April 1, 1854. Archives, Medical Department, Transylvania University, loaned by Professor Eric H. Christianson, University of Kentucky, Lexington.

Payne, John Morton, Marion County, 1835-1887

Dr. Payne, son of George Morton and Eliza D. Payne, was born in Virginia about 1835.[1] In his early youth he moved with his family to Marion County where they purchased a large tract of land on the southwest shores of Orange Lake, a portion of which they developed into orange groves. They called the place "Lochbie." It was situated around the present site of Orange Lake Post Office.[2]

Young Morton doubtless received an early education from private teachers. When he chose to begin the study of medicine, he placed himself under the guidance of Dr. George B. Payne, a cousin of his father, who had earlier settled at Micanopy a few miles north of "Lochbie." He entered the Medical College of the State of South Carolina in 1857 from which he was graduated the following year having chosen as his thesis topic, "Anaesthesia."[3]

After graduation Dr. Payne returned to Florida to practice medicine and assist his mother in the operation of the plantation, his father and younger brother, Robert, having died in the meantime.[4] The Civil War was already well under way when in March 1862 he enlisted in the Confederate Army. He entered as a private and was assigned to Company G, 7th Florida Infantry. After approximately three months of basic training at a temporary base in Marion County he was transferred to Co. C, 2nd Florida Cavalry, then quartered at Camp Finegan just west of Jacksonville. It was only in February 1863 that his medical training and skill were recognized. He was then assigned to the role of medical examiner of army recruits arriving at Camp Finegan. Finally, in July 1863, he was discharged from the cavalry regiment, appointed assistant surgeon and sent to Gainesville as medical examiner, a duty which he carried out later at Lake City.[5]

On his return to "Lochbie" in 1865 Dr. Payne offered the property for sale, describing it as "the beautiful and fertile estate...eight miles south of Micanopy, containing between 900 and 1000 acres...considered to be the richest and prettiest place in the County." He would sell for $5,000 in gold or an equivalent in currency or cotton.[6] When the sale did not materialize as expected, it was announced on March 1, 1866, that the land as well as the farm stock and equipment would be sold at public auction on March 15 following.[7] In this instance the estate was offered for sale by Dr. Payne's mother, Mrs. E.D. Payne, who announced that she was moving to Fernandina immediately.

Meanwhile Dr. Payne had purchased a hotel in Fernandina, a place known as "Coy House." This was noted in the Gainesville newspaper with the following statement: "Dr. Payne is a gentleman who understands the wants and wishes of the travelling public and will doubtless make his hotel a useful as well as ornamental establishment in the 'Island City.'"[8] Still the sale of "Lochbie" was delayed, and in April 1866 it was announced by Dr. Payne that Capt. George Houston had been appointed as agent to take charge of the estate of Mrs. Payne and the minor children of George M. Payne, deceased.[9] Still later in the year it was announced that "Dr. Payne has not been able to open Coy House as planned."[10] Not long afterward, however, the Fernandina *Courier* reported a visit to Fernandina by Governor David S. Walker, who was entertained sumptuously at "Fernandina House" by Dr. Payne, whose taste and skill "elicited flattering encomiums." It is, therefore, inferred that Dr. Payne had indeed opened Coy House, but under a more felicitous name.[11]

The Nassau County census of 1870 shows Dr. Payne as a resident of Fernandina and his occupation as "hotel keeper." His hotel was called "Virginia House." His property was valued at $73,000 which in those reconstruction years was a fortune of considerable size.[12]

At some time in the 1870s Dr. Payne gave up his Florida career and moved to Richmond, Virginia, where he was married and where he resumed the practice of medicine. Still later he moved to Roanoke, Virginia, where he continued practice and lived out the balance of his days. He died in Roanoke on August 3, 1887, and was judged to have been a "true Christian gentleman." He was the last of the Payne male line. Dolly (Payne) Madison, wife of the President, was of the same family.[13]

1. U.S. Census, 1850, Marion County, Florida, item 123. Although John Morton Payne was not included in this census, probably because of a temporary absence from his home, his identity as a member of the George M. Payne family is incontrovertably established in subsequent censuses and elsewhere.
2. Jacksonville *Florida News*, April 1, 1854.
3. Archives, Waring Historical Library, MUSC, Lists of Graduates of MCSSC.
4. See note 2 supra for obituary of Robert Payne.
5. NA, Service Records, CSA, M251, Roll 79; for his cavalry and medical records see ibid., Roll 11.
6. Gainesville *New Era*, October 21, 1865.
7. Ibid., March 3, 1866. Here the name of the seller is erroneously given as Mr. E.D. Payne instead of Mrs. Eliza D. Payne.
8. Ibid.

9. Ibid., April 7, 1866.
10. Tallahassee *Tri-Weekly Florida Sentinel*, August 2, 1866. This was a reprint of the Savannah *News*, June 30, 1866.
11. Gainesville *New Era*, July 13, 1866, reprinted from the Fernandina *Courier*.
12. U.S. Census, 1870, Nassau County, Florida, p. 42, it. 423.
13. Fernandina *Florida Mirror*, August 20, 1887. In Dr. Payne's obituary it is noted that three of his sisters still lived in Fernandina: Mrs. Downie, Miss Celia Payne, and Miss Susan Payne.

Peacock, Calvin, Suwannee County, 1813-post 1870

Dr. Peacock, physician and farmer of Suwannee and Lafayette Counties in the latter half of the 19th century, arrived in Florida about 1857 from North Carolina. He purchased land near the village of Houston a few miles east of Live Oak and in 1860 his real and personal properties were valued at $14,000 and $18,000 respectively.[1] Extrapolating from the census data of that year the date of his birth was about 1813. His children, nine in number, were born in North Carolina with the exception of the youngest, Elbert, who was born in Florida. At some date prior to 1870 Dr. Peacock moved to New Troy, located in Lafayette County, on the west side of the Suwannee River. The ravages of war are reflected in the Census of 1870 which shows that his property had dwindled in value to $5,500.[2] As for Dr. Peacock's medical education and practice nothing is currently known.

Dr. Peacock was twice married, his first wife, a North Carolina native named Elizabeth, died prior to 1870. After her death Dr. Peacock married Georgia-born Ann whose age in 1870 is said to have been 44. Both she and Dr. Peacock were still living in 1880.

1. U.S. Census, 1860, Suwannee County, Florida, p. 26.
2. U.S. Census, 1870, Suwannee County, Florida, pp. 666, 668.

Pearson, Benjamin, St. Johns Section, 1819

There is only a fleeting glimpse of Dr. Pearson and this on the occasion of his appearance before the Spanish authorities in St. Augustine on January 18, 1819, to take an oath of allegiance to the Spanish crown. He stated that he was a native of Plymouth, England, and unmarried. He gave his age as 37, religion as Protestant and profession as physician.[1]

The compilers of *Spanish Land Grants in Florida* have identified a Captain Pearson, commander of the Schooner *Florida* engaged in the slave trade, as Benjamin Pearson. The documentation is missing, however.[2]

1. EFP., Reel 163, Bundle 350-U4, p. 5000. Seen in P.K. Yonge Library of Florida History. Information courtesy of Bruce S. Chappell.
2. SLGF, I. D-4. See ibid., Index, p. 364.

Peck, Seth S., St. Augustine, 1790-1841

The arrival in St. Augustine of Dr. Peck and his family in mid-October 1834 was an event of more importance than indicated by the local newspaper which relegated it to the shipping news.[1] The Pecks were people of quality and cultivation who soon established themselves as social and cultural leaders in the community. Although Dr. Peck was doubtless in delicate health when he came to

Florida and destined for an early death, his son John, also a physician, took his place as an outstanding practitioner and citizen for many years.

Local tradition has it that Dr. Peck had come to St. Augustine as early as 1832, possibly in search of a healthful climate, and bought an ancient house at the corner of St. George and Treasury Streets, now known as the Peck House, whose walls dated back to the late 17th century.[2] Well-documented, however, is Dr. Peck's entry into medical practice in the city in 1833. It was announced on November 27, 1833, that Dr. S.S. Peck, "having concluded to make this City his future residence, offers his services in the practice of medicine and surgery to the citizens and visitors of St. Augustine." It was further stated that he had opened an office in "the south room of the City Hotel" and also that he had a supply of drugs and medicines of the best quality.[3] It augured well for him that simultaneously the popular Dr. Andrew Anderson was retiring from active practice and was pleased to recommend "Dr. S.S. Peck of New York as a gentleman, whose liberal attainments, long experience and extensive practice" entitled him to the "patronage of the Public."[4]

In the latter part of 1834 Dr. Peck returned to his home in Whitesboro, N.Y., to arrange for his family to join him in St. Augustine. They arrived aboard the Schooner *Topic* on October 16. Included were his wife, Sarah, daughters, Mary, Lucy (later to become the wife of George Burt) and Sarah (who died only two years later at the age of six), as well as his only son John, a lad of 16. Not included in the passenger list was the other daughter, Rebecca.[5]

In addition to a substantial investment in his house Dr. Peck purchased other properties in the north part of the City, some 31 lots in all, which would provide his children with a munificent legacy.[6] He also became a stockholder in the Southern Life Insurance and Trust Company, serving for a time on its board of trustees.[7]

Either through his own cultural interests or those of his wife the Peck house was made available for the teaching of classes in French and German by Professor J.J. Delissa, an enterprise supported also by Dr. Peter Porcher, a Charleston physician living in St. Augustine, who offered his house for the afternoon sessions.[8]

Beyond the day-to-day practice in which most physicians engaged, the onset of the "sickly season" coming usually about the end of August and ending in November, bringing a variety of fevers the most deadly being the "yellow" type, imposed exceptional demands on the medical practitioners of Florida. A few glimpses of Dr. Peck's labors in such crises are preserved in the writings of Dr. Benjamin B. Strobel, a Charleston doctor who had spent four years in Key West (1829-33) and was inspired to make extensive investigations into the origins and transmissibility of the disease. Hearing of a very serious outbreak of yellow fever in the fall of 1839 Dr. Strobel hurried there to obtain first-hand information. He sought out Dr. Peck and other St. Augustine physicians interrogating them on every conceivable aspect of the epidemic. Dr. Peck was able to provide useful data and well-considered theories, having himself kept records of the local outbreak. These became an important segment of Dr. Strobel's book. It was Dr. Peck's opinion that yellow fever was not endemic to the area but instead was introduced by visitors or seamen arriving from other parts. He also noted that the ailment was generally of a milder form among the natives than among "strangers." He reported to Dr. Strobel that he had attended upwards of 300 cases in the current season among whom he had recorded 15 deaths. Dr. Peck was obviously not a mere dilettante physician.[9]

Dr. Peck died in St. Augustine on July 21, 1841, aged 50 years and 11 months, after a lingering illness.[10] An informative obituary notice bears citing:

> Died.......Doctor Seth S. Peck, a native of Connecticut, and for many years previous to his removal to Florida, a resident of Whitesboro, N.Y. For several years past he has been known to this city, as in the place of his former abode, as a faithful and skillful physician, and a man of strict integrity. He was a man of few professions (possibly a reference to casual concern with formal religion), but the tenor of his daily life proved the sincerity and depth of his attachment to the principles of religion and morality, of which he was ever the steadfast friend and advocate. The memory of this just and good man will long be revered, and to the bereaved family, over which as the kind husband, the watchful and affectionate parent, he has presided with a firm, gentle and wise spirit, the warmest sympathies of this community are respectfully tendered.[11]

Dr. Peck and his wife, Sarah, who lived on until August 16, 1879, when she died at the age of 88, were buried in the Huguenot Cemetery in St. Augustine.[12]

1. St. Augustine *Florida Herald*, October 16, 1834.
2. WPA, Writers Program, St. Augustine (Four Parts), typescript, unpaginated. Pt. II, sketch by Darran Bridges. In the early part of the 20th century the house belonged to Miss Anna Burt, granddaughter of Dr. Peck. In 1931 she gave the house to the city of St. Augustine.
3. St. Augustine, *Florida Herald*, December 5, 1833.
4. Ibid., November 27, 1833.
5. Ibid., October 16, 1834.
6. Ibid., April 2, 1844.
7. Ibid., August 3, 1838.
8. Ibid., June 3, 1835 and subsequent issues.
9. B.B. Strobel, *An Essay on the Subject of Yellow Fever, Intended to Prove Its Transmissibility*, Charleston, 1840, p. 163. Dr. Strobel also sought opinions from other physicians, including Dr. Frederick Weedon, Dr. Charles Byrne and Dr. Richard Weightman.
10. It was recorded by the *Florida Herald*, July 23, 1841, that he had died of "pulmonary consumption."
11. St. Augustine *News*, July 23, 1841. Whitesboro, Oneida County, N.Y.
12. The gravestones of Dr. and Mrs. Peck are among the few which are well preserved and whose inscriptions are quite legible.

Peeler, Anderson, Jefferson County, 1818-1893

Dr. Peeler was one of four members of the Peeler family who left their native Georgia and settled in Florida in the mid-19th century. Two of them, James and William, were clergymen instrumental in the propagation of Methodism throughout Florida while the third, Joseph, spent his adult life as a Jefferson County farmer. Although he does not appear in the Jefferson County Census of 1850,[1] Dr. Peeler was a resident of the state as early as 1845 when he attended the first annual meeting of the Florida Methodist Conference which convened at Tallahassee on February 6 of that year. He was one of 12 men ordained as elders at that session.[2] A year later when the conference met at Monticello, he was "located," that is admitted to preach whenever his services were needed.[3]

Meanwhile Dr. Peeler had carried on a medical practice at Bailey's Mill, later to be known as Lloyd. He was "readmitted" to the Conference in 1850 and appointed to serve as pastor in Brunswick, Georgia.[4] The following year he was assigned to Albany, Georgia, as a regular preacher,[5] while in 1852 both Dr. Peeler and his brother, James, were appointed to the Madison circuit.[6]

For the next few years Dr. Peeler's whereabouts are unknown but at some juncture he appears to have shed his clerical robes and resumed medical practice. He announced on January 9, 1858, that he was moving to Waukeenah, a village some 14 miles southwest of Monticello, where he would join Dr. J.C. Bates in a medical partnership.[7] He remained there for the next two years, moving into Monticello in January 1860. According to his professional card he expected to "continue his practice of medicine in all acute and chronic diseases" and could be found "at his residence on the southwest corner of the public square, west of Col. (Elias E.) Blackburn's Hotel."[8]

As the Civil War drew near Dr. Peeler came forward as a champion of states' rights and an opponent of the Abolitionists. When the election of Lincoln was assured, a wave of anger engulfed Middle Florida, a land of plantations supported by slave labor. On November 7, 1860, a meeting was convened at the Jefferson County Court House presumably to calm the anxiety and caution against rash action by the citizens. It appears to have produced the opposite reaction. Col. Blackburn took the podium and railed against the Abolitionists; he was followed by Dr. Peeler who labeled Lincoln's election a disaster. Any union with Lincoln was unthinkable. He saw secession as inevitable and urged Florida to join the movement[9] which the people proceeded to do just four weeks later.

Dr. Peeler appears to have remained in Monticello throughout the war although nothing is known of his activities. There is no doubt, however, that he gained the confidence and respect of local citizens for in November 1865 he was elected to represent Jefferson County in the Florida House of Representatives, in which he served for the sessions of 1865 and 1866.[10] As far as is known Dr. Peeler continued medical practice without interruption until December 1874 when for reasons by no means clear he returned to the church as a regular pastor. According to the Reverend John C. Ley, for many years a Florida Methodist, Dr. Peeler was "readmitted" at the Live Oak meeting of the Conference (1874) "returning to spend his remaining strength in the service."[11] His death occurred in 1893 at the age of 75. The Reverend Mr. Ley remembered him as "a clear reasoner, and his sermons partook of a doctrinal type."

Dr. Peeler spent his last years in Orange County where his second son, James P., had settled in the practice of medicine.[12] His eldest son, Wilber, also a physician, practiced at Mount Tabor, Columbia County, in the latter part of the 19th century.[13]

1. An anecdotal account of the early history of Methodism in Florida can be found in John C. Ley, *Fifty-Two Years in Florida*, Nashville, 1899, which contains numerous references to the Peeler family. It is to be borne in mind that throughout its early history Methodism, especially in the frontier areas of America, demanded little by way of formal preparation for its ministry. Outward manifestations of piety, grace, and devoutness as well as a gift with words were often sufficient to qualify a person for the pulpit. Novices were usually admitted "on trial," ordination being withheld if they were judged unworthy of trust. As for the Florida Conference, at its inception, and for many years afterwards, it embraced all of Middle and East Florida as well as that portion of Georgia lying south of Ft. Gaines, Albany and the Altamaha River, roughly the southern fifth of the state.

2. Ibid., p. 60.

3. Ibid., p. 61.

4. *Minutes of the Annual Conference of the Methodist Episcopal Church, South*, 1845-1853 (n.p., 1845), p. 260. For Dr. Peeler's appointment to the Brunswick District, see Tallahassee *Floridian and Journal*, February 11, 1850. At this meeting he was also appointed an agent for the Fletcher Institute, an academy located in Thomasville, Georgia.

5. *Minutes*, p. 366.

6. Ibid., p. 421.

7. Tallahassee *Floridian and Journal*, January 16, 1858.

8. Monticello *Family Friend*, February 18, 1860.

9. Ibid., November 8, 1860. Soon thereafter Dr. Peeler was a member of a Committee of Fifteen charged with preparing an agenda for a second mass meeting soon to follow. Ibid., November 17, 1860.

10. Florida, House Journals, 1865, 1866, passim.

11. Ley, Fifty-Two Years, p. 104.

12. After completing his medical training Dr. James P. Peeler settled in Kissimmee located in that portion of Orange County which was to become Osceola County in 1887. He was a member of the Florida Medical Association until his death in 1891. At the time of his death he was President of the Osceola County Medical Society. See *Proceedings, Florida Medical Association*, 1891, p. 8. See also ibid., 1893, p. 46.

13. U.S. Census, 1880, Columbia County, Florida, Dist. 8, item 97.

Peeples, William Lewis, Hamilton County, 1833-1896

Dr. Peeples, second son of Isam and Mary Peeples, was born in Camden County, Georgia, on September 18, 1833.[1] After obtaining a basic education in local schools and presumably serving his medical apprenticeship in the office of a St. Mary's doctor, he entered Oglethorpe Medical College in Savannah in the fall of 1857 and was graduated on May 1, 1859, after submitting a thesis entitled "The Human Body."[2] Soon after graduation he settled in Hamilton County, where his sister Mary and her husband, Lemuel Taylor, had previously homesteaded. For a brief period Dr. Peeples shared their house. He married Sarah Hartford Tuten on September 11, 1861, daughter of a family originating in South Carolina.[3]

In the course of time the Peeples lived at two different locations in Hamilton County, both rural. They settled first at Belmont some 14 miles northeast of Jasper near the Suwannee River; later they moved to Marion Station, six miles south of Jasper on the Savannah, Florida and Western Railroad. Through his integrity and service to the people of his county he became a highly respected and trusted citizen, and in 1877 was elected to the Hamilton County Commission in which he served for two years. A decade later he was elected to the Florida House of Representatives, in which he served for two terms, 1885, 1887.[4]

Although he was never a member of the Confederate armed forces, he is known to have attended Confederate soldiers wounded in the Battle of Olustee in February 1864. He lived out his life in Hamilton County, dying there on September 2, 1896.

1. The biographical information was supplied for the most part by Vernon E. Peeples of Punta Gorda, a grandson of Dr. Peeples. The Hamilton County Censuses for 1860, 1870 and 1880 include entries for the Peeples family.

2. See Savannah *Daily Morning News*, March 3, 1859, for an account of the commencement exercises of Oglethorpe Medical College, held at St. Andrew's Hall on March 1, 1859. This includes a list of graduates and topics of their respective theses.

3. Information, Vernon E. Peeples.

4. Allen Morris, *The People of Lawmaking in Florida*, 1977 ed.

Pelot, James D., Nassau and Duval Counties, 1816-1840

Dr. Pelot, member of a prominent Georgia family of Swiss extraction, was born about 1816[1] on Amelia Island, Nassau County. He received a medical degree from Jefferson Medical College, Philadelphia, in 1836.[2] His earliest professional notice appeared in the Jacksonville *East Florida Advocate* of August 4, 1840, but he appears to have been in practice in Jacksonville a year or so earlier for in April 1840, Dr. Abel S. Baldwin announced that he was moving into "rooms previously occupied by Dr. Pelot."[3]

Dr. Pelot's career ended tragically in December 1840 the result of a duel with a man named Babcock, the sequel to a drinking bout in a Jacksonville tavern.

The "affair of honor" took place on Cumberland Island, Georgia. Rifles were the weapons agreed upon by the antagonists and with the simultaneous firing by the two men Dr. Pelot was struck in the stomach, the bullet penetrating his body and severing his spine. Death, however, was not instantaneous. Duval County records show that he was given medical treatment for about a week before his death on or about December 31. The duel had apparently taken place on or about the 24th.[4]

Dr. Pelot was the grandson of James Pelot Sr., first of the family to settle in America. His father, James Jr., had settled on Amelia Island and married Susan Marion Cooper.[5] He was survived by two brothers, John Cooper and Charles H., the latter becoming an attorney in Fernandina. His nephew, John Crews Pelot, son of John Cooper Pelot, enjoyed a long and distinguished career in medicine and politics.

1. This date is a deduction from the date of his medical degree which he received in 1836. The average age of medical degree recipients of that era appears to have been about 20.

2. Archives, Jefferson Medical College, Philadelphia, Lists of Graduates.

3. Jacksonville *East Florida Advocate*, April 21, 1840.

4. Information provided by Mrs. Julia Pelot Colket, Cleveland Heights, Ohio, a direct descendant of Dr. Pelot's brother, John Cooper Pelot (1809-1879). See also T. Frederick Davis, *History of Jacksonville, Florida, and Vicinity*, facsimile ed., Gainesville, 1964, p. 83.

5. From information provided by Mrs. Colket. See note 4, supra.

Pelot, John Crews, Nassau and Manatee Counties, 1831-1917

Dr. Pelot, member of a family of property and social prominence in North Florida, spent the greater part of his professional career in Manatee County.[1] The date of his arrival there is undetermined, but it seems reasonably certain that it occurred in late 1865. A conveyance of 1,147 acres of land on the Manatee River, known as the Dr. Joseph Braden tract, from Daniel Ladd and wife to Mary E. Pelot, wife of Dr. Pelot, is a matter of record, the indenture bearing the date August 8, 1867.[2] For their residence the Pelots bought the Griffin home in the village of Manatee, which was located in the second block east of the Methodist Church. They then proceeded to plant a number of orange groves on portions of their land.

Dr. Pelot came from Swiss stock, his earliest American ancestor having settled at Purysburg, South Carolina, some 15 miles upriver from Savannah. His grandfather, James Pelot Jr., moved from South Carolina to Amelia Island in Florida shortly after 1790 and acquired land there in 1793. He married Susan Marion Cooper in 1806. Their son was John Cooper Pelot[3] who married Sarah Crews of St. Mary's, Georgia, and their son was John Crews Pelot who was born March 29, 1831, at his grandfather's plantation on Amelia Island. Soon afterwards, however, the family purchased land in Columbia County, Florida, and it was there that he grew up.

Education of the Pelot children was entrusted to private tutors. In due time young John Crews matriculated at Jefferson Medical College in Philadelphia, where in the spring of 1858 he received the M.D. degree.[4] By that time his father had bought land in the Newnansville section of Alachua County and settled there. So it was that the young physician returned to Florida and established his practice near Newnansville. On December 22, 1858, at Battle Bluff, Amelia

Island, he married Mary Elizabeth Cooper, daughter of James G. Cooper.[5]

With the Civil War already in progress Dr. Pelot, at age 31, enlisted in the Confederate Army as a private in Capt. Harrison's Company (K), 2nd Florida Cavalry, and was mustered in at Callahan on May 16, 1862. For several months his company remained in Nassau County although Amelia Island had fallen to Union troops. He was sent on a special mission by General Joseph Finegan on November 19, 1862, to accompany supplies to the Florida Hospital in Richmond. The following spring he participated in a daring mission to Amelia Island to determine the strength and location of the occupying Union troops. On December 31, 1863, he was "discharged by promotion" to the rank of assistant surgeon, although he had previously (May-June, 1863) been "detailed as company surgeon" of his unit.[6]

In the spring of 1864 Dr. Pelot was assigned as medical officer at the recently-established Andersonville prison in Georgia. He arrived in time to assist in processing the first shipment of Union prisoners to be incarcerated there. It was his fate to remain there for the duration of the war. His letters from Andersonville detailing some of his experiences are now in possession of his descendants in Bradenton. Notable is his commentary on the improper trial, unwarranted conviction and subsequent execution of Capt. Henry Wirz, which he regarded as an outrageous miscarriage of justice.[7]

Family tradition holds that the Cooper and Pelot families arrived in Manatee in 1866; so they were there prior to the purchase of the Braden property. In any event Dr. Pelot quickly settled down to the practice of his profession. He was probably the first qualified physician to practice in the county. Dr. Joseph Braden, who had arrived there in the 1840s, never actually practiced medicine. Dr. Pelot is said to have traveled great distances in Manatee and adjoining counties to treat those who required his services. In 1886 he demonstrated his concern for the poor quality of medical practice in the state by joining the Florida Medical Association.[8] Although his attendance at annual meetings was irregular, he retained his membership for many years. In conjunction with his medical practice he and his son, John James Francis Pelot, established a drug store, The Pelot Pharmacy, which is still in existence.

Throughout his adult life Dr. Pelot maintained a vital interest in Florida politics. As the secession issue became acute he was one of the Manatee County citizens who went to Tallahassee on June 4, 1860, to confer with Governor Perry on a course of action. In the following year he represented Manatee County at the Secession Convention which met in Tallahassee on January 3, 1861. In the emotionally charged atmosphere of Reconstruction politics he entered vigorously into public affairs of Manatee County, becoming involved in the bitter Tilden-Hayes campaign of 1876. As president of the Manatee Democratic Club it was his function to supervise the election machinery of the county.

The state government, then under Republican control, sought to prevent the holding of an election in Manatee County. In defiance of the Tallahassee authorities, however, Dr. Pelot proceeded to arrange an election, meticulously observing all the legalities and proprieties. The ballots from Manatee County were carefully tabulated and presented to the officers in Tallahassee, at that time a Carpetbagger element, who promptly refused to admit them. It was largely through the persistence of Dr. Pelot that the matter was brought to the attention of the Florida Supreme Court, which validated the ballots, thus giving the Democrats a majority in the gubernatorial race, ensuring the election of George F. Drew,[9] a Democrat. A decade later Dr. Pelot was a member of the Constitutional Convention of 1885 and served as Manatee's representative in the Florida House for the sessions of 1887, 1889 and 1899.[10] It should be added that he was equally vigorous and effective in local affairs.

One son was born to Dr. Pelot and his first wife, Mary Elizabeth Cooper, who died in 1873. He was christened John James Francis Pelot. Six years later Dr. Pelot married Katie Gates, daughter of Judge Josiah Gates, one of the first white settlers in the Manatee area. To this marriage were born two sons, Charles Edward and Josiah Crews, the latter dying at an early age.

Dr. Pelot was without doubt a man of superior intelligence and cultivation. He was greatly respected as a reliable practitioner of medicine and responsible citizen. Beyond his medical and political skills he was a gifted musician, being especially proficient with the violin and flute. His piano, said to have been a massive, square, rosewood instrument, is thought to have been the first to be brought to Manatee County. Dr. Pelot died on May 2, 1917.[11]

1. The author gratefully acknowledges the assistance of two of Dr. Pelot's grandchildren, Julia Pelot Colket, Cleveland Heights, Ohio, and John Crews Pelot, Bradenton, in the preparation of this sketch. Additional information has been gleaned from Rowland W. Rerick, *Memoirs of Florida*, 2 vols., Atlanta, 1902, II, 651-652; James B. Whitfield, comp. *Florida State Government, 1885*, Tallahassee, 1885; Lillie B. McDuffie, *The Lures of Manatee*, 2nd ed., Bradenton, 1961; and James W. Covington, *The Story of Southwestern Florida*, 2 vols., New York, 1957, II, 555-556.

2. McDuffie, *Lures*, p. 182.

3. Ex info, Mrs. Colket. Letter to E.A. Hammond, July 1, 1979.

4. Archives, Jefferson Medical College, Philadelphia, List of Graduates.

5. See note 3, supra.

6. NA, Service Records, CSA, M 251 Roll 11.

7. Civil War Articles by Dr. Pelot. Originals in possession of his descendants in Bradenton. Only photocopies have been examined.

8. *Proceedings, Florida Medical Association, 1886*, Jacksonville, 1886, p. 6.

9. Rerick, *Memoirs, II, 652.*

10. Allen Morris, *The People of Lawmaking in Florida*, Tallahassee, 1977.

11. Covington, *Southwestern Florida*, p. 556.

Penny, George A., Gainesville and Cedar Keys, 1840-1878

Dr. Penny, a South Carolina native, was a resident of Gainesville in 1870. The census of that year lists him as "physician," residing in the home of real estate agent S.F. Halliday.[1] He was 30 years of age at the time. A few years later, probably about 1872 or 1873, he moved to Cedar Keys where, in addition to his regular practice, he held the post of Port Inspector, presumably a federal appointment. It was his responsibility to board, examine and inspect all ships entering the port. It was also his duty to enforce such ordinances and regulations as the town's Board of Health, consisting of the Mayor and Aldermen, ex officio, might enact or impose. This was especially important when quarantines were in effect.

Dr. Penny's remuneration for such services was not always promptly forthcoming, as in early 1878 when he found it necessary to employ a lawyer and sue the New Orleans, Florida and Savannah Steamship Company for $154 owed him for his services in "boarding steamships Margaret and William P. Clyde."[2]

The Florida Medical Association, meeting at the Yacht Club in Jacksonville, elected Dr. Penny to membership in the organization on April 16, 1878. His nomination was presented by Dr. R.D. Murray of Key West. Unfortunately Dr. Penny did not live to enjoy the affiliation and prestige which could accrue to the membership. He died on October 28, 1878, at his home in Cedar Keys.[3] At its annual meeting the following year Dr. Penny was honored when Association members ordered that a full page in their *Proceedings* for 1879 be devoted to his memory. It is recorded that Dr. Murray and Dr. R.P. Daniel of Jacksonville made "appropriate remarks.[4]"

So far as is known, Dr. Penny was never married.

1. U.S. Census, 1870, Alachua County, Florida, item 126.
2. S.E. Gunnell, *Search for Yesterday, A History of Levy County, Florida*, Bronson, Levy County Archives Committee, 1977, Chapter 6, p. 8
3. Florida Medical Association, *Proceedings*, Jacksonville, 1879, pp. 8, 11.
4. Ibid.

Perrine, Henry, Florida Keys, 1797-1840

Dr. Perrine,[1] an adventurous and restless type of man, was born in Cranbury, Middlesex County, New Jersey, on April 5, 1797, son of Peter and Sarah (Rosengrant) Perrine. Little is known of his early education and professional training. It is assumed that he studied medicine as an apprentice to a local physician, but there is no evidence that he attended an established college of medicine. As a young man he taught school at Rocky Hill, New Jersey, for a brief period before beginning the study of medicine. He began his professional practice in Ripley, Illinois, where he remained for five years. In 1822 he married Anne Fuller Townsend, daughter of a Denham, New York, clergyman.

By an unfortunate accident, which may have been fortuitous, Dr. Perrine's health was seriously impaired by an intake of arsenic in 1821. The consequences of this mishap forced him to seek a mild climate which he found in Natchez, Mississippi, where he practiced medicine for six years. Upon receiving an appointment, probably through influence, as United States Consul to Mexico in 1827, he spent the next six years in Campeche on the east coast of the Yucatan Peninsula.

It cannot be determined at what point in his life Dr. Perrine began his study of flora. It seems certain, however, that the abundance of tropical plants he found in Yucatan became a constant fascination. He began collecting botanical specimens which eventually found their way into the New York Botanical Garden. This interest, once his consular service was terminated, led him to Florida, where he introduced numerous tropical plants. For their cultivation he was able to obtain substantial financial support from the United States government, a portion was a tract of land south of Miami in the vicinity of the town which bears his name.

Dr. Perrine, after exploring the chain of Florida Keys, chose to establish a residence on Indian Key[2] about 1830 attracted by its natural beauty and the great variety of tropical flora. There his wife and children joined him, perhaps not expecting to remain there permanently but for the duration of the Seminole War then being waged. Indian Key, because of its beauty, began to attract settlers, some of whom were unfortunately of unsavory character. It did enjoy briefly, however, the distinction of being named the seat of Dade County.

The lovely island paradise was doomed to virtual extinction, however. Its Indian inhabitants and kinsmen from other nearby Keys joined in an assault on the white "intruders" on August 7, 1840, killing many and burning their buildings and homes. Dr. Perrine was among the victims.[3] It is apparent that his fame rests more securely on his enormous contribution to the science of botany than on medical practice. He was noted for his use of massive doses of quinine in the treatment of fevers.

1. Every major biographical dictionary and encyclopedia contains a sketch on the life and career of Dr. Perrine. The present brief account is drawn chiefly from the *Dictionary of American Biography*. Another very important essay is that prepared by Jacksonville physician Dr. Edward Jelks and presented as the Presidential Address at the Florida East Coast Medical Association meeting in Miami, October 27, 1933, and later delivered before the Jacksonville Historical Society.

2. Indian Key gained a somewhat odious reputation in the late 18th and early 19th centuries as the rendezvous for "Freckers" who plied their enterprise among the Florida Keys. A subject of controversy, often they saved the lives of ships' crews whose vessels had been dashed on the reefs and rocks along the main routes leading to the Caribbean Islands and the Gulf of Mexico. On the other hand they were known to have salvaged many cargoes of the wrecked ships and were said on occasion to have tampered with warning lights set at dangerous shoals and rocks. Some who visited Indian Key found its residents honorable people, engaged in humanitarian services.

3. See note 1 above. The other major source is the account of the massacre at Indian Key and the death of Dr. Perrine written by his daughter, Hester Perrine Walker, who was present at the tragic event, and miraculously escaped with her life. The manuscript in the form of a journal was written in 1885. It was published in the *Florida Historical Quarterly*, Vol. V, No. 1, July 1926, pp. 18-42.

Perry, John J., Jackson County, 1864

Information concerning the career of Dr. Perry is derived almost entirely from his military record as Assistant Surgeon in Company D, 6th Florida Infantry Regiment, commanded by Colonel J.J. Finley. A resident of Jackson County, Dr. Perry was mustered into the Confederate Army at Mt. Vernon Arsenal, Gadsden County, on March 17, 1862, and began his actual service at Jacksonville on March 18, committing himself to three years of service or duration of the War. He was 35 years of age at the time. Although he was a physician approaching middle age, he was inducted as a private. A month later, however, this absurdity was corrected and he was commissioned Assistant Surgeon.[1]

The month of May 1862 found Dr. Perry in service at Cumberland Gap, Tennessee, where he remained until early 1864 when he was granted a leave of absence for two months. It is apparent from his military record that this leave was granted because of poor health. His record shows that by June 1864 he was a patient at the Confederate General Hospital, No. 9, in Richmond, having been admitted on June 30.

Dr. Perry was a native of Sumter County, Georgia, born in 1836. He was five feet, nine inches tall, of fair complexion, dark hair, and by civilian occupation, a farmer. Although the date of his death has not been determined it is a safe assumption that, given his chronic health problems, he died at a fairly early age.

1. The list of graduates from the Medical College of Georgia, Augusta, contains the names of five native Georgians but Dr. Perry's name is not among them.

Perry, Joseph Milton, Alachua, Polk and Escambia Counties, 1837-1911

Dr. Perry, a well-regarded physician, arrived in Florida soon after the Civil War. He was born at Liberty Hill, Kershaw County, South Carolina, in April 1837[1] into a family of Irish extraction. He received an early education at Liberty

Hill Academy, said to have been an institution of excellent reputation. In the fall of 1858 he matriculated at the Medical College of the State of South Carolina, Charleston, from which he was graduated in March 1860 after submitting a thesis entitled "Yellow Fever."[2]

With the onset of the Civil War in 1861 Dr. Perry interrupted his professional practice and volunteered for military service in the Second South Carolina Volunteer Regiment which was soon incorporated into the famous Kershaw Brigade,[3] commanded by the indomitable Joseph B. Kershaw. After a short period as a private, he was transferred to the Medical Department in which he remained for the duration of the conflict. His regiment engaged in heavy fighting in both Virginia and Tennessee, but it is not clear that Dr. Perry was present at all of its battles.

Near the end of the War Dr. Perry married Emma Long,[4] also a South Carolinian. Soon after the War was concluded the couple moved to Florida, arriving at some time in 1866 and settling in the village of Waldo, Alachua County. On September 13, 1866, Dr. Perry and Dr. George W.A. McRae announced the formation of a professional partnership,[5] an unusual arrangement in that Dr. McRae, who had settled in Florida about 1853, was living in Clay County at McRae's Mills,[6] some 15 miles from Waldo. Their professional card included the following expectation: (We) "hope by moderate charges and strict attention to business to merit the liberal patronage bestowed upon us. Consultation fees are on occasions gratis."

Dr. Perry entered vigorously into the public life of Waldo. He was among the leaders of the effort to incorporate the village and bring order into its development, a move opposed by many who feared the probable imposition of taxes. Not until 1876 were the efforts successful. On December 15 a call was issued to all registered voters of the community to meet at the school house for the purpose of electing officers and organizing a municipal government. Dr. Perry was chosen secretary and subsequently elected to serve on the town council.[7] The following January Dr. Perry, a staunch Democrat, was authorized by Governor George F. Drew to represent the Democratic Club of Waldo and cast a vote in the nomination of Alachua County officers.[8] Four months later he was present and active at a meeting called for the purpose of promoting a canal connecting Waldo with Lake Santa Fe. He became a member of a committee charged with pursuing the effort further.[9]

Meanwhile, Dr. Perry had not remained in professional obscurity. He had evinced interest in the Florida Medical Association organized in Jacksonville in 1874 and in 1875 was elected to membership by unanimous vote of members although he was not present at the meeting.[10] Irregular in attendance at annual meetings, he continued his membership in the Association at least until 1896. He was elected 2nd Vice President in 1877 and again in 1888.[11] He was also chairman of the Committee on Accounts in 1878.[12] In 1877 Dr. Perry opened a drug store in Waldo. The Fernandina newspaper, in announcing the event, added: "The Doctor is a jolly good fellow and we wish him success."[13]

Three children were born to Dr. and Mrs. Perry, a daughter, Winnie, and two sons, Robert and Charlton, all born in Florida.[14] About 1885 the family left Waldo for what appeared to have been a more favorable situation in Lakeland, then only a village overshadowed by the Polk County seat, Bartow. There the doctor resumed private practice in addition to becoming local physician to the Plant

System of railways, later to become a part of the Atlantic Coast Line System. On Dr. Perry's retirement from active practice in 1901, he and his wife moved to Pensacola where they resided with their daughter, Mrs. Charles S. Bonacker, and her husband, former Lakeland residents. Dr. Perry died at the Bonacker residence on September 19, 1911, and was buried in Lakeland with full Masonic honors. In addition to Mrs. Perry and their daughter, he was survived by his son, Charlton, then living in Richmond, Virginia. The other son, Robert, had died earlier.[15]

1. Much of the information in this sketch was gleaned from Dr. Perry's obituary notice written by his close friend, General E.M. Law, of Lakeland, who had settled in the town soon after the Civil War. His eulogy, somewhat personalized, has not been included. See Bartow *Courier-Informant*, September 28, 1911.
2. Charleston *Daily Courier*, March 14, 1860.
3. See note 1, supra.
4. Ibid.
5. Gainesville *New Era*, September 14, 1866.
6. In addition to his medical practice Dr. McRae operated a grits mill and sawmill near his residence. The location shown on some modern maps simply as "McRae" is near Gold Head Branch State Park.
7. Bettee V. DeSha, *East of Eden*, Gainesville, 1977, p. 71.
8. Gainesville *Times*, January 20, 1877.
9. Ibid., May 5, 1877.
10. *Proceedings, Florida Medical Association*, 1874-75, Charleston, S.C., 1875, p. 8.
11. Ibid., 1893, Jacksonville, 1893, p. 46.
12. Ibid., 1878, Jacksonville, 1878, p. 17.
13. Fernandina *Florida Mirror*, May 3, 1879.
14. U.S. Census, 1880, Alachua County, Florida, p. 15.
15. U.S. Census, 1900, Polk County, Florida, p. 98. Here the date of Dr. Perry's birth is shown to have been April 1837.

Perry, Robert Jasper, Key West, 1900

Dr. Perry was born in Virginia about 1838. No information concerning his youth and education has been discovered. He apparently arrived in Key West soon after the end of the Civil War. At some unknown date he married a Pennsylvania lady, Ann Elizabeth Brown, and their first child was William, born in late 1869.[1] For the first year or two after their marriage the Perrys lived in the home of the eminent Jefferson Beale Brown.

Dr. Perry was obviously a man of superior intelligence and high principle, qualities much needed in the Key West of those early years. He immediately established himself as a trusted physician and druggist. Moreover, he assumed an important role as leader in civic affairs. In 1887 he became Monroe County's Superintendent of Public Instruction while simultaneously serving as Mayor of Key West.[2] In the latter role he made a trip to Washington in 1899 to investigate charges made by the Cuban government that certain citizens of Key West had violated federal labor laws regarding employment of Cuban citizens. Accompanying him were two other prominent citizens of Key West, George W. Allen and Jefferson Beale Brown, the latter to become the author of the extremely valuable *Key West, the Old and the New.*[3]

Two of Key West's most prominent families were joined by the marriage of Dr. Perry to Ann Elizabeth, daughter of Joseph Beverly Brown and Mrs. Brown, the former Mary Nieves. To this union were born two sons, William and Sidney, and a daughter, Genevieve.[4] The date of Dr. Perry's death has not been determined. It is known, however, that he was still living in the year 1900 at the age of 62.

1. Vital data are drawn from Monroe County Censuses of 1870, 1880 and 1900.
2. Jefferson B. Browne, *Key West, the Old and the New*, St. Augustine, 1912, p. 23.
3. Ibid., pp. 126-127.
4. U.S. Census, 1880, Monroe County, p. 224.

Perry, Thomas Alexander, Madison County, 1835-1862

Dr. Perry's professional career had scarcely begun when it was suddenly terminated by his death at the Battle of Seven Pines near Richmond, Virginia, on May 31, 1862. He was born in South Carolina in 1835, son of Samuel and Margaret, who moved to Madison County about 1842 and settled on a farm outside the town of Madison.[1] Apparently young Thomas was returned to South Carolina to begin the study of medicine under preceptors.[2] In the fall of 1856 he matriculated at the Medical College of the State of South Carolina, Charleston, from which he was graduated in the spring of 1858. His doctoral thesis bore the title "Erysipelas."[3]

Soon after graduation Dr. Perry returned to Madison where, in late summer, he began practice in partnership with Dr. Henry J. Parramore. Their office was located "one door north of the post office;" they offered free consultations.[4] Dr. Perry, still unmarried, resided in the home of his brother, William L. Perry, editor of the Madison newspaper, *The Southern Messenger*, whose family consisted of his wife and one child.[5]

With the outbreak of war in 1861 Dr. Perry was an immediate enlistee, joining the "Madison Rangers" which was to become Company "L" of the 2nd Florida Infantry Regiment. He was accorded the rank of first lieutenant. After being mustered in on July 13, 1861, Dr. Perry spent the following eight or nine months in Jacksonville. In the spring of 1862 his unit moved into the war zone near Richmond where he received a captaincy on May 11. Just 20 days later he was killed at the Battle of Seven Pines near Richmond in the encounter in which Confederate General Joseph F. Johnston was seriously wounded.[6]

In October 1862, Samuel J. Perry appeared before Probate Judge G.M. Brinson in Madison to file claim for such pay as was due his deceased son. In the process he deposed that he was indeed the father of the physician, who had died leaving neither wife nor child, stating further that William L. Perry, then of Richmond, was acting as his attorney.[7]

1. U.S. Census, 1850, Madison County, Florida, p. 210.
2. This statement is conjectural in that none of young Perry's preceptors, four of whom are named, appears to have been Florida residents.
3. Archives, Medical College of the State of South Carolina, Waring Historical Medical Library, Medical University of South Carolina, Charleston.
4. Madison *Southern Messenger*, December 25, 1858, 1st printed on September 25.
5. U.S. Census, 1860, Madison County, Florida, item 12.
6. NA, Service Records, CSA, M 251, Roll 40. Dr. Perry's service record is informative, stating his age as 26 in the summer of 1861, but it fails to indicate the nature of his military service, whether medical or otherwise. See Tallahassee *Floridian and Journal*, July 26, 1862, for Dr. Perry's obituary.
7. Ibid. The Perry Family eventually received $131, the pay due their departed member.

Peters, Francis Marion, Santa Rosa County, 1823

Dr. Peters, a South Carolina native, was practicing medicine in Milton in the late 1850s.[1] The Santa Rosa County Census of 1860 lists him at age 37, unmarried, and a resident in the home of L.B. Owens, a Milton civil engineer. With the Civil War already under way, he enlisted for Confederate service at Quincy on March 12, 1862, committing himself for three years of service. He was mustered in nine days later and assigned to Company A, 6th Florida Infantry Regiment.[2]

When the war ended Dr. Peters returned to Milton and resumed his medical career. Soon thereafter he married a widow, known only by her Christian name, Susan, a native of Alabama, with a 14-year-old daughter, named Alabama.[3] A list of physicians practicing in Florida in 1869 compiled by the Medical College of the University of Pennsylvania indicates that Dr. Peters settled briefly in the village of Knox Hill, Walton County, situated near the Washington County line but by 1870, however, he had returned to Milton where he would live out the last years of his life. It appears that the Peters family enjoyed a comfortable living, having been able to employ two household servants in 1870.

Living as he did in one of Florida's more rural areas, the activities of Dr. Peters remain unchronicled. The date of death is unknown.

1. U.S. Census, 1860, Santa Rosa County, Florida, p. 45.
2. National Archives, Confederate Records, Sixth Florida Infantry.
3. U.S. Census, 1870, Santa Rosa County, Florida, p. 555, item 60.

Pettus, John G., Monticello, 1810-1870

Dr. Pettus, a native of Georgia, settled in Jefferson County in the 1830s when he was still in his early 20s.[1] He appears to have settled in Monticello although he purchased farmland outside the town and, like many of the physicians of the times, divided his energies between medicine and agriculture. He is known to have followed the common practice of contracting his medical services on a yearly basis to other plantation owners for attendance upon their slaves. The papers of the estate of the well-known Abraham Bellamy contain an item showing that in 1845 Dr. John G. Pettus "received $24.50 for twelve visits during the year" to treat the slaves on the Bellamy Plantation.[2]

Although he could not have been considered a wealthy planter, Dr. Pettus was nevertheless "well off." Slave schedules of 1840 show him owning 20 slaves while that of 1860 lists for him 29 of whom six were house servants in his Monticello home, the others farm laborers. In 1860 his real property was valued at $20,000 and personal property at $40,000.

Throughout his career Dr. Pettus remained conservative in politics and active in the Whig Party.[3] Predictably he found Reconstruction measures imposed by federal authority objectionable, especially the dicta of the Freedmen's Bureau. He vehemently resisted the order of the Bureau to provide annual accountings or settlements with his erstwhile slaves, now sharecroppers. Shofner refers to him as "the most difficult planter with whom the Bureau had to deal" in Jefferson County.[4] His resentment was no doubt intensified by the deep personal loss he had suffered when both his sons, John G., Jr., and Thomas, were killed in action in the course of the war.

A few items of random evidence point to Dr. Pettus as a respected medical practitioner. He is said to have been the doctor of the family of Darius Williams, a prominent Monticello merchant. The story is told that upon the birth of

Williams' first daughter by his second wife, Pamelia Palmer, in 1935, Dr. Pettus not only presided at the delivery but planted a magnolia tree in the Williams yard to which he assigned the name given to the baby at her christening, Rose Amelia.[5] More important, however, is the interest he demonstrated in the improvement of the standards of medical practice. Having observed the failure of a small group of colleagues, including his fellow townsman, Dr. John L. Call, to obtain through legislative action a viable medical regulatory body in 1849, he joined Dr. E.S. Gaillard of Waukeenah and other Jefferson County physicians in establishing a county medical society in 1856. Dr. Pettus himself presided over the organizational meeting in Monticello on January 11, 1856.[6] This group antedated the state medical association by 18 years and pledged itself to work toward a state organization.

Very little is known about the Pettus family. His wife, Margaret, was a native of South Carolina; the older son, John G., Jr., was born about 1836. In addition to the two sons, there were three daughters, Margaret, Anna and Lucy. Margaret Antonia (her full name) was married on May 10, 1859, to the Rev. Franklin A. Branch of Tallahassee.[7] Since no listing for Dr. Pettus appears in the Census of 1870 for Jefferson County, it is assumed that he had died prior to that date.

1. U.S. Census, 1850, Jefferson County, p. 1. Here Dr. Pettus' age was said have been 41.
2. Julia Floyd Smith, *Slavery and Plantation Growth in Antebellum Florida*, Gainesville, 1973, p. 97.
3. Jacksonville *Florida Republican*, June 10, 1852.
4. Jerrell H. Shofner, *History of Jefferson County*, Tallahassee, 1976, p. 287.
5. Mary Oakley McRory and Edith Clarke Barrows, *History of Jefferson County, Florida*, Monticello, 1935, p. 33.
6. Shofner, *History*, p. 203.
7. Monticello *Family Friend*, May 17, 1859.

Phillips, Ethelred, Marianna, 1801-1870

Dr. Phillips was born in North Carolina on January 11, 1801.[1] Nothing is known of his education but he is presumed to have prepared for medical practice through the apprenticeship system prior to moving to Florida about 1830. He married Susan Gautier, daughter of Peter W. Gautier on April 30, 1840. She was some 23 years his junior.[2] To this marriage were born three sons, Charles, Frank (later Col. Frank Phillips of the Confederate Army and subsequently Judge of the Jackson County Circuit Court), and Ethelred. Dr. Phillips was among the founders of St. Luke's Episcopal Church in Marianna and a member of its first vestry which, incidentally, included two other physicians, E.C. Bellamy and Simmons J. Baker. Early in 1839 Dr. Phillips was a delegate at the Second Diocesan Convention meeting at St. John's Church in Tallahassee.[3]

Random gleanings from various sources indicate that Dr. Phillips was a typical practitioner in a rural town, attending the sick over a wide rural area at any hour of the day or night and undergoing many hardships for modest remuneration. Dr. Charles A. Hentz, for several years a resident of Jackson County, related an incident growing out of a beef-shooting match during which liquor-laden participants turned their guns on each other. He was called to the scene well after midnight to treat the wounds of an antagonist, "Honorable Wm. C. Neel," while Dr. Phillips had been summoned to treat the wounds of the other participant, a Colonel Irving.[4] On another occasion Dr. Phillips received through legislative action $25 for assisting a colleague in the postmortem examination of a slave, property of Benjamin A. Dickens. Presumably, however, the greater part of his practice was of a routine kind. At any rate remuneration was sufficient to establish him as a prosperous citizen. In the county tax rolls of 1845 he is shown as declaring an income of $1,500 and owning town lots assessed at $2,000.

During the troubled times of the 1850s and 1860s Dr. Phillips' outspoken political opinions on several issues provoked criticism. He expressed his opposition to secession urged by the local paper, the Marianna *Patriot*, which unequivocally stated: "The only question is Secession or Submission...We opt for speedy secession for Florida from this unhallowed Union."[5] To this intemperate statement Dr. Phillips replied: "They think the South can whip all creation, that cotton is king and separation will bring peace and happiness—a fatal delusion." Such Unionist sentiments did not endear him to the majority of Marianna's residents. Even his son, Charles, Marianna's telegrapher, became suspect and was accused of having turned over to occupying Union troops "all the telegrams exchanged between the Marianna defenders and the Confederate headquarters in Quincy, from which relief was being dispatched."[6] Dr. Phillips remained a unionist to the end of the conflict.

Dr. Phillips did not long survive the hard times of war and reconstruction which had left him physically and financially reduced. He died in Marianna on June 29, 1870, some six months short of his 70th birthday. He was buried in St. Luke's Cemetery. In his reminiscences Dr. Charles Hentz remembered him thus: "...Dr. Phillips was the old doctor of the place; a delicate, frail old gentleman who could not stand much exposure, who practiced there (Marianna) for many years."[7]

1. The dates of Dr. Phillips' birth and death are recorded on his gravestone in St. Luke's Cemetery, Marianna.
2. St. Joseph *Times*, May 5, 1840. See also J. Randall Stanley, *History of Jackson County*, Marianna, 1950, p. 60n.
3. Ibid., p. 77.
4. Charles A. Hentz, "My Autobiography," Unpublished, Southern Collection, University of North Carolina, Chapel Hill, p. 175.
5. Jerrell H. Shofner, *Jackson County, Florida—A History*, Marianna, The Jackson County Heritage Association, 1985, pp. 215-216. In this voluminous work Dr. Shofner has included many references to the Phillips family.
6. Ibid, p. 246.
7. Hentz, "*Autobiography*," p. 276.

Pickard, Adoniram Judson, Pensacola, 1838-1882

Dr. Pickard, who spent only a few years of his career in Pensacola, was born in Hampden, Maine, on December 24, 1838. He attended Bowdoin College, Brunswick, Maine, for a couple of terms but left without a degree in 1863 to enter military service. After the war he attended the Homeopathic Hospital College in Cleveland, from which he was graduated in 1872, and later made his way to Pensacola where he practiced from 1872 until 1879 when he moved to Carmel, Maine, where he died on December 26, 1882.[1]

1. "Medical Obituaries."

Pinckney, Theodore A., Key West, mid-19th century

Dr. Pinckney was born in Phelps (earlier known as Vienne), Ontario County, New York, about 1810. Little is known of his early life and education but it may be assumed that he enjoyed traditional exposure to the classics, considered essential for an educated person in those times. It is also assumed that he attended a medical school in the North, possibly leaving without a degree. He arrived in Key West in October 1836, his decision to settle there having been influenced by Judge William Marvin, whose sister, Sybil, was the wife of Dr. Pinckney.[1]

There is abundant evidence that Dr. Pinckney was a popular and successful physician. Moreover, he benefited in some degree from his kinship with Judge Marvin. In his autobiography Judge Marvin wrote: "I, having been successful in my efforts to get him (Pinckney) appointed to the post of Inspector of Customs and Surgeon in the Marine Hospital, he continued these employments for three or four years, at the end of which time he had accumulated some ten to twelve thousand dollars."[2]

Having become financially independent Dr. Pinckney decided to return to the place of his birth with the intention of practicing medicine. He soon abandoned the idea, at least as a full-time occupation, turning instead to storekeeping, having formed a partnership with his brother, Isaac. The two men also purchased a flour mill in Unionville (Ontario County), New York, having paid for the property, according to Dr. Pinckney, "much too large a sum of money."

As far as can be determined the Pinckneys never returned to Key West, at least not for professional reasons. Judge Marvin, however, refers to his niece, Dora Pinckney, with pride and affection, indicating that there had been family visits. As for Dr. Pinckney, it is doubtful that he ever resumed his medical practice in Unionville, turning instead to running his mill and perhaps other business enterprises.

1. Data have been derived entirely from the "Autobiography" of Judge William Marvin, published in the *Florida Historical Quarterly*, XXVI, January 1958, No. 3, pp. 179-222.

Plummer, Joseph W.V.R., Key West, 1842-post 1900

Dr. Plummer, who spent the latter part of his life in Key West, was born in Maryland in March 1842.[1] The Special Florida Census of 1885 states that his father was a native of the Bahamas while his mother was born in Key West.[2] Although no information concerning Dr. Plummer's childhood and youth has been located, it seems probable that he was trained for his profession in either England or Scotland.[3]

By 1870 Dr. Plummer was a practicing physician in Key West, aged 28 and married to a native of Key West known by her Christian name, Anna. Her parents were natives of the Bahamas.

In the local Key West election of 1872, said to have been a very spirited affair, Dr. Plummer was a candidate for the office of mayor. He lost to L.W. Bethel by a very narrow margin. Jefferson B. Browne, the well-known historian of Key West, recalled that the Doctor had overplayed his hand in his political zeal, which manifested itself in torch light processions, and the organizing of "respectable white Republicans to block the vote of the Negroes, the scalawags, and other undesirables, to prevent their take over of the Party."[4] Browne remembered the subsequent election as "a turbulent affair."

Dr. Plummer was later to voice his disapproval of the tactics of his Party.

He found its affiliation with carpetbaggers, Negroes and scalawags repugnant, and attempted to purify it by reorganization, a tactic which led to the formation of a "Liberal Republican Party." When its members met at the County Court House, a group of Negroes, led by carpetbaggers, assembled in force and attempted to break up the meeting. Just when a riot seemed to be developing a group of old-time Whigs and a few young men, many of whom had been in politics, came forward hoping to organize a "respectable White Republican Party." Its purpose appeared futile, however, when its leader, Dr. Plummer, wisely called upon his friends to stand together and resist the threatened violence of the Negroes. Peace was soon restored.

Dr. Plummer was twice married. His first wife, Anna, lived on past the year 1900. His second wife, Cora L., is listed in the Census of 1910, age 35. Four sons were born to this marriage. They were, in order of birth, George, Joseph Jr., Lionel, and Mark. The date of his death has not been determined.

Census data, the principal source of material for this sketch, are not totally reliable. For example, the 1870 Census, Monroe County, gives Dr. Plummer's birthplace as Maryland; that of 1885 indicates he was a native of the Bahamas, while that of 1910 shows him to have been born in Florida. There are other inconsistences.

1. U.S. Census, 1870, Monroe County, p. 332.
2. This data appears to be correct.
3. This risky surmise is based on the fact that his name does not appear in the lists of graduates of any of the major medical colleges of the United States for the period under consideration. It is to be recalled that his father was English-born; his mother was born in the Bahamas.
4. A full account of this turbulent affair is found in Jefferson B. Browne, *Key West, the Old and the New*, facsimile edition, Gainesville, University of Florida Press, 1973, p. 135.

Pointevin, Anton, Pensacola, 1846

Dr. Pointevin, a native of France, practiced medicine for only a brief period in Pensacola. In February 1846 he announced his services to the citizens of the town, presenting impressive qualifications. He claimed to have been a member of the Medical Faculty of the University of Montpellier, a surgeon in the French Navy, a disciple of the Midwifery Hospital of Marseilles, etc. He had established his office at the corner of Government and Baylen Streets.[1] In October of the same year he advertised at length his vast assortment of fresh drugs and medicines, the greater part of them from the establishment of Messrs. Thiboumery and Dubose, Chemists of Paris. His stock included: "Ipecac in Chocolate, very useful for chest afflictions, also could be used as an emetic or expectorant, a calming medicine." He also offered Pills in Chocolate (for asthma), Digestive Paste of Darcet (?) for indigestion, and French Vermifuge (for intestinal worms). He also claimed to have had six years experience on French vessels of war, and in civil and military hospitals in Toulon and Marseilles, experience which "renders it in his power to be able to put up any prescription entrusted to his care." His office was located on Goverment Street in the house of Sebastian Barrios and finally, he "would treat the poor gratis."[2]

Dr. Pointevin's rhetoric, however, does not appear to have impressed the citizens of Pensacola. He had departed the town prior to 1850.

1. Pensacola *Gazette*, September 12, 1846.
2. Ibid., October 31, *et seq.*, 1846.

Polhill, Augustus James, Hamilton County, 1825-post 1883

There is only slender evidence to show that Dr. Polhill actually practiced medicine in Florida while there is substantial evidence that he was a successful farmer and politician who spent the latter years of his life in the Bellville community of Hamilton County. Born in Richmond County, Georgia,[1] on May 30, 1825, he moved with his family to Hawkinsville, Pulaski County, Georgia, at the age of eight. There he spent the greater part of his youth. After attending the common schools he enrolled at Dunham's Academy in nearby Perry and at some juncture began the study of medicine in the office of a local physician, presumably in Hawkinsville. Succumbing to the gold fever of 1849-50 he joined the rush to California where he remained for seven years before returning to the East and settling in Hamilton County.[2]

Meanwhile, prior to settling in Florida, Dr. Polhill had married Mrs. Virginia P. Davies (nee Bracewell), also of Georgia, a union to which no children were born, although her nephew, James Bracewell, was a member of the Polhill household in 1870 and 1880.[3]

Although Dr. Polhill was a relative newcomer to Hamilton County, he was elected to the Florida House of Representatives for its 12th session, 1862-63, one of the stormiest of its history. Again 20 years later he represented the Eleventh District in the Florida Senate in the sessions of 1881 and 1883, having aided in healing the schism within the Democratic Party which had split into two wings, the Regulars and Independents.

Dr. Polhill made his last census appearance in the enumeration of 1880 when he was listed at the age of 55 (obviously an inaccurate figure) living with his wife, Virginia, and two nephews, James Bracewell and Joseph Polhill. He was designated "farmer."[4]

1. A brief but inaccurate sketch of Dr. Polhill appeares in J.V. Drake, *The Florida Legislature: An Official Directory of State Government*, Jacksonville, 1883, p. 41. This half-page biography is to be used with caution.
2. Since Dr. Polhill does not appear in the Hamilton County Census of 1860, he is presumed to have moved to Florida after that date; nevertheless, he was sufficiently well-known to be elected to the Florida House in 1862.
3. U.S. Census, 1870, Hamilton County, Florida, p. 12, Bellville community; ibid., 1880, p. 281.
4. Dr. Polhill's nephews, both aged 20, are listed as farm laborers.

Pope, John Hunter, Jefferson and Madison Counties, 1815-1878

Dr. Pope, a highly respected physician in Middle Florida, was born in Washington, Wilkes County, Georgia, in 1815. His father, who bore the same name, was a Virginian from Prince William County who had received his medical degree from the University of Pennsylvania in 1808 and soon thereafter moved to Georgia, where he practiced medicine until his death in 1851.[1] The younger Pope matriculated at the University of Pennsylvania in the fall of 1835 and was graduated as M.D. in 1837.[2] Soon afterward he returned to Georgia for a year or two of practice before moving to Monticello where he established his office in May 1840 over William Denham's General Store.[3] A little more than a year later his medical school friend, Dr. James S. Robinson, invited him to become his professional partner in Tallahassee. The two young physicians purchased a drug store which had belonged to Dr. R.L. Baker and on August 13, 1841, announced that their office would henceforth be located in the drug store.[4]

This joint venture was unhappily terminated by the untimely death of

Dr. Robinson in August 1842.[5] For reasons which are not clear Dr. Pope did not long remain in Tallahassee, choosing instead to move his practice to Madison; the actual date is unknown. It was, however, the beginning of a long and successful practice which continued until his death on September 28, 1878.[5] Occasional references suggest a routine professional career mingled with numerous civic activities. As an active Democrat he found time to attend regional meeting of the party.[6]

During his sojourn in Tallahassee Dr. Pope married Eliza Smith, daughter of Aaron P. Smith, a Leon County planter.[7] Their children were sons Aaron, John Hunter, Francis and Randolph, and daughter Eva. Aaron was killed in the Battle of Missionary Ridge at the age of 19. John Hunter became a distinguished member of the Florida Bar, while Francis (Frank), a fine orator, had a successful career as lawyer and politician, having practiced in both Madison and Jacksonville. He represented District Ten in the Florida Senate in 1883 and Duval County in the House in 1897. These and other descendants have been prominent in public life of Florida for more than a century.[8]

1. Much of the biographical data included here has been made available through the courtesy of F.J. Dallett, Archivist, University of Pennsylvania Archives.
2. Ibid.
3. Jerrell H. Shofner, *History of Jefferson County, Florida*, Tallahassee, 1976, p. 62.
4. Tallahassee *Sentinel*, September 24, 1841.
5. Tallahassee *Star of Florida*, February 16, 1843; 1st printing August 26, 1842.
6. "Parish Records, St. John's Episcopal Church, Tallahassee, Florida," a typescript of which is found in the P.K. Yonge Library of Florida History, University of Florida, Gainesville, Burial Section. See also Tallahassee *Weekly Floridian*, October 1, 1878.
7. "Parish Records," Marriages.
8. Typescript, Biographical Box "P," P.K. Yonge Library of Florida History, University of Florida, Gainesville.

Pope, William Henry, Madison County, 1830-1890

Dr. Pope was born in Washington, Wilkes County, Georgia, in 1830. His father, Dr. John H. Pope, was also a physician.[1] According to the Wilkes County Census of 1850 Dr. Pope began his professional career as an attorney but later turned to medicine. Although nothing is known of his medical education it can be established that in April 1858 he joined his older brother, Dr. John Hunter Pope, in a medical partnership in Madison.[2]

Soon after settling in Madison Dr. Pope entered politics, running successfully for the Florida House of Representatives as a representative of Madison, Lafayette and Taylor Counties. He demonstrated qualities of leadership as chairman of the Committee on Elections while serving as a member of four other committees.[3] Before opening of the adjourned session in November 1859, however, he submitted his resignation and was replaced by Stephen R. White.[4] Various entries in the House Journals show Dr. Pope to have been a man of moderation and good judgment. On the matter of his resignation the Madison newspaper noted his action with regret that the state "will be deprived of his valuable service," adding that "it will be no easy matter for his late constituents to place in his stead one who will be so well qualified to fill the high, honorable and responsible position."[5]

The partnership of Dr. Pope and his brother was terminated early in 1862 when Dr. Pope enlisted in the Confederate Army. He was appointed Surgeon in the

First Florida Cavalry Regiment. His military service was brief, however, for in November 1862 he resigned his appointment and returned to private practice in Madison.[6]

There is no indication that the Pope brothers resumed their professional association. In February 1863 Dr. William Henry Pope received from the state of Florida $21.60 for performing postmortem examinations and $40 for "maintenance of lunatics."[7]

At some unknown date in the 1870s Dr. Pope moved with his family to Fernandina where he would spend the remainder of his life. He purchased a home on Fifth Street between Centre and Ash and maintained an office at Clay's Drug Store.[8] He was elected mayor of Fernandina in April 1885, running on the Republican ticket and defeating his two opponents, S.L. Duchette and G.F. Avery.[9] It appears that Dr. Pope had allied himself with the radical party controlled by the federally-appointed John W. Howell, Collector of Customs, and his black colleague, Samuel Petty, Customs Inspector. At any rate, when James M. Griffin won the mayor's office the following year the Florida *Times-Union* hailed his victory over "Howell bossism which has controlled Fernandina for so long."[10] The heavy white vote explained the Griffin victory.

Dr. Pope married Charlotte, from a well-to-do South Carolina family and niece of John C. McGehee, one of Madison County's wealthiest planters, on April 13, 1859.[11] After her death (date unknown) he married a native Virginian whose given name was Celia. Several children were born to the first union but only one child, a daughter christened Lulu, was born to the second.[12] Dr. Pope died suddenly in Fernandina on September 30, 1890. He was extolled as "a gentleman of sterling qualities."[13]

1. U.S. Census, 1850, Wilkes County, Georgia, item 724. Newspaper sources for Madison County in the 19th century are meagre and biographical detail, even for prominent families, is scarce.
2. Madison Southern *Messenger*, December 25, 1858; 1st printing, May 22, 1858.
3. Florida House Journal, 1858, p. 43.
4. Ibid., adjourned session, 1859.
5. Tallahassee *Floridian and Journal*, August 27, 1859, reprinted from Madison *Southern Messenger*, August 20, 1859 (not extant).
6. NA, Service Records, CSA, M251m, Roll 2. This record is incomplete, providing little more than dates of appointment and resignation. During the 3rd Seminole War Dr. Pope had spent six months, August 10, 1857—February 10, 1858, as Assistant Surgeon, Regiment of Florida Volunteers. He was mustered in at Ocala, reached Ft. Brooke on August 13, left for Ft. Myers on September 2 and was assigned to duty at Regimental Headquarters. NA, Records, Adjutant General's Office, Group 34, M 1086, Roll 51.
7. Tallahassee *Sentinel*, February 24, 1863.
8. U.S. Census, 1880, Nassau County, Florida, item 21; Fernandina *Express*, April 23, 1881.
9. Jacksonville *Florida Times-Union*, April 7, 1885. It is clear from numerous sources, e.g., his signature to city ordinances, etc., that Dr. Pope had won the election.
10. Ibid., April 7, 1886.
11. In the Census of 1860, McGehee's properties were estimated to have been worth $115,000; his slaves numbered 100.
12. U.S. Census, 1880, Nassau County, Florida, p. 302, it. 21.
13. Jacksonville *Florida Times-Union*, October 1, 1890; Madison *Recorder*, October 3, 1890.

Porcher, Peter, St. Augustine, 1829

Dr. Porcher, member of a prominent Huguenot family of South Carolina, first appeared in the historical records of Florida when he announced to the citizens of St. Augustine and vicinity that he "would attend to the duties in the several departments of his profession." This card, first printed on April 1, 1829, also gave his residence as the house formerly occupied by Fleischman.[1] At some time, either prior to coming to Florida or shortly thereafter, Dr. Porcher had purchased what was known as the Buyck (Byke, Byck) plantation some 10 miles south of St. Augustine near the head of the Matanzas River and had set up a farming operation carried on with 44 slaves.[2] This enterprise was doubtless managed by an overseer since Dr. Porcher continued to maintain his St. Augustine residence.

In the early 1830s Dr. Porcher appears to have lived the life of a well-to-do practitioner, lending his support to various political and civic causes. In 1831, for example, he joined a large group in endorsement of Joseph L. Smith for reappointment as judge of the Eastern District of Florida.[3] The following year he joined other members of the St. Augustine Presbyterian Church in their effort to maintain the old Huguenot Cemetery for the use of all Protestant denominations,[4] while in 1833 he lent his support for the reconstruction of the sea wall.[5] In late 1833 he endorsed a protest to Congressional Delegate Joseph M. White concerning the delay in completing a road from Jacksonville to New Smyrna.[6]

With intensification of Indian hostilities along the east coast of Florida in 1835 came efforts to strengthen and augment the territorial militia. A group, designated as the Second Regiment (a part of the Second Brigade), was activated with Col. Joseph S. Sanchez in command. Dr. Porcher became the regimental surgeon.[7] His actual role in this capacity remains unclear, however.

Before the Second Seminole War had run its course Dr. Porcher had abandoned Florida and returned to Charleston where he established practice. In January 1836 he had been present at a public meeting in St. Augustine called to discuss the Indian threat to life and property. A nine-member committee was appointed to prepare a report on the situation; it included Dr. Porcher. On the following day the committee met again with Dr. Frederick as chairman and prepared the report which was subsequently printed in the local newspaper.[8] It is possible that Dr. Porcher together with his family left St. Augustine soon thereafter. On March 23, 1836, the list of letters being held by the postmaster included five for Dr. Porcher, the list appearing in several subsequent issues of the newspaper.[9] At any rate the Charleston census of 1840 includes the doctor, his wife and three children as residents. His reasons for moving may have been the profitless plantation, insufficient income from medical practice, or perhaps concern for the safety of his family.

No effort is made to trace Dr. Porcher's career after his return to South Carolina. In 1861 he volunteered for medical service with a military unit located on Sullivan's Island.[10] A single bizarre incident, discovered by Prof. John K. Mahon, bears repeating. An English pharmacist's mate, John Bemrose, while still a teenaged lad, had made his way to America at about the time the Second Seminole War got under way. He proceeded to Florida and because of his brief apprenticeship in pharmacy was welcomed in the medical department of the militia. He came to know Dr. Peter Porcher.

Many years later, after the Civil War, Bemrose was awarded a bounty grant of 160 acres of land in Kansas in recognition of his service in Florida. He had no wish to retain the grant. In the meantime he had been in touch with Dr. Porcher who through age and economic disasters had come upon difficult times. Bemrose referred to him as "my dear old friend, whom age and poverty has made wretched" and was moved to help ameliorate his situation by conveying to him his bounty grant. Through the intervention of General William T. Sherman this was accomplished and it was recorded that an army officer on duty in Charleston was ordered by Sherman to deliver the warrant into the hands of Dr. Porcher. It is also a matter of record that on June 18, 1875, Dr. Porcher sold the grant.[11]

1. St. Augustine *East Florida Herald*, April 1, 1829. This was Dirk Fleischman listed in the 1830 census of St. Augustine in the entry following that of Dr. Porcher.
2. T.P., XXIV, 593. This plantation had earlier belonged to Augustine Buyck, husband of Ann Buyck. She was the daughter of Josiah Dupont who claimed large holdings south of St. Augustine. See *Spanish Land Grants in Florida*, I, D, 52; I. B, 31-35; III. F, 22, 58.
3. T.P., XXIV, 602.
4. Ibid., p. 685.
5. Ibid., p. 871.
6. Ibid., p. 936.
7. St. Augustine *Florida Herald*, January 13, 1836.
8. Ibid.
9. Ibid., March 25, 1836.
10. *War of the Rebellion, Compilation of Official Records*, Ser. I, Vol. I, 42.
11. John K. Mahon, "Postscript to John Bemrose's Reminiscences," *Florida Historical Quarterly*, XLVII, No. 1, July, 1968, pp. 61-62.

Porter, John Bliss, St. Augustine, 1869

Dr. Porter, a surgeon in the United States Army, was born in Connecticut in the early 19th century.[1] On December 1, 1833, he enlisted in the United States Army with the rank of Assistant Surgeon and on October 4, 1846, was promoted to the rank of Major Surgeon. He appears to have been assigned for a portion of his career to St. Augustine where on May 23, 1842, he married Anita A. Smith, the wedding taking place in St. Augustine's Trinity Episcopal Church.[2] Nothing is known of his subsequent professional career. Army records show that he retired from active service on August 27, 1862, and died on June 15, 1869.[3]

1. Francis B. Heitman, *Historical Register and Directory of the United States Army*, Vol. I, Washington, Government Printing Office, 1903, p. 799.
2. "Parish Register, 1821-1904, Trinity Parish, St. Augustine, Fla." (Unpublished). List of Marriages.
3. Heitman, loc. cit. Dr. Porter's death is presumed to have occurred at his home in Connecticut.

Porter, Watson, Gainesville, 1840-1911

Although the medical career of Dr. Porter appears to have been negligible, if indeed he ever practiced medicine at all, his role in the development of postwar Gainesville was significant. He and his wife, Olivia A., natives of Centreville, Nova Scotia, arrived in the town in late 1886,[1] along with many other Northerners who flocked into the state of Florida in the early days of reconstruction. Since Dr. Porter's service to the community was performed unselfishly and generally for the public good one hesitates to brand him with the depreciatory label, "carpetbagger," although it cannot be denied that he benefited substantially from the opportunities available to him during those early days after the War.

Dr. Porter received appointment as postmaster of Gainesville on January 29, 1867, the first of several public offices he was to hold.[2] In September, it was announced that "Dr. Porter is putting up a new building on Era (?) Street, designed for a postoffice. The Doctor proposes to have all the modern arrangements...and make it worthy of the City."[3] At about the same time the military authority of Gainesville appointed him "superintendent of the town," the equivalent of acting mayor.[4] Two years later, with termination of military rule and partial resumption of civil government, Dr. Porter (with many citizens still without the voting privilege) was elected alderman (one of eight) under the mayoralty of S.Y. Finley.[5]

Meanwhile, a United States Land Office, one of several in the state, was established in Gainesville with Dr. Porter as one of the three clerks in charge of land transactions. Given the political situation of the times such office personnel were advantageously positioned for making profitable investments. It appears very probable that Dr. Porter was able to invest to his personal benefit.[6] At any rate, by the end of the century the Porters were among Gainesville's more affluent landowners, having bought property at several locations within the town and outside its limits. Besides their residence at 214 West Liberty Street (now with the second block of West University Avenue), they owned valuable property on what is today the one hundred block of Northeast First Street, which came to be known as the Porter Block. Presently this is parking lots serving Gainesville's City Hall and Public Library.[7]

A school for black children was established in Gainesville in 1866, sponsored by the Republican government of the town with the blessing of the Freedmen's Bureau. In the early 1870s Dr. Porter became principal of the school, known as Union Academy, and without doubt he was a capable and benevolent schoolman. In 1873, however, he came under attack from Leonard G. Dennis, a Massachusetts carpetbagger and Republican boss of Alachua County, and William K. Cessna, an Ohioan who had gained power in the Republican administration of the town. As the Tallahassee newspaper reported the incident:[8]

> Trouble arose...when Dennis and Cessna attempted to interfere with the operation of the school, and to displace the regularly appointed principal, Dr. Watson Porter. The attempt was boldly made to oust Porter, but Dennis and Cessna were defeated and no damage resulted save a few hours interruption of school operations.

This affair was apparently the result of a rift within the ranks of the Alachua County Republicans, Cessna and Dennis leading one faction and Congressman Josiah T. Walls, black congressman from the Alachua district (1870-76) and also an influential trustee of the Academy.

A few weeks prior to the Academy incident a meeting of Gainesville Republicans occurred on August 27, 1873, at which Dr. Porter was nominated by acclamation for mayor of the city to fill the vacancy occasioned by resignation of Walls.[9] By the mid-1870s, however, the Democrats were gradually regaining control of public offices in the county, and Dr. Porter was among the Republicans who retired to private life, spending his later years in the operation of his business.

Both Dr. Porter and his wife were active parishioners in Holy Trinity Episcopal Church. Mrs. Porter was one of the chief benefactors of the church, having donated its beautiful altar. She had in the earlier years of her residency in Gainesville been one of the principal organizers of the Women's Auxiliary. In his last will and testament Dr. Porter bequeathed the Porter Block to his wife with the stipulation that certain income go to foreign missions.[10] Upon her death the property was bequeathed to the Church, a munificent benefaction indeed.

Dr. Porter died on March 13, 1911, at the age of 71. It is odd that the local newspaper published a brief notice of the event, stating only the time of the funeral, with the following brief eulogy: "Dr. Porter was one of Gainesville's oldest and best citizens." Then "heartfelt sympathy goes out to his beloved widow in her loss and bereavement."[11] Although he had been a Mason from 1867 until his death, there is no indication that Masonic rites were accorded him. The service was held at Holy Trinity Church in which he had served for many years as warden and vestryman.

Mrs. Porter died on October 1, 1920, at the age of 75. It is stated in her obituary that she had been a resident of Gainesville for 53 years. She was survived by two brothers, Robert Kinsman of Centreville, Nova Scotia, and Amos Kinsman of Danvers, Mass.[12]

1. In the Alachua County Census of 1900, it is shown that Dr. Porter had moved to the United States in 1863, in which year he had become naturalized. He did not arrive in Florida, however, until 1867.
2. Jess G. Davis, *History of Alachua County, Florida*, Gainesville, 1966, p. 59.
3. Gainesville *New Era*, September 20, 1867.
4. Ibid., November 30, 1867.
5. Charles H. Hildreth, and Merlin G. Cox, *History of Gainesville, Florida*, Gainesville, 1980, p. 42.
6. U.S. Census, 1880, Alachua County, Florida, p. 107. Here Dr. Porter is designated as "Clerk in Land Office." His total wealth 10 years earlier (1870 Census) was estimated at $11,000.
7. The Porter Block is shown on George V. Arnow's, "Map of Gainesville, Florida, 1893," as the property of Mrs. Porter. It was situated on the east side of what is now Northeast First Street in the 100 block, bordered on the south by East University Avenue and on the north by Northeast First Avenue. The location of Dr. Porter's farmland has not been determined although it is thought to have been south of the town.
8. Tallahassee *Weekly Floridian*, November 11, 1873.
9. Gainesville *New Era*, August 30, 1873.
10. Frank W. Pisani, *Holy Trinity Church—Its Story*, Gainesville, 1951, p. 9.
11. Gainesville *Daily Sun*, March 15, 1911.
12. Ibid., October 2, 1920.

Powell, James L., Marianna, 1907

Dr. Powell is known only because he was buried in Riverside Cemetery at Marianna. His gravestone indicates that he was born in 1847 and died in 1907. No further information regarding him has been discovered.

Power, Edward R., Alachua and Lafayette Counties, 1820

Dr. Power, a native of New York State, arrived in Florida at the end of 1853 and settled in Newnansville, Alachua County. There he joined Dr. Craven Lassiter in establishing a drug store in early 1854.[1] At approximately the same time the following notice appeared in the Tampa *Herald*:[2]

> Dr. E.R. Power, having located in Newnansville, Florida, respectfully tenders his professional services to the citizens of this place and the surrounding country, hoping that by strict attention (after a successful practice of eight years) to give general satisfaction.

The decision to settle in Newnansville was ill-timed, although at the time it was a thriving town whose only rival was Micanopy on the other side of the county. In the summer of 1854 an election was held to determine the permanent county seat. Although Gainesville was little more than a sawmill on Hog Town Creek, its location near the center of the county was the determining factor and the seat was removed from Newnansville to Gainesville. Henceforth Newnansville declined and eventually disappeared as a viable municipality.

By 1860 Dr. Power had transferred his practice to the village of Fayetteville in Lafayette County.[3] The Census of 1860 lists him as 38 years of age (probably an error), living with his five-year-old son, Edward R. Power Jr., in the home of George W. Martin. His occupation was "physician" his properties, real and personal, were valued at $6,000.

With the coming of the Civil War in 1861 Dr. Power enlisted as a private in a special battalion of Florida volunteers which became a unit of the 10th Florida Infantry. He entered service at Fernandina on December 12, 1861, committing himself for 12 months. His military experience appears to have been uneventful, disturbed only by a siege of illness in the fall of 1862, after which he applied for discharge. This was promptly granted, since he was "a twelve months man" and "over forty-five years old." He resumed civilian status on February 15, 1863. His discharge papers include these personal facts: 46 years old, five feet ten inches tall, florid complexion, hazel eyes and dark hair, occupation: physician.[4]

Subsequent to his discharge nothing further is known of Dr. Power. It is worth noting, however, that in the Alachua County Census of 1870, City of Gainesville,[5] the entry for Robert W. Campbell, farmer, aged 25, in addition to his wife, Fanny, and their two daughters, there was also Edward R. Power Jr., aged 15. One can only speculate concerning the relationship of young Power to the Campbells.

1. Tampa *Herald*, February 22, 1854.
2. Ibid.
3. U.S. Census, 1860, Lafayette County, Florida, item 6. Here it is indicated that Dr. Power was a widower, but there is nothing to suggest that there were ties of kinship between him and the Martin family. The Fayetteville settlement was situated on the west bank of the Suwannee River about 10 miles south of Branford. It would have been in the northwestern corner of present-day Dixie County.
4. Dr. Power was a native of Ontario County, N.Y., possibly of the town of Canandaigua. See NA, Service Records, CSA, Microcopy 251, Roll 97. There is no explanation as to why Dr. Power's experience as a physician was not properly utilized by the Confederate Army.
5. U.S. Census, 1870, Alachua County, Florida, p. 207.

Preston, Francis, Suwannee County, 1870

Dr. Preston, a native of Virginia, was a practicing physician in the Wellborn community of Suwannee County in 1870.[1] The census of that year lists him as 45 years of age. Other members of his household were his wife, Amanda, and four children, all born in Florida. His real property was valued at $3,000, personal property at $150. Since no further information on this family has emerged it is assumed they left Florida prior to 1880.

1. U.S. Census, 1870, Suwannee County, Florida, p. 692, item 478. Mrs. Preston's age was 27. The children were Ann, nine; Walter, six; Mary, four; and Josephine, two.

Price, William D., Leon, Gadsden and Franklin Counties, 1827-1844

Dr. Price, probably a native of Virginia, was a resident of Tallahassee as early as 1827. With establishment of a Medical Board for the Territory by enactment of the Legislative Council on December 31, 1827, he was one of the three Tallahassee practitioners to be named to the nine-member Board,[1] an indication that he was already a physician of good repute.

Dr. Price married Marcia Duval, daughter of Governor William Pope Duval, on April 25, 1828, an event which brought him under the patronage of the

Governor and secured for him a place in Leon County's highest social circle.[2] This is borne out in an account of an elegant dinner given in Tallahassee on September 30, 1828, honoring Col. Joseph M. White, the Territory's representative in Congress. Present at the affair were several of the most notable political figures of the Territory. The arrangements were handled by Dr. Price and Dr. Frederick Weedon.[3]

Although none of his professional notices have survived, it is still evident that Dr. Price was a respected physician in Tallahassee from about 1827 until 1831. He purchased a lot in the town in 1829, presumably with the intention of building a home,[4] but Tallahassee during those years was overstaffed with doctors and without other income (which several enjoyed from their farming operations) some found their medical fees inadequate. Dr. Price seems to have been one of them. Nevertheless he was the son-in-law of the Governor who was incidentally the ex officio Superintendent of Indian Affairs for the Territory, so Dr. and Mrs. Price were encouraged to move to the newly-developed town of Aspalaga on the Apalachicola River in Gadsden County. He served as an unofficial medical officer to the Apalachicola tribe rounded up there preparatory to resettlement in the West.[5]

Governor Duval was not averse to using his position to the advantage of his son-in-law. When the decision was made to vaccinate the entire Seminole tribe which had been collected in the Alachua settlement near Ft. King and Dr. John Hamilton, citizen-surgeon serving the area, refused to undertake the task because of the poor pay, Governor Duval wrote in a letter to Lewis Cass, Secretary of War:[6]

> If you have not appointed a physician to inoculate the Indians, I recommend Dr. William D. Price of Florida for that service. He resides near the Apalachicola Indians and his smile, standing and knowledge in his profession is not surpassed by any in the faculty in Florida. His post office is at Aspalaga on the Apalachicola River. (Signed) W.P. Duval.

Due largely to the failure of the War Department to fund the vaccination project, however, nothing came of Duval's effort on behalf of Dr. Price, although on February 12, 1832, the Governor's appointment list for Franklin County included the name of Dr. Price for notary public and auctioneer.[7] In the following year the notary public appointment was renewed. In the meantime Dr. Price had been brought to the attention of the Postmaster General and the Secretary of the Treasury which resulted in his appointment as postmaster of Apalachicola and inspector of customs at its port.[8] While residing there he appended his name to several petitions and memorials requesting federal assistance in developing the commercial potential[9] of the town as well as the improvement of mail service and judicial agencies.[10]

Dr. Price encountered difficulty in 1833 when a postal inspector discovered that the postmaster was also the customs inspector and proceeded to so inform the postmaster general, W.J. Duane. The principal complaint was that Dr. Price in this dual capacity was neglecting his customs duties, i.e., failing to inspect properly all the ships which came into port. In an attempt to save his job he appealed to his friend, Andrew Stevinson (sic), congressman from Virginia, requesting that he intercede with Duane, explaining that the meager incomes accruing from even two jobs were inadequate for his needs.[11]

Duval left office in 1834 but his successor, John H. Eaton, renewed Dr. Price's notary appointment.[12] He was replaced, however, in his federal offices in Apalachicola and moved in down-graded situation to the inspectorship in St. Joseph, a position which he held until early 1844 when, in spite of numerous protests, the Treasury Department decided to terminate the office.[13]

In the summer of 1841 while her husband was in Washington Mrs. Duval, Mrs. Price's mother, went to St. Joseph to spend part of the summer in the hope that the gulf breezes would benefit her health. Instead she became one of the first victims of the yellow fever epidemic, which beset the community about the first of July. She died on July 14, 1841. The epidemic one of the deadliest ever to strike a Gulf Coast town, blighted the once-thriving community and no doubt influenced the decision to discontinue St. Joseph as a port of entry. With the closing of the port in 1844 Dr. Price and his family abandoned their hopes for a good life in Florida and migrated to Texas to live out the remainder of their lives.[14]

Unfortunately no records remain to inform us of Dr. Price's medical practice during the last decade of his Florida residence. It is reasonable to assume, however, given the meager income accruing from his public offices, and the dearth of practitioners in both Apalachicola and St. Joseph, that he continued to practice whenever his services were required.

1. *Acts, Florida Legislative Council*, 6th Session, 1827-28, Tallahassee, 1828, pp. 46-49. In the following year the membership of the Board was increased to 15. Other members from Leon County were Drs. Lewis Willis and Thomas Munroe.

2. Pensacola *Gazette*, May 2, 1828. This is a reprint from an issue of the Tallahassee *Florida Advocate* no longer extant.

3. Pensacola *Florida Argus*, October 21, 1828.

4. Leon County, Florida, Records, compiled by Daughters of the American Revolution, typed copy, Tallahassee, 1937, p. 109.

5. This ugly episode in the history of the Florida Indians is described in John K. Mahon, *History of the Second Seminole War*, Gainesville, 1967, Chapters IV and V.

6. NA, Letters Received, Office of Indian Affairs, 1823-81. Microcopy 234, Roll 288.

7. TP, XXIV, 660.

8. Ibid., 902-3.

9. Ibid., 533, 924.

10. Ibid., 986, 1001.

11. Ibid., 902-3. Dr. Price explained that he knew of several instances in which postmasters held other jobs simultaneously, citing cases at Tampa and Tallahassee. He stated that his salary as Inspector was $750 per annum and as postmaster $200.

12. Ibid., XXV, 104.

13. Ibid., XXVI, 889. Letter, Secretary of Treasury J.C. Spencer to President John Tyler.

14. Their imminent departure is mentioned in a diary kept by Master Edward C. Anderson, USN, published as *Florida Territory in 1844*, W. Stanley Hoole, ed., Tuscaloosa, University of Alabama Press, 1877, p. 33. The entry for May 11, 1844, St. Joseph, is: "Met at this place a Dr. Price and his wife, acquaintances of Mrs. Jones; they were on the eve of departure for Texas." Other members of the Duval family had already gone to reside in Texas. One of these was Mrs. Price's brother, Thomas, who had settled in the San Antonio area.

Quina, Desiderio, Pensacola, 1817-1891

Dr. Quina, son of Desiderio and Margaret Quina, was born in Pensacola on February 5, 1817. He apparently qualified for medical practice by serving an apprenticeship in the office of a local physician. Immediately thereafter he began the practice of his profession in Pensacola and continued to practice until the debility of old age necessitated his retirement. He was married to a local girl, Emma Patterson, and they became the parents of a daughter and four sons. His death occurred at the home of his son, Marion, on October 13, 1891. He was buried in the family plot in St. Michael's Cemetery, Pensacola.[1]

1. Obituary notice, Pensacola *Daily News*, October 15, 1891.

Randolph, Arthur Lee, Leon County, 1848-1884

Arthur Lee Randolph, fourth child of Dr. James Henry Randolph[1] and his first wife, Margaret Hayward, was born in Tallahassee in 1848 and christened at St. John's Episcopal Church on March 25 of that year.[2] He spent his youth in Tallahassee where he received his early education. He entered the University of Virginia in the fall of 1868 but remained for only one term before going elsewhere for his medical degree.[3] Soon after graduation Dr. Randolph married Genevieve Valle of St. Louis, returning with her to Tallahassee where they lived in the old Beard House at 319 N. Monroe Street. His office was located a short distance away at the corner of E. Park Avenue and Calhoun Street where the Cherokee Hotel later stood.[4]

Dr. Randolph's success as medical practitioner was assured from the start. His highly respected father was at the height of his career at the time the son began practice, and the two are known to have combined their knowledge and skill in treating numerous cases. The younger Randolph, however, given his superior intellect and dedication to medicine, would have succeeded without the sponsorship of his popular father.

The Tallahassee Weekly Floridian on August 3, 1875, reported a "panicky reaction" in the city to a rumor that a yellow fever epidemic was raging in nearby St. Marks. Dr. Randolph decided to investigate. Arriving at St. Marks he discovered one case aboard a ship anchored in the St. Marks River eight miles south of town. On returning to Tallahassee he was able to put the rumor to rest and the newspaper was critical of those "who exaggerate and spread false rumors, causing unwarranted anxiety."

Both Randolphs were elected to membership in the Florida Medical Association at its organizational meeting in Jacksonville in January 1874 although neither was in attendance nor were they present at the meeting of 1875. In 1876 Dr. Arthur made his initial appearance at the meeting in Tallahassee and was elected secretary and member of the Necrology Committee. The following year he was reelected secretary and also chosen to replace his father as chairman of the Committee on Endemic Disease.[5] He became First Vice President in 1878 and the next year while vice president and orator read a paper entitled "Report on Cases of Conservative Surgery,"[6] which was in essence a plea for extreme caution in making the decision to resort to major surgery, especially in cases seeming to require amputation. He cited in considerable detail several cases out of his own experience in which limbs were saved through careful and attentive medication.

Dr. Randolph's active participation in the affairs of the Association continued on into 1881 when he was once more secretary. At the meeting that year in Tallahassee, he was selected as a delegate to the annual meeting of the American Medical Association; however, by 1882 his health had begun to fail and when the group met in Pensacola he sent his regrets and resigned from the Association.

Dr. Randolph had also made his presence felt in Leon County politics. He embraced the Democratic Party (by the 1870s the conservative party) as benefited a man of his background and like other Southern Bourbons abhorred "Carpetbagger Rule." As a Leon County delegate to the State Democratic Convention in Quincy in June 1876,[7] he ardently supported the Tilden-Hendricks ticket. He felt profound outrage at the rascality involved in the vote counting in certain Florida counties which resulted in the election of Hayes. Dr. Randolph was also a member of the Executive Committee of the Democratic Party in Leon County.[8]

Dr. Randolph's death came on July 31, 1884,[9] when he was only 36. He was survived by his wife and three small children (a fourth child had died in infancy). Dr. Henry Palmer regarded him as "brilliant" while his eulogist recalled his "easy bearing, bright mind and polite demeanor." There can be no doubt that his premature death was a tragic loss to the Tallahassee community.[10]

1. Randolph Whitfield and John Chipman, comp. "The Florida Randolphs, 1829-1978." Photocopy of typescript, 1978, P.K. Yonge Library of Florida History, genealogical tables.
2. Archives, University of Virginia, Charlottesville, Lists of matriculants and graduates.
3. The medical college from which Dr. Randolph received his degree has not been identified, although it appears to have been one of the Philadelphia schools.
4. Henry E. Palmer, "Physicians of Early Tallahassee and Vicinity," Apalachee, 1944, p. 32.
5. Information relating to Dr. Randolph's affiliation with the Florida Medical Association has been gleaned from the annual Proceedings, published in Jacksonville. For unknown reasons Dr. James Henry Randolph, although elected to membership in the Association in 1874, never attended a meeting, not even that held in Tallahassee in 1876. He resigned from the Association in 1878.
6. In these case histories Dr. Randolph mentioned his consultations with medical colleagues, including his father. Proceedings, FMA, Jacksonville, 1879, pp. 93-102.
7. Tallahassee *Sentinel*, June 10, 1876.
8. Tallahassee *Weekly Floridian*, May 2, 1876.
9. Ibid., August 5, 1884. He was buried in St. Johns churchyard.
10. Whitfield and Chipman, "The Florida Randolphs," p. 69. Here the surviving children of Dr. Randolph are identified as Valle Joseph, Mary Page and Arthur Lee Jr., all of whom reached adulthood and married.

Randolph, Arthur Moray, Leon and St. Johns Counties, 1815-1867

Dr. Randolph,[1] youngest of the eight children of Thomas Eston and Jane Cary Randolph, arrived in Leon County at the age of 13 in company with his sister Mary Elizabeth Cleland Eppes, her husband, Francis Eppes, and two younger sisters in June 1829. They were the first contingent of their family to make the long and hazardous trip overland from their birthplace in Albermarle County, Virginia. The elder Randolphs, with their son, James Henry, also to become a doctor, and the remainder of the family, made the trip from Norfolk, arriving at Magnolia—then a river port on the St. Marks River—in mid-November 1829.

Dr. Randolph was born on August 23, 1815. In the fall of 1836 he entered the Medical College of the University of Pennsylvania and in the spring of 1838 was graduated M.D., having submitted a doctoral thesis entitled "Neuralgia."[2] He had earlier studied engineering for which he was later to abandon medicine as a source of livelihood. Shortly after graduation Dr. Randolph returned to Leon County and in late May 1838 offered his professional services to the citizens of Tallahassee and vicinity.[3] He announced that he would share an office with his brother James Henry already a practicing physician in Tallahassee. Two years later the brothers formally announced their professional partnership[4] with offices in the home of Dr. James Henry Randolph. Dr. Randolph was married to Laura H. Duval,[5] daughter of William P. Duval, Florida's governor from 1822 to 1834, on January 15, 1840, and to this union eight children were born.

The Randolphs, having been a family of wealth, cultivation and lofty social position in Virginia, purchased extensive acreage in Leon, and with their numerous slaves set about developing their land into profitable plantations. On the death of Thomas Eston Randolph in 1842 his properties passed into the hands of his children. Thus Arthur came into possession of a plantation which encompassed the old Spanish mission of San Luis, some three miles northwest of Tallahassee on Mission Road. He is said to have developed this into a successful farming enterprise in the boom years for cotton growers, the 1840s and 1850s.

Dr. Randolph had the misfortune early in his professional career to contract tuberculosis, or consumption, as it was commonly known. Virtually abandoning medical practice he turned instead to civil engineering, a more healthful occupation. On January 1, 1842, it was announced that the "medical partnership heretofore existing between J.H. and A.M. Randolph is dissolved by mutual consent,"[6] however, one week later Dr. Arthur, "residing two and a half miles northwest of Tallahassee, near the Bainbridge Road," offered his professional services to the public, the last reference to his medical practice.[7]

At about this time the General Land Office, now that the Second Seminole War had ended, pressed toward the completion of surveys in the Florida Peninsula. The office of the surveyor-general, Valentine Y. Conway, was located in Tallahassee. Dr. Randolph contracted with Conway on November 12, 1842,[8] to become a deputy surveyor and in this capacity went immediately to Tampa Bay to survey the lands around Ft. Brooke. He spent the next few months there. When the surveyor general's office was relocated in St. Augustine in March 1844,[9] Dr. Randolph moved with his family to that city where he would remain for some eight years. The 1850 Census for St. Johns County designates him only as "Surveyor."[10]

In the early 1850s Dr. Randolph and family resumed their residence at the Leon County plantation where he would spend the remainder of his life, faced with failing health and personal grief brought on by the Civil War. When the call for volunteers came in 1861, his two eldest sons, Thomas Eston and William Duval, enlisted, though William Duval was only 16 years of age.[11] When Eston was fatally wounded in the fall of 1862 while serving with his Regiment, First Florida Infantry, in Virginia, Dr. Randolph made the difficult journey, sometimes through enemy lines, to the bedside of his dying son near Culpepper, an experience which he recorded in his diary. In late 1864, in disappointment mingled with anger, Dr. Randolph was moved to write to President Jefferson Davis bringing to his attention the unfair treatment his son William had received and imploring the President to intercede on his son's behalf for a lieutenant's commission. He pointed out that William had enlisted when still a schoolboy without a professional education, that he had served faithfully and well for more than three years, and that he had by virtue of this earned a junior lieutenant's commission.[12] It is recorded that the President referred the request to his Secretary of War who, in turn, instructed a member of his staff to state that the laws of the confederacy would not permit the granting of such a request, adding that junior lieutenancies could only be conferred after election by the soldier's company, which in this case was Company D, Second Florida Cavalry. Four months later the war ended and William returned home safely.

Dr. Randolph died in Marietta, Georgia, and was buried there in the St. James Episcopal Cemetery on October 19, 1867. His death is thought to have occurred while he, in very weakened health, was making his way to the more salubrious climate of the Carolina mountains.

1. Unless otherwise indicated the biographical data are derived from the splendid genealogical work on the Randolph family compiled and narrated by descendants of Thomas Eston Randolph of Dungeess, Randolph Whitfield and Dr. John Chipman. See Randolph Whitfield and John Chipman, "The Florida Randolphs, 1829-1978," 3rd. ed., 1978, photocopy of typescript, P.K. Yonge Library of Florida History, University of Florida.

2. Archives, University of Pennsylvania, Lists of Matriculants and Graduates.

3. Tallahassee *Floridian*, December 1, 1838; 1st printing in ibid., May 26, 1838.

4. Tallahassee *Star of Florida*, May 20, 1840.

5. Parochial Records, St. John's Episcopal Church, Tallahassee, 1832-1880. Typescript, P.K. Yonge Library of Florida History. Mrs. Randolph died in Tallahassee on November 8, 1907, at the age of 87 and was buried in St. John's churchyard.

6. Tallahassee *Star of Florida*, January 5, 1842.

7. Ibid., January 12, 1842.

8. See Letter, Randolph to Conway, May 8, 1843. TP, XXVI, 655-656.

9. Ibid., pp. 758-759, 871-872.

10. U.S. Census, 1850, St. Johns County, Florida, p. 405. Parish Records, Trinity Episcopal Church, St. Augustine, contain entries relating to baptism of two of Dr. Randolph's children, William Duval and James Henry.

11. NA, Service Records, CSA, M 251, Roll 29. The service record of Thomas Eaton is incomplete.

12. Ibid., Roll 11. William Duval spent his first two years in the Confederate Army as a private. On March 1, 1863, he was promoted to corporal and between the date of Dr. Randolph's letter to President Davis, December 7, 1864, and his discharge on May 17, 1865, he became a sergeant. Dr. Randolph's letter, a well-written plea on his son's behalf, is included in the service record of Company D, Second Florida Cavalry.

Randolph, James Henry, Leon County, 1809-1892

Dr. Randolph, one of Leon County's most eminent citizens, was born at Bunkershill, Albermarle County, Virginia, on July 3, 1809. He was the son of Thomas Eston and Jane Carey Randolph, who migrated to Leon County in November 1829 and settled on a plantation called "Ashton" some four miles north of Tallahassee.[1] After preparatory schooling in Virginia he entered the Medical College of Ohio, now a division of the University of Cincinnati, at the age of 18. Learning that he could not be awarded a degree before age 21 he transferred to the Medical College of the University of Virginia in the fall of 1828 only to have his studies interrupted before the end of term by a typhoid fever epidemic. In the following year he matriculated at the Medical College, University of Pennsylvania, from which he received his medical degree in the spring of 1831. His thesis bore the title "Haemoptysis."[2]

Soon after graduation Dr. Randolph joined his family near Tallahassee and on June 2, 1831, announced the beginning of practice in an office at the corner of Clinton and Adams Street.[3] A short time later he moved to a new location on the southeast corner of Duval and Brevard. Except for brief intervals of service elsewhere he remained in Tallahassee for 50 years,[4] attending patients throughout Leon and adjoining counties.

After settling in Leon County Dr. Randolph joined Dr. W.W. Waddel and Benjamin C. Lewis in establishing a drug store in Tallahassee,[5] a venture from which Dr. Waddel soon withdrew. The other partners continued to operate the store until August 1841 when they sold out to D.H. Ames.[6] In the meantime, on January 1, 1840, Dr. Randolph had been joined by his brother Arthur Moray Randolph, an 1838 graduate of the Medical College, University of Pennsylvania, in a professional partnership,[7] an association which endured until 1842 when Dr. Arthur, for reasons of health, abandoned the medical profession to become a civil engineer with the General Land office.

Throughout his career Dr. Randolph was a popular and successful physician. His illustrious lineage (the Randolphs occupied a lofty position among Virginia's aristocracy, and both his parents were Randolphs) assured him high social position in Tallahassee, while his intelligence and compassion gained for him the trust and devotion of a wide circle of friends and acquaintances. In 1843 his medical colleagues chose him chairman of the medical faculty of Tallahassee,[8] and in 1845 he represented Leon County in the Florida Legislative Council, the last session prior to statehood.[9] Years later, in 1876, he was elected Mayor of Tallahassee. In politics he was a staunch Whig, maintaining his allegiance to the party until its demise in the 1850s.[10] From the earliest days of his residence in Florida he was a true pillar of St. John's Episcopal Church, having served for many years as Senior Warden.[11]

With the outbreak of the Civil War in 1861 Dr. Randolph was among the first to offer his services to the Confederate cause. Although 52 at the time, with a wife and several minor children, he was commissioned Surgeon by the Secretary of War on September 13, 1861, and appointed Medical Director of the military district of Middle Florida. His duties were essentially those of coordinator of medical services within his district but by virtue of position the important responsibility of presiding over the District Medical Examining Board developed upon him.[12]

With the end of the war in 1865 Dr. Randolph resumed private practice in Tallahassee and in 1867 was joined in partnership by Dr. Zachary B. Herndon,[13] also a Virginia native. This association was terminated by the death of Dr. Herndon a few years later. In 1875, upon solicitation of a legislative committee, Dr. Randolph prepared an article dealing with conditions of health in that part of Florida lying between the Apalachicola and Suwannee Rivers. Printed in the House Journal, it reveals not only a high degree of literacy but also an extensive knowledge of climate, topography and disease.[14]

In 1881, at age 72, Dr. Randolph accepted the position of Superintendent and Physician-in-Charge, State Insane Asylum, Chattahoochee. He held the post for four years, returning to Tallahassee in 1885.[15] The last years of his life were spent in the home of his son, Thomas Hayward Randolph, a local merchant. He died on May 23, 1892, at the age of 83.[16]

Although he was 65 years of age at the time of its founding in 1874, Dr. Randolph was elected to membership in the Florida Medical Association in absentia, presumably on the recommendation of Tallahassee colleagues, Drs. G.W. Betton and R.B. Burroughs, who were among the founders. He resigned from the Association in 1878 without ever attending a meeting, not even the session in Tallahassee in 1876. His son, Arthur Lee Randolph, also a physician, elected to membership in 1874 along with his father, was active in the affairs of the Association for several years.[17]

Dr. Randolph married Margaret Estelle Hayward of Cambridge, Maryland, in 1840. To this marriage were born Jane Carey (Mrs. Wm. N. Whitner), Mary Lucia (1842-49), Thomas Hayward, Arthur Lee, and James Henry Jr. Mrs. Randolph died on May 12, 1851, and a year later Dr. Randolph married Elizabeth Beard, a North Carolina native and resident of Tallahassee. To this marriage were born Maria Beard (Mrs. John Chipman), Elizabeth (Mrs. John Cook), Mary Lucia (her namesake by the first marriage had died earlier), Constance, John and Lucy Beverly (Mrs. Theodore D. Bratten).[18]

1. Two descendants of Dr. Randolph, Dr. John Chipman and his cousin Randolph Whitfield, have compiled a splendid genealogical work, "The Florida Randolphs and Some Related Families," now in its 3rd edition (1978), from which some of the data included in the present sketch have been gleaned. The work exists in typescript and photocopies. See also Henry E. Palmer, "Physicians of Early Tallahassee and Vicinity," *Apalachee*, Tallahassee, 1944, p. 32. Dr. Randolph's father, Thomas Eston Randolph, was married to his cousin, Jane Carey Randolph. He was appointed U.S. Marshal, Middle District of Florida, by President Andrew Jackson in 1831.

2. Archives, University of Pennsylvania, Lists of Graduates. Haemoptysis: expectoration of blood usually resulting from lung hemorrhage.

3. Tallahassee *Floridian and Advocate*, June 2, 1831.

4. Palmer, "Physicians." In 1861 his office was located in the Drug Store of Gregory, Tatum & Co., Tallahassee *Floridian and Journal*, January 26, 1861.

5. Tallahassee *Florida Watchman*, February 17, 1838.

6. Tallahassee *Floridian*, December 4, 1840. After the departure of his brother, Dr. Randolph was joined by his brother-in-law, Dr. Wm. R. Hayward, recently arrived from Maryland.

7. Tallahassee *Star of Florida*, May 21, 1840.

8. In this capacity he presided over the meeting of the faculty convened to honor Dr. William Woodson Waddel, his former colleague, who had died on November 15, 1843. Tallahassee *Sentinel*, November 21, 1843.

9. Florida *House Journal*, 23rd Session, 1845, Tallahassee, 1845, p. 4, et passim.

10. Jacksonville *Florida Republican*, June 10, 1852. He also served as Mayor of Tallahassee in 1876. Palmer, "Physicians."

11. *Semi-Centennial, Diocese of Florida*, 1888, Jacksonville, 1889, pp. 15-16.

12. Palmer, "Physicians." Dr. Randolph actually had brief military service as Medical Officer aboard the USS Grampus in 1838. To, XXV, 484.

13. Tallahassee *Sentinel*, May 14, 1867.

14. Florida *Assembly Journal*, 8th Session, 1875, App., pp. 135-139.

15. Palmer, "Physicians."

16. Ibid.

17. *Proceedings, FMA*, 1874, Jacksonville, 1874, p. 6; ibid., 1893, p. 47.

18. "Parish Records, St. John's Episcopal Church, Tallahassee, Florida." Typed copy in P.K. Yonge Library of Florida History, University of Florida.

Randolph, Richard H., Quincy, 1834-1878

Dr. Randolph, second son and fourth child of Thomas P. and Jaxintha Randolph, was born in Quincy in 1834.[1] His father had arrived in Gadsden County in the 1820s, purchased land outside the town of Quincy, and settled into the life of a moderately well-off planter. According to the Census of 1830 his slaves numbered 54. He was influential in the establishment of the widely known Quincy Academy and served on its first board of trustees.[2] He was also one of the founders of St. Paul's Episcopal Church of Quincy.[3] His death in the 1840s left the major family responsibilities on the shoulders of his elder son, Thomas.

It is assumed that Dr. Randolph received his basic education at the Quincy Academy, and it is probable that he began medical studies under the preceptorate of his brother-in-law, Dr. John Screven Bond, to whom his sister Louisa was married in 1848.[4] In 1853 he entered the Medical College of the State of South Carolina, Charleston, from which he was graduated in the spring of 1855,[5] having submitted a thesis entitled "Inflammatory Process." Immediately thereafter he returned to Quincy and began practice.

When war appeared inevitable in the spring of 1861 Southern leaders hastened to assemble a military force. Dr. Randolph was among the Gadsden volunteers who enlisted on April 4 for a year's service in the company assembled by the Quincy physician, Capt. John H. Gee, which became Company "G," 1st Florida Infantry Regiment. He was 28 years old at the time and an experienced physician, but he enlisted as a private which he remained for the term of his enlistment. For reasons not explained in his military record, however, he was granted an honorable discharge in November 1861 and returned to Quincy. But with intensification of the conflict he reenlisted on May 10, 1862, again as a private, and was assigned to Company "B," 8th Florida Infantry. Before the end of the year he was assigned to the Ordnance Department, and on January 1, 1863, he was promoted to sergeant.[6]

It is not known how long Dr. Randolph remained an ordnance sergeant. Eventually, however, probably in mid-1863, when the need for an increased medical staff became urgent, he was removed from Ordnance and given his proper assignment in the Confederate Medical Department. For the remainder of the war he served as a medical officer in the Richmond area, and during the last months of the conflict he was surgeon in charge of the Jackson Hospital in Richmond, a position he held for several months after conclusion of the war.[7]

Subsequent to his discharge, Dr. Randolph returned to Florida and for a brief time resumed practice in Tallahassee. Within a few months, however, he moved to New York City where he practiced until his death on July 4, 1878, at the age of 44. For much of his adult life he was troubled with a heart ailment which doubtless accounts for his discharge from the army in November 1861 and, according to his obituary notice, accounted for his untimely death.[8]

1. U.S. Census, 1850, Gadsden County, Florida, p. 390, item 360.
2. Miles K. Womack Jr., *Gadsden, A Florida County in Word and Picture*, Gadsden County Historical Commission, 1976, p. 40.
3. Ibid., p. 52.
4. Tallahassee *Floridian*, January 6, 1849. Although Dr. Bond spent the greater part of his professional life in Tallahassee, he and his wife were residents of Quincy in 1850, living in the home of her mother, Mrs. Randolph.
5. Archives, MCSSC, Waring Historical Library, MUSC, Charleston. See also Charleston *Mercury*, March 16, 1855.
6. NA, Service Records, CSA, M251, Rolls 29 and 85.
7. Ibid. The official entry for Richard H. Randolph ends with his promotion to sergeant of ordnance in January 1863. Additional information concerning his army medical service is derived from his obituary notice in the New York *Herald*, July 9, 1878, and reprinted in the Tallahassee *Weekly Floridian*, July 16, 1878.
8. Ibid.

Rascoe, John T., Marianna, 1850

Florida sources allow only a fleeting glimpse of Dr. Rascoe. A legislative act of the Florida Assembly in its session of 1850-51 authorized payment of $100 to Dr. Rascoe and Dr. Franklin Hart for examining the body of James Durden "lately murdered in Jackson County." This act obtained Senate approval on January 20, 1851, House approval two days later, and was signed by Gov. Thomas Brown on January 24.[1]

The Marianna newspaper published his professional card on April 26, 1852.[2] The Jackson County Census of 1850 lists Dr. Rascoe, John T., "physician," age 29, North Carolina-born, living in the household of Dr. Franklin Hart.[3] It may be assumed that the two physicians had known each other in North Carolina.

1. *Acts and Resolutions, General Assembly*; Florida, 5th Session, 1850-51. No. 450.
2. Marianna *Florida Whig*, April 26, 1852.
3. U.S. Census, 1850, Jackson County Florida, p. 619. Here his name appears as Roscoe.

Rasky, J., Fernandina, mid-19th century

The death of Dr. Rasky, for several years a citizen of Fernandina, was announced in the Tallahassee *Semi-Weekly Sentinel* of February 5, 1867.

> Dr. J. Rasky—The sudden death of this old citizen of Fernandina, at Columbia, S.C., is announced in the Fernandina *Courier*.[1]

He was said to have been an old citizen of Fernandina although his death occurred in South Carolina. Unfortunately, Fernandina newspapers which might have taken notice of his death with some biographical information have not survived.

1. Tallahassee *Sun-Weekly Sentinel*, February 5, 1867.

Raysor, A.W., Jefferson County, 1832

Only minimal information concerning Dr. Raysor has emerged and it cannot be shown with certainty that he actually practiced medicine in Florida. Born in Abbeville District, South Carolina, about 1832, he was brought to Florida by his parents,[1] Alfred and Mary Raysor, prior to 1850. He received his preparatory education at the Cokesbury Institute located in Abbeville District and one of the most reputable schools in the state. His medical preceptor was Dr. John May of Monticello. In the fall of 1850 he was enrolled at the Medical College of the State of South Carolina from which he received his medical degree in March 1852 after submitting a doctoral thesis entitled "Cathartics."[2] No record of his medical practice has been discovered.

1. Several members of the Raysor family settled in the Williamsburg community of Jefferson County in the mid-19th century. Their lands lay along the Aucilla River southeast of Monticello. The name Williamsburg was discontinued before the end of the century, being replaced by the name, Aucilla, which exists today.
2. Lists of Students and Graduates, Medical College of the State of South Carolina, Catalogue, 1851-52. Waring Historical Library, Medical University of South Carolina, Charleston. See Charleston *Mercury*, March 18, 1852.

Redfield, Achilles Mansfield, Tampa, 1811-1853

The Florida residence of Dr. Redfield was tragically brief. There remains some doubt that he ever actually practiced in the state. He was born in Claremont, New Hampshire, on October 1, 1811.[1] After attending local schools he enrolled at the Vermont Medical College, Woodstock, Vermont, where he remained for one term before transferring to Berkshire College, Pittsfield, Massachusetts, from which he received his medical degree in 1838. He is presumed to have begun professional practice in either Vermont or Massachusetts.

Dr. Redfield's professional career was interrupted in the early 1850s by an illness, presumed to have been tuberculosis, which forced him to seek a more benign climate. He chose Tampa but the change came too late; he died there on October 24, 1853. His gravestone in Oak Lawn Cemetery bears the following inscription:[2]

ACHILLES MANSFIELD REDFIELD, A native of New Hampshire
Died, October 24, 1853. Age 42.

1. Brief biographical data on Dr. Redfield is found in *The Story of a Country Medical College*, by Frederick Clayton Waite, Vermont Historical Society, Montpelier, 1945, p. 193.
2. The location of Dr. Redfield's gravestone and the inscription was provided by Dr. Paul J. Schmidt, Director of the Southwest Florida Blood Bank, Tampa.

Reeves, John W., Gadsden County, 1827

Dr. Reeves, a native of Georgia and possibly a graduate of the Medical College of Georgia, Augusta,[1] settled in the Concord community of Gadsden County in 1852. In late December that year he married Mrs. Carolina Gouldin, a widow and also a Georgia native.[2] For the next 10 years or more he was Concord's leading medical practitioner, sharing the practice with Dr. Thomas Henley. The 1870 census shows Dr. Reeves and his wife sharing their home with William Gouldin, probably Mrs. Reeves' child by her first marriage, and two young women.[3] In the latter stages of the Civil War Dr. Reeves joined Company I, First Florida Reserves, in which he served until the end of the conflict in 1865.[4]

Beyond the year 1870 nothing is known of Dr. Reeves' activities. It may be assumed that he continued to practice as a country doctor. Of his extraprofessional activities it is only known that he was a member of the Concordia Lodge (Mason), No. 28.[5] The date of his death remains unknown.

1. In the list of graduates of the Medical College of Georgia there is the name, W.J. Reeves, native of Georgia, class of 1852.
2. Floreda Duke Varick and Phyllis Rose Smith, comps., "Gadsden County, Florida, Marriage Records, 1849-76," Tallahassee, 1980, Mimeographed, p. 59.
3. U.S. Census, 1870, Gadsden County, Florida, p. 708.
4. *Soldiers of Florida*, Board of State Institutions, Live Oak, 1903, p. 312.
5. *Records, Grand Lodge of Florida, 1860-1866*, date and place of publication unknown, p. 428.

Reid, Jeremiah D., Madison County, 1802-1856

Notwithstanding his wealth and social prominence in Madison County, biographical information on Dr. Reid is not abundant. He was born in South Carolina, probably in the vicinity of Beaufort, in 1802, received his medical education at an unidentified school and moved to Madison County in the mid-1830s.[1] Apparently he arrived with sufficient funds to purchase extensive acreage southwest of the Town of Madison, having doubtless brought with him some of his 45 slaves whom he set to work improving his newly-acquired estate.[2] Thus he settled into the life of a well-to-do plantation master. The evidence suggests that he was more planter than physician.

Dr. Reid appears to have lived a somewhat circumscribed life, content to manage his plantation and help in the establishment of a vigorous Baptist Church in Madison.[3] On one occasion he was persuaded to offer himself as a candidate to represent the Middle District of Florida in the Territorial Legislative Council for the session of 1838. It was a dismal experience: he placed eighth in a field of eight.[4] Only the top four recipients were elected. Four years later he was present at a public meeting at the Madison County Court House on September 2, assembled for the dual purposes of discussing the continuing threat of the Seminole Indians and nominating candidates for the Legislative Council. He was a member of the committee elected to draw up a statement to be forwarded to federal authorities.[5]

By an odd inadvertence the Madison County censuses of 1840 and 1850 do not include entries for Dr. Reid although the slave schedule of 1850 lists him as the owner of 45 slaves. We are, therefore, deprived of important information concerning the Reid family. The Census of 1860 (Dr. Reid had died four years earlier), however, lists his widow, A.B. Reid, as aged 40, owning property valued in excess of $30,000. Also listed is the Reid daughter, Sarah, owner of real property valued at $2,400. In addition, William Reid, probably a brother of Dr. Reid, owned property valued at $25,700.[6]

Dr. Reid died at his home on June 5, 1856, after a protracted illness. According to his obituary he was survived by "a devoted wife and an idolized daughter and numerous relatives and friends." The notice continued: He was "an affectionate and devoted husband and father, a warm and sincere friend, a kind and indulgent master...a Baptist."[7] He was buried in the Old Oakland Cemetery located about seven miles southwest of Madison.

1. Although the relationship has not been verified, evidence suggests that Dr. Reid was a cousin of Robert Raymond Reid, Territorial Governor of Florida, 1829-41. See Robert E.H. Peeples, "A Miles Genealogy," *South Carolina Historical Magazine*, LXVII, January 1966, p. 36.

2. The slave schedule for Madison County, 1850, listed Dr. Reid as the owner of 45 slaves, while 10 years later the combined number owned by widow and daughter was 58.

3. Edwin B. Browning, *First Baptist Church, Madison, Florida, A Historical Sketch*, Tallahassee, 1956, p. 8.

4. Dr. Reid actually received only three votes; the leading candidate William P. Duval received 341. Tallahassee *Floridian*, September 1, 1838; October 13, 1838.

5. WPA, Madison County Writers' Project, "County Commissioners," Typed Copy, P.K. Yonge Library of Florida History.

6. U.S.Census, 1860, Madison County, Florida, p. 169.

7. Tallahassee *Floridian and Journal*, June 14, 1856.

Renault, Leon, Alachua County, 1828

Dr. Renault, a native of Paris, France, and member of the Medical Faculty of Paris,[1] was approaching the age of 50 when he made his appearance in Waldo. He had previously practiced medicine in St. Louis, Missouri, and even earlier in Illinois where his four children were born. In the style of the times his professional notice made extravagant claims as to his proficiency.[2] His professional card, which was included in the advertising section of Carl Webber's book, *The Eden of the South*, said the doctor:

> I have made a specialty of female and chronic diseases for the past thirty years with great success, having cured many diseases which have been incurable by other physicians. The number may be learned by inquiring abroad. Such diseases as Prolapsus, Tumors, Ulcerations, Retroflexions, Retroversions, Etroversions, and Displacement of the Womb; and also Chronic Diseses of the Liver, Dropsy and Heart Disease will, if neglected, prove fatal. My charges are reasonable, and I want the sufferers to receive the benefit of my success. Yours, with Respect. D.L. Renault, M.D.

Census data of 1880 show Dr. Renault residing on his farm a mile and a half east of Waldo; his age was 52. Included in his household were his wife, Susanna, aged 48, also born in Paris; children, George, aged 15; daughters, Alice, aged 13, and Leonie, nine, all born in Illinois.

The date of Dr. Renault's death has not been determined. There is no gravestone to indicate that he was buried in Waldo's cemetery.

1. Webber, Carl, *The Eden of the South*, New York, 1883, p. 181.

Renshaw, Francis (Frank) B., Pensacola, 1815-1867

Dr. Renshaw was born in Pennsylvania on May 23, 1815. In the late 1840s he arrived in Pensacola and assumed his assignment as physician at the Pensacola Navy Yard.[1] Soon thereafter he married Florida J., daughter of Dr. John

Brosnaham, a marriage terminated by her death on November 25, 1851. He subsequently remarried and became the father of three children, twins, Fannie and Frank Gayle, and Georgia Ella.[2] No evidence has been discovered which would indicate that Dr. Renshaw was ever a civilian practitioner in Pensacola, although his son, Frank Gayle, a graduate of the Medical College of Louisiana in 1880, was a prominent physician in the city until his death in 1935.[3]

Dr. Frank Renshaw died in Pensacola on June 9, 1867, and was buried in St. Michael's Cemetery. He was survived by his three children and his sister, Mary B., born in Philadelphia in 1810 and died in Pensacola on May 14, 1900.[4]

1. U.S. Census, 1850, Escambia County, Florida, p. 243.
2. The name of Dr. Renshaw's second wife has not been ascertained. Data relating to his children derives from St. Michael's Cemetery records.
3. Elizabeth Dwyer Vickers and F. Norman Vickers, M.D., "Notations on Pensacola's Medical History, 1873-1923," *Journal, Florida Medical Association*, January 1974, p. 87.
4. Pensacola *Daily News*, March 14, 1900. This obituary requests that Philadelphia newspapers reprint the death notice which suggests that Dr Renshaw was probably a native of that city.

Ribble, George W., Jefferson County, 1830-1876

Although he was styled "physician" by the census enumerator in 1870, it is doubtful that Dr. Ribble ever practiced medicine in Florida, except perhaps on a very limited scale. He arrived in Jefferson County about 1868[1] apparently with financial resources sufficient to purchase or rent considerable acreage on which he planted cotton. He also built a cotton gin which, in addition to his own requirements, accommodated other farmers of the community.[2] Searches in Jefferson County mortgage books of the postwar period reveal that he maintained substantial credit with the Savannah brokerage firm of William B. Brookridge.[3] His residence was located south of the town of Waukeenah.

Dr. Ribble was born in Roanoke, Virginia, on May 15, 1830. His wife, Virginia, and only son, George Jr., were also native Virginians. Census data suggests that the Ribbles were able to live comfortably, employing two "live-in" household servants and numerous farm workers. Dr. Ribble died at his home on August 26, 1876,[4] at the age of 46. He was buried in Grantham Cemetery just south of Waukeenah.

1. This date is an extrapolation from the Census of 1870 which lists the age of the Ribble son as four, and his birthplace as Virginia.
2. Jerrell H. Shofner, History of Jefferson County, Tallahassee, 1976, p. 324.
3. Ibid., p. 326.
4. Gravestone inscription, Grantham Cemetery, Jefferson County.

Rice, John A., Marion and Hillsborough Counties, 1818-1858

Except for data included in the Marion County Census of 1850[1] very little is known of the early years of Dr. Rice. He was born in South Carolina in 1818, lived for a brief time in Georgia where he met and married Elizabeth, and where his eldest child, Benjamin, was born. Records of the Medical College of South Carolina indicate that he was a student there in 1839-40[2] but did not return for the second year. His preceptor had been a Dr. McDowell. In those days a medical degree was not a requirement for obtaining a license to practice in Florida.

About 1843 Dr. Rice moved to Marion County, settling west of Ocala in a part of the county soon to be inhabited by numerous migrants from South Carolina. He carried on his practice until the summer of 1854 when he moved to Hillsborough County, establishing his residence in the village of Ichepuksassa, situated some 15 miles east of Tampa.[3] He entered practice in partnership with Dr. M.M. Weissinger, a tuberculosis patient who had come to Florida seeking a more benign climate. The association was of brief duration when in early 1855 Dr. Weissinger became too ill to continue practice. Dr. Rice announced his intention to continue alone on April 7, 1855. Dr. Weissinger died in January 1856.[4]

Dr. Rice soon discovered that medical practice in rural Florida was not a lucrative occupation. His wife and children must be provided for, so he proceeded to build both a grist mill and sawmill near his home. In April 1855, he informed the public that he had "completed his saw and grist mills and can fill bills for lumber and turn off meal with dispatch."[5]

Dr. Rice remained in Ichepuksassa, milling and practicing medicine until early 1858 when he moved to Tampa and joined Dr. William J. Oliver in a partnership. Their office was located in Capt. McKay's Building on Franklin Street.[6]

At about this juncture Dr. Rice's fortunes took a turn for the better. On April 28, 1858, the Tampa City Council drew up a set of ordinances of which number 13 announced the appointment of Dr. Rice as Inspector of the Port of Tampa and named a Board of Health composed of Drs. John F. Crichton, S.B. Todd, and John A. Rice.[7] Dr. Rice was elected to the City Council on September 20 that year.[8]

The fall of 1858 was a tragic time for the people of Tampa and a bewildering one for the physicians. By mid-September yellow fever had appeared, spreading alarm throughout the city. The responsibility for coping with the epidemic and reassuring the populace weighed heavily upon the Board of Health. On October 2 the Board informed the public that there were indeed "some cases of yellow fever, though in a mitigated form; we do not think that there is any danger that the disease will become epidemic."[9] But epidemic it was and on October 16 the editor of the Tampa newspaper defended his cautious stance in response to reader impatience with the following statement: "For the information of such persons we will state that we are dependent upon our physicians for the truth of our reports. When Doctors disagree...when their views are diametrically opposed...what chance have we to arrive at a correct conclusion?" The paper then proceeded to name six persons who had succumbed to yellow fever during the preceding week.[10]

The epidemic continued to spread, and within a month Dr. Rice had become a victim of the disease at the age of 40.[11] On November 16 J. Darling was elected "Councilman of this city...to fill the unexpired term of Dr. John A. Rice, deceased."[12] The Census of 1860 for Hillsborough County lists Mrs. Elizabeth Rice and her five children, ages 17 to five, as residents of Tampa. Her occupation: "Seamstress."[13]

1. This date is an extrapolation based on data in the Census of Marion County, Florida, 1850, p. 265.
2. *Catalogue, Medical College of the State of South Carolina*, Session of 1839-40.
3. Tampa *Herald*, October 25, 1854. Ichepuksassa is now Plant City.
4. "Diary of William C. Brown," December 24, 1855-April 9, 1856. P.K. Yonge Library of Florida History, University

of Florida. Entry for Sunday, February 10. Brown, ill at the time, wrote: "I slept most of the day. This morning we sent for Dr. Rice and he came in this evening." Dr. Weissinger had become totally disabled in early 1855, whereupon Dr. Rice announced the termination of the partnership on April 7, 1855.

5. Tampa *Florida Peninsula*, April 7, 1855, Brown, "Diary," entry for February 20, 1856.

6. Tampa *Florida Peninsula*, April 3, 1858. First printing, not extant, March 20, 1858, James McKay was a successful Tampa merchant.

7. Ibid., November 27, 1858. These ordinances had been drafted on April 28, 1858, and continued to appear in the paper throughout the year.

8. Ibid., September 25, 1858.

9. Ibid., October 2, 1858.

10. Ibid., October 16, 1858.

11. Several issues of the *Peninsula* between October 16 and November 20 are not extant. Dr. Rice died during this period.

12. Ibid., November 20, 1858.

13. Mrs. Rice's eldest son, Benjamin, entered the Confederate Army on October 31, 1861, and was assigned to the Fourth Florida Infantry (Capt. Mitchell's Company). He was killed in the Battle of Murfreesboro, Tenn., on January 2, 1863. A claim for pay due him at the time of his death was filed in Thomasville, Ga., on August 4, 1863, by H.H. Tooke, attorney for Mrs. Rice. This suggests that she had returned to her native Georgia during the war.

Rice, William S., Madison and Hamilton Counties, 1840-1878

Dr. Rice was born in Georgia in early 1840. At some unknown date in the 1850s he moved with his family to Madison County settling on land outside the county seat usually designated Madison Court House. His family appears to have been one of considerable means. While still a resident of Georgia he matriculated at the Oglethorpe Medical College in Savannah from which he was graduated M.D. on March 3, 1860.[1] Soon thereafter he began practice in Madison County, having obtained lodging in the home of George Hammock, a native of Georgia[2] and a comparatively wealthy planter.

With the coming of the Civil War Dr. Rice was of an age to be recruited for service in the Confederate Army. He had endeared himself to the people of the community as a good citizen and reputable physician, however, and the local recruitment agency was persuaded to allow him to remain in Madison. A short time later he moved to Jasper, the seat of Hamilton County, where he soon came to be regarded as an indispensable citizen. About 1863 when the Southern military situation began to deteriorate and medical replacements were desperately needed, Dr. Rice received orders to report for duty. The reaction of the Jasper community was expressed in the following response from the Hamilton County Commissioners to the Confederate recruitment board:[3]

> Dr. William S. Rice, the only physician in Jasper for the first two years, has been ordered to the Camp of Instruction to be placed in service. Dr. Rice is of more service to the community than to the army and they want him restored to the community.

The request was granted and Dr. Rice remained in practice in Jasper and its environs for the duration.

In 1865, with peace more or less restored, Dr. Rice married Eugenia Self (Selph) and by 1870 two daughters, Ada and Selma, had been born. Before Dr. Rice's untimely death three additional children, a son, William, and two daughters, Rosa and Bethulea, had blessed the union.[4]

Dr. Rice was not one to shun civic responsibilites. In 1866 he was elected Treasurer of Hamilton County, an office to which he was reelected two years later.[5] In 1875 the Florida Commissioner of Lands and Immigration, Dennis Eagan, collected information on economic resources, industrial development, health conditions, etc., by a questionnaire to each county. The task of responding for Hamilton County fell to Dr. Rice. His report was a well-constructed document, reflecting good judgment and honesty. The final paragraph, relating to health, bears quoting here:[6]

> Our water is principally freestone, though some is sulphur, some lime, and some rotten lime, which is rare. We have one physician to 4000 population, whereas in other states and counties the ratio is one to every 700 or 1000. Our principal diseases are fever and ague and remitting and bilious fever. Some years they prevail almost all over the county, but again we have but a very light sprinkling of them. A wet winter and a dry summer to follow it, will cause these diseases. To persons of ordinary information they are manageable, rarely requiring a physician, and scarcely ever producing death if uncomplicated with any other disorder. Occasionally I have seen these fevers assume one or the other of the following types, viz.: Malignant, congestive, inflammatory, and typhus. I can't say that, during fifteen years' residence and practice of medicine here, that I have ever seen a genuine case of typhoid fever to originate in the county. Once or twice, in winters, I have seen pneumonia to prevail endemically, i.e., in particular localities. Mosquitoes and fleas are quite troublesome for a few months in summer. Respectfully, W.S. Rice, M.D.

Dr. Rice died in 1878 at the age of 38; the date of his death remains unknown.[7] His widow, Eugenia, was only 31 at the time. In 1880, she and her five children were living in the home of Jasper merchant Samuel Register, whose wife is thought to have been a sister of Mrs. Rice.[8]

1. Savannah *Daily Morning News*, March 5, 1860. Dr. Rice is listed as a resident of Georgia, which he was at the time of matriculation. Prior to 1860, however, his family had moved to Madison County.
2. U.S. Census, 1860, Madison County, Florida, p. 207.
3. Cora Hinton, comp., *A Brief History of Hamilton County, Florida*, Jasper, Florida, 1976, p. 82.
4. U.S. Census, 1870, Hamilton County, Florida, p. 1, item 2; Ibid., 1880, p. 301.
5. Hinton, *Brief History*, p. 29.
6. *Journal of Proceedings of the Assembly of the State of Florida*, 8th Session, 1875, Tallahassee, 1875, App., pp. 124-126.
7. Notes of Olin Norwood, in possession of Mrs. Cora Hinton, courtesy of Miss Melanie Barr, Gainesville.
8. In 1880 Mrs. Rice was the proprietress of a rooming (or boarding) house in Jasper. Living with her were her daughters, Ada and Bethulea, and her aunt, Mrs. H.M.C. Selph.

Rich, John S., Marion County, 1860

Dr. Rich was born in Sumter District, South Carolina, about 1813. He began the study of medicine under the preceptorate of local physician Dr. J.B. Weatherspoon and in the fall of 1834 matriculated in the Medical Department, Transylvania University,[1] where he appears to have spent only one term. No evidence of further medical study has been discovered. Only a year or two prior to the outbreak of the Civil War he moved with his family to Florida, settling in the Wacahoota community of Marion County.[2] His wife, L.B., and their four sons and one daughter, aged one to eight, were natives of South Carolina.[3]

Almost nothing is known of Dr. Rich's professional service. Presumably because of his age, 47 in 1860, and domestic responsibilities he was exempt from military duty in the army of the Confederacy. He was still a resident of Marion County as late as the spring of 1867 when he was one of three local citizens involved in settling the estate of Dr. George Baxter Hunter of Wacahoota whose untimely death had occurred in late 1865.[4] Since he does not appear in the Florida Census of 1870 it is assumed that he had departed the state by that year.

1. Transylvania University, Lexington, Kentucky, List of matriculants, 1834-35.
2. The village of Wacahoota was situated near the northern boundary of Marion County. It had obtained a post office in 1842, only to lose it when nearby Flemington was assigned a post office in 1847.

3. Since the youngest Rich child, one year old in 1860, was born in South Carolina, it appears that the family did not move to Florida before 1859.

4. Gainesville *New Era*, May 18, 1867.

Richardson, John G., Gainesville, 1836-1864

Dr. Richardson, eldest son of James Richardson, a well-to-do planter of Alachua County, was born in South Carolina in 1836. Much of his youth, however, was spent in Mississippi where his family had settled about 1847. About 1856 they moved to Alachua County and acquired land north of Gainesville. Their properties were estimated to have been worth about $36,000 in 1860.[1]

It is not known where Dr. Richardson received his medical education,[2] but by 1860 he had joined his family and entered medical practice. His professional career was brief, however, for with the approach of war and the secession of Florida in early 1861 he became one of the early enlistees, offering his services to the Confederacy on March 24, 1861, committing himself for a period of 12 months. Nine days later he was mustered in as a private in Company H, (Gainesville Minute Men), 1st Florida Infantry, and sent to Camp Magnolia, near Pensacola, where he spent the next year.[3]

Immediately after his discharge in April 1862, Dr. Richardson reenlisted for a term of three years and was assigned to Company D (Alachua Rebels), 7th Florida Infantry, with the rank of 4th sergeant.[4] The following 18 months he spent at Camp Lee, Florida. By early 1863 he had been promoted to 1st sergeant but on December 1 of that year for unknown reasons he was demoted to 3rd sergeant.

By early 1864 the 7th Florida Regiment had been assigned to the Army of Tennessee under the command of General Joseph E. Johnston, who had recently replaced General Braxton Bragg. One of the preliminary engagements of the Atlanta campaign occurred near Resaca on May 13-16, 1864, with the Florida 7th participating. In the encounter Dr. Richardson was killed at the age of 28.[5]

1. U.S. Census, 1860, Alachua County, Florida, item 598.

2. The records of the Medical College of the State of South Carolina do not mention Dr. John G. Richardson. James P. Richardson, his younger brother, who had begun medical study under the preceptorate of Dr. Thomas W. McCaa of Gainesville, received his medical degree from the Charleston school in 1861.

3. NA, Service Records, CSA, m251, Roll 29.

4. Ibid., Roll 79.

5. No further information concerning Dr. James P. Richardson has emerged. The 1870 Alachua County Census indicates that the father was deceased but several younger members of the Richardson family still resided in the county.

Richardson, Thomas J., Columbia County, 1860

Dr. Richardson, a native of Georgia, appeared in the Columbia County census of 1860 as a resident in the home of Nathan and Alpha Bryan, a young couple living outside Lake City. His age was 40, while the ages of the Bryans were 21 and 17 respectively. Nothing further is known of the physician.[1]

1. U.S. Census, 1860, Columbia County, Florida, p. 182.

Richburgh, William L., Santa Rosa and Walton Counties, 1827

Dr. Richburgh, scion of a Charleston family of note,[1] was born in South Carolina about 1827. Nothing is known of his earlier years and professional training. It is assumed, however, that he had been apprenticed to a practicing physician, probably in Mobile. At some undetermined date he married an Alabama native, Margaret, and their first five children, Jefferson, John, William, Frances, and James, were natives of Alabama.[2]

About 1858 the Richburghs removed to Santa Rosa County where he resumed his practice and where two daughters, Mary and Sarah, were born.[3]

Census data indicate that the Richburghs lived only slightly above the poverty level. In 1860 their property, all personal, was valued at a mere $150. For the next decade, after settling in the Shoal River District, they were far from affluent, their total properties, real and personal, being appraised at only $300.[4]

By 1880 the family had been reduced, presumably by the marriages of several of their children, leaving only Dr. and Mrs. Richburgh, two daughters, Mary and Sarah, and son William, apparently a widower, and his five-year-old son, William.[5] They were still residing in the Shoal River District of Walton County in 1885.[6] The date of Dr. Richburgh's death has not been determined.

1. Dr. Richburgh is presumed to have been a descendant of the eminent French Huguenot clergyman, Charles Phillippe de Richebourg, who had arrived in Charleston, South Carolina, as a missionary about 1710. He was assigned to St. James Santee Parish, the most remote from Charleston, where he, his wife and five children suffered from depredations attending the Indian wars about 1715. See *South Carolina Historical and Genealogical Magazine*, XXXII, 259, 262-263.
2. U.S. Census, 1860, Santa Rosa County, Florida, p. 701.
3. Ibid., 1870, Walton County, Florida, p. 811.
4. Ibid. The Shoal River District, then in Walton County, became a part of Okaloosa County after its formation in 1915 from portions of Walton and Santa Rosa Counties.
5. U.S. Census, 1880, Walton County, Florida.
6. Special Census, Florida, 1885. Shoal River District, Walton County, p. 71.

Ridley, E.B., Wakulla County, 1860

Except for the data contained in the Census of 1860, nothing is known of Dr. Ridley, a brief sojourner in Wakulla County. He was a native of Georgia, as were his wife, Martha, daughter, Mary A., and son, Imma. They were residents of Newport, apparently having arrived about 1859. Dr. Ridley's property was valued at about $4,000. His age was 44.[1] It is likely that he returned to Georgia as the war ensued.

1. U.S. Census, 1860, Wakulla County, Florida, p. 1.

Rives, James H., Gadsden County, 1812

The only information concerning the Florida career of Dr. Rives derives from the Census of 1850 which indicates that he was born in Georgia, was married to Nancy, a Florida native 17 years his junior, and that they were the parents of a daughter, Mary, one year old. Included in the household was G.S. Rives, aged 26, probably a brother.[1]

1. U.S. Census, 1850, Gadsden County, Florida, p. 216, item 569.

Roberson, William, Gadsden County, 1870

Dr. Roberson, native of Virginia, was on the staff of the Florida State Hospital for the Insane in 1870. The census of that year lists him at age 50. Other members of the family were Mrs. Mary Roberson, aged 51, and a daughter, Cornelia, aged 11, born in Florida. This would indicate that the Robersons had arrived in Florida prior to 1860, although they are not listed in the Census of 1860. In the same item is listed the name of the Commander of the Institution, Col. Malachi Martin, aged 45, a native of Ireland.[1]

1. U.S. Census, 1870, Gadsden County, Florida, p. 781.

Roberts, Cornelius O.O., Columbia County, 1843-1875

Dr. Roberts, son of Arthur and Rebecca Roberts, both natives of Georgia, was born on the family farm near Lake City in 1843.[1] He received an early education in Lake City and presumably served an apprenticeship under the preceptorate of a physician of the town. In 1865 he entered the Medical College of Georgia in Augusta from which he was graduated in the spring of 1867.[2] Returning to Florida he began practice in Lake City and soon thereafter married a local girl, Mary.

From the beginning of his professional career Dr. Roberts exhibited the professional qualities which would assure him a successful practice and the respect of his colleagues. At the second annual meeting of the Florida Medical Association held in Jacksonville in February 1875, his name was presented for membership and he was elected by the unanimous vote of those present.[3] At the business of the following day, February 18, he was appointed to the Committee on Accounts.[4] His promising career came to a tragic end later in 1875 when he died at the age of 31. At its next meeting, held in Tallahassee, the Association took note of his death with an expression of regret and sympathy for his grief-stricken family.[5] He was survived by his widow, his father, and several brothers and sisters.[6]

1. U.S. Census, 1850, Columbia County, Florida, p. 89.
2. Medical Department, University of Georgia, "List of Graduates from 1829 to 1891," Augusta, 1891, p. 24.
3. *Proceedings, Florida Medical Association*, Charleston, S.C., 1875, p. 8.
4. Ibid., p. 11.
5. *Proceedings, Florida Medical Association*, Jacksonville, 1877, p. 7.
6. Meanwhile Arthur Roberts' first wife had died, after which he married Levinia, and they had four children. U.S. Census, 1880, Columbia County, Florida, p. 376.

Roberts, John W, Tampa, 1801

Dr. Roberts, for several years a physician in Tampa and its vicinity, lived about the middle of the 19th century. The evidence, although rather limited, suggests that his professional career fell somewhat short of success and he found it necessary to eke out a living in other pursuits. Certainly he never enjoyed the popularity and prestige achieved by several of his professional contemporaries who formed the nucleus of the local medical faculty, Drs. Franklin and Darwin Branch, William A. Lively, and John P. Crichton.

Nothing is presently known of Dr. Roberts' education and professional training, but it is conjectured that he learned medicine under the preceptorate of a local physician. He first appears in Florida records in 1848 when he was elected clerk of court for Hillsborough.[1] The Census of 1850 lists him as "doctor," aged 49, living with his wife, Ann Maria, four years his junior and a native of Connecticut. She was the proprietress of a boarding house, her assets valued at $1,500.[2]

With renewal of hostilities between the remnant of Seminole Indians in South Florida and the whites pressing ever southward by mid-century, residents of Hillsborough and Polk Counties became involved in the conflict. In response to the call for volunteer troops, Dr. Roberts was among those offering his services. On January 27, 1856, he enlisted for a period of six months, joining the company being assembled at Ichepuksassa (now Plant City) in the northeastern corner of Hillsborough County by Captain Simeon L. Sparkman.[3] He provided his own horse, valued at $135, doubtless the animal he had used in his medical practice.[4] Within a few weeks after expiration of his term of service Dr. Roberts reenlisted for an additional six months, the date of enlistment being August 23, 1856, continuing in service until he was mustered out at Ft. Brooke on February 17, 1857.

Financially, Dr. Roberts' year of military service availed him little. At the time of mustering out he was still owed pay from the date of his enlistment. On return to civilian status he resumed medical practice, his professional card first appearing in the local newspaper on January 1, 1858, to be discontinued after the issue of May 28, 1859. Meanwhile he had run successfuly for the office of justice of the peace and, in addition to the pittance he derived therefrom, was able to garner occasional fees for performing marriage ceremonies.[5] Beyond the summer of 1857 no record of his career has been located.

Two diaries still extant provide a few glimpses of Dr. Roberts activities. That of William C. Brown,[6] covering the months December 1855 to April 1856 gives some information on his military service, while the other, that of George F. Thompson,[7] gives some insight into his less-than-happy marriage. It appears almost certain that the marriage had ended prior to 1860.[8] Dr. Roberts does not appear in any Florida Census of 1860, and it is assumed that he had either died or departed the state by that date. Mrs. Roberts, on the other hand, continued to operate her boarding house, at least until 1870, when she is shown at the age of 65 still in charge of a "private boarding house and possessing assets valued at $2500.[9]

1. See "Diary of William Charles Brown," transcribed with notes by Theodore Lesley, 1956. Typed copy in P.K. Yonge Library of Florida History, p. 7, n.3. The original diary is also among the manuscripts of the same.

2. U.S. Census, 1850, Hillsborough County, Florida, p. 486.

3. Records of Adj. Gen. Office, Record Gp. 94, Compiled Service Records, Volunteer Soldiers, Florida Indian Wars, 1835-58, 112-B, Microcopy 1086, Roll 63. He is also mentioned in the Brown "Diary."

4. Dr. Roberts' horse died of lockjaw on April 26, 1865. Ibid.

5. Tampa *Florida Peninsular*, July 16, 1859; June 25, 1859.

6. See note 1, supra.

7. "Journal of George F. Thompson," P.K. Yonge Library of Florida History, pp. 101-102. The following excerpt, sad but somewhat amusing, reveals something of the relationship:

> Mrs. Roberts "was formerly a Connecticut woman...when young probably marrying a Southerner with the high expectation of being a lady. But her experience proves to her and to others that misfortunes happen to the best of people, and her experience shows the effect of slavery upon conjugal relations sometimes to be anything but conducive to harmony and happiness. Dr. Roberts acquired the habit of spending his evenings at home, where a man of domestic feelings should, and the result was an internecine war, the Dr. coming out second best in the contest, concluded to divide the house with his spouse, giving her the inside

and himself taking the outside, since which time Mrs. Roberts has lived a sort of widowhood, said by some to be of the vegetable species."

This is presumably a reference to the expression, "grass-widow," designating a woman, separated from her husband, but not divorced.

Robertson, William, St. Augustine, 1823

Dr. Robertson, a native of Glasgow, Scotland, who began practice in St. Augustine during the Second Spanish period, was a resident there at the time of the cession by Spain in early 1821. He was among the signers of a memorial to Congress, dated January 28, 1822, expressing their joy and gratitude that the cession had been accomplished.[1] In the general naturalization of citizens which occurred on November 20, 1822, he declared himself to be a subject of the English king, stating also that his occupation was that of planter.[2] Dr. Robertson's wife, Ann, was also Scottish, having been born in Inverness.[3]

Dr. Robertson died in St. Augustine on September 29, 1823, of fever which had become epidemic in the city. On the following day J.N. Glenn, also a resident of the city, made the following entry in his "Journal."[4]

> This evening (afternoon) I acted as Chaplain to the Masonic burial of Dr. William Robertson of this City, and after the Masonic cerimony (sic) Borson Lothrop concluded the service by a Prayer.

Dr. Robertson was survived by his widow, Ann, who remained in St. Augustine until her death on April 9, 1850,[5] and his only child, Margarette A., who on November 4, 1844,[6] became the wife of Lt. Lafayette Bowyer Wood, an officer in the United States Army, who was stationed at St. Augustine.[7]

1. Clarence E. Carter, *The Territorial Papers of the United States*, Vol. XXII, "The Territory of Florida, 1821-24," Washington, 1956, p. 350.
2. Ibid., p. 434.
3. St. Augustine *The Ancient City*. From the obituary of Mrs. Robertson.
4. J.N. Glenn, "Journal of the First Part of My Life," Microfilm, 161-E, P.K. Yonge Library of Florida History, University of Florida.
5. See note 3 supra.
6. St. Augustine *Florida Herald and Southern Democrat*, November 5, 1844.
7. Captain Wood, a graduate of the United States Military Academy in 1843, was decorated for bravery in the Mexican War. He died on October 19, 1858. See Francis B. Heitman, *Historical Register and Dictionary of the U.S. Army*, Washington, 1903, vol. I, p. 1055.

Robertson Jr., William Fitzgerald, Leon County, 1840-1905

Dr. Fitzgerald Jr., son of Dr. William Fitzgerald Sr., was born in Terrebonne Parish, Louisiana, on January 27, 1840.[1] The elder Robertson, a Virginia native, had practiced in Louisiana before moving to Leon County in 1846 and settling near Lake Iamonia[2] where William Fitzgerald Jr. was born. He is presumed to have begun the study of medicine under the guidance of his father. At any rate he was accepted for admission into the Medical College of the State of South Carolina in the fall of 1857 and was graduated as Doctor of Medicine in the spring of 1859, having submitted a thesis bearing the title, "Yellow Fever."[3]

Soon after graduation Dr. Robertson returned to Florida and in December 1860 announced the beginning of his practice at the plantation of his father near Centreville.[4] He discontinued the practice on April 19, 1862, and joined the Army of the Confederacy, enlisting in Capt. R.H. Gamble's (later to become the company of Capt. Charles E.E. Dyke) Light Artillery Company. Within a few weeks he came down with an illness which caused him to be hospitalized at the General Army Hospital in Tallahassee, from which he was discharged on September 15, 1862, upon a surgeon's certificate of disability. In the following year, however, he reenlisted, receiving an appointment as assistant surgeon, dated July 7, 1863. Thereafter, for almost two years, nothing is known of his service, the final item of his record being a requisition bearing his signature, dated at Anderson(ville), Georgia, on April 1, 1865. The assumption is that he was paroled in the mass parole action later in that month.[5] Incidental data describe him as "five feet, ten inches tall, of light complexion, light hair, and by profession a physician."

At the conclusion of the war, Dr. Robertson resumed his practice at Iamonia where he also carried on small-scale farming. At age 50 he married Katherine Player Bannerman,[6] daughter of his wealthy neighbor, Charles W. Bannerman. She was only 28. Soon after their marriage the couple moved into Tallahassee where they remained for the rest of their lives and where their three children, William Fitzgerald III, Mary and Charles Archibald, were born.[7]

Dr. Robertson died at his Tallahassee home on May 15, 1905,[8] leaving his widow and three children, ages 14, 13 and 10. He was buried, not in St. Johns churchyard with his parents but, because he had become a Presbyterian, in the Old City Cemetery. Mrs. Robertson lived until July 10, 1937. In his brief sketch of Dr. Robertson, the well-known Tallahassee physician, Dr. Henry E. Palmer, wrote: "Dr. Robertson is said to have been a most successful practitioner, a kindly, generous gentleman."[9]

The eldest Robertson child, William Fitzgerald III, settled in Savannah and became the father of three daughters and one son. The second child, Mary, became the wife of William L. Baker of Tallahassee. Two sons were born to their marriage.[10] The youngest child of Dr. and Mrs. Robertson, Charles Archibald, became Professor of English and later Chairman of the Department of English at the University of Florida, Gainesville. He died in 1975.[11]

1. Gravestone, Old City Cemetery, Tallahassee. Some uncertainty persists as to Dr. Robertson's place of birth. In his Civil War Service Record, both Terrebonne Parish and Claiborne Parish, Louisiana, are given as his birthplace. The former seems more likely to be correct. See NA, Service Records, CSA, M251, Roll 22.

2. See obituary of Dr. William F. Robertson Sr., Tallahassee *Weekly Floridian*, February 19, 1885.

3. Charleston (S.C.) *Courier*, March 16, 1859.

4. Tallahassee *Floridian and Journal*, July 26, 1862; 1st printed December 1, 1860.

5. Additional information concerning Dr. Robertson's war record is found in a letter, Adjutant General E.S. Adams, War Department, to the Comptroller, Department of Pensions, State of Florida, Tallahassee, February 17, 1942. Photocopy in MSS Box 69, P.K. Yonge Library of Florida History.

6. Obituary for Mrs. Katherine Player Robertson in Tallahassee *Daily Democrat* July 11, 1937.

7. For dates of birth of the three children see Bannerman Papers, genealogical data, MSS in Box 73, P.K. Yonge Library of Florida History.

8. See note 1, supra.

9. Henry E. Palmer, M.D., "Physicians of Early Tallahassee and Vicinity," *Apalachee*, Tallahassee Historical Society, Tallahassee, 1944, p. 39.

10. Obituary for Mrs. Robertson, note 6, supra.

11. *The University Record*, University of Florida, Gainesville, 1977-78, Gainesville, 1977, p. 363.

Robertson Sr., William Fitzgerald, Leon County, 1814-1885

Dr. Robertson, one of Leon County's most esteemed citizens, was born in

Virginia on February 27, 1814.[1] Nothing is known of his parentage nor of his early education. He was, however, a student at the University of Virginia in 1837 and 1838 but there is no evidence that he was a graduate of that institution.[2] Instead there is indirect but nevertheless credible evidence that he received his medical degree from the University of New York.[3] Then, for reasons not clear, he elected to settle in Louisiana to enter the practice of his profession. It is possible that he practiced both in Homer (Claiborne Parish) and Houma (Terrebonne Parish).[4]

Dr. Robertson moved to Leon County in 1846,[5] purchased land in the vicinity of Centreville, and settled into the life of planter-physician. In both enterprises he enjoyed a fair degree of success. In 1860 his properties were valued at $57,000 while his slaves numbered 27.

In the spring of 1857 Dr. Robertson traveled to Charleston, S.C., probably to arrange for admission of his son, William Fitzgerald Jr., to the Medical College of the State of South Carolina. While there he attended the commencement exercises of the College at which he was awarded an honorary degree *ad eundem gradum*, Doctor of Medicine, presumably in recognition of his reputation as a practitioner, but certainly on the basis of his earlier degree from the University of New York.[6]

The earliest reference to Dr. Robertson's Leon County practice is found in the Tallahassee *Sentinel* of September 2, 1851, in which the public was notified that Drs. Robertson and Robert W. Fisher had formed a professional partnership in medicine and surgery and "could be found at their respective residences near Centreville when not attending patients." The notice concluded with information that the senior partner (Robertson) "has had much experience in the profession, having practiced for some years near New Orleans."[7]

The association of the two was dissolved a few years later when Dr. Robertson acquired a home in Tallahassee, where in 1858 he joined Dr. John Screven Bond, recently returned to Tallahassee after practicing for 10 years in Quincy. Their office was located "over the store lately occupied by Betton and Higgs."[8] This association was terminated after only a year, Dr. Robertson announcing on February 6, 1859, that he would continue his practice with both office and residence "at Dr. (J.H.) Randolph's old stand."[9] He remained there for the duration of the Civil War and for a few years thereafter, after reassuring his patients in January 1862 that he would continue to practice notwithstanding the uncertainties of the times.[10]

As was true of most planters the years of war and reconstruction were trying times; Dr. Robertson was no exception. His slaves were gone, his lands greatly depreciated in value, and the gracious style of living to which his family had become accustomed could no longer be maintained. But Dr. Robertson did not sulk in bitterness. Instead he appears to have faced the future with courage and hope, lending his talents to the efforts to rebuild the shattered institutions of his state. In the summer of 1866 the National Union Convention was held in Philadelphia in an effort to heal the schism between North and South. The proposals emanating from the gathering were firm with respect to maintaining the integrity of the U.S. Constitution, but somewhat conciliatory in other areas of concern. When the recommendations of the Convention were submitted to the states for action the various counties were asked to record their responses. In

Leon County Dr. Robertson was the chairman of the committee organized to respond to the question. The statement set forth by the committee was a solid endorsement of the Philadelphia proposal. Of course, it came to naught when radical reconstruction soon prevailed, but the stand of Dr. Robertson and his committee was noteworthy for its courage and wisdom.[11]

By the mid-1870s Dr. Robertson had moved once more, returning this time to his land north of Tallahassee.[12] The early 70s had seen the dominance of the radical reconstructionists with government in many parts of the South falling into the hands of carpetbaggers and other opportunists. Florida was no exception. A glimmer of hope appeared, however, as the two political parties met in June 1876 for the presidential nominating conventions. This hope increased as the party platforms were enunciated and nominees were announced. Such hopes gave rise to a series of Democratic Reform Clubs in several states. One of the first in Florida was organized at Holland Place, Iamonia District, on July 15 with Dr. Robertson as its president and Edward Van Brunt as secretary. It was known as the Drew and Hull Democratic Reform Club, George F. Drew and Noble A. Hull being the nominees for Governor and Lt. Governor respectively. The resolutions which followed were strongly worded, denouncing the rottenness and corruption which had characterized recent Florida administrations. The final resolution was simply an endorsement of the Tilden-Hendricks Democratic presidential ticket.[13]

This was probably Dr. Robertson's last major public service. A few years later he and Mrs. Robertson returned to Tallahassee to the home of their son, Dr. William Fitzgerald Robertson Jr. He died there on February 11, 1885, Mrs. Robertson having died a few months earlier. Both were buried in St. John's churchyard, Tallahassee, near the church of which they had been long-time members.

Life for the Robertsons had been sometimes difficult, but generally happiness and good fortune had prevailed. A few lines from his obituary seem adequately to summarize their lives together:[14]

> Early in his life he (Dr. Robertson) had married a beautiful and accomplished lady, who but recently preceded him to the grave. She was a lady of lovely character and manners and of high literary attainments, the Doctor being not only a learned and skillful physician, but also a man of general reading, with excellent character, temper and address. They were a congenial and happy pair. During the palmy days of Tallahassee their house was the resort of many fine literary people...They dispensed a truly elegant hospitality...But now, after the happiness, the misery, the prosperity and adversity of many years, they are gone....

Dr. Robertson was survived by his daughter, Amanda Harris, wife of Henry Rutledge Shine, and his son, Dr. William Fitzgerald Robertson Jr. In addition, there were several Shine grandchildren.

1. Obituary notice, Tallahassee *Weekly Floridian*, February 19, 1885. Some uncertainty exists regarding the place of Dr. Robertson's birth in that the University of Virginia records give his birthplace as Courtland, Alabama. The fact that Courtland is located near the Tennessee border and that Mrs. Robertson was a native of that state seems to support the University of Virginia document. The obituary notice and census schedules, however, indicate that he was born in Virginia.

2. Again the evidence is in conflict. Virginia records indicate only that he was a student in the sessions of 1837 and 1838. Other evidence shows that he was a graduate of the University of New York Medical College. See Charleston (S.C.) *Daily Courier*, March 20, 1857, for a list of degrees awarded at the recent commencement of the Medical College of the State of South Carolina.

3. The University of New York Medical College was doubtless the institution which existed under that name from 1841 till 1898 when it merged with Belleview Hospital Medical College to become the University and Belleview Hospital Medical College.

4. The obituary states only that he went to Louisiana to begin practice. There again is conflicting evidence. Civil War records state that his son, William F., Jr., was born in Terrebonne Parish, Louisiana, the seat of which is Houma, while another item in his war record indicates his birthplace as Claiborne Parish, whose seat is Homer. One can only state with assurance that he practiced in Louisiana.

5. See note 5, supra.

6. Charleston (S.C.) *Daily Courier*, May 20, 1857.

7. This would support the claim that he practiced in Houma, Terrebonne Parish.

8. Tallahassee *Sentinel*, March 2, 1858.

9. Ibid., December 25, 1860. 1st printed February 6, 1859, not extant.

10. Tallahassee *Florida Sentinel*, January 14, 1862.

11. Tallahassee *Tri-Weekly Sentinel*, September 11, 1866.

12. Centreville lost its post office in October 1874 and henceforth, until February 1877, was served by the Iamonia post office. Therefore some communications emanating from the Centreville community would have borne the Iamonia postmark.

13. Tallahassee *Weekly Floridian*, August 8, 1876.

14. Ibid., February 26, 1885.

Robinson, Henry, Marianna and Jacksonville, 1838-1924

The remarkable career of Dr. Robinson, who spent the greater part of his professional career in Jacksonville, had an unusual beginning. Born in central Europe and adopted at the age of two by an uncle who brought him to America and settled in Laurens County, South Carolina, he spent his childhood and early youth on a farm outside the town of Laurens. The date of his birth is said to have been March 6, 1838.[1] In 1859 he matriculated at the University of Pennsylvania School of Medicine from which he was graduated on March 14, 1861. Immediately thereafter he returned to Laurens and in the following August enlisted in a local unit of South Carolina Volunteers known as the James Battalion. In a fairly short time he was commissioned Assistant Surgeon in the Army of the Confederacy with the military rank of captain.

Dr. Robinson was ordered by General P.T.G. Beauregard to report to Marianna, Florida, in 1863 and establish a Confederate Hospital, a much needed facility at this stage of the war. Having accomplished this mission he returned to service in the field and participated in several of the battles waged on Florida soil. At the conclusion of the struggle he was paroled in Quincy after taking the oath of allegiance to the United States.

Dr. Robinson married Margaret Amelia Dickson of Marianna on December 14, 1865, having already begun his medical practice in the town. Three years later, for reasons quite unknown, he moved to Jacksonville where he was to spend the balance of his life, first as a medical practitioner, but later as the proprietor of a thriving wholesale and retail drug business on Bay Street, an enterprise which brought him a good income and which he relinquished only late in life.[2]

As a public figure in Jacksonville and Duval County Dr. Robinson enjoyed a high degree of success and acclaim. During the era of reconstruction he was an activist in the struggle to rid the state of "carpetbag" rule and restore it to Democratic control. His activities projected him into the center of the local political scene and resulted in his election to the office of mayor of Jacksonville.[3] Even earlier he had been elected to the Duval County Commission, of which he was chairman in 1886-87. For 18 years he was president of the

Commercial Bank of Jacksonville and upon retirement from that position he was accorded life membership in the Florida Bankers Association. In a somewhat different type of enterprise Dr. Robinson was largely responsible for building the Jacksonville Home for Confederate Soldiers and Sailors of which he was president for several years. He also provided significant assistance in the struggle against the deadly yellow fever epidemic which devastated the town in 1888.

In addition to these activities Dr. Robinson served the local Masonic Order as treasurer for several years. In 1913 he was elected treasurer of the Florida Historical Society, another prominent local man, George C.M. Chapin, having become president at the same time.[4] His interest in maintaining the integrity of druggists and their profession throughout the state led him to organize the Florida Pharmaceutical Society, of which he became the first president. As for his interest in the medical profession, he became a member of the Florida Medical Association at its second annual meeting held in Jacksonville in February 1875. He attended the meeting at the Jacksonville Yacht Club in April 1878 at which he was appointed to the Committee on Publications. He did not attend the meeting in Jacksonville the following year, however, but the treasurer's report indicated that he paid his dues for the three previous years, which were overdue. Later in the year he resigned from the Association. This may possibly be explained by the fact that he was becoming less active in medicine and more active in pharmacy. He obviously left in good standing.[5]

Mrs. Robinson died on September 2, 1911. The doctor lived on until November 6, 1924, dying at his home at 328 Ocean Street where his funeral services were held. He was survived by four daughters, Mrs. George W. Wilson, Mrs. A.W. Fritot and Mrs. W.W. Frazier, all of Jacksonville, and Mrs. A.H. March of Pittsburgh, Pennsylvania, and several grandchildren. Dr. Robinson was buried in Jacksonville's Evergreen Cemetery.

1. The principal sources of biographical detail on Dr. Robinson were his obituary which appeared in the Jacksonville *Florida Times-Union*, November 10, 1924, and a brief sketch in Webster Merritt's, *A Century of Medicine in Jacksonville and Duval County*, Gainesville, 1949, pp. 128-129. A puzzling conflict of statement should be noted in that Merritt cites Dr. Robinson's place of birth as "Central Europe," while the *Times-Union* states that he was born in Laurens District, South Carolina. Since Merritt cited the *Times-Union* obituary in his sketch he was aware of the conflict of evidence. He also acknowledged having received biographical information from one of Dr. Robinson's daughters which apparently convinced him that the European birthplace was correct. It should be added that census data are also in conflict. The 1870 Duval County Census (p. 475) gives Dr. Robinson's birthplace as South Carolina as does the Census of 1880 (p. 566). It adds gratuitously that both of Dr. Robinson's parents were born in Germany. Therefore it is assumed that Dr. Robinson was German-born.

2. It should be noted that in both censuses, 1870 and 1880, Dr. Robinson was designated "Druggist" not "Physician."

3. Several of Dr. Robinson's numerous achievements, listed in his obituary notice, have been omitted.

4. For Dr. Robinson's association with the Florida Historical Society, see Watt Marchmann, "The Florida Historical Society, 1856-61, 1879, 1902-1940," *Florida Historical Quarterly*, XIX, No. 1, July 1840, pp. 17, 25, 27.

5. Proceedings of the *Florida Medical Association*, Sessions of 1875, p. 9; 1878, Erratum Sheet and p. 17, and of 1879, p. 26.

Robinson, James S., Leon and Calhoun Counties, 1812-1842

The life span of Dr. Robinson was tragically brief; in fact, it may even be said to have begun in tragedy. His father, English-born James Robinson, had become a seaman around the turn of the 19th century and on the eve of the conflict with England in 1812 had risen to the rank of ship's captain. In this capacity he went to Liverpool in 1811 and met and married Maria Clement. With the outbreak of war the following year he was conscripted into naval duty, leaving his pregnant wife to be cared for by others. A few weeks after the birth of her baby she had word that her husband would be in Philadelphia at a certain time and if she were able to come to Philadelphia with the baby he would be able to see them there. She went but arrived too late. Her husband's ship was just leaving the harbor. Shortly thereafter he was killed in one of the early engagements of the war and his widow and little son were left to fend for themselves.

Mrs. Robinson knew that her husband had relatives living in Halifax County, North Carolina. She was able to find a refuge with them although they had become somewhat impoverished by the privation of war. It happened that two wealthy and socially prominent families owned plantations nearby. These were the Bradfords and the Branches. On one of his visits from Raleigh to his plantation near Enfield, John Branch, governor of North Carolina,[2] accompanied by Mrs. Branch, met Mrs. Robinson and her small son. They were searching for a suitable governess for their children and impressed by the charm and cultivation of Mrs. Robinson they engaged her services. She was thus able to provide her son with the best educational opportunities.

In the fall of 1832 young James S. Robinson entered the Medical School of the University of Pennsylvania and two years later he was graduated M.D.[3] At about this time the Branch and Bradford families decided to move to Florida. Purchasing large tracts of inexpensive land in Leon County north of Tallahassee, they proceeded to clear the acreage and settle down to planter life. Accompanying the Branch family was Mrs. Robinson. In 1834 Branch became governor of Florida, an office he was to hold until statehood was achieved in 1845. In the same year Dr. Robinson joined his mother in Tallahassee where they became householders and he began medical practice. Having been, in a sense, sponsored by Governor and Mrs. Branch, the Robinsons were cordially received by Tallahassee society and young Dr. Robinson became a most eligible bachelor. On March 20, 1838, he married Mary H. DuVal, daughter of former governor William P. DuVal.[4]

Probably shortly after their marriage the Robinsons settled in St. Joseph, then a thriving commercial town. In due time the couple was blessed by the birth of a daughter, Ellen Frances, who was christened in St. John's Episcopal Church, Tallahassee, on July 12, 1840.[5] Their happiness, however, was of brief duration. In the summer of 1841 St. Joseph was visited by one of the deadliest yellow fever epidemics ever to strike a Florida town. Among its first victims was Mrs. Robinson's mother, Mrs. Nancy DuVal, who died on July 14.[6] The total death toll was exceedingly high and "Old St. Joe" was virtually finished.

The Robinsons returned to Tallahassee and on August 27, 1841, the following professional card appeared: "Having associated themselves in the practice of medicine, Drs. J.S. Robinson and J.H. Pope offer their professional services to the people of Tallahassee and adjacent country. Office at their drug store."[7] A few weeks later they announced that they had bought the drug business formerly belonging to Dr. R.L. Baker.[8]

This partnership was soon to be dissolved, however. Dr. Robinson died suddenly on August 22, 1842, at the age of 30.[9] On that day the medical faculty of Tallahassee met to pay their respects to their departed colleague and to frame their expressions of grief and sympathy. One of their resolutions included the following: "...we take this occasion to express our admiration of his character as a highly talented man, a learned and skillful physician, and a most amiable and high-minded gentleman."

With the loss of her son the elder Mrs. Robinson found herself in a situation similar to that which she had faced 30 years earlier.[10] This time she joined the household of Dr. Edward Bradford at Pine Hill plantation as governess for his daughters, having served similarly for their mother when she was a daughter in the Branch household. Mrs. Robinson, called Auntie Robinson by the Bradford daughters, was reputed to have been a strict disciplinarian.[11]

1. Some of the information used in this sketch was gleaned from Susan Bradford Eppes, *Through Some Eventful Years*, Macon, 1926, pp. 24-26, et passim. Although many of Mrs. Eppes' statements may be open to question, her recollections of the Robinson family appear to be credible. As the governess of Mrs. Eppes, Mrs. Robinson doubtless related to her many of her memories of earlier years.

2. Branch was governor of North Carolina from 1817 to 1820. He was later U.S. senator from that state, then Secretary of the Navy under Andrew Jackson, and for one term a congressman from North Carolina (1831-1833).

3. Archives, University of Pennsylvania, List of Graduates.

4. Parochial Records, St. John's Episcopal Church, Tallahassee. Carbon copy of transcription, p. 47.

5. Ibid., p. 14.

6. Tallahassee *Florida Sentinel*, August 20, 1841.

7. Some confusion exists as to when the Robinsons returned to Tallahassee. Dr. Robinson announced on June 4, 1841, that he "has not relinquished the practice of medicine, but may be found in the Senate Chamber of the New Capitol, ready to attend to all professional business." Ibid., June 4, 1841. He had served as Chief Clerk of the Legislative Council, session of 1838. For the next four sessions, 1839, 1840, 1841 and 1842, he was Secretary to the Senate. He had apparently left his wife and young daughter in St. Joseph with Mrs. DuVal while he went about his business in Tallahassee. But almost certainly after the yellow fever disaster in St. Joseph and the death of his mother-in-law he brought his family back to Tallahassee, hence the Robinson-Pope card of August 27 announcing their partnership.

7. Ibid., August 27, 1841.

8. Ibid., August 13, 1841.

9. Ibid., August 26, 1842.

10. No attempt has been made to discover the fate of Dr. Robinson's widow and daughter. Since she was the daughter of former Governor DuVal it appears likely that they were cared for by the DuVal family. Governor DuVal lived on until 1854.

11. One additional problem remains: the place of death and burial of Dr. Robinson, Mrs. Eppes states that he died in St. Joseph and was buried there. No gravestone for him has survived, however. The Tallahassee papers made no mention of place of death or burial.

Robinson, William, Gadsden County, 1820

Dr. Robinson, a native of Virginia, probably migrated to Florida in the early 1850s, establishing practice in Quincy but later removing to Chattahoochee. Although his identity is not well established, he is thought to have been the William Robinson who, in April 1854, married Mary Ann Barber.[1] He does not, however, appear in the Gadsden County Census of 1860. Ten years later he was a resident of Chattahoochee, owning property valued at $8,500.[2] In his household were his wife, Mary, aged 50, and daughter, Cornelia, aged 11. Another resident was Colonel Martin Malachi, the Irish-born superintendent of the State Penitentiary.[3] Nothing further is known of this physician.[4]

1. Gadsden County, Florida, marriage records.

2. U.S. Census, 1870, Gadsden County, Florida, p. 781, item 1147.

3. The old Arsenal, established during the Second Seminole War, was later converted into a penitentiary.

4. Dr. William Robinson mentioned in David A. Avant's revised edition of J. Randall Stanley, History of Gadsden County, Tallahassee, Florida, 1985, p. 68, as having been confirmed and admitted into St. Paul's Episcopal Church, Quincy, may have been the Dr. Robinson here under consideration.

Rogers, Lucious D., Hillsborough County, 1820

Dr. Rogers was born in South Carolina in 1820.[1] Nothing is known of his parentage, childhood and early education. In 1841 he matriculated at the Medical College of Georgia, Augusta, from which he received his degree in medicine in March 1843.[2] Soon thereafter he moved to Florida, settling in Tampa, probably in the vicinity of Ft. Brooke, where he launched his professional practice. Aware of the need for a drug store in the area, he proceeded to established one and appears to have been successful both as druggist and physician. In 1849 the Jacksonville *News* (Tampa had no newspaper at the time) published the following notice:

> Dr. L.D. Rogers has in stock in his Tampa Drug Store a supply of patent medicines and other medical supplies, for example, shoulder braces, supporters, etc.

In addition to his professional activity Dr. Rogers became actively involved in the politics of Hillsborough County. In May 1850 he was present at a public meeting in Tampa, assembled to discuss plans for participating in the upcoming Nashville Convention, scheduled to consider a proper response to the growing number of Northern diatribes against slavery. Dr. Rogers was the recording secretary. Although no report of transactions has survived, the participants probably expressed strong support for the continuation of Negro slavery, a stand which was to be presented at the Nashville meeting.[3]

During the early years following his move to Tampa Dr. Rogers had lodging and board at a rooming house managed by Mrs. Elizabeth Matair, a widow and native of Georgia. Among the other residents was Dr. Robert J. Kendrick.[4]

1. This date is a deduction from the Census of 1850, Hillsborough County, Florida, which gives his age as 30.
2. Phinizy Spalding, A *History of the Medical College of Georgia*, Athens, University of Georgia Press, 1987.
3. Jacksonville *Florida Republican*, May 9, 1850.
4. U.S. Census, 1850, Hillsborough County, p. 251, item 30. Dr. Rogers is presumed to have returned to South Carolina about 1860. His name does not appear in the Florida Census of that year.

Rogers, William J.C., Ocala, 1850

Dr. Rogers, native of Tennessee, had practiced medicine in Alabama for a few years before moving to Ocala in 1850 at the age of 32. His wife, Emma, was a native of North Carolina while his three children were born in Alabama.[1] He first offered his services to the people of Ocala and Marion County on June 4, 1851.[2] Shortly after arriving he was appointed postmaster of the town, possibly an inducement to obtain his services.

In addition to medical practice which he pursued with apparent success, Dr. Rogers was active in the public affairs of the town and county. He assisted in organization of the Ocala Academy, the first school of its kind in the area.[3] He gave financial support and served on its board of trustees. In August 1852 he was a nominee for the state Senate, although John Scott was the ultimate nominee of the County Convention.[4] As the need for a railroad in Marion County became more critical in the 1850s, Dr. Rogers joined planters and businessmen in an effort to promote such an enterprise which, it was assumed, would connect Ocala with existing transportational facilities on both Florida coasts.[5]

Dr. Rogers established his office on Main Street in Ocala, while his residence was located just east of the Methodist Church. He formed a partnership with a Dr. Peck in 1854 but little is known of the arrangement beyond the fact that their office was located "west of Bullock's Hotel."[6] Since so few Ocala newspapers of the mid-1850s have survived, it is impossible to trace the year-to-year activities of Dr. Rogers from 1854 to 1857.

As the Third Seminole War, which had begun on December 20, 1855, dragged on into 1857, state and federal authorities finally decided to intensify their efforts toward conclusion of the conflict. In August 1857 Samuel St. George Rogers, brother of Dr. Rogers, was authorized to assemble a regiment of cavalrymen for service on the Caloosahatchee River and among the enlistees was Dr. Rogers who was mustered in along with the main cadre at Ocala on August 10. The term of enlistment was six months; Dr. Rogers' rank was assistant surgeon. He was present for duty in Ft. Myers in early September and a month later, as surgeon, he was in charge of the makeshift hospital at Ft. Deynaud, a few miles upriver from Ft. Myers. When the term of enlistment expired in February 1858, he was mustered out to return to Ocala.[7]

No sooner was Dr. Rogers back in Ocala than he received an order from Governor Perry that he organize another mounted volunteer regiment to be sent to the war zone. The following notice appeared in the Ocala paper:[8]

> Who'll enlist? Dr. W.J.C. Rogers has received an order from the Governor to raise a Company of Mounted Volunteers to serve in the Seminole War. His Company is to be mustered into service at Ocala, which will be quite an inducement to those who wish to enlist in this vicinity.

Before the order could be complied with, however, the beleaguered Indians gave up the hopeless resistance and additional troops were not required.

Subsequent to this notice Dr. Rogers disappeared from the Marion County scene. In 1858 he would have been 38 years of age. It is conjectural to suggest that he returned to his native Tennessee.

1. U.S. Census, 1850, Marion County, Florida, p. 220. The children with their respective ages are: William R., six; Sarah, three; Samuel, one.
2. Ocala *Conservator*, October 22, 1851; 1st printing, June 4, 1851.
3. Ibid., February 11, 1852. The Ocala Academy is considered to have been the lineal ancestor of the present University of Florida.
4. Jacksonville *Florida Republican*, August 12, 1852.
5. Ibid., July 21, 1853; Ocala *Florida Mirror*, August 19, 1853.
6. This Dr. Peck, whose Christian name is not given, was very probably John E. Peck, who spent most of his professional life in St. Augustine. Ocala *Southern Sun*, April 8, 1854.
7. NA, Records, Adj. Gen Office, Record Group 94, Service Records. Volunteer Soldiers, Florida Indian Wars, 1835-1858. M 1086, Roll 51.
8. Ocala *Florida Home Companion*, February 23, 1858. Although scattered remnants of the Seminole tribe took refuge in the Florida Everglades, the resistance was virtually ended with the surrender of their Chief, Billy Bowlegs, in early March.

Roland, William A., Hamilton County, 1832

Although Dr. Roland (Rowland) is designated "physician" in the Census of 1870,[1] there is no evidence that he was more than a part-time practitioner of medicine, while it appears that in the latter part of his life he abandoned medical practice completely. About 1866 he moved from his native Georgia[2] with his wife, Sallie, and young son, Robert, and settled in the Bellville community of Hamilton County. Some 10 years later he is shown to have been a dry goods merchant, very probably in the town of Bellville.[3] By this date (1880) the Roland household included Mrs. Roland's parents, William and Martha Hudson, aged 64 and 61, respectively. Among the black residents living on the Roland land were Anderson Rowland (sic), his wife, Jennett, and their four children, which probably indicates that they had earlier been slaves owned by the Roland family. Nothing further is known of Dr. Roland.

1. U.S. Census, 1870, Hamilton County, Florida, p. 5.
2. Evidence points to Camden County, Georgia, as the place of Dr. Roland's birth. At least two families named Roland are listed in the 1850 census of Camden County. In one instance, that of Needham Roland, the eldest son was Robert, the name being also that of Dr. Roland's eldest child. See U.S. Census, 1850, Camden County, Georgia, item 308.
3. U.S. Census, 1880, Hamilton County, Florida, p. 284.

Royall, E.M., Marion County, 1850

Dr. Royall appears to have been a brief sojourner in Florida about 1852. Of his Florida practice it is only known that he first offered his services to the citizens of Marion County on February 4, 1852, stating that he had established his residence "seven miles south of Ocala."[1] He is not listed in the Florida censuses of 1850 and 1860.

1. Ocala *Conservator*, issues of March 24 and June 23, 1852.

Russell, James, St. Lucie County, 1860

Dr. Russell's tour or duty in Florida was brief. A native of New York State, probably Syracuse, he was mustered into the United State Army with the rank of assistant surgeon on June 22, 1839.[1] He was in St. Lucie County in 1860 at a critical time. The Indians were engaged in a losing effort to protect their hunting and fishing rights from the encroaching whites. The Census of 1850 lists only 82 white persons in the entire County. Of this number 68 were army personnel.

Dr. Russell did not long continue to practice in such an unrewarding situation. Having fulfilled his commitment to the Army, he resigned his commission, effective as of March 1, 1853, and returned to his home in upstate New York.[2]

1. Francis B. Heitman, *Historical Register and Directory of the United States Army*, Washington, 1903, p. 853.
2. *Medical Department of the United States Army*, Harvey E. Brown, comp., Washington, 1872, p. 293.

Russell, James S., Jefferson County, 1815-1870

Dr. Russell, far better known for political activities than medical practice, was a native of Georgia.[1] He moved to Florida with his wife, Theresa, and the four eldest of his eight children in the mid-1840s, settling in the Waukeenah community some 12 miles south of Monticello.[2] There he purchased a small plantation which he appears to have operated with the help of his two older sons, Benjamin and William, and eight slaves. As was true of many Southern physicians in the antebellum period he was both farmer and medical practitioner.[3]

Dr. Russell's presence was being felt in political circles of the county by 1850.

In July he addressed a public meeting at Bunker Hill northwest of Monticello assembled to consider the recently-adopted Compromise of 1850 and to discuss the southern reaction as expressed at the Nashville Convention of the previous June.[4] On September 7, he was present at a Monticello meeting called for similar purposes.[5] In June 1854 he was prominently involved in a meeting of Jefferson County Democrats, serving as a member of the Resolutions Committee.[6] Dr. Russell was sufficiently known and respected by 1859 to become one of the nominees for a seat in the state House of Representatives. He won rather handily[7] and was returned in 1861. He was elected to the state Senate for the session of 1862 and reelected for the sessions of 1863 and 1864.[8] A casual perusal of the Journals of the House and Senate indicates that he was a vocal and influential member. It was a time when the problems and issues confronting the legislative body were never more critical and perplexing.

With his legislative service finished and the Civil War concluded, Dr. Russell returned to the privacy of his Waukeenah farm, devoting, it is thought, more of his time than ever to the practice of medicine. The Census of 1870 shows him to have been in much-reduced circumstances, his properties being valued at a mere $500. It also lists an additional child, a daughter named Jessie, born in 1863. Since the doctor is not listed in the Census of 1880, it is assumed that he had died prior to that date. Cemetery surveys of the county did not disclose a grave marker for him. His widow, Theresa, and daughter, Jessie, are included in the 1880 Census, however.[9]

1. U.S. Census, 1850, Jefferson County, Florida, p. 47.
2. The Russell children, as listed in the Census of 1860, were Benjamin, aged 22; William and Susan, twins, aged 18; Elizabeth, aged 14; Martha, aged 11; Lucy, aged nine; Mary, aged seven; and Aurelia, aged three. Ibid. 1870, Jefferson County, Florida, p. 937.
3. In 1860 the Russell property was valued at about $13,000.
4. Tallahassee *Floridian and Journal*, August 10, 1850.
5. Ibid., September 21, 1850.
6. Ibid., June 24, 1854.
7. Allen Morris, *The People of Lawmaking in Florida*, Tallahassee, 1977, no pagination. There were five candidates for the three seats assigned to Jefferson County. Dr. Russell finished in third place, B.W. Bellamy and D.B. Bird in first and second places respectively.
8. Morris, *People of Lawmaking*.
9. U.S. Census, 1880, Jefferson County, Florida, p. 144.

Russell, Joseph Pynchon, U.S. Army, 1849

Dr. Russell was born in Vermont during the last decade of the 18th century. As a young man he enlisted as surgeon's mate in the Fourth Infantry Division, United States Army, his date of enlistment having been May 24, 1814. The following year on May 17 he was transferred to the Fifth Infantry. Three years later he was promoted to post surgeon and on January 28, 1820, to the rank of surgeon. In August 1836, with establishment of a General Hospital in St. Augustine, Dr. Russell was assigned to that post as the physician in charge.

With the outbreak of the Mexican War he was among the medical officers ordered to Texas in 1845, serving there for a brief period. At about this time his health began to decline and he died at Ft. Columbus, New York, in September 1849. He was survived by his wife and several children. It is a matter of record that his death left his wife and children impoverished, although he had served in the U.S. Army for more than 35 years. A number of his Army colleagues, upon learning of the plight of the family, collected more than $4,000 for their relief.

1. Data are found in Francis B. Heitman, *Historical Register and Directory of the United States Army*, Washington, 1903, p. 853.

Rutherford, Walter, Santa Rosa County, 1825-1892

Very little is presently known about the career of Dr. Rutherford. A native of Scotland, he had arrived in the United States prior to the Civil War. As a resident of the North, he had enlisted for service in the Union Army and only in the latter part of the century did he move to Florida and settle in Santa Rosa County. In the mid-80s he was living in the vicinity of what is today Gulf Breeze. The Census of 1885 lists him at age 55, physician, sharing his home with his son, David, and daughter, Molly, both natives of Alabama.[1] His gravestone in the Rutherford Cemetery bears this inscription in addition to his name: "Vet. Union Army in Civil War. 1825-1892."

1. Florida Special Census, 1885, Santa Rosa County, p. 106.
2. See *Santa Rosa Cemeteries*, Richard Earl Jernigan, comp. and ed., Pensacola: The West Florida Genealogical Society, 1987, p. 614, for the exact location of the Rutherford Cemetery.

Sabal, Emil T., Jacksonville, 1835-1907

Among the more prominent physicians who practiced in Jacksonville in the latter half of the 19th century, Emil Talvande Sabal was one of the most admired and most successful. The son of Cuban-born parents, Adolph and Cephisa Sabal,[1] who had immigrated to Augusta, Georgia, he enjoyed the advantage of growing up in a family of above average means who provided their sons with the advantage of good education. Two sons became successful physicians. After completing his basic education in Augusta schools, Dr. Sabal matriculated at the Long Island Medical College, Brooklyn, New York, from which he was graduated as Doctor of Medicine.

Dr. Sabal began practice in Jacksonville in 1859. He had scarcely established his professional reputation when the war began in 1861. He volunteered for Confederate service in July and was assigned to Company K, 2nd Florida Infantry, a unit known as the Davis Guards. He went with the company to Virginia and soon after arriving there was placed on duty at the Confederate Hospital in Richmond,[2] where he remained for the duration of the conflict. Upon his release he returned to Jacksonville where he practiced medicine until his death on October 11, 1907, at age 72.[3]

Throughout his career Dr. Sabal obviously exhibited concern for the quality of medical practice among members of the profession. Though not present at the organizational meeting of the Florida Medical Association, held in the Jacksonville office of Dr. Abel S. Baldwin on January 14, 1874, he was among those nominated and elected to charter membership.[4] He was elected President for 1884, but at the meeting that year at the Florida Yacht Club, Jacksonville, he was too ill to attend. He did , however, sign the official report of the meeting with the signature, "E.T. Sabal, M.D., Pres." Although he did not attend any meetings, he continued to pay his annual dues almost to the time of his death.[5]

Although Dr. Sabal married fairly soon after completing medical school, no information about his wife has been found. To the marriage was born one daughter, Clara, who survived him. Jacksonville City Directories of the late 19th century list him as a resident of 45 West Monroe Street in 1880, the other resident of the house being his mother, Mrs. Adolphus A. Sabal. In 1907, the year of his death, he was living with his daughter, Clara, at 29 West Monroe where he died. He was buried in Jacksonville's St. Joseph Cemetery.[6]

1. Some of the data included in this sketch is derived from Webster Merritt, M.D., *A Century of Medicine in Jacksonville and Duval County*, Gainesville, University of Florida Press, 1949, pp. 59-61.
2. Civil War Records, CSA, Co. K, 2nd Florida Infantry Regiment.
3. Obituary, Ocala *Evening Star*, October 12, 1907.
4. *Proceedings, Florida Medical Association*, 1874-75.
5. Ibid., Annual Issues, 1876-1907.
6. *Grave Markers of Duval County*, 1808-1916, Lucy Ames Edwards, comp., 1955.

Sample, Caleb D., Assistant Surgeon, Eleventh Florida Infantry, 1863

Perhaps Dr. Sample should not be included in a register of 19th century Florida physicians. He was, however, mustered into the Tenth Florida Infantry Regiment in September 1863 at Thunderbolt, St. Simon's Island, Georgia, remaining there for two months before being transferred to Savannah where he spent November and December 1863. The next year he was in Petersburg, Virginia.

His army rank from the beginning of his service appears to have been that of captain. Early in 1865 he was taken prisoner by Union troops, spending the last months of the War in prison. He was paroled on April 9, 1865, at Appamattox, Virginia. There is no evidence that he returned to practice in Florida after the War.

1. Knowledge of Dr. Sample is derived entirely from his military record, Field and Staff Muster Rolls, Tenth and Eleventh Infantry Regiments.

Sams, Francis W., St. Joseph, Apalachicola and Palatka, 1819-1855

Dr. Sams, a native of Georgetown, South Carolina, was graduated from the Medical College of the State of South Carolina, Charleston, on March 13, 1839.[1] He began practice in April 1840 in St. Joseph. Unmarried, he took up residence at Mansion House.[2] In September 1840 he moved to the neighboring town of Apalachicola, leasing the office previously occupied by Dr. T.H. Thompson, recently deceased.[3] In the following December he joined Dr. D.J. Harrison in a professional partnership, the two occupying an office at the corner of Centre and Market Streets.[4]

It is not known how long Dr. Sams continued to practice in Apalachicola; it is known, however, that at some date in 1850 he moved to Palatka. The Putnam County census of that year lists him as physician, aged 34, sharing his abode with his wife, Cornelia, and their four-year-old son, Francis W. Sams Jr.[5]

Dr. Sams' promising career was tragically terminated by sudden death on July 15, 1855, at age 39. He was survived by his wife and three small children. The public notice of his death stated simply that "He died as he had lived, an honest man...with only a few surpassing him professionally."[6]

1. Charleston *Courier*, March 21, 1839. The list of graduates of the College that year included two other men who were later to practice in Florida, Jacob Cohen and John H. Verdier. The list gives Dr. Sams' address as Florida.
2. St. Joseph *Times*, April 7, 1840.
3. Ibid., July 21, 1840. See also the Apalachicola *Commercial Advertiser*, September 12, 1840. Dr. Thompson had died on August 1.
4. Apalachicola *Commercial Advertiser*, December 26, 1840.
5. U.S. Census, 1850, Putnam County, Florida, p. 387.
6. Jacksonville *Florida News*, July 28, 1855. See also the Jacksonville *Florida Republican*, August 2, 1855. Subsequent to her husband's death Mrs. Sams went to live in Jacksonville, where in 1858, tragedy again struck when her six-year-old son, Charles, was drowned in the St. Johns River on December 17. See Tampa *Florida Peninsular*, December 25, 1858, and the Jacksonville *Republican*, December 18, 1858.

Sanders, R.A., Jackson County, 1860

An entry in the Jackson County Census of 1860 identifies Dr. Sanders as a resident and practitioner in Marianna. He was a native of North Carolina, aged 35, owning real property valued at $15,000. Considering the economy of the times he would have been considered "well-off." His wife, Ann, was the daughter of Dr. Simmons J. Baker of Greenwood, a village some 10 miles north of Marianna. Professor Shofner has determined that he arrived in Marianna in 1857.[1] Also in the Sanders household was John L. Finlayson, a medical student, for whom Dr. Sanders was doubtless preceptor.[2] Dr. Charles A. Hentz, who appears to have known Dr. Sanders personally, did not hold him in high esteem. He described him as "...a rough, uncouth man, full of whisky, priding himself on a brusque, unpolished bearing; as he had married Miss Ann Baker, a wealthy young lady of Greenwood, he had a strong influence in his favor."[3]

Since Dr. Sanders is missing from later censuses as well as the Confederate military records for Florida, it is assumed that he had left the state by the beginning of the Civil War.

1. Jerrell H. Shofner, *Jackson County, Florida—A History*, Marianna, Jackson County Heritage Association, 1985, p. 185.

2. U.S. Census, 1860, Jackson County, Florida, p. 7.

3. Charles A. Hentz, "Autobiography," Southern Historical Collection, University of North Carolina, Chapel Hill. Dr. Hentz, a somewhat egotistical sort of fellow, did not hesitate to criticize his professional associates.

Sargent, G., Pensacola, 1822

Dr. Sargent entered the practice of medicine in Pensacola about the first of June 1822 with an office "one door east of G.W. Barkley's store on the public Green."[1] He continued practice at least until the outbreak of the severe yellow fever epidemic in late August that year. His professional card which first appeared on June 8, continued to be published until suspension of the newspaper on August 17. Beyond that date nothing is known of him.[2]

Of medical interest is the fact that the Pensacola newspaper for several weeks carried Dr. Sargent's quarter-column endorsement of Sedlitz Powders, a popular panacea of the times "prepared and sold at the Soda Fountain on the public Green."[3]

1. Pensacola *Floridian* June 8, 1822.

2. The *Floridian* ceased operation with the issue of August 17, 1822, due to the outbreak of fever and resumed publication on March 8, 1823. Since it was the only newspaper published in West Florida, and one of only two published in Florida in 1822, the other being the St. Augustine *East Florida Herald*, of which no issues for 1822 are extant, we are deprived of information on the critical latter months of 1822 in Pensacola. In its first issue of 1823, on March 8, the *Floridian* carried numerous notices of administration of estates of yellow fever victims, including three physicians. Dr. Sargent's name does not appear. This invites conjecture that if he had indeed survived the fever he had elected to leave Florida forever.

3. Ibid., June 8, 1822, and subsequent issues.

Satterlee, Richard Smith, Tampa Bay, 1880

Dr. Satterlee, one of the most eminent surgeons to serve in the Army of the United States in the 19th century, was a native of New York State. No information regarding his youth and professional training has been located. On February 25, 1822, he was commissioned Assistant Surgeon in the Army of the United States, a rank which he held until July 13, 1832, when he achieved the rank of Major Surgeon.

With the Second Seminole War well under way, Dr. Satterlee was assigned to duty in Florida as Surgeon and Medical Director for the area south of the Withlacoochee River. He was there when the Battle of Okeechobee occurred. On January 5, 1838, while on duty at Ft. Brooke, Tampa Bay, he submitted a report to the Surgeon General: "Lacking a hospital in which to treat the wounded, I deemed it proper to bring them immediately to this place (Tampa). I arrived with them last evening, and have now the satisfaction to say they are in comfortable quarters." Dr. Satterlee continued with an explanation of how he improvised litters by attaching blankets and "the raw hides of cattle we found along the way." He continued: "the medical officers with me (Adam Neill McLaren and Josiah Simpson) as well as myself were fully occupied night and day with the wounded...The wounded including volunteers amounted to one hundred and eleven. These have been placed in a hospital under the care of surgeons."

In due time Dr. Satterlee's skill and diligence were rewarded with promotion to the rank of Lieutenant Colonel and Chief Medical Officer (July 10, 1866). He eventually achieved the rank of Brigadier General. His death occurred on August 10, 1880.[1]

1. Francis B. Heitman, *Historical Register and Directory of the United States Army*, Washington, 1903.

Saunders, John Bartlet, Apalachicola, 1838

Dr. Saunders practiced for a brief time in Apalachicola about 1838. His professional announcement first published in the Apalachicola *Gazette* of October 26, 1837, read as follows:

Dr. J.B. Saunders has settled in Apalachicola. He may be found at E. Wood's Store, unless out on professional business. Dr. Saunders is the oldest practicing physician in Middle Florida.

No further information on Dr. Saunders has been discovered.[1]

1. The records of the Medical College of Transylvania University, Lexington, Kentucky, indicate that a John Bartlet Saunders was a matriculant in the class of 1828-29. He was probably the Dr. Saunders mentioned herein.

Saxon, Benjamin W., Hernando County, 1861

Dr. Saxon, a native of Newberry District, South Carolina, is thought to have arrived in Florida about 1858-59, settling in Hernando County, probably in the village of Brooksville.[1] His educational background and professional skills were quickly recognized and appreciated in what was at that time a sparsely settled and somewhat backward area of the state. The threat of abolition of slavery was already a burning national issue whose repercussions were felt in Hernando County. Florida's political leaders, many of whom were slaveholders, called for a meeting in Tallahassee to come into session on January 3, 1861, to organize resistance against the threat of abolition. Dr. Saxon attended as Hernando's representative in what was immediately known as the Secession Convention. When the question of Florida's secession from the Union came up for vote on January 10, Dr. Saxon was among the 62 who favored taking Florida out of the Union. Only seven were opposed.

Even before Dr. Saxon left Brooksville for Tallahassee he was ailing. The strain of traveling to Tallahassee combined with the subsequent emotional drain on his constitution during the Convention were too much. He died on January 22. The immediate cause of death was said to have been diphtheria.[2]

Dr. Saxon's death brought immediate emotional reaction on the part of the Florida Senate. At its session on January 23, Senator James T. Magbee of Hillsborough County and personal friend of Dr. Saxon delivered a touching eulogy, or what may better be described as an effusive eulogy, on the departed doctor. He then offered the resolution "that the Senate do now take a recess until half past three p.m., and then to meet here and repair as a body to the

Planters' Hotel to attend the funeral ceremonies...and that the Senate shall stand adjourned for today."

It was then resolved that as a token of respect for the deceased who was a signer of the Ordinance of Secession that each senator "wear the usual badge of mourning for thirty days." It is regrettable that no further information relating to Dr. Saxon's early life and professional career has come to light.

1. Stanaback, Richard J., *A History of Hernando County*, 1840-1976, Brooksville, Florida, p. 30.
2. The greater part of present knowledge of Dr. Saxon is the *Florida Senate Journal*, Session of 1860-61, pp. 134-135.

Scales, Absolem W., Tallahassee, 1808

Dr. Scales, sometime physician in Tallahassee, was a migratory type whose movements are difficult to trace. Records of Transylvania University, Lexington, Kentucky, list him as a medical student in the fall of 1826, giving his place of origin as Patrick County, Virginia.[1] After submitting a thesis bearing the title "On the Uses of the Bandage in Gunshot Wound" he was graduated as Doctor of Medicine in the spring of 1828. Soon thereafter he appears to have begun his practice in North Carolina[2] where he remained for 12 years.

In May 1840, Dr. Scales appeared in Tallahassee where he resumed practice. The following professional card appeared in the Tallahassee *Floridian* of May 4, 1840:

Dr. A.M. Scales, from North Carolina, presents himself to the patronage of the inhabitants of Tallahassee and vicinity, in the practice of the various branches of the profession. A regular graduation and the experience of twelve years' practice are his recommendations to confidence. Persons requiring surgical assistance and those suffering under chronic and protracted disease would do well to test his skill.

No basis for judging the degree of success Dr. Scales enjoyed in Tallahassee has been found. It is only known that three years later, motivated perhaps by a lack of clientele, by a desire for futher education, or possibly by sheer restlessness, he abandoned Tallahassee and returned to Transylvania University for additional study. In this instance the University record listed him as "Practitioner, M.D." and a resident of Harrodsburg, Kentucky.

In the fall of 1847 Dr. Scales was once more in Florida but probably as a visitor. On Saturday, September 17, he joined a party of Wakulla County hunters from St. Marks for a hunting expedition, returning to Newport the same evening for a "splendid Ball at the Wakulla Hotel."[3] Nothing further is known of his professional career.

1. Archives, Transylvania University, Lists of Matriculants and Graduates.
2. Patrick County is situated on the North Carolina border.
3. Others in this deer-hunting party were Col. Hawley; George Brockenbrough, a Wakulla County lawyer; Squire Coleman, a well-to-do farmer, and Count D'Orsay, unidentified.

Scott, Ira, St. Joseph, 1840

Dr. Scott, assumed to have been a native of South Carolina, began medical practice in St. Joseph in the latter part of 1838.[1] In April 1839 he had apparently made a loan of $100 to Captain E.J. Wood of St. Joseph for which Wood had signed a promissory note. Dr. Scott had lost or misplaced the note, however, and advertised the loss.[2] By early 1840, Dr. Scott had returned to South Carolina, settling in the town of Aiken, where he died later that year. On December 16, 1840, the St. Joseph *Times* published the following announcement:[3]

Married, in Aiken S.C., 26 November, 1840, Capt. E.J. Wood, of Florida, to Annette, eldest daughter of the late Dr. Ira Scott, late of St. Joseph.

1. St. Joseph *Times*, February 23, 1839, first printed in December 1838, not extant. St. Joseph, commonly referred to as Port St. Joe, enjoyed an era of prosperity in Florida's Territorial Period, only to be overshadowed later by Apalachicola which had the commercial advantage at the mouth of the Apalachicola River connecting it with the agricultural areas of southeast Alabama and southwest Georgia as well as the Florida settlements along the River.
2. Ibid., April 20, 1839.
3. Ibid., December 16, 1840.

Scott, John G., Pensacola, 1809-1874

Dr. Scott, a native of London, England, began practice in Pensacola in the late 1850s. Census data indicate that he had arrived in the United States about 1849 accompanied by wife Eliza and two children, daughter, Florence, and son, E.M. They settled in Tennessee where their son, Thomas K., was born but later moved to Alabama where another son, Bernard, was born.[1]

The extent of Dr. Scott's practice is not known, but it is clear that he was overshadowed by popular native-born physicians such as R.B.S. Hargis, James S. Herron, and Frank G. Renshaw. It is known that on occasion he performed postmortem examinations for the state.[2]

Yellow fever epidemics were a common occurrence in Pensacola in the latter part of the 19th century, attributable in large measure to the frequent arrival in its port of vessels from Caribbean ports. When a particularly deadly epidemic of fever occurred in the fall of 1874, Dr. Scott chose to leave Pensacola. His departure in the midst of the onslaught prompted Dr. William Henry Davison, obviously with a touch of bitterness, to make the following entry in his diary: "Dr. Scott left his fever-stricken people for the more salubrious climate of New York."[3] Three weeks later he included the following: "Dr. Scott, and other runaways are arriving."[4]

It appears that Dr. Scott did not long remain in Pensacola. His subsequent whereabouts are not known.

1. U.S. Census, 1860, Escambia County, Florida, p. 52.
2. Tallahassee *Florida Sentinel*, February 24, 1863. A list of this date, provided by the State Treasurer's Office, indicates that Dr. Scott received $20.
3. "Diary of William H. Davison," entry of October 12, 1874.
4. Ibid., entry of November 8, 1874.

Scott, Robert, Jefferson County, 1832-1886

Dr. Scott, third child and second son of James and Margaret Bailey Scott, was born in Jefferson County in 1832. His parents, both natives of Georgia, had moved from Camden County about 1820, settling first on lands between Lloyd and Waukeenah. In the late 1830s, when Indian hostilities intensified, they moved to land nearer Monticello. After the death of his father in 1852 Dr. Scott's mother moved into the town, having her country home rebuilt and enlarged. Young Scott received his early education at the Jefferson Academy, said to have been one of the best schools in all of Florida.[1] In 1854 he entered Jefferson Medical College in Philadelphia from which he was graduated M.D. in 1856;[2] soon thereafter he returned to Monticello and entered the dual vocations of physician and druggist.[3]

In the feverish activity which followed Florida's secession from the Union in January 1861, sons of many of Florida's most prominent families answered the call for volunteers from the Confederate Army. By mid-May three volunteer companies had been assembled in Jefferson County. At a meeting in Monticello on April 26, one of these known as the Jefferson Beauregards was organized with Daniel B. Bird as captain and Dr. Scott as first lieutenant.[4] The company was mustered into service on May 15 and ordered to rendezvous in Monticello prepared to encamp on May 18.[5] Their first assignment took them to the lighthouse south of St. Marks which was thought to be an immediate target for Northern gunboats. After a few days devoted to constructing entrenchments and fighting mosquitoes and sand fleas they returned to Monticello. On June 6 the company was ordered to Fernandina and in mid-July to St. Augustine. In the meantime Dr. Scott was replaced as first lieutenant by M.J. Clark.[6] No explanation for this change is given but it apparently brought no discredit or dishonor to Dr. Scott who immediately resumed practice in Monticello and continued throughout the war.[7]

In the confusing and difficult postwar years Dr. Scott was involved in numerous transactions which reflect the breadth of his interests. In 1868, for example, when the Jefferson County Tax Collector, S.V. Neely, defaulted in his accounts, Dr. Scott, Junius Turnbull and others who had bonded Neely were called upon to pay for the shortages. In January 1869 when General Patton Anderson was unable to settle his accounts with a Monticello business firm, Dr. Scott, who had been operating Anderson's farm, interceded with the merchants for an extension of credit for an additional year. In 1879, after Alonzo B. Crumwell, former Union Army officer, was appointed administrator of the Freedmen's Bureau in the county, Dr. Scott was able to persuade him to mitigate some of his demands on local farmers.

Throughout his career Dr. Scott appears to have remained on the periphery of town and county politics although showing keen interest in many public issues; however, he never ran for public office.[8] In the difficult days of Reconstruction he seems to have controlled his emotions and maintained an agreeable relationship with administrators.

Dr. Scott was twice married, first to Mary E. White and second to Rebecca, a widow, daughter of Robert P. Johnson, whose first husband, William Simkins, had died in 1870. To the first marriage were born five daughters;[9] the second marriage was childless. The first Mrs. Scott died in the 1870s, the second lived well into the 20th century.[10] Dr. Scott continued his medical practice until near the end of his life. The mortality records of 1885 for Jefferson County indicate that he was among the most active physicians. He died on January 8, 1886.[11]

1. A portion of the information relating to the Scott family is derived from a Jefferson County WPA Writers' Program typescript containing an assortment of sketches on various aspects of history. Much of the material is unpaginated.

2. Archives, Jefferson Medical Colleges, Lists of Students.

3. Monticello *Family Friend*, March 22, 1859. Dr. Scott's professional cards for both his medical practice and drug store appeared first in the second issue of the newspaper, Vol. I, No. 2, dated March 1, 1859.

4. Ibid., May 4, 1861.

5. Ibid., May 18, 1861.
6. Ibid., September 28, 1861.
7. Lacunae in the file of the Monticello newspaper make it impossible to follow Dr. Scott's career during the war years, only the issue of February 8, 1862, having survived. An item in the Tallahassee *Florida Sentinel* of February 24, 1863, listing him as the recipient of a $25 payment from the State Treasurer "for post mortem examinations" indicates that he had continued his practice.
8. Jerrell H. Shofner, *History of Jefferson County, Florida*, Tallahassee, 1976, pp. 312, 323, 324. Dr. Scott was vice president of an assembly of Jefferson County Democrats in Monticello in 1880. He was also among the organizers of the County Truck Farmers Association in 1883. Ibid., pp. 339, 380.
9. U.S. Census, 1870, Jefferson County, Florida, p. 27. The daughters were listed as Lizzie and Henrietta (elsewhere known as Nettie), R. Adam (sic), Minnie and Julia.
10. Shofner, op. cit., p. 423. The U.S. Census, 1900, Jefferson County, Florida, p. 2., lists Mrs. Scott, aged 58, head of a household and operating a boarding house. Other residents were India Johnson, sister of Mrs. Scott, aged 37; and Mamie Linton, niece of Mrs. Scott, aged 20, a schoolteacher.
11. Dr. Scott was buried in Roseland Cemetery, Monticello.

Screven, Benjamin S., Tallahassee, 1840

The Screven family was prominent in both Beaufort and Georgetown Districts of South Carolina. Its members were a prolific family in which certain Christian names were repeated in several generations. Dr. Screven is thought to have been the son of the Rev. Benjamin S. Screven, a Baptist minister, who died in Beaufort on September 5, 1826.

He was a native of Georgetown District, Prince Frederick Parish, and hardly more than a sojourner in Florida. He came to Tallahassee about 1845 and was employed to provide medical service for prisoners confined to the Leon County jail, for which the State Legislature authorized payment of $69.75 on the last day of its 1846-47 session.[1]

Dr. Screven married Cornelia A. Archer, daughter of Hugh Archer, a successful Tallahassee turpentine distiller and businessman on August 3, 1848, in a ceremony performed in St. John's Episcopal Church.[2] They had one child, Mary Hamilton Screven, who became the wife of Thomas P. Myers on February 20, 1873.[3]

In 1849 Dr. Screven became infected with the gold rush fever leaving his wife and child with her family as he made his way to California where he died a short time later.[4]

1. *Acts and Resolutions, General Assembly, State of Florida*, 2nd Session, 1846-47, Tallahassee, 1846, p. 94.
2. Parochial Records, St. John's Episcopal Church, Tallahassee. Copy in P.K. Yonge Library of Florida History, University of Florida, p. 48.
3. Ibid., p. 51. A daughter, Maud Hamilton Myers, became the wife of Dr. Henry E. Palmer of Tallahassee. See Henry E. Palmer, "Physicians of Early Tallahassee and Vicinity," *Apalachee*, 1944, p. 35.
4. This entry in the Leon County Census of 1850, p. 82, item 184, is baffling: "B.S. Screven, aged 30, physician, born in S.C." The listing of the Archer family in ibid., p. 66, includes Screven, Cornelia, aged 20, born in South Carolina. The Screven child, Mary Hamilton, aged one, is listed as Mary Hamilton Archer. This suggests an estrangement between Dr. and Mrs. Screven and may explain his departure for California.

Scull, C.B., Gadsden County, 1848-1900

Due to the ups and downs of mid-19th century Chattahoochee, located on the east bank of the Apalachicola River just south of the confluence of the Flint and the Chattahoochee, steady progress was slow in arriving. Such early importance as it may have enjoyed derived from its arsenal constructed at the beginning of the Second Seminole War in 1835. The facility came into use again during the Civil War. Only in 1876, however, when the arsenal became the nucleus of the Florida State Hospital for the Insane did the town begin to experience a period of prosperity. Dr. Scull, a Pennsylvania native, who had spent some time in Virginia, arrived in Chattahoochee in 1870 with his wife, Margaretta. His decision to settle in the remote community was doubtless determined by earlier arrival of his father, the Reverend William Dundas Scull, in the Midway community as an Episcopal clergyman.[1]

Chattahoochee and its adjoining village, River Junction, did not present a very inviting appearance in 1870. One traveler, recalling the scene, wrote: "there were only three dwelling houses, no churches or schools for the whites, but the negroes had two churches. Dr. Scull was the only physician and H.H. Spear was the postmaster."[2] Notwithstanding its dismal prospects Dr. Scull chose to remain and was to spend the balance of his life attending to the medical needs of the community. Judging from the mortality schedules for Gadsden County in 1885, as set forth in the special census of that year, he found adequate work if perhaps not adequate pay.[3] Of the patients whom he attended between May 31, 1884 and May 31, 1885, 10 did not survive. Only Dr. Joseph Wragg lost more—12. These statistics are cited not to derogate Dr. Scull's skill but to indicate the extent and popularity of his services.

Beyond his medical practice very little is known of Dr. Scull's activities. He served as postmaster of Chattahoochee for a time. As an enlightened professional man and son of a well-educated[4] father, he doubtless contributed much to the early development of Chattahoochee. It is unfortunate that nothing is known of his association with the physicians of the Insane Asylum such as Dr. William Foreman.

The date of Dr. Scull's death is not known. He was living in 1892 when a roster of Florida practitioners was prepared by the Florida Medical Association but had died prior to the enumeration of the census in 1900 when his wife, Margaretta, is listed as a widow.[5] The Sculls were childless.

1. The Reverend Mr. Scull was received into the Diocese of Florida by Bishop F.H. Rutledge in 1859. He had arrived with a letter of dismissal from the Diocese of Maryland. At the Diocesan Convention at St. John's Church, Tallahassee, in May 1860, he was officially received. His first assignment was that of rector of St. Luke's Parish, Marianna. From that time on until his death in 1871, he was active in the affairs of the Diocese, devoting the greater part of his energies to missionary work among the Negroes of Gadsden and adjoining counties. He was their teacher as well as pastor, having established a school for them at Midway. For details of his service see *Diocese of Florida, Convention Journal*, Tallahassee, 1860, and subsequent years.

2. J. Randall Stanley, *History of Gadsden County*, Quincy, 1948, pp. 196-197. See Miles Kenan Womack Jr., Gadsden, *A Florida County in Word and Picture*, Quincy, 1976, p. 235.

3. Special Florida Census, 1885, Mortality Schedule. See Randall, *History*, p. 197.

4. The Reverend Mr. Scull's reports to the Diocese reveal a high degree of literary skill.

5. U.S. Census, 1900, Gadsden County, Florida, item 343.

Scull, William Jasper, Chattachoochee, 1838-1879

Dr. Scull was born in Prince William County, Virginia, in 1838, son of the Reverend William Dunbar Scull, Episcopal clergyman. He was the older brother of Dr. Charles B. Scull whose career ran parallel to his own. He matriculated at the University of Pennsylvania's Department of Medicine in October 1859 and was graduated Doctor of Medicine on March 14, 1861. It is recorded that he had earlier attended a college "somewhere in the South."[1]

Dr. Scull enlisted for service in the Army of the Confederacy shortly after the firing on Ft. Sumter on April 12, 1861. In early 1862 he was commissioned Acting Assistant Surgeon and assigned to field service in Captain J.L. Dunham's Light Artillery Company, retaining that position throughout the War.[2]

With establishment of the Florida State Prison at Chattahoochee in 1868 Dr. Scull became a member of its medical staff with the title "Prison Physician." When instructions for the operation of the prison were set forth it was stipulated that no member of the staff would be allowed to be otherwise employed "with the exception of the surgeon," Dr. Scull being permitted to supplement his prison pay through private practice.[3]

Mr. Martin in 1875, Warden of the Prison, included in his report: "The Almighty has vouchsafed to protect us from any epidemic during the past year. There has been but two deaths since my last report. I respectfully refer you to the report of the Prison Surgeon, W.J. Scull, M.D."[4]

In Dr. Scull's report, submitted on December 31, 1874, from the Office of the Surgeon, State Prison of Florida, the Doctor requested that the state build a prison hospital. He further reported that "he had treated 1500 cases and made 2210 prescriptions." The diseases he had treated included intermittent fever, remittent fever, rheumatism, dysentery, diarrhea and catarrh as the main ailments.

Dr. Scull died at Chattahoochee on May 9, 1879.

1. Biographical data obtained from the Archives, University of Pennsylvania.
2. *Soldiers of Florida*, published under auspices of Board of State Institutions, Tallahassee 1903, p. 320.
3. C. Ray McDaniel, "History of the Florida Prison System," paper prepared for a Legal History Seminar under the supervision of Professor Francis McCoy. Copy in P.K. Yonge Library of Florida History, p. 3.
4. "Surgeon's Report," *Journal of the Proceedings of the Assembly of the State of Florida*, 8th Session, 1875, pp. 109-110.

Sessions, Abner M.R., Leon and Madison Counties, 1823

Dr. Sessions was a native of Georgia but at the time of admission to the Medical Department of the University of Georgia in Augusta he was a resident of Monticello where he had read medicine under the direction of Dr. B. Waller Taylor.[1] He entered medical school in 1842 and received the M.D. degree in the spring of 1844.[2] Upon graduation he returned to Florida, settling in Leon County. The Leon County Census of 1850 lists him as 27 years old, married, wife's name, Camelia, with one son, David.[3] Apparently he continued to practice in Leon County throughout the 1850s. The "Journal of Charles Bannerman," owner of Iamonia Plantation, includes entries recording the visits of Dr. Sessions to attend members of the Bannerman household.[4]

Dr. Sessions had moved to the town of Madison by 1860 and his household included a second son, George W., aged five.[5] Records indicate that he spent the remainder of his life in Madison County. The Madison County census of 1870 lists two additional children, a daughter, Martha, and a son, Abner.[6] Indications are that Dr. Sessions enjoyed a large, though not necessarily lucrative, practice. The Special Census of 1885 for the county suggests that he and two colleagues, Drs. Joseph F. Bythewood and James P. Peeler, were handling more than 50% of the cases for the entire county.[7]

No date of death for Dr. Sessions has been located.

1. Information in letter, Dorothy Mims, Reference Librarian, Medical College of Georgia, to E.A. Hammond, August 9, 1976.
2. *List of Graduates From 1829 to 1891*, Medical Department, University of Georgia , Augusta, 1891, p. 24.
3. U.S. Census, 1850, Leon County, Florida, p. 94.
4. James D. Glunt, *Plantation and Frontier Records of East and Middle Florida*. Ph.D. dissertation, University of Michigan, 1930, II, 69, 77. Typescript in P.K. Yonge Library of Florida History.
5. U.S. Census, 1860, Madison County, Florida, p. 10.
6. Ibid., 1870, p. 56.
7. Special Census, 1885, Florida. Schedule of deaths and physicians attending deceased.

Shaffer, Robert W., Madison, 1819

Little information has emerged concerning the career of Dr. Shaffer who practiced medicine in Madison just prior to the Civil War. Records of the Medical College of the State of South Carolina list him as M.D., class of 1839, after having submitted a doctoral thesis on the subject, "Revulsion." He had entered the College from Columbia, South Carolina, where his preceptor had been a Dr. Nott.[1] His whereabouts for the next 15 years remain unknown, but the fact that his older children were born in South Carolina indicates that he was a practitioner in that state.[2] By 1854 he had become a resident of Madison. The following year the Florida legislature authorized the comptroller to pay to Dr. R.H. Shaffer $25 "for his attendance on the Coroner's inquest at an examination held on the body of Mitchel Allen in the year 1854."[3] The bill had originated in the Senate on the motion of William A. Brinson, Senator from Madison County. Among arrivals at Buffington House, Jacksonville's leading hotel, on February 12, 1855, was Dr. R.H. Shaffer.[4]

Dr. Shaffer's professional card appeared in the Madison newspaper in 1858. His office was located "in a building formerly occupied by O.M. Lee," from which he expected to serve Madison and the vicinity.[5]

The Census of 1860 listed Dr. Shaffer, his wife, Elizabeth, and their seven children aged 16 to one month as residents of Madison. His property was valued at more than $25,000, an indication that he was "well-to-do."[6] Beyond this point no information of Dr. Shaffer has been located. Civil War records show, however, that his two older sons, Michael and Frederick, volunteered for military service. Michael enlisted in 1860 when he was only 17 years old. He was captured at Missionary Ridge in November 1863 and spent the rest of the conflict in a Northern prison.[7] Frederick enlisted on April 23, 1864, at the age of 18 and was among the troops surrendering at Baldwin, Florida, on May 17, 1865,[8] Of the entire Schaffer family only Frederick appears in the Madison County census of 1870.[9]

1. Archives, Medical College of State of South Carolina, "Lists of Matriculants and Graduates."
2. U.S. Census, 1860, Madison County, Florida, p. 152.
3. *General Assembly, State of Florida*, 7th Session, 1855, *Acts and Resolutions*, p. 48. The Act was passed by the Senate on December 10, 1855; passed by the House on December 11, 1855; approved by Governor Broome on December 14, 1855.
4. Jacksonville *Florida Republican*, February 15, 1855.
5. Madison *Southern Messenger*, December 25, 1858, 1st printing, October 24, 1858.
6. See n. 2, supra.
7. NA, Service Records, CSA, M251, Roll 57. Michael had been assigned to Co. C, 4th Florida Infantry Regiment.
8. Frederick Shaffer was assigned to Capt. Kilcrease's Light Artillery Battery; Ibid., Roll 23.
9. U.S. Census, 1870, Madison County, Florida, p. 5. He is listed as a wheelwright, age 23, married to Mary M. Shaffer, age 24.

Shafter, Adolph, St. Augustine, 1850

The only information which has come to light on Dr. Shafter is that found in the Census of 1850 which shows him to have been a resident of St. Augustine. He was a native of Switzerland, aged 38. His wife, Anna, aged 25, was born in Florida as were his two daughters, Lucy and Louisa, eight and six respectively, and his son Charles, aged one.[1]

1. U.S. Census, 1850, St. Johns County, Florida, p. 425, it. 260.

Sharp, John S., Hamilton County, 1821-1853

Dr. Sharp, who practiced medicine for a short time in Hamilton County, was born in North Carolina, was married to a native Georgian named Martha and was the father of three sons, James, Stephen and John, aged 11, 10 and eight, respectively, in 1860.[1] He appears in the 1850 Census as physician,[2] aged 29. His widow, five years his junior, was still living in Hamilton County in 1860. Her properties were valued at approximately $5,000.

1. U.S. Census, 1860, Hamilton County, Florida, p. 597, item 252.
2. Ibid., 1850, p. 224, item 4.

Shelby, William A., Orlando, 1835-1889

Dr. Shelby, a native of Georgia and 1856 graduate of the Atlanta Medical College,[1] practiced his profession for several years prior to moving to Orlando in the 1870s. He was a popular and successful practitioner from the time of his arrival in Orlando. He built a home just east of Lake Eola near the intersection of Sumerlin and Robinson Avenues and maintained an office in the Blus Drug Store located near his residence. Indications are that he carried on an extensive practice and was highly regarded by professional colleagues.

Dr. Shelby's death came tragically and ironically on March 2, 1889, after he mistakenly took a dose of gelsemine, a poisonous crystalline alkaloid concocted from the root of jasmine. He had apparently mistaken it for a concoction of chincona bark, a specific used for treating malaria.[2]

Dr. Shelby was survived by his wife, Mary Louise, a daughter, Anne (familiarly known as Fannie), and a son, William. In 1885, their ages were 40, 22, and 17, respectively. All were natives of Georgia.[3]

1. *Atlanta Medical College*, Annual Announcement, Session of 1878-79, Atlanta, 1978, p. 12.
2. Madison *Recorder*, March 8, 1889.
3. Florida, Special Census, 1885.

Shelton, Vardy H., Alachua County, 1830

Dr. Shelton, who practiced medicine in Alachua County for more than a decade, was born in South Carolina about 1830.[1] He was graduated from the Medical College of University of Georgia in Augusta in 1856 and within a year or two moved to Florida, settling in the town of Waldo.[2] The evidence indicates that he had entered medical school at a more advanced age than most students.[3] Soon after arrival in Florida he purchased a tract of land south of Waldo from

Madison Sparkman, one of the more affluent landowners of the area.[4] On this land, which records indicate to have been about 80 acres, Dr. Shelton is said to have planted 20 acres in seedling China oranges and in 1860 his properties had an estimated value of $3,000.[5]

Very little is known of Dr. Shelton's role in the Waldo community, but a single reference suggests that he was involved in the public issues of the times. When a group of Waldo citizens met in August 1865 to discuss postwar conditions and the means of restoring a normal way of life, Dr. Shelton was a member of the committe chosen to draft a public statement. The resulting resolution urged speed in returning to a normal situation and early acceptance of federal authority. The committee also drafted a memorial to Acting Governor William Marvin asking him to call for conventions in every Florida county for the purpose of "getting on with the business of returning the State to civil law."[6]

At the beginning of January 1866, Dr. Shelton moved to Micanopy and on January 20 the following notice appeared in the Gainesville *New Era*:

> The undersigned, a graduate of the Medical College of Georgia, of thirteen years experience in the practice of his profession, seven of which have been in the State of Florida, has removed from his former residence near Waldo to Micanopy, Florida, and now occupies the late residence of the Rev. J.C. Ley.

There followed a list of fees: mileage, 50 cents per mile by day, $1 by night; common obstetrical case, $10, instrumental obstetrical case, $25; amputation of a limb, $50; setting broken limb, $10; extraction of a tooth, $1. He also announced that he would keep on hand a good selection of drugs and would fill his own prescriptions.

Dr. Shelton's family included his wife, Sarah, four daughters and three sons. Only the youngest, Julia, aged seven in 1870, was born in Florida. The other members, including Mrs. Shelton, were natives of Georgia.

Subsequent to 1870 nothing is known of the Shelton family. They do not appear in the Alachua County census of 1880. It may be assumed that they had departed the state by that date.

1. This is an extrapolation from census data of 1860 and 1870, both of which are patently erroneous.
2. U.S. Census, 1860, Alachua County, Florida, item 68. See Medical Department, University of Georgia, *List of Graduates from 1829 to 1891*, Augusta, 1890, p. 24.
3. If Dr. Shelton was indeed 38 years old in 1860, as is shown in the census of that year, or 45 in 1870, as shown in the census of that year, he would have been somewhat older than most graduates. Also he stated in a public notice of January 1, 1866, in the Gainesville *New Era*, January 13, that he had practiced for 13 years, seven in Florida.
4. F.W. Buchholz, *History of Alachua County, Florida*, St. Augustine, 1926, p. 176. See also Alachua County, Deed Book E, pp. 349-350.
5. See note 2, supra. Real estate valued at $1,200, personal property at $1,800. The Slave Schedule, 1860, shows him owning one slave.
6. Gainesville *New Era*, September 2, 1865.

Sheppard, Lyman, Gadsden County, 1890

Dr. Sheppard, a native of Georgia, apparently moved to Gadsden County in the 1840s. The sole reference to his presence in Florida is found in the Census of 1850 which lists him as 60 years of age, a physician, whose wealth was estimated at $1,000. Sharing his household was 20-year-old Arionna Smith, possibly a granddaughter.[1]

1. U.S. Census, 1850, Gadsden County, Florida, p. 206. It should be noted that in mid-19th century there resided

in Leon and Gadsden Counties several families of the name Sheppard (the spelling varies), most of them originating in Georgia.

Shields, James L., Quincy, 1820

Dr. Shields was hardly more than a brief sojourner in Florida. Born in the Darlington District of South Carolina about 1820,[1] he matriculated at the Medical College of the State of South Carolina in the fall of 1838 and was graduated on March 19, 1840.[2] His Darlington preceptor had been a Dr. Dargan; his doctoral thesis bore the title, "Sympathy."[3] He is thought to have arrived in Quincy in the mid-1840s, a supposition suggested by the fact that he was sufficiently known and respected to have been elected to the Florida House of Representatives in the fall of 1847. It is noteworthy that he ran for office as a Democrat, the minority party at the time.[4]

In his role as legislator Dr. Shields exhibited a progressive and enlightened position. As a member of the Standing Committee on Schools and Colleges he worked diligently for passage of an act which would establish a system of common schools in every Florida county. It passed the House on December 31, 1847.[5] He was less successful as a member of a Select Committee which included two other physicians, John L. Crawford and Daniel Bradwell, in his effort to persuade the Legislature to establish a Registry of Births, Marriages and Deaths, a much-needed state agency. The effort had been prompted by a communication from the National Medical Convention held in Philadelphia in May 1847.[6] The proposal, as drafted by the Select Committee, was a sensible one but the conservative and niggardly body defeated it by a vote of 21 to 12. Florida must wait another 71 years before a viable Bureau of Vital Statistics would be added to the functions of the State Board of Health.[7]

In May 1848 Dr. Shields joined eight other physicians from Gadsden and neighboring counties, all men of integrity, concerned about the low quality of medical practice and loose procedures for licensing physicians in the state. Meeting in Quincy,[8] it was their purpose to lay plans for establishment of a state medical association. Dr. Shields as a member of the Corresponding Committee undertook to contact all other licensed practitioners in the state, urging them to be present in Tallahassee on the first Monday of January 1849. It was assumed that by late December the Legislature would have granted a charter for the proposed organization and that by early January they would proceed to organize the Association. It was not to be. The bill which would have approved the charter was killed by a House vote of 18 to 12 on December 28. This action stunned the little group of worthy physicians.[9]

Dr. Shields was reputed to be a skillful surgeon. Dr. Charles A. Hentz, never hesitant about expressing his opinion on his medical colleagues, recalled the case of the young son of an Ochesee (Calhoun County) planter, Jason Gregory, both of whose arms were badly mangled in a cotton gin accident. Dr. Shields, who lived 25 miles away, was sent for. He answered the call, amputated the left arm, but was able to save the right arm with only the loss of three fingers. So successful was the operation that the lad was able "to write a very good hand." Wrote Dr. Hentz: "Shields was the leading popular doctor of Quincy."[10]

Beyond this point very little is known of Dr. Shields. In March 1851 he is known to have performed a postmortem examination on the body of a John White. At about the same time he attended a prisoner in the Gadsden County jail. For these services the State Legislature awarded him $76 in January 1853.[11] It may be conjectured that he had left Florida by the mid-1850s, possibly discouraged by the failure of the state's political leaders to enact progressive legislation.

1. Archives, Medical College of the State of South Carolina, Waring Historical Medical Library, Charleston.
2. Charleston *Courier*, March 26, 1840.
3. There is no accounting for the medical implications of the subject.
4. Tallahassee *Floridian*, September 11, 1847. Ibid., October 16, 1847.
5. *Florida House Journal*, 3rd Session, 1847, p. 170.
6. Ibid., p. 167.
7. The first Bureau of Vital Statistics for Florida was authorized in 1913 but did not become a fully functioning agency until 1924.
8. Quincy *Times* May 20, 1848. In addition to Dr. Shields the physicians were: William Booth, John M.G. Hunter, and David White, all of Gadsden, John L. Call of Jefferson, John S. Bond of Leon, E.D. de Graffenreid of Jackson.
9. For an account of this effort see E. Ashby Hammond, "Medical Regulation and Organization in Florida, 1821-74," Journal of the Florida Medical Association, January 1974, pp. 62-70.
10. Charles A. Hentz, "Autobiography." Unpublished manuscript, Southern Historical Collection, University of North Carolina, Chapel Hill, I.225.
11. *General Assembly of Florida, Acts and Resolutions*, 1852-53, p. 162.

Shine, William Francis, Tallahassee and St. Augustine, 1835-1910

Dr. Shine was born in Tallahassee on January 9, 1835, the son of R.A. Shine Sr., wealthy Leon County planter and slaveowner.[1] After receiving his medical degree probably from the University of Virginia, he entered practice in Tallahassee in May 1858 occupying an office opposite the court house.[2] With the coming of the Civil War Dr. Shine enlisted in Lt. Col. D.P. Holland's Battalion of Florida Volunteers, 10th Florida Infantry Regiment, as regimental surgeon, having received his commission from Governor Perry on September 28, 1861, and entered active duty at Ft. Clinch, Nassau County, on November 12, 1861.[3] Although no record of his discharge from active service remains he is presumed to have served throughout the war.

Dr. Shine appears to have returned to medical practice in Tallahassee about 1865.[4] In December of that year he married Maria Jefferson Eppes,[5] daughter of the socially prominent Francis Eppes, by his second wife, Susan Margaret Ware. Francis Eppes was a grandson of Thomas Jefferson.

Dr. Shine had transferred his practice to St. Augustine by 1870 and he lived there until his death on October 21, 1910.[6] The registers of Trinity Episcopal Church, St. Augustine, contain numerous entries relating to him and his family, including a record of his own belated confirmation in March 1875. Recorded in these registers are the baptisms of the two Shine children, Francis Eppes Shine, born January 13, 1871,[7] and a daughter, Mildred, baptized on May 29, 1874.[8]

William S. Branch of Orlando, who had access to family records, describes Dr. Shine as "a large man in physique and in his later years...considerably overweight." As for his medical interests, Branch further states: "Years before the Army experiments in the cause of yellow fever, Dr. Shine was convinced that a mosquito carried the fever germs. His theory was unpopular and those who heard of it considered him 'crazy' until Dr. Walter Reed proved the facts, following the Spanish-American War."[9]

Both Dr. Shine and his wife are buried in the Eppes-Shine plot in Greenwood Cemetery, Orlando.

1. William S. Branch, *The Eppes-Shine Families of Orange County, Florida*, Orlando, 1949. This brief genealogical study provides useful information on the two families, especially those members who migrated from Tallahassee. It is somewhat extraordinary that three Shine brothers, all Tallahassee-born, were married to three Eppes sisters, daughters of Francis Eppes. Two of these brothers, Capt. Thomas Jabez Shine and David Shepard Shine, were among the early settlers in Orlando. The third, Dr. William Francis Shine, elected to settle in St. Augustine. A fourth brother, R.A. Shine Jr., remained in Tallahassee.
2. Tallahassee *Florida Sentinel*, May 18, 1858.
3. NA, AGO, Service Records.
4. Tallahassee *Semi-Weekly Floridian*, January 9, 1866. His professional card appeared in this issue.
5. St. John's Episcopal Church, Tallahassee, Records, Unpublished, marriages, p. 51.
6. USCO, 8th Census, Leon County, Florida. Here Dr. Shine, aged 22 and resident of Tallahassee, is shown as living in the household of John Sharpless, a merchant. The 9th Census, St. Johns County, lists him as a resident of St. Augustine.
7. Trinity Episcopal Church, St. Augustine, Records, Unpublished, baptisms. This son also became a physician, identified as Dr. Frank Shine, who eventually settled in Arizona, where he was chief surgeon for the Southern Pacific Railroad.
8. Ibid. It is apparent that Dr. Shine was not a member of Trinity Church at the time of these christenings. Sponsors for the son were Francis Eppes, W. Call and Susan M. Eppes. Sponsor for the daughter was her mother, Mrs. Shine.
9. Branch, op. cit. This work is not paginated, therefore no specific pages are cited.

Shomo, David T., Pensacola, 1850

Dr. Shomo practiced medicine in Pensacola for a brief period about 1850. He was born in Alabama about 1824, the eldest child of Joseph Shomo, a native of Pennsylvania who had moved to Alabama in early manhood, married there and reared five of his six children, only the youngest, a son named Francis, having been born in Florida.[1] Since his name does not appear in the Florida census of 1860, it is assumed that he had departed the state by that date.

1. U.S. Census, 1850, Escambia County, Florida, p. 233. The youngest child of the Shomos was born in Florida in 1848.

Sierra, Eugenio Antonio, Pensacola, 1750-1849

Dr. Sierra, for many years a prominent citizen and physician of Pensacola, was born in Salamanca, Spain, in 1750. Upon deciding to prepare for a career in surgery he became an apprentice to a surgeon, presumably in Salamanca. After some five years of training he went to Madrid where he became surgeon for the city jail and later a *practicante* at a Madrid hospital.[1]

Dr. Sierra made his way to the New World in 1785, settling for a brief period in Havana, Cuba, as surgeon to the sugar manufactory of Miguel de Peñalver. For what has been explained as "reasons of health" he soon moved to Pensacola to become *practicante de aparato* at the Pensacola Royal Hospital.[2] His professional relationships, however, appear to have been unsatisfactory, due possibly to a contentious nature or conflicts of personality, and he soon moved to the Apalachee Settlement which encompassed much of present-day Wakulla and Leon Counties and whose main channel of ingress was the Apalachee River, now St. Marks River. There he was surgeon to the Spanish settlers.[3]

After a few years Dr. Sierra moved once more to Pensacola, assuming the title of senior practitioner *practicante mayor* or possibly general practitioner. Again things did not go well. In spite of years of apprenticeship and practice he was denied a permit to practice in Pensacola by Governor Vizente Folch. It appears that Dr. Sierra appealed this decision to higher authority, for on April 7, 1817, Folch wrote to Baron de Carondelet, Governor of Louisiana, explaining that it was Dr. Sierra's lack of formal medical education, i.e., a university diploma, which had prompted his denial, adding gratuitously that "Sierra's ministrations are responsible for many unjustified cemetery residents."[4]

Folch's appraisal was probably unjust in that shortly after the cession of West Florida to the United States in July 1822, Dr. Sierra became a well-respected physician of Pensacola, actually succeeding Dr. James C. Bronaugh, for years Andrew Jackson's personal physician and president of Florida's first Legislative Council, as President of the Pensacola Board of Health, subsequent to Dr. Bronaugh's untimely death from yellow fever in September 1822. It is worthy of note that in this newly-assigned capacity his public notice regarding the erection of facilities to house persons subjected to quarantine in Pensacola, he signed himself, "E.A. Sierra, M.D., Resident Physician and President of the Board of Health."[5] He was still serving as President of the Board as late as September 1827 when he responded to a request from the Pensacola *Gazette's* editor, W. Hasell Hunt, for a health report on the City with assurances that the situation was by no means serious although the "sickly season" had arrived.[6]

Evidence relating to the last two decades of Dr. Sierra's life is sparse. It is not known how long he continued in practice. As late as 1837, at the age of 86, he was among the petitioners of Pensacola requesting that Congress provide a more satisfactory mail service for the community.[7]

Dr. Sierra was married to Francesca Dauphin, who died in Pensacola on September 6, 1833, at the age of 56. Several children were born to this union, including a daughter, Irene, who was married on December 18, 1823, to Lt. P. Morrison of the United States Army,[8] and Isabella Eugenia, who became the wife of Dr. Juan Brosnaham, for many years one of Pensacola's leading physicians and citizens.[9] Dr. Sierra died in Pensacola on March 12, 1849, at the age of 99.

1. The medieval notion that surgery was a craft rather than a profession and therefore inferior to medicine lingered on until the early 19th century in much of western Europe. Surgery, unlike medicine, was not taught in universities but had to be learned through an apprenticeship system. The biographical information on Dr. Sierra prior to 1821 is derived from "Papeles de Cuba," Legajo 35, Reel 438, p. 748. Microfilm, P.K. Yonge Library of Florida History, University of Florida, Gainesville. It was brought to my attention by Bruce S. Chappell, Archivist. The original document may be found in the Archivo General Indias, Seville, Spain.

2. *Practicante de aparato*, i.e., practitioner who employs surgical instruments. Note that Dr. Sierra is not designated *medico* or *cirujano*.

3. See note 1 supra.

4. No doubt Dr. Sierra was frequently at odds with the Spanish administrators in Pensacola and probably with other medical practitioners of the settlement.

5. Pensacola *Gazette and West Florida Advertiser*, August 14, 1824.

6. Pensacola *Gazette*, September 7, 1827. Dr. Sierra's residence was on Intendencia Street.

7. TP, XXV, p. 365.

8. Pensacola *Floridian*, December 20, 1823.

9. Descendants still reside in Escambia County: Henry A. Brosnaham Jr., great-grandson of Juan and Isabella Bronsnaham, who graciously provided extensive information on the Brosnaham-Sierra families. Letter, Henry A. Brosnaham Jr., to E.A. Hammond, February 21, 1979. Isabella Eugenia was born at St. Marks on March 6, 1799, during the period when her parents resided at the Apalachee Settlement.

10. This date appears on his gravestone in St. Michael's Cemetery, Pensacola.

Simkins, James Lawrence, Jefferson County, 1814-1887

Dr. Simkins, physician and farmer of Jefferson County, was born in Edgefield District, South Carolina, on May 6, 1814, of a family of prominence—politics, agriculture and military.[1] Although sources relating to his early life are not at hand, there is evidence that as a young man he migrated to Mississippi where he married and his first child, William, was born.[2] He was a widower at the time he moved to Florida in the mid-1850s. Dr. Simkins married Emily Scott, daughter of Capt. James Scott of Edgefield on July 25, 1857. She was 23 years his junior.[3] They had six children, James, Margaret, Jesse, Emily, John L., and Parker.[4] Mrs. Simkins died about 1868-69 and Dr. Simkins hastily married a local girl known only as Ella M.[5] This marriage produced three sons, Arthur, Eldred and Willie, the first two being namesakes of Dr. Simkins' Edgefield forebears, Cols. Arthur and Eldred Simkins.

The third Mrs. Simkins died on September 5, 1883, at the age of 35 and four years later, on March 3, 1887, she was followed in death by her husband.[6]

On arriving in Florida Dr. Simkins purchased farmland of considerable value near Monticello, although he appears to have resided within the limits of the town. He also came well supplied with farm and domestic labor, owning 42 slaves in 1860. His properties that year were estimated to have a value of about $70,000 which would have established him, if not the wealthiest, as one of the substantial citizens of the county.[7]

As far as military service in the Army of the Confederacy was concerned, the Simkins family were of ages not to be involved, the father being too old, the sons too young. As was the experience of most Southern slave-holding landowners, however, Dr. Simkins suffered considerable losses in property and income, although in 1880 his household servants (all black) numbered five,[8] and five years later he was said to have employed 50 black laborers to whom he paid $1,100 wages in the production of salable farm products worth $2,250.[9] It is assumed that these farm workers lived in houses formerly occupied by slaves.

It is obvious that the practice of medicine, at least after the beginning of his Florida residence, was not his major occupation. Even at the prime of his life, about 1858-1861, for which period some issues of the Monticello *Family Friend* have survived, his card does not appear among the professional notices. It is assumed, however, that with numerous children and 42 slaves he engaged in "family" practice.

1. At the beginning of the 19th century the Simkins brothers, Arthur and Eldred, were men of wealth and influence in Edgefield District. They owned valuable lands just east of the town of Edgefield. See Robert Mills, *Mill's Atlas of South Carolina*, 1825, revised by Charles E. Lee, and published in limited edition, Columbia, 1965, "Map of Edgefield District."
2. The evidence here is tenuous, based solely on the listing of William, aged 13 and native of Mississippi, a resident of the household of Dr. James L. Simkins, U.S. Census, 1860, Jefferson County, Florida, p. 907.
3. Ibid.
4. U.S. Census, 1870, Jefferson County, Florida, p. 313.
5. U.S. Census, 1880, Jefferson County, Florida, p. 86.
6. The vital statistics are found in Cemetery Survey of Jefferson County, Florida, compiled by Mrs. Theo Frances Rowe Delp, and published in Monticello in 1966 under the title, *God's Acre of Jefferson County, Florida.*
7. Slave Schedule, Jefferson County, Florida, 1860.
8. U.S. Census, 1880, Jefferson County, Florida, p. 86.
9. Special Florida Census, 1885, Jefferson County, Dist. 6.

Simmons, Alfred A., Monticello, 1841

Dr. Simmons announced the opening of his practice in Monticello on December 4, 1841. His office and residence were located at the Barrington Hotel. In his public notice he cited previous professional success and hoped for a liberal patronge in the town. He named as references five physicians: Richard McGoldrick, Macon, Ga., A. Norfleet Lightfoot, Columbus, Ga., Cuthbert G. Hudson, Lafayette, Ala., Alexander Caine, Florence, Ga., and William E. White, Whitesville, Fla. It would appear that these were men with whom he had been acquainted in medical school. This notice was first printed on September 28, 1841.[1]

1. Tallahassee *Floridian*, December 4, 1841.

Simmons, G.M.T., Sumter County, 1897

Notwithstanding the enormous growth of population in Florida in the latter half of the 19th century some areas of the state remained predominantly rural, for instance, Sumter County. It had lost substantial land and people by the establishment of Lake County in 1887 by legislative enactment and two of the most thriving towns, Leesburg and Tavares. The resulting situation did not encourage many of the best-trained and qualified physicians to choose the county as a place of opportunity. There were, however, a few who chose to settle and practice there.

Probably the best known was Dr. George McIntosh Troupe Simmons, a native of Alabama, who settled some two miles northwest of the site which would later become Bushnell. He is thought to have been the first well-trained physician to practice in Sumter County.[1] That he was highly regarded is borne out by his election as Clerk of the County Court in 1873. He held the office for four years. Availing himself of the cheap land in that part of Florida, he invested in real estate and planted a portion in citrus, which proved a good investment.[2]

A search of the rosters of students at the better medical colleges of the South in the mid-19th century failed to verify the fact that Dr. Simmons attended any one of them. This leads to the supposition that either he attended for only one term—satisfactory performance for two terms being the normal requirement for a degree—or more probably qualified for a professional license through the apprenticeship system. By whatever route, he seems to have acquitted himself well and gained the confidence of the people of Sumter County.

With the Civil War well under way, Dr. Simmons enlisted for duty in the Coast Guard Artillery at Fernandina on December 1, 1861,[3] and was mustered in at Midway, Gadsden County, on May 17, 1862, committing himself for the duration. Not surprisingly, his whereabouts were unknown for a brief period in 1862, during which he was reported "absent without leave." It was soon discovered, however, that he had joined the staff of the Confederate Hospital in Talladega, Alabama, with the rank of Assistant Surgeon.[4]

At some point between the War's end and the year 1870 Dr. Simmons settled in Sumter County. The census of that year lists him simply as "farmer."[5] He spent the last years of his life on his farm "two miles northwest of Bushnell."[6]

Soon after his return from military service in 1865 Dr. Simmons married a Georgia native known only as Annie E. To this union were born six children: Mary, James, Felix, Susan, Annie A. and a daughter of four months unnamed when the 1880 census was taken, but later called Augustina.[7]

Dr. Simmons died in 1897 at the age of 61 and was buried in the Bushnell Cemetery located about three tenths of a mile from the Sumter County Court House.[8]

1. The principal source of information of Sumter County's history is the small but very valuable volume, *Looking Back: Sumter County*, sponsored by the Sumter County Historical Society and published in 1981 by the Sundial Print Shop, Bushnell. The U.S. Censuses of Sumter County have been used extensively for vital data.
2. Ibid., p. 14.
3. National Archives, Service Records, CSA, 8th Infantry Regiment.
4. Ibid.
5. U.S. Census, 1870, Sumter County, Florida.
6. *Looking Back*, p. 14.
7. U.S. Census, 1870, Sumter County, Florida, p. 251.
8. Gravestone, Bushnell Cemetery.

Simmons, John, Taylor County, 1835

Very litle is known of the presence of Dr. Simmons in Florida. The Census of 1870 lists him as a resident of Rose Hill, Taylor County.[1] He is designated "physician," owning property, personal and real, valued at a mere $400. In his household were his wife, Lora, native of North Carolina, aged 28, and four children, Leoni, five; John, four; Achele, three; and Louisa, two.[2]

1. Dr. Simmons remains an obscure figure. In the first place, Rose Hill is shown on the Florida place-name list only for a village in Citrus County. There was, however, a Rose Head in Taylor County, which was possibly the locality in which Dr. Simmons lived.
2. U.S. Census, 1870, Taylor County, Florida, p. 713. Here Dr. Simmons is shown to have been 35 years of age.

Simmons, Samuel E., Marion County, 1860-70

Dr. Simmons, native of Georgia, is known to have practiced medicine in Marion County during the latter part of the 19th century.[1] The Marion County Census of 1860 lists him as 45 years of age; his occupation: "preacher." Both Dr. Simmons and his wife, Martha, were natives of Georgia. Sharing their home was George Simmons, aged 37, presumed to have been the doctor's brother. He was without occupation. Ten years later Dr. Simmons is listed in the Marion Census as 55 years of age. His wife, Martha, was 40. The Simmons home was in the Flemington community in northwest Marion County.[2]

1. U.S. Census, 1860, Marion County, p. 279.
2. U.S. Census, 1870, Marion County, p. 193. Included in the census item was one black female servant, Maggie Morgan.

Simmons, William Hayne, St. Augustine, 1784-1870

Dr. Simmons, one of the most prominent political and social figures to participate in the complex transfer of the Florida Territory from Spain to the United States, was born in Charleston, South Carolina, in January 1784.[1] After receiving a classical education in Charleston schools he matriculated at the University of Pennsylvania Department of Medicine in the fall of 1804 and was graduated as Doctor of Medicine in the spring of 1806.[2] Possessing acceptable literary skill he is known to have published at least four items.[3] Meanwhile he had a brief exposure to South Carolina politics, having served one term (1816-1818) in the state legislature where he was a colleague of the well-known Robert Y. Hayne.

Soon after the end of the Spanish occupation of Florida in 1821 Dr. Simmons, doubtless stirred by an adventurous spirit, made his way to St. Augustine, arriving there just as the town was suffering through an epidemic of yellow fever. In his book on yellow fever, Dr. B.B. Strobel, a fellow Charlestonian, makes frequent mention of Dr. Simmons, who has "resided in Florida for more than fourteen years, with only an occasional absence."[4]

Dr. Simmons, given his intelligence and educational background, could not avoid an active role in the procedures by which Florida was transferred from Spain to the United States. It was not a simple procedure. Spanish officials, being forced to abandon St. Augustine, were by no means cooperative in transferring public documents and archives to the new occupants. In the Introduction to Volume I, *Spanish Land Grants*, pp. vii and viii, the editors include a brief account of the Archives at the time of cession:

> The Archives were forcibly taken from the Spanish Secretary's Office in St. Augustine by American authority...and stored in the Old Customs House. A commission was appointed to examine them and select those claimed by the United States under the terms of the Treaty of Cession.

In the process some of the papers passed into the hands of Dr. Simmons and his colleague, Dr. Edward B. Gibson.

As expected, one of the first acts of the newly-installed government was appointment of a Board of Health for St. Augustine and St. Johns County. Dr. Simmons was chosen as president but promptly declined the position. Dr. Micah Stone was appointed in his stead but his tenure was brief, terminated by death on December 3, 1821. Again the position was offered to Dr. Simmons, who promptly declined to serve.

After an interval of six years the Legislative Council of Florida created a Board of Health for the entire Territory. Dr. Simmons was named to the Board and in this instance he accepted.[5]

The principal health problem which plagued St. Augustine during much of its early days was the annual recurrence of fevers, especially the strain designated as yellow. At the time microbiology was in its infancy and various theories as to its cause and origins were proposed by various physicians. Dr. Simmons and Dr. Strobel offered their theories. In the summer of 1821 a particularly virulent form of the disease occurred in St. Augustine and Dr. Simmons attributed the onslaught to the utterly "filthy conditions left by the Spaniards" as they were "about emigrating to Cuba, having for some years neglected all police regulations." He continued: "The season was hot and rainy without thunder and lightening (which could have destroyed the atmospheric impurities?), alternations of heat and showers. The fever broke out in September...the disease was the genuine yellow fever, most of the cases terminating fatally....First came the death of Lt. Washburn of the U.S. Artillery. Many officers and soldiers died."[6]

Dr. Strobel, on the other hand, believed the sickness to have been brought in from other tropical and subtropical areas. It was a friendly difference of opinion, however, both had known each other since their early years in Charleston. It remained for microbiologists of a later period to settle the dispute.

Meanwhile Dr. Simmons was increasingly fascinated with Indian culture. The Seminoles of Florida and their treatment at the hands of the white "invaders" touched him deeply. His response was expressed in two lengthy poems: *Onea* (Charleston, 1820) and *Alasco* (Philadelphia, 1867). His prose works, published independently, were: *Notices of East Florida* (Charleston, 1822), 105 pp., and *An Essay on Some of the Effects of Contusions of the Head* (Philadelphia, 1806)

27 pp.[7] In addition he published numerous essays on a variety of subjects.

1. George E. Buker, facsimile edition *Notices of East Florida*, p. xi. See also *Appleton's Biographical Encyclopedia*.
2. University of Pennsylvania Archives. Lists of Graduates.
3. In addition to the works mentioned herein Dr. Simmons contributed several items to a number of periodicals of the 19th century.
4. B.B. Strobel, *An Essay on the Subject of the Yellow Fever*, Charleston 1840, p. 139.
5. *Territorial Papers of the United States*, Vol. XXII, 1821-24, pp. 359.
6. Ibid., p. 197.
7. Buker, op cit. This book is part of the Bicentennial Floridiana Facsimile Series, Gainesville, University of Florida Press, 1973.

Simons, John Hume, St. Augustine, 1818-1876

Having spent only the last years of his life in Florida, Dr. Simons scarcely qualifies for inclusion in the list of Florida physicians. He was born in Charleston, South Carolina, in 1818[1] and is thought to have begun the study of medicine in the office of a Charleston physician. Since there is no record of his having attended either of the two medical schools in Charleston in the 1830s, it is assumed that he went out of the state for his medical degree. He attended the College of Charleston in 1840-41 from which he received "a second degree in liberal arts" at its commencement on February 23, 1841.[2]

Dr. Simons published a medical handbook, *The Planter's Guide and Family Book of Medicines* in 1848 which Dr. Waring states was popular with the planters of South Carolina and adjacent states. At any rate it was printed in a second edition in 1850.[3] Meanwhile he carried on an extensive practice in Charleston and vicinity. With the coming of the Civil War in 1861 Dr. Simons served as an assistant surgeon in the Confederate army and after the war moved to St. Augustine. His professional card, published in the St. Augustine *Examiner* of August 14, 1869, states that he "was bred to the medical profession and practiced extensively for many years. He is authorized to refer to the physicians of St. Augustine, and to Dr. H.S. Phillips, United States Army."[4]

Meanwhile Dr. Simons supplemented his income by turning schoolmaster in St. Augustine. Announcing the discontinuance of school for the summer months in June 1869, he called attention to its reopening on October 1 with "male and female Departments, entirely separate...rigid discipline...full course in English studies, mathematics, Belles Lettres, Latin, Greek, French, Spanish...etc." Signed "J. Hume Simons, A.M., M.D."[5]

So far as is known Dr. Simons remained unmarried. The St. Augustine census of 1870 shows him, aged 52, the sole resident of his household.[6] He died in St. Augustine in 1876.[7]

1. A brief biography of Dr. Simons is found in Joseph I. Waring, *A History of Medicine in South Carolina, 1825-1900*, Charleston, South Carolina Medical Association, 1967, pp. 292-293. He was only one of several members of the Simons family who were prominent in medical circles in South Carolina.
2. Charleston *Courier*, February 23, 1841.
3. Waring, *History*, loc. cit.
4. St. Augustine *Examiner*, August 14, 1869.
5. Ibid., June 19, 1869.
6. U.S. Census, 1870, St. Johns County, Florida, p. 623.
7. Waring, *History*, p. 292.

Simonton, Alfred A., Monticello, 1841

Dr. Simonton announced the beginning of his practice in Monticello on September 28, 1841. His professional card included the names of five physicians who, he asserted, would vouch for his character and professional competence.[1] There is no indication that he was more than a brief sojourner in Florida.

1. Tallahassee *Floridian*, December 11, 1841.

Simpson, Josiah, Surgeon, U.S. Army, 1815-1874

Dr. Simpson was born in Lambertville, New Jersey, in 1815.[1] Although very little information concerning his early life and education has emerged, it is probable that he entered the medical profession by way of the apprenticeship route. On July 11, 1857, he was commissioned Assistant Surgeon in the United States Army, a rank he held for 18 years before receiving promotion to the rank of Surgeon, which was conferred on August 13, 1855. His bravery in action at the Battle of Okeechobee (Florida) earned for him a citation of merit which he received from General Zachary Taylor himself.

Dr. Simpson was a member of the contingent of the United State Army which established a position on the Rio Grande in 1845, during the conflict with Mexico. He remained with his unit as it participated in the final stages of the War and finally made its way into Mexico City on September 6, 1847.

Having gained control of the Capital City, the invaders occupied the Archiepiscopal Palace at Tacubaya, converting it into a hospital, with Dr. Simpson as its chief medical officer. Records indicate that the responsibilities devolving upon him were enormous, owing to the fact that all Americans wounded in action were brought to that hospital.

In April 1848 Dr. Simpson and his medical staff were assigned the troublesome task of removing all sick and wounded Americans, some 600, to hospitals in New Orleans.

His valiant service as an army physician was rewarded by periodic advancement in military rank. On August 12, 1855, he was promoted to Major Surgeon and on March 13, 1865, he became a Colonel "for faithful and meritorious service during the War."

Dr. Simpson died in Baltimore on March 3, 1874, at the age of 59. His funeral was held at Lambertville, New Jersey. On March 6, the *New York Times*, in its announcement of his death, suggested that those "wishing to attend the funeral can travel by train, leaving Pennsylvania Station (New York City) at eight-thirty a.m."

1. The greater portion of the present sketch has been drawn from Francis B. Heitman, *Historical Register and Directory*, Vol. I, Washington, Government Printing Office, 1908, p. 888.

Skrine, Thomas C., Key West, 1858-61

Dr. Skrine, a native of Edisto, South Carolina, began medical training under the preceptorate of the eminent Charleston physician and anatomist, Dr. Eli Geddings, and in 1840 entered the Medical College of the State of South Carolina from which he was graduated in the spring of 1842, having submitted a thesis on "Insanity."[1] After some years of practice in his native state he moved to Key

West where on March 6, 1858, he announced his professional services to the citizens of the town.[2] His residence and office were located at the corner of Front and Carolina Streets, only a couple of blocks from the Marine Hospital which had opened in 1845.

Upon the resignation of Dr. George Troup Maxwell as surgeon and health officer at the Marine Hospital in late 1857,[3] Dr. Skrine was appointed in his stead after a lapse of a few weeks and was still serving in this capacity in early 1861. In late November 1860, the Key West newspaper was "happy to learn in confirmation of the health, not only of our own city, but that of the surrounding neighborhood, that the United States Marine Hospital, under the professional charge of Dr. T.C. Skrine, has for three or four days been untenanted by a single invalid."[4]

With the secession of Florida from the Union in January 1861, it is apparent that Dr. Skrine, who held a federal appointment but whose sympathies remained firmly with the secessionists, was facing a dilemma. By late May the fate of Key West had been determined. The United States Navy had secured the two fortifications on the Florida Reef, Ft. Taylor at Key West and Ft. Jefferson at the Tortugas. Secessionist sentiment, lacking leadership and organization, began to fade while unionist support diminished.[5] At some juncture, precise date unknown, Dr. Skrine left Key West, presumably for Charleston. The Florida segment of his career had ended.

1. Lists of Matriculants and Graduates, Medical College of the State of South Carolina, Library, Medical University of South Carolina, Charleston.

2. The Skrines were a family of prominence in and around Charleston. In the antebellum period they had extensive holdings on the Santee River. Dr. Skrine was a man of considerable means, owning property valued at $15,000 in 1860. See U.S. Census, 1860, Monroe County, Florida, p. 129, where he is listed as the sole member of his household. For his professional card see Key West *Key of the Gulf*, March 6, 1858.

3. Tallahassee *Floridian and Journal*, December 12, 1857.

4. Key West *Key of the Gulf*, November 24, 1860.

5. For a very able discussion of this period of political and social turmoil in Key West see Rodney E. Dillon Jr., *The Civil War in South Florida*, unpublished doctoral dissertation, University of Florida, 1980, pp. 59-101.

Slade, Edwin D., Washington County, 1806-1853

Knowledge of Dr. Edwin D. Slade is from his obituary which appeared in the Tallahassee *Floridian and Journal* of September 24, 1853. He was born in Warren County, North Carolina, in 1806. After completing medical studies at a school not identified he practiced in his native state for a brief period before moving to Mississippi and thence to Alabama where he practiced briefly before moving to Florida. He was said to have been of a sedate and retiring disposition, "little given to display." In addition to having been "deeply skilled in medical," his attainments as a scholar were said to have been extensive. His Florida practice ended with his death on September 1, 1853. "After an illness of thirteen days.[1]

1. Tallahassee *Floridian and Journal* reprinted the obituary which appeared in the Tuscaloosa, Ala., *Monitor*, September 15, 1863.

Smith, Aaron P., Bradford County, 1833-post 1900

Dr. Smith, who spent the greater part of his professional life as a medical practitioner in Bradford County, was born in Coosahatchee, South Carolina,[1] in 1833. He appears to have spent a part of his youth in Madison, Florida, where he began the study of medicine under the preceptorate of Dr. John H. Pope, one of the town's most prominent citizens. In the fall of 1856 he matriculated at the Medical College of South Carolina, Charleston, where he studied for only one term departing without a degree.[2] He may have completed the requirements for his degree at another college, although at that time it was not a prerequisite for obtaining a license to practice.

With the outbreak of the War Between the States Dr. Smith volunteered for service in the Confederate Army. He was mustered in as a private at Fernandina on September 28, 1861, at the age of 28 and two days later began active duty at Starke.[3] By early 1862 he had been assigned to the First Florida Special Battalion which, for administrative purposes, was a unit of the Tenth Florida Cavalry Regiment. Soon thereafter he was stationed at Rickoe's Bluff on the Apalachicola River below Bristol in what is now Liberty County.

Dr. Smith had been in the army only a few weeks when he was disabled by a broken left leg which necessitated his discharge issued at Rickoe's Bluff on May 14, 1862. He was allowed $26.76 for transportation to Starke.[4]

Dr. Smith's military career was not finished. As the Confederacy faced a desperate situation in 1863, he was recalled to duty and on March 18 commissioned Assistant Surgeon. In this capacity he served at several posts in North Florida including Lake City and Palatka.[5] At a date not indicated in his military record, he was taken prisoner by Union troops. In an official record of May 26, 1864, and designated "Report of Prisoners of War, Deserters, etc., arriving in Jacksonville for the week ending on May 20, 1865," the name Dr. A.P. Smith appears. The war had actually ended on May 4 but General Kirby-Smith did not surrender his Trans-Mississippi units until May 26.

Dr. Smith was practicing medicine in Sanderson, Baker County, by 1870. Meanwhile he had married Elizabeth, a woman 10 years his junior. The Census of 1870 shows the Smiths as parents of three children, daughter Mary, and two sons, Robert and Frank.[6]

In his later years Dr. Smith turned increasingly to farming. His orange grove attracted much attention,[7] especially among those who doubted that the trees could survive an uncommonly cold winter. The grove was presumably damaged by a freeze in 1886 and destroyed by a more severe freeze on the night of December 29-30, 1894, when the temperature dropped to 12 above zero.[8]

The date of Dr. Smith's death has not been ascertained. The Census of 1900 indicates that he was living in the Pine Hill District of Bradford County at the age of 70. His wife's Christian name is recorded as Mary E., perhaps Elizabeth.

There is no record of Dr. Smith's ever having been affiliated with the Florida Medical Association. The directory of physicians practicing in Florida, published by the Association in 1898, includes Dr. Smith. His post office was New River, a town some nine miles west of Starke.

1. The greater part of the vital data relating to Dr. Smith is derived from his military record as a soldier in the First Florida Special Battalion, a unit of the Second Florida Cavalry Regiment.

2. Records, Medical College of South Carolina, Waring Historical Medical Library, Charleston. Dr. Smith's place of birth, Coosahatchee, never more than a village, is located in Jasper County, South Carolina, a few miles north of Ridgeland. In earlier days it was in Beaufort County.

3. NA, Service Records, CSA, Second Cavalry Regiment.

4. Ibid.

5. Ibid.

6. U.S. Census, 1870, Bradford County, Florida, item 39.

7. Webb, Wanton S., *Webb's Historical, Industrial and Biographical Florida*, New York, W.S. Webb & Co., Pt. I, 1885, p. 32. The 1885 Agricultural Schedule, Bradford County, Florida, lists Dr. Smith as owner of 160 acres of land, only 10 acres were under cultivation. It is assumed that this was his orange grove. The total value of his farm was $4,100.

8. Although the freeze of January 8-10, 1886, was destructive (the Jacksonville *Florida Dispatch* of January 8 reported that the oranges were frozen solid, the trees survived), it was not so devastating as that of the night of December 28, 1894. The Jacksonville *Daily Florida Citizen* of December 30, 1894, reported these temperatures for the previous night: Palatka, 12 above; Titusville, 10 above; Callahan, 12 above; and Fernandina, 10 above.

Smith, Andrew Kingsbury, New Smyrna, 1899

Dr. Smith, a native of Connecticut, attended Jefferson Medical College, Philadelphia, from which he was graduated in the spring of 1849.[1] The summer of 1853 found him in Florida. When Dr. Robert Southgate, surgeon at the Army post in New Smyrna, was ordered to Texas in early 1853, Major Allen Lowd, commander of the post, notified the Surgeon General that as a replacement he had made a contract with Dr. A.K. Smith "to attend the troops here."[2] It appears that Dr. Smith was a civilian but on June 26, 1853, he was appointed Assistant Surgeon, U.S. Army.

It is not known how long Dr. Smith remained in Florida but he subsequently went on to a successful career as an army physician. He was on active service with the Union Army during the Civil War and was promoted to Major Surgeon on June 11, 1862. Twenty years later on July 2, 1884, he was named Lieutenant Colonel Surgeon and, finally, on July 10, 1889, Colonel Surgeon. He retired from the Army on February 9, 1890, but lived for another nine years, dying on August 14, 1899.[3]

1. List of Graduates, Jefferson Medical College, Philadelphia, p. 87.

2. National Archives, Surgeon General Records, Letter: A. Lowd, Brevet-Major, U.S. Army, Commanding, New Smyrna, to Lt. A.J. Lock, Asst. Adj. Gen.

3. Francis B. Heitman, *Historical Register and Dictionary of the United States Army*, Washington D.C., Government Printing Office, 1913, p. 894.

Smith Daniel A., Marion County, 1830-1909

Dr. Smith, who did not settle in Florida until after the Civil War, was born in Richard County, South Carolina, on October 14, 1830.[1] The medical school he attended remains unidentified, although his obituary implies that he was indeed a graduate of a medical school. After graduation it is said that he settled in Georgia in the early 1850s and began his practice there. In 1856 he married Mary Wadsworth. With the outbreak of the Civil War he enlisted in the 22nd Georgia Regiment with the rank of captain and served as Regimental Surgeon.

At the close of the War Dr. Smith returned to Georgia, settling in Butler, county seat of Taylor County, about 30 miles southwest of Macon. He did not arrive in Florida until 1884, when he settled in Anthony, a farming community in Marion County northeast of Ocala. Soon after he was elected mayor. Given his experience and popularity it is not surprising that in 1895 he was elected to the Florida House of Representatives, in which he served for one term. Soon thereafter, although he had enjoyed rugged, robust good health he suffered a paralytic stroke. He died at Anthony on September 24, 1909, and was accorded full Masonic funeral service. He was survived by his son and daughter-in-law, Mr. and Mrs. W.W. Smith, and a sister who lived in Texas.

1. The Ocala *Banner*, September 24, 1909.

Smith, James, Tallahassee, 1836

The Tallahassee *Floridian* of July 7, 1836, had the announcement that Dr. Smith had permanently located in Tallahassee. His office was located at Franklin Place on Madison Street. He had apparently employed the term "Permanently" loosely. He does not appear in the Florida Census of 1840 nor in later censuses.

Smith, John Patrick, Leon County, 1839

Dr. Smith was born in the Miccosukee community of Leon County in 1839. His father, Patrick Smith, a North Carolina native, was a farmer of above average means, his property having been valued in excess of $40,000[1] in 1860. As a young man Dr. Smith began the study of medicine under the preceptorate of Dr. Flavius A. Byrd of Miccosukee, a popular physician who had obtained professional training at Jefferson Medical College in Philadelphia before settling in Miccosukee.[2] In the fall of 1859 he was enrolled at the Atlanta Medical College but remained for only one term, leaving without a degree.[3] He returned to Miccosukee where he began the practice of medicine.

With the Civil War well under way Dr. Smith enlisted for Confederate service. Four days later, on December 15, he was mustered in as a corporal and assigned for duty in Company A, Fifth Florida Infantry Regiment.[4] Although his military record is quite incomplete, he apparently went with his unit to Virginia and participated in the Second Battle of Manassas (or Bull Run) in late August 1862. His record shows that he was promoted to sergeant on August 19, 1862. All information is missing relating to his whereabouts for the next two years. In July 1864 he is listed as First Sergeant and "detailed for duty as Assistant Surgeon." The final entry on his record for September-October 1864 shows him "absent on furlough."[5]

With the war experience behind him Dr. Smith returned to Miccosukee to resume medical practice[6] and operate the family farm. Census data indicate that he married a local girl, Alice, in 1864. Eight children were born: Edwin, Carolina, Thomas, Annie, Patrick, Mary, Charles and George. Thomas died prior to 1885. There is no evidence that Dr. Smith ever engaged in medical practice as a full-time occupation.

1. U.S. Census, Leon County, Florida, p. 50.
2. Dr. Byrd was one of the most eminent physicians of antebellum Florida. Prior to attending Jefferson Medical College, he had graduated from the University of Alabama.
3. See *Annual Announcement of the Atlanta Medical College*, Atlanta, Georgia, 1859.
4. National Archives, Confederate Records, 5th Florida Infantry Regiment.
5. Census data and Confederate Records indicate that Dr. Smith was married while on furlough in late 1864.
6. It is obvious that after return to civilian life Dr. Smith was more farmer than physician. A "List of Medical Practitioners in 1870," compiled by the University of Pennsylvania Medical Department, lists Dr. P. Smith of Miccosukee as an active practitioner.

Smith, William F., Marion County, mid-19th century

Except for the fact that he was born in Tennessee about 1820, nothing is presently known of the early years and education of Dr. Smith, a resident of Marion County in the mid-19th century. In October 1853, a notice of the sale of a farm in Marion County, 320 acres, located six miles from Silver Springs, appeared in the Ocala *Florida Mirror.* It was reputed to be "good land, with good water." Persons interested in purchasing the property were advised to inquire of Dr. Wm. Smith, "now residing there."[1]

In 1860 the census enumerator noted his presence there, designating his occupation as "planter" and his properties, real and personal, valued at $7,600. As for the family, Dr. Smith was a widower. His household included five children, all natives of Tennessee. They were: James, 21; Mary E., 18; Martha L., 16; Juliett, 12; and William F. Jr., 10.[2]

Notwithstanding his apparent domestic responsibilities, Dr. Smith succumbed to the pressure of his convictions and offered his professional services to the Confederate cause and was mustered into Company "G," Ninth Florida Infantry Regiment at Gainesville on March 5, 1863, reporting for duty at Bronson on March 17, committing himself for "three years, or the War."[3] His military record is only partially legible. It includes an item from the office of the Judge Advocate certifying that "William F. Smith is entitled to pay as a witness before the court martial, for a period from December 21, 1863, to January 4, 1864." The case involved a soldier who had deserted, but was apprehended.

Since Dr. Smith's named does not appear in the Florida census of 1870, it is conjectured that he moved from Florida prior to that date, possibly to return to his native state.

1. Ocala *Florida Mirror*, October 7, 1853.
2. U.S. Census, 1860, Marion County, p. 275.
3. Military Records, Confederate States of America, Ninth Florida Infantry.

Smoke, Samuel D., Newnansville, Micanopy and Ft. Ogden, 1837

Dr. Smoke, a native of Orangeburg, South Carolina, where his medical preceptors were Drs. Powell and Templeton, spent the greater part of his professional career as a rural practitioner in Alachua County. He was graduated from the Medical College of South Carolina[1] in the class of 1859, his doctoral thesis was entitled "The Abuse of Tobacco," and shortly thereafter established his practice in Newnansville, a town already declining in population due to transfer of the county seat to Gainesville in 1854. In 1860 he was living in the home of a Newnansville farmer, W.H. Kennedy.[2] Census schedules indicate that Dr. Smoke was married about 1862; his elder son Samuel was born that year. It is possible that the Smoke family sojourned briefly in Lake City for the local newspaper of March 22, 1865, printed an appeal to all persons indebted to Dr. Smoke to make payment immediately to Mrs. Smoke, "his legal attorney during his absence."[3]

Soon afterward the Smoke family, including another son, Wallace, and daughter, Sallie, moved to Micanopy where they remained for a couple of decades and Dr. Smoke became the town's "leading physician." They lived there at the time of the daughter's marriage to James S. Lewis Jr. on June 25, 1889.[4] Mrs. Smoke's death apparently occurred in the early 1890s.

Dr. Smoke remarried about 1898 a woman some 32 years his junior and moved to Ft. Ogden in DeSoto County[5] where he lived out his life. The date of his death remains unavailable.[6]

1. MCSC, "List of Graduates," Archives, Medical University of South Carolina, p. 127.
2. U.S. Census, 1860, Alachua County, Florida, Item 352.
3. Lake City *Columbian*, March 22, 1865. There is no record of military service for Dr. Smoke.
4. Caroline B. Watkins, *The Story of Historic Micanopy*, Gainesville, 1976, p. 47. See also Carl Webber, *The Eden of the South*, N.Y., 1883, p. 126.
5. The destruction by fire of most of the census schedules of 1890 has created an unfortunate hiatus in vital statistical information. The schedule, however, for 1900 is a valuable source which provides actual dates and places of birth, family relationships, occupations, and time spans of marriages. U.S. Census, 1900, DeSoto County, Florida, p. 362. Dr. Smoke is shown to have been married for two years and still practicing his profession.
6. The *Catalogue of the Physicians of the State of Florida*, Jacksonville, 1898, p. 13, lists Dr. Smoke as a practitioner in Ft. Ogden. Records of the Florida Medical Association do not show that he was ever a member. Dr. Smoke's son, Wallace H., also became a practicing physician in the village of Luraville, Suwannee County. See Catalogue mentioned supra, p. 13.

Snipes, William T., Leon County, 1838-1899

Dr. Snipes, a native of Georgia, was born on April 6, 1838.[1] Evidence points to the probability that he was a graduate of the Southern Botanico-Medico College in Macon, Georgia,[2] about 1858. He moved to Leon County in 1859 and established his practice, having taken residence in the home of John Grambling, a farmer living in the northern part of the county.[3] He gave up practice in March 1862, enlisted in the Army of the Confederacy and was assigned as a private to Company K, Fifth Florida Infantry Regiment.

Although Dr. Snipes was doubtless a man of intelligence and good judgment he was never given a medical assignment during his army career nor promoted to officer's rank, although he had become a sergeant by early 1863. This is strange since the commanding officer of Company K was Richmond N. Gardner, also a Leon County physician.[4]

The Fifth Florida Regiment had scarcely completed its organization before it was sent to the combat area of Northern Virginia, participating in the Second Battle of Manassas and the Maryland campaign. Back in Virginia it fought in the Battle of Gettysburg where Captain Gardner lost an arm and where 1st Lieutenant Joel C. Blake of Leon was killed.[5] The following year the Fifth was involved in the Battle of the Wilderness and at the engagement near Spottsylvania Court House on May 3 Dr. Snipes was taken prisoner, not to be released until June 23, 1865. Confederate records include this personal data: "William Snipes, M.D., Place of residence, Thomasville, Ga., florid complexion, red hair, blue eyes, height, 5 ft. 7½ inches."

By late 1865 Dr. Snipes was once more in Florida. On January 5, 1866, a Tallahassee paper carried this announcement:[6]

Dr. W.T. Snipes—Reform Medical Practice.
Having permanently located at Centreville, offers his services.

Thus he introduced his botanico-medico variant of Thomsonianism to the people of Centreville, notwithstanding the fact that by mid-century it was already under attack by leaders of the medical profession.

Dr. Snipes married Mary Ann Willis of Leon County in the late 1860s, daughter of Mrs. Sarah Willis, already a widow at age 25.[7] To this union were born three daughters, Mamie, Sadie and Maud, and two sons, Roscoe and Clarence.[8] The Snipes family continued to live in the Centreville community throughout the century. As late as 1885 Dr. Snipes was an active practitioner[9] but little is known of his participation in community affairs. Death came on Christmas Day, 1899. He was buried in nearby Pisgah Church Cemetery.

1. Dates of his birth and death are from his gravestone in Pisgah Church Cemetery near Centreville. Joy Smith Paisley, "The Cemeteries of Leon County, Florida," a compilation sponsored by Tallahassee Chapter, DAR, Tallahassee, 1978, p. 108.

2. This conjecture is based on the fact that the Macon college was the only institution of its type prior to the Civil War in the State of Georgia. Dr. Snipes was a Georgia native.

3. U.S. Census, 1860, Leon County, Florida, Sheet 77, Item 442.

4. NA, Service Records, CSA, M251, Roll 67.

5. Soon after Lt. Blake's death members of his company, "The Dixie Yeomen," met near Culpepper, Va., and drew up a statement expressing their esteem and respect for the fallen leader. Dr. Snipes helped draft the statement. Tallahassee *Florida Sentinel*, August 18, 1863.

6. Tallahassee *Semi-Weekly Floridian*, January 5, 1866.

7. U.S. Census, 1850, Leon County, Florida, p. 54. Her husband, Jessie R. Willis, had died on April 24, 1850, at the age of 34. He was buried in Pisgah Church Cemetery. See note 1, supra.

8. Florida, Special Census, 1885, Leon County, p. 144.

9. Ibid., Mortality schedule, p. 2. Dr. Snipes is shown to have been the attending physician of six persons who had died in the year 1884-85.

Snowden, Peter Gaillard, Gainesville and Ocala, 1823-1889

Dr. Snowden, son of William and Lydia Gaillard Snowden, was born in Charleston, South Carolina, in 1823.[1] Nothing is known of his early years but it may be assumed that he enjoyed the advantages common to members of the slave-owning aristocracy of tidewater South Carolina. In 1842, at the age of 19 he matriculated at the Medical College of the State of South Carolina, Charleston, from which he was graduated in March 1844.[2] On November 20, 1845, he married Laura Stephens, daughter of a prominent family of St. Stephen's Parish, Charleston district.[3] Having inherited, probably through his mother, a fairly large plantation in the northern part of St. John's Parish, Berkeley (Charleston District), in the vicinity of Black Oak, Dr. Snowden and his bride repaired to their estate and settled down to the life of the gentry. Their neighbors and friends included members of well-known families: Porcher, Sinkler, Cordes, Gourdin, and Gaillard. Most of them were of French Huguenot extraction, all members of the Episcopal Church.[4]

It is not known when Dr. Snowden began the practice of medicine but since the Census of 1850 designated him "physician,"[5] it is likely that he had begun practice prior to that date. It appears certain, however, that he was also a planter, as identified in the Census of 1860.[6] Inevitably he also entered into the social and religious life of the community. In 1856, for example, he was a member of the Pineville Jockey Club, contributing to the purse to be awarded to the winner of one of the major horse races.[7]

As the late 1850s came on the tranquil existence of the planters of Black Oak and Pineville communities, whose welfare was tied to a slave-based economy, was seriously threatened. Their anxiety reached its peak with the election of Lincoln in November 1860. In early December the South Carolina Legislature called for a Secession Convention to meet on December 17. On December 20 a "secession ordinance" was adopted, South Carolina being the first state to declare itself. Present at the Convention were two delegates from St. John's Berkeley. One of them was Dr. Snowden, owner of 50 slaves and total property valued at $42,000.[8]

From this point nothing is known of the South Carolina phase of Dr. Snowden's career. By the outbreak of the War in 1861 he was a widower, aged 38, with five children whose ages ranged from 13 to two. Consequently he would hardly have been subject to conscription for military service. It is likely that he remained in his home community trying to eke out a living for his family. With emancipation of his slaves in 1863 and dissipation of his other resources he was doubtless left in considerably reduced circumstances.

The date of Dr. Snowden's move to Florida is not known but it is thought to have occurred in 1871.[9] The earliest extant announcement of his medical practice in Gainesville is that of March 1873 when he announced his services to the citizens of Gainesville.[10] Like many other physicians of the times he also became the proprietor of a drug store; in fact, the Census of 1880 designates him only as "druggist." He is also known to have invested modestly in land at the western end of the Alachua Lake (Payne's Prairie), an area which lent itself to prosperous vegetable farms and orange groves.[11]

Little public notice attended Dr. Snowden's professional activities, but occasional references to his medical practice suggest that he was a capable practitioner and a beloved human being. Far better known is his role as a religious leader in Gainesville's Holy Trinity Church, then known as Trinity Church. A devout Episcopalian since youth, his services to Holy Trinity during the difficult years of Reconstruction and later are incalculable. For months at a time the Church was without a priest. During these intervals Dr. Snowden was always there as lay reader to conduct services and hold the little congregation together. Wrote the historian of the Church, B.P. Richards, "The high morale during these trying conditions was undoubtedly due in part to Dr. P.G. Snowden...who kept the parish in working condition."[12] Not to be overlooked was the service of Dr. Snowden's wife, Mrs. Lilla Snowden, to Holy Trinity. In 1877 she was President of the Woman's Auxiliary.[13]

Dr. Snowden left Gainesville for Ocala in 1881 where he was to spend the remainder of his life. He resumed the practice of medicine. His son, Rene, had established a drug store in Ocala and Dr. Snowden had lived there for a year during the mid-1870s. He continued to practice medicine until near the end of his life. He died in October 1889.[14]

Dr. Snowden was twice married. His second wife, a native of North Carolina, is known only by her Christian name, Lilla. Born to the first wife, Laura, were five children: Charles Stephens, who became an Episcopal clergyman;[15] Lydia Gaillard, Edwin, Mary B., and Rene.[16] To his second wife, Lilla, were born Susan, Sally, Bolivar and Laura.[17]

1. For the Gaillard family connections see *South Carolina Historical and Genealogical Magazine*, XLIII, 1942, 222.
2. Charleston *Mercury*, March 19, 1844.
3. *South Carolina Historical Magazine*, LXXVI, 1975, 172.
4. The Parish Church of St. John's, Berkeley, better known as the Biggin Church, was located about seven miles south of Black Oak post office. See Robert Mills, *Atlas of South Carolina*, originally published in 1820, revised in 1825, revised again, Columbia, 1965.
5. U.S. Census, 1850, Charleston District, St. John's Parish, South Carolina, p. 403, item 163.

6. Ibid., 1860, p. 149, item 1.

7. Pineville, located in the extreme northern part of Berkeley County, has survived up to the present, though still a small village. The horse races were an annual affair. No betting was permitted, although members of the Jockey Club were expected to contribute a dollar each to a purse to be awarded to the winners of certain races, notably the one-mile race. Other members of the Club included the Ravenels, Porchers, Gaillards and Sinklers, all notable Huguenot families, South Carolina Historical Magazine, LXXXI, 1980, 182.

8. Ibid., LV, 1944, 192.

9. Dr. Snowden probably moved to Florida in late 1870. He is not listed in the Florida Census of 1870 nor has his name been located in the South Carolina Census of that year. See B.P. Richards, "History of Holy Trinity Episcopal Church, Gainesville." Typescript; 3 bound volumes, unpublished. Richards cites vital information concerning Dr. Snowden provided by two granddaughters, Mrs. Nelson of Tampa and Mrs. W.A. Shands of Gainesville. According to them Dr. Snowden established his residence in Gainesville in 1871.

10. Gainesville *The New Era*, March 22, 1873.

11. Jess G. Davis, *History of Gainesville Florida*, Gainesville, 1966, p. 30. According to the Snowden granddaughters, Dr. Snowden had traveled to Gainesville before the Civil War and purchased "a plantation" outside the town. This is probably accurate. During the later antebellum days innumerable South Carolinians invested in Florida land.

12. Richards, "History" contains numerous references to Dr. Snowden services to the Church.

13. Ibid., I. 63.

14. Ibid., I. 98. Professor George R. Bentley, who prepared a history of Holy Trinity Episcopal Church, Gainesville, has provided the following information concerning Dr. Snowden's Ocala years. (1) The parochial report for Grace Church, Ocala, for the year ending May 1883 was submitted by "R.R. Snowden, Secretary." Diocese of Florida, Annual Journal, 1883, p. 54. R.R. Snowden was almost certainly Dr. Snowden's son, Rene R., the Ocala Druggist. (2) P.G. Snowden, M.D., was a lay delegate from Grace Church, Ocala, to the annual diocesan convention of 1887 held at Holy Trinity, Gainesville. Diocese of Florida, Annual Journal, 1887, p. 12. (3) Dr. Snowden was also a delegate from Grace Church at the diocesan convention of 1888 held at St. John's Church, Jacksonville, p. 10.

15. Charles Stephens Snowden, Dr. Snowden's eldest child, became an Episcopal clergyman. He occasionally held services at Holy Trinity when the Church was without a rector, journeying from his parish in Ellaville, Columbia County. In the mid-1880s he was parish priest and missionary at Macclenny, Baker County, where he died during the yellow fever epidemic in 1888. Richards, "History," I, 16.

16. U.S. Census, 1860, Charleston District, S.C., St. John's Berkeley Parish, p. 149, item 1.

17. U.S. Census, 1880, Alachua County, Florida, p. 64, item 520.

Snyder, Martin, Apalachicola, 1840

Dr. Snyder practiced medicine in Florida for a brief period about 1840-41. His professional card of December 23, 1840, announced that he was returning to Apalachicola after an absence and that his services were available "at 33 Water Street, upstairs."[1] His announcement continued to appear in the early part of 1841.[2] Nothing further has been discovered concerning him.

1. Apalachicola *Florida Journal*, December 23, 1840.
2. Ibid., March 21, 1841.

Sondag, Francois J., St. Mary's River Settlement, 1799

Dr. Sondag, surgeon, is known only through the record of his having taken an oath of allegiance to the Spanish crown on January 26, 1799. He was born in Alsace, obviously into a family of German origin. He was of Roman Catholic faith, a resident of St. Mary's district and swore that he was bringing in only movable property. It is a matter of speculation that he was a kinsman of Dr. Karl Sontag who resided in Fernandina "Old Town," c. 1810.[1]

1. E.F.P., Bundle 350 U4, Reel 163.

Sontag, Karl, Fernandina, 2nd Spanish Period

Very little is known about Dr. Sontag beyond the facts that he was of German birth and after coming to Fernandina during the Second Spanish Period he was granted lots in the "Old Town" on which he built a house and a hospital.[1] The date of construction of these edifices appears to have been 1810.[2] The hospital was probably the first nonmilitary hospital established in Florida. There is little doubt that it was much needed since the Fernandina settlement was in the grip of a lawless and depraved element. Stabbings and other bodily injuries were commonplace.[3] One observer noted "the frequent brawls among the sailors along the Paseo de las Damas," and the casualties which "were cared for by Dr. Sontage, or by quiet burial parties."

1. From "Spanish Land Grants in Fernandina" compiled by WPA researchers, in this instance probably Louis J. Mendelis. A bound copy of these unpublished and unclassified materials is in the P.K. Yonge Library of Florida History, University of Florida. See supra, Francois J. Sontag.

2. The grant included half lots 3 and 4, Square 7, corner of Calles San Fernando and Commandante. See 1811 map of Fernandina by George I.F. Clark, surveyor-general of Florida, P.K. Yonge Library of Florida History, Map, 1911, 232. A modern map, prepared by Franz and Maria Dollheimer and based on Clark's notes, locates actual holdings of various residents of Fernandina as of 1810. See Helen R. Pink, "Amelia Island: Resource Unit for Teacher in Secondary Schools," unpublished dissertation, University of Florida, 1949, facing p. 221.

3. S.C. Hood, "The St. Mary's, A River of Turmoil," mimeographed copy of unpublished, manuscript, p. 77, MS, Box 60, James Hall Folder, P.K. Yonge Library of Florida History.

Southgate, Robert, military surgeon, 1815

Dr. Southgate was born in Virginia about 1815.[1] Nothing is presently known of his early education, either general or professional. In 1836, at the age of 21, he was commissioned Assistant Surgeon in the United States Army.[2] It is not known where he spent the next 14 years but in 1850 he was at Ft. Brooke, Tampa Bay, his rank unchanged. Two years later he was stationed at the army post in St. Augustine. On January 17, 1852 the local newspaper, *The Ancient City*, printed the following announcemnt:

> Dr. Southgate, U.S. Army, has requested us to state that he will hereafter decline private practice among the inhabitants of St. Augustine. To strangers and visiters (sic) in the City his professional services are respectfully tendered.

Dr. Southgate did not long remain in St. Augustine. In early 1853 Major Allen Lowd, Commander of the New Smyrna Army Post, wrote to the Surgeon General: "Assistant Surgeon Southgate, having been ordered to leave this post for Texas, I have made a contract with Dr. A.K. Smith...to attend the troops here." Upon receipt of the order sending him to Texas, Dr. Southgate immediately resigned his commission effective on May 31, 1853. Nine months later on February 22 he was reappointed to his former rank only to resign once more on March 31, 1856.[3] He subsequently entered private practice in Virginia.

With the outbreak of the Civil War Dr. Southgate's services were required by the Confederate Headquarters in Richmond. His appointment was an important one: Senior Surgeon and ex officio Medical Director of the Confederacy. At a meeting of the Advisory Council, State of Virginia, a panel which included Judge John J. Allen, Col. Francis H. Smith, Captain M.T. Maury, and presided over by the Lieutenant Governor of Virginia, Dr. Southgate's services in the Confederate cause were discussed.[4] His role as medical officer at Yorktown during a critical phase of the War is a matter of record. On August 21, 1861, Brigadier General J. Bankhead, Commander at Yorktown, wrote to General Samuel

Cooper, then in Richmond, calling attention to the shortage of quinine for treating the Yorktown troops suffering from malaria. He pointed out that Dr. Southgate's order for a hundred ounces of this medicine had received no response from Richmond headquarters. He pointed out also that in the lowlands about Yorktown and Williamsburg fevers were endemic, and only by an adequate supply of quinine could they be effectively dealt with.[5]

Dr. Southgate, however, did not survive the War. The date of his death is given as 1864.[6]

He was a superbly literate and scholarly practitioner. "An Essay Read before the Medical Association of the State of Georgia, at their Annual Meeting at Rome, Georgia, April 11, 1860," has survived. It is a thorough examination of the practice of blood-letting as a therapeutic procedure and was printed at the office of the Augusta *Constitutionalist* in 1860.

1. U.S. Census, 1850, Hillsborough County, Florida, p. 492, item 80.
2. Francis B. Heitman, *Historical Register and Directory of the United States Army*, Washington, Government Printing Office, 1903, Vol. I, p. 908.
3. Ibid.
4. *War of the Rebellion* Washington, Government Printing Office, 1891, Ser. I, 51, Vol. 2, p. 55.
5. Ibid., p. 246.
6. Heitman, loc. cit.

Spann, Willis J., Ocala, 1819-1849

Dr. Spann, a native of Sumter District, South Carolina, was born in 1819.[1] In the fall of 1836 he entered the Medical College of the State of South Carolina, Charleston, from which he was graduated in the spring of 1838 after submitting a thesis titled "Acute Hepatitis."[2] He appears to have returned to his home district for a few years of practice before moving to Ocala in the spring of 1846. On July 3, 1847, he announced his services to the citizens of Marion, Alachua, St. Johns, Levy and Benton (later Hernando) Counties,[3] a preposterous undertaking given the primitive conditions prevailing in much of the area. His Ocala office was located at the corner of Professional Street and Merchants Row. In May 1848 he announced the opening of a drug store in connection with his office.[4]

Dr. Spann is thought to have been the first physician to settle in Ocala.[5] This may, in part, account for his immediate success in building up a substantial clientele, but more likely it was his gentle spirit and high level of intelligence which attracted patients. He died quite suddenly of a heart attack on December 31, 1849, while on a visit (possibly professional) to Indian River (City), Brevard County. The following remarks were included in an obituary notice which appeared in the St. Augustine newspaper.[6]

> From his first settlement in Florida the writer of this notice was acquainted with him. There soon grew up between them an intimacy and friendship which was never disturbed, and which was strongly cemented by the high qualities of the deceased. Intellectually and morally Dr. Spann was very happily gifted, and those who enjoyed his confidence and witnessed his professional skill are mournfully admonished of the uncertainty of the brightest prospects and hopes of life.

1. St. Augustine *The Ancient City*, January 12, 1850. The 1840 Census of Sumter District contains upward of a dozen entries of the name Spann including one Willis Spann, possibly the father of the doctor.
2. Charleston, S.C., *Mercury*, March 19, 1838.
3. Ocala *Argus*, February 1848; 1st printing July 3, 1847.

4. Ibid., May 25, 1848.
5. Eloise R. Ott and Louise H. Chazal, *Ocali Country*, Oklawaha, Florida, 1966, II, 48.
6. See note 1, supra.

Speer, Algernon Sydney, Orange and Volusia Counties, 1818-1857

Dr. Speer (Spear) was born in Abbeville District, South Carolina about 1818.[1] His parents were Alexander and Elizabeth (Middleton) Speer,[2] whose families were of substance and good social standing in that state. Virtually nothing is known of Dr. Speer's early education nor medical training although it is assumed he served an apprenticeship under an Abbeville physician.

The passage in August 1842 of the congressional Armed Occupation and Settlement Act was a significant event in the history of Florida. It encouraged white settlers to homestead in those parts of the state most vulnerable to renewal of Indian hostilities following cessation of the Second Seminole War earlier in the year. The lure of free land prompted the immediate migration of scores of settlers mostly from South Carolina and Georgia. Of particular importance was settlement of the territory now encompassed by Orange, Seminole, Volusia and Brevard Counties. An added inducement was assurance that the settlers would receive protection against any possible renewal of Indian attacks. Dr. Speer was among a group of South Carolinians who accepted the challenge and acquired land on the southern shore of Lake Monroe which is now within the corporate limits of the City of Sanford.

In spite of the recent defeat of the Indians they still posed a threat to the land-hungry migrants as they were pushed farther southward and westward. In 1844 many settlers who had arrived in late 1842 and early 1843 discovered that the lands on which they had settled were unsuitable for agriculture. Flooding was a major problem. Even safe drinking water was unobtainable in some parts. In March 1844 60 heads of families petitioned Congress for a revision of the Settlement Act which would allow them to abandon their earlier homesteads and move to more desirable lands. Dr. Speer was among the petitioners;[3] he had arrived in Florida in 1843.

The renewed pressure against the Indians, of course, provoked retaliation. The renewed threats prompted the white settlers to make appeals to Governor Thomas Brown for the promised protection. Arthur Ginn, Dr. Speer's father-in-law, informed the Governor on January 13, 1852, that the Mellonville area was especially vulnerable, and in case of raids he expected the Governor to provide protection. The following postscript was appended to his letter:[4]

> Dr. Spear informs me that in your communication made to him some twelve or eighteen months ago that you promised him in case of any difficulties, that you would give us full protection....we will therefore depend upon you in such an event.

Throughout the years 1843 until the time of his death in 1857 Dr. Speer's medical career appears to have been overshadowed by his success in citrus growing. He had homesteaded on good land and had built an imposing two-story frame house of many rooms from which he is known to have offered hospitality to occasional travelers in the area. John Cole Ley, a well-known Methodist clergyman, wrote in his diary:[5]

May 7, 1846—This afternoon we reached Ft. Melon (sic) having seen no man or human habitation during the day. We were the guests of Dr. Speer, and comforts and luxuries we relished.

So widely publicized were his citrus groves that in April 1852 he was one of five Florida physicians chosen by Governor Brown to attend an important industrial convention in New Orleans in early May. It is not known whether he attended.[6]

Inevitably, given his intelligence and qualities of leadership, Dr. Speer was drawn into public life. From April 1 to December 1, 1854, he served as postmaster of Mellonville and that year was appointed judge of the probate court of Orange County.[7] In the fall of 1854 he was elected to the Florida House of Representatives from Orange County, serving also in the adjourned session the following year. As a legislator his principal committee assignment was as chairman of the Indian Affairs Committee.[8]

As for Dr. Speer's medical career very little is known. Under threat of Indian attacks formation of a militia unit from Orange County was ordered by Governor Brown and placed under the command of Major General Benjamin Hopkins of the 2nd Division of Florida Militia. Among his instructions to General Hopkins, Governor Brown wrote: "I will suggest the name of Arthur Ginn, Esq., of Enterprise, as qualified for the duties of Quarter Master...and Dr. A.S. Spear, of the same place as Surgeon. Dr. S., I believe, acted in the same capacity in the last Indian disturbance... .He is an estimable gentleman, and stands high in his profession."[9] In a dispatch to Governor Brown on June 26, 1852, General Hopkins reported from his headquarters at Ft. Mellon: "I thought it advisable...to detach Dr. Spear from the command, and directed him to accompany the sick to Ft. Capron,[10] at which place he arrived safely in two days. He was kindly received by the United States officers, and every attention rendered the sick."[11]

One further incident establishes Dr. Speer as a continuing medical practitioner, notwithstanding his nonmedical enterprises. In June 1852 Major Thomas W. Jones, a member of the Mellonville militia, was stabbed by Private George M. Grouard, a Jacksonville enlistee, at the store of H.A. Crane. Whereupon "Dr. Speer was sent for, but he could be of no service to the unfortunate man who was stabbed to the heart."[12]

Dr. Speer was twice married. His first wife, Mary, was the daughter of Arthur Ginn, a native of Ireland, who was also an early settler in the Mellonville area. To this marriage were born five children: Arthur (1839-1889), Mary C. (1843-1920), Algernon S. (1845-1919), Catherine and Frederick, both of whom are thought to have died in childhood, and finally, Ella (1850-1912). After the death of Mrs. Speer in the early 1850s, Dr. Speer married Julia A. Hart of Jacksonville, to whom a daughter, Lula Josephine Middleton Speer, was born in 1856.[13]

As was true of most physicians in 19th-century Florida, Dr. Speer did not find medical practice a lucrative occupation and like many others turned to other pursuits. Besides citrus groves, which seem to have yielded substantial income, he turned to shipping on the St. Johns River. By the early 1850s his boats were plying the river from Lake Monroe to Jacksonville. He was able to capitalize on the militarization of the area in 1852 by the "hire of lighters, boats, etc." for the sum of $216, and for the "transportation of supplies" for $240.[14]

It was while engaged in such work in 1857 that Dr. Speer met a tragic death, an account of which appeared in the Jacksonville *News* about the first of September 1857. There is an unfortunate lacuna among the preserved issues of that newspaper but the account was reprinted in the Tallahassee *Floridian and Journal* of September 12, 1857.

> FATAL AND MELANCHOLY ACCIDENT—Our community experienced deep sorrow at the receipt of the intelligence, by the Darlington, on its last trip down, of the drowning of Dr. A.S. Spear, of Orange Co. He was being towed across Lake George in a small steamer owned by him, in company with his little son, Mr. Peter Eveleth, and a negro boy belonging to the Doctor. While being thus towed, and while going on, as far as was observed by those on the Darlington, in safety, the little craft was seen suddenly to capsize, capsize, or go under, leaving those on board to struggle for life. The boat of the Darlington was lowered at once, and her engine checked, but before the Doctor could be reached, he sank to rise no more, and with him his negro boy. His little boy clung to a floating box, and was picked up. Mr. Eveleth, also by swimming, kept himself up until he was reached and rescued, though he was found in a nearly exhausted condition.

The craft referred to was the Steamer Hancock which had plied the Savannah River from Savannah to Augusta for some time. It was purchased by Dr. Speer on September 15, 1853.[15]

Family tradition says Dr. Speer's young son was saved by two empty jugs tied together and attached to his body, enabling him to remain afloat until rescued. This account, doubtless coming from the boy himself, is probably correct.

1. This date is an extrapolation from the Census of 1850 which gives Dr. Speer's age as 32.
2. The genealogical data is derived chiefly from Mr. and Mrs. G. Andrew Speer of Sanford. Letter, Mrs. Speer to E.A. Hammond, January 26, 1979. Their kindness is gratefully acknowledged. Among the Marriage and Death notices gleaned from various South Carolina newspapers and published in the *South Carolina Historical Magazine*, Vol. XLVIII, p. 115, appeared the following notice: "Married: on Friday 13, (1813), Mr. Alexander Spears, student of law of Abbeville District, to the amiable and accomplished Miss Eliza Middleton, daughter of Major Hugh Middleton, deceased, of Edgefield District."
3. TP., Vol. XXVI, Territory of Florida, 874-876.
4. Letter, Arthur Ginn to Gov. Thomas Brown, January 13, 1852. MSS, Box 37, P.K. Yonge Library of Florida History, University of Florida,. Gainesville.
5. John C. Ley, *Fifty-two Years in Florida*, Nashville, 1899, p. 67.
6. Tallahassee *Florida Sentinel*, April 20, 1852.
7. Letter referred to in note 2 supra.
8. *Journal, Florida House of Representatives*, Tallahassee, 1854, p. 3, et passim.
9. Ibid., Tallahassee, 1852, Appendix, p. 63. Gov. Brown to Gen. Hopkins, February 29, 1852.
10. Ibid., p. 84. Gen. Hopkins to Gov. Brown, June 26, 1852. Ft. Capron was located on the west bank of Indian River, three miles north of Ft. Pierce.
11. Given the terrain and the unbridged streams which had to be crossed this two days was a remarkably short time for such a movement.
12. Jacksonville *Florida Republican*, June 17, 1852.
13. Ex info Mrs. Speer. See note 2 supra.
14. *Journal*, House of Representatives, 1852, App., p. 139.
15. Ex info Mrs. Speer, see note 2, supra.

Spence, William Alexander, Duval County, 1816-1893

Dr. Spence,[1] whose Florida career spanned the last 19 years of his life, arrived in the state in 1874, settling first in Orange County from which he moved to Jacksonville in 1880. He was born in Westmoreland County, Virginia, near the town of Montross on November 26, 1816, son of Edmund and Sally Hackney (nee Sisson) Spence who belonged to the planter aristocracy. His father had been an artillery officer in the War of 1812. In his early youth Spence attended Benjamin Holland's (Quaker) school in Alexandria, Virginia, and later Dickinson College in Carlisle, Pennsylvania, but did not remain to earn a degree.

While in Alexandria young Spence was frequently in the company of

Washington socialites. In a letter dated at Alexandria on November 11, 1834, addressed to his sister, he related the exciting experience of witnessing a balloon ascension, following which he made the acquaintance of "many of the young ladies of Washington, among whom was the beautiful Miss Woodbury, daughter of the Secretary of the Treasury (Levi Woodbury), under whose hospitable roof I spent several hours and met several ladies of the District."[2]

At one of the social functions he was introduced to Dr. Cousins, "the most eminent physician of the City." He added:

> During my stay there we (i.e., Dr. Cousins and I) discovered some relationship which made his friendship for me almost unbounded. He has offered to assist me in the study of medicine which I have determined shall be my profession so that I may become a useful member of society.

Thus was Spence's professional goal set and in October 1837 he matriculated at the Medical Department, University of Pennsylvania, from which he was graduated Doctor of Medicine on April 6, 1839. His doctoral thesis was entitled "Secale Cornutum."[3]

Dr. Spence began practice at the village of Tidewater, Virginia, some 15 miles from the place of his birth. Soon after the outbreak of War he enlisted (in May 1861) as a private in the Confederate Army but within a matter of weeks was elevated to the rank of surgeon and assigned to field service. His rise in the military was rapid. He was soon promoted to the rank of major with the medical rank of Brigade Surgeon. He later became Chief Surgeon, First Division, 10th Army Corps, under the command of General A.P. Hill (in the Army of Northern Virginia) and after the death of General Hill in April 1865, serving in the Division of General Henry Heth (Heath).

Dr. Spence stood so high in the estimation of General Robert E. Lee that the General appointed him medical examiner for the exchange of prisoners at Charleston, South Carolina, in 1864. Later, when his health became impaired from too much exposure in the field, he was assigned to duty in Richmond where, at the time of the surrender of the Confederacy, he was in charge of sick prisoners at Libby Prison.

At the conclusion of the War Dr. Spence resumed medical practice in Baltimore. In 1870 he moved to Savannah, practicing there for four years before moving to Orange County in 1874. There he planted an orange grove and encouraged others to do likewise. During his brief stay he was an active member of the Fruit Growers Association of Orange County.

In 1880 Dr. Spence made his final move, settling into medical practice in Jacksonville, to find that his professional reputation had preceded him. He immediately became a member of the Duval County Medical Society before which he read several professional papers. In 1883, at its meeting in Jacksonville, the Florida Medical Association elected him to membership and at the same session chose him to represent the Association at the annual meeting of the American Medical Association, and also at the upcoming meeting of the Georgia Medical Association.[4] He was present at the 1884 meeting of the Association, again held in Jacksonville, but in subsequent meetings at other towns there is no record of his attendance, although he continued to pay annual dues.

In his politics Dr. Spence was a staunch States' Rights Democrat, having been very active in Virginia and continuing his participation in Florida. In Orange

County he was Chairman of the Party. He was proud of his Scottish heritage and in Jacksonville was President of the Scottish Association, presiding over the celebration of the 128th anniversary of the birth of Robert Burns.

There can be no doubt that Dr. Spence was an outstanding member of the medical profession as well as a distinguished and beloved citizen. The following excerpts from eulogies elicited by his death indicate the general esteem in which he was held:

> Dr. Spence was a large-hearted man. He possessed in an eminent degree all those qualities of head and heart that attach men to each other. He was an unflinching friend where one was needed, showing by his action that no sacrifice of personal comfort must stand in the way of serving a friend. The warm grip of his hand, the genial smile, the work of tender interest, all bespoke his sympathy with his fellow man. Of magnificent physique, replete with vigorous life, a heart that knew no fear, and yet, I have seen the tear-drop gather in his eye when some case of destitution was brought to his notice, and no such appeal was made in vain. "His pity gave where charity began."
>
> He was a good son and brother, an affectionate husband and father, and a valuable citizen. He was a member of the Protestant Episcopal Church, a vestryman of St. James Church, Montross, Virginia, and later of St. John's Church, Jacksonville, Florida, for several years.

Dr. Spence was twice married, first to Cornelia Green of Columbia, Pennsylvania, daughter of Evan Green, a merchant of the town. They had seven children: daughters Sally, Cynthia and Mary; and sons Edward Evan, William Alexander, Evan, and Jasper Green. His second wife was Mrs. Archie White, daughter of Benjamin P. Gaines[5] of Gaines Landing, Arkansas. No children were born to this union.

Dr. Spence died in Jacksonville on April 11, 1893. He had suffered a paralytic stroke a few years earlier and spent his last two years in almost constant pain which, it was said, he bore with heroic patience. He was buried in Jacksonville's Evergreen Cemetery.[6]

1. Abundant biographical material relating to Dr. Spence exists in the Archives of the University of Pennsylvania. It was made available by the kindness of Maryellen C. Kaminsky, Archival Specialist. No effort has been made to identify each of the various items included in the Spence folder.

2. A photocopy of this letter, in a very legible hand, has been made available for the present study. It was written by Dr. Spence to his sister, Mrs. Mary Hungerford.

3. The term, *secale cornutum* as it appears in the list of medical theses submitted by candidates for graduation at the Medical Department, University of Pennsylvania, is not clear. The Latin *secale* designates a kind of grain, pro-rye, and would appear to have a pharmaceutical application. It may possibly have been intended as *sacral*, the adjective referring to the sacrum, the lowest bone of the spine, which, if true, would have a medical connotation.

4. *Proceedings, Florida Medical Association*, 1883, Jacksonville, 1883, passim.

5. The identity of Mrs. White's father, Benjamin P. Gaines, has not been determined. Such evidence as is available points to the probability that he was a son of James Gaines (1742-1830), who was twice married and sired seven children by each of his wives. If so, Benjamin Gaines would have been a brother or half-brother of the well-known Edmund Pendleton Gaines. Some information relative to this is found in a letter: Joe Ingraham, U.S. District Judge, Houston, Texas, to U.S. District Judge, Sidney O. Smith, Gainesville, Georgia, dated July 3, 1968. Copy in MSS. Collection, P.K. Yonge Library of Florida History, University of Florida, Gainesville.

6. The obituary notice of Dr. Spence lists only one surviving member of the family, a daughter. A tabulation of the grave markers in Evergreen, compiled and published in 1955 by Lucy Ames Edwards, contains two errors: the name is spelled Spenser, the date of death, 1898.

Spencer, Samuel W., Apalachicola, 1807-1865

Dr. Spencer, a native of Maryland and graduate of the University of Maryland School of Medicine in the class of 1828,[1] made his first appearance in Florida when he arrived in Apalachicola aboard the *Roanoke* from Columbus, Georgia, in December 1840.[2] In all probability he had previously practiced medicine in Georgia where his elder child, Ann Elizabeth, was born in 1839.[3] Lacunae in local newspapers make it impossible to construct a year-by-year calendar of his activities, but his professional card printed on August 12, 1843, implies prior practice in Apalachicola, stating that "Dr. Spencer, having returned to the City, offers his services..."[4] His office and residence were located on Live Oak Street in a house previously occupied by C. Rogers.[5] A few weeks later he obtained office space upstairs in the Baltzell Building but continued to live on Live Oak Street.[6] In April 1844 he advertised the receipt of a new shipment of fresh medicines.[7]

For about a year Dr. Spencer served as physician of the Marine Hospital in Apalachicola, having replaced Dr. John Gorrie in that position. He is said to have become dissatisfied with the meager pay attached to the job, wishing to relinquish the duties and turn them over to Dr. Gorrie, but when Dr. Gorrie refused to consider returning, he remained until June 30, 1846, but received no pay for either his services or the medicines he dispensed.[8] He remained a close friend of Dr. Gorrie until his death in 1855, having actually witnessed Dr. Gorrie's will.[9]

Random references indicate that Dr. Spencer took an active interest in local civil and political matters. In 1846, for example, he and Dr. Gorrie were members of a committee to remedy the lack of military defenses for the port and town of Apalachicola.[10] In 1852 he represented Franklin County Democrats at the State Convention held at Madison Courthouse,[11] at which he and Dr. John Westcott were selected to represent Middle Florida at the National Democratic Convention in Baltimore.[12] In 1854 he ran for the State Senate, losing by a narrow margin to Whig candidate Thomas G. Eppes.[13] In 1861 he represented his county at the famous Secession Convention which convened in Tallahassee on January 3. He was among the majority voting for secession.[14]

Dr. Spencer is known to have died prior to 1870, although the exact date has not been determined. The census schedule of 1870 shows his widow, Henrietta, still living in Apalachicola, the only other members of the household being two black servants. Neither of the Spencer children, Ann Elizabeth and Samuel Jr., appears in the Franklin County census of that year.[15]

1. E.F. Fauntleroy, *Historical Sketch of the University of Maryland*, 1807-90, Baltimore, 1891, p. 198.
2. Apalachicola *Florida Journal*, December 23, 1840.
3. U.S. Census, 1850, Franklin County, Florida, p. 328.
4. Apalachicola *Watchman of the Gulf*, August 12, 1843.
5. Ibid.
6. Apalachicola *Commercial Advertiser*, January 8, 1844, first printing December 4, 1843.
7. Ibid., April 20, 1844.
8. Raymond B. Becker, *John Gorrie, M.D.*, New York, 1972, p. 74.
9. Ibid., p. 137.
10. Apalachicola *Commercial Advertiser*, May 30, 1846.
11. Ibid., April 19, 1852.
12. Tallahassee *Floridian and Journal*, May 22, 1852.
13. Jacksonville *Florida News*, October 14, 1854.
14. *Florida Historical Quarterly*, "Notes and Comments," V, No. 2, April 1926, p. 118.
15. U.S. Census, 1870, Franklin County, Florida, p. 703.

Spotswood, Narborne Dandridge, Pensacola, mid-19th century

Very little information has been forthcoming on the Florida career of Dr. Spotswood. He was the brother of the well-known William Augustine

Spotswood,[1] naval surgeon who served several tours of duty at the Hospital of the Pensacola Navy Yard. He made his first recorded appearance in Pensacola in August 1848 when he tendered his "professional services to the citizens of Pensacola and vicinity, in the several departments of his profession,"[2] stating that he had some years of experience. His office was located "in the room adjoining the office of the *Florida Democrat*." At a slightly later date he established a drug store, known as Spotswood and Company on Palafox Street opposite the Winter's House, from which he carried on his medical practice.[3] He apparently continued his practice until the beginning of the Civil War, at which time he entered service as a Confederate surgeon.[4]

Dr. Spotswood is thought to have received his medical education at Kemper Medical School (later to be called Missouri Medical School) in St. Louis.[5] Since no further information about him has turned up in Florida sources, it is assumed that he did not return to the state after the War.

1. Dr. W.A.W. Spotswood spent a major part of his long career in Pensacola, which may account for his brother's decision to settle there.
2. Pensacola *Florida Democrat*, August 17, 1848.
3. Pensacola *West Florida Times*, March 17, 1857.
4. Dr. W.R. Chitwood to Prof. E.A. Hammond, December 2, 1976. Dr. Chitwood made an exhaustive study of the Spotswood Family out of which emerged his article, "Dr. Spotswood and the Confederate Navy," *Virginia Medical*, October, 1976, pp. 728-733.
5. Ibid.

Spotswood, William Augustine Washington, Pensacola, 1806-1891

Dr. Spotswood,[1] who spent the greater part of his professional career as a navy surgeon, was born in Orange County, Virginia, on October 3, 1806, of distinguished lineage. An early ancestor, Alexander Spotswood (1676-1740), was Governor of Virginia and two generations later another Alexander Spotswood, the doctor's grandfather, was a renowned general in the Revolutionary War. Dr. Spotswood's paternal grandmother, Elizabeth Washington, was a niece of President Washington. His father, George Washington Spotswood, served in the War of 1812 as a member of the Orange County company of the 2nd Virginia Regiment. He married his cousin, Lucy Spotswood.

When he was 19 years of age Dr. Spotswood's family moved to Charlottesville where the University of Virginia had recently been established and where he began medical studies. Records of the University show him to have been a mediocre student, ranking tenth in a class of 13. Probably discouraged by his unimpressive record he left the University without a degree in the summer of 1828. Before the end of the year, however, he was commissioned Assistant Surgeon in the United States Navy.[2] With or without the proper professional credentials Dr. Spotswood was an impressive looking man, of adequate intelligence, and the bearing of a natural leader. The Confederate Secretary of the Navy, Stephen R. Mallory, described him as a "brawny, gray-haired, six-footer, rough and ready in ways and looks, but a gentle-hearted man."[3]

Dr. Spotswood's first assignment, aboard the USS St. Louis, ended in December 1831 when he was assigned to Norfolk, Virginia, just in time to face a severe epidemic of cholera, a disease entirely new to his experience. By way of experiment he is said to have abandoned the regimen of emetics and bleeding in favor of opium, calomel, brandy and water with slightly better results.

He arrived in Pensacola, probably in late 1832, to assume the position of chief medical officer of the hospital at the Navy Yard where he remained for about three years before being reassigned to sea duty on ships of the West Indies Station. In 1837 he received the significant promotion to surgeon and in 1842 returned to the Pensacola Navy Yard. Shortly thereafter he married Mary R. Eastin, daughter of Col. Thomas Eastin of Mt. Vernon, Alabama.

After three years at Pensacola Dr. Spotswood was returned to sea duty. With the Mexican War under way he was sent to a naval station in the vicinity of Vera Cruz, thence back to Pensacola. In 1857, however, he became Fleet Surgeon to the East Indies Squadron composed of four steam frigates and three sloops. He was again assigned to the Pensacola Naval Station in 1860. When Florida seceded from the Union in January 1861, he faced a dilemma. After more than 30 years in U.S. naval service he doubtless had regrets about leaving but within a few days he cast his lot with the Confederacy. In recognition of his extensive experience as a navy surgeon he was appointed Chief of the Bureau of Medicine and Surgery by Confederate Secretary of the Navy, Stephen R. Mallory, himself a Pensacolan and erstwhile friend of Dr. Spotswood. Before assuming duties in Richmond he moved his family for safety sake to Monroeville, Alabama, some hundred miles north of Pensacola.

Due to the destruction of war records in the burning of Richmond not much is known of Dr. Spotswood's war years. Such evidence as has survived, however, indicates that he was an efficient and successful administrator, notwithstanding the enormous difficulties in obtaining medical supplies, particularly quinine, so much needed in the treatment of malaria from which great numbers of Confederate soldiers suffered.

At the war's end Dr. Spotswood went to Monroeville but by 1870 he had returned to Pensacola with his family where the census enumerator found them that year. His older children having left the home, the schedule included, besides the doctor and his wife Mary then 46, a daughter, Lutie 18, and three sons, Barclay, Charles and Dillon, 15, 12 and nine respectively.[4] The doctor himself is designated only as "physician." His properties were valued at $700.[4] It is known, however, that during this last residence in Pensacola he held the post of Quarantine Officer. His final years were spent in Mobile, Alabama, where he died on September 7, 1891. Since he was not listed in the Escambia County Census of 1880, it is assumed that he had moved to Mobile prior to that date. Mrs. Spotswood's death had occurred seven years earlier. Both were buried in Mobile's Magnolia Cemetery.

1. In 1976 Dr. W.R. Chitwood of Wytheville, Virginia, published a lengthy and well-documented biographical sketch of Dr. Spotswood. See W.R. Chitwood, M.D., "Dr. Spotswood and the Confederate Navy," *Virginia Medical*, October 1976, pp. 729-733. The present sketch is condensed from Dr. Chitwood's work.

2. It was not at all uncommon that medical students with minimal professional study obtained licenses to practice. Especially was this true in rural and remote areas. Prior to organization of the American Medical Association in Philadelphia in 1847, and for many years thereafter in some regions, measures for the regulation of the medical profession were few and seldom rigidly enforced. There is no reason to assume, however, that Dr. Spotswood, even without a medical degree, was not a good and conscientious physician.

3. Joseph T. Durkin, S.J., *Stephen R. Mallory, Confederate Navy Chief*, Chapel Hill, University of North Carolina Press, 1954, p. 143.

4. U.S. Census, 1870, Escambia County, Florida, p. 163.

Staggers, John G., Marion County, 1860

Dr. Staggers, one of several South Carolinians who settled in Marion County in the antebellum period, was apparently more planter than physician.[1] The Census of 1860 lists him at age 29 owning property valued at $75,000, a portion of which represented his investment in slaves, who numbered 63. It is assumed that the Civil War dealt him a disastrous blow. He does not appear in any subsequent Florida census schedules, which indicates that he had left prior to 1870.

1. U.S. Census, 1860, Marion County, Florida, item 85.

Staley, John W., Jackson County, 1850

Dr. Staley appears to have practiced medicine in Jackson County for a brief period about the year 1860. The census of that year lists him as 33 years of age, native of South Carolina.[1] He appears to have been a restless type, having married a native of North Carolina, Rebecca, by whom he had three children: Benjamin, born in Alabama, aged eight; Sarah, aged five, born in Georgia; and Emma, aged two, born in Florida. He is assumed to have departed the state prior to 1860.

1. U.S. Census, 1850, Jackson County, Florida, item 178.

Stanfill, James T., Calhoun County, 1828-1899

Dr. Stanfill[1] or Stanfield, as it appeared in the Census of 1860, was born in South Carolina in 1828.[2] He was the firstborn of Thomas and Martha Stanfill who moved to Georgia soon after his birth. They later moved to Alabama where they lived for a few years before settling in Calhoun County about 1847.[3] The Stanfills were among the earliest inhabitants of the Long Cane precinct situated on the west side of the Apalachicola River some 10 miles north of present-day Blountstown. Long Cane enjoyed the distinction of having its own post office from 1856 to 1859.

Nothing is known of Dr. Stanfill's early education or medical training.[4] There is no evidence that he was a medical practitioner until he was of middle age; instead, he appears to have been engaged in farming, as were his father and brothers. In the late 1850s he was elected sheriff of Calhoun County[5] and in 1860 owned properties valued at more than $3,000 which meant that he was comparatively "well off" in a county which could boast of not more than a dozen families of substantial means. Ten years later in 1870 the census enumerator listed him as "farmer" with property valued at $1,400.[6]

At some time in the 1870s Dr. Stanfill moved to the village of Marystown[7] located some 10 miles south of Blountstown and four miles west of the Apalachicola River. There is evidence that he was indeed a medical practitioner. The Census of 1880 designated him "M.D." and the list of recognized Florida physicians compiled by the State Board of Health and published in 1898 by the Florida Medical Association[8] includes him as a properly licensed member of their faculty. He continued medical practice in Marysville until his death in 1899. He was buried in the Shiloh Cemetery.

Although the record of Dr. Stanfill's militry service is incomplete, he is known to have enlisted for service in the Confederacy on May 1, 1863, furnishing his own horse. He was assigned to Company "A," 2nd Florida Cavalry. He was among the troops who surrendered to Union authorities on April 26, 1865. He was paroled at Baldwin, East Florida, on May 17 following.[9]

Census schedules indicate that Dr. Stanfill was thrice married. To his first wife, Sarah, a South Carolina native, was born one child, a son named William.[10] To his second wife, Mary, were born three children, Daniel, Mary and Henry.[11] To his third wife, Jane, were born Elizabeth, Margaret, Jane and Sarah.[12]

1. Notwithstanding its proximity to prosperous Jackson County and the navigable Apalachicola River, which formed its eastern boundary, Calhoun County's economic development was slow. Much of its territory, which included all of what would later become Gulf County, did not lend itself to the development of a plantation system. Its sparse population and lagging economy meant that historical records, especially for the antebellum period, were few. The first newspaper published in the county, the Altha *Times*, appeared in 1946. The searcher must therefore rely heavily on census schedules for information concerning the county's 19th century history.

2. Works Projects Administration, Florida #7, Calhoun County. Veterans' Graves Registration, St. Augustine, 1940-41, p. 13. The dates of Dr. Stanfill's birth and death were found on his gravestone in Shiloh Cemetery.

3. U.S. Census, 1850, Calhoun County, Florida, p. 76, items 138 and 139.

4. Dr. Stanfill is thought to have been trained as an apprentice to an established physician but this cannot be verified. His name does not appear in the lists of graduates of any of the well-known medical colleges which flourished in the South in the antebellum period.

5. U.S. Census, 1860, Calhoun County, Florida, Jacksonville, 1898, p. 120.

6. Ibid., 1870, Calhoun County, Florida, p. 301.

7. Ibid., 1880, Calhoun County, Florida, p. 295.

8. Florida Medical Association, *Catalogue of Physicians in the State of Florida*, pp. 13, 18.

9. It cannot be explained why Dr. Stanfill, a physician, at the age of 35, did not receive an officer's rank. He remained a private for the two years of service. He received $24 per month for the "use and risk" of his horse. National Archives, Service Records, CSA., M251, Roll 12.

10. See note 3, supra.

11. See note 6, supra.

12. See note 7, supra.

Starke, James Douglas, Volusia and Alachua Counties, 1820-1903

Dr. Starke, a competent physician but better known for his public service, was born in Fairfield District, South Carolina, on March 31, 1820.[1] Son of Thomas Starke, who owned a plantation near Lynch's Creek, Dr. Starke had the advantage of being born into a family of comparative wealth. He received the best education available in the state, graduating from South Carolina College, later to become the University of South Carolina in Columbia. He then proceeded to Charleston and in 1845 was graduated from the Medical College of the State of South Carolina. His doctoral thesis bore the title "Hysteritis."[2]

About 1850, probably in 1849, the father of Dr. Starke and John S. Stark left his South Carolina plantation and purchased a large tract of land which had been a part of the old Spanish grant to Paul Dupon on the north side of Lake Monroe and including the site of old Enterprise about a mile east of the present town of that name. The tract also included Garden Springs, presently known as DeLeon Springs. He brought with him 60 slaves.[3]

Soon Dr. Starke also settled in the area, purchasing the property previously owned by Cornelius Taylor near Enterprise on which he built a fine home to which he gave the name Bueno Retiro,[4] said to have been the finest home in the area. It still stands today.

In 1860 Dr. Starke ran successfully for the Florida Senate and was present at the opening session on November 26. His committee assignments were Federal Relations, Claims and Accounts, and Schools and Colleges. He was returned to the Senate in the following year, serving on the Committees on Engrossed Bills, Claims and Accounts, Schools and Colleges. He appears in most instances to have voted with the majority. Only once was he in a conspicuous minority, that being a bill to be entitled "An Act to Reduce the Pay of the Surgeon." The vote was 16 to one for passage, the lone vote against having been cast by Dr. Starke.[5] Thirteen years later he was elected to the Florida Assembly (lower House) and distinguished himself by efforts to establish public schools in all areas of the state so that no child would be deprived of the opportunity to obtain a basic education.[6]

With the Civil War already well under way, Dr. Starke enlisted in the Army of the Confederacy on October 15, 1863, and was commissioned Captain and assigned for duty as Commanding Officer of Company H, Fifth Florida Cavalry Battalion. His duties never took him out of Florida. He first served at Headquarters, Outpost Army of Florida, near Jacksonville, and later with the same unit at Waldo. Apparently feeling that his maturity and medical skills were being wasted he wrote a letter of resignation to General Samuel Cooper on December 20, 1864, setting forth the following:[7]

> My military capacity is limited, while that of my successor has eminently qualified him for the position. I believe that I can serve my country more efficiently in some other department.

His request for termination of assigned service was granted although he was apparently not reassigned for further military duty. Doubtless, at age 44, retirement was a proper decision. At any rate he returned to private medical practice at Bueno Retiro which was then in Volusia County after the remaking of county lines.

At some time in the later 1880s Dr. Starke moved to Gainesville settling in a house at 405 East Orange Street, now 303 Northeast 2nd Avenue, where he and his family immediately endeared themselves to the people of the town. They were devout members of the Presbyterian Church. Dr. Starke died at his home on Sunday morning, June 14, 1903. He was buried in Evergreen Cemetery.

Dr. Starke was survived by his wife, Selina, for whom he was a second husband. Her first husband was a Mr. Ferber, by whom she had two sons. Her third and only child by Dr. Starke was a daughter, Margaret (Mrs. Perry).[8]

1. A lengthy obituary for Dr. Starke appeared in the Gainesville *Daily Sun*, June 16, 1903; it was headed, "Death of a Noble Man." Then followed an elegaic paragraph: "Gainesville is mourning today over the death of one of Florida's oldest and most beloved citizens—Soldier, Statesman, Gentleman—in the person of Dr. J.D. Starke, who passed away at his home on Sunday Morning."

2. Charleston, S.C., *Courier*, March 12, 1845.

3. U.S. Census, Orange County, Florida, Slave Schedule.

4. A house on the same location had been built earlier by Cornelius Taylor who named it "Bueno Retiro," good retreat. He had been living there a short while when his young daughter, an only child, had died of typhus fever, whereupon he decided to abandon the place. Soon thereafter Dr. Starke bought it and restructured the house. The gravestone of the Taylor child still stands near the house.

5. See *Florida Senate Journal*, 11th Session, November 1861, p. 150.

6. *Florida House Journal*, 1874.

7. NA, Service Records, CSA, Co. H., 5th Battalion, Florida Cavalry. Dr. Starke enlisted on October 15, 1863, at Volusia for the duration with rank of captain. His letter was written at Waldo.

8. See note 1, supra.

Staten, W.F., Hamilton County, 1847-1893

Dr. Staten was born near Stockton, Lowndes County, Georgia, on February 25, 1847.[1] He was the eldest son of Capt James W. and Caroline Malloy Staten. He received his medical degree from the University of Louisville Department of Medicine and settled in Jasper where he quickly gained a fine reputation as physician and citizen. On February 16, 1876, he married Ella E. Goodbread, daughter of A.S. Goodbread, a prominent Hamilton County planter, and they had two sons and two daughters.

Through the inheritance of Mrs. Staten the family came into possession of a tract of land outside the town of Jasper, some 326 acres, most uncleared.[2]

Toward the end of the 1880s the Statens moved back to Lowndes County, settling in Valdosta, where Dr. Staten resumed his practice.[3] His health soon began to fail, however, and he sought relief by spending winters at Charlotte Harbor, Florida, but it was to no avail. He died in Valdosta on June 21, 1893, survived by his aged mother, his wife and the four children.

1. Jasper *News*, June 23, 1893, obituary notice. This was followed in ibid., July 28, 1893, by a lengthier eulogy.
2. Florida Special Census, 1885, Hamilton County, Agricultural Production Schedule, Dist. 2, p. 7.
3. Ibid. Mortality Schedule, p. 2. This schedule shows him to have been one of the most active physicians of the county.

Steele, Holmes, Jacksonville, 1820-1867

Although his Florida career spanned a mere 10 years, Dr. Steele's influence in the fields of medicine, journalism, military service and politics was of tremendous importance. A man of exceptional intelligence, superior education, unwavering honesty and humanitarianism, his untimely death in Jacksonville on May 9, 1867, at age 47 stunned the community and evoked from many quarters expressions of sorrow and esteem.

Notwithstanding his prominence and popularity only a few details of his early life have survived. Dr. Steele was a native of Charleston, South Carolina, where he spent his childhood. His youth and early manhood he spent in Georgia.[1] Upon completion of his medical education (even the medical college he attended has not been identified)[2] he returned to Georgia and entered practice. In October 1865 he joined the faculty of Oglethorpe Medical College, Savannah, as Professor of Obstetrics and Diseases of Women and Children, a position he held for two sessions.[3] At the close of the term in March 1858 he relinquished his chair at Oglethorpe.[4] In the fall of the previous year, he had visited Florida, passing through Jacksonville, doubtless with the thought of returning and settling there upon completion of his Oglethorpe contract.[5] In April 1858, the Savannah *Republican* reported:[6]

> Dr. Holmes Steele, M.D., for some time back favorably known in Savannah as one of the professors at the Oglethorpe Medical College, has returned to Jacksonville where he contemplates establishing himself professionally. Dr. Steele is a gentleman of very superior ability in his profession, having assiduously devoted his mind to the same for the love thereof. On all medical subjects his skill will deserve the confidence and patronage of our friends in Jacksonville.

In November 1858, a Jacksonville hotel, Judson House, seeking to attract winter visitors, advertised in the Charleston *Courier*, including among its inducements, the following: "Dr. Holmes Steele, Editor of the *Standard*, is a

Charlestonian, and I know would greet you warmly."[7]

The medical faculty of Jacksonville in the 1850s included several outstanding physicians, some of whom were notable in fields other than medicine. Drs. Abel Baldwin, Richard P. Daniel, John S. Murdoch, and William J. L'Engle were men of broad education whose contributions to the general development of the community were significant. They were also prime movers in establishment of the Duval County Medical Society in 1863. In this fraternity Dr. Steele was quite at home. His superior qualifications were recognized and their welcome for him appears to have been warm. Even when he strayed well beyond the bounds of medical practice to serve in other areas their respect from him was undiminished.

Still unmarried at the time of his arrival in Jacksonville Dr. Steele took a room at the Holland House, a small hotel across from the post office and near the more pretentious Buffington House.[8] His office was also located at the Holland House. In the fall of 1859 he was married at St. Helena, a village in Columbia County, to Rebecca Summerlin, the wedding having taken place at the home of Capt. Thomas D. Dexter, a local merchant, on October 20.[9]

Meanwhile, Dr. Steele, probably motivated by the need to earn a better living but more likely from the desire to gain an instrumentality through which to publicize his political opinions and lend support to the Democratic Party, entered the field of journalism. In July 1858, he joined Ramon Canova in launching the Jacksonville *Standard* with himself as editor. The first issue evoked this comment from the Tallahassee *Floridian and Journal*: "We welcome into the Democratic brotherhood this new candidate for public favor...The first number gives earnest promise of vigorous support of Democratic men and measures. We commend it to the party throughout the State."[10] When Canova withdrew from the enterprise Dr. Steele was joined by Aristides Doggett and the paper continued to be published until December 1860 but during the last months it was plagued by financial losses due chiefly to the failure of advertisers and subscribers to pay their bills.[11]

As the interests of North and South came increasingly into conflict it was inevitable that Dr. Steele, a man of the press, should be drawn into political controversy. Foreseeing the probability of civil disorder and the possibility of military restraint he organized the Jacksonville Light Infantry on April 30, 1859, assuming the position of captain and commanding officer.[12] In October of the following year in a letter to the Tallahassee *Floridian and Journal*, he called attention to the number of volunteer units being organized in Florida, citing with pride the Jacksonville Light Infantry and urging the various units to associate into a Volunteer Battalion and obtain a charter from the State Legislature.[13] In February 1861, one month after Florida's secession from the Union, he offered his Jacksonville unit to Governor Perry.[14]

Meanwhile Dr. Steele had emerged as a civic and political leader while continuing medical practice.[15] Upon completion of the railroad connecting Jacksonville with Lake City he joined Dr. Baldwin in addressing a large gathering in the latter town in celebration of the event.[16] In April 1860, he represented Duval County at the State Democratic Assembly in Tallahassee. He was elected assistant secretary and by an interesting coincidence served with the famous Dr. John M. Gorrie who was secretary.[17] Dr. Steele was also a member of the Committee on Resolutions.

Four months later following the split in the national Democratic Party, Dr. Steele addressed the Duval County Democrats asembled in Jacksonville to ratify the nominees of the Southern wing, John C. Breckenridge and Joseph Lane. He is reported to have seized the opportunity to denounce the Northern nominee, Stephen A. Douglas.[18]

On January 8, 1861, the day following Florida's act of secession, Dr. Steele, although 40 years of age, enlisted for military duty. He was mustered in on August 10 when the Jacksonville Light Infantry became Company A of the Third Florida Infantry Regiment. He resigned his commission in November and returned to Jacksonville, only to reenter service in May when the Third Regiment was reassembled at Wartrace in Gadsden County. He was Adjutant at Regimental Headquarters. Soon thereafter he moved with his Regiment into the Chattanooga area where in August the unit was assigned to the brigade of General John C. Brown. The Regiment saw action in Tennessee and Kentucky, suffering severe losses at the Battle of Perryville, Kentucky. Shortly thereafter Dr. Steele was transferred to the Medical Department, spending the last year of the War as hospital surgeon at Ockmulgee Hospital in Macon.[19]

Upon his return to Jacksonville in the spring of 1865 Dr. Steele not only resumed medical practice but ventured once more into newspaper work. He was present at a meeting of the Duval County Medical Society on November 4, 1865, at which the eight physicians in attendance passed a series of resolutions relating to their professional policies.[20] In February 1866 Dr. Steele announced that he had returned to the city from service in the Florida Legislature and was available for professional consultations at his home "on Forsythe Street, between Market and Newnan Streets."[21] Soon thereafter he moved his office to City Hall, immediately over the Engine House on Bay Street, "where calls may be left at all hours of the day...at night at his residence."[22] Finally, in January 1867, he announced that he could be found at St. John's House, "first door to the right, where calls may be left."[23]

In July 1865, Dr. Steele assumed editorship of the Jacksonville *Herald*, a weekly paper published by E.H. Reed, who was also Jacksonville's postmaster. In less than a month, however, he gave up the position, his departure prompting the Gainesville *New Era* to remark: "the valedictory of the noble and brave Dr. Steele...whose editorial career, we regret, was so short."[24] But his editorial career was not finished. The rival Jacksonville *Florida Union* lost the services of W.C. Morrill in April 1865 and in the issue of September 30 Dr. Steele's name appeared in the masthead as associate editor with J.K. Stickney as editor and proprietor. This association continued through July 1866 after which Dr. Steele was no longer affiliated with Stickney. The termination of the partnership had not resulted from animosity, however, for the two men remained close friends up to the time of Dr. Steele's death. It appears to have been determined by his involvement in other matters; namely, medical practice, excursion into politics and acceptance of the office of mayor of Jacksonville.

Florida was placed under martial law on May 10, 1865. The negotiations leading to return of the state to more or less normal conditions were slow and troublesome. The way was cleared for elections to state offices in November 1865 and the election was held on the 29th. Dr. Steele was persuaded to run for Duval County's seat in the Senate. Duval and Clay Counties were paired for one seat. He won easily over the other candidate, Osias Buddington, a resident of Clay County, the resulting vote being 215 to 48.[25]

Dr. Steele's presence in the Senate was immediately felt. His committee assignments were Judiciary,[26] Public Lands (chairman), Executive, and the most challenging of all, the Committee on all Subjects Connected with the Colored People of the State. In that role he demonstrated his statesmanship and sound judgment by leading the fight against oppressive legislation which would have virtually reenslaved the Negro by rendering him punishable by pillory and lashing for crimes for which whites would have received only fines or brief imprisonment. His arguments were persuasive. "The Freedmen," he declared, "were committed to the care, to the guidance, and the tutelage of the Southern legislator. Let that master and friend legislate in the light of Christian charity." The bill passed, however, in spite of his plea.[27]

Later in the session Dr. Steele was chief spokesman in opposition to a bill which would have encouraged immigration of large numbers of Europeans to Florida "to revive her industry and develop her great resources." As chairman of the joint committee (Senate and House) charged with processing the bill, he argued that "in the present crippled condition of the financial resources of the State, and in view of the experiment which she is now making through legislation, to direct and utilize the class of laborers already in her midst, the Committee can see no means at her command to be used to advantage in the encouragement of immigration."[28] The proposal was never formulated into a bill.

In the second session of the 14th General Assembly Dr. Steele was equally active. His statements, such portions of which have survived in the printed *Journal*, are remarkable for their cogency and clarity. It is to his credit that he introduced into the Senate a bill which would have established a much needed State Medical Board. It appeared to have an excellent chance of passing, especially with its referral to a special committee composed of Dr. Steele, Dr. D.W. Whitehurst of Key West and Joseph Finegan who reported it favorably, but even with Drs. Steele and Whitehurst joined by a third physician-senator, Dr. John L. Crawford, all favoring it, the bill lost by a vote of 13 to 11. Dr. John M. Gorrie, for unknown reasons, had been excused from the voting.[29]

With adjournment of the Legislature on January 16, 1866, Dr. Steele returned to Jacksonville and on February 3 announced that he had resumed his professional duties at the Forsyth Street residence.[30] At about this time Jacksonville's incumbent mayor, Halstead H. Hoey, then in his third term, came under fire and was ousted from office. He was immediately replaced by Dr. Steele.[31]

Henceforth, until the beginning of the second session of the Fourteenth Legislative Assembly on November 14, 1866, Dr. Steele was mayor, physician, and associate editor of the Jacksonville *Florida Union*. As mayor his problems were many. As radical reconstructionists gained control of Congress and took advantge of the ineptitude of President Johnson it was virtually impossible for any Southern official to please his local constituents and still comply with federal mandates. Dr. Steele, a man of moderation, probably managed the dilemma as well as any could have done. Even on such a minor matter as publication of city ordinances he came under the fire of the Republican paper, the Jacksonville *Florida Times*, for having published a set of City Ordinances in the *Union*.[32] He survived this attack as well as subsequent ones on other issues with dignity and aplomb.

Dr. Steele returned to Tallahassee in November 1866 for the Legislative Assembly, the session ending on December 14. On January 8, 1867 he announced that he had resumed practice and could be found at "St. John's House, first door to the right, where calls may be left for him."[33] His remaining days were few, however. If he were indeed in failing health in those early months of 1867, the fact was never publicized. When death came suddenly on May 9 even his close associates appear to have had no warning and were duly shocked. The outpourings of sorrow were unprecedented. The Jacksonville medical faculty met and took appropriate action as did the Masonic Lodge, Solomon No. 20. Obituary notices appeared in the newspapers of Florida, Georgia and South Carolina, none more touching than that written by his older brother, Major John H. Steele.[34] He was survived by his widow and small daughter.

1. The biographical information is derived chiefly from the elegy which appeared shortly after his death in the Atlanta *Intelligencer*, of which Dr. Steele's older brother, Major John H. Steele, was editor. It read in part: "He was the youngest brother of the editor of this journal; South Carolina his native State; Georgia, during many years of his youth and early manhood; his residence, Florida, in the later years of his life, his home... The immediate family connections of the deceased in Georgia and South Carolina mourn the sad event." The elegy was reprinted in the Tallahassee *Sentinel* of May 28, 1867.

2. There is no record of Dr. Steele having attended the Medical College of the State of South Carolina nor any of the four medical colleges existing in Georgia in the mid-19th century.

3. Oglethorpe College of Medicine began its brief existence in November 1855 with Dr. E. LeRoy Anthony holding the chair of obstetrics. Savannah *Morning News*, September 27, 1855. For the session of 1856-57 during which Dr. Steele was Professor of Obstetrics, see Jacksonville *Florida News*, October 11, 1856.

4. Oglethorpe medical college existed for only four terms and throughout it was torn by internal strife, arrogance and jealousy on the part of its faculty. It opened in the fall of 1856 and closed in the spring of 1861. At one point Dr. Steele served as Dean of the faculty, having been chosen as the member most likely to bring a peaceful settlement to the conflict. His efforts were unavailing. The entire sordid affair was reported in detail in the Savannah *Daily Morning News* issues of March 17 and 18, 1859. The statement that Dr. Steele had spent five years as Professor at Oglethorpe, repeated by Dr. Webster Merritt in his *A Century of Medicine in Jacksonville and Duval County*, Gainesville, 1949, p. 50, is apparently an error.

5. In the fall of 1857 it was reported in Savannah that a sickness, presumably yellow fever was raging in Jacksonville. *The Savannah Morning News*, in an effort to ascertain the facts, solicited opinions from several Jacksonville physicians as well as Dr. Steele. He concurred with them to wit: IT WAS NOT YELLOW FEVER. He mentioned his recent trip to Florida and his visit to Jacksonville in mid-October. *Savannah Morning News*, November 3, 1857.

6. This item from the Savannah *Republican* was printed in the Fernandina *Florida News*, April 14, 1858.

7. Ibid.

8. Jacksonville *Standard*, March 17, 1859.

9. Fernandina *East Floridian*, November 3, 1859.

10. Tallahassee *Floridian and Journal*, July 31, 1858.

11. In the last issue on December 6 Dr. Steele offered his half interest in the paper for sale, adding that he was giving up editorial work.

12. Richard A. Martin, *The City Makers*, Jacksonville, 1972, p. 30.

13. Tallahassee *Floridian and Journal*, November 3, 1860. The letter ended on a gloomy note: "The times, gentlemen, are ominous, and while viewing the signs, let us in 'peace prepare for war,' for though no evile may come, yet it is imperative for the State to arm."

14. Martin, *City Makers*, p. 32.

15. When Samuel C. Emery, a young Jacksonville medical student matriculated at the Medical College of the State of South Carolina in the fall of 1861, he indicated that his preceptor had been Dr. Holmes Steele. See Archives, Waring Historical Medical Library, MUSC, Charleston, S.C.

16. Fernandina *East Floridian*, March 22, 1860.

17. Ibid., April 19, 1860.

18. Ibid., August 2, 1860.

19. Regrettably, the Civil War record of Dr. Steele has not been preserved. The data offered here are drawn from National Archives, Service Records, CSA, M251, Roll 52, and from the brief data in *Soldiers of Florida*, Board of State Institutions, Live Oak, 1903, pp. 99-103, which provide a brief history of the Third Florida Infantry Regiment.

20. Present were Drs. Abel S. Baldwin, Holmes Steele, E.T. Sabal, H.C. Vaughn, George E. McPherson, J.A.S. Todd, M.J. Murphy and R.P. Daniel. The chief matters under discussion were charity work, patients who were delinquent in paying bills and how they might most effectively be persuaded to remit payment. Jacksonville *Florida Union*, December 2, 1865.

21. Ibid., February 3, 1866.

22. Ibid., July 26, 1866.

23. Ibid., January 6, 1867.
24. Gainesville *New Era*, September 2, 1865.
25. Jacksonville *Florida Union*, December 2, 1865.
26. Serving on the Judiciary Committee of the Senate with Dr. Steele was his earlier companion-in-politics, Dr. John M. Gorrie.
27. *Florida Senate Journal*, 14th General Assembly, 1st Session, 1865-66, pp. 145-147.
28. Ibid., pp. 183-184.
29. Ibid., 2nd Session, 1866 m, pp. 35, 38, 41, 43, 47, 48.
30. Jacksonville *Florida Union*, February 3, 1866.
31. Martin *City Makers*, p. 90.
32. The Florida *Times*, established in Jacksonville by Ossian B. Hart and Harrison Reed and edited by W.H. Christy, became the mouthpiece of the radical constructionists and "scalawags." It was eventually consolidated with the Jacksonville *Florida Herald*. See *Times* issue of December 14, 1865.
33. Jacksonville *Florida Union*, May 18, 1867. The notice was first printed in the issue of January 8, 1867, not extant.
34. See note 1, supra. The reaction of the Jacksonville City Council to Dr. Steele's death was remarkable. It may be regarded as a true measure of the esteem in which he was held. After lamenting his death and expressing sympathy to his widow and orphan, they invited all citizens to his funeral. Council members were to wear mourning bands for 30 days; all businesses were requested to close from 2 to 7 p.m. on the day of the funeral "out of respect." Tallahassee *Sentinel*, May 14, 1867.

Stevenson, Henry, St. Marks, 1822

Dr. Stevenson, a native of Virginia, was commissioned assistant surgeon in the Medical Department, United States Army, on July 16, 1821. He had actually begun his military service on November 13, 1818, as surgeon's mate in the Sixth Infantry. He was serving at St. Mark's Hospital in 1822 when he was called upon to treat a case of ileus (severe blocking of the intestine resulting in constipation) on July 11, a soldier of the Fourth Regiment. The account gives the details of the treatment.[1] It was reported that the patient was recovering, "but slowly." Dr. Stevenson resigned his commission on August 31, 1833, presumably to engage in private practice.

1. American State Papers, Class V, Vol. II, 516, "Military Affairs."

Stewart, Charles F., Jackson County, 1840

Dr. Stewart was among the early settlers in the Webbville community of Jackson County. He first appears in the records as a participant in a Fourth of July celebration in Chipola in 1826 when he offered a toast to Joseph M. White, Florida's delegate in Congress.[1] He was one of the trustees of the Webbville Academy which was opened on February 27, 1827.[2] He was one of the most adamant supporters of the establishment of Webbville as the seat of Jackson County and when Lackland M. Stone announced his candidacy for reelection to the Legislative Council in 1828 (he had supported the Marianna proposal) Dr. Stewart actively campaigned against him.[3]

Very little is known of the Stewart family. The Census of 1830 offers little information beyond establishing Dr. Stewart's age as between 30 and 40 and his slaves as numbering four.[4] Since he does not appear in subsequent census schedules for Jackson County it may be assumed that he had died or moved to other parts before 1840.

1. Tallahassee *Florida Intelligencer*, September 1, 1826.
2. J. Randall Stanley, *History of Jackson County*, Marianna, 1950, p. 88.
3. Ibid., p. 50. The Webbville group angered by Stone's support of the Marianna group refused to support him and offered Dr. Stewart as their substitute candidate. The move, however, was unsuccessful for Stone was reelected.

4. U.S. Census, 1830, Jackson County, Florida, Sheet 83. The Stewart entry is confusing since only the head of the household is listed by name while the ages of the other male members range from under five to between 20 and 30. This seems to suggest that some of them were brothers of either Stewart or his wife.

Stewart, J. Edwin, Tallahassee, 1838

The medical career of Dr. Stewart was of short duration and tragic ending. A native of Cambridge, Dorchester County, Maryland, he arrived in Tallahassee with his wife, Charlotte Hodson Stewart, in the early 1830s.[1] Parish records of St. John's Episcopal Church show him to have been a parishioner as early as 1832.[1] Not until late 1833, however, did he give public notice that his services were available to the citizens of the city and vicinity from his office on Jefferson Street next door to Mr. Perkins' Drug Store.[2] For the next two years he appears to have gone quietly about his work. On January 2, 1836, he announced that he was moving to the "west end of Major Wyatt's New Brick Building, adjoining the new Post Office." To this he added an urgent plea that those "who are indebted to him for medical services for 1834 and 1835...make immediate payment."[3]

In May 1836 Dr. Stewart announced the opening of a new Drug Store in connection with his office, the enterprise to be run by a Mr. Lewis, "a well-educated and experienced druggist."[4] The arrangement continued for more than a year but was terminated when Dr. Stewart formed a copartnership with Edward Barnard Jr. and opened a new drug store "opposite the Market House, to be known as Stewart and Barnard."[5]

On June 4, 1838, Dr. Stewart, his wife and small son, brother William A. Stewart, and a servant girl, in company with five other Tallahasseans,[6] made the overland journey to Savannah, Georgia, where they boarded the recently commissioned steamer, Pulaski, for the voyage to Baltimore. The Stewarts were returning to Cambridge for a visit with relatives. The Pulaski left Savannah on the morning of July 13 and reached Charleston before nightfall. Sixty additional passengers came aboard and next morning the ship continued on to Baltimore. In late afternoon it ran into heavy seas off the South Carolina-North Carolina border, the over-pressurized starboard boiler exploded, virtually tearing the ship apart. Some passengers were saved in the four lifeboats, others by hanging on to the debris from the ship, but the majority of the more than 150 plus the crew members were lost. Among the casualties were Dr. Stewart, who had been in poor health before leaving Tallahassee and was too weak to hang on to a makeshift raft, his wife and small son. Of the Tallahassee group only William A. Stewart and the servant girl survived.[7]

Only the legalities of settling the Stewart estate remained. On September 15, the administrator, Joseph A. Richardson, made the customary requests that those with claims or obligations come forward and settle, while simultaneously Edward Barnard Jr. declared the copartnership dissolved "by the death of the senior partner."[8]

1. Parish Register, St. John's Episcopal Church, Tallahassee, typed copy, P.K. Yonge Library of Florida History, p. 9. Dr. Stewart was a member of the St. John's Church Building Committee.
2. Tallahassee *Floridian*, November 23, 1833.
3. Ibid., January 2, 1836.
4. Ibid., May 28, 1836.

5. Ibid., August 5, 1837.

6. Subsequent to the disaster several accounts appeared in numerous newspapers. Perhaps the most reliable is that of Dr. Stewart's brother, William, written on July 5, three weeks after the tragedy, and published in ibid., July 28. He identified the other Tallahasseans as "my relative, Samuel H. Hodson, the Rev. Mr. Woart (Rector of St. Johns), Mrs. Woart, a Dr. Ash (of Philadelphia), and F. McCrea."

7. St. John's Records show that the Stewart's firstborn, a son named Samuel was baptized on August 15, 1834, and died July 22, 1835. The second son, who was lost at sea, was christened Samuel Hodson on May 21, 1837. Parish Records, St. Johns, p. 12, 13.

8. Tallahassee *Floridian*, September 15, 1838.

Stewart, James A., Micanopy, 1823-1871

Dr. Stewart, one of six physicians practicing at Micanopy in Alachua County in 1860, was born in South Carolina in 1823.[1] He appears to have moved to Micanopy about 1852 accompanied by his wife, Angelina, and small daughter, Mary.

From the beginning Dr. Stewart was active in the public life of the village. As a member of the Democratic Party he was a delegate to the Alachua County Democratic Convention in Newnansville in 1856.[2] A year later he joined Col. George Leitner, who lived on nearby Lake Wauberg, in obtaining a commitment to extend the Florida Railroad from Hatchet Creek, thus bypassing the recently established county seat in Gainesville.[3] A short time later he was a member of the Micanopy delegation at a meeting in Ocala, their purpose being to block a reconsideration of the plan demanded by a delegation from Gainesville.[4] He was a sponsor for a series of lectures on the "Science of Geology" in 1860 given by Professor Augustus V. King, a member of the faculty of Hanover College, Hanover, Indiana.[5] In 1858, however, he was among the Micanopy voters opposing incorporation of the town, an act which, if passed, would have increased property taxes.[6]

Dr. Stewart became a property owner in Micanopy soon after his arrival, having purchased a plot of land from fellow physician, George B. Payne, in 1855. On a portion he built a two-room office at the south end of Main Street which he later enlarged into a residence.[7] In 1872 this property passed by purchase into the hands of William Edwards when Mrs. Stewart, then a widow, decided to return to her native state of South Carolina.[8]

Dr. Stewart's Florida career was marred by tragedy. His daughter, Mary, died on January 15, 1854, at the age of two, while his wife, Angelina, died on March 22, 1860, at the age of 29.[9] His second marriage, to Emma Fleming of Laurens, S.C., took place on November 6, 1867. It was, however, of brief duration, the doctor himself dying at some unknown date in 1871.[10]

1. U.S. Census, 1860, Alachua County, Florida, item 242. Although the medical college which Dr. Stewart attended has not been identified, it is possible that he may be identified as the James H. Stewart of Chester Court House, S.C., an 1848 graduate of the Medical College of the State of South Carolina. See Charleston *Courier*, March 23, 1848.

2. Jacksonville *Florida News*, March 29, 1856.

3. Tampa *Florida Peninsular*, May 1, 1858.

4. Ibid. The efforts of the Micanopy delegation came to naught. The divergence off the Fernandina-Cedar Key Line built years later bypassed Micanopy and later a spur off the Waldo-Ocala Line had no direct connection with either Gainesville or Ocala.

5. Fernandina *East Floridian*, February 9, 1860.

6. James L. Glunt Papers, II, MSS, P.K. Yonge Library of Florida History.

7. Caroline B. Watkins, *The Story of Historic Micanopy*, Gainesville, Alachua County Historical Commission, c. 1976, p. 74. This transaction is recorded in Alachua County Deed Book, 84, under the date January 26, 1855.

8. Ibid., pp. 74, 75.

9. Gravestones, Oak Ridge Cemetery, Alachua County. This cemetery is off State Road 234 between Micanopy and Rochelle.
10. Area newspapers of Ocala and Gainesville of this period contain many lacunae, making a search for an obituary fruitless.

Stone, Andrew, Orange County, 1847

The sojourn of Dr. Stone in Florida was brief and marked by tragedy. Natives of Indiana, Dr. Stone and his wife Harriet made their way to Florida in October 1847 seeking a benign climate for their young son, M. de Felenburg, and daughter, Harriet, both suffering from an illness diagnosed as "inflammation of the brain."[1] According to the Jacksonville *News* of November 12, 1847, the son died at Enterprise in Volusia County on October 31 at the age of four years and six months. In the style of the times the *News* added: "It is a severe dispensation of Providence which strikes down in the family of a stranger those who can alone enliven the hours of hardship and adversity."

Enterprise was the county seat of Orange County during this period. On May 31, 1924, its name was changed to Benson Springs; in 1937, however, it was changed back to Enterprise.

Devastated by the loss of their son, Dr. and Mrs. Stone elected to leave Florida. In mid-November 1847 they took passage on the schooner, *Hannah and Jane,* bound for New York. Before the ship cleared the St. Johns River their daughter, Harriet, suddenly became ill, dying after three days. She was five years old.[2]

Nothing further is known of this unfortunate family; they are presumed to have departed the state.

1. This was not an uncommon diagnosis of ailments of the head in those times.
2. Jacksonville *News,* November 19, 1847.

Stone, James B., Leon County, 1820-1842

The professional career of Dr. Stone was brief, lasting less than four years, most of which he spent in Florida. A native of Jefferson County, Virginia, he attended the Medical College of the University of Pennsylvnia from which he was graduated in the spring of 1839.[1] Soon thereafter he contracted his services to the United States Army,[2] practicing in Florida where the Second Seminole War was being waged.[3] In May 1840 he announced the opening of his practice in Leon County, stating that he would be residing in the home of Henry Branch on Lake Iamonia in the northern part of the county.[4] In December, however, he moved to Tallahassee renting office space in the store of J.B. Hall. His announcement included the statement, "Dr. Stone hopes from the considerable experience he acquired in the treatment of Southern diseases during his late connection with the U.S. Army to merit a share of patronage."[5]

Nothing further is known of Dr. Stone until February 1842 when he announced removal of his office "to the building lately occupied by General Searcy as a post office."[6] His untimely death came on December 26, 1842. He was buried in the churchyard of St. John's Episcopal Church, Tallahassee. His epitaph reads, in part: (He died) "in his twenty-third year, far from home of his nativity...son and brother."

1. Archives, Medical College of University of Pennsylvania, list of graduates. His doctoral thesis was entitled "Ventriculus Stomachus."

2. See note 5, infra.

3. Dr. Stone's name does not appear in the roster of Medical Department, U.S. Army, 1775-1873, which doubtless means that he was never commissioned but instead served as a civilian under contract.

4. Tallahassee *Star of Florida*, May 21, 1840.

5. Ibid., December 29, 1840.

6. Tallahassee *Florida Sentinel*, March 4, 1842. Gen. Searcy was Joshua G. Searcy, for a short time postmaster of Tallahassee, who was removed from the position by Postmaster General Francis Granger within two weeks after John Tyler assumed the presidency. TP, XXVI, 301.

Stone, Micah, St. Augustine, 1821

It has not been determined when Dr. Stone, a native of Massachusetts,[1] arrived in Florida. That he was not among those required to take the oath of naturalization after the secession of Florida to the United States would suggest that he had arrived at about the time the negotiations with Spain were under way, i.e., in the early summer of 1821.

When the ceremony of transfer of St. Augustine from Spain was completed on July 10, 1821, the Acting Governor of East Florida, W.G.D. Worthington, proceeded to appoint a full complement of public officials for his province. He forwarded his list to John Quincy Adams, Secretary of State, on February 1, 1822, with the note that these appointments had been completed as of August 20, 1821. The Board of Health for St. Johns County was composed of Dr. Stone, President (Dr. Wm. H. Simmons having declined the post), Dr. Richard Murray, Health Officer, with the St. Augustine Board of Aldermen to serve as ex officio members.[2]

Dr. Stone's term of office had scarcely begun when he and the Board faced altercations with the military establishment of the city, commanded by Capt. John R. Bell. The trouble sprang from two sources, refusal of Capt. Bell to relinquish to civil authorities any of the public buildings within the city and the resolution passed by the Board of Health demanding in the name of the safety of the citizens that the old Spanish hospital be removed from the center of the city to the so-called South Common on the southern fringe of the settlement. This demand, in the form of a resolution, had been drafted and signed by Dr. Stone with the concurrence of the Board.[3]

Capt. Bell, doubtless a capable military leader, took umbrage to the demands of the civil authorities, apparently regarding them as a threat to his own position as military commander. At any rate the dispute was intensified by Capt. Bell's overreaction and was brought to the attention of Governor Jackson and ultimately to the office of President Monroe who judiciously stated the opinion that "the military ought to yield every accomodation (sic) in their power to civil officers..."[4]

In connection with the bickering there developed a conflict of medical opinion relating to removal of the hospital. The army surgeon under Capt. Bell's command was Dr. Charles N. McCoskry who had advised the removal of all troops from St.Marks and the quartering of those who were ailing in the Old Spanish Hospital. It was also Dr.McCoskry who had endorsed Capt. Bell's contention that location of the hospital presented no hazard to the health of the civilian population since only a single soldier had died at the hospital since his arrival in the city. Inquired Capt. Bell, "does this look like a malignant disease? The disease I fear as it respects the hospital was only imaginary with the Hon(ora)ble Council." Hence a conflict between the two ranking physicians of the city. Looking back the folly of Capt. Bell's position is obvious. He adamantly defended it just as the most destructive yellow fever epidemic of the century was about to reach its peak in St. Augustine.[5] Dr. Stone's days were numbered, however. He died in St. Augustine at the age of 55 on December 3, 1821.[6]

1. St. Augustine *Florida Gazette*, December 10, 1821.
2. TP, XXII, 354-362. This volume contains numerous letters relating to the controversy, one of the most acrimonious being that of September 27, 1821, in which Capt. Bell stated his case. Ibid., pp. 215-217.
3. For the resolution as drafted by Dr. Stone, see ibid., p. 219.
4. Ibid., p. 246, No. 70. President Monroe to John C. Calhoun, Secretary of War, October 11, 1821.
5. Ibid., p. 197; ibid, pp. 216-217.
6. St. Augustine *Florida Gazette*, December 10, 1821.

Addendum: The Hospital, known as the Old Spanish Hospital, was located on the east side of Aviles Street, just off the public plaza. It was in use during the Second Spanish Period, 1781-1821.

Stonelake, A.B., Leon County, 1860

Although he was designated Doctor of Medicine in newspaper items relating to his activities, there is no evidence that Dr. Stonelake actually practiced in Florida. Instead he held an appointment as Registrar of the United States Consolidated Land Office in Tallahassee subsequent to the closing of the regional offices at St. Augustine, Newnansville and Tampa. In his capacity Dr. Stonelake announced that henceforth all applications for obtaining public land should be addressed to the Tallahassee office "where, in obedience to the above order I desire to state that I shall be ready to receive applications from all parts of Florida, on and after May 20, 1867." Signed: A.B. Stonelake, M.D.[1] A similar announcement appeared in the Gainesville *New Era*, June 8, 1867. Dr. Stonelake is not listed in the Florida Census of 1870. As a federal employee he did not long remain in Florida.

1. Tallahassee *Sentinel*, May 24, 1867.

Stork, William, St. Johns River Area, mid-18th century

In his researches on North Florida during the British Period, 1764-1784, Professor Daniel L. Schafer discovered a considerable amount of information relating to Dr. Stork, an adventurer who publicized the great opportunities open to settlers bold and adventuresome enough to stake their futures in the St. Johns River area.[1] Dr. Stork was a traveler and publicist of German birth who made his way into North Florida in the 1760s, was impressed with the possibilities of settling along the St. Johns and lost no time in publicizing through the London press the beautiful future for those willing to invest in that part of Florida.

He was no doubt a "slick" salesman and was successful in persuading several Englishmen of wealth to buy land in the area. He is presumed to have studied medicine in Germany and qualified as a practitioner but there is no evidence that he was ever a regular practitioner in Florida.

1. See Daniel L. Schafer, "Early Plantation Development in British North Florida," El Escribano, vol. 19, pp. 37-53.

Storrow, Samuel Appleton, Fort Jefferson, Dry Tortugas, 1831-1879

Only a few biographical details for Dr. Storrow have been discovered. Born in Virginia in 1831 he matriculated at the Jefferson Medical College, Philadelphia, in 1850[1] and was graduated Doctor of Medicine in the spring of 1852. After a few years in private practice, probably in the vicinity of Washington, D.C., he was commissioned Assistant Surgeon in the Army of the United States on August 5, 1861.[2] In spite of his Virginia heritage he remained in the service of the Union Army throughout the Civil War.

In 1869, Dr. Storrow appeared on the roster of an Army unit, a part of the 5th United States Artillery, at Ft. Jefferson, Dry Tortugas, as Post Surgeon, a rank equivalent to that of major. He remained at this post until March 1872 with frequent leaves of absence on some of which he overstayed his allotted time and was carried on the Post returns as "absent without leave." He can hardly be censured for such remisses, however, given the isolation of the Fort and the inevitable monotony which must have prevailed. He disappears from the Post returns in March 1872 when he was replaced by Dr. Van Buren Hubbard.[3]

Dr. Storrow was promoted to Major Surgeon for faithful and meritorious service on June 26, 1876. He died on July 12, 1879.[4]

1. Jefferson Medical College, Philadelphia, *List of Dead or Lost Graduates in Classes from 1826 to 1879*, Philadelphia, p. 88.
2. *Medical Department of the Army, from 1775 to 1879*, Harvey E. Brown, Compiler, Washington, Surgeon General's Office, 1873, p. 295.
3. U.S. Army, Returns from Ft. Jefferson, Dry Tortugas, 1869 to 1875, microfilm.
4. Francis B. Heitman, *Historical Register and Directory of the United States Army*, Vol. I, Washington, Government Printing Office, 1903, p. 930.

Stringer, Sheldon, Brooksville and Tampa, 1833-1903

Dr. Stringer, generally considered Hernando County's premier 19th century physician and certainly among the top-ranked physicians of Florida, was a native of North Carolina, having been born in that state in November 1833.[1] After obtaining his early education and serving a medical apprenticeship, presumably in North Carolina, he was admitted to the Medical School of Tulane University in New Orleans in the fall of 1857. He was graduated Doctor of Medicine in the spring of 1859.[2]

Following graduation Dr. Stringer began practice in Tampa where his widowed mother, Mary, and sister, Laura, joined him about the beginning of 1860. They appear to have been people of modest means, the total family wealth having been estimated at about $2,000 in 1860.[3] Mrs. Stringer established a boarding house in the town while young Dr. Stringer attempted to get his professional career under way. Before the end of the year 1859, however, the family left Tampa to settle in the village of Ichepoksassa in the northeastern section of Hillsborough County later to be known as Plant City. Dr. Stringer's professional card first appeared in the Tampa *Florida Peninsular* of October 20, 1860, announcing his services to the citizens of Ichepoksassa, Alafia and the Pease Creek settlements, a rather vast rural area. His undertaking was given a significant boost by the editor of the Tampa newspaper who called attention to Dr. Stringer's move, adding gratuitously, "We commend Dr. Stringer to the citizens of that locality as a promising young physician, and trust they will extend to him a living support."[4]

For about two and a half years Dr. Stringer practiced with apparent success in the rural area which would have acquainted him with many of the families who inhabited what are now parts of Hernando and Polk Counties.

With the Civil War already under way Dr. Stringer was commissioned surgeon in the Confederate Army on July 13, 1862. Good fortune became his lot, however, when instead of being dispatched to the Army of Virginia or Tennessee, he was appointed Surgeon General of the Florida State Troops, a post he held for the duration of the War.[5]

At the conclusion of his military service Dr. Stringer settled in Brooksville where he was to remain for the rest of his life. In 1873 he married a native South Carolinian known only by her Christian name, Mary. She was 11 years his junior. To this marriage were born three children: Frederick L., 1874, Marguerite, 1879, and Sheldon Jr., 1883.[6]

Dr. Stringer's professional career was marked by success and popularity. A man of compassion, common sense and good humor he was held in high regard by the people of Hernando County. In 1877 he was elected Superintendent of Public Instruction for the county, an office he held for four years,[7] relinquishing it when he was elected to the Florida House of Representatives in 1881.[8]

Meanwhile Dr. Stringer continued to practice medicine and operate a commercial enterprise, the City Drug Store, in Brooksville. In May 1888,[9] at the age of 55, he made his first appearance at a meeting of the Florida Medical Association held that year in Gainesville. He was elected to membership along with six others including the distinguished Dr. Thomas P. Gary of Ocala. His influence on the proceedings was soon felt. Two years later he was elected first vice president as well as chairman of the Committee on Gynecology and delegate to the next annual meeting of the American Medical Association.[10] Henceforth he exercised considerable influence over the proceedings of the group, often speaking extemporaneously on matters of concern to him, such as inferior medical education and lax standards of licensing which still prevailed in the state. At the meeting of the Association in Key West and Havana, Cuba, in 1892, he urged drastic measures against illegal practice and licensing. At the final session of the meeting in Havana Dr. R.A. Lancaster of Gainesville placed Dr. Stringer's name in nomination for the presidency of the Association. He won handily.[11] His speech of acceptance was brief and modest, an expression of surprise and gratitude.

Although Dr. Stringer was a general practitioner, as were nearly all physicians of the time, he was particularly well known as a gynecologist. He was apparently well acquainted with the literature on gynecology, as demonstrated in his first published paper, "A New Instrument in the Operation for Vesico-Vaginal Fistula," sprinkled with references to earlier efforts to treat the ailment.[12] In 1895, as Chairman of the Section on Gynecology, he read a paper, "Occlusion of the Entire Cervical Canal," written by Dr. Theodore Turnbull of Monticello who was unable to attend the meeting.[13]

In the course of his daily practice Dr. Stringer inevitably encountered an assortment of ailments and accidents, often unusual and demanding inventiveness on his part. Some of these he brought to the attention of his colleagues, as in 1895 when he reported a case of "Unusual Complications in the Compound

Fracture of the Humerus"[14] and another in 1894, "Report on Two Cases of Foreign Bodies in the Air Passages."[15]

Dr. Stringer was reputed to possess a very fine sense of humor which could at times relieve tensions and restore calmness in excited situations. There can be no doubt that his colleagues found him genial, intelligent and trustworthy. This trust was evident at the time of his election to the presidency of the Florida Medical Association when seven of the 20 votes were cast for Dr. Frank Caldwell of Sanford and Dr. Joseph Y. Porter moved for a unanimous vote for Dr. Stringer. The motion was carried.

Dr. Stringer continued to attend the annual meetings of the Florida Medical Association through the session of 1902 held in Tampa. He failed to appear a year later, however, at the meeting in St. Augustine, doubtless because of increasing infirmity. His death came on August 6, 1903, at his Brooksville home. He was 70. He was buried in the Lykes Cemetery in Brooksville.[16]

Of the Stringer sons who survived their father, Frederick, the older, became a successful Brooksville lawyer who served four terms as Mayor of Brooksville (1909-1912), and five terms in the Florida Legislature, three in the House (1910, 11, and 12), and two in the Senate (1913 and 1915). The younger son, Sheldon, followed in his father's footsteps, choosing medicine as a profession and practiced throughout his career in Tampa.

1. U.S. Census, 1900, Hernando County, Florida, p. 26, item 144.
2. *Transactions, Florida Medical Association*, 1903, p. 33.
3. U.S. Census, 1860, Hillsborough County, Florida, p. 504.
4. Tampa *Florida Peninsular*, October 22, 1859. His office, at least temporarily, was located in the country store of David Hughes, Esq.
5. Board of State Institutions, *Soldiers of Florida*, Rev. Ed., Macclenny, 1983, p. 320.
6. See note 1, supra.
7. James H. Jones, ed., *Governmental Guide to Hernando County, Florida* (n.d., n.p.), p. 37.
8. Ibid., p. 44.
9. *Proceedings, Florida Medical Association*, Jacksonville, 1888, p. 5.
10. Ibid., 1890, p. 12.
11. Ibid., 1892, p. 5. Dr. H.K. DuBois of Port Orange nominated Dr. Frank H. Caldwell of Sanford who received seven of the 20 votes.
12. Ibid., 1891. The paper was read at the Pensacola meeting.
13. Ibid., 1895.
14. Ibid., Appendix 13, pp. 92-93.
15. Ibid., 1894, Appendix 9. Paper read at meeting in Tampa.
16. An obituary for Dr. Stringer appeared in ibid., 1903, p. 33. His place of burial is recorded in WPA, "Register of Decreased Veterans," Hernando County, St. Augustine, Veterans' Graves Registration Project, 1940-41, p. 13.

Stringfellow, William Hall, Alachua County, 1818-1869

The Florida career of Dr. Stringfellow[1] spanned only 14 years and yet his leadership in civic affairs and his humanitarianism were significant in the early development of Alachua County and the town of Gainesville. He was born in Chester, South Carolina, on July 31, 1818, the son of William and Patience Buford Stringfellow. After receiving his early education in the schools of Chester he attended the University of South Carolina from which he was graduated as Bachelor of Arts in 1838. After an interval of a year he enrolled in the Medical Department of the University of Pennsylvania where he received his medical degree in the spring of 1841.[2] His doctoral thesis was entitled "The Non-Existence of Congestive Fever."

Returning to Chester after graduation Dr. Stringfellow began his professional practice. A year or so later he married Julia Eliza Rainey, a union to which two children, William Jr. and Eliza, were born.[3] Mrs. Stringfellow, however, did not long survive the birth of her second child. Within a year or so after her death Dr. Stringfellow married a widow, Mrs. Sarah Dogan Wright, who had two children by her first husband, Richard Simpson Wright.

Family documents do not clearly indicate the date of Dr. Stringfellow's move to Florida, although 1856 is the year usually cited. There is evidence, however, that he had been in Alachua County as early as 1854 and that he had attended a Fourth of July celebration at Dr. Anderson's mill at the head of Sweetwater Branch where he had given "a firey speech." He is also reported to have attended a meeting at Boulware Springs, a mile south of Gainesville, at which a vote was taken to locate the county seat in Gainesville. It appears likely that he was in Alachua prospecting for suitable land on which he might settle.

Whatever the date of his arrival, 1854 or 1856, Dr. Stringfellow purchased a tract of land at Ft. Clark, six miles west of Gainesville, where he developed the Stringfellow Plantation. His first years in the new location bode well for the future as he carried on the dual roles of physician and planter achieving success in both. In 1860 his slaves numbered 35 and other property was valued at $8,000.[4] He also entered vigorously into the life of the community and is said to have been responsible for bringing the eminent South Carolina Presbyterian minister, the Reverend W.J. McCormick, to Alachua County and establishing the Kanapaha Presbyterian Church, the first such church in the county.[5]

Meanwhile Dr. Stringfellow was establishing himself as a trusted and dedicated physician whose services were much in demand over a wide area of Alachua County. His daughter, Sallie, in her reminiscences, wrote:

> My father was a very fine man, a wonderful doctor dearly beloved by all who knew him. One of our slaves, Jane Gaines, told me a lot about "Marse William;" she took care of him in Chester, S.C. She told me of his going on horseback to visit his patients, and in winter he would come in from his visits, his feet almost frozen, and Aunt Jane would get a foot tub full of warm water and "thaw out" his feet.

The disruptions brought on by the War (1861-65) prompted Dr. Stringfellow to leave his plantation and move into Gainesville where he continued to practice medicine. In 1869 he returned to his native state for a visit. He became ill and died in Aiken but his remains were taken to Union, S.C., for burial.[6] He was survived by his wife, Sarah, and five of the six children who had been born to the couple.[7]

1. The greater portion of the information here was provided by Mrs. Hart S. Stringfellow Jr. of Gainesville whose husband is a direct descendant of Dr. Stringfellow. Many other descendants still live in Alachua County. Unless otherwise indicated the data included are derived from this source. Additional sources are: Jess G. Davis, *History of Alachua County, Florida*, Gainesville, 1970, p. 13; and Webster Merritt, "Physicians and Medicine in Early Alachua County and Gainesville, Florida," *Journal of the Florida Medical Association*, Vol. XI, No. 4, October 1955, p. 301.

2. Archives, University of Pennsylvania, Lists of Matriculants and Graduates.

3. U.S. Census, 1850, Chester County, S.C., p. 136. Here it is indicated that Dr. Stringfellow was practicing medicine in Chester. His property was valued at $5,000.

4. U.S. Census, 1860, Alachua County, Florida.

5. Mr. McCormick later assisted in the establishment of the First Presbyterian Church of Gainesville.

6. Prior to his departure for South Carolina in 1869 Dr. Stringfellow processed a deed by which he gave 600 acres of land to his wife. This deed, recorded in Gainesville on April 29, 1869, is the last extant record of his residence in Florida. It possibly suggests that he had a promonition that he might not return. See Alachua County Deed Book, "G," p. 746.

7. The surviving children were Joseph Dogan, Thornton B., Robert Lee, Clarence, and a daughter, Sallie. See U.S.

Census, 1880, Alachua County, Florida, p. 62, ite, 494. A son, James Lawrence, had died earlier. The five surviving children were destined to play important roles in the social and business life of the Gainesville community.

Strong, C.B., Gadsden County, 1852

Dr. Strong was a brief sojourner in Florida. He arrived in Quincy in late September 1852 and departed after a few months. In its issue of October 5, 1852, the Tallahassee *Sentinel* announced his arrival, stating that he was offering his services to the public and could be found at his office in the Drug Store of J.F. Jordan and Company. A similar announcement appeared simultaneously in the Tallahassee *Florida and Journal* of October 30, 1852. Since his name does not appear in the Florida census of 1860, it is assumed that he had departed the state prior to that year.

Subers, Jacob J., Quincy, 1838

Dr. Subers, styled in the Census of 1860 as "M.D., Reformed," was born in Bibb County, Georgia, (seat, Macon) about 1838. In all probability he was a graduate of the Southern Botanico-Medico College, a Macon institution which enjoyed more than a modicum of success in the antebellum period. It existed from 1839 until 1881.[1] He arrived in Quincy in time to be included in the Census of 1860 which gave his age as 22.

His professional card appeared in the Quincy *Republic*, on March 3, 1861:

> Dr. J. J. Subers, having returned, again offers his professional services to the citizens of Quincy and surrounding country...Thankful for past favors, he solicits a continuance of the same. Office over F.M. Smith's New Clothing Store....Those afflicted with chronic diseases of long standing especially might do well to test the virtues of his peculiar (illegible) which rarely fail to effect permanent cure...

It is clearly implied, therefore, that he had been away from Quincy for a few weeks, possibly months.

Dr. Subers had scarcely resumed his practice when the call to arms came. Like most, able-bodied young white men he responded, enlisting on April 4, 1861, as a private in Company "G", 1st Florida Infantry, a unit commanded by Dr. (Capt.) John H. Gee of Quincy. The company was mustered in at Camp Magnolia on April 19 and from that date until December 21 he was regularly present for duty.[2]

Before the end of December, however, Dr. Subers applied for a discharge so that he might join the light artillery company of Capt. Robertson.[3] Capt. Gee offered no objection but wrote an affidavit supporting the request for discharge dating it December 21, 1861, at Warrington, near Pensacola. This document provides some information as to Dr. Subers' appearance:

> This certifies that Jacob J. Subers, a private of Capt. John H. Gee's Co. (G), First Regular Florida Volunteers, born in Bibb County, Ga., age 23; 5'10" tall, light complexion, hazel eyes, black hair, and by profession a physician, was enlisted by Capt. John H. Gee, at Quincy, Fla., on April 4, 1861, to serve for one year, and is now entitled to a discharge by reason of reenlisting for the War.[4]

Further military information shows that Dr. Subers shortly thereafter saw duty with Capt. Robertson's battery near Knoxville, Tennessee, where he was disabled. On November 21, 1862, he was given terminal pay in the amount of $52.50. Although no documentation can be located it appears likely that he returned to practice as soon as recovery was complete. Only in September 1865 did his professional notice reappear in the local newspaper. In this instance he offered his services with the claim that he was "especially able to treat chronic diseases of females."[5]

Dr. Subers married Zilla Innis in January 1869.[6] The census of the following year shows the couple residing in a boarding house in Quincy.[7] Beyond this date, however, nothing is known of Dr. Subers.

1. U.S. Census, 1860, Gadsden County, Florida, p. 519. The term "reformed" as applied to the medical profession may designate any one of several types of practice which were developed in the 19th century, each basically a departure from the orthodox system of the so-called allopaths, who relied heavily on calomel and the lancet. Most of the reformed practitioners relied to some degree on vegetable substances, or botanicals, as they were called. Of these deviators the Thomsonians were perhaps the most notable. Others advertised themselves simply as botanic physicians, or, as Dr. Subers, "reformed physicians." By mid-19th century the homeopaths emerged onto the medical scene with some success and in many parts of the western world still flourish.

2. NA, Service, Records, CSA, M251, Roll 30.

3. It is not known why Dr. Subers chose to change his branch of service; possibly out of boredom or perhaps with the expectation of finding an outlet for his medical skills.

4. V. note 2, supra.

5. Quincy *Commonwealth*, May 15, 1866. The notice first appeared in the issue of September 9, 1865, not extant.

6. Floreda D. Varick and Phyllis R. Smith, comp., *Gadsden County, Florida, Marriage Records, 1849-1876*, Quincy, 1980, p. 71.

7. U.S. Census, 1870, Gadsden County, Florida, p. 825.

Sullivan, Wade, U.S. Army, 1838

Dr. Sullivan was one of several medical practitioners who enlisted for service in the Army of the United States during the Second Seminole War in Florida. Beyond the fact that he was a native of Virginia and resident of that state at the time of enlistment, on November 21, 1836, nothing is known of his professional training or previous practice. His death came, not from Indian arrows, but from natural causes, presumably fever, on May 15, 1838.[1]

1. Tallahassee *Florida Sentinel*, September 16, 1842. Francis B. Heitman, *Historical Register and Directory of the United States Army*, Volume I, Washington, Government Printing Office, 1903, p. 935.

Sutton, William J., Monticello, 1842

The Monticello sojourn of Dr. Sutton was brief, lasting scarcely one year. He announced opening of his practice on January 5, 1842, indicating that he could be found either at his office or at his residence in the Florida Hotel, adding "unless professionally engaged," a *pro forma* phrase of the times.[1] His professional notices continued to appear as late as December 22, 1842, but disappear after that date and nothing more is known. Historian Jerrell H. Shofner, after identifying him as a Monticello physician of 1842, dismisses him tersely with the words, "but he soon moved on."[2]

1. Tallahassee *Star of Florida*, January 5, 1842. His professional notice appeared a few days earlier in the Tallahassee *Sentinel*. See issue of January 14, 1842.

2. Jerrell H. Shofner, *History of Jefferson County*, Tallahassee, 1976, p. 62.

Tabb, Thomas, Madison County, 1855

Dr. Tabb, son of William A. Tabb of Sandy Ford, later known as Greenville, was graduated from the Medical College of Georgia, Augusta, in 1855. His preceptor had been Dr. T.S. Mims, who had practiced medicine for a brief period in Madison County.[1] As far as can be determined, however, Dr. Rabb did not return to practice in Florida.

1. Records of the Medical Department of the University of Georgia.

Talbird, John H., Orange County, 1870

Dr. Talbird, a native of Beaufort District, South Carolina, was only a brief sojourner in Florida, having practiced for a few years in Orange County. Annals of the Savannah Medical College, Savannah, Georgia, show that he was graduated from that institution in the spring of 1855.[1]

1. U.S. Census, 1870, Orange County, Florida, p. 435. Dr. Talbird was 40 years of age. The other member of his household was John Hickman, a farm laborer native of North Carolina.

Taylor, Benjamin Rush, Tallahassee, 1818-1840

Dr. Taylor, son of Dr. John Bradford Taylor, for many years a Tallahassee medical practitioner, was born in Maryland in 1818. Having been christened Benjamin Rush, namesake of the famous physician and signer of the Declaration of Independence, he seemed destined from birth for a career in medicine. He moved to Florida with his family in 1832, but a few years later returned to the East for his medical education. In 1839 he came back to Florida to launch his professional career, his card first appearing on November 30, 1839.[1] It simply announced that "Dr. Benjamin R. Taylor offers his services to the citizens of Tallahassee and Vicinity, office at the residence of his father, north side of Washington Square." Two months later the partnership of the two was announced.[2]

Dr. Taylor's career was tragically brief. On September 19, 1840,[3] he succumbed to congestive fever at the age of 22. His death was a shock to the Tallahassee community, calling forth from his eulogist a sorrowful reflection on the cruel fate which had "struck down this worthy and noble young man who had just stepped forth on the verdant lawn of life." He concluded: "Heavy indeed has the hand of affliction fallen upon his devoted father and sisters."[4] He was buried in Tallahassee's Old City Cemetery on September 20, 1840.

1. Tallahassee *Floridian*, February 8, 1840; 1st printing, November 30, 1839.
2. Ibid., January 18, 1840.
3. Ibid., October 3, 1840.
4. Dr. John Bradford Taylor's first wife, Sarah, had died prior to removal of the family to Florida. Of his three daughters, Grace Augusta, Janette, and Eliza, Grace Augusta had died in 1836. Dr. Taylor remarried in 1846 and one son and two daughters were born to the second marriage.

Taylor, Benjamin Waller, Tallahassee and Monticello, 1815-1891

Dr. Taylor was born in Mecklenburg County, Virginia, in 1815, the son of Major John Taylor who moved to Leon County in the 1820s and purchased land a few miles north of Tallahassee off the Centreville Road. The Taylors were apparently a family well above average means; the Census of 1840 shows them as owners of 26 slaves.[1] Nothing is known of Dr. Taylor's early education. He matriculated at the Medical College of the University of Pennsylvania in the fall of 1833 and was graduated in the spring of 1835. His doctoral thesis entitled "Dysmenorrhea" is extant.[2]

On his return to Florida Dr. Taylor entered medical practice in Monticello where he was joined in 1842 by his brother, Littleton, a practitioner of dubious qualifications. This association was terminated following a scandalous incident in which the younger doctor publicly beat his wife on a Monticello street.[3] In 1844 Dr. Taylor was joined in partnership by Thomas M. Palmer who was destined to become one of Florida's foremost physicians. This partnership was dissolved by mutual consent on January 1, 1861.[4]

Very little information concerning Dr. Taylor's day-to-day practice has survived but apparently he attracted many patients and enjoyed a fine reputation throughout Jefferson County. His concern for the improvement of medical practice in Florida was demonstrated by his appearance at the Medical Convention in Quincy on May 15-16, 1848, in support of the effort to establish a state medical association.[5] Occasional references show that he was retained by certain plantation owners for the medical needs of their families and slaves.[6] In 1851 the Florida Assembly authorized payment of a hundred dollars to Drs. Taylor and Palmer for medical and surgical services for a prisoner in the Jefferson County jail.[7]

As was true of many doctors of the times Dr. Taylor was active in the political affairs of his county and state. He was a regular participant at Independence Day celebrations, sometime revealing his sectional bias, as on the occasion in 1838 when he spoke on the proposition that "Southern Education be Obtained from Southern Teachers."[8]

When Indian troubles beset Middle Florida in the late 1830s he hurriedly joined the Ninth Regiment as regimental surgeon. This unit was composed principally of men from Jefferson County.[9] A decade later, when sectional feelings deepened because of "infractions on the part of the people of the North" Dr. Taylor was one of the six delegates from his county to attend the Nashville Convention proposed by John C. Calhoun.[10]

Soon after receiving his medical degree Dr. Taylor married Elizabeth Simkins, member of a prominent Leon County family which had originated in South Carolina. Her sister Emily or Emmala, as it appears in census schedules,was the wife of William Bellamy, wealthy Leon planter. The Bellamy offspring consisted of four daughters;[11] the Taylors were childless. With the early death of their parents the Bellamy daughters became the wards of relatives, two of them, Emily and William (sic), lived with the Taylors. The oldest daughter, Elizabeth, whose legacy was a plantation near Bel Air, became the wife of Dr. George W. Parkhill.[12]

With the onset of war in 1861 most younger physicians of Middle Florida offered their services to the Confederate cause. Dr. Taylor, 46 at the time, remained in Monticello as the town's sole physician. When Dr. Parkhill became an early casualty in a skirmish at Gaines Mill near Richmond in June 1862, Dr. Taylor made the long journey to Virginia to escort Mrs. Parkhill and her two small children back to Bel Air.[13]

The later years of Dr. Taylor's life were not uneventful. His wife died in the early 1870s and he lost little time remarrying, in this instance, Mariah B. Bailey, widow of Capt. William Bailey Jr., a casualty at Gettysburg on July 2, 1863.[14] Three children had been born to the Bailey union, William M., John B., and Mary. To Dr. Taylor's second marriage, which occurred in 1873, were born two children, Waller, a son, age six in 1880, and a daughter, age five. The household that year also included Mrs. Taylor's daughter by her first marriage.[15] Dr. Taylor was an active practitioner in Monticello as late as 1885.[16] Local records indicate that his death occurred in 1891 at the age of 76.[17] He was buried in Monticello's Roseland Cemetery.

1. *The Cemeteries of Leon County, Florida,* Joy Smith Paisley, comp. and ed., Tallahassee, 1978, p. 141. John Taylor died December 15, 1842, at age 63. He is buried in Whitaker Cemetery, five miles north of Tallahassee off Centreville Road.
2. Archives, University of Pennsylvania, List of Graduates.
3. Jerrell H. Shofner, *History of Jefferson County, Florida,* Tallahassee, 1976, p. 62.
4. Monticello *Family Friend,* August 5, 1861.
5. Tallahassee *Southern Journal,* May 22, 29, 1848. A total of 13 physicians representing the counties of Gadsden, Leon and Jefferson attended the conference. Besides Dr. Taylor, Jefferson was represented by Dr. John L. Call.
6. Shofner, History p. 143. Retainer fees from well-to-do planters were probably the most reliable source of income for many physicians of Middle Florida during the 1830s and 1840s. Most found collections difficult.
7. Laws of Florida, General Assembly, 5th Session, 1850-51, chap. 458, no. 147.
8. Tallahassee *Floridian and Advocate,* July 7, 1838.
9. Shofner, History, p. 82.
10. Ibid., p. 183.
11. "Old Plantations Near Monticello," typescript, P.K. Yonge Library of Florida History, no author; no date, pp. 57-61.
12. Ibid.
13. Shofner, History, p. 265.
14. William Bailey Jr., son of the wealthy and prominent business leader, William Bailey of Jefferson County, was one of the early enlistees. He had been an officer in the Aucilla Guards which was absorbed by the Fifth Florida Infantry Regiment in March 1861 and was assigned to command Company G with the rank of captain. Seriously wounded at Gettysburg on July 2, 1863, he never made a complete recovery. Still a prisoner of war at Hilton Head, S.C., he died on March 5, 1865, of "inflammation of the lungs," apparently a complication related to a chronic consumption from which he had suffered. Dr. Taylor's first wife died in Monticello on September 22, 1871, at age 57. Tallahassee *Weekly Floridian,* October 10, 1871.
15. U.S. Census, 1880, Jefferson County, Florida.
16. Special Census of Florida, 1885, Jefferson County. Here Dr. Taylor is listed as attending physician of several persons deceased within the previous 12 months.
17. WPA, Writers Project, Jefferson County, Florida, Typescript, P.K. Yonge Library of Florida History, p. 133. Here appears the following statement: "The Dixie Hotel was formerly the house built by B. Waller Taylor, old time doctor, who was born in Virginia in 1805 and lived in this house until he died in 1891." The census schedules for 1860, 1870, and 1880, which are consistent, show that Dr. Taylor's year of birth was 1815, not 1805.

Taylor, John Bradford, Tallahassee, 1785-1864

Dr. Taylor, who practiced medicine in Tallahassee from 1832 until his death in 1864, was born in Maryland, quite probably Dorchester County.[1] His professional card, first appearing on May 8, 1832, identified him as a previous resident of Baltimore.[2] In the practice of the times he offered his services in Medicine, Surgery and Midwifery from an office located next door to the Drug Store of E.B. Perkins. He also advertised that he had on hand a supply of "genuine vaccine matter." Apparently his change of air and water required some adjustment for on August 1, 1832, he announced that his health was "sufficiently improved to permit him to resume his practice."[3]

About a year after becoming a resident of Tallahassee Dr. Taylor joined four other local physicians in drafting a schedule of fees they agreed to charge which was published in the *Floridian* on February 2, 1833. This provoked a storm of protest from the citizens and prompted a hurried response from Dr. Taylor and two of his colleagues, assuring the public that the rates were intended only as maximal charges and that physicians might, if they chose, charge less and, furthermore, no indigent person would be denied their services.[4]

Little can be said of Dr. Taylor's extraprofessional activities. Presumably he was apolitical, nor does he appear to have been particularly religious, beyond observing the conventional rites of baptism for his children. He maintained a loyal devotion to the Order of Freemasons, however, and for his service was honored by election to the office of Grand Master of the State of Florida.[5]

Dr. Taylor appears to have been the typical small-town doctor, relying heavily on commonplace remedies, common sense, and the natural proclivity of the human body to heal itself. A few entries in the diary of Dr. Thaddeau Hentz, dentist, who during a visit to Tallahassee in 1863 became ill and sought Dr. Taylor's help, bear quoting:[6]

> May 11th---violent headache, sick stomach, and fever. Dr. Taylor, an excellent old gentleman, came to see me...I had Blue Mass, an opium; he prescribed more opium...
>
> May 12th, Dr. Taylor called again...prescribed brandy, but said there was none in the place fit to drink, and what there was cost $15 a bottle.
>
> May 13th, Better this a.m...Saw Dr. Taylor...offered to pay him, but he positively refused, said I was a brother physician.

As has been true of physicians throughout history, Dr. Taylor often found collecting professional fees difficult. In May 1842, he addressed his delinquent patients as follows:[7]

> Dr. Taylor is compelled to request all persons indebted to him to come forward and settle the same, forthwith. Those neglecting this notice are informed that no message from them will be attended to in the future.

Dr. Taylor was twice married. His first wife, Sarah, was a native of Maryland. It appears that four children were born to this marriage, Benjamin Rush, who became a physician; Grace Augusta, who died in 1836 at the age of 19 and was buried in the Old City Cemetery; Eliza and Janette, both of whom were baptized at St. John's Episcopal Church, Tallahassee, on May 16, 1839.[8] Dr. Taylor married Mrs. Mary Lockerman Chandler, widow of Edward Chandler of Tallahassee on July 16, 1846. To this union were born a son, James Lockerman, who had a successful career as a railroad executive,[9] and two daughters, Adele and Anna, aged 10 and five respectively in 1860.

Soon after his son, Benjamin Rush, began practice in Tallahassee, a partnership was formed. The announcement of this association first appeared in the Tallahassee *Floridian* on January 18, 1840. It read: "Dr. John B. Taylor has associated himself with his son, Benjamin R. Taylor." The arrangement was terminated by his son's untimely death on October 19 that year at the age of 22.[10] Many years later Dr. Taylor joined Dr. John S. Bond in a medical partnership located, according to their notice, "at Dr. Taylor's Old Stand."[11] This ended with Dr. Taylor's death in late 1864.[12] An inscription on his gravestone in the Old City Cemetery in Tallahassee provides this incidental information: "Surgeon's Mate, 5th Regiment, Maryland Militia, War of 1812."

Mrs. Taylor survived her husband by only 13 months, dying on February 20, 1866, at the age of 63.[13]

1. Troublesome lacunae in documentation make it impossible to provide a complete account of Dr. Taylor's career.
2. Tallahassee *Floridian,* May 8, 1832.
3. Ibid., August 1, 1832.
4. Ibid., February 9, 1833.
5. Ibid., December 11,1847; ibid., February 26, 1852. See also *Proceedings of the Grand Lodge, 1860-66,* Tallahassee, 1866, p. 257.
6. Hentz Ms. property of J.D. Smith, Marianna; typed copy in P.K. Yonge Library of Florida History, University of Florida, Gainesville.
7. Tallahassee *Sentinel,* May 13, 1846.
8. "Parochial Records, St. John's Episcopal Church, Tallahassee, Florida," typed copy, P.K. Yonge Library of Florida History, University of Florida, Gainesville. The baptismal rite took place on May 16, 1839. Since Mrs. Sarah Taylor's name does not appear in either St. John's Church Records or Leon County cemetery records, it is assumed that she had died prior to the family's move to Florida in 1832.
9. For notice of marriage see Tallahassee *Florida Sentinel,* July 21, 1846. For information on James Lockerman Taylor see Henry E. Palmer, "Physicians of Early Tallahassee and Vicinity," *Apalachee,* Tallahassee Historical Society, 1944, p. 33.
10. Tallahassee *Floridian,* October 3, 1840.
11. Tallahassee *Floridian and Journal,* January 12, 1861. First printed in ibid., February 1, 1859.
12. *Proceedings of the Grand Lodge,* 1860-66, Tallahassee, 1866, p. 257. Dr. Taylor is said to have died after a long and painful illness.
13. The second Mrs. Taylor was also a native of Maryland, having been born in Cambridge, Dorchester County, on February 20, 1813. Tallahassee *Semi-Weekly Floridian,* March 13, 1866.

Taylor, Junius Littlepage, Leon County, 1827-1890

Dr. Taylor was born in Brunswick County, Virginia,[1] on February 20, 1827.[2] In the early 1830s at about the age of five, he was brought to Tallahassee by his father, Major John Taylor, and on February 12, 1832, he and his two brothers were christened at St. John's Episcopal Church.[3] Very little is known of Dr. Taylor's youth and early manhood, but it is assumed that he was provided with the best education available in Tallahassee. Circumstances point to the probability that he became a student of medicine under the preceptorate of Dr. Miles Nash Sr., prominent physician and druggist of the town. At the age of 23 Dr. Taylor was a resident in the Nash household.[4] The census of 1850 for Leon County designates him "physician."[5] His obituary notice, however, states that in "1848 Capt. Taylor was associated with Dr. Miles Nash in the firm of Nash and Taylor, apothecaries and druggists."

On October 3, 1850, Dr. Taylor married Sarah A. Bradford, second daughter of Dr. Edward Bradford of Pine Hill Plantation north of Tallahassee and the following year a daughter, Martha, familiarly known as Mattie, was born.[6] On November 21, 1852, occurred the sad and untimely death of Mrs. Taylor at the age of 22.[7] In the meantime Dr. Taylor had disposed of his interest in the Tallahassee drug business, purchased a plantation northeast of Tallahassee which he named "Neck-a-Nothing" and settled down to the life of a farmer. In all probability, however, he and his little daughter spent much time in the home of Dr. Bradford whose Pine Hill Plantation lay only three or four miles west.[8]

Leaving his daughter in the care of the Bradford family Dr. Taylor enlisted in the Confederate Army on February 20, 1862. He was commissioned second lieutenant and assigned to Company K, 5th Florida Infantry Regiment. He was with his regiment in Virginia later in 1862, participating in some of the encounters around Richmond. After being promoted to the rank of first lieutenant in September 1863, he served for a time in the Department of the Quartermaster but near the end of the War, on order of General Lee himself, he was assigned to the Medical Department. Before discharge in April 1865, he was promoted to a captaincy, the title he bore for the rest of his life.[9]

Susan Bradford Eppes, Dr. Taylor's younger sister-in-law, has recorded with tenderness of feeling the homecoming of Dr. Taylor and two other soldiers to Pine Hill on April 19, 1865. She relates the tearful reaction of his daughter upon seeing her war-weary father; how he refused to greet even his daughter before retiring to "the room which was always known as his," bathing thoroughly, having one of the black servants cut his hair and then, after ordering his be-raggled military clothing burned, donning immaculate linen with silk tie and coming down to a joyful homecoming.[10] He recalled to the assembled family the details of General Lee's surrender which he had witnessed.

Shortly thereafter Dr. Taylor returned to his own plantation where, except for the desertion of one of his most trusted slaves, he found things in fairly good order.[11] He lived out his life there in modest circumstances. He died on December 14, 1890, at the home of his son-in-law, W.A. Demilly, in Tallahassee and was buried in the Demilly lot in the Old City Cemetery.[12]

1. Preston A. Demilly of Tallahasse, great-grandson of Dr. Taylor, provided some of the biographical data.
2. Obituary notice for Dr. Taylor, Tallahassee *Weekly Floridian*, December 17, 1890.
3. "Parochial Register, St. John's Episcopal Church, Tallahassee, Florida, 1832-1880." Typed copy, P.K. Yonge Library of Florida History, University of Florida, p. 8.
4. U.S. Census, 1850, Leon County, Florida, p. 74.
5. Ibid. There is little doubt that in his earlier adult years Dr. Taylor was a medical practitioner, although later he was certainly more planter than doctor. Susan Bradford Eppes, *Through Some Eventful Years*, facsimile ed., Gainesville, 1968, pp. 293, 313. On at least two occasions in 1865, Mrs. Eppes, Dr. Taylor's sister-in-law, referred to him as "brother doctor" or "doctor brother."
6. "Leon County, Florida, Records," Tallahassee Chapter, DAR, comp., typed copy, P.K. Yonge Library of Florida History.
7. Tallahassee *Floridian and Journal*, November 27, 1852.
8. See n. 2, supra. The Leon County Census, 1860, shows Martha Taylor as a member of Dr. Bradford's household.
9. National Archives, Service Records, CSA, M 251, Roll 67. Unfortunately some of the original documents relating to Dr. Taylor's war record are faded to the point of being illegible.
10. Eppes *Eventful Years*, p. 274 et seq.
11. Dr. Taylor's plantation was situated about three miles northeast of Centreville.
12. At the time of Dr. Taylor's death the road from Tallahassee was impassable due to heavy rains. This accounts for his burial in Tallahassee rather than in the Bradford Cemetery at Pine Hill where his wife was buried. Ex info., Preston A. Demilly.

Taylor, William Ford, Tallahassee and Monticello, 1834-35

In spite of apparent prominence as physician and civic leader, very little is known of the career of Dr. Taylor. Upon arriving in Florida he practiced briefly in Tallahassee, having announced his services to the citizens of Leon County on March 30, 1833.[1] On December 14, 1833, however, he announced the formation of a professional partnership with Dr. Benjamin Mellichamp in Monticello, where they would be found at the office occupied during the previous summer by Dr. Taylor.[2] At the Fourth of July celebration the following year in Monticello Dr. Taylor, as orator for the occasion, delivered an address "in a masterly manner, sustaining himself throughout in a style of eloquence that Cicero himself would not disown."[3] In October 1834, he announced that he would be a candidate to represent Jefferson County in the Florida Legislative Council but there is no evidence that he actually ran for the office nor is he listed in the register of members.[4] Nothing is known of his subsequent career.

1. Tallahassee *Floridian*, March 30, 1833. His office was located "two doors east of the Planters' Hotel." Incidental information suggests that he may have been previously a sojourner if not a native of Charleston, S.C. See ibid., April 6, 1833. Alexander Shine, a recent arrival in Tallahassee from Charleston, cited Dr. Taylor as one who could vouch for his good reputation.
2. Ibid., December 21, 1833.
3. Ibid., July 12, 1834. Dr. Taylor was asked to submit a copy of his speech for publication.
4. Ibid., October 4, 1834.

Teague, Isaac G., Jefferson County, 1830

Dr. Teague's Florida career was of short duration. He had left his native South Carolina in the late 1820s and settled in Jefferson County where he purchased real estate, "lands, houses, town lots," of considerable value[1] and entered into the public life of the community.

In early 1829, Dr. Teague announced his candidacy for a seat in the Florida Legislative Council to represent the counties of Jefferson, Madison and Hamilton.[2] He ran against the incumbent, Abraham Bellamy, and made a poor showing.[3] Probably motivated by pique, Dr. Teague addressed a public letter to the people of the three counties accusing James Dunlap, the candidate from Gadsden, of false and malicious statements which had affected the outcome of the election. He pointed out that at the time of the election he had been in New Orleans on business, returning to find these damaging lies being circulated. Particularly offensive was the statement that he was a fugitive from justice in South Carolina and had been driven out of the state.[4]

To the letter Dunlap replied claiming he had been urged by "several gentlemen from Jefferson County" to look into Dr. Teague's background. He had found it unsavory and had reported only what he had verified. He professed no animosity toward Dr. Teague.[5]

Within a year Dr. Teague was dead. A notice of administration of his estate appeared in mid-July 1830, the administrators being Lucy Teague, his widow, and William Blackburn.[6] In September a notice of public sale of the Teague belongings was announced. It was to be held in Monticello on November 10, 1830,[7] but due to a legal prohibition concerning the alienation of such property, the sale was cancelled.

Meanwhile Mrs. Teague and her infant son had returned to her relatives in South Carolina awaiting Legislative Council action which would permit the sale. This finally came in January 1832.[8] The act also stipulated that a guardian for the small son should be appointed in South Carolina.

Dr. Teague's activities as a medical practitioner cannot be documented. It is probable that he had entered into medical practice upon his arrival in Florida and had continued it until the time of his death. Legal notices suggest that he was a man of moderate means. His listing in the Census shows him to have been the owner of three slaves.[9]

1. Florida (Territory), Acts of Legislative Council, 10th Session, 1832, Tallahassee 1832, pp. 9-10.
2. Magnolia *Advertiser*, April 24, 1829.
3. Abraham Bellamy, an established political figure, had represented Duval County in the Council in 1824 and St. Johns County in 1825 when he was the presiding officer. He had represented Jefferson, Madison and Hamilton Counties in 1829, 1831 and 1832, and Jefferson in 1833 and 1835.
4. Magnolia *Advertiser*, July 3, 1829.

5. Ibid., July 14, 1829.
6. Tallahassee *Floridian and Advocate*, July 20, 1830.
7. Ibid., September 7, 1830.
8. Florida Acts of Legislative Council, loc. cit.
9. U.S. Census, 1830, Jefferson County, p. 162. The listing for Dr. Teague shows both him and his wife in the age bracket, 20 to 30 years; the son is listed as under five. In the household there was also an older woman between 60 and 70, obviously the mother of Dr. Teague or his wife.

Teasdale, Henry R., Palatka, 1870

Although Henry R. Teasdale appears in the list of physicians practicing in Putnam County in 1869-70,[1] evidence in support of such a claim in missing. The census of 1870 for Putnam County lists him as merchant living in Palatka with his wife and five children. He was born in Georgia but his wife, Estamislada, and all children were Florida born.[2] The following notice, which appeared in the Palatka newspaper in 1873, casts further doubt on his role as a medical practitioner.[3]

> RECEIVING AND FORWARDING
> Henry R. Teasdale
> Having superior Steamboat Warehouse and Wharf facilities will be pleased at all times to attend to the business of their friends and the public generally.

1. University of Pennsylvania, "List of Medical Practitioners in the Year, 1869-70," University of Pennsylvania Archives, MS, UPC 2.3 No. 16.
2. U.S. Census, 1870, Putnam County, Florida, p. 518, Town of Palatka.
3. Palatka *Eastern Herald*, April 5, 1873, 1st printed in issue of Mar. 17, 1869.

Telfair, David A., Gadsden and Wakulla Counties, 1827-1867

Knowledge of Dr. Telfair derives from the "Autobiography" of Dr. Charles A. Hentz who was closely associated with him as friend and colleague for several years.[1] He was a native of North Carolina. Accompanied by his mother he migrated to Florida in the late 1840s and found lodging in the household of William T. Stockton who appears to have been a relative.[2] After a few years of practice in Quincy he moved to Wakulla County, locating in New Port and advertising his servies on April 29, 1857.[3] Simultanously he joined John Madden in opening a drug store in which he located his office.[4] His endorsements for certain patent medicines, Life Pills, Phoenix Bitters and Pain-Killer, also appeared in the local paper.[5] In August 1858, however, the sale of his stock of "Drugs, Medicine, etc." was announced, the purchaser being J.W. Skipper. Local citizens were assured, however, Mr. Madden would continue to run the store.[6]

By the end of 1859, at the latest, Dr. Telfair was again settled in Quincy. A few weeks prior to his return, however, he had demonstrated a weakness which had shaken the confidence of Dr. Hentz. Dr. Talfair's wife, Louisa, was a sister of Dr. Milton McBride, who also practiced in New Port. Dr. McBride had become desperately ill in October 1859 and it was assumed that Dr. Telfair would attend to his medical needs. Unfortunately, however, Dr. Telfair was at the time on one of his "sprees" and quite unable to come to the aid of his brother-in-law, so Dr. Hentz was summoned from Quincy. His assistance came too late. In his diary he wrote: "Poor Dr. McBride was evidently sick unto death; his mind was unhinged; he smuggled chloroform into his room and inhaled it until he was crazed." Besides Dr. Telfair had earlier given him an enormus amount of calomel. He became maniacal before he died. "Subsequently, Dr. Telfair, ashamed made an effort to stop drinking.[7]

The census schedule of 1860 indicates that Dr. Telfair was a man of substance. At the age of 33 his property was valued at more than $20,000. His wife was then age 30 while his only child, Milton Stuart, was a boy of six.[8] For the next few years he was closely associated with Dr. Hentz who made frequent mention of him. In 1860 he assisted Dr. Hentz in a major surgical operation — amputation of a man's leg above the knee.[9] In the same year he attended Dr. Hentz' sister Carolina, wife of Dr. J.W. Keyes, at her accouchement. During the latter years of the Civil War Dr. Telfair was a member of the Board of Examiners for the Militia of Gadsden County.[10] In 1867 he again aided Dr. Hentz in a serious operation, this one requiring excision of a large tumor in the breast of Mrs. Shidor, wife of a Gadsden County judge. Others observing the surgery were "an unfledged doctor, Will Forman" and Dr. Telfair's young son, Stuart. Dr. Hentz recalled that "Dr. Telfair assisted me admirably, in holding the arteries as they were cut."[11]

Dr. Telfair's remaining days were few, however. He had apparently resumed drinking. While driving in his buggy near Bristol his horse was startled and lurched forward throwing him, intoxicated as he was, from the vehicle. Dr. Hentz reported that in the fall he sustained broken bones one of which severed an artery. Although his companion, a fellow named Tom Jones, was able to place him in the buggy and get him home, he died soon thereafter, it was assumed, from loss of blood.[12]

1. Dr. Hentz wrote his "Autobiography" some years after the events described had transpired. Although his memory was prodigious and his descriptions of persons and events probably fairly asccurate, his chronology is at times utterly confusing, with the dates of many occurrences being totally omitted. For example, although he describes the death of Dr. Telfair and recalled that he refused all medical assistance offered by Dr. John H. Gee, he provides no hint of the month or year of Dr. Telfair's death.
2. U.S. Census, 1850, Gadsden County, p. 342.
3. New Port *Wakulla Times*, June 23, 1858. 1st printed in issue of April 29, 1857 (missing).
4. Ibid.
5. Ibid., April 14, 1858.
6. Ibid., August 7, 1858.
7. Hentz, "Autobiography," I, 324.
8. U.S. Census, 1860, p. 60.
9. Hentz, "Autobiography," I, 329.
10. Quincy *Semi-Weekly Dispatch*, March 15, 1865.
11. Hentz, "Autobiography," II, 40. Included here is an interesting description of the mastectomy technique employed by Dr. Hentz. Incidentally, his fee was $250.
12. Ibid., II, 77.

Tennille, Alexander S., Jackson County, 1838

Dr. Tennille, a native of Georgia, was a resident of Jackson County in 1870. The census of that year gives his age as 31, his occupations as "M.D. and Farmer," while his real and personal property was valued at $7,000.[1] He was the sole occupant of the house. The single reference to his Florida sojourn, found in one of the few surviving newspapers of the period, indicates that he found Radical Reconstruction a bitter pill. In the elections of November 8, 1869, he joined with other citizens of the county in an effort to thwart the democratic process and prevent the election of Josiah T. Walls, a black, to the U.S. Congress.[2]

More than two years elapsed before federal authorities arrested Dr. Tennille and his fellow conspirator, Col. J.P. Coker on charges of "disturbing the election of the 8th of December, 1869," the arrest being made in early December 1871. According to the newspaper accounts, Col. Coker and the U.S. Deputy Marshal who arrested him were to leave immediately for Jacksonville to appear before United States Commissioner Acosta. But, added the editor whimsically, "Dr. Tennille has taken a circuitous route, if any, to the same city, but will not probably reach it within the same time as the first-named gentleman."[3]

Unfortunately, nothing more is known of this sometime Florida man of medicine.[4]

1. U.S. Census, 1870, Jackson County, Florida, item 384.

2. The resistance to federal authority during the early days of Reconstruction was particularly bitter in Jackson County, resulting in a series of murders before order was restored.

3. Marianna *Courier*, December 14, 1871, as reprinted in the Tallahassee *Sentinel*, December 23, 1871.

4. Dr. Tennille does not appear in the Confederate War Records pertaining to Florida. If he indeed had been in Confederate service it would probably have been with a Georgia unit. Confederate Records for Florida do, however, include the name William Tennille, also of Jackson County, a private in the 5th Battalion of Florida Cavalry, likely a relative.

Thomas, Gabriel Philip, Gainesville, 1827-1890

Dr. Thomas, one of Gainesville's most highly esteemed citizens, was born in Laurens District, South Carolina, on September 8, 1827.[1] He was the second son of Reuben and Malvina Thomas, and older brother of Dr. Robert Y.H. Thomas, also a Florida medical practitioner. Available records do not identify the medical school which he attended but it may be inferred from the census schedule that he had entered medical study at a more advanced age than was the case with most physicians.[2]

Dr. Thomas is said by local historians to have arrived in Gainesville in 1855,[3] but the earliest documentation for his presence in Gainesville is a land sale record of October 10, 1856, relating to purchase of a lot on the west side of the courthouse square.[4] On July 4 the following year he attended a celebration in Gainesville at which he offered a toast to "the Pulpit, the Press, and Hoops, the three ruling powers of the day, the Pulpit spreads morality, the Press knowledge, and Hoops spread considerably."[5] On January 20, 1858, he married Omera Brazile Fraser of South Carolina. Their first child, a son christened Thomas Fraser Thomas, was born in February 1860.[6]

Dr. Thomas came to Gainesville soon after the town had been selected to replace Newnansville as the county seat. He appears to have recognized its growth potential, responding by purchasing valuable real estate. He was the first to establish a drug store, an enterprise which he later shared with Thomas R. Kennedy. This was eventually expanded into a general merchandise establishment, although it retained a department of "medicine and drugs."[7] He was soon to build his residence at the northwest corner of North Main and Church Streets, presently the site of the Williams-Thomas Funeral Home.[8]

Notwithstanding his business interests Dr. Thomas was an active and highly reputable physician. He occasionally served as preceptor for students expecting to enter medical schools.[9] With the arrival in Gainesville of young Dr. James F. McKinstry in 1866, the two men entered into a professional partnership which was to last for almost two decades.[10] When a cholera scare disturbed the community in the summer of 1866, Dr. Thomas responded by publishing two lengthy articles on the disease, describing its symptoms and prescribing treatments. These were presented, of course, as an effort to relieve the rampant anxiety which had spread among the populace but they survive as useful documents setting forth contemporary theory and practice with respect to the dreaded ailment.[11] It may be assumed from random notices that his practice ran the gamut of demands facing most rural practititoners in those times, including attention to the trivial aches and pains as well as the hopeless cases, and often postmortem examinations.[12]

Dr. Thomas also found time to engage in nonprofessional activities although he seems to have kept himself aloof from local politics. He was, for example, one of the founders of the Gainesville Literary Association, organized on May 25, 1866. He became its first treasurer and with Dr. T.M. Colbert and Judge J.C. Gardner served as a committee to arrange future programs.[13]

It is not known just when Drs. Thomas and McKinstry dissolved their partnership. It is a matter of record, however, that Dr. Thomas spent his last years as a partner with his son, Dr. Thomas F. Thomas, who returned to Gainesville in 1884.[14] Dr. Thomas died in Gainesville on September 8, 1890, his 63rd birthday. He was survived by his widow who lived on until New Year's Day of 1901,[15] a daughter and three sons.[16]

1. U.S. Census, 1850, Laurens District, S.C., p. 281. The Thomases were a farming family whose real estate was valued at $5000. There were 10 children in the family. Their ages ranged from 24 to three, the youngest being three-year-old twin daughters.

2. Ibid. In this schedule Gabriel Philip Thomas' age is stated as 22 and his occupation as farmer.

3. F.W. Buchholz, *History of Alachua County*, St. Augustine, 1929, p. 193.

4. Chas. H. Hildreth, "A History of Gainesville," Ph.D. dissertation, University of Florida, 1954. Revised and published by Hildreth and Merlin G. Cox, Gainesville, Alachua County Historical Society, 1981, p. 12.

5. Jacksonville *Florida News*, July 25, 1857.

6. Marriage Records, Alachua County, Book III, p. 2.

7. Hildreth, "History of Gainesville," p. 18. See Gainesville *New Era*, September 27, 1866.

8. The Thomas House was one of the first to be built in Gainesville. Orange Street is now 4th Avenue, N.E. and N.W.

9. Lists of Graduates and Matriculants, Medical College of the State of South Carolina, Waring Historical Medical Library, Charleston, S.C.

10. Gainesville *New Era*, February 23, 1867.

11. Ibid. Issues of September 21 and 28, 1866.

12. Ibid., February 10, 1866.

13. June 1, 1866. Dr. Thomas did not, however, shun civic responsibility. In 1876 he helped organize the Alachua Club. As its president he led discussions designed to find solutions to some of the woes of Reconstruction. Gainesville *Times*, July 28, 1876. Three weeks later he was chairman of a meeting called to select delegates to a County Convention and to nominate a senator from the local district. Ibid., August 10, 1876. In early January 1877, Governor Drew appointed Dr. Thomas Collector of Revenue for Alachua County. This action was greeted with a rumble of resentment at the Convention a week later. Several delegates considered the Governor's action premature, claiming that he should have waited until the Convention had made the nomination. The altercation was settled peacefully, however, with a majority voting to accept the Governor's choice. Dr. Thomas, however, incurred some resentment when he published a list of delinquents who had failed to pay their taxes. Ibid., August 20, 1877.

14. Rowland H. Rerick, *Memoirs of Florida*, Atlanta, 1902, II, 723.

15. Gravestones, Evergreen Cemetery, Gainesville.

16. In addition to Dr. Thomas F. Thomas, mentioned supra, the other children of Dr. Thomas were William Reuben, who became mayor of Gainesville; Omera, who married M.F. McCook of Brunswick, Georgia; and Samuel J., who became a furniture dealer in Gainesville.

Thomas, Patrick H., Gadsden County, 1838-1863

Dr. Thomas, son of James and Mary Ann Thomas, both natives of Georgia, was born in Gadsden County in 1838. He was the fourth of nine children. The elder Thomas was apparently a comparatively prosperous farmer.[1] Young Thomas entered the Medical College of the State of South Carolina in the fall of 1858 and was graduated as M.D. in the spring of 1860. The records of the College show his home town as Quincy and his preceptors as Drs. John H. and Charles Gee. His doctoral thesis was entitled simply "Pleurisy." He was said to have had a classical education before entering upon the study of medicine.[2]

Dr. Thomas had scarcely begun the practice of medicine in Quincy when his medical service were required by the Confederate Army. The actual date of his enlistment is presently unknown. In the summer of 1863 he was surgeon in the Fifth Battalion, Florida Cavalry, stationed at Camp Anderson, "near Ft. Gadsden, Fla."[3] On September 3, he recommended a sick leave of 25 days for Private William Gatlin, appending his signature as P.H. Thomas, Surgeon. But for Dr. Thomas himself death came shortly therafter. The following item documents his demise:

> Camp Anderson, Near Fort Gadsden, Fla., Sept. 7th 1863.
> Sergeant G.B. Poppell is Detailed to carry Dr. P.H. Thomas Corpse to Quincy and Return on Saturday Night 12 inst.
> By Order of Capt. A.C. Smith, Comdg Inspr Cav Co. by A.W. Smith, 2nd Lieut, said Company.[4]

1. U.S. Census, 1850, Gadsden County, Florida, p. 377.
2. Catalogue, Medical College of the State of South Carolina, Lists of Students, pp. 399, 420, 425.
3. Ft. Gadsden, dating back to the war of 1812, was located on the east bank of the Apalachicola River some 10 miles from the present town of Apalachicola. It is located in Franklin County. A state park commemorates its historical significance.
4. For the two items cited here I am indebted to E. Wilson Hinson Jr., of Quincy, who discovered them among the papers of William Gatlin, now in the possession of his grandson, Lester Gatlin, also of Quincy.

The military record of Dr. Thomas is missing from the official documents preserved in the National Archives, Service Records, CSA. This omission suggests that he may have retained his civilian status while serving as an army surgeon by contractual arrangement.

Thomas, Robert, Hamilton County, 1820

Dr. Thomas, who practiced medicine for about a decade in Florida, was born in North Carolina in 1820.[1] As a young man he moved to Georgia, settling in Camden County, probably in what was known as the St. Mary's River Settlement outside the town of St. Mary's. When still in his early 20s he married Elizabeth Lang, daughter of wealthy planter, Isaac Lang, of Camden County. The census of 1850 designated him "merchant"[2] but since the slave schedule of that year indicates that he was the owner of 12 slaves, it is assumed that he also engaged in farming.

Apparently weary of his occupation, and at an age more advanced than that of most medical students, Dr. Thomas enrolled at the Savannah Medical College in the fall of 1855 and in the spring of 1857 received his medical degree, having presented a doctoral thesis entitled "Bilious Remittent Fever."[3] Soon thereafter he moved to Hamilton County and entered practice at White Springs, a popular spa on the Suwannee River. By this stage of his life, either through inheritance or marriage, he had become of person of considerable means. The Slave Schedule of 1860, Hamilton County, shows him as owner of 44 slaves while the regular census of that year estimates his total assets at $33,000.[4] His slave holdings strongly suggest that he was still both physician and planter.

As was true of most planters, the War Between the States, emancipation of slaves, and disruptions of Reconstruction profoundly altered the life-style of Dr. Thomas and his family. These events, combined with the death of his wife, prompted Dr. Thomas to move to Valdosta, Georgia, where he operated a drug store in partnership with H.Y. Tillman. In contrast to his assets of 1860, the census of 1870 lists his total property value at $2,300.[5] Soon after settling in Valdosta he married Katherine Wyche. About 1890 Dr. Thomas sold his interest in the drug store to his partner, Tillman,[6] and lived out his retirement in Valdosta.

Several children were born to the two marriages of Dr. Thomas. Two sons, Robert and David, became druggists, while his eldest son, William, was a businessman in Valdosta. A grandson, Joseph Thomas, after graduation from Auburn (Alabama Polytechnic Institute) and the Medical College of the University of Virginia, returned to Valdosta to practice medicine.[7]

1. All census schedules, 1850 through 1880, indicate that Dr. Thomas was born in 1820.
2. U.S. Census, 1850, Camden County, Georgia, p. 382, item 87.
3. Savannah Medical College, "Circular & Catalogue," Session of 1857-58; also ibid, Session of 1875-76, which lists all graduates up to that date.
4. U.S. Census, 1860, Hamilton County, Florida, p. 603.
5. U.S. Census, 1870, Lowndes County, Georgia, p. 316.
6. *History of Lowndes County, Georgia, 1825-1941.* Prepared by Daughters of the American Revolution, Valdosta Chapter, Valdosta, 1942. Reprint, Spartanburg, S.C., 1978, pp. 239, 326.
7. Ibid., p. 329.

Thomas, Robert Young Hayne, Marion, Alachua and Levy Counties, 1834-1892

Robert Y.H. Thomas, namesake of the famous Senator, Robert Young Hayne of South Carolina, remembered for his debate in 1830 with Daniel Webster, was born in Laurens District, South Carolina, on September 24, 1834, son of Reubin and Malvina Thomas.[1] He entered Jefferson Medical College, Philadelphia, Pennsylvania, in the fall of 1857, and in the spring of 1855 received his medical degree.[2]

Soon after graduation Dr. Thomas moved to Florida, doubtless persuaded by his brother, Dr. Gabriel Philip Thomas, who had begun medical practice in Gainesville about 1855. Dr. Robert, however, elected to settle in adjoining Marion County where he purchased land and entered into the dual roles of planter and physician.[3] He appears to have arrived in the winter of 1857-58.[4] His professional notice of May 15, 1860, implies that he was already a well-established physician. It states: "Dr. Robert Y.H. Thomas, being thankful for past favors, continues to practice medicine, Surgery and Obstetrics in Marion and surrounding counties...Same liberal terms, office and residence twelve miles northwest of Ocala."[5]

With the Civil War already under way Dr. Thomas enlisted for service in the 7th Florida Infantry Regiment, an Alachua County unit, on April 12, 1862. He was mustered in at Camp Lee near Gainesville and assigned to Company H with the rank of sergeant, having committed himself for "three years, or the duration."[6] He had scarcely become oriented to military duty, however, when he was beset by a pulmonary ailment which was diagnosed as chronic bronchitis. A medical board judged him unfit for further service and he was discharged on July 28 after spending a month in an army hospital. The recommendation for discharge signed by his commanding officer included this description of Dr. Thomas: "five feet, ten inches tall, of light complexion, blue eyes, light hair, and by profession a physician."

Upon his return to Marion County, and with the improvement of his health, Dr. Thomas was persuaded to run for a seat in the Florida House of Representatives. He won handily and took his seat in the House in November 1862 serving for two terms.[7]

About 1863 Dr. Thomas married a South Carolina girl, Mary R., daughter of Thomas Fraser. It is not known how long the Thomases remained in their Marion County home, known as Pine Hill. They were there as late as October 1865 when Dr. Thomas was administrator of the estate of Kitchen W. Syms, deceased. In the settlement process he found it necessary to bring charge against another Marion County physician, Dr. C.W. Lesesne, who was indebted to the Syms estate.[8]

By 1870 Dr. Thomas had moved to Gainesville where he joined his brother, Gabriel, in a professional partnership. In addition to medical practice the two men maintained an active interest in the social and political life of the county and state. Dr. Robert found the radical reconstruction of the Republican Party abhorrent and embraced with fervor the Democratic or Conservative policies. In July 1876, he called the Democrats of Alachua County into convention for the purpose of selecting candidates for the approaching elections, himself serving as secretary of the meeting.[9] He was promptly nominated for the Florida Senate but in the voting lost to Judge Thomas F. King by the one sided margin of 34 to four.[10] In the ensuing gubernatorial race he was an active supporter of George F. Drew who won the election.[11]

In September 1876, Dr. Thomas was appointed Health Officer for Gainesville,[12] a post he resigned a year later to accept an appointment as Port Physician and Inspector of Cedar Keys in lieu of Dr. George A. Penny, who had resigned because of unacceptable restrictions imposed upon him by the town's Board of Health.[13] The Gainesville *Times* of September 22, 1877, announced: "Dr. Thomas is now in Cedar Keys." Before the end of the year he had joined Dr. Andrew E. Hodges, widely known Levy County physician and businessman, in a partnership.[14] In the city elections held the following spring Dr. Thomas was elected City Marshal.[15]

For the next few years Dr. Thomas appears to have carried on the typical practice of a small town physician of the times. The Mortality Schedule for Levy County for the year ending May 31, 1885, indicated that he was one of the most active practitioners of the county.[16]

In the summer of 1892 Dr. Thomas was one of three nominees for Levy County's seat in the Florida Senate, the others being Newton A. Blitch and N.R. Carter.[17] The elections were set for October 4 but death came for Dr. Thomas on September 6. His body was brought to Gainesville for burial in the family plot in Evergreen Cemetery.[18] Besides his wife, Dr. Thomas was survived by three daughters, Hattie (Mrs. William H. Anderson), Belva and Julia, and one son, Robert.

1. U.S. Census, 1850, Laurens District, S.C., p. 281.

2. Jefferson Medical College, *List of Graduates*, Philadelphia, 1879, p. 88.

3. Several physicians and others from South Carolina settled in the northwestern part of Marion County in the 1840s and 1850s. Dr. Thomas' holding was hardly a plantation in the usual sense, however, having been operated with only five slaves.

4. Ocala *Florida Home Companion*, February 16, 1858. Guests arriving at Ocala House on February 8 included Dr. R.Y.H. Thomas of Pine Hill.
5. Ibid., June 5, 1860. 1st Printing May 15.
6. National Archives, CSA, M. 251, Roll 80.
7. Allen Morris, *The People of Lawmaking in Florida*, 1977 ed.
8. Letter, Chas. A. Northrop, Lieut., 34th U.S. Army Command Post, Ocala, to Dr. C.W. Lesesne, October 24, 1865, P.K. Yonge Library of Florida History, Mss. Box 720.
9. Gainesville *Times*, July 27, 1876. Ibid., July 6, 1876.
10. Ibid., August 17, 1876.
11. Ibid., September 14, 1876.
12. Ibid., September 21, 1876.
13. Ibid., September 22, 1877.
14. Ibid., December 22, 1877.
15. Ibid., March 6, 1878.
16. Special Florida Census, Levy County, 1885.
17. Gainesville *Sun*, July 15, 1892. Blitch was the winner.
18. The dates of Dr. Thomas' birth and death are found on his gravestone.

Thomas, William J., Newnansville, 1860-70

Although Dr. Thomas was a member of the Thomas family of South Carolina, several members of which migrated to Florida in the antebellum period, he never achieved the prominence which accrued to those who settled in Gainesville. This is possibly explained by the fact that Newnansville where he settled was declining in importance after 1854. He came to Florida about 1860 but not in time to be included in the official census of that year. According to the census of 1870 he was married to a Florida-born wife, Mary, about 1861 and their family included four sons, Julius, Brantley, Henry and William, aged eight, six, four and two, respectively. His worldly goods were of negligible value, a mere $200. Nothing further is known of him.[1]

1. U.S. Census, 1870, Alachua County, Florida, p. 346.

Thompson, J.C., Madison County, 1870s

Of Dr. Thompson it is only known that he was a medical practitioner in the Moseley Hall district of Madison County in the 1870s. The Census of 1880 lists him as physician, aged 50, a native of South Carolina. His wife, R.B., was a native of North Carolina while their two daughters, Eliza and Maggie, aged 17 and six respectively, were natives of Florida. Dr. Thompson is not listed among the graduates of the Medical College of the State of South Carolina.[1]

1. U.S. Census, 1880, Madison County, Florida, p. 10.

Thompson, John H., Quincy, mid-19th century

Dr. Thompson, who practiced medicine for a few years in Quincy, was a native of Calhoun District, South Carolina. Records of the Medical College of the State of South Carolina, at which he matriculated in the fall of 1848, indicate that he was a resident of the town of St. Matthews. He was graduated as Doctor of Medicine in March 1850 having submitted a thesis entitled "Pneumonia."[1] No trace of his early practice has been found. By 1870 he was a resident of Quincy, the census of that year stating his age as 42. Other members of his household were daughters, Eleanor, aged 12; Claudia, aged 10; Eliza, aged six, and son, Paul, aged eight.[2] Since all the children were born in Florida it is assumed that Dr. Thompson had moved to the state as early as 1857-58. No further information has been discovered.

1. Archives, Waring Historical Library, Medical University College of Medicine, Charleston, S.C.
2. U.S. Census, 1870, Gadsden County, Florida, p. 830, item 120. Paul Thompson later studied law and became a county judge of Gadsden County.

Thompson, Thomas H., Apalachicola, 1804-1840

Since all that is presently known of Dr. Thompson is found in an obituary notice published in the St. Joseph *Times* of August 6, 1840, it seems fitting and adequate to reproduce it here.

> Died in this city on Saturday, 1st of August, Thomas H. Thompson, M.D., of Apalachicola, aged 35. Dr. Thompson was a native of Charleston [Charlestown], Massachusetts, and came to Apalachicola in the fall of 1837. Skillful as a physician, a kind friend and an accomplished gentleman, he soon ingratiated himself into the esteem, confidence and love of the circle in which he moved. But a few weeks before his decease Dr. Thompson became, with Mr. Baltzell, a joint editor of the Apalachicola *Advertiser*, and the profession particularly may deplore the loss of a highly gifted member whose chaste and classical mind would have imparted unusual interest to the topics within his department. He was removed to this City [St. Joseph] a few days before his decease. Every attention, medical and otherwise, was shown to his comfort....

The notice ends with a further eulogy couched in deeply sentimental language.[1]

1. The Mr. Baltzell was George F. Baltzell. See J.O. Knauss, *Territorial Florida Journalism*, Deland, 1926, p. 120. Although Baltzell had studied medicine there is no indication that he ever practiced.

Todd, James A.S., Marion and Duval Counties, 1837

Dr. Todd, fourth child and eldest of the three sons of Dr. Patrick H. Todd, was born in Lexington District, South Carolina, in 1837.[1] He entered the Georgia Medical College in Augusta in 1856 and was graduated as Doctor of Medicine the following spring.[2] In the winter of 1857-58 his family moved to Marion County and settled on a farm in the southern part of the county.[3] Dr. Todd joined them in early 1858 and on April 13 announced his services to the citizens of adjoining Sumpter County, giving his residence and office address as Col. Thomas' Hotel in the village of Adamsville[4] situated some 25 miles south of Ocala.

Dr. Todd's sojourn in Adamsville appears to have been brief, however, for in November 1859 he moved to Ocala, announcing on November 30 his decision to settle permanently in the town. His office was located above the store of Dickinson and Harn from which his services were available.[5] In the following year he relocated at the hotel run by E.J. Harris, at which three other physicians had also obtained lodgings.[6]

With the outbreak of war in 1861 Dr. Todd joined his younger brother, Patrick, also a graduate of the Georgia Medical College, in enlisting in the Confederate cause. His enlistment is dated July 5, 1861. Both men were assigned to Company E, Second Florida Infantry Regiment. Soon after induction both were transferred to Camp Virginia in Jacksonville where Dr. James Todd remained for at least a year. Meanwhile he was detailed as Acting Hospital Steward and on May 21, 1862, was promoted to Steward and designated "Company Physician." He was still serving in this capacity on September 30, 1862, the final item included in his military service record.[7]

On September 22, 1865, Dr. Todd announced the opening of his professional office in Jacksonville, located "upstairs in C. Nichols Building, Bay Street."[8] In June the following year he moved to the corner of Adams and Ocean Streets.[9] Beyond this date, however, nothing further is known of the man. He either moved to another locality or was deceased. He was not included in the Duval County census of 1870.

1. This date of birth is an extrapolation from the Marion County, Florida, census of 1860 which gives his age as 23.
2. Medical Department, University of Georgia, Augusta, *List of Graduates from 1829 to 1891*, Augusta, 1891, p. 26.
3. Ocala *Florida Home Companion*, February 2, 1858; March 6, 1858.
4. Ibid., April 13, 1858.
5. Jacksonville *Florida Times*, December 7, 1865. 1st printed September 22, 1865, issue not extant.
6. These were Drs. H.C. Vaughan, Emile T. Sabal and E.S. Aldrich.
7. NA, Service Records, CSA, M251, Roll 42.
8. Jacksonville *Florida Times*, December 7, 1865.
9. Jacksonville *Florida Union*, September 29, 1866.

Todd, Patrick H., Marion County, 1810-1880

Dr. Todd, a native of Lexington District, South Carolina, and medical practitioner there until the late 1850s, was one of many South Carolinians who settled in Marion County during the two decades prior to the Civil War. The Lexington census of 1850 shows him to have been a physician of moderate means, operating a farm in the predominantly rural part of the District.[1] In early 1858, following the lead of some of his neighbors, he made his way to Florida, arriving at Ocala House, Ocala, on January 28.[2] It was obviously a prospecting trip for having made preliminary arrangements he returned to South Carolina and in early March arrived in Ocala accompanied by his wife, Mary Ann, and five of his six children.[3] The Census of 1860 lists him a "planter-doctor" with property valued at $21,000. The slave schedule of that year numbered his slaves at 15.[4]

As it did for many, the War of Secession and the accompanying emancipation of slaves brought disaster for Dr. Todd. Meanwhile, the death of his wife was an additional blow, and to compound his unhappiness his second son and namesake, Patrick P.L. Todd, an 1858 graduate of the Georgia Medical College, Augusta, and an early enlistee in the Confederate cause, was mortally wounded at Mine Run, Virginia, in November 1863.[5]

Dr. Todd married his second wife on September 3, 1874, Mrs. Mary E. Brown, a widow some 20 years his junior[6] and also a native of South Carolina. From this point onward little is known of Dr. Todd. The 1880 census shows him living with his wife and stepson, Adison Brown,[7] nor is much known of Dr. Todd's children by his first wife. In addition to Dr. Patrick Todd Jr., there were two other sons: Joseph A.S. Todd, like his brother a graduate of the Georgia Medical College and sometime practitioner in Jacksonville, and John C. Calhoun Todd. There were also daughters Laura, Louisa and a third known only as "Miss B.A." Todd.[8] Biographical information on them is missing. Since the date of Dr. Todd's death is unknown it can only be said that it occurred after 1880.

1. U.S. Census, 1850, Lexington District, S.C., p. 374, it. 513.
2. Ocala *Florida Home Companion*, February 2, 1858.
3. Ibid., March 6, 1858.
4. U.S. Census, 1860, Marion County, Florida, p. 526.
5. NA, Service Records, CSA, Co. E, 2nd Florida Infantry.
6. Ocala *East Florida Banner*, September 5, 1874.
7. U.S. Census, 1880, Marion County, Florida, p. 137.
8. The Christian names of the Todd daughters were gleaned from various census listings.

Todd, Patrick P.L., Marion County, 1841-1863

Except for his military career in the Confederate Army little is known of the life of Dr. Todd. He was a native of Lexington District, South Carolina, the son of physician, Dr. Patrick H. Todd, and his wife Mary Ann.[1] Following in the steps of his father and older brother, James, he elected to go into medicine. He matriculated at the Medical College of Georgia, Augusta, in the fall of 1856 and was graduated in the spring of 1858.[2] From Augusta he went directly to Ocala where he is thought to have begun medical practice, although no actual confirmation of this has been discovered. Other members of his family had settled in Marion County at about the same time, March 1858.[3]

With the coming of the War in 1861, Dr. Todd was among the first to enlist, having enrolled in Company E, Second Florida Infantry, at Ocala, on July 5, 1861. He was sent shortly thereafter to Camp Virginia in Jacksonville where he remained in various capacities until the summer of 1863. Meanwhile he was promoted with regularity from private which he remained for only about six weeks to a captaincy July 3, 1863, and company commander. He went with his regiment to Virginia in the summer of 1863 and in the following November was wounded at Mine Run. He was taken to the General Hospital at Charlottesville which was at the time under the command of another Floridian, Dr. T.M. Palmer. Young Dr. Todd died there on December 9, 1863 from a "wound of the chest traversing his lungs," thus terminating what appears to have been a promising medical career.[4]

1. U.S. Census, 1850, Lexington District, S.C., p. 374.
2. Medical Department, University of Georgia, *List of Graduates, 1829-1891*, Augusta, 1891, p. 26.
3. Ocala *Florida Home Companion*, March 16, 1858.
4. NA, Service Records, CSA, M251, Reel 42.

Todd, Samuel B., Hillsborough County, 1820

Few traces of the earlier and later years of the life of Dr. Todd remain. He was born in Vermont about 1820 but he does not appear in the records of either of the medical schools existing in Vermont in the mid-19th century. The earliest reference to his presence in Florida is found in a letter, Governor Thomas Brown to Major David E. Twiggs, Commander, 2nd Division, U.S. Army, Headquarters, Tampa Bay, dated October 7, 1849, in which Brown called the attention of Twiggs to two companies of militia from Hillsborough County recruited a few months earlier by ex-Governor Moseley. These troops were encamped on the Caloosahatchee River at a site soon to be called Ft. Myers. Brown suggested that the troops be discharged or, if needed, inducted into the regular United States Army. Included in the letter was the following:[1]

> I am informed that Dr. S.B. Todd was elected surgeon to these companies and that he has not only devoted his services as physician to the troops, but that he has attended the sick of the destitute families in the forts, to which they have been driven for protection and security, along the frontier for the distance of some thirty miles, and furnished medicines from his own resources. If it is not inconsistent with army regulations I hope he may be received into the United States service with the troops as surgeon.

Apparently nothing came of this, however, for in the following year the census schedule for Hillsborough County lists Dr. Todd and his wife, Martha, a Georgia native, as residents of the Simmons Hammock community of the county. He was 30; his wife 18. His occupational designation was "Protestant minister and doctor of medicine."[2]

Almost from the time of his arrival in Florida Dr. Todd was involved in the problems and issues of his community. He was among the Hillsborough citizens who came together in Tampa on December 15, 1851, to take action against the threat emanating from recent Indian hostilities.[3] As a member of the Resolutions Committee he read the draft which demanded the removal of all Indians from the state. On several occasions he lent his support to efforts to obtain a railroad connecting Tampa with Ocala. He represented his county at a meeting in Ocala called for that purpose in March 1858.[4] He not only addressed the group but delivered subscriptions for stock amounting to $225,000 collected mostly from Tampa subscribers.[5] In 1859 the Fernandina newspaper published a letter from Dr. Todd to Governor Perry telling of the inconveniece he had in going by steamship from Cedar Key to Tampa because of the shallow channel at Cedar Key.[6]

As for Dr. Todd's medical career only occasional data appear. In a professional notice of March 10, 1855, it was announced that "S.B. Todd, M.D., *still* offers his professional services to the citizens of Tampa...He will keep on hand a large and choice assortment of Drugs and Medicines...also a valuable and well-selected stock of books, stationery, maps, pictures, etc."[7] With the appearance of Dr. Sheldon Stringer in Tampa about 1860 the two physicians joined in a medical partnership, first advertised on February 3 that year. Their offices were located at the Tampa Book and Drug Store, Dr. Todd's establishment.[8]

The census of 1860 for the City of Tampa indicates that Dr. Todd was a man of modest means, his properties being valued at $8,992. Mrs. Todd was then 27. Their five children were listed as Martha, 10; Samuel Jr., eight; Frances, six; Charles, four; and Mary, nine months.[9]

In 1858 Dr. Todd made a formal request to the Florida Legislature for compensation for service performed for the state. The request was presented to the House by Tillman Ingram of Alachua County and eventually approved by a vote of 35 to one, only to come to naught when the Claims Committee of the Senate rejected it as "unjustified."[10]

Information is vague concerning Dr. Todd's military service in the Civil War. It derives from a single entry in the compilation, *Soldiers of Florida,* and appears as follows: "S.M.E. *(sic),* surgeon, Field Service; Camp Instruction; dead."[11] It may be conjectured that as a physician, aged 40, he was not drafted but instead had contracted his services for instruction in hygiene or sanitation in an army camp. It seems likely that he died during the period of the War. No member of the Todd family appears in the Hillsborough County Census of 1870.

1. Two medical schools existed in Vermont: Castleton, 1818-62, and the Vermont Medical College at Woodstock, 1827-56. *Florida Senate Journal*, 1850-51, App., p. 22.
2. U.S. Census, 1850, Hillsborough County, Florida, p. 497.
3. Jacksonville *Florida Republican*, January 2, 1852.
4. Tampa *Florida Peninsular*, March 20, 1858.
5. Fernandina *Florida News*, March 31, 1858. At a Tampa meeting on June 9, 1858, the railroad, known as the Florida Peninsula Railroad Co., was organized and Dr. Todd was elected as president. Tampa *Florida Peninsular*, June 19, 1858.
6. Fernandina *Florida News*, March 17, 1859.
7. The insertion of the word "still" suggests that Dr. Todd was simply resuming his advertising but had not ceased practice. Tampa *Florida Peninsular*, March 10, 1855.
8. It was very common for physicians of the times and well into the 20th century to own and operate drug stores.
9. U.S. Census, 1860, Hillsborough County, Florida, item 521.
10. *Florida House Journal*, 1858, p. 205 et passim; Florida Senate Journal, 1858, pp. 311-12, 359.
11. *Soldiers of Florida*, Tallahassee, 1903, p. 320.

Toland, Elihu, Quincy, 1834

One of the most titillating yet reproachable affairs ever associated with a 19th century Florida physician involved Dr. Toland, who for a few years practiced medicine in Quincy, becoming a trusted citizen and a member of the Medical Examining Board of the Middle Florida District during the Civil War. This Board was charged with determining the fitness of recruits for entering military service.

Dr. Toland was a native of Laurens District, South Carolina, the son of Hugh Toland, a wheelwright and farmer, who lived near the town of Clinton.[1] Scarcely any information about his childhood and education has survived, nor has the medical college which he may have attended been identified. The best that can be said of him is that he was without doubt a charming rascal; the worst, that he was an inveterate and unscrupulous liar, capable of outrageous and irresponsible behavior.[2]

The Civil War was already under way when Dr. Toland arrived in Florida. He claimed, however, to have seen some service in a South Carolina regiment but that has not been verified. He is thought to have begun his Quincy residence in 1863. Whatever the date he quickly ingratiated himself with the people of the town. With his appointment to the State Examining Board his status as a respectable citizen was assured. While serving in this capacity he was introduced into the home of Isaac C. Jeffress and soon gained the trust and confidence of the family. He quickly became enamored of daughter Linda, and apparently his sentiments were reciprocated, and proceeded to propose marriage, urging his bride to go to Brazil with him, explaining that he was financially well-off, but that his life would be in jeopardy should he return to South Carolina. He hinted that he had been active in tracking down South Carolina "Tories," the term applied to those Southerners who embraced the Union cause.

The two were married in Quincy on May 11, 1865. Four weeks later Dr. Toland left for South Carolina, having explained to his bride that he was going to prepare his sumptuous house for the arrival of new wife, the Brazil plan having apparently been abandoned.

Meanwhile Dr. Toland revealed an earlier marriage in South Carolina to Linda Lowry of a fine Edgefield, South Carolina, family. He also told of the two children born to that marriage and, with tears streaming from his eyes, he related the death of both wife and children, referring to the first Mrs. Toland as "my sainted wife." For the trip back to South Carolina he borrowed a team of horses and a buggy from his new father-in-law, Mr. Jeffress. In due time he returned to Quincy, not with the borrowed team and buggy, but by public conveyance, explaining that a hired man would be arriving soon with the horses and buggy. Apparently his fabricated story aroused little if any suspicion.

Back in Quincy Dr. Toland resumed medical practice for several months, still boasting of his extensive and valuable holdings in various towns including Charleston, Columbia, and Augusta, meanwhile borrowing money from Mr. Jeffress. His secretive behavior regarding his mail, however, began to arouse suspicion. He instructed the Quincy postmaster that under no circumstances was his mail to be delivered to anyone except himself. One day, however, his new wife ventured to open a packet of his mail, discovering letters from his wife in South Carolina. When confronted with this discovery Dr. Toland explained that the letters were from his sister-in-law, also named Linda.

Forthwith, Colonel Samuel B. Love of Quincy was dispatched to South Carolina to investigate Dr. Toland's background. There he met the first Mrs. Toland, whom he found to be a nice, respectable woman of good family, still wearing a breast pin with Dr. Toland's picture. Colonel Love also discovered that Dr. Toland had sold the horses and buggy for cash. But even with the disclosures brought back by Love, Dr. Toland maintained his innocence, claiming that he was never married to Linda Lowry, that she had only been his concubine. It had been confirmed, however, that the two children born of that first union were deceased. Furthermore, the postmaster of Clinton, S.C., well acquainted with the Toland family, recalled that Dr. Toland during his brief residence in Clinton had seduced a local girl who had become the mother of his child.

The tangled web of Toland lies was further extended and threatened to enmesh him. In desperation he tried to persuade his Quincy wife to escape to California with him. There, he claimed, he had a wealthy cousin willing to endow them. She rejected his every proposal, however.[3]

A warrant for arrest was issued in Quincy and on May 31, 1866, he was apprehended in Tallahassee, taken in hand by the Gadsden County sheriff and the following day returned to Quincy to face charges of bigamy. His trial, which took place during the first week of July, resulted in a verdict of guilty. A fine of $1,000 was imposed but unable to raise the amount he was returned to jail. While he languished there he made one unsuccessful attempt to escape. Meanwhile Sheriff Jordan advertised from the Court House door the services of the prisoner, presumably manual labor, but no employer came forth and he was returned to jail, or as the Gainesville *New Era* of September 28, 1866, phrased it, he was "sent back to his rooms in the 'public hotel.'"

The Tallahassee *Tri-Weekly Sentinel* of September 27, 1866, pondered the severity of Dr. Toland's punishment as required by Florida law, wondering whether "even in these hard times the penalty bears any sort of just proportion to the enormity of the crime. Only $1,000 for wrecking happiness for life." It concluded, however, that "the punishment is not too severe," adding that it is "another warning to girls in marrying strangers before knowing their whole history."

The final public notice concerning the affair appears in the Quincy *Commonwealth* of September 25, 1866, in which it was stated that since no one wished to hire Toland, he was "bid in by the County of Gadsden for five years for $1,127, the amount of the fine and cost of prosecution. He was remanded to the jail and there awaits the command of the County Commissioners." Nothing further has come to light about this clever but unfortunate physician.

1. The Hugh Toland of this sketch is not to be confused with another of the same name, a South Carolina physician of some distinction whose sexual appetites were similar to those of the subject of this sketch. His affair with a married lady of Newberry, S.C., a Mrs. Boozer, who later joined him in Columbia, inspired gossip. Also it is probable that the "cousin" referred to by Dr. Elihu Toland as a resident of California was Dr. Hugh Toland. See Thomas H. Pope, *The History of Newberry County, South Carolina,* Vol. 1, 1749-1860, p. 102. See also Joseph I. Waring, *A History of Medicine in South Carolina, 1825-1900,* Charleston, 1967, p. 311. The South Carolina Census, 1850, Laurens District, lists Elihu Toland, age 16, third son of Hugh Toland.

2. The whole sordid story of Dr. Toland's Florida escapade is set forth in a series of items in various newspapers, beginning with the account of his arrest in the Tallahassee *Semi-Weekly Floridian* of September 27, 1866.

3. The most damaging testimony against Dr. Toland was contained in a letter, Isaac C. Jeffress to the Editor of the Tallahassee *Tri-Weekly Sentinel* and published in the issue of July 5, 1866. The item contains a catalog of Toland's misdeeds, while revealing the anguish of Jeffress from the wrongs committed against his daughter.

Tommy, Oliver P., Hamilton and Marion Counties, 1850s

Dr. Tommy (Tommey), sometime medical practitioner in Hamilton County, appears in the Census of 1850 as a resident of Bellville, a village in the northwestern part of the county. In that year he was 33 year of age. A native of Georgia, he is thought to have moved to Florida about 1848. Both his wife, Mary, and son, George, aged five, were born in Georgia.[1] Ten years later, however, the Marion County census lists him as a resident of Ocala, employed as a "railroad agent." By that date an additional son, Walter aged seven, had been born to the Tommys. Nothing further is known of the family.[2]

1. U.S. Census, 1850, Hamilton County, Florida, p. 440, item 55.
2. Ibid., 1860, Marion County, Florida, p. 5.

Towers, J.A., Gadsden County, 1820-1850

Information relating to the career of Dr. Towers is not plentiful. It is reasonably clear, however, that he was born in Georgia about 1820 and that in the later 1830s he made his way into Florida where he began his medical study as an apprentice in the office of Dr. John Malone of Quincy.[1] In the summer of 1842 he was among the group of Gadsden citizens who signed a petition urging Senator John C. Calhoun of South Carolina to press for statehood for the Florida Territory.[2]

A few weeks later Dr. Towers matriculated at the Medical College of South Carolina, Charleston. At the completion of the term in March 1843, he returned to Florida and appears to have offered medical services to the military unit remaining at Fort King, Marion County, after cessation of the Second Seminole War. His signature was the first to be attached to a petition of September 1, 1843, and circulated at the Fort, requesting that Congress aid in construction of a road linking St. Augustine and Palatka. In this instance his signature appears as "J.A. Towers, M.D."[3] It was not uncommon for practitioners of medicine to arrogate the designation M.D. regardless of their formal medical training.

In the fall of 1843, Dr. Towers returned to Charleston, resuming his studies and graduating in March 1844. His thesis topic was "Tetanus."[4]

No date of death for Dr. Towers has been discovered. Since he does not appear in the Florida census of 1850, it is assumed that he had died prior to the tabulation of that year.[5]

1. U.S. Census, 1850, Gadsden County, Florida, pp. 345-46. This entry lists Mrs. Maria Towers, presumably the widow of Dr. Towers, and her two children, Charles, aged six, and Nancy, aged five. Her age was 21. Marriage records of Gadsden County show Mrs. Towers remarrying in 1866. In this instance her husband was Robert Holloman.

2. Clarence Edwin Carter, ed. & comp., *The Territorial Papers of the United States*, vol. XXVI, "The Territory of Florida, 1839-1845," Washington D.C., 1965, p. 500. This petition was referred to Congress on August 10, 1840.

3. Ibid., p. 736.

4. *Catalogue of Students, Medical College of the State of South Carolina, 1842-43*, p. 141. Ibid., 1843-44, p. 152.

5. The census data leaves many questions unanswered. It appears, however that Mrs. Towers and her two children were living in the home of her mother, Mrs. Mary Attoraber, her son William, and daughters Elizabeth and Sarah. The Towers son Charles served in the Civil War and at the conclusion of the War married Margaret Woodbury also of Gadsden County.

Tradewell, William, Leon County, 1847

Dr. Tradewell (Tradwell, Tredwell, Treadwell), probably a native of South Carolina, arrived in Tallahassee early in 1833, doubtless having been urged to come to Florida by his friend, Dr. John McLemore, who had established a medical practice in Tallahassee in December 1831.[1] Whatever the inducements, Dr. McLemore announced "with pleasure that Dr. Tradewell, a gentleman of fine talents and first rate medical reading, has been engaged for a few months until the practicing season to superintend his drug store."[2]

Within weeks after this notice appeared a complete professional partnership between Drs. Tradewell and McLemore was formed "to practice physics in Leon and adjacent counties."[3] Before the end of that year, however, the partnership had been dissolved and Dr. Tradewell advertised that he had recently purchased the residence of Capt. John Taylor outside Tallahassee and would, beginning on January 1, 1834, carry on his practice from the new location. He also stated that he would charge mileage in addition to the usual fees.[4]

For the next decade Dr. Tradewell appears to have prospered and found his niche in both professional and social circles in the capital city. In September 1838, he won a seat as a Leon County representative in the House of the Territorial Legislative Council[5] and served in the session of 1839.

In 1843, however, tragedy befell the Tradewell household. On February 9 Dr. Tradewell's wife, Eliza Ann, died at the age of 27, leaving four small children.[6] Then on September 13 a devastating hurricane swept in from the Gulf of Mexico dealing destruction to a large area around Apalachee Bay. The Tradewell children and their black nursemaid were visiting in the village of Port Leon and in the tidal wave which accompanied the hurricane the youngest of the children was drowned while another narrowly escaped death.[7]

Within the following year Dr. Tradewell married for the second time. His bride was 19-year-old Anna Maria Hayward, daughter of socially prominent Leon County planter, Richard Hayward.[8]

Dr. Tradewell continued his medical practice in Leon County until the summer of 1847 when he was persuaded either by his own conscience or the insistence of Capt. Robert G. Livington to contract his services as surgeon to Livingston's company of Florida Volunteers about to depart for the Mexican War. He had obviously gained local fame for his success in the treatment of yellow fever, the prime health hazard of the war. Even while en route from St. Marks to New Orleans on the first leg of the journey he was credited with having successfully treated several cases of the fever including one case of black vomit which, reported Capt. Livington, "is fatal in almost every case."[9]

While marking time in camp on the outskirts of New Orleans, Dr. Tradewell was summoned to come into the camp of a Louisiana company then ravaged by the fever. So skillfully did he serve and with such success that his reputation spread about the city and, said Livingston, he was invited to remain to practice in New Orleans "with most flattering assurances of an immediate and extensive practice."[10] But, concluded Livingston, "he prefers to stand by the Florida Volunteers, and will proceed with us to Mexico under a contract which, I hope, will soon be changed to a regular appointment."[11]

Dr. Tradewell's career as an army surgeon was unfortunately of short duration. Soon after arrival at Vera Cruz he became a victim of the fever he had so successfully treated in others. He had probably arrived in Mexico about the first of October; he died on October 24, 1847.[12] There can be no doubt about the high esteem in which he was held by his army associates and the people of Leon County. Upon receiving confirmation of his death the physicians of the Tallahassee community convened to honor him and draft an appropriate tribute to his memory. Of the several resolution approved by the group it is fitting to quote the following:

> (Resolved) that the distinguished success which attended the practice of our lamented friend in the treatment of the Scourge of the South, the Yellow Fever, gave us the greatest satisfaction, and that we are proud of the fame he acquired.[13]

1. Tallahassee Floridian, December 27, 1831.
2. Ibid., March 9, 1833.
3. Ibid., May 4, 1833; 1st printing, April 27, 1833.
4. Ibid., November 16, 1833. 1st printing, August 17, 1833.
5. Tallahassee *Florida Watchman*, September 8, 1838. Allen Morris, *The People of Lawmaking in Florida*, unpaginated.
6. Tallahassee *Star of Florida*, March 2, 1843. This notice assigns her death to February 8 while the Tallahassee *Florida Sentinel* indicates February 9. She was a native of Edgefield District, S.C.
7. This hurricane, one of the most severe to strike the area during the 19th century, completely destroyed the shipping port of Port Leon which had been established a few years earlier to accommodate cotton planters and brokers. It was located down the St. Marks River about two miles from the town of St. Marks but on the east side of the river. The tidal wave, totally unexpected, seems to have made it impossible for residents to take refuge in the nearby lighthouse, about the only structure left standing. The best available account of the tragedy is that of the Tallahassee *Sentinel*, September 19, 1843. Recognizing the risks involved in rebuilding the town, the survivors elected to build farther inland, the new settlement being called Newport. See W.T. Cash, "Newport as a Business Center," *Apalachee*, 1944, p. 20.
8. St. John's Episcopal Church, Tallahassee, Records, "Marriages" February 1, 1844.
9. Most of what is known of the last weeks of Dr. Tradewell's life is found in a lengthy letter, Captain Livingston to the *Sentinel*. This letter, written at New Orleans on September 14, 1847, and published in the newspaper on October 5, contains important information on the incidence of yellow fever then raging not only in the army camps but in the city as well. It hints at the general inefficiency of the entire military operation.
10. Ibid.
11. Ibid., See Francis B. Heitman, *Historical Register and Dictionary of the United States Army*, I, 969. Heitman states, without documentation, that Dr. Tradewell was officially Assistant Surgeon as of August 25. This obviously implies a contractual arrangement and not an army commission.
12. Heitman, loc. cit. No obituary notice can be found in the extant Tallahassee newspapers and a lacuna exists in the files of the *Sentinel* for the latter part of 1847. A letter of October 26 from an unnamed member of Capt. Livingston's company at Vera Cruz includes this statement: "I am sick, and only able to write you a few lines. You will hear of the death of Dr. Tradewell by a letter which I wrote to Major Hayward on yesterday." Tallahassee *Floridian*, November 20, 1847.
13. Ibid., December 11, 1847.
14. Scarecely any information has been discovered which might reveal the fate of the surviving children of Dr. Tradewell and his first wife. The St. John's Episcopal Church Registers, Tallahassee, contain this entry: 1866, Feb. 1, Marriage, William S. Hogue & Elizabeth Geraldine Tredwell. By his second wife Dr. Tradewell had one daughter,

Eliza, shown in the 1850 Leon County Census as living with her mother in the home of her grandfather, Richard Hayward. She was six years old. The St. Johns Church Records noted the death of Mrs. Tradewell on October 5, 1860, at the age of 35.

Travers, Thomas, St. Augustine, 1788

A single reference indicates that Dr. Travers, a citizen of Ireland, was probably a brief sojourner in St. Augustine. On March 22, 1788, he was given permission to travel to St. Augustine. It is assumed that he made the trip, but there is no evidence that he settled there.[1]

1. East Florida Papers, Reel 38, doc. 10158, 1788-91.

Treadwell, B.F., Monticello and Madison, 1836-1866

Dr. Treadwell (Tradewell) first appeared in Florida records in 1859 although he had probably arrived in the state a year or two earlier.[1] He came into public view in March 1859 when he attended a Democratic meeting in Monticello,[2] assembled for the purpose of making plans for the upcoming Democratic State Convention. He was chosen as one of three delegates from Beasley's Precinct or voting precinct No. 8, the other two being David S. Walker, later to become governor of Florida, and William Bailey. In the Census of 1860, Dr. Treadwell, aged 24, was listed as a resident in the household of M.A. Beasley, a farmer of the Waukeenah community, some 10 miles south of Monticello.[3]

As the year 1860 moved on, political tensions were rapidly building up, especially in the rich plantation counties of Middle Florida. With the election of Lincoln on November 6 anxiety became desperation. A series of almost frenzied political gatherings ensued. Secession was, of course, the principal issue. Cool heads did not prevail. With South Carolina leading the march out of the Union the states of the deeper South soon followed. Swift military action occurred, with hastily assembled troops from Florida and Alabama being ordered to Pensacola to seize its military installations. On January 12, 1861,[4] the combined troops under the command of Major W.H. Chace of Pensacola moved into the Navy Yard and other installations, most of them already abandoned by Federal personnel. Only Ft. Pickens, the strongest fortification, resisted the seizures. Some two weeks later Pickens surrendered to the make-shift army.[5]

Throughout these operations Dr. Treadwell was the surgeon to the Jefferson County contingent.[6]

In the more orderly reorganization of the Jefferson County troops which followed, Dr. Treadwell was appointed Assistant Surgeon but in the second reorganization which came some two months later he was not included as either officer or enlisted man.[7] One can only wonder why.

At this juncture Dr. Treadwell disappeared from view, not to reappear until the spring of 1866 when the newspaper at Madison printed a professional card announcing the partnership of Dr. Treadwell and Dr. John Hunter Pope.[8] This association ended tragically six months later with the suicide of Dr. Treadwell. On September 29, 1866, a Tallahassee newspaper printed this announcement dated at Madison on the previous day:[9] "Dr. B.F. Treadwell of this place attempted suicide yesterday afternoon by shooting himself in the head. He is alive this morning but cannot live long." This was followed three days later on October 1 by another Madison dispatch: "Dr. Treadwell died yesterday after noon (Sept. 30th). He continued insensible up to the time of his death."[10]

One can only speculate on the probable cause of Dr. Treadwell's suicide. It could have been failure to fulfill satisfactorily his military obligations; since he never married, it could have been disappointment in love; possibly an unfortunate incident in his professional life. No clue has been discovered.

1. There remains a possibility that Dr. Treadwell was a son of the better-known Dr. William Tradewell (Treadwell), a Leon County physician of the late 1830s and 1840s who died of yellow fever while on duty with American troops in Mexico in 1847. Dr. Tradewell is known to have had a son who survived him. Such a connection has not been established, however.
2. Monticello *Family Friend*, April 7, 1860.
3. U.S. Census, 1860, Jefferson County, Florida, p. 889.
4. Ibid., January 20, 1861.
5. Ibid., January 26, 1861.
6. Ibid., February 2, 1861. Here is printed a list of officers and men involved.
7. Ibid., March 30, 1861.
8. Madison *Southern Messenger*, April 20, 1866; 1st printing March 29, 1866.
9. Tallahassee *Sentinel*, September 29, 1866.
10. Ibid., October 2, 1866.

Tripler, Charles Stuart, Army Surgeon, 1866

Dr. Tripler,[1] who served as a medical officer in Florida during the Second Seminole War, was born in New York State during the first decade of the 19th century. Nothing is presently known of his youth and education. He was commissioned Assistant Surgeon in the United States Marine Corps on October 30, 1830.

By the middle 1830s the white encroachment on erstwhile Indian lands in Florida aroused their hostility and led to the conflict known as the Second Seminole War. Indian resistance proved to be far more formidable than had been expected and resulted in a major military response from the United States. Among the Army physicians dispatched to the Florida scene was Dr. Tripler who had been appointed Assistant Surgeon on October 30, 1830. On May 22, 1837, he was ordered to report for duty at Tampa Bay to relieve Surgeon John A. Kearney of the Navy as chief physician of the Army Hospital at Ft. Brooke. His order further stated that he would have direction of "the Medical Department South of the Ouithlacoochee (Withlacoochee)."

In the following year, 1838, Dr. Tripler received a promotion to the rank of Surgeon, the commission dated July 7, 1838. He is thought to have remained at the Tampa post for the duration of the War which ended in 1842.

Dr. Tripler's military career was by no means terminated with the end of the War. He served in the Union Army as medical officer during the Civil War, having been promoted to the rank of Brevet Colonel on November 29, 1864, and to Brigadier General on March 13, 1865. Death came for him on October 20, 1866.

1. The biographical data are derived almost entirely from Major Edwin North McLellan, *Indian Campaigns, 1835-1842*. Copy in P.K. Yonge Library of Florida History, pp. 69-70, et passim.

Trippe, Henry, Jackson County, 1830

Only a few scattered facts relating to the Trippe family of Jackson County have come to light, although it is known that several members were landholders in the northern part of the county in the 1820s and 1830s between present-day Malone and Campbellton. Records of land acquisitions in the Jackson County area indicate that Dr. Trippe was the son of John L.T. Trippe about whom nothing further is known.[1]

Such evidence as has survived suggests that the Trippes were a family of above average wealth and importance in the Welch community. Although the Census of 1830 provides only meagre information about such matters, it does show that Dr. Trippe was the owner of 13 slaves, a figure which implies a fairly substantial planting enterprise.[2] In December 1824, he was one of four justices of the peace appointed for Jackson County.[3] In several instances his name appears as a signatory to petitions relating to the development and improvement of the County.[4] For at least two terms he was a member of the grand jury of Jackson County.[5]

Dr. Trippe first appeared in the role of practicing physician when, on April 17, 1832, he and Dr. Harris B. Crews announced the opening of their professional office in Webbville.[6] This partnership was one of brief duration, however, for by the end of the year Dr. Crews was engaged in other pursuits which were presumably more lucrative. Nothing further is known of Dr. Trippe. Since no families of that name are listed in the Florida Censuses of 1840 and 1850, it is assumed that Dr. Trippe had left Florida in the late 1830s.[7]

1. Perhaps the Trippe family entered Florida from the State of Georgia where the name Trippe was not uncommon. The roster of graduates of the Medical Department, University of Georgia, included the names of three Trippes who were graduated between 1848 and 1852.
2. U.S. Census, 1830, Jackson County, Florida, sheet 88.
3. Pensacola *Gazette*, February 5, 1825.
4. *Territorial Papers*, XXIII, 99, 398, 949, 1009.
5. J. Randall Stanley, *History of Jackson County*, Marianna, 1950, p. 28. *Territorial Papers*, XXIV, 609.
6. Tallahassee *Floridian*, April 17, 1832.
7. On May 27, 1858, the Alligator (now Lake City) *Columbia Democrat* printed a list of Georgians recently graduated from Jefferson Medical College of Philadelphia. The list included Henry W. Trippe, who may have been a son of the Dr. Trippe here under consideration.

Troutman, Lessee B., Walton County, mid-19th century

Dr. Troutman, born in Georgia about 1820, was a medical practitioner in Walton County in 1860. The census of that year indicates that he had been twice married, first in Georgia where his two eldest children were born and later in Alabama where his wife, Martha, and five additional children were born. It is apparent that he had only recently settled in Florida at the time of the census enumeration. The family located at the village of Almirante, which in 1915 was incorporated into Okaloosa County.[1]

1. U.S. Census, 1860, Walton County, Florida, p. 55.

Tryon, James Rufus, Pensacola, 1837-1912

Dr. Tryon scarcely qualifies as a Florida physician, having spent only a few months of his distinguished career in the state.[1] Born in New York on September

24, 1837, he attended Union College in Schenectady from which he received both the Bachelor and Master of Arts degrees. He then enrolled in the medical college of the University of Pennsylvania from which he was graduated Doctor of Medicine in 1861. His whereabouts for the next two years are unknown, but it is probable that he began practice in New York, probably remaining there until 1863 when he received appointment as Assistant Surgeon in the United States Navy.

Soon after enlistment Dr. Tryon was assigned to duty as a medical officer in a squadron operating in the Gulf of Mexico under the command of Admiral David Farragut. Following the Battle of Mobile on August 5, 1864, he was placed in charge of those wounded, who were transferred to the Naval Hospital in Pensacola.

At the conclusion of the War in April 1865, Dr. Tyron was ordered to report to the Bureau of Medicine and Surgery in Washington where he was assigned to the challenging task of writing a "Naval History of the War," which he proceeded to accomplish. It is unfortunate that Congress refused to appropriate the necessary funds for its publication. The manuscript was subsequently lost.

Subsequently Dr. Tryon served tours of duty in Asian and North Pacific waters and in 1884 was named Fleet Surgeon of the so-called "White Squadron," serving on the first steel ship in the United States Navy.

As the crowning achievement of his lengthy naval career Dr. Tryon was named Surgeon General, a post to which he brought numerous innovations, one of the most notable being the assigning of a hospital ship to the fleet. He also advocated the assignment of women nurses to naval hospitals.

Commodore Tryon retired from active duty in September 1899. He lived out the last years in Coxsackie, New York, where he died on March 20, 1912.

1. The present sketch has been taken almost entirely from an article, "A Surgeon General of the Navy," by Dr. Louis H. Roddis and published in *Medical History* and from his obituary in the New York *Times* of March 22, 1912. His Florida residence was limited to a tour of duty at the Naval Hospital in Pensacola. The esteem in which he was held is indicated by his selection as the representative at two international medical congresses: Copenhagen in 1884 and Madrid in 1888.

Tucker, Edmund, Tallahassee, 1826

Dr. Tucker informed the citizens of Tallahassee on April 28, 1826, that he "still devotes his entire attention to the practice of medicine." By day he could be found in the home of Col. (Charles) Pindar; by night at the office of Major Ward.[1] Dr. Tucker was one of five Tallahassee physicians who met with their counterparts from Gadsden County in Tallahassee on March 25, 1826, when they drew up a fee rate to which all of them affixed their signatures.[2] Three weeks later the local newspaper announced the dissolution of the partnership which had been formed by Dr. Tucker and Dr. C.A. Watkins.[3]

At some time following formation of this partnership Dr. Tucker apparently left Tallahassee. In early January 1830, he announced that he had returned, "which he intends to make his permanent residence," and again offered his professional services to the citizens of the community.[4] Nothing more is known of Dr. Tucker.

1. Tallahassee *Florida Intelligencer*, April 28, 1826.

2. Ibid., April 14, 1826.
3. Ibid., May 19, 1826.
4. Tallahassee *Floridian and Advocate*, January 8, 1830.

Turnbull, James Theodore, Jefferson County, 1811-1854

Dr. Turnbull, one of Jefferson County's most eminent citizens, was born in Abbeville, South Carolina, in 1811.[1] In his youth he began the study of medicine under the preceptorate of Dr. William Tennant of Abbeville.[2] In 1831 he entered Transylvania University in Lexington, Kentucky, where he remained for one academic term.[3] In 1834 he received his medical degree from the Medical College of the State of South Carolina in Charleston, having submitted a thesis on the subject, "Bilious Remittent Fever."

Soon after graduation Dr. Turnbull moved to Jefferson County, purchasing a plantation which bordered on Lake Miccosukee near the Leon County line. He married Caroline Parish, a native of Wilmington, North Carolina, and daughter of Colonel Richard Parish, a union to which several children were born.[4] After a year or so Dr. Turnbull moved again, this time to a plantation three miles south of Monticello to which he gave the name, *Sunrise.* The Turnbulls lived there until their sons were of an age to be educated beyond the capacities of the Jefferson Academy in Monticello; they then moved to Oxford, Georgia, home of Emory College, which several Turnbull sons attended.[5]

After a few years Dr. Turnbull's health began to fail, which prompted him to return to *Sunrise* where he lived out the balance of his life.

Dr. Turnbull is said to have possessed an inquiring mind which led him to experiment with cures and regimens. Family tradition has it that he was a pioneer in the use of quinine in the treatment of malaria, trying various dosages on his slaves with ultimate success. He is known to have been a diligent and dutiful practitioner, responding to calls throughout Jefferson County from the Georgia line to the Gulf of Mexico. Being frequently away from home he left the burden of rearing a large family to his capable wife. Again family lore holds that she was a stern but devoted mother, arriving at the breakfast table each morning with a Bible and a switch.[6]

The Turnbulls were a family of substance and social prominence. Although the doctor himself had little time for politics and social intercourse, his influence was considerable. Having suffered financial losses in the Union Bank debacle of the 1830s he joined a Jefferson County group in protesting the Territory's refusal to accept the banknotes of the defunct Union Bank in payment of taxes.[7] The lighter aspect of his personality is revealed in a letter of 1839 describing the ball following the wedding of Margaret Livingstone and William Moseley, at which "Dr. Theodore attracted attention by 'cutting the pigeon wing!"[8]

Dr. Turnbull's career was terminated by his untimely death in 1854 at the age of 43.[9] He was buried in the family cemetery at *Sunrise.* The Turnbull house, known today as the Turnbull-Ritter house, still stands, though in need of extensive repair. Several of Dr. Turnbull's descendants were destined to play important roles in the public affairs of Jefferson and Leon Counties. His son, Richard, who married Margaret Bellamy in 1859,[10] was Jefferson County's representative in the Florida House in 1864. His grandson, Theodore, son of

Samuel Turnbull, was a well-known physician of Monticello and Jacksonville. His great-grandson, Samuel J. Turnbull, M.D., was a much-decorated medical officer in the United States Army in World Wars I and II.[11]

1. Much information derives from Mary Oakley and Edith Clark Barrows, "History of Jefferson County, Florida," produced as an FERA Project under the direction of R.C. Simpson, Monticello, 1935. A typed copy has been consulted in P.K. Yonge Library of Florida History.
2. Archives, MUSC, Lists of Matriculants and Graduates, Medical College of the State of South Carolina, Charleston.
3. Archives, Transylvania University, Lists of Students, Microfilmed copy.
4. See note 1, supra.
5. The Turnbulls are said to have had 11 children but the number who died in infancy or childhood is not known.
6. See note 1, supra.
7. Jerrell H. Shofner, *History of Jefferson County, Florida*, Tallahassee, 1976, p. 170.
8. Letter, Catharine Wirt to her sister, November 30, 1839, cited in ibid., p. 38.
9. Some confusion exists as to the date of Dr. Turnbull's death. Shofner gives "about 1845." Since he appears in the Leon County Census of 1850, this is incorrect. Theresa Yaeger Palmer, *The Palmer Physicians*, 1966, App. gives the date of death as 1858. McRory and Barrows, "History of Jefferson County," assign the date, 1854, which appears to be correct.
10. Tallahassee *Floridian and Journal*, October 29, 1859. It was partially through this marriage that Richard Turnbull became a wealthy man, owning 144 slaves in 1860.
11. *The Magnolia Monthly*, "The Palmer Physicians," XII, No. 2, February 1974, genealogical section.

Turnbull, Junius, Jefferson County, 1840

Dr. Turnbull, second son of Dr. James Theodore and Carolina Parish Turnbull, was born in Monticello in 1840. He was enrolled in 1860 at the University of Virginia and is said to have begun the study of medicine there.[1] With the Civil War in progress and the need for army physicians acute, he was commissioned Acting Assistant Surgeon in the Confederate Army on August 28, 1864, and assigned to field service with the light artillery battery of Capt. Henry F. Abell.[2] At the end of the War he returned to Monticello and settled down to the life of a planter. There is no evidence that he pursued a medical career beyond that date.

Dr. Turnbull was married to William (sic), youngest daughter of William and Emily Simkins Bellamy whose dowry added substantially to the family's wealth.[3]

1. Archives, University of Virginia, Lists of Students.
2. *Soldiers of Florida*, Tallahassee, 1903, 320.
3. "Old Plantations Near Monticello," typescript, P.K. Yonge Library of Florida History. The references to Junius Turnbull, found in J.B. Whitfield, comp., *Official Directory of the State Government*, Tallahassee, 1885, p. 11, are obviously in error.

Turner, George F., Army Surgeon, 1854

Dr. Turner, a native of Massachusetts, was commissioned assistant surgeon in the United States Army on July 23, 1833. Nothing is known of his early life and education.[1] His first post of duty was Fort Mackinac on Mackinac Island, Michigan, where he remained until 1836 when he was transferred to Castle Pinckney, located in Charleston Harbor, South Carolina.[2] In late 1837 or early 1838 he transferred to Florida as surgeon to the troops fighting in the Second Seminole War. He managed to survive the hazards of fever endemic to the Florida Territory as well as enemy action. On Januay 1, 1840, he was promoted to surgeon and continued to serve in the Army until his death which occurred at Corpus Christi, Texas, on October 17, 1854.

1. The dates of Dr. Turner's commissions and place of birth are found in *Medical Department of the Army, from 1775 to 1873* compiled by Harvey E. Brown, Washington, D.C., Surgeon General's Office, p. 292.
2. Castle Pinckney was located on Shutes Folly Island about one mile from the East Battery, Charleston.

Turnstall, Peyton R., Pensacola, 1795-1847

Dr. Turnstall, a native of Spottsylvania County, Virginia, practiced medicine for a brief time in the vicinity of Pensacola. He received his education in eastern Tennessee and for 10 years was surgeon at the U.S. Arsenal at Mt. Vernon, Alabama. During the two years of his residence in Florida he apparently earned the confidence and respect of his professional colleagues as well as the general public. He was said to have had much concern for the poor and to have rendered much of his service gratuitously. He died at his home on the night of September 23, 1847, "in the 52nd year of his age."[1]

1. Pensacola *The Live Oak*, October 6, 1847.

Tyng, Anita E., Duval County, late 19th century

Dr. Tyng, a competent and dedicated physician, arrived in Jacksonville in the early 1880s, having accepted an appointment as resident physician at St. Luke's Hospital. Her identity and an account of her role as "angel of mercy" have been preserved in the Jacksonville *Times-Union* of September 25, 1888. Having been on constant duty at the Hospital for several months she was granted a leave of absence which was long over due. This she chose to spend at her home in the North, departing from Jacksonville on the "crack" train, the *Seminole,* on August 6th.

Soon after her departure Jacksonville was struck by a deadly epidemic of yellow fever, about which Dr. Tyng had no knowledge until August 24. Upon receiving word she immediately decided that her services were much needed. After much difficulty and considerable expense she returned to Jacksonville on August 30. Only then did she learn that St. Luke's was under the management of the County Board of Health. She immediately reported for duty, but was advised to return to her home for much needed rest. On September 4 she again offered her services which were readily accepted. She was ordered to report to the Board, which she did the following day.

On September 14 the President of the Board appointed her as physician for the Chaseville community. She reported that only a single case of the fever had occurred there.

It is unfortunate that no further information relating to Dr. Tyng has emerged. A careful perusal of the Duval County Censuses of 1885 and 1900 yielded no trace of the remarkable woman.

Underwood, William H., Hamilton County, 1843-1870

Dr. Underwood, Jefferson Medical College,[1] Class of 1868, had hardly begun his professional practice in Jasper when his career was tragically ended by death. He was born in Lowndes County, Georgia, on April 4, 1843,[2] son of John J. Underwood and Sarah King Cauthon, who were among the early settlers in the county, having migrated there from Laurens County, Georgia, by 1825. When young William was six his family moved to Hamilton County, Florida, where he spent the rest of his brief life except for two winters in Philadelphia in medical study. The census schedule of 1870[3] lists him as a resident in the home of his mother, his father having died in 1865. Also in the household were three of his sisters, all of whom later married. Before the end of 1870 Dr. Underwood was dead. A manuscript in the Archives of the University of Pennsylvania lists him as an active practitioner in the year 1869.[4]

1. Archives, Jefferson Medical College, Philadelphia, List of Graduates.
2. *Brief History of Hamilton County, Florida*, Cora Hinton, comp., Jasper, 1976, p. 82. Vital statistics cited here are from Mrs. Hinton's book.
3. U.S. Census, Hamilton County, Florida, 1870.
4. Archives, University of Pennsylvania, MS, UPC 2.3 No. 16.

Ury, Joseph, Jackson County, 1835

Dr. Ury, a native of Tennessee, had practiced medicine for several years prior to his death in Jackson County on February 16, 1835. Nothing is known of his early education and professional training. His obituary, which was published in the Tallahassee *Floridian* of March 7, 1835, is the only source of biographical information and includes the following eulogy:[1]

> For some years past he had resided in this (Jackson) County where his worth had won universal esteem. Regret for his death will not soon pass away, for we have lost a useful physician and an excellent citizen —one who combined in his character many valuable qualities...A kind husband, a tender father, an affectionate brother, a faithful friend...esteemed and beloved.

1. Since Dr. Ury's name does not appear in the Florida Census of 1830, it is assumed that he did not move to Florida until after the enumeration of that year.

Valentine, Jesse M., Newnansville, 1827-1862

Dr. Valentine, Medical College of the State of South Carolina in the class of 1854, was born in North Carolina about 1827.[1] Before beginning the study of medicine he had become a minister in the Methodist Church and in that capacity had settled in St. Mary's, Georgia, as a resident in the home of Dr. Francis O. Curtis, a South Carolinian, where the census enumerator found him in the summer of 1850.[2] His age was then 23. At some point he began the study of medicine under the direction of Dr. Curtis and in 1852 was accepted as a student at the Charleston institution. He wrote a doctoral thesis on "Intermittent Fever."[3]

His medical college record indicates that he began the practice of medicine at Alligator (after 1859, Lake City), but in early 1858 he moved to Newnansville where he and Dr. Philip W. Cato formed a professional partnership.[4] It is an item of minor interest that at the marriage of Dr. Cato's daughter, Ophelia, to Joseph Warren on May 29, 1859, the "Reverend Jesse M. Valentine, M.D.," was the officiating clergyman.[5]

Beyond the routine medical practice in which he was engaged not much is known of Dr. Valentine's activities. He was, however, a dedicated member of the Democratic Party, and as the sectional tensions developed in 1860 he asserted his role as a political leader. At the county-wide meeting of Democrats in Gainesville on August 14 he was the presiding officer.[6] Later in the year, November 22, 1860, he was secretary at a gathering of Alachua County citizens to consider secession proposals. He addressed the group and reported to area newspapers.[7]

With the outbreak of the War Dr. Valentine appears to have stuck by his practice for a few months, but on March 20, 1862, he enlisted for military service and was assigned to Company C, 7th Florida Infantry, not as surgeon but as a private. His unmarried status was obviously a factor in the decision.[8]

He entered the Confederate Army at Camp Lee near Tallahassee for a term of three years; his days were numbered, however. In less than five weeks after enlistment he died in Gainesville of an unspecified illness on April 25.[9]

Ironically, in February 1863, he was among physicians receiving payments from the State Treasury for having performed postmortem examinations. His posthumous windfall amounted to $25.[10]

1. U.S. Census, 1850, Camden County, Georgia, p. 391, item 246. His age, here listed as 23, is probably correct. The entry in the Census of 1860, Alachua County, Florida, item 682, listing his age as 38 appears to be in error.
2. Here Dr. Valentine's occupation is given as "Methodist Minister."
3. *Catalogue of Students, 1853-54, MCSSC*, pp. 297, 314.
4. Alligator *Columbia Democrat*, March 27, 1858.
5. Fernandina *East Floridian*, June 16, 1859.
6. Ibid., August 23, 1860.
7. Ibid., November 28, 1860.
8. NA, Service Records, CSA, M251, Roll 80.
9. Ibid.
10. Tallahassee *Florida Sentinel*, February 24, 1863.

Van Wyck, Cornelius C., Tallahassee, 1819-1868

The medical career of Dr. Van Wyck as it relates to Florida was brief but not totally insignificant. He was born in Fishkill Landing, New York, a river village south of Poughkeepsie, on August 9, 1819, the son of Peter Schenck and Sarah

Wickham Van Wyck. He attended Princeton College, then known as the College of New Jersey, from which he was graduated in 1838 with the Bachelor of Arts degree. In the fall of that year he enrolled at the Medical College of the University of Pennsylvania and in the spring of 1841 was graduated Doctor of Medicine, having submitted a thesis entitled "Creosote in Dyspepsia."[1] Soon thereafter he began practice in Philadelphia which he continued until 1847 when he became Professor of Surgery at the recently-organized Franklin College of Medicine in Philadelphia.[2]

In the summer of 1848 Dr. Van Wyck arrived in Tallahassee where he joined Dr. John Thomas Jefferson Wilson in a professional partnership.[3] Soon after the launching of their joint practice in medicine and surgery, the two men notified the public that, in addition to their regular practice, they were prepared to offer instruction to medical students. Their prescribed course of study was probably typical of that offered throughout the country under the apprenticeship system of medical education. They promised prospective students "Books, Plates, Anatomical and Other Preparations" as well as "Instruction in Compounding and Dispensing Medicines, as well as the everyday duties of the Surgeon—Bleeding, Cupping, Bandaging, etc." Their public announcement closed with the promise that, as soon as possible, "an Infirmary for Reception of both Medical and Surgical Patients will be opened (where) the students will have the opportunity for practically studying diseases."[4]

That nothing came of such a well-intentioned plan was unfortunate, especially when it appears that both Drs. Van Wyck and Wilson were, by the standards of the times, physicians of competence. It is possible, though not ascertainable, that they in some way aroused the hostility of the medical faculty of the town. The plan was soon abandoned and both men left Tallahassee, Dr. Wilson to his plantation near Tallahassee and Dr. Van Wyck to Cuba where he settled in the town of Cardenas a few miles east of Matanzas. He died there on October 14, 1868. His wife, the former Ann Eliza Forbes of Philadelphia, is thought to have survived him. The couple left no heirs.[5]

1. Biographical details are from Archives, University of Pennsylvania, Philadelphia.

2. Dr. Van Wyck's professional notice first appeared in the Tallahassee *Floridian*, June 10, 1848. He stated that he had taken up residence in Tallahassee. His office was located "South of Bartlett's Building." He identified himself as "Erstwhile Professor of Surgery in the Franklin Medical College of Philadelphia." Since this College had only been organized in 1847 (it became defunct in 1852) he could have taught there for only one session.

3. Ibid., July 22, 1848. The announcement also appeared in the Jacksonville *News*, August 5, 1848, and ran for four issues.

4. Notices of this kind seldom appeared in the antebellum newspapers of Florida.

5. See note 1, supra.

Vann, Henry W., Gadsden County, 1816

Dr. Vann, a resident of rural Gadsden County in 1850, was a native of South Carolina. Nothing is known of his educational background or professional training. He is listed in the Census of 1850 as the owner of property valued at $2,500. His wife, Elizabeth, was a Georgia native. Another Vann (William T.), doubtless his brother, was a neighbor.[1]

1. U.S. Census, 1850, Gadsden County, Florida, p. 199, item 307.

Verdier, George L., Fernandina, 1832

Very little is known of the career of Dr. Verdier, a sojourner and practitioner in Fernandina just prior to the Civil War.[1] He was a son of Dr. James R. Verdier of Beaufort, South Carolina, a wealthy planter and physician and cousin of Dr. John H. Verdier, for many years a Florida practitioner. He seems to have arrived in Fernandina in late 1859 when the local newspaper announced the arrival of "Dr. G.L. Verdier, his lady, and servant."[2] The Census of 1860, which gives his age as 28, shows him to have been a resident of a Fernandina hotel.[3] It is a reasonable conjecture that with the coming of the War he returned to his home state.

1. In the Census of 1850, Beaufort District, S.C., St. Helena Parish, item 76, he is shown as the second child of Dr. James R. Verdier, who owned more than a hundred slaves.
2. Fernandina *East Floridian*, December 8, 1859.
3. U.S. Census, 1860, Nassau County, Florida, item 125.

Verdier, John H., Leon and Gadsden Counties, 1819-1881

Dr. Verdier was born to a prominent Huguenot family of Beaufort, South Carolina, about 1819.[1] His father, John M. Verdier, was a lawyer-planter of means, owning 29 slaves in 1850, while his uncle, James R. Verdier, a planter-physician, was similarly situated. Young John H. is thought to have received his early education in the local schools of Beaufort. At a fairly early age he was enrolled at Bristol College, Pennsylvania, from which he was graduated with honors.[2] He returned to Beaufort and served an apprenticeship under the preceptorate of his uncle, James R. Verdier. In the fall of 1837 he matriculated at the Medical College of the State of South Carolina from which he received his degree in the spring of 1839, after submitting a thesis entitled "Traumatic Fever (sic)."[3]

Dr. Verdier moved to Florida in late 1839. The earliest record of his residence is his signature to a petition signed by numerous citizens protesting the arbitrary removal from office of Governor Richard Keith Call in November 1839.[4] The signatures on the document were those of residents of Middle Florida. Dr. Verdier had apparently already settled in Tallahassee at that time as is indicated by his professional notice which appeared in the local newspaper in early 1840.[5] He remained in Tallahassee for about two years.

In 1842 Dr. Verdier transferred his practice to Gadsden County where he was immediately successful as a physician and gained local prominence as a leader of the temperance movement. To this cause he devoted much effort, first as President of the Salubrity Marshall Temperance Society[6] and later as the movement assumed statewide dimensions as an officer in Florida Sons of Temperance.[7]

Other public matters also claimed Dr. Verdier's attention ranging from organizing Independence Day celebrations[8] to ardent support of the Southern states' rights movement. With the latter issue he gained sufficient acclaim to be named a Gadsden County delegate to the Nashville Convention held in November 1850.[9] On his return from that mission he was invited to make a report to the Florida Legislature where he was honored by being seated "within the bar" of the House of Representatives.[10] Shortly afterward he joined the influential David L. White, also a Gadsden physician, in organizing the Southern Rights Association of Gadsden County.[11] Both were elected vice presidents, with C.H. Dupont as president.

Although Dr. Verdier had been reared almost in the shadow of St. Helena's Episcopal Church in Beaufort, in whose churchyard many of his relatives were buried, he had apparently never been confirmed. Hence on December 27, 1844, he was confirmed at St. Paul's Church, Quincy, and on March 23, 1845, admitted to membership.[12]

Some obvious errors appear in census data relating to the Verdier family, but the information included in the Gadsden County schedule of 1850 appears to be reliable. Here Dr. Verdier is shown as 30 years of age, a physician, owning property valued at $10,000, and a resident in the home of Eastman McIver. His brother, Meade, was also a resident of the household.[13] In 1853 he married Corinne Crawford, daughter of the Honorable Joel Crawford of Sparta, Georgia.[14] The following year he was appointed military aide to Governor James E. Browne.[15]

By 1856, and for unknown reasons, the Verdiers had departed Gadsden County and taken up residence in Putnam County where they purchased a plantation some 10 miles north of Palatka.[16] There, with a labor force of about 50 slaves, they carried on a farming operation which evidence indicates was lucrative.[17]

With the change of residence Dr. Verdier also changed his politics. He had obviously been comfortable in the Whig atmosphere of Middle Florida but in Putnam County he chose another standard, as the following report of a Democratic meeting indicates:[18]

> An important and interesting incident connected with the proceedings of the Palatka meeting is the appearance of the name of Dr. J. H. Verdier, old line Whig, as its chairman. This announcement will occasion feelings of agreeable surprise with the Doctor's new political friends in this quarter.

It is unlikely that the Verdiers actually resided on their plantation north of Palatka for it is known that in the late 1850s they occupied a house in the village of Welaka, upriver from Palatka where they were neighbors of the Hopkins, Bryant and Stephens families. Octavia Stephens (nee Bryant), in that portion of her diary covering the years 1858 and 1859, made numerous references to the Verdiers, with whom her family regularly exchanged social courtesies.[19] Octavia, at that time an impressionable girl, regarded Mrs. Verdier as somewhat shrewish and much given to quarreling with her husband. The Putnam County Census of 1860 lists Verdier as "M.D. and farmer," owning property valued at about $50,000. The names of two children, a daughter Wille T., aged three, and a son J. Crawford, aged one, are also included.[20]

The activities of the Verdiers during the Civil War remain obscure. They doubtless suffered financial disasters similar to those of other planters dependent upon slaves to cultivate their crops. Whatever the reasons, they abandoned Putnam County for nearby Alachua and in 1870 Dr. Verdier was a resident of Gainesville, no longer a planter but a physician.[21] By 1880, however, he had moved again, in this instance to Tampa where he resumed the practice of medicine.[22] By the end of that year, however, he was practicing in Bartow, seat of Polk County, where he died on September 25, 1881.[23] He was buried with the highest honors of the Masonic Order.

Even in the somewhat scant details of the life of Dr. Verdier can be detected overtones of sadness, even tragedy. He was unquestionably a man of intelligence and splendid character. His political convictions were those of the planter aristocracy. In his earlier years he was a highly regarded physician, one of 12 men of his profession who assembled in Quincy in 1848 to organize a Florida Medical Society. Subsequently, however, he appears to have allowed medicine to become a secondary interest, subordinating it to his agricultural interests. When those failed in the 1860s he seemed to have been unable to cope with the adversities, incapable of recapturing a medical practice which would have provided a living. Besides, in his last years he was plagued by "a disease that had affected his health seriously for years."[24] In his final tribute to the deceased physician the editor of the Bartow *Informant* wrote: "In his death the community has lost a strong advocate of all that is virtuous and ennobling."

1. The date of birth is an extrapolation from the Census of 1850, Gadsden County, Florida, p. 346.
2. Bartow (Fla.) *Informant*, September 29, 1881. Bristol College in Bristol, Pennsylvania, 20 miles northeast of Philadelphia, is long since defunct.
3. Archives, Waring Historical Medical Library, Charleston, S.C. Lists of Matriculants and Graduates, Medical College of the State of South Carolina.
4. *Territorial Papers, Florida*, Clarence E. Carter, comp., XXVI, 86.
5. Tallahassee *Star of Florida*, May 21, 1840. His office was located at 200 Foot Street just off Monroe Street.
6. Tallahassee *Florida Republican*, June 24, 1842; ibid., October 3, 1843.
7. Jacksonville *Florida Republican*, December 13, 1849.
8. Tallahassee *Florida Sentinel*, July 11, 1843.
9. Tallahassee *Sentinel*, December 3, 1850.
10. Ibid., January 14, 1851.
11. Edward B. Gearhart, "St. Paul's Church in Quincy, Florida, During the Territorial Period," FHQ, XXXIV, No. 4, April 1956, 363.
12. Ibid., p. 364.
13. U.S. Census, 1850, Gadsden County, Florida, p. 346.
14. Tallahassee *Floridian and Journal*, December 24, 1853.
15. Jacksonville *Florida News*, February 11, 1854.
16. The Verdier property lay on the left bank of the St. John's River some 10 miles north of Palatka, southwest of Federal Point which lies on the right bank. There is still a site on the river known as Verdier Point, near where the Verdier post office stood.
17. Slave Schedule, 1860, Putnam County.
18. Tallahassee *Floridian and Journal*, September 20, 1856.
19. Stephens Papers; MSS, P.K. Yonge Library of Florida History, University of Florida, Gainesville; entires of 1857-58.
20. U.S. Census, 1860, Putnam County, Florida, p. 327.
21. Ibid., 1870, Alachua County, Florida, item 99.
22. Ibid., 1880, Hillsborough County, Florida, p. 414, item 133.
23. M.F. Hetherington, *History of Polk County, Florida*, St. Augustine, 1928, p. 40.
24. A poignant and laudatory obituary appeared in the Bartow *Informant*, September 29, 1881.

Villeret, Francis F., Tallahassee and Jacksonville, 1867-1889

Among the unorthodox practitioners of medicine who periodically appeared on the Florida scene was Dr. Villeret who settled in Tallahassee just after the Civil War. His professional card, which first appeared on April 9, 1867, offered services as follows:[1]

> ELECTRICITY—Dr. F.F. Villeret, from Paris, France—Medical Electrician engaged exclusively in the treatment of Nervous and Chronic Diseases, Rheumatism, Neuralgia, Paralysis, Spinal Diseases, Dyspepsia, Torpidity of the Liver and General Prostration of the Nervous System, by his new and successful mode of applying electricity; besides, he will attend to any kind of diseases. Apply to his office at Dr. Stonelake's residence.

Three years later, in 1870, Dr. Villeret was a resident of Jacksonville, living in the suburb of La Villa at 111 Monroe Street. The Census of that year gives his age as 52, while his recently acquired wife, Julienne, a native of Cuba, was 30.[2] Their children, Francisco, aged four, and Anneta, aged two, were Florida-born.

The Villerets were still living in Jacksonville as late as 1889. The Jacksonville City Directory of 1889 shows them as residing at the same location,[3] but their names do not appear in later directories.[4]

1. Tallahassee *Sentinel*, April 9, 1867.
2. U.S. Census, 1870, Duval County, Florida.
3. Webb's *Jacksonville Directory*, 1889, pp. 240, 273. At this date the son, Francis, was working as a baggagemaster at 109 Cedar Street.
4. The *Catalogue of the Physicians of the State of Florida*, prepared under auspices of the Florida Medical Association in 1892 and published in January 1893, includes Dr. Villeret. He was still living at that date.

Vogt, Daniel A., Marion County, 1823-1883

Dr. Vogt, one of several physicians who settled in Marion County in the mid-19th century, was born in St. Matthew's Parish, Orangeburg District, South Carolina, in 1823. His father, Michael Vogt, was a native of Switzerland. After reading medicine and observing medical procedures in the office of Dr. J.H. Felder of St. Matthews he enrolled at the Medical College of the State of South Carolina, Charleston, from which he was graduated on March 14, 1843, having submitted a doctoral thesis entitled "Intermittent Fever."[1] Thereafter he returned to his home district and began practice, residing for a brief time in the home of his brother, Jesse.[2]

In the early 1850s Dr. Vogt, following the lead of numerous other South Carolinians, moved to Marion County, purchasing a tract of land a few miles southwest of Ocala on which he engaged in a farming operation while continuing medical practice. He appears to have been a man well above average means; in 1860 he owned 15 slaves, his total properties having been valued at $17,000.[3]

Dr. Vogt was a man of strong convictions which he did not hesitate to express. Imbued with the prevailing opinions of his class regarding such issues as states' rights and slavery, he was comfortable in the company of numerous South Carolinians who were his neighbors. In 1856 he was nominated for a seat in the Florida House of Representatives, winning by a very substantial majority of votes.[4] He was returned to the House for the sessions of 1858, 1860 and 1861.[5] He was among the leaders of the secessionist movement in Marion County and in late November 1860 was present at a meeting of concerned citizens at the Marion County Court House at which he assisted in drafting the much-publicized "Ocala Resolution" which urged Governor Madison Starke Perry to call the State Legislature into session to consider "dissolving our connection with the Federal Union."[6] Although he was not a member of the Secession Convention which met in Tallahassee on January 3, 1861, he had on December 1, 1860, as a member of the House, read the "Ocala Resolution" before that body.[7]

With the Civil War already under way Dr. Vogt, prompted by his strong convictions, enlisted for military service on March 8, 1862, at the age of 39, committing himself for a period of three years. Four days later he was mustered in as a private and assigned to Company "G" of the Seventh Florida Infantry Regiment. Three months later he was found to be physically unfit for active duty and on June 12, 1862, was honorably discharged from the Regiment.[8]

On returning home to Marion County and resuming operation of his farm, Dr. Vogt found his professional services much in demand, there being a scarcity of physicians at that time. Mrs. Mary Baker Taylor, his neighbor and friend, in that portion of her "Diary" covering the years 1863-67, makes frequent mention of his services in the community.[9]

The latter years of Dr. Vogt's life appear to have been comparatively uneventful. As was true of most Southern plantation owners, especially those who had relied on slave labor for the cultivation and harvesting of their crops, the postwar years were difficult. The Census of 1870 lists the value of Dr. Vogt's property at $3,400.[10] For the years following conditions improved slowly. With failing health and financial anxieties his last years could not have been free from care. It becomes apparent from available data that by the late 1870s Dr. Vogt had almost ceased to practice medicine, devoting his energies for the greater part to management of his farm. In fact, the Census of 1880, Marion County, designates him only as "farmer." He died at his Marion County home on February 26, 1883.[11]

1. Centennial Memorial of the College of Medicine of the State of South Carolina, Charleston, S.C., 1924, p. 120.
2. U.S. Census, 1850, Orangeburg District, South Carolina, item 536.
3. Ibid., 1860. Marion County, Florida, item 677. The Vogt plantation was located about half way between Ocala and Dunnellon. See also the Slave Schedule, Marion County, 1860.
4. Jacksonville *Florida News*, August 23, 1856.
5. See *House Journals*, Florida General Assembly, for the aforementioned years.
6. Eloise Robinson Ott, "Ocala Prior to 1868," *Florida Historical Quarterly*, VI, No. 2, October 1927, p. 104.
7. *Florida House Journal*, 1860, pp. 52-54. Text of the Resolution.
8. National Archives, Service Records, CSA, M251, Roll 80.
9. See note 3, supra.
10. Following the untimely death of his brother, Jesse, Dr. Vogt became the foster parent of his brother's two children Albertus and Elizabeth Roxanne. Albertus eventually became a wealthy businessman by developing the phosphate industry in the vicinity of Dunnellon. See J. Lester Dinkins, *Dunellon, Boomtown of the 1890s*, St. Petersburg, Great Outdoors Publishing Co. 1969. Mr. Dinkins has provided abundant biographical information on members of the Vogt family.
11. The date of Dr. Vogt's death was kindly provided by his great niece, Mrs. James D. DuVal, recently of Atlanta but currently residing in Banner Elk, North Carolina.

von Balsam, Henry, Jacksonville and St. Augustine, 1850s and 1860s

Mystery surrounds the origin and early life of Dr. von Balsam. Available evidence points to the probability that he arrived in Florida about 1845 and settled in Jacksonville with his wife, Caroline, a Maryland native, and their three sons, Fredric, born in Georgia; Guardo, born in Alabama; and Isadore, born in Georgia. The fourth son, Robert, was born in Florida and in 1850 was four years of age.[1] By early 1855 he had been appointed Port Physician at Jacksonville, and on May 1 that year reported on his activities to the Jacksonville City Council.[2] A month later, however, he had been replaced by Dr. J.S. Hankins.[3] At its meeting on June 5, the Council instructed its clerk to notify Dr. Hankins of his election and "also Dr. Balsam, former Port Physician, of the discontinuance of quarantine at Dames Point."[4]

It appears that Dr. Balsam (the German **von** no longer appeared in the references to his practice) had not been fully paid for his services at the time of his dismissal for the City Council at its meeting on February 17, 1858, agreed to pay a bill for $10 from Dr. Balsam "as Port Physician for medical attention to the sick."[5]

The year 1870 found Dr. von Balsam living in St. Augustine. Presumably his first wife was deceased. He was married to French-born Mary J. Bourguardy (Bogardy), whose aged mother was also in the household.[6] His age was given as 68. He had died prior to the census enumeration of 1880, although his widow and mother-in-law still lived.[7]

1. U.S. Census, 1850, Duval County, Florida, p. 103. von Balsam was born in Prussia.
2. Jacksonville *Florida Republican*, May 3, 1855.
3. Ibid., June 14, 1855.
4. Ibid.
5. Ibid., March 24, 1858.
6. U.S. Census, 1870, St. Johns County, Florida, p. 617. Listed also in this schedule is his son, Robert, a grocer and auctioneer in St. Augustine. Ibid., p. 618.
7. U.S. Census, 1880, St. Johns County, Florida, p. 142.

Voorhees, John V.D., Pensacola, 1822

Dr. Voorhees, a native of New Jersey, arrived in Pensacola in July 1821 at about the time of the Spanish cession.[1] It is probable that he was already suffering from tuberculosis which may explain his decision to migrate to the more salutary climate of the Florida Territory.[2] He immediately came to the attention of territorial officials and on July 21, 1821, Governor Andrew Jackson announced his appointments to public office, which included that of Dr. Voorhees as Health Officer of Pensacola.[3] Shortly thereafter he became a member of the Board of Health and at its organizational meeting on July 23 he presented his medical diploma from "the University of New York" and was licensed to practice medicine in the Territory.[4]

On September 1, 1821, the Pensacola newspaper published the professional card of Drs. Voorhees and James C. Bronaugh announcing their partnership and the location of their office next door to the Governor's House.[5] A cruel fate awaited this professional union, however; on April 23, 1822, death of "a pulmonary ailment" came for Dr. Voorhees and less than five months later on September 2, 1822, Dr. Bronaugh was one of the early victims of the particularly deadly yellow fever epidemic of that year.[6] Dr. Voorhees age was stated as 27. An extremely laudatory obituary notice suggests the high esteem in which he was held in Pensacola.

1. In his obituary notice it is stated that Dr. Voorhees "had resided in this place since the occupation...by the American authorities." The Pensacola *Floridian*, April 27, 1822.
2. This is implied in the same obituary notice which identified his ailment only as "a pulmonary disease." Ibid.
3. TP, XXII, 131; also the Pensacola *Floridian*, August 18, 1821.
4. Ibid. The "University of N.Y." mentioned here is almost certainly the Columbia University College of Physicians and Surgeons organized in 1807. King's College, closed during the American Revolution, reopened as Columbia College in 1784. Its medical adjunct, known as the College of Physicians and Surgeons, was opened in 1807.
5. Ibid., September 1, 1821. Dr. Bronaugh, close associate and personal physician of Andrew Jackson was Resident Physician and President of the Board of Health. He was also president of the Territorial Legislative Council at the time of his death.
6. Ibid., April 27, 1822. For date of Dr. Bronaugh's death see TP, XXII, 73n.

Waddel, William Woodson, Tallahassee, 1807-1843

Few physicians have been so beloved and respected as Dr. Waddel who spent the last nine years of his life in Tallahassee. His death in 1843 at the age of 36 cast gloom over the city and evoked extraordinary eulogies. He was born in Abbeville, South Carolina, on March 22, 1807, the third son of the Reverend Moses Waddell, D.D., for several years president (chancellor) of the University of Georgia at Athens. His mother was Elizabeth Woodson Pleasants.[1]

From early childhood Waddel displayed unusual talent, so much indeed that he was permitted to enter the University of Georgia at the age of 13. He was graduated in 1823 with the A.B. degree and remained to take a master's degree in 1826. In the fall of that year he entered the Medical Department of the University of Pennsylvania from which he received his degree in the spring of 1828 after submitting a thesis entitled "The State of Biliary Secretion in Fever."[2]

Upon graduation Dr. Waddel returned to Athens and entered practice. He is presumed to have remained there until late 1833 when he moved to Tallahassee, having declined a professorship at the Medical College of Georgia in Augusta. In December 1828, he married Mary Louisa Hilliard, daughter of Dr. Joseph R. Hilliard. Three children, two daughters, Mary Louisa and Rosas, and a son, Moses, were born to this marriage.[3]

On January 4, 1834, Dr. Waddel announced his services to the people of Tallahassee and vicinity, adding that he had "taken the office formerly occupied by Dr. Aiken (Edward, d. 1831), and more recently by Dr. Craig (John A.)."[4] A few years later he joined fellow-physician, James Henry Randolph, and a young druggist from New York named Benjamin C. Lewis, in opening a New Drug Store on Monroe Street, one door north of Mr. Birge's.[5]

Dr. Waddel quickly established himself as a trusted physician and respected citizen. When the Indian threat to Middle Florida brought terror to the people of Leon and adjoining counties and the federal government failed to provide protection Dr. Waddel made the long journey to Columbia, South Carolina, to beseech Governor McDuffie to raise a body of volunteers for what came to be known as the Second Seminole War. He returned to Tallahassee with a letter from the Governor promising immediate assistance. The latter was placed in the office of the editor of the *Floridian*, William Wilson, and local citizens were urged to come and read it for themselves, "inasmuch as it contains expressions of good feelings toward the people of Florida."[6] Dr. Waddel further demonstrated his concern by enlisting in the Sixth Regiment, First Brigade of the Florida Militia, as regimental surgeon.[7] When the great fire of May 25, 1843, swept through the business section of Tallahassee Dr. Waddel was active in organizing relief for its victims.[8] He was an elder in the Tallahassee Presbyterian Church.[9]

Dr. Waddel died quite unexpectedly on November 15, 1843, at his Tallahassee home soon after suffering an attack of la grippe. While not completely recovered he had returned to work only to have a relapse which was fatal. Rarely has the death of a citizen produced such shock and outpouring of sorrow. The medical faculty of the city met to do him honor. Both newspapers published lengthy notices extolling his virtues and lamenting his death. The *Sentinel* devoted more than two columns to eulogizing his professional skill as well as his humanitarianism. The Athens (Ga.) *Southern Whig* remembered, among other achievements, his eminence as a musician and Biblical scholar. The Tallahassee

Star of Florida of November 17, 1843, considered his death "a great public calamity, as well as a private and individual loss.[10]

1. Archives, University of Pennsylvania, Medical Department, List of Graduates. His date of birth from this source, said to have been 1802, is in error.
2. Ibid.
3. Ibid. Here only the two daughters are shown. In the Tallahassee *Floridian*, August 22, 1835, however, is found the following: "D., 18th August, 1835, Moses, only son of Dr. W.W. Waddel, age 4." There is contradiction in the sources concerning Dr. Waddel's association with the Augusta institution. It was the claim of the Tallahassee *Sentinel* of November 21, 1843, that he had actually served as Professor of Medicine. The Tallahassee *Floridian*, however, stated that he had declined the offer.
4. Tallahassee *Floridian*, January 4, 1834.
5. Ibid., December 30, 1837. Dr. Waddel's patients included some of Leon County's most affluent citizens including Prince Achille Murat who in 1839 paid him a four-year bill in the amount of $331 for service to himself and his servants. Henry E. Palmer, "Physicians of Early Tallahassee and Vicinity," *Apalachee*, 1844, p. 31.
6. Tallahassee *Floridian*, June 25, 1836.; Ibid., December 1, 1838.
7. Tallahassee *Sentinel*, November 21, 1843.
8. Fred P. Ley Jr., "The Tallahassee Fire of 1843," *Apalachee*, 1848-50, p. 14.
9. See note 7, supra.
10. The issue of the *Floridian* containing the lengthy obituary is not extant but it was reprinted in the *Sentinel* of November 21, as was the obituary from the Athens (Ga.) *Southern Whig*.

Wade, James M., Tallahassee, 1857

Although Dr. Wade spent several winters in Florida, it is doubtful that he ever practiced medicine on a regular basis in the state. Born in Louisa, Louisa County, Virginia, about 1830, he was graduated from the Medical College of the University of Virginia[1] "with high distinction" in 1848. He began practice in Scottsdale, Virginia, a town some 15 miles south of Charlottesville, but shortly thereafter began to suffer hemorrhage of the lungs. He was forced to suspend practice and seek "the mild and balmy atmosphere of the almost tropical climate of Florida," where he spent several successive winters. In spite of the handicap and the imminence of death he gained a splendid reputation in his profession. As the winter 1857-58 drew on he left Florida to return to his Virginia home where he died in December.[2]

1. *The General Catalogue of the University of Virginia* for 1880 contains a list of all medical graduates from 1828 through 1880. Dr. Wade is listed among the graduates of 1848.
2. Tallahassee *Floridian and Journal*, February 6, 1858. The appearance of the obituary in the Tallahassee newspaper suggests that Dr. Wade had spent his winters in the vicinity of Tallahassee.

Waggoner, G.J., Monticello, 1859

Only a fleeting glimpse of Dr. Waggoner is permitted by Florida sources. He appeared in Monticello in the spring of 1859, entered practice in partnership with Dr. Archibald Campbell McCants for the practice of homeopathy. They announced their intention to maintain two offices, one in the home of Dr. McCants in Monticello, the other in the City Hotel at Tallahassee,[1] their professional card first appearing in the local newspaper on April 9, 1859. The partnership was apparently dissolved about the first of October when Dr. Waggoner's name was discontinued in their advertisement.

1. Monticello *Family Friend*, May 10, 1859, 1st printing, April 9, 1859.

Wakefield, Adoniram Judson, Jacksonville, 1823-1911

Dr. Wakefield, for four decades one of Jacksonville's most beloved citizens, was born in New Hartford, Litchfield County, Connecticut, in September 1823.[1] He is thought to have been a graduate of Harvard Medical School and prior to moving to Florida is known to have been a member of the Harvard Medical Society.[2] It has not been determined just when he arrived in Florida, but it appears to have been very soon after the Civil War. Although an obituary notice states that he had practiced in Florida for 48 years, this would have placed his arrival in 1863, an unlikely year for migrating from Massachusetts into the South.

Dr. Wakefield was a man of exceptional intelligence and compassion. He appears to have quickly gained the confidence and friendship of a large number of patients as well as colleagues in the medical profession. When the Florida Medical Association was organized in the office of Jacksonville physician, Dr. Abel S. Baldwin, on January 14, 1874, Dr. Wakefield, though not present, was one of 14 physicians to be nominated and elected to membership by unanimous vote of the organizers. From that date until almost the time of his death he was a constant and loyal member of the Association, frequently in attendance at its annual meetings, even that of 1910 when he was 86 and in poor health.[3] For several years in the 1880s he was a member of the medical and surgical staff of St. Luke's Hospital.[4]

Prior to moving to Florida Dr. Wakefield was married. His wife, known only as Catherine, was a native of Massachusetts. For many years the childless couple resided at 61 Ocean Street, a short distance from the business part of the city. Having been members of the Congregational Church in New England and finding no such church in Jacksonville, they proceeded to help organize the Union Congregational Church of which they were charter members.[5]

Dr. Wakefield died on March 28, 1911, at the age of 87 at the home of Mrs. Katherine McCallum at 34 Ashley Street. After a funeral at the Congregational Church he was buried in Jacksonville's Evergreen Cemetery on June 1. His pallbearers included three members of the Duval County Medical Society of which he was a long-time member.[6]

Mrs. Wakefield died in Boston on April 28, 1923. Her remains were brought to Jacksonville and buried by the side of her husband.[7]

1. Dr. Wakefield's obituary notice appeared in the Jacksonville *Florida Times-Union*, March 29, 1911. Some uncertainty remains as to the date of his birth, the newspaper notice states it as September 10, 1824, while it is shown on his gravestone as September 20, 1823. A similar discrepancy occurs regarding the date of his death; the gravestone has it March 26, 1911, while the obituary of March 29 begins: "Dr. A.J. Wakefield, one of Jacksonville's oldest citizens, died last night at 10:45 p.m." (the 28th)

2. *Transactions, Florida Medical Association*, 1911, Jacksonville, 1911, p. 28. It is interesting that Dr. Wakefield's unusual Christian name, Adoniram, appears only in the obituary notices of himself and his wife. In the census of 1880, it appears as Andrew J. and in the census of 1885 as Albert J. It is likely that he was known to his intimates as Judson.

3. Ibid., 1910, Jacksonville, 1910, p. 11.

4. Webster Merritt, *A Century of Medicine in Jacksonville and Duval County*, Gainesville, 1949, p. 89.

5. This is suggested in the obituary for Mrs. Wakefield, Jacksonville *Florida Times-Union*, April 29, 1923.

6. The three physicians were Cary P. Rogers, H.R. Drew and James Douglas.

7. A question arises concerning the relationship of Dr. Wakefield and his wife. His obituary indicates that he had no surviving relatives while the account of her death 12 years later mentions her burial by the side of her husband. She was obviously not in Jacksonville at the time of his death.

Waldo, Benjamin, Madison and Marion Counties, 1816-1871

Dr. Waldo was born in Edgefield District, South Carolina, on December 11, 1816, son of Joseph Warren and Elizabeth Lamar Waldo.[1] The Waldos, a family of cultivation and substance, traced their ancestry to a 17th-century Englishman, Cornelius Waldo, who emigrated to America. Family tradition has it that when Benjmin was a mere lad his father, not pleased with the local schools in Edgefield, took him north to be educated. In due time he matriculated at Jefferson Medical College in Philadelphia.[2] There is no evidence, however, that he remained there for more than a term. Records of the Medical College of the State of South Carolina indicate that he matriculated there in the fall of 1836 and was graduated as Doctor of Medicine in the following spring.[3] His thesis topic was "Intermitting (sic) Fever." The same sources show that as a postdoctoral student he returned for an additional year of study, not uncommon for medical students of the times.

On completion of medical study Dr. Waldo returned to Edgefield where he practiced for a short time. One of his early patients was Sarah Lipscomb whom he later married. Soon thereafter the doctor and his wife moved to nearby Newberry where he practiced for several years.

In 1847 Dr. Waldo moved with his family to Madison County where he purchased a plantation and settled down to the life of a planter. Significantly the census schedule of 1850 designates him not as physician but as farmer.[4] Surviving records throw very little light on his Madison county experience, but it appears that his poor health dictated that he virtually abandon medical practice. A Tallahassee newspaper reporting the First Annual Leon County Agricultural Fair, held in the fall of 1852, states that Dr. Waldo was one of the livestock judges.[5]

In the late 1850s Dr. Waldo, for unknown reasons, decided to leave his Madison County holdings and move to Marion County. He purchased lands in the northwest part of the county near the village of Flemington in an area already settled by several prominent South Carolinians.[6] The last antebellum decade was a time of comparative prosperity for slave owners engaged in the production of cotton and Dr. Waldo appears to have prospered. The census of 1860 lists him as "planter," owning real property valued at $15,000 and other properties valued at $28,000. His slaves numbered 38.[7] Besides the cultivation of cotton Dr. Waldo was one of the first in the area to experiment with citrus culture.

Soon after arriving in Florida Dr. Waldo became acquainted with David Levy Yulee, U.S. Senator, land dealer and exponent of internal improvements. The two men became close friends. In 1853 Yulee incorporated the Florida Railroad Company, authorized to build a railroad from Fernandina to Cedar Key. As the project progressed, Dr. Waldo , aware of the importance of a railroad to Marion County, led a group of local planters and Ocala businessmen in an effort to obtain a branch line connecting Ocala with the Fernandina-Cedar Key line near Waldo, the village which Yulee is said to have named for his friend, the doctor. At one of the meetings of the group Dr. Waldo, in support of the project, was said to have spoken "clearly, logically, and in an enlightened manner," stressing the importance of an Ocala terminus,[8] explaining the alternatives of subscribing stock for the enterprise, or purchasing free land bonds.

For the last few years of his life, Dr. Waldo appears to have lived quietly on his plantation, making occasional journeys back to his native state and now and then participating in matters of public concern. Three children, two sons and a daughter, were born to the Waldos. The elder son, Joseph Warren, the namesake of his grandfather, too young for enlistment at the beginning of the war, volunteered for service in the Confederate Army on March 4, 1863, though only 16. He was assigned to Company C, 2nd Florida Cavalry, but spent much of his time on detached service driving beef cattle from place to place for army consumption. He was paroled at Baldwin on May 17, 1865,[9] and returned to the plantation which he would operate after his father's death.

Mrs. Waldo died at her Marion County home on September 11, 1867. Dr. Waldo survived her by nearly four years, dying on April 4, 1871.[10]

1. Much of the biographical information included in the present sketch was provided by Mrs. Bettee V. DeSha, writer and genealogist of Waldo. Her assistance is gratefully acknowledged.

2. There remains some doubt about Dr. Waldo's association with Jefferson Medical College. The archives of the College do not list him as a graduate.

3. Archives, Medical University of South Carolina Library, Lists of Students and Graduates.

4. U.S. Census, 1850, Madison County, Florida, p. 215. For the date of his removal to Florida see Thos. H. Pope, *History of Newberry County, South Carolina*, Columbia, 1973, vol. I, p. 267. At the time of his leaving for Florida Dr. Waldo was serving in the S.C. House of Representatives from Newberry District.

5. Tallahassee *Sentinel*, October 26, 1852.

6. Flemington is situated in north Marion County, five miles west of Orange Lake.

7. U.S. Census, 1860, Marion County, Florida, p. 83. It is odd that Dr. Waldo is listed as the only member of his household. Possibly Mrs. Waldo and her children had remained for a while in Madison County. Included in the Waldo property were 13 lots in Fernandina and four lots in Nassau County outside Fernandina. See Fernandina *Florida Mirror*, December 21, 1878.

8. Fernandina *Florida News*, February 17, 1859.

9. NA, Service Records, CSA, M251, Roll 13.

10. No newspaper which might have contained an obituary of either Dr. Waldo or his wife has survived. Besides their son, Joseph, Dr. and Mrs. Waldo were survived by their daughter, Susan, and their younger son, Albert.

Waldron, Daniel, Putnam County, mid-19th century

Although Dr. Waldron was born in Florida, he apparently spent only a small part of his life there. His father was a native of New Hampshire, his mother a native of Georgia. Census data suggest that the doctor and his wife were living in Florida when their first child, a daughter named Mary, was born in 1859. On November 16, 1866, the Tampa *Florida Peninsular* printed this item: "Dr. Daniel Waldron, formerly of Polk and Hernando Counties, we learn, is now settled in the practice of Medicine in Washington, D.C." This is verified by the fact that the only son of Dr. Waldron was born in the District of Columbia in 1867.

The final note on the Waldrons stems from the Putnam County Census of 1880, in which it is shown that the Waldron household included his grandson, Charles F. Allen, aged two and Florida-born, obviously the son of Mary Waldron, who had married an Allen, who is shown to have been a native of New Jersey.

Walkup, Henry Clay, Marion County, 1843-1907

Dr. Walkup, a native of North Carolina, spent the greater part of his professional career in the McIntosh community of Marion County. It is apparent that he enjoyed a fine reputation both as physician and community leader. His obituary, which appeared in the Ocala *Evening Star* of October 16, 1907, included the following: "He had resided in McIntosh between thirty-five and forty years, one of the best known and highly respected citizens in the County, and was said to be the most skiled and successful county doctor in this part of Florida."

As an avocation Dr. Walkup spent much of his time in agricultural pursuits. In 1885 he owned 70 acres of land, of which 20 acres were under cultivation, the value of the land having been estimated at about $6,000. In addition he owned 50 acres of woodland.[1]

Dr. Walkup was twice married, his first wife, known only as Nannie, was born in 1846 and died in 1889. Not long after her death he married a Floridian of South Carolina parentage, Ida Wood, who was born on July 5, 1852, and died on June 12, 1922. To each marriage were born several children, some of whom lived well into the 20th century.[2] The Ocala newspaper, in reporting Dr. Walkup's death, simply stated that "he leaves a large family of grown-up children and a wide circle of friends." The doctor was buried in Center Point Cemetery, located about a mile and a half north of McIntosh.[3]

Dr. Walkup was never a member of the Florida Medical Association. He would doubtless have been pleased to know, however, that his son, Adam Clay, followed his footsteps and became a successful physician in Marion County. He was a member of the Marion County Medical Society, eventually affiliating with the Florida Medical Association.[4]

1. The Special Florida Census of 1885 indicates that Dr. Walkup was an active physician that year. The Mortality Schedule of 1885 lists the deaths of three patients of Dr. Walkup: one who died of diphtheria, one of "bilious fever," the third, a one-year-old child, of gastritis.

2. Marion County Census, 1900, lists the following Walkup children and their ages: Lillis, daughter, born August 1883, and Rosa L., twin sister; Adam Clay, born January 1886; Mary C., born February 1888.

3. *Transactions, Florida Medical Association*, 1912, p. 243.

Wall, John Perry, Tampa, 1836-1895

Few if any Florida physicians of the 19th century achieved greater eminence within the ranks of their profession and more esteem among the general public than Dr. Wall. Fortunately, biographical data on this remarkable man abound; these remarks do little more than present a resume of the work of others.[1]

Dr. Wall was born in Hamilton County on September 17, 1836. His parents, Perry G. and Nancy Hunter Wall, natives of Liberty County, Georgia, had arrived in Jasper a short while earlier and in 1845 when their son was nine years old they moved to Benton (after 1850, Hernando) County, settling in the rural community known as Pierceville.[2] Such early education as the boy received was doubtless gained in a local rural school.

When young Wall turned his attention to medicine he was apprenticed to a local doctor named Mayo, about whom scarcely any knowledge has come to light. In 1856 he was enrolled at the Medical College of the State of South Carolina, Charleston,[3] from which he was graduated in March 1858 after satisfying the college requirements. His doctoral thesis bore the title *Morbus Coxarius*, which is translated loosely as ailment of the hip.[4]

Soon after graduation Dr. Wall returned to Florida, settling in Brooksville, which had become the seat of Hernando County, where he joined another young physician destined to make his mark in medicine, Dr. Thomas P. Gary. The two formed a professional partnership,[5] an arrangement announced in February 1859[6] but dissolved after a few months. In January 1860 Dr. Gary offered his services to the people of Hernando County,[7] thanking them for past favors. Meanwhile Dr. Wall had departed for Fernandina where on March 8, 1860, he offered his services to the people of that town.[8] He announced the location of his office in the Pioneer Hotel. A little later that year the census enumerator found him residing in a rooming house which he shared with five other men including Dr. Edmund Seabrook, an 1853 graduate of the Charleston medical school.[9] He apparently remained in Fernandina until the outbreak of war in 1861.

Irksome lacunae in the Confederate Army records in the case of Dr. Wall render their information almost worthless. These records indicate that Dr. Wall was mustered into the 9th Florida Infantry Regiment as a member of a company calling itself the Gulf Coast Rangers organized at Bay Port on the Gulf Coast of Hernando County. Family records which appear to be more reliable indicate that Dr. Wall enlisted in the Confederate Army at the outbreak of war and after a brief stint as assistant surgeon in the 9th Infantry, he was transferred to a Confederate Hospital, probably the Chimborazo, in Richmond where he remained until 1863 when, at his request, he was assigned to field duty. In 1864 he was promoted to the rank of surgeon, serving in that rank until the end of the War.[10]

Dr. Wall obtained permission to absent himself from his hospital duties in 1862 for a trip back to Florida to marry his beloved Pressie E. Eubanks whom, in spite of the difficulties of travel, he was able to take back to Richmond.

Upon the conclusion of the War Dr. Wall and his wife returned to Brooksville where in 1866 their son, John P. Wall Jr., was born. They shared the home of Mrs. Wall's mother, Mrs. Sarah Eubanks,[11] who, like her daughter, was a native of South Carolina.

In 1871 Dr. Wall moved with his family to Tampa to resume a career which brought him fame and a fair degree of fortune. His medical practice was sufficiently successful to elevate him to the top rank of the profession, but the year 1871 was also one of tragedy. He was called to attend a young seaman aboard a ship in Tampa harbor. It was a case of yellow fever which Dr. Wall transmitted to his wife and two-year-old daughter, both of whom died of the disease. Henceforth Dr. Wall devoted much of his time to the concerns of public health, becoming a member of the American Public Health Association in 1875 and the American Medical Association in 1879. Although he was not present at the launching of the Florida Medical Association in Jacksonvile in 1874 he was present at the meeting in February 1875 where his presence was immediately felt. He was elected to membership and responded with a paper entitled "Preventive Medicine," a subject to which little attention had been given. It provoked considerable interest among his colleagues.[12]

By request Dr. Wall was asked to read a report of several of his interesting cases. These were puerperal convulsions, fracture of the humerus, gunshot wound of the heart, and stricture of the esophagus. Immediately after this presentation he was elected Second Vice President of the Association and appointed a delegate to the next meeting of the American Medical Association.

Throughout his career Dr. Wall worked diligently for establishment of a State Board of Health, joining Dr. Joseph Y. Porter of Key West in the effort. He was one of the first to be convinced that yellow fever was spread by mosquitoes. Although he had difficulty convincing his fellow physicians, he was able as Health Officer of Tampa to enforce rigid quarantine regulations and thus to some degree stem the rapid spread of the disease. The efforts of Drs. Porter and Wall were finally successful when in 1889 Governor Francis P. Fleming virtually ordered a reluctant State Legislature to authorize the State Board of Health.

Dr. Wall's numerous papers on disease and health, many of which were published, reveal not only a mastery of diction and accuracy of expression but a firm understanding of scientific observation and procedure. In them is courageous exposure of the ignorance and superstition which lingered on among many Florida practitioners. His opinions were generally well-considered. Never was he intractably dogmatic. Wrote his eulogist: "He was a man of convictions and he dared to have the courage of his convictions, and yet born of a tenderness tempered by the grace of God had a kindly regard for opinions different from his own."[13]

At its meeting in Jacksonville in 1884, Dr. Wall was elected President of the Florida Medical Association and a year later at Sanford delivered his presidential address, "On the Medical Profession—Its Achievements and Responsibilities," an eloquent statement of his heart-felt convictions.[14] As a medical scholar and practitioner he was active until the very hour of his death, which occurred at the annual meeting of the Florida Medical Association in Gainesville. At the morning session in a lecture hall of the East Florida Seminary on April 19, 1895, he collapsed a few minutes after he began reading his paper, "Public Hygiene in the Light of Recent Observations and Experiments." His colleagues who rushed to attend him were helpless to resuscitate him. There was a difference of opinion as to the cause of his death, one thought it had been heart failure, another was certain it was brain hemorrhage. The paper, typical of his careful research and inquiring mind, was published later that year in the *Proceedings* of the organization.[15] It is significant that up to the very time of his death, Dr. Wall's professional notices were appearing in the Tampa *Tribune*, of which he had earlier been editor.

The review of Dr. Wall's civic, social and religious activities is left to others. He entered enthusiastically into the life of the Tampa community. He was mayor for a term, served on the Hillsborough Board of Education for a term, during which he had serious altercations with the State Superintendent of Public Instruction, who threatened to remove him from the Board and, perhaps just as important, was Assistant Editor of the Tampa Sunland *Tribune* and later Editor of the Tampa *Tribune*.

Needless to say his sudden death was a severe shock not only to his immediate family but to the whole City of Tampa and the State of Florida.[16] Probably there has never been a lengthier or more laudatory obituary in the State of Florida than that which appeared in the Tampa *Tribune* on April 25, 1895, filling four full columns.

Dr. Wall was three times married, first to Pressie Eubanks. Of that marriage to which several children were born, only a son, John Perry Wall Jr., survived to live out his adult life in Tampa. To the second marriage to Matilda McKay, one son, Charley McKay Wall, of several children born to the union, survived to manhood. After the death of Matilda in November 1893, Dr. Wall married Louisa Williams, who survived him. Dr. Wall's aged father also survived him and was among the throng present at the funeral services. Also present were Dr. Wall's four sisters: Mrs. Mary Frierson and Mrs. Susan Hendry of Ft. Myers, and Mrs. S.L. Clark and Mrs. Julia Friebele of Tampa; and two half brothers, General J.B. Wall of Tampa and Charles F. Wall of Seaside.

1. Of special importance is James M. Ingram, "John Perry Wall, A Man for All Seasons," *Journal, Florida Medical Association*, August 1966, pp. 709-717. See also Karl H. Grismer, *Tampa*, St. Petersburg, 1950, p. 330; *Florida State Government*, 1885, An Official Directory of State Government, J.B. Whitfield, Tallahassee, 1885, p. 18. This sketch was compiled when Dr. Wall was a delegate at the Florida Constitutional Convention of 1886. Additional data are to be found in the various issues of the *Journal of the Florida Medical Association*, 1875-1896.

2. Pierceville was little more than a crossroads with perhaps a store or two. It had a post office from 1854 to 1871 when it lost the facility and disappeared from the map.

3. *Catalogue, Medical College of the State of South Carolina*, 1856-57. List of Students.

4. Charleston *Mercury*, March 22, 1858.

5. The two men apparently became acquainted in Charleston when both were students. Dr. Gary was graduated in 1857 and later gained prominence in Marion County.

6. Tampa *Florida Peninsular*, February 5, 1859.

7. Ibid., July 10, 1860.

8. Fernandina *East Floridian*, August 23, 1860; first printed March 8, 1860, issue not extant.

9. U.S. Census, 1860, Nassau County, Florida, p. 5.

10. Dr. Ingram was allowed access to Dr. Wall's logbook covering his Civil War experiences in Richmond.

11. U.S. Census, 1870, Hernando County, Florida, item 355.

12. *Proceedings*, Florida Medical Association, 1875, pp. 9-13.

13. Tampa *Tribune*, April 25, 1895.

14. *Proceedings*, Florida Medical Association, 1885, pp. 14-20.

15. *Proceedings*, Florida Medical Association, 1895, pp. 112-128.

16. Tampa *Tribune*, April 25, 1895.

In addition to the numerous articles written by Dr. Wall and published in the *Proceedings*, following are a few which appeared in other professional journals: "Congenital Absence of Eyeballs," *Medical Record*, New York, 1881, p. 9; "Observation on Yellow Fever, with Special Reference to Diagnosis, Prognosis and Treatment, *Journal American Medical Association*, Chicago, 1888, XI, pp. 691-695; "The Yellow Fever in Tampa, Plant City, Manatee and Palmetto," *Report, Surgeon General Marine Hospital*, Washington, 1889, pp. 60-76; "The Climate of Florida," *Climatologist*, Philadelphia, 1891, I, pp. 164, 210; "Continued, or Typhoid(?) Fever of the South," *Gaillard's Medical Journal*, N.Y., LV, pp. 531-539; "Public Hygiene in the Light of Recent Observations and Experiments," *Virginia Medical Monthly*, Richmond, 1895-96, pp. 161-176.

Waterhouse, Henry S., Key West and Indian Key, 1786-1835

Dr. Waterhouse, believed to have been a native of Vermont,[1] established his medical practice in Key West in August 1828.[2] He was a medical student at the Dartmouth Medical School, Hanover, New Hampshire, in 1806 and apparently earned his medical degree there a couple of years later.[3] He had established a practice in Vermont remaining there until his health deteriorated to the point that he sought a more favorable climate in Key West. William A. Whitehead, writing 40 years later, recalled Dr. Waterhouse at the time of his arrival as "a slightly framed individual...with a sallow complexion and cadaverous expression of countenance...peculiar mouth...false teeth, which he was wont to assure his friends were manufactured from 'a tusk of the hippopotamus or sea horse.'"[4]

Dr. Waterhouse, according to Whitehead, had left his wife and small son in Vermont but with improvement of his health sent for them to come to Florida. The rigors of the journey were such that Mrs. Waterhouse became ill and died soon after arriving in Key West, leaving her husband to care for the child. By this time he was no longer a young man, being between 45 and 50.[5]

From the beginning of his residence in Key West Dr. Waterhouse was much concerned with the public affairs of the Island. In January 1829 he joined a number of citizens in petitioning Congress for establishment of regular postal service for the town.[6] When Congress responded favorably a short time later Dr. Waterhouse was named the first postmaster, the appointment having been made on February 18, 1829. He continued to hold the position until April 11, 1833, when he was replaced by Alexander Patterson.[7]

Other public responsibilities were soon entrusted to him. In 1830 he was a member of the Monroe County Grand Jury;[8] early in 1831 he was named a justice of the peace.[9] He seems to have continued to carry on his other tasks ably and vigorously, however. Being dissatisfied with the postal service he worked toward its improvement. Early in 1831 he sought the support of Florida's congressional representative, Joseph M. White, in his efforts to obtain a decent post office and more frequent and reliable deliveries. Calling the attention of the Post Office Department to the increasing importance of Key West in federal matters he pointed out that it was requiring three months or more for dispatches from Washington to reach federal employees in the Keys.[10]

Meanwhile Dr. Waterhouse was practicing medicine and manifesting serious concern for the public health of the town. The winter of 1828-29 saw the outbreak of an epidemic of smallpox in Havana causing alarm in Key West. In its issue of March 19, 1829, the Key West *Register* carried the following notice: "...our worthy fellow-citizen, Dr. H.S. Waterhouse, has procured from the Government Hospital in Havana a supply of pure fresh vaccine, or Cow Pock Matter, and intends devoting Saturday, the 21st to inoculation of all desiring it. The *Register* recommends..."[11] A few months later Dr. Waterhouse advertised that "he has for sale and will keep constantly on hand Drugs and Medicines of the best quality, suitable for diseases of warm climates," adding that individuals, families, and crews of vessels would be supplied on reasonable terms.[12]

Dr. Waterhouse's concern for public health is evinced in two lengthy letters. The first was calculated to dispel unfavorable rumors, abroad in northern states and cities, about the dangerously unhealthy climate of Key West. The second, printed in the Key West *Gazette*, July 18, 1832, responding to a communication from a reader employing the pseudonym "Lacon," was originally addressed to the Town Council of Key West in April 1829. In it Dr. Waterhouse presented a commonsense approach to the problems of public health, emphasizing the importance of sanitation, personal hygiene, and restraint in the use of alcohol in combating disease.

In 1827 the Florida Legislative Council established a regulatory body known as the Medical Board of the Florida Territory with a membership of nine physicians. In the following year its membership was increased to 15 and among those added was Dr. Waterhouse.[13]

For reasons not totally clear, Dr. Waterhouse gave up the post office in Key West on July 11, 1833, and moved with his young son to Indian Key, Whitehead says "anticipating a more extensive practice and new openings for business."[14] Once there he immediately received Governor Duval's nomination for justice of the peace and was duly approved by the Legislative Council.[15] Soon a new post office was established and Dr. Waterhouse was named its first postmaster. It was at Indian Key that a tragedy claimed the life of Dr. Waterhouse on January 17, 1835. On the evening of the 17th, which was a Saturday, Dr. Waterhouse and his son had gone out in a boat on a fishing excursion. On the following morning it was discovered that they had not returned home. Search parties were sent out and before long the overturned boat was located. Before the day was over the body of Dr. Waterhouse was found, brought ashore on Indian Key and there interred. The body of the boy was never located. It was the opinion of the Islanders that the boat had capsized in a severe squall.[16]

Whitehead, who knew Dr. Waterhouse well, wrote of him as follows:

> The writer will not venture any opinion as to his skill as a physician, but he was a man of some reading, had quite a collection of books, larger than any other on the island, and his intelligence combined with his eccentric manners and well developed disposition to look after his own interests made him quite a marked man in the little community.

Whitehead also recalled that he was gifted at repartee and in his small wooden house near Clinton Place often played the violin, but that he was ready "to put the instrument aside at any moment to receive a guest or discuss the news of the last mail."[17] His two published letters are those of a man of good education and literary style.

1. In his *Dartmouth Medical School: The First 175 Years*, Hanover, N.H., 1973, Carleton B. Chapman has included a page from the College catalogue of 1806 which is a list of medical students in 1806. Henry S. Waterhouse is listed, but his home residence was Stillwater, N.Y., a town on the Hudson River in Saratoga County, some 20 miles north of Albany. His obituary notices say only, "The Doctor was, we believe, a native of Vermont." Whitehead thought he was from Vermont.
2. Key West *Register*, March 19, 1829. In a letter, Dr. Waterhouse to Rev. B.B. Smith of Philadelphia, he says he had arrived in Key West in "August last" (1828).
3. Chapman, *Dartmouth Medical School*, p. 17. Here he is shown only as a student.
4. Thelma Peters, ed., "William Adee Whitehead's Reminiscences of Key West," *Tequesta*, XXV, 1965, p. 14.
5. Ibid., p. 16.
6. TP, XXIV, 136. Document dated January 10, 1829.
7. Walter C. Maloney, *A Sketch of the History of Key West, Florida*, Newark, N.J., 1876, p. 79.
8. TP, XXIV, 418.
9. Ibid., p. 485. Nominations of January 18, 1831.
10. Ibid., pp. 625, 681.
11. Efforts to determine a possible kinship between Dr. Waterhouse and the eminent New England physician, Benjamin Waterhouse who first employed vaccine in America (1800) have been fruitless.
12. Key West *Register*, May 30, 1829.
13. *Acts, Legislative Council, Territory of Florida*, 6th Session, 1827-28, Tallahassee, 1828, pp. 46-49. For second enactment see ibid., 7th Session, 1828, Tallahassee, 1828, pp. 258-60.
14. Whitehead's "Reminiscences," p. 16.
15. *Journal, Proceedings, Legislative Council of Florida*, Tallahassee, 1834, p. 79.
16. Key West *Enquirer*, January 24, 1835.
17. Peters, "Whitehead's Reminiscences," p. 16.

Watson, William J, Jackson County, 1834

Dr. Watson, born in South Carolina about 1796, was one of the earliest white settlers in Jackson County, having settled there in the early 1820s.[1] Like many of his fellow citizens he had purchased land and slaves, pursuing the dual roles of physician and planter. His ownership of 29 slaves would establish him as well-to-do.[2] His lands, located between Marianna and Webbville, amounted to approximately half a section, in township 5 north, range 11 west.[3]

Several items to be found *passim* in the *Territorial Papers* for Florida indicate that Dr. Watson was held in high regard by the people of Jackson County. He was, for example, appointed Justice of the Peace by the Governor in February 1827,[4] and in the following year he was Judge of the County Court.[5] In 1833 he was among eminent Floridians designated as appraisers of the ill-fated Union Bank,[6] while his name appeared as signer of several memorials and petitions relating to public issues and personalities.[7]

On a more localized scene Dr. Watson was one of the overseers, named by court order, of the poor of the county, whose responsibility was their relief.[8] He was also a member of a court-appointed commission to contract for the erection of a cupola on the Jackson County courthouse which would house the court bell, although these duties were expanded to include supervision of the general maintenance of the building.[9]

Although the records are so often silent on such matters as the day to day practice of physicians, an obituary notice provides assurance that Dr. Watson was a trusted and beloved practitioner.[10] It read, in part:

> In all his varied relations in life, Dr. Watson had uniformly deported himself in such manner as to secure the approbation and esteem of all who knew him... .As a physician he was learned and skillful without ostentation. As a man his kindness and benevolence were limited only by his means.

Dr. Watson's death occurred on August 26, 1834, when he was only 38. A widow, Mary, and five children survived him.[11] His descendants still live today in Marianna. Stanley tells us that one of his daughters, Mrs. Carolina M. Whitehead, was living in the old Watson residence north of the city at the time of the Battle of Marianna in 1864,[12] and also cites the financial disaster which befell Dr. Watson's youngest son, Hinton, during reconstruction days as being typical of the troubles which beset so many families during those troubled years.[13]

1. This place of birth is conjectural. The 1830 Census for Jackson County shows Mrs. Watson to have been South Carolina-born.
2. U.S. Census, 1830, Jackson County, Florida, Sheet 84.
3. For location and extent of his acreage see T.P., XXV, 180.
4. Ibid., XXIII, 779.
5. Ibid., p. 1005. The nomination was dated September 11, 1828.
6. Ibid., XXIV, 814.
7. Ibid., XXIII, 949, 1009.
8. J. Randall Stanley, *History of Jackson County*, Marianna, 1950, p. 31.
9. Ibid., p. 33.
10. Pensacola *Gazette*, September 13, 1834.
11. U.S. Census, 1850, Jackson County, Florida, p. 616. Mrs. Watson's age is here shown to be 56.
12. Stanley, op. cit., p. 22.
13. Ibid., p. 201.

Wauchope, Samuel Augustine, Tallahassee, 1822-1907

Dr. Wauchope, a native of Virginia, was born on June 28, 1822, and died in Selma, Alabama, on February 3, 1907.[1] He appears to have practiced medicine in several localities, one of those having been Tallahassee. It is not known when he arrived in Florida nor is it clear as to when he may have departed. His professional notice, which appeared in the Tallahassee *Weekly Floridian* of February 24, 1887, claimed for him 30 years' experience, two degrees, Master of Arts and Doctor of Medicine. He was still a resident of Tallahassee as late as 1897-98.[2]

Dr. Wauchope was twice married, first to Louise Banks of Virginia and after her death to Mary Marion Gerry of White Springs, Florida. To his second marriage were born three children, daughters Jessie and Marie Maud,[3] the former having been a school teacher in Centreville for several years, and a son, J.A. Wauchope, who settled in Selma, Alabama.

Dr. Wauchope was a member of the Masonic Order. Dr. Henry E. Palmer, an early 20th century Tallahassee physician and medical historian, recalled that

Dr. Wauchope had practiced "in Tallahassee before he moved to Carrabelle and Apalachicola."[4] He died in Alabama, presumably at the home of his son. A gravestone to his memory was placed in the Old City Cemetery in Tallahassee.

1. Dates from the gravestone, Old City Cemetery, Tallahassee.
2. *Catalogue of Physicians of the State of Florida*, Jacksonville, Florida Medical Association, 1898, p. 14.
3. Jessie, born August 26, 1837, died December 1, 1865. Marie Maud was born March 21, 1872, and died March 9, 1886. Mrs. Wauchope was born April 18, 1832, and died March 21, 1886.
4. Henry E. Palmer, "Physicians of Early Tallahassee and Vicinity," *Apalachee*, Tallahassee, 1944, p. 42.

Weademann, Philipp, St. Johns County, 1822

Dr. Weademann (Wiedemann) was a resident of St. Johns County during the last decade of the Spanish occupation. On July 4, 1815, he took the oath of allegiance to the Spanish crown, indicating that he was a planter and practitioner of medicine. He gave his age as 36, his religion as Catholic, stating also that he was married.[1] After cession of the Florida Territory to the United States Dr. Weademann appeared before James G. Forbes, Mayor of St. Augustine, and took the oath of naturalization to the new government on March 4, 1822. In this instance he was identified only as physician. He gave his age as 42 and claimed to be the head of a family of eight. He gave his birthplace as Mainz, Germany, and is shown to have been a subject of the Duke of Mainz.[2]

Spanish land grant records show that in 1815 Dr. Weademann petitioned for 400 acres in the St. Johns area, land bounded on the west by Turnbull Creek and on the south by the main road from St. Augustine to Picolata. Governor Estrada granted him only 150 acres, however. In his petition Dr. Weademann stated that he had been a militiaman serving the Spanish crown in the revolution of 1812-13. He finally received royal title to the land on July 3, 1819.[3] Since Dr. Weademann is not listed in the Florida Census of 1830, he is presumed to have left the Territory by that date.

1. East Florida Papers, Reel 163, Bundle 350 U4, p. 500. Microfilm in the P.K. Yonge Library of Florida History. This information provided by the courtesy of Bruce S. Chappell, Archivist, University of Florida.
2. *Territorial Papers, Florida* XXII, 434.
3. *Spanish Land Grants, Florida* (Confirmed), V. W-15.

Weatherly, Dr., Gadsden County, 1843

Dr. Weatherly (patronymic unknown) practiced medicine for a brief period in Quincy as the partner of Dr. John Henry Gee. Their professional notice first appeared in a Tallahassee newspaper on January 20, 1843, and was continued for several months.[1] Nothing further is known of him.

1. Tallahassee *Florida Sentinel*, January 20, 1843.

Weedon, Frederick, Leon, St. Johns and Monroe Counties, 1784-1857

Dr. Weedon,[1] one of the more colorful medical figures in antebellum Florida, was born in Baltimore on October 28, 1784, the son of Colonel William and Sarah Sands Weedon. After completing medical training, probably at the medical division of the University of Maryland in Baltimore, he moved to Huntsville,

Alabama, where he set up practice. It was there that he married Mary Wells Thompson in 1817, a native of Elbert County, Alabama, and sister of General Wiley Thompson of Seminole War fame. Dr. Weedon soon gained the trust and support of the citizens of Huntsville who elected him to the legislature for the sessions of 1819, 1820, and 1821.[2]

The precise date of Dr. Weedon's move to Florida is not known, but family papers indicate that the first six of his 10 children were born in Alabama, the youngest in 1828. He had arrived in Leon County by the summer of 1828; however, for on September 30 he attended a public dinner honoring Col. Joseph M. White, Florida's territorial delegate in Congress. The doctor not only assisted in the duties of master of ceremonies but also offered a toast, "To the memory of the citizen-soldiers who fell in the defense of Baltimore," memorializing an heroic event of the War of 1812 in which he had probably participated.[3] The Weedon family settled just southeast of the City of Tallahassee on a 320 acre tract which they had purchased in November 1829 from Joseph Harley.[4]

Not much is known of Dr. Weedon's activities in his five years of residence in Leon County. In the summer of 1829 he made a trip to Havana, leaving his business in the hands of James W. Ringgold.[5] It may be assumed, however that he divided his time between medicine and planting, an assumption borne out by the census schedule of 1830 which shows him owning 39 slaves.[6] On one occasion the Tallahassee newspaper called attention to his success in growing pineapples.[7]

For reasons which remain obscure Dr. Weedon stayed in Leon County only until 1834 when he decided to transfer his practice to St. Augustine. He purchased at public auction on June 16, 1834, a parcel of land "with the groves and houses thereon, said lot containing about six acres and bounded on the West by the St. Sebastian River, on the South by a street leading to Veil's Ferry, on the north and east by lands of John Drysdale," for which he paid $2,821.[8] Here he would remain for the next 20 years and become a comparatively successful practitioner of medicine and public figure of some note.

Dr. Weedon's first professional notice appeared in the local newspaper on June 3, 1835, with the announcement that he could be reached at his home on Charlotte Street, the house previously occupied by Dr. W.H. Simmons.[9] For the next few years he was an active participant in the civic affairs of the Territory. In August 1835 he was appointed a justice of the peace for St. Johns County in place of the departing John Lee Williams.[10] Later in the same year he was elected mayor of the city of St. Augustine for a 12-month term. Numerous items among the Florida Territorial papers as well as in the local newspaper reflect his continued interest in both local and state politics as well as his deep concern for the public health of St. Augustine.[11]

With intensification of Indian hostilities following the Dade Massacre of December 1835, numerous volunteer groups of citizen-soldiers were organized to complement the regular militia for an impending conflict. Among these was the battlion of Florida volunteers under the command of Major Benjamin A. Putnam. Within this battalion was Company C under the command of Dr. Weedon who was mustered in with the rank of captain. He appears to have served locally as a home guard officer, although on at least one occasion he led his company a few miles south to Matanzas Inlet to bolster the security of St.

Augustine. The company was mustered out on June 2, 1837.[12]

The most widely publicized event of Dr. Weedon's medical career resulted from a contract into which he had entered with the Office of Indian Affairs. By the agreement drawn up by Capt. Pitcairn Morrison of the U.S. Army, Superintendent of the Seminole Immigration project on January 13, 1838,[13] Dr. Weedon would accompany a group of Indians then being held at Ft. Marion, St. Augustine, to Ft. Moultrie, Charleston, S.C. He was to receive $150 for each month of service in addition to his expenses as surgeon. He would bear the rank of acting assistant surgeon. In order to justify the high cost of Dr. Weedon's services Capt. Morrison wrote to the Office of Indian Affairs: "It was the best contract I could make as no experienced Physician could be had for a less sum." In his dispatch Morrison also certified that "the persons entitled to medical attendance at Ft. Moultrie...is Forty soldiers, Three Company Women and two hundred and thirty Indians" and that no physician could be obtained at a lower rate.[14]

The Indian contingent which had been corraled in St. Augustine and shipped to Charleston Harbor included several of the most eminent of Seminole leaders, among them Osceola, Micanopy, Cloud and King Philip. Weeks of confinement, improper food, crowded conditions and indifference toward sanitation had reduced many of the prisoners to a weakened state and rendered them susceptible to illness. Even before they arrived at Ft. Moultrie on January 1 several had fallen ill. The most notable victim was Chief Osceola himself who became desperately ill on the night of January 26. Dr. Weedon was in attendance. Estimating the seriousness of the case, he summoned Dr. B.B. Strobel, formerly a resident of Key West but then Professor of Anatomy at the Medical College of South Carolina, to examine the patient and give an opinion. The following report, prepared by Dr. Weedon and printed in the Charleston *Courier* on February 6, 1838, provides a few details of the case.

> On the night of the 26th of January, ultimo, he was attacked in the night with a violent Quinsy, of which I was informed very soon, and hastened to his room. He was then laboring under considerable difficulty of deglutination and respiration, accompanied with pain and inflammation of the tonsils. To prevent suffocation it was necessary to support him nearly in an erect position. His pulse was full, quick and hard. Blood was instantly drawn, and an emetic and blister prescribed. At this moment an Indian entered the room, who as I afterwards understood, was held in high esteem as a Prophet and Doctor. From the moment of his entrance there was a refusal to take anything. Finding myself debarred from the administration of a suitable remedies and feeling the responsibility devolving on me, I requested Professor B.B. Strobel to visit the patient with me. He attended and used his best exertions to prevail on the patient to submit to treatment, such as sacrification, leeching, etc.—but he pertinaciously refused; not but what he would have been disposed to acquiesce, had he not been overruled by the influence of his family.
>
> F. Weedon, Asst. Surgeon
> Ft. Moultrie, Sullivan's Island, Feb. 5th.

Immediately following this report was a statement from Dr. Strobel corroborating Dr. Weedon's account.

There is a widely circulated story concerning the decapitation of Osceola's corpse by Dr. Weedon. It was by no means uncommon in those times for the bodies or parts of bodies of anatomical interest to be preserved for medical exhibits. The impulse or whim of Dr. Weedon to preserve the head of Chief Osceola should provoke no particular surprise or horror. It is perhaps unfortunate that the incident was brought to the attention of Dr. Andrew Welch, an English physician who resided for about two decades in Duval and St. Johns Counties as a medical practitioner and real estate promoter, and who published an account of his American experiences. Dr. Welch, who was outraged by the injustice and brutality inflicted upon the Seminoles by the white man, claimed to have been appalled by Dr. Weedon's act which he described as a violation of the "sacred remains of the dead," motivated, said Dr. Welch, by "foul, mercenary" considerations.[15]

Following his brief service in Ft. Moultrie Dr. Weedon returned to his regular practice in St. Augustine. In the fall of 1839 Dr. Strobel was gathering information for a forthcoming book on yellow fever. Having learned that St. Augustine was experiencing one of its worst epidemics of the disease he arrived there in November and immediately sought out both Dr. Weedon and Dr. Seth Peck, soliciting their opinions concerning the spread and nature of the fever, interrogating them about its transmissibility. Their observations are included in the Strobel text published in 1840. He wrote: "Dr. Weedon has resided here for nearly seven years... .The Doctor has seen the Yellow Fever for 20 or 30 years at Havana, Baltimore, Natchez & Baton Rouge." There followed Dr. Weedon's description of what he had witnessed in St. Augustine. Concerning Dr. Peck's opinions Dr. Strobel wrote, "...he does not believe Yellow Fever to be contagious, but will not pretend to say but what under certain circumstances the disease may be transmitted from one place to another."[16]

Random gleanings from the St. Augustine newspapers of the 1840s indicate Dr. Weedon's continued interest in the major public concerns of the times such as treaties with the Seminoles, statehood for Florida, and road construction. Incidentally among claims presented to Congress by Charles Downing, Florida's representative, were two on behalf of Dr. Weedon, one for the recovery of property taken from him by the military, the other for compensation for medical services rendered to the military.[17]

At some juncture during his residence in St. Augustine Dr. Weedon and family moved from Charlotte Street to Bridge Street. A business directory for the City, published in 1851, shows only Dr. Weedon and Dr. John Peck practicing medicine there.[18]

Death struck frequently in the Weedon household. Of his 10 children three died in infancy; his eldest daughter, Mary Euphrasia Teresa, died in 1838 at age 20 and his fourth daughter, Julia, died the following year. On November 2, 1849, Mrs. Weedon died in St. Augustine. Only three of the Weedon children produced offspring: Henrietta who married Dr. Daniel Winchester Whitehurst; William Henry Harrison who married Augusta Ann Renfroe of Georgia, and Hamilton M. who married Molly Dent of Alabama. Two of the sons, Hamilton and George B., followed their father into the medical profession.

In 1850 the censustaker found only two members of the family living at the home—Dr. Weedon and his son, Frederick, then aged 23. Their slaves numbered seven and were apparently of a single family.[19] The real estate was valued at $1,000, probably a conservative estimate. By 1853 Dr. Weedon began disposing of his property in preparation for leaving St. Augustine. An indenture, preserved in the St. Johns County Courthouse and executed on December 30, 1853, records the gift by Dr. Weedon of all his slaves to his daughter, Henrietta, with the stipulation that she pay to her brothers, George and Frederick, $550 each and that she agree to pay annually to Dr. Weedon himself "the sum of one hundred dollars and take care of and provide for the said party of the first part (Dr. Weedon) a home, food, clothing, and the necessaries of Life so long as he shall live."[20]

In the meantime, the Whitehursts had departed from St. Augustine prior to 1850 and taken up residence in Key West, and subsequently at Fort Jefferson in the Dry Tortugas where the censustaker located them in 1850. It was there that Dr. Weedon joined them probably in 1824. He died there in March 1857 at the age of 73.[21]

1. Much of the biographical information has been gleaned from the Weedon Family Papers in the possession of Mrs. Mary Weedon Keen, Tallahassee, and her brother, Dr. Frederick R. Weedon, Jamestown, N.Y., which Mrs. Keen kindly allowed me to examine. Mrs. Keen and Dr. Weedon are great-grandchildren of Dr. Weedon. Two other great-grandchildren, Mrs. May McNeer Ward, Leonia, N.J., and Col. James Weedon McNeer, Alexandria, Va., also possess family papers which I have not seen.
2. William Garrett, *Reminiscences of Public Men in Alabama for Thirty Years*, Atlanta, 1872, p. 757.
3. Pensacola *Florida Argus*, October 21, 1828.
4. Clerk of Court Office, Leon County, Florida, Deed Book B, Pt. 2, p. 565.
5. Tallahassee *Floridian and Advocate*, August 1, 1829. The Key West *Register*, August 13, 1829, also took notice of his arrival there aboard the *James Webb*.
6. U.S. Census, 1830, Leon County, Florida, p. 238.
7. Tallahassee *Floridian and Advocate*, November 16, 1830.
8. Weedon Family Papers.
9. St. Augustine *Florida Herald*, June 3, 1835.
10. Ibid., August 5, 1835.
11. TP, XXV, pp. 132, 326, 330, 376, 413, 428, 451.
12. St. Augustine *Florida Herald*, January 28, 1837; ibid., March 15, 1837; ibid., June 1, 1837.
13. NA. Microcopy, 234, Roll 290. Letters Rec'd., Office Indian Affairs, Emigration, 1828-38. Due to illness of Capt. Morrison during the negotiation of the contract there was a delay in formalization of the agreement and in getting it into the Office of Indian Affairs in Washington. In the meantime Dr. Weedon and the party of soldiers had arrived in Charleston Harbor on January 1. Charleston *Courier*, January 3, 1838.
14. Ibid.
15. Andrew Welch, *A Narrative of the Early Days and Remembrances of Osceola Nikkanochee, Prince of Econchatti*, Facsimile Ed., Frank Laumer, ed., Gainesville, 1977, pp. 201-202. George Catlin, the famous 19th century writer on American Indian lore, was at the deathbed of Osceola but departed Charleston the day prior to his death. Dr. Weedon wrote to Catlin describing Osceloa's last hours. Although Catlin probably knew of the decapitation he made no mention of it in his account. See George Catlin, *Manners, Customs, and Condition of the North American Indians*, London, 1844, II, 218-222. The incident was revived with further documentation by Mrs. May McNeer Ward, great-granddaughter of Dr. Weedon in an article published in 1955. See May McNeer Ward, "The Disappearance of the Head of Osceola," *Florida History Quarterly*, XXXIII, Nos. 3 and 4, January and April, 1955, pp. 193-201.
16. B.B. Strobel, *An Essay on the Subject of Yellow Fever Intended to Prove Its Transmissibility*, Charleston, 1840, pp. 162-63.
17. St. Joseph, Florida, *Times*, March 4, 1840.
18. St. Augustine *Ancient City*, July 19, 1851.
19. U.S. Census, 1850, St. Johns County Florida, p. 406. See also Slave Schedule for St. Johns County for same year.
20. Office, Clerk of Court, St. Johns County, Florida, Book A, p. 57.
21. The date of death is provided in the Weedon Family Papers. It agrees with Dr. Weedon's gravestone in Key West. Each generation of decendants of Dr. Weedon included at least one member of the medical profession.

Weedon, George B., Jacksonville, 1830

The professional career of Dr. Weedon is documented by only a single notice appearing in a Jacksonville newspaper in the summer of 1855 in which he announced that he was establishing his practice in the city. It read, in part, "He will also perform surgical operations, having had considerable experience in this branch of his Profession."[1] His card appeared in only two issues of the paper which suggests that he probably reconsidered his decision. He does not appear in the Duval County Census of 1860.

The Weedon family papers, however, provide a few biographical items relating to his early life.[2] He was born in Quincy in 1830, the third son and seventh child of Dr. Frederick Weedon and Mary Wells Thompson Weedon, who had recently arrived from Alabama. His first years were spent in Leon County where his father was a practitioner from about 1829 to 1834. The Weedons moved to St. Augustine in 1834 and there young George spent his youth. In the final disposition of the property of the elder Weedon in 1853 preparatory to his moving to Key West, it was stipulated in an indenture that for certain considerations his daughter, Henrietta, married to Dr. D.W. Whitehurst, was to receive his real property in St. Augustine but that she was bound to pay to her brothers, George B. and Frederick, $550 each. Dr. Weedon signed a statement dated at Ft. Jefferson, the Dry Tortugas, Monroe County, on April 27, 1855, that he had received that amount. In a similar document of the same date and same place he appointed Major Benjamin A. Putnam of St. Augustine his attorney and legal agent to handle his other interests in St. Augustine property, "particularly that known as the Orange grove." These were transactions executed four months before his card appeared in the Jacksonville paper.

1. Jacksonville *Florida Republican*, August 23 and 30, 1855.
2. Weedon Family Papers in possession of Mrs. Mary Weedon Keen, Tallahassee.

Weedon, Hamilton M., Key West, 1834-1919

Dr. Weedon,[1] ninth child of Dr. Frederick Weedon, was born in Tallahassee on March 15, 1834. While an infant the Weedon family moved to St. Augustine where he spent his youth.[2] Following his father and brother, George, he chose to become a physician and completed medical study about 1854 just as his father was retiring from practice and disposing of his St. Augustine properties preparatory to moving to Key West where young Hamilton's sister and her husband, Dr. Daniel W. Whitehurst, were living. Documents among the Weedon family papers indicate that in the division of family property Hamilton came into possession of seven slaves, five of whom he sold to the Whitehursts for $3,000 in May 1861.[3] Apparently he received none of the family real estate.

Although the records are not clear on the matter it appears that Dr. Weedon established his first practice in Key West about 1855 or 1856. The Key West Census of 1860 lists him as aged 26, a resident of the Whitehurst household, and owner of property valued in excess of $5,000.[4]

With the coming of the Civil War Dr. Weedon entered the Confederate Army with the rank of assistant surgeon. He joined the medical staff of the Fourth Infantry Regiment of Florida Volunteers in the early summer of 1861. During the earlier months of its existence, July 1861-May 1862, the various units within the Fourth Regiment were scattered about the state. During this period Dr. Weedon was medical officer for Companies G and H, stationed first at Fernandina but after the town's capture was assigned to Camp Langford, Jacksonville, and Camp Ward, Escambia County. With reorganization of the Regiment in May 1862 he was reassigned to Camp Ward. By early fall, 1862, the Regiment had moved as a unit to Tennessee where it became a part of General Bragg's Army and saw action at Nashville. Later it was to be involved in fierce fighting at Chickamauga and Murfreesboro. In May 1863 Dr. Weedon was with the brigade under General M.A. Stovall sent to relieve Vicksburg then under siege. Although the records do not provide the essential details it may be assumed that Dr. Weedon remained with the Fourth Regiment until its surrender in North Carolina in 1865.[5]

Dr. Weedon obviously was not pleased with his original rank as assistant surgeon. With discharge of the regimental surgeon near the end of 1861 he was given the temporary rank of acting surgeon but did not regard this as adequate recognition. He then proceeded to take the bold step of applying directly to the Secretary of War, Judah P. Benjamin, requesting promotion to surgeon. He enclosed supporting letters from regimental commander, Col. Edward Hopkins, and other officers. Impatient at not hearing from the Richmond headquarters, he wrote another letter from Fernandina on January 7, 1862, this one to General John M. Winder in Richmond restating his case and suggesting that "someone is trying to defeat me." He further added, "Would you as a friend speak to the Secretary of War for me, if opportunity occurs..." He concluded with the informative statement, "Last May I left a lucrative practice and considerable property in Key West to join this cause."[6] By July 1862 his commission had been approved. With the end of the War Dr. Weedon returned to Key West only long enough to settle business affairs before moving to Eufaula, Alabama, where he would spend the rest of his life.[7] He married Mary E. Dent, known as Molly, and they had five children. The fourth of these, Hamilton Weedon Jr., was to become a practicing physician in Alabama. Dr. Weedon Sr. died in 1919.

1. Part of this information was made available by Mary Weedon Keen, of Tallahassee, whose grandfather, William H. Weedon, was a brother of Dr. Hamilton M. Weedon.
2. Dr. Frederick Weedon moved to St. Augustine about mid-year, 1834.
3. This transaction executed on May 5, 1861, in Key West was done in preparation of Dr. Weedon's imminent departure for military service. Two other slaves, both children, who had been given to him by his father, had been sold to Henrietta Whitehurst, already in Key West, on December 13, 1853. Document in Clerk of Court Office, St. Johns County.
4. U.S. Census, 1850, Monroe County, Florida, p. 424.
5. *Soldiers of Florida*, Tallahassee, 1903, pp. 118-119.
6. NA, Service Rec., CSA, Fla., M251, Roll 58.
7. No date of marriage has been located. Family records show that his death occurred in 1919.

Weems, Gregory, Key West, 1829

Dr. Weems, a brief sojourner and practitioner in Key West, probably arrived in the Island city no earlier than 1828. He was in Havana with other Americans who gathered at the establishment of a Mrs. Howard "who has kept a house of entertainment for many years in Havana" on February 22, 1822, to honor the first American president. It was reported that Col. Pardon C. Greene of Key West offered a toast to General Lafayette which was followed by a toast by Dr. Weems to Andrew Jackson.[1] The Key West *Register* of April 2 reported the arrival of the Revenue Cutter Pulaski from Havana on March 29 with, among others, Dr. Weems aboard.

Dr. Weems apparently had planned to leave Key West prior to the outbreak of yellow fever in the summer of 1829 but before he could depart the fever, one of the worst onslaughts ever to attack Key West, was prevailing and he was persuaded to remain. On August 13 he announced that "through the solicitations of many of the inhabitants of Key West, and in consequence of the many cases of disease now prevailing here, I have just been induced to remain on the Island a short time; and I beg leave to tender my professional services to the residents and visitors"[2]

Before the end of the year Dr. Weems was dead, most probably a victim of the fever. On December 24, Algernon S. Thurston, administrator of his estate published the customary legal notices to debtors and creditors of the deceased doctor.[3] The final accounting, audited by R.B. Stanard and Edward Chandler, showed him to have been a man of meager means. The total value of the estate was estimated at $178.56¼. The most valuable item was a pair of gold buckles worth $25; the least valuable, one earring worth 6¼ cents.[4]

1. Key West *Register*, March 12, 1829.
2. Ibid., August 13, 1829. Dr. Weems' Christian name is here George, but corrected in subsequent issues to Gregory.
3. Ibid., December 31, 1829.
4. Deed Book, A., Monroe County, Clerk of Court's Office, pp. 197-198.

Weibley, J.C., Jacksonville, 1854

Dr. Weibley, a native of Virginia, appeared in Jacksonville in January 1854 and for a brief period was a partner of Dr. Henry D. Holland, one of the city's most popular physicians. The professional card of the two men, which appeared in local newspapers, announced the practice in Medicine, Surgery and Obstetrics. Dr. Holland could always be found at his office or his home. Dr. Weibley, on the other hand, resided temporarily at Buffington House, Jacksonville's leading hotel. As the junior partner, Dr. Weibley would handle all the country practice except for cases requiring consultations which would be handled in Dr. Holland's office.

The partnership appears to have been of brief duration. Dr. Weibley withdrew and is believed to have left Jacksonville prior to 1860.[1]

1. Jacksonville Florida *Republican*, January 12, 1854, and subsequent issues.

Weightman, Richard, St. Augustine, 1793-1841

Dr. Weightman, a native of Washington, D.C., and army surgeon, arrived in Florida early in 1821 while negotiations for transfer of the Territory to the United States were still in progress. In his quarterly statement on health conditions at military posts throughout the country, Surgeon General Thomas Lawson cited Dr. Weightman's report on Fernandina for the first quarter of 1821. He pronounced the health of Fernandina as excellent. In his own condensation of the report Lawson wrote: "This happy result is attributed by Asst. Surgeon Weightman to the attention given to cooking and the establishment of regular messes, and the commutation of the ration of whiskey (which was voluntarily relinquished) for tea, coffee, and sugar... .Cleanliness is the life of an army. The Jewish code, enjoining ablutions and purifications as religious rites, has been quoted as a system adapted to a camp..."[1]

A month or so later Capt. John R. Bell, in command of the detachment of troops enroute to occupy St. Augustine when the cession should be effected, wrote from Fernandina on May 18, 1821, three days after his arrival in the harbor: "Dr. Weightman came in last evening from Pablo and states from information that three days ago the Gov. of St. Augustine (Jose Coppinger) rec'd. despatches via Pensacola, supposed to relate to the delivery of the province."[2]

Henceforth, except for brief intervals, Dr. Weightman was a resident of St. Augustine in what appears to have been a dual role of military surgeon and civilian physician. In 1823, for example he purchased 200 acres of land on the east side of Lake George from George W. Clarke[3] at the cost of $1 per acre. In succeeding years his signature was affixed to a number of petitions and recommendations relating to civil affairs in East Florida.[4] When the Florida Legislative Council in its session of 1827-28 created a Medical Board for the Territory December 31, 1827, Dr. Weightman was named to the Board.[5] In 1826 he found himself an antagonist in a duel with Edgar Macon who had recently been dismissed from his office as U.S. attorney for east Florida by presidential order. The dispute which provoked this encounter almost certainly had political overtones,[6] but the court action launched against both participants did nothing to tarnish Dr. Weightman's reputation as a respected civil leader. The 1830 census schedule for St. Augustine lists him as physician, aged between 30 and 40, without family but the owner of two slaves and resident of "Barracks Ward."[7]

As for his military career, Dr. Weightman was commissioned post surgeon on August 21, 1818. He appears to have retired briefly from this position on March 2, 1821, only to return as assistant surgeon on June 1 of the same year.[8] He was never promoted beyond this rank. His birthplace as well as his residence at the time of his first commission was the District of Columbia.

Dr. Weightman found himself performing an unusual mission of mercy in 1825 when the commanding officer at Ft. Marion, Lt. Edwin R. Alberti, dispatched him to attend a wounded member of an Indian raiding party. The incident is recorded in a letter from Alberti to General Edmund P. Gaines, Commander of the Eastern District, U.S. Army. Alberti wrote: "...believing that it was due to the wounded man to afford him the benefit of Dr. Weightman's...valuable assistance, and that it would have a salutary effect, in convincing the Indians of our friendly disposition toward them, and as he (Weightman) could without injury leave those of our men who were on the sick list, I thought it advisable to direct him...to give such assistance as was practicable."[9]

A few years later Dr. Weightman served as judge advocate in a court-martial session in St. Augustine, the case involving a Lt. Tuttle of the U.S. Corps of Engineers.[10]

As the Indian hostilites intensified in 1835 Dr. Weightman reappears as a full-time military surgeon serving under Brevet Brigadier General Duncan L. Clinch at Ft. King. When Clinch found it necessary to redeploy his meager troops he wrote to his Washington superior, General Robert Jones, explaining his plight and mentioning reassignment of his three assistant surgeons. Dr. Weightman, he said, was being sent back to Ft. Marion with Co. D, 2nd Artillery,[11] where he was destined to remain until the following summer when the tempo of the war increased and garrison soldiers were pressed into actual combat. Among these were Dr. Weightman, who was wounded in the battle of Welika Pond in July 1836.[12] Neither the seriousness of his wound nor the extent of his recovery is a matter of record. It is known, however, that he continued to live in St. Augustine for another five years, dying there on October 30, 1841.[13] A local newspaper stated that his death resulted from "dropsy in the chest" and recalled that except for a brief interval, he had been stationed at Ft. Marion since 1822. He was praised as "a superior physician, amiable and benevolent in disposition...lamented by all."[14] He may perhaps be regarded as representative of the better class of military medical men of his times.

1. Lawson, *SRSMAUS*, p. 28.
2. TP., XXII, 47. Letter to John C. Calhoun, Secretary of War. Pablo was a small settlement some five miles from the mouth of the St. Johns River, near the point at which Pablo Creek enters the River.
3. *Spanish Land Grants in Florida*, V, W. 18. A transaction of September 14, 1823.
4. TP., XXII, 985; XXIII, 55; XXIV, 486, 569.
5. *Acts, Florida Legislative Council*, 6th Session, 1827-28, pp. 46-49.
6. St. Johns County, Florida, Office of Clerk of Circuit Court, Misc. File, Drawer T-3. Dr. Weightman's second in this encounter was his fellow physician, Richard Murray.
7. Fifth U.S. Census, 1830, St. Johns County.
8. *MDUSA*, pp. 283, 290.
9. TP., XXIII, 275. Letter dated at Ft. Marion, June 28, 1825.
10. St. Augustine *East Florida Herald*, July 3, 1834.
11. TP, XXV, 130. Letter dated April 24, 1835.
12. MDUSA, p. 290.
13. St. Augustine *Florida Herald and Southern Democrat*, November 5, 1841. The St. Augustine *News*, November 6, 1841, was equally laudatory. See also "Parish Register," 1821-1904, Trinity Parish (Episcopal), St. Augustine. In its list of burials for 1841 Dr. Weightman is shown as Asst. Surg., USA, age 48, and burial on October 31, 1841.
14. Although the final settlement of Dr. Weightman's estate was announced as complete on August 19, 1844 (St. Augustine *Florida Herald and Southern Democrat*, October 1, 1844), there is evidence that as late as 1846 litigation for the collection of medical fees long overdue from the estate of George T.F. Clarke was still pending. See Louise Biles Hill, "George T.F. Clarke, 1773-1838" FHQ, XXI, January 1943, 197-253.

Weissinger, M.M., Tampa, 1856

The medical career of Dr. Weissinger was tragically brief. A native of Marion, Alabama, he began his medical study under the direction of a local Marion physician, Dr. H. S. Levert. In 1851 he entered the Medical College of the State of South Carolina and was graduated in the spring of 1853. His doctoral thesis was titled "Uterine Haemorrhage." At a meeting of the students of the College prior to the 1853 commencement Dr. Weissinger and Dr. John H. Blake of Florida were elected secretaries which suggests that they were above average students.[1]

In the fall of 1854 Dr. Weissinger appeared in Tampa as the professional partner of Dr. John A. Rice.[2] He was doubtless suffering from tuberculosis at the time, which probably explains his decision to settle in Florida. In the diary of a Tampa resident, William C. Brown, appears the following entry (January 12, 1856): "Dr. Wysinger (sic) died this evening. He did like many of them do, stayed here until he was most well and then went north again and took a relapse and came back here but too late to save himself."[3]

1. Archives, Medical University of South Carolina, Lists of Matriculants and Graduates.
2. Tampa *Herald*, October 25, 1854.
3. "Diary of Wm. C. Brown, Dec. 24, 1855-Apr. 9, 1856." MS., P.K. Yonge Library of Florida History.

Welch, James Andrew, Duval and St. Johns Counties, 1797-1852

Dr. Welch was born in Nazeing, Essex, England, on March 20, 1797.[1] He was admitted to the College of Surgeons, London, on April 3, 1818, and at about the same date established his residence at Kingsland Place, St. Leonard's Parish, Middlesex, Shoreditch, London. On May 8, 1819, he married Jane Glidden and in 1821 obtained a licentiate of Apothecaries Hall.

After several years of practice in London Dr. Welch, apparently intrigued by what he heard of the culture of America, especially the southern portion, elected to observe for himself the ongoing struggle of the Seminole Indians to resist encroachments of the white man and have a closer look at Negro slavery as it existed in the Southern States. He arrived in Florida in July 1838 and purchased land on the south bank of the St. Johns River some five miles from the Atlantic and about 35 miles from St. Augustine where he developed a village which he called St. Johns. He became enchanted by Indian culture and was touched by the relentless encoachment and cruelty with which the white man was destroying the Indian and his culture. Slavery he also found inhumane and openly expressed his opposition to it. James M. Gould, editor of the St. Augustine newspaper, *The Florida Herald and Southern Democract*, on hearing of remarks made by Dr. Welch before a London audience, remarks critical of the institution of slavery, was incensed and proceeded to blast Dr. Welch in his columns.[2]

Dr. Welch attracted much attention when he virtually adopted an Indian boy, Nikkonuchee, and took him to London to be educated. Gould was relentless in his attack on Dr. Welch. He examined his Florida ventures, all of which he found fraudulent, including the land deal on the St. Johns, and preying on "an innocent woman," a Mrs. Johns, whom Dr. Welch had treated after she had been scalped by an Indian raiding party. It was claimed that Dr. Welch had introduced the boy as the son of Indian chieftain Econchattimico, chief of a tribe located in Jackson County, Florida. This assertion was promptly refuted by Joseph Clisby, a Tallahassee publisher and printer, who claimed that the chieftain had no children.

Meanwhile, Dr. Welch had become a member of the Royal College of Surgeons. He gained lasting fame through the publication of three brief books, *A Narrative of the Life and Sufferings of Mrs. Jane Johns; A Narrative of the Early Days and Remembrances of Oceola Nikkonochee,* and a *Narrative of the Life of Benjamin Benson*, the ordeal of a Negro slave who had been brought from Gambia and sold into slavery in Alabama and Louisiana. Through these books which became well-known and widely read in England, Dr. Welch became well known. He died in London on January 20, 1852, and was buried in the churchyard of St. John-at-Hackney.

1. Frank Laumer, *A Narrative of the Early Days and Remembranes of Oceola Nikkonochee*, Bicentennial Floridiana Series, Gainesville, University of Florida Press, 1977.
2. James M. Gould, *Florida Herald and Southern Democrat*, St. Augustine, July 24, 1843.

Weller, Frederick S., St. Augustine, 1844

Dr. Weller, a New Jersey native, was a resident of St. Augustine in the 1840s. As was true of many 19th-century physicians, he combined medical practice with operation of a drug store.[1] On December 5, 1844, he married a widow, Mrs. Elizabeth Loving, the ceremony taking place at Trinity Episcopal Church, with the Reverend F.H. Rutledge presiding.[2] Since the Wellers did not appear in the Census of 1850, it is assumed that they had departed the state by that date.

1. St. Augustine *Florida Herald and Southern Democrat*, May 6, 1845. Notices of his Drug Store appeared in several issues of the local paper.
2. Parish Register, 1821-1904, Trinity Parish, St. Augustine, Unpublished.

Wellford, Francis Preston, Jacksonville and Fernandina, 1829-1877

Seldom in the history of Florida medicine did the passing of a physician evoke such an outpouring of genuine sorrow and affection as did the death of Dr. Wellford on October 10, 1877. With the outbreak of yellow fever in Fernandina in September 1877, he left his Jacksonville home and volunteered his services to the citizens of the stricken town where he became an early victim of the dreaded disease. He need not have gone. Being of delicate constitution he could have with impunity remained at home and possibly delayed his death for many years. But he never weighed the risks and, as a result, died a virtual martyr.

Dr. Wellford was born in Fredericksburg, Virginia, on September 12, 1829,[1] into an old and honored family. As a child he suffered poor health. Denied the usual pastimes of youth, he was given every encouragement toward development of his mental capacities. He appears to have been a gifted student. After completing his baccalaureate course at the University of Virginia[2] he enrolled at the Medical College of the University of Pennsylvania from which he was graduated with distinction in 1852. Returning to Fredericksburg he began professional practice in which he is presumed to have been eminently successful.

With the coming of the War in 1861 Dr. Wellford enlisted in the service of the Confederacy and spent the war years as surgeon in the Medical Department, "carrying relief alike to friend and foe, in battlefield and hospital from the waters of the Potomac to the hills of Georgia."[3]

When the War was finished Dr. Wellford returned to Fredericksburg, only to find his "family scattered, his health broken and his fortune gone." Valiantly he resumed medical practice but after five years, and the further deterioration of his health, he was advised to seek a warmer climate. He chose Jacksonville where for the next seven years he devoted his diminishing energies to healing the sick, "rich and poor alike." His splendid qualities were quickly recognized by his medical colleagues and he readily established himself as a respected member of the medical fraternity. He became a member of the Duval County Medical Society and in 1874 was among the founders of the Florida Medical Association, of which he became the first secretary and treasurer.[4] He continued as secretary until 1877 when, although unavoidably absent from its sessions in Jacksonville, he was elected president of the Association.[5]

When yellow fever appeared in Fernandina in the late summer of 1877, news of its presence was suppressed by local authorities or, if revealed, it was dismissed as merely intermittent fever and no cause for alarm. On September 4, 1877,[6] Dr. J. Denham Palmer, local physician, wrote to Dr. Emile T. Sabal, of Jacksonville: "There is most emphatically, no yellow fever here. The mild remittent type which exists, yields most promptly to treatment...If not satisfied with this will you, Dr. Wellford and Dr. Daniel, not come over today and see for yourselves." On September 7, however, Mayor Samuel T. Riddell admitted that yellow fever was indeed present in the town.[7]

Within a week the fever was reaching epidemic proportions. Whole families were evacuating the town. Neighboring towns such as Jacksonville hastily established quarantines. The Duval County Medical Society was busily taking precautions. On September 10 it reported the following action: "The petition asking permission for Dr. Wellford to visit Fernandina and return after treating the family of Capt. Joseph Smith is refused."[8] By mid-month the situation was becoming critical. With two of the town's three physicians, Dr. Palmer and Dr. W.H. Pope, lying ill with fever, only Dr. C.W. Horsey was left to cope, calls went out for help. Doctors, nurses and supplies began to arrive. By September 24 Dr. Wellford was among them. A report of that date, but printed on the 29th, stated: "Dr. Welford (sic) who so nobly volunteered to come to our aid, is hard at work, and his cheery smile and pleasant voice bring comfort and hope to many a patient."[9]

Within a week Dr. Wellford also had fallen to the fever. On October 2, U. Sinclair Bird, Secretary of the Sanitary Commission of Fernandina, reported: "Dr. Wellford, from Jacksonville, was taken down with fever last night."[10] Bird wrote on October 8: "Dr. Wellford is dying. How sad! He came promptly at the call of duty, not counting his life dear if he might do the will of God by devoting his time and talents and attainments to the victims of the devouring scourge..."[11] Two days later, at ten o'clock in the morning of the 10th he died. Although he had been a life-long Presbyterian, his funeral services were held in St. Peter's Episcopal Church, Fernandina, with burial thereafter in the Church cemetery.[12]

The esteem in which he was held is indicated by the following excerpt from his obituary which appeared in the Jacksonville *Daily Sun and Press*, written by his friend and colleague, Dr. Albion W. Knight.

> The closing act of his life was but an epitome and crowning illustration of his useful and self-denying career. When the cry for help came from the plague-stricken city of Fernandina, he at once claimed the privilege, by reason of his office as President of the State Medical Association, to answer the call in person. With a perfect sense of the terrible risk, he calmly set his house in order that death might not find him unprepared, and then went boldly to the discharge of what he conceived to be a sacred duty.[13]

1. The biographical material in this sketch is derived chiefly from Dr. Wellford's obituary notice which appeared in the Jacksonville *Daily Sun and Press*, October 14, 1877. See also Webster Merritt, *A Century of Medicine in Jacksonville and Duval County*, Gainesville, 1949, pp. 103-105, for additional biographical data.
2. Ibid.
3. Ibid.
4. *Proceedings, Florida Medical Association*, Session of 1874, Jacksonville, 1875, pp. 3, 5.
5. Ibid., Session of 1877, pp. 11, 18.
6. Jacksonville *Daily Sun and Press*, September 4, 1877. The page cited appears as a single sheet inserted between the issues of September 12 and September 13 in the microfilm copy consulted.
7. Ibid., September 8, 1877.
8. Ibid., September 11, 1877.
9. Ibid., September 29, 1877.
10. Ibid., October 3, 1877.
11. Ibid., October 12, 1877. This letter was dated October 8th.
12. The obituary notice, cited in note 1, states that Dr. Wellford was buried in the churchyard of St. Peter's. Webster Merritt states (*A Century of Medicine*), on the authority of a letter from the rector of St. Peter's Church, Fernandina dated September 10, 1944, that he was buried in Fredericksburg, Virginia. This has not been verified. It is known, however, that Dr. Baxter Upham of Boston, Massachusetts, donated a splendid stained glass window for the west end of St. Peter's Church as a memorial to Dr. Wellford and his colleague, Dr. James C. Herndon, of Savannah, Ga., both of whom died of the fever in Fernandina. Dr. Herndon was also a native of Fredericksburg, Virginia.
13. It should also be noted that at its subsequent meeting, on April 16, 1878, in Jacksonville, the Florida Medical Association paid fitting honor to the memory of the departed President. Dr. Thomas M. Palmer of Monticello was elected to preside. *Proceedings, Florida Medical Association*, 1878, pp. 5-9.

Wells, Richard M., Hillsborough County, 1839

Dr. Wells, a native of Mississippi, moved to Hillsborough County soon after the end of the Civil War, settling in the Alifia community, some 23 miles from Tampa. Nothing is known of either his early life or medical training. The census of 1870 lists him as "physician and farmer," owning property valued at

$1,600.[1] Soon after arrival in Florida he married a Florida native, known only by her Christian name, Jane. They had three children, a son John Samuel, and two daughters, Fanny and Lucy.[2]

There is evidence that he was among the more active physicians of the county. That he was the attending physician of several patients who died during the 12 months prior to July 1, 1885, is not to be construed as an indication that he was less competent than his professional associates in the county.[3]

1. U.S. Census, 1870, Hillsborough County, Florida, p. 148.
2. Ibid., 1880, p. 431.
3. Special Florida Census, 1885, Hillsborough County, Mortality Schedule.

West, Edwin F., Hamilton County, 1833

Dr. West, a physician of Jasper, Hamilton County, was born in South Carolina about 1833.[1] When he was still a youth his family moved to Jacksonville where his widowed mother became a seamstress and sons Edwin and William entered the carpenter's trade.[2] Edwin entered the Savannah Medical College in 1855 from which he was graduated in the spring of 1857 after submitting a doctoral thesis on "Gun Shot Wounds."[3]

By 1860 Dr. West had begun his practice in Jasper. He was scarcely established when war began and on August 15, 1861, he enlisted in the Confederate cause, and on September 28 was mustered in with the rank of First Lieutenant and assigned to Company C, Tenth Florida Infantry Regiment. After brief service in Fernandina, where he came favorably to the attention of Colonel (later General) Joseph Finegan, he was stationed with his company at Ricco's Bluff on the east bank of the Apalachicola River.[4] When Captain William Frink failed to gain reelection as the commander of Company C in May 1862, Lt. West was moved up to a captaincy and elected to command the company.

Later in 1862 Dr. West was selected by General Finegan to command a special battalion and ordered to Lake City on special assignment. At some unspecified date in 1864 he was ordered to the Virginia war front; an inspection report dated September 30, 1864, indicated only that he was "in the trenches near Petersburg." The rigors of winter and constant exposure to cold caused him to contract pneumonia, however, and the last two months of 1864 found him a patient at the 1st Division General Hospital at Howard's Grove, near Richmond. Failing to make a satisfactory recovery resulted in his being transferred to the hospital at Farmville, Virginia, where he appears to have remained until the end of the War.

Upon his return to medical practice in Jasper in the summer of 1865, Dr. West gained immediate popularity. He had been cited by General Finegan for his exemplary "conduct and spirit."[5] He was forthwith nominated for a seat in the Florida House of Representatives and served for the terms of 1865 and 1866, in both instances as chairman of the Committee on Engrossed Bills and member of the Committee on Corporations.[6]

Very little is known of Dr. West's activities subsequent to the legislative session of 1866. The census of 1870 shows him living in the home of Mrs. Mary A. Bryant, a Jasper school teacher, and her son, Lawton.[7] Later Hamilton County censuses do not include him.

1. This date is an extrapolation from Dr. West's military record which gives his age as 28 at the time of enlistment. Ages supplied by census schedules are inconsistent and unreliable.
2. U.S. Census, 1850, Duval County, Florida. This schedule includes also a daughter, Penelope, aged 16.
3. Savannah Medical College, "Circular and Catalogue," Session of 1857-1858; also ibid., Session, 1875-1876.
4. NA, Service Records, CSA, M251, Roll 98. Dr. West's service record is somewhat garbled, although the chronological sequence seems fairly accurate.
5. *War of the Rebellion, Records of Union and Confederate Armies*, prepared under direction of Lt. Col. Robt. N. Scott, Washington, 1885, Series I, Vol., XIV, p. 235.
6. *Florida House Journal*, Sessions of 1865, 1866, passim.
7. U.S. Census, 1870, Hamilton County, Florida, p. 2.

West, Theophilus, Jackson County, 1836-1923

Dr. West was born in Leon County on September 5, 1836. His parents, C.B. and Zipporah (Tapping) West, had migrated to Florida from their native state of Virginia about 1825.[1] In the fall of 1857 he enrolled at the Oglethorpe Medical College in Savannah and in the spring of 1859 was graduated Doctor of Medicine, having submitted a thesis entitled "Menstruation."[2] Immediately thereafter he returned to Jackson County and launched his practice in Marianna, residing for a time in the home of Mrs. Rebecca C. Russ, a well-to-do matron and landowner of the town.[3]

With the outbreak of war in 1861 Dr. West enlisted for service on May 13, 1862, and was assigned to Company E, 8th Florida Infantry Regiment, with the rank of First Sergeant. A short while later he was promoted to the rank of 2nd Lieutenant and transferred to Field and Staff Headquarters as Assistant Surgeon, the assignment occurring in July 1862. The Regiment at that time was located outside Petersburg, Virginia. He remained with the unit until the summer of 1864 when he became Assistant Medical Officer, Office of Inspector of Hospitals, located at Orange Court House, Virginia. He continued in this service until General Lee's surrender at Appomattox on April 9, 1865.[4]

Returning to Marianna at the close of the War, Dr. West settled down to the career of a small town practitioner and civic leader. From time to time his professional notices appeared in the local newspaper with the information that he could be found during the day at his drug store, at other times at his residence which was formerly the home of Captain John Davis.[5] Meanwhile he had become Superintendent of the Marianna Methodist Sunday School, a position he held until his death in 1923. In 1868 he became Superintendent of Schools of Jackson County, the first person to hold that position.[6] In addition to these services he was for one term mayor of Marianna and for several terms a town councilman.

Dr. West was first married to Mrs. Rebecca Spears, widow of Hugh Spears and daughter of John Davis. To that marriage was born one son, who, according to Rerick, traveled for a drug firm and later became an insurance salesman. A few years after her marriage to Dr. West, Mrs. West died. A year or so later Dr. West married again, to Annie Louise Slade, of Columbus, Georgia.[7]

Dr. West continued medical practice well into the 20th century, at the same time operating his plantation outside Marianna. His death occurred on April 10, 1923.[8]

1. Some biographical data are drawn from Roland H. Rerick, *Memories of Florida*, 2 vols., Atlanta, 1902, I, 719.
2. *Annual Circular, Oglethorpe Medical College*. Session of 1861-62, p. 3. See also Tampa *Florida Peninsular*, March 19, 1859.
3. U.S. Census, 1860, Jackson County, Florida, item 257.

4. National Archives, Service Records, CSA, Microcopy 251, Roll 86.
5. See Marianna *Courier*, July 6, 1876.
6. J. Randall Stanley, *History of Jackson County*, Marianna, 1950, p. 75.
7. Ibid., p. 91, 202n.
8. Date obtained from the cemetery survey of Jackson County, compiled by Doris E. Pamphilon, 1984.

Westcott, John, Madison and St. Johns Counties, 1803-1888

Dr. Westcott, a man of exceptional learning and intelligence, was born in New Jersey about 1803.[1] After graduating from West Point where his specialty had been civil engineering he migrated to Middle Florida where his older brother, James Diament Westcott, had already risen to prominence in Territorial politics. Dr. Westcott is said to have studied medicine, probably under private preceptors, and is presumed to have practiced in the early years of his Florida residence in Madison.[2] It is also claimed that he served as army surgeon during the Second Seminole War, although records of the Medical Department of the U.S. Army make no mention of such service. Nevertheless, the Madison County Census of 1840 styles him "physician," aged 45.

In politics Dr. Westcott was a Democrat. He ran successfully for the Florida House of Representatives in 1846, one of Madison County's two representatives. In 1852 he was one of the Florida delegates to the Democratic National Convention in Baltimore.[3] When Franklin Pierce, the Democratic nominee, won the presidential election, Dr. Westcott's party service was rewarded with an appointment as Surveyor-General of Florida, a position he held from 1853 till 1858. The appointment required that he become a resident of St. Augustine. His arrival there on May 22, 1853, was viewed with some misgiving when it was announced that he had "dispensed with the services of all employees under the late administration."[4]

Dr. Westcott was vigorous and innovative in discharging the duties of the surveyor's office. In a major undertaking he attempted to produce a series of maps depicting locations and identifying claims of all Florida lands. In one of his dispatches to the General Land Office in Washington he claimed to have traveled, mostly on foot, more than 750 miles often through uncharted wilderness.[5]

In the later 1850s, as political tensions mounted and party realignments occurred, Dr. Westcott found that he could no longer support the main body of Florida Democrats. In the congressional elections of 1858, after refusing to endorse the Party's candidate for the House, Judge George S. Hawkins, Dr. Westcott announced his candidacy for the office as an "Independent Democrat." This brought the wrath of Democratic leaders and subjected him to scurrilous denunciations from Democratic newspapers. He was branded "traitor," "know-nothing," and "medical quack." Stated the Fernandina *Florida News* on August 25, 1858: "After all Dr. Westcott could speak learnedly about quackery, having earned his title of Doctor by peddling quack pills and bitters."[6] In spite of such attacks and the lack of substantial party support, Dr. Westcott received approximately one third of the votes, however, his federal job was lost.

It appears that Dr. Westcott had been able to accumulate sufficient assets to purchase a pleasant house on Bay Street in St. Augustine so he elected to remain there as a practicing civil engineer. His natural scientific bent combined with his vast knowledge of Florida topography gained for him the esteem of the city. During his years as Surveyor General he had become intrigued by the Florida adventures of Hernando de Soto. Having previously read Theodore Irving's work on de Soto, Dr. Westcott used his Florida wanderings to verify the de Soto legends and accounts. In an address before the St. Augustine Historical Society in 1860 he publicly criticized the Irving work, stated prefatorily that he had himself traveled most of de Soto's route "on foot."[7]

In June 1862 with the Civil War already well along, Dr. Westcott enlisted in the Confederate cause. He was given the rank of captain and assigned to the 10th Florida Infantry Regiment. After some two years of service in Florida as commander of Company I of his Regiment he was, in spite of his age, promoted to the rank of major (July 1864) and ordered to the combat zone near Petersburg, Virginia, as a regimental officer. The rigors of life "in the trenches" were too exacting, however. He was taken sick in August, admitted to the General Hospital at Howard's Grove near Richmond on September 9 where he was immediately furloughed to Madison and recommended for retirement by the local Medical Examining Board. He was paroled in April 1865 returning forthwith to St. Augustine.[8]

Except for brief trips Dr. Westoctt spent the remainder of his life in St. Augustine. His consuming interest was internal improvement. He was the driving force behind the building of the St. Johns Railroad which connected St. Augustine with the St. Johns River at the river village of Tocoi, thereby providing easy transportation with Palatka and the towns to the west.[9] In the meantime he had envisioned an intracoastal waterway which would run from the mouth of the St. Johns River to Key West, a project to which he devoted much time and work, the completion of which was an achievement of the 20th century.

In 1879, when he was in his 70s, Dr. Westcott was elected to represent St. Johns County in the Florida House of Representatives,[10] just 33 years after he had served Madison County in the same capacity. In 1885 he was a delegate to the Constitutional Convention in Tallahassee, holding the distinction of being the oldest man present. Meanwhile his fertile mind remained active in pursuit of internal improvements and technological advancement which would bring remote Florida into the mainstream of American industry and transportation.

Very little information is available concerning Dr. Westcott's family and domestic life. The Madison County Census of 1840 lists him with wife and small daughter as residents of Madison. Ten years later his wife, presumed to have been born in Bradford in South Carolina, was no longer living while his daughter, Rachel, was living in the home of Dr. Theodore Hartridge, a Madison physician, and Dr. Westcott was a resident in the home of Daniel G. Livingston, recently come to Florida from South Carolina. The 1860 Census for St. Johns County lists Dr. Westcott as a resident of St. Augustine. In his household was his sister, Emma,[11] who died in St. Augustine on January 9, 1900. Daughter Rachel was the wife of Andrew J. Miller. She died in St. Augustine on October 22, 1854. Another daughter became the wife of Henry Gaillard.[12] Dr. Westcott died in St. Augustine on December 31, 1888, and was buried in the New St. Augustine Cemetery.[13]

1. Some confusion still exists as to the date of his birth. Although his gravestone bears the date 1807, obituary notices state that he was in his 86th year. Madison *Recorder*, January 11, 1889; Jacksonville *Times-Union*, January 1, 1889. See also Greville Bathe, *The St. Johns Railroad*, St. Augustine, 1958, p. 57, where the date of his death is stated to have been June 16, 1887.

2. Rowland P. Rerick, *Memoirs of Florida*, 2 vols., Atlanta, 1902, II, 157.

3. Tallahassee *Floridian and Journal*, May 22, 1852.

4. Dr. Westcott was replacing Benjamin A. Putnam, an eminent local citizen, who had been active in the Whig Party, Jacksonville *Florida News*, May 7, 1853; St. Augustine *Ancient City*, May 28, 1853.

5. *Report 1855, House Document*, new series, 34th Congress, 1st Session, Pt. I, 266-273.

6. Fernandina *Florida News*, August 4, 25, 1858; Tallahassee *Floridian and Journal*, July 31, 1858.

7. Theodore Irving, *The Conquest of Florida by Hernando de Soto*, 2 vols., Philadelphia, 1835. This work was based on two sources, one Spanish, one Portuguese, neither of which Dr. Westcott deemed totally reliable. Theodore Irving was a nephew of Washington Irving.

8. NA, Service Records, CSA, M251, Roll 98. There are regrettable lacunae in the official record of Dr. Westcott's military service.

9. Bathe, St. Johns Railroad, cited supra.

10. Allen Morris, *The People of Lawmaking in Florida*, Tallahassee, 1977.

11. Parish Register, Trinity Episcopal Church, St. Augustine, "Burials." See also the obituary notice, St. Augustine *Evening Record*, January 9, 1900. Her age as recorded in the St. Johns County Census of 1860 (26) is obviously in error.

12. Obituary, cited in note 11.

13. Parish Register, Trinity Episcopal Church, "Burials." Here Dr. Westcott's age at time of death is recorded as 86. See also Madison *Recorder*, January 11, 1888.

Whaley, James E., Alachua County, 1860

Dr. Whaley, member of a South Carolina planter family, arrived in Florida about 1861 bringing with him a number of slaves. His move is said to have been prompted by the occupation of the sea islands of South Carolina by federal troops.[1] Upon arrival he obtained land either by purchase or lease on Orange Creek in the vicinity of Hawthorne and settled there to engage in planting.[2]

Dr. Whaley had achieved sufficient prominence in Alachua County by 1865 to be nominated as a delegate to the Florida Constitutional Convention scheduled for October 25 in Tallahassee. In the elections of October 10, however, he received 12 of the 792 votes which were cast, placing him sixth in the field of six[3] in spite of his having campaigned actively prior to the election.[4] In its preelection appraisal of the candidates the Gainesville newspaper said of him: "He is a gentleman of fine educational ability and generous to a fault."[5]

Dr. Whaley's wife, Jesse, was born in Georgia, while his three children, two daughters and one son, were born in South Carolina. His age in 1870, according to the census of that year, was 44, while his property, real and personal, was valued at $2,500.[6] There is no evidence, however, that Dr. Whaley ever practiced medicine as a paid profession in Florida.

1. Gainesville *New Era*, October 7, 1865.

2. F.W. Bucholz, *History of Alachua County*, St. Augustine, 1929, p. 134.

3. Gainesville *New Era*, October 14, 1865.

4. Ibid., October 7, 1865.

5. Ibid.

6. U.S. Census, 1870, Alachua County, Florida, p. 306. The children are listed: Carrie, aged 14; Thomas R., aged 12; Elizabeth, aged 10.

White, David L., Gadsden County, 1781-1862

Dr. White, a man of varied interests and one of the most respected and influential of the early settlers of Middle Florida, was born in Bladen County, North Carolina, in 1781. Nothing is known of either his early education or professional training but both appear to have been sufficiently sound to qualify him for the variety of positions he held after arriving in Florida. He is known to have served as sheriff of Bladen County prior to leaving North Carolina.[1] At an undetermined date he moved with his wife, Elizabeth (neé Kennon), to Putnam County, Georgia, where he lived for a few years and where his three eldest children, David L. Jr., Pleasants Woodson, and Ann, were born.[2] He moved to Gadsden County in 1822 and shortly thereafter acquired land at different locations within the county.[3] Although he never became one of the areas most affluent plantation owners, he is said to have owned more than a thousand acres of land and 30 slaves at the beginning of the Civil War.[4]

From the start of his Florida residence Dr. White's intelligence and good judgment were recognized by his peers and he emerged as a leader in several fields, notably civil service and religion as well as medicine. In 1824 he was appointed justice of the peace;[5] in 1825 he was appointed to a commission to locate a county seat and plat the town which would evolve around it.[6] In the latter year he was appointed county judge, within whose authority was the granting of licenses to practice law and medicine and, incidentally, it was at this juncture that he was licensed to practice both professions.

Although he had originated in an area of North Carolina heavily populated with Scottish settlers committed to Presbyterianism, Dr. White embraced Methodism and upon settling in Florida served the Methodists as a steward and from time to time as a local preacher. His son, David L., became a regular preacher in the Florida Methodist Conference. In the first Conference meeting, held in an encampment near Little River, Gadsden County, both the doctor and his son were in attendance.[7]

In these early Florida years Dr. White appears to have had little time for the practice of medicine. With a large family the income from medical practice was inadequate and he was forced to seek opportunities elsewhere. He accepted an appointment from the U.S. Treasury Department in January 1826 to replace Charles J. Jenkins as collector of customs and inspector of revenue at the port of Apalachicola.[8] In 1827 he was appointed notary public and justice of the peace for Washington County[9] and a few years later, in 1832, he became judge of the County Court of Franklin County.[10] When the Dade Massacre of late December 1835 prompted hasty organization of a Florida militia, Dr. White was offered a commission; he declined.[10]

After returning to his residence in Gadsden County and the practice of medicine Dr. White could not remain apart from the intruding issues and events of the times. As the demand for statehood status grew, especially in Middle Florida, he became involved, presenting himself as a candidate to represent his county at the St. Joseph Convention of 1838.[11] He did not win election, although two of his medical colleagues from Quincy, Drs. Banks Meacham and John W. Malone, were among Gadsden's four representatives.[12] As a leader of the Gadsden Whigs in 1840 he was the prime mover at a countywide meeting on September 17, called to promote the Whig platform and elect Whigs to public office.[13] Two years later he was the presiding figure at a joint meeting of Whigs from both Leon and Gadsden Counties.[14] Later as the Abolition Movement gained headway, he was chairman of a nonpartisan assembly in Quincy called to discuss means of coping with "aggressive liberalism from the North."[15] Only his advanced age prevented him from accepting more vigorous roles.

Meanwhile Dr. White demonstrated his profound concern for the lowly condition of medical practice in Florida by joining a small group of physicians from Jefferson, Leon, Jackson, Calhoun and Gadsden Counties meeting in Quincy on May 14-15, 1848, for the purpose of organizing a statewide medical society. Of the 13 doctors in attendance five were from Gadsden. As vice president and corresponding secretary he wrote an eloquent and impassioned statement on the wretched condition of the medical profession in Florida and called on all qualified physicians to meet in Tallahassee on the first Monday in January 1849 for the purpose of organizing a Florida Medical Society. His statement inveighed against the quackery and charlatanry abroad in the land and lamented the absence of a regulatory body. It was dated November 18, 1848, and sent to several newspapers around the state. At least three published it. The effort failed, however, when very few physicians showed up for the meeting and when the State Legislature, by a very narrow margin, failed to grant a charter for the Society.[16] Florida must wait 26 years before a similar effort was successful.

Dr. White lived out his life near Quincy, dying on his plantation "about four miles from the Court House" on April 5, 1862, at the age of 81.[17] He was thrice married. His first wife, Elizabeth, had died in Georgia. He married Catharine Pope of Jackson County on December 4, 1824,[18] and after her death (date unknown) he took as his third wife a widow, a Mrs. Wade, whose maiden name was Charlotte Booth, a sister of the well-known Dr. William Booth of Quincy.[19] He was survived by his widow and several children, at least one of whom, Edward B., served in the Confederate Army.

Of Dr. White it can be said that he exemplified the finest element among early 19th century Florida settlers. He appears to have been industrious, trustworthy, civic-minded and, if we may judge from his statement regarding the medical profession, intelligent.

1. Rowland H. Rerick, *Memoirs of Florida*, Atlanta, 1902, I, 722. As a preface to his biographical sketch of Pleasants W. White, eminent Florida judge, Rerick has included brief biographical data on Dr. White, the Judge's father.

2. Florida Censuses of Gadsden County 1850 and 1860 indicate that these three children of Dr. White were Georgia natives.

3. See land grants Nos. 76, 2456, 4748 and 4749, in "Alphabetical List of Tallahassee and Newnansville Land Office Receiver's Receipts," II, W13-14.

4. Julia Floyd Smith, *Slavery and Plantation Growth in Antebellum Florida*, Gainesville, 1973, p. 216.

5. J. Randall Stanley, *History of Gadsden County*, Quincy, 1948, p. 24.

6. Ibid., p. 31.

7. Miles Kenan Womack Jr., *Gadsden, A County History in Word and Picture*, Quincy, 1976, p. 7. See also Stanley, *History*, p. 63.

8. *Territorial Papers*, XXIII, p. 170n.

9. Pensacola *Gazette and West Florida Advertizer*, February 9, 1827. At this date Washington County included what was later to become Franklin County.

10. *Territorial Papers*, XXIV, 292.

11. Tallahassee *Florida Watchman*, May 19, 1838.

12. F.W. Hoskins, "The St. Joseph Convention," *Florida Historical Quarterly*, XVI, 41.

13. Quincy *Sentinel*, August 28, 1840.

14. Tallahassee *Florida Sentinel*, August 19, 1842.

15. Jacksonville *Florida Republican*, March 1, 1849. In June 1851 Dr. White assisted in organizing a Southern Rights Association of which he was elected vice president. Tallahassee *Sentinel*, June 10, 1851.

16. For an account of this effort to organize a Florida Medical Society see E. Ashby Hammond, "Medical Regulation and Organization in Florida, 1821-1874," *Journal Florida Medical Association*, Centennial Issue, 1974, pp. 62-69. Included is the letter drafted by Dr. White.

17. Charles A. Hentz, "Autobiography." Typed copy of original MS in Southern Collection, Wilson Library, University of North Carolina, Chapel Hill, I, 338. Dr. Hentz attended Dr. White in his last illness.

18. Pensacola *Gazette*, December 25, 1924.
19. Hentz, "Autobiography," loc. cit.

White, E.K., Alachua and St. Johns Counties, 1840

Notwithstanding his prominence and public activity in both Alachua and St. Johns Counties, biographical data on Dr. White are not abundant. Nothing is presently known of his youth and professional training.[1] His earliest known appearance in the public records of Florida identifies him as a resident of Alachua County in 1838 when he represented the county at the St. Joseph Convention, assembled to produce a constitution for the Territory.[2] The meager records of the Convention, however, provide almost no insight into his convictions and contributions but his presence indicates that the people of his home community, Newnansville, held him in fairly high regard. He had earlier shown his concern for the welfare of the community when he signed a petition calling for establishment of a public school to be called the Dade Institute,[3] honoring the memory of Major Francis L. Dade who had been slain by Indians three years earlier.

In another area of civic concern Dr. White was instrumental in drafting a petition to Congress requesting the establishment of a Land Office in Newnansville, then the most populous community of the county. Dr. White argued that the great distance of Alachua County from the Land Office in St. Augustine placed a burdensome expense and inconvenience on persons living between the St. Johns and Suwannee Rivers who wished to purchase land in Alachua and Columbia Counties. Under the prevailing arrangement, any purchase or sale must be recorded in the Land Office in St. Augustine. The petition carried a large number of signatures, among them E.K. White, M.D.[4]

In the latter part of 1840, for reasons not presently known, Dr. White left Newnansville for St. Augustine where he joined Dr. Seth Peck in a professional partnership. This move was certainly advantageous to Dr. White in that Dr. Peck had been a resident of the town since 1834 and was highly regarded both as physician and civic leader. In his obituary notice of a few months later particular mention was made of his sincerity and his "attachment to the principles of religion and morality."[5]

The Peck-White partnership was destined for a brief duration, however, Dr. Peck died on July 21, 1841. A week later Dr. White announced his intention to continue his "practice of medicine and surgery, in all its branches" from his office "at the residence of the late Dr. Peck."[6]

It is not known how long Dr. White continued to live in St. Augustine nor has the date of his death been determined. His name does not appear in the Florida Census of 1850.

1. Dr. White's name does not appear in the lists of students of any of the major medical colleges existing in the United States prior to 1845. He was probably trained for his profession through the apprenticeship system so common at that time.

2. A full account of the St. Joseph Convention by F.W. Hoskins was published in the *Florida Historical Quarterly* in four installments, vols. XVI and XVII, 1837-1938. The other Alachua County delegates were Isaac Garrison and Edmund Bird. By 1840 Dr. White's political reputation was sufficiently praiseworthy to win for him an appointment as Judge of the Court of Alachua County. *Territorial Papers*, XXVI, 60.

3. Ibid., XXV, 456-457. The proponents of the measure to incorporate the Dade Institute of Florida envisioned this as the first step toward estblishment of a state university.

4. *Territorial Papers*, XXVI, 12.

5. St. Augustine *Florida Herald*, July 23, 1841.
6. Ibid., July 30, 1841.

White, Robert Catlett, Pensacola, 1832-post 1900

Dr. White was a native of Kentucky and a graduate of the Medical Department of the University of Louisville in the class of 1853.[1] Soon after receiving his medical degree he began practice in Louisiana where he appears to have remained for some 15 or 20 years. His wife, known only by her initials, F.B., was a native of that state as were their five children. It is not known just when Dr. White moved to Florida but he is thought to have arrived at some time in the 1870s.

Although Dr. White was a respected physician, his professional career was somewhat overshadowed by those of Drs. Hargis, Herron, and Renshaw, all of whom were much involved in operation of Pensacola hospitals. On the other hand Dr. White held the post of Port Physician of Pensacola, which doubtless yielded lesser fees than those accruing to some of the other physicians.

At the meeting of the Florida Medical Association in Pensacola in April 1891, Dr. White was one of five local physicians elected to membership, Dr. Herron having been a member of the Nominating Committee or Committee on Credentials as it was called.[2] A year later he attended the meeting of the Association in Key West and Havana but there is no record of his having attended any subsequent meeting. He was dropped from membership in 1897 for nonpayment of dues.[3]

Dr. White was still practicing medicine in Pensacola in 1900 at the age of 68. His household that year included his wife, aged 60, whom he had married in 1858, his elder daughter, Susie Lyman, then a widow, her three young children; his son, Robert White Jr., a clerk in a timber company office, and his younger daughter, Stella, unmarried.[4]

No date of death for Dr. White has been discovered nor has his place of burial been found in any survey of Pensacola cemeteries. A splendid picture of the doctor appeared in Charles H. Bliss' Quarterly, "Pensacola Today," issue of January 1897 which depicts him as a man of strong features and a long flowing, white beard.

1. The records of the Board of Medical Examiners, First Florida Judicial District (date uncertain), cite these credentials.
2. *Proceedings, Florida Medical Association*, Session 1891, Jacksonville, 1891, pp. 4-5.
3. Ibid., 1897. Given the remoteness of Pensacola from other populated parts of the state as well as the difficulties of transportation, it is not surprising that many members of the Association allowed their membership to lapse. The fact that some did not maintain their membership does not necessarily indicate their indifference.
4. U.S. Census, 1900, Escambia County, Florida, p. 341, item 322.

White, Stuart, Leon County, 1860

Dr. White, about whom very little is known, arrived in Leon County in the latter part of 1859. His first professional notice appeared on November 29. He found lodging at the home of J.J. Chaires[1] which was located about one mile from Station No. 1 known as the Chaires Station on the Pensacola and Georgia Railroad. His card continued to appear in the Tallahassee *Florida Sentinel* for more than a year,[2] last appearing in the issue of December 25, 1860. No information concerning his birthplace and education has been located nor is his whereabouts known subsequent to 1860.

1. J.J. Chaires, member of the wealthy family of landowners who moved into Leon County from their native Georgia prior to the Civil War. Dr. White had probably departed from the county prior to arrival of the census enumerator in 1860.
2. Only a few issues of the Florida *Sentinel* of 1860 have survived.

Whitehead, Edwin, Jackson County, 1803-1852

Dr. Whitehead was born in Virginia about 1803[1] and received his professional training at the University of Maryland School of Medicine from which he was graduated in the spring of 1823.[2] At some unknown date in the 1830s he moved to Florida and established his practice in Marianna.[3] On February 2, 1843, he married Carolina Watson, daughter of Dr. William J. Watson.[4] Dr. Whitehead appears to have been a man of modest means, the census enumerator of 1850 having estimated the value of his properties real and personal at only $900. On the other hand Mrs. Whitehead's family, the Watsons, were people of moderate wealth.[5]

Dr. Whitehead died in 1852.[6] The census of 1860 lists his widow as a resident in the home of her mother, Mrs. D. Watson. Mrs. Whitehead died on November 10, 1891.[7]

1. This date is an extrapolation from the Jackson County Census of 1850 which gives his age as 47.
2. Eugene Fauntleroy Cordell, *Historical Sketch of the University of Maryland School of Medicine, 1807-90*, Baltimore, 1891, p. 204.
3. U.S. Census, 1840, Jackson County, Florida.
4. Information derived from the obituary of Mrs. Whitehead. Jacksonville *Florida Times-Union*, December 1, 1891.
5. U.S. Census, 1860, Jackson County, Florida, p. 741.
6. See note 4, supra.
7. Ibid.

Whitfield, John W., Brevard County, mid-19th century

Only sparse data on the Florida career of Dr. Whitfield, or Wittfeld as it appears in the U.S. Census of 1880, has been located in Florida sources. Prussian-born and for several years a resident of Pennsylvania, he arrived in Florida just prior to outbreak of the Civil War, leaving his family in Pennsylvania. The Florida Census of 1860[1] lists him at the age of 29 residing in the home of well-to-do farmer, William F. Russell, located in or near the village of Sand Point, later to be known as Titusville. His family had joined him by 1870 in Sand Point: wife Clara, aged 31 and a Pennsylvania native, and sons William and John, aged 12 and 10 respectively, both born in Pennsylvania.[2] The date of his death has not been discovered nor is his gravestone listed in the Vera G. Langlais, *Cemetery Census of Brevard County, Florida*.

1. U.S. Census, 1860, Brevard County, Florida, item 32.
2. Dr. Whitfield is presumed to have been the brother of Dr. William H. Whitfield.

Whitfield, William, Brevard County, 1827-1913

Dr. Whitfield, born Wilhelm Wittfeld in Germany in 1827, was a pioneer settler in Brevard County. He is presumed to have studied medicine in his native country prior to emigrating to America about 1860.[1] As was true for many German immigrants arriving in America, he settled in Philadelphia where he remained a few years before making his way to Florida to join his brother, John W. Whitfield, who had settled in Brevard County in the late 1850s. Dr. Whitfield settled first in Sand Point, later to be named Titusville. He later took up a homestead at Georgiana where he built a home to which he gave the name, "Fairyland." With his new bride, known only as Clara, a native of Philadelphia, his life at Georgiana appears to have been indeed idyllic. With his spacious grounds, his wife, Aloretta,[2] his sons, William and John, and four daughters, Edna, Ella, Julia and Ora, he could not have asked for a better life.

After becoming a resident at Georgiana it seems certain that Dr. Whitfield gave up the practice of medicine except possibly on a very limited scale. His death occurred on July 27, 1913, while he was visiting in the home of his neighbors, Mr. and Mrs. John Frey, of Bonaventure. His eulogy, which appeared in the *Cocoa-Indian River Florida Star* of August 1, 1913, suggests the esteem in which he was held. "The doctor was a gentleman of the old school—kind, courteous, genial, honest in his dealings, beloved by all who knew him." He was survived by a son, William and four daughters, his wife, a native of Maryland, having died in 1900.

1. The vital data are derived from two sources, the Brevard Censuses of 1860, 1870, 1880, 1885, and 1900, and the obituary notice.

2. The spelling of Mrs. Whitfield's Christian name is possibly in error. It appears that Dr. Whitfield was twice married for no other satisfactory explanation can be offered. The Census of 1870 clearly designates her as Clara. In subsequent censuses, however, the name Aloretta or possibly Amoretta appears. No obituary of Clara has been located nor any grave marker. It is also unusual that no mention of a surviving wife is included in his obituary notice.

Whitehurst, Daniel Winchester, Key West, 1807-1872

Dr. Whitehurst, one of 19th century Florida's most distinguished physicians and public servants, spent the greater part of his adult life in Key West. Born in Norfolk, Virginia, on September 29, 1807, he received his early education in that city. As he approached manhood he read law and actually began his professional life as a lawyer in St. Augustine at some time in the 1840s. Finding the legal profession dull and unremunerative he sought other paths for his energies, one of which was working for the African Colonization Society, an organization which sponsored the deportation of Negroes to Africa. He made a trip to Liberia to investigate the feasibility of such a project. Another cause which gained his support was that of ousting the Seminole Indians from Florida, an activity which is said to have earned for him the rank of major in the United States Army.[1]

From 1838 to 1841 Dr. Whitehurst was publisher of the St. Augustine *News* but this occupation apparently soon began to pall. Therefore in the fall of 1841 he went to New York and enrolled in the medical department of New York University from which he received his degree in March 1843. He had finally found his proper niche. For the next two years, however, all trace of him is lost, but in the latter part of 1845 he appeared in Key West and accepted the position of Post Surgeon at Fort Jefferson located on a tiny island known as the Dry Tortugas some 60 miles due west of Key West.

During his brief stay in St. Augustine he had met and married Henrietta, the only daughter of Dr. Frederick Weedon, a physician who had practiced in St. Augustine and gained certain fame, or possibly infamy, by cutting off the head of the Indian chieftain, Osceola, and displaying it publicly as though it were a hunting trophy. The Whitehursts apparently made the most of their years at Ft. Jefferson, beguiling their boredom and loneliness by occasional trips to Key West. The end of their residence came in 1861 just as the Civil War began. Federal troops had seized and occupied Ft. Jefferson. In the presence of their chief officer Mrs. Whitehurst spoke freely of her Southern sympathies, whereupon the Whitehursts were expelled from the Island.[2]

With the war years behind them the Whitehursts resumed their residence in Key West, although the Doctor did make occasional trips back to Ft. Jefferson for professional purposes. During the outbreak of yellow fever at the Fort in 1867, for example, he went to the assistance of the famous Dr. Samuel A. Mudd. From his home at the corner of Eaton and Duval Streets Dr. Whitehurst, in addition to his occasional medical practice, was involved in numerous civic activities, such as providing housing facilities for the first group of Catholic nuns to arrive in Key West until they could make permanent arrangements. He also donated the first rectory for the Catholic Church to be built on the Island.

Dr. Whitehurst's eulogist remembered him as "a jovial man with a beautiful disposition...often times curing his patients with quips and jests instead of physics." He continued his medical practice almost to the time of his death which occurred on January 12, 1872.

1. "Dr. Daniel Whitehurst," *Martello*, Key West Art and Historical Society, No. 4, 1867, pp. 21-22.
2. Ft. Jefferson is best remembered as the place of imprisonment of Dr. Samuel A. Mudd, accused of complicity in the assassination of Abraham Lincoln.

The literature relating to Dr. Mudd is abundant. Notable is Nettie Mudd, *The Life of Dr. Samuel A. Mudd*, containing his Letters, etc., edited by his daughter, New York and Washington, 1906. A recent edition published by the Continental Book Co., Marietta, Georgia, in 1955 is still in print.

Whiting, John Cary, Pensacola, 1834-1883

Dr. Whiting who spent the greater part of his professional career in Pensacola was born in Hampton, Virginia, on July 3, 1834.[1] His family had established roots in Virginia prior to the American Revolution and are presumed to have been members of the planter aristocracy. As a youth Dr. Whiting was probably privately educated, later attending William and Mary College in nearby Williamsburg from which he received a baccalaureate degree.[2] About 1854,[3] for reasons unknown, he moved to Mobile, Alabama, where for a brief time he worked in a drug store. He matriculated at the Medical College of the University of Pennsylvania in 1857[4] and was graduated Doctor of Medicine in the spring of 1859 after submitting a thesis on the subject, "Yellow Fever," probably inspired by his observations of the disease during his residence in Mobile.

Soon after receiving his medical degree Dr. Whiting returned to Mobile where he entered medical practice and, it is thought, resumed his association with the drug store. In 1860 he married Clara Regina Hyer, daughter of Henry Hyer, a native of Bavaria,[5] who had settled in Mobile several years earlier. With the outbreak of war in 1861 Dr. Whiting offered his services to the Confederacy and presumably served in an Alabama military unit.[6]

At some unknown date but probably in late 1865, Dr. Whiting moved with his family to Pensacola where he resumed the practice of medicine. By late 1866, however, he had established a drug store, its first public notice appearing in the Pensacola *West Florida Commercial* of November 15, 1866. He designated himself as "Druggist and Pharmaceutist, dealer in French, English and German Chemicals." He also offered for sale "Pure Wine and Brandy, for Medical Purposes." Sometime later Dr. Robert B.S. Hargis, probably Pensacola's premier physician, joined him as co-proprietor of the drug store.

Throughout his brief career in Pensacola Dr. Whiting displayed an interest in civic matters. In 1867 he sponsored the establishment of a school emphasizing classical subjects, to be directed by Everard Meade.[7] Perhaps more important, however, was his interest in public health, periodically threatened by epidemics of yellow fever. In his capacity as Secretary and Inspector of the Pensacola Board of Health, of which Dr. Hargis was President, he was vigilant in enforcement of quarantine measures for the City and Harbor of Pensacola. A short time before his death he assisted in drafting a directive setting forth the duties of the quarantine officers of the Port of Pensacola.[8]

Dr. Whiting died at his Pensacola home on April 16, 1883, only two months prior to his 49th birthday. His eulogist wrote: "Dr. Whiting has been a citizen of Pensacola since the War and has occupied a leading position as a man and as a physician. His death is a severe blow to our community." His residence was located at 75 West Romana Street. His was a large household, including in 1880, in addition to Dr. and Mrs. Whiting, 10 children ranging in ages from 19 to six months, and five servants. One daughter, Alberta, had died in early childhood.[9]

1. Gravestone, St. Michael's Cemetery, Pensacola.
2. Obituary notice, Pensacola *Commercial*, April 17, 1883.
3. Ibid.
4. Information, University of Pennsylvania Archives, courtesy of Maryellen Kaminsky, Archival Specialist.
5. During the antebellum period Mobile had attracted a large number of immigrants from Germany. After Dr. Whiting moved to Pensacola the Hyer family also settled in Pensacola. The Hyer burial lot is located in St. Michael's Cemetery.
6. This statement is conjectural, based on the cemetery listing of Dr. Whiting as a Confederate veteran. Since his name does not appear in Confederate records of Florida it is assumed that he had enlisted in an Alabama unit.
7. Pensacola *West Florida Commercial*, November 25, 1867. The "Select School" would offer instruction in Latin, Greek, English and Mathematics, for a limited number of students. Further details could be obtained at Whiting's Drug Store.
8. Pensacola *Commercial*, May 9, 1882. This notice employed a full column, specifying the duties of the Quarantine Physician in detail.
9. Data on names and ages of Whiting children are found in the Escambia County Censuses of 1870 and 1880.

Whitlock, Isaac W., Madison County, 1833

Dr. Whitlock, a native of South Carolina, was graduated Doctor of Medicine at the Medical College of Georgia, Augusta, in the spring of 1852.[1] At some date prior to 1860 he married Mary E. Griffin, a Georgian by birth, and settled in the Sandy Ford community of Madison County[2] where he was practicing his profession in 1860. His professional career was tragically brief, however, having been terminated by death prior to 1870. Two daughters, Lutia (Lucia) and Hattie, aged 10 and seven respectively in 1870, were born to the Whitlocks.[3]

The census of that year shows them living in the home of Mrs. Whitlock's mother, Mrs. Rachel Griffin, aged 76.

1. *Medical Department, University of Georgia,* "List of Graduates, 1829-1891," Augusta, 1891, p. 27.
2. U.S. Census, 1860, Madison County, Florida, item 345. Here Dr. Whitlock is shown to have been 27, his wife 25. The date of his birth by extrapolation is calculated to have been 1833.
3. U.S. Census, 1870, Madison County, Florida, p. 99.

Whitner, Elias E., Madison, 1840

Dr. Whitner, whose brief medical career was spent in Madison, was born in Pendleton District, South Carolina, about 1840. His grandfather, Joseph Whitner, a native of Germany, had emigrated to South Carolina in the latter part of the 18th century and had become a substantial landowner. By trade he was a surveyor,[1] a calling which seems to have provided the opportunity to obtain valuable land from which he was able to build a modest fortune. His son, J.N. Whitner, studied law and eventually was appointed to a circuit judgeship encompassing various South Carolina districts.[2] He too became a comparatively wealthy man, owning 43 slaves in 1860 as well as other properties whose total value was estimated to have been upwards of $200,000.[3] He made one unsuccessful venture into politics when in 1838 his good friend John C. Calhoun persuaded him to run for a congressional seat. He was soundly defeated by the other candidate, Waddy Thompson.[4]

Dr. Whitner was the third son and fourth child of Judge Whitner. In the late 1850s his older brother, William, a young lawyer, had moved to Madison and launched his practice. Dr. Whitner appears to have joined him there and begun a medical apprenticeship in the office of Dr. John Hunter Pope. The outbreak of war interrupted his study, however, and before he could finish formal training the Medical College of the State of South Carolina had closed for the duration. With reopening of the College in November 1865, he enrolled and in March 1867 was graduated M.D.[5] Soon thereafter he returned to Madison where he began medical practice.

The failure of Madison newspapers of the 1860s to survive,[6] as well as the absence of family diaries and letterbooks, deprives us of the details of Dr. Whitner's career. It is known, however, that in December 1869 he married a Madison girl, known through the census records as Stevie Duvall. She was seven years his junior. They had a daughter, Berta, and son, Elias E., aged 10 and seven respectively in 1880.[7] Dr. Whitner is believed to have died in 1876. By 1880 his widow had remarried, taking Walter A. Baker, a Madison druggist, as her second husband.[8] To this second union was born one son, enrolled in the census of 1885 as "baby."

1. *South Carolina Historical Magazine*, LXI, 221n.
2. Ibid., L: 148, 149, 153.
3. U.S. Census, 1860, Anderson District, S.C., Item 23. In the reordering of District lines Pendleton District was absorbed by Anderson District.
4. *South Carolina Historical Magazine*, LIX, 31.
5. Charleston *Daily Courier*, March 4, 1867.
6. For the period under consideration only three issues of the newspaper, Madison *Recorder*, those of December 25, 1858, April 20, 1866, and April 27, 1866, have survived.
7. U.S. Census, 1880, Madison County, Florida, 1880, p. 6.
8. Special Florida Census, 1885, p. 16, item 137.

Whitted, Levi P., Orlando, 1870

Dr. Whitted was among the earliest settlers in the community which was to become Orlando and is considered to have been the area's first regular physician. He was a native of North Carolina, having been born there about 1826. He was accompanied by his wife, Sallie, also a North Carolinian.

Miss Kena Fries, writing in the 1940s, recorded his arrival:[1]

> One day in the sixties a man riding an old black mule stopped in front of Ed Spier's store. Saddle bags were well filled; both rider and saddle bags received a warm welcome. The rider was Dr. Whitted from Volusia County, Orlando's first physician. The saddle bags held drugs and simple surgical instruments. Until his arrival home remedies were all that stood between life and death. Soon Spier opened a drug store in the little one-room log store which was also the post office.

The Orange County Census record of 1870 lists the following members of the Whitted family with other pertinent information:

Whitted, Levi	44	Physician $500-$400	born	N.C.
Whitted, Sallie	30		"	N.C.
Whitted, William	8		"	N.C.
Whitted, Joseph	7		"	N.C.
Whitted, Lizzie	4		Alabama	
Whitted, Mary	1		Florida	

It is clear from this entry that subsequent to the Civil War, Dr. Whitted had resided briefly in Alabama, and that the family moved to Florida about 1868-70.

1. Fries, Kena, *Orlando in the Long Long, Ago. . .And Now*, Orlando, Tyn Cobb's Florida Press, 1938, p. 56.

Wilcox, Samuel Andrew, Taylor County, 1824-1887

Dr. Wilcox,[1] who spent the last 28 years of his life in Taylor County, was born in or near Augusta, Georgia, on August 9, 1824. He was the son of Martin and Mamie (neé McIntyre) Wilcox, both Virginia natives, who settled near Augusta. He received his early education at the Augusta and Sand Hill Academies and spent his next four years in a mercantile establishment in Augusta. At the outbreak of the Mexican War in May 1846, he joined Company C, 1st Regiment, Georgia Volunteers, commanded by Col. Henry R. Jackson. At the end of the War he returned to Georgia and began working in a mercantile business in Atlanta where he remained until 1852.

Dr. Wilcox was determined to become a physician and in 1852 began reading medicine. After a few months he enrolled at the Medical College of Georgia in August[2] from which he was graduated in 1854. Forthwith he made his way to southwest Georgia and began the practice of his profession. In 1859 he moved to Perry and soon established himself as a reputable physician. The Census of 1860 for Taylor County, a document not totally trustworthy, lists him as physician, owning property valued at more than $3,000.[3]

Dr. Wilcox was still in practice when the Civil War began. For reasons not altogether clear but probably because of his age, family responsibilities, and the necessity of having one physician remain on the home front, he did not become a military surgeon. In 1864, however, at the age of 40 he contracted his professional services to the Union Army unit, the Second Florida Cavalry, then in control of Cedar Keys,[4] which from the standpoint of supply was a port of considerable importance. The appointment as Contract Surgeon, however, turned out to be an unfortunate move for Dr. Wilcox.

The Cedar Keys post was commanded by Major Edmund C. Weeks, by some accounts an arrogant, short-tempered man, given to strong drink. On or about September 9, 1864, Weeks arrived at Depot Key (one of the Cedar Keys) in an inebriated condition. It was a dark night and the private who was on sentry duty at the dock, not recognizing him, demanded that he halt and identify himself. This the Major refused to do. Instead he fired his musket in the direction of the sentry, penetrating his side. Private Joseph L. White was taken to the Post Hospital and placed under the care of Dr. Wilcox. Meanwhile Weeks was held under arrest pending the recovery of Private White. He had resisted arrest and attempted to shoot the arresting officer, Lt. William H. Stebbins.

Within a few days after the incident Private White died, whereupon Major Weeks was taken to Key West for court-martial. Dr. Wilcox was ordered to Key West as a key witness for the prosecution of Major Weeks.

The trial, conducted by Lt. Col. John Wilder, was a nasty affair. The commander of the Key West Post was Brigadier General John Norton, who ordered the composition of the court-martial, one major and four captains, in addition to Wilder. The thrust of the defense was to discredit Dr. Wilcox completely by attacking his professional competence and thus proving that White's death was due to that incompetence rather than Weeks' outrageous act, thus shifting the blame for the soldier's death from Weeks to Dr. Wilcox. The official account of the trial suggests that the witnesses for the prosecution were intimidated and in some instances reduced to admitting that they had no knowledge other than what they had heard from other soldiers. For Dr. Wilcox it was an ordeal. His professional credentials were questioned; the effort was to humiliate him in any way possible. The result of the affair was the exoneration of Major Weeks and cancellation of Dr. Wilcox's contract.[5]

Following the trial Dr. Wilcox returned to Perry and resumed his medical practice. Shortly thereafter he moved on to the political scene, winning the office of Circuit Court Clerk. He developed an interest in law, reading it in his spare time, and by 1870 was able to gain admission to the Florida Bar. In 1882 he was elected to the Florida House (Assembly), serving in the session of 1883. His committee appointments were: Legislative Expenses (Chairman), Engrossed Bills, Enrolled Bills, and Education. His term of office expired in 1885.[6]

Dr. Wilcox again turned to the practice of medicine. The Florida Census of 1885 lists him as "Physician and Farmer," owning 75 acres of land, 30 of which were under cultivation.

Dr. Wilcox was thrice-married, first on October 10, 1851, to Virginia Swift of Augusta, Georgia. A son, John, was born on November 12, 1852.[7] Mrs. Wilcox died on August 7, 1853. On February 14, 1857, Dr. Wilcox married Elsie Loudusky Parramore of Thomasville, Georgia, who died on November 20, 1862, leaving two daughters, Elsie Loudusky and Mary. Dr. Wilcox married his third wife, Miley Delilah Humphrey of Taylor County, on March 31, 1863. To this union were born five daughters, Moulton, Leilah, Ella, Ida and Emma, and two sons, Willie M. and Boss H.[7]

Dr. Wilcox's services to Taylor County and the Town of Perry went beyond those mentioned. As a member of the Pisgah Methodist Church, the parent church of the present First Methodist Church of Perry, he had been lay reader. He was also a regular Sunday School teacher. At the time of his death on April 6, 1885, he was Superintendent of the Taylor County Schools. Many descendants of Dr. Wilcox live in Taylor County and elsewhere. He was buried at his home site on West Wilcox Street in Perry.[8]

1. Much of the biographical data was provided by two descendants of Dr. Wilcox, Mrs. Thyrza Bolton and Mrs. Janie Hamilton, both residents of Taylor County. Their assistance is gratefully acknowledged. Some additional facts were gleaned from J.V. Drakes' *An Official Directory of the State Government*, Jacksonville, 1883, p. 43.

2. The fact of Dr. Wilcox's graduation from the Augusta school has not been verified. The "List of Graduates from 1829 to 1890," Augusta, 1890, does not include his name. It is to be recalled, however, that in mid-19th century Florida it was not uncommon for a medical student to attend a medical school for one session (after having served an apprenticeship under a practicing physician) and without further study obtain a license to practice.

3. U.S. Census, 1860, Taylor County, Florida, p. 835, item 76.

4. Cedar Keys had been seized by units of the 2nd Florida Regiment, U.S. Army, in 1862. Major Weeks was the commanding officer assigned to the post. On more than one occasion he had exhibited dubious judgment in defending the post against forays of Confederate soldiers attempting the retake of Cedar Keys.

5. A detailed account of the Weeks trial is preserved in the National Archives, Washington, D.C. The account is labeled RG 153, Records of the Office of the Judge Advocate General (Army), General Court Martial Record of Major Edmund C. Weeks.

6. *Journal of the Proceedings, The Assembly of the State of Florida, 1883*, Tallahassee, 1883, pp. 42-43.

7. John Wilcox grew up in Augusta, where he married and reared a family. Ex info, Letters, Mrs. Janie Hamilton to E. Ashby Hammond, April 1, 1985.

8. Ibid.

Wiley, Evan S., Hamilton County, 1836

Dr. Wiley, a native of North Carolina, practiced medicine briefly in Jasper, Hamilton County. He is listed in the 1860 Census as aged 24, owning property valued at $4,000.[1] He was a member of the Jasper Masonic Lodge.

He enlisted in the Confederate Army on March 14, 1862, and was assigned to Company F, Fifth Florida Infantry Regiment, with the rank of first lieutenant. Before the summer of 1862 was over his unit was ordered to the Virginia zone of combat where he became ill and was admitted to the Confederate Hospital at Culpepper, Virginia. On October 1 he was sent to the General Hospital near Richmond. His condition continued to worsen, however, and on March 3, 1863, he submitted his resignation on the basis of a medical report which stated that he was in a "considerably advanced state of consumption." He was discharged on the following day. The statement from the Medical Examining Board gave phthisis as the reason for his termination.[2]

Dr. Wiley apparently did not return to practice in Jasper, although nothing is known of his career subsequent to his discharge.

1. U.S. Census, 1860, Hamilton County, Florida, p. 1.

2. NA, Serv. Recs., CSA, M251, Roll 68.

Williams, James Alexander, Newnansville, 1836-1895

Dr. Williams was born in Liberty County, Georgia,[1] on October 23, 1836. Within a year after receiving his medical degree at Savannah Medical College, Class of 1856,[2] he migrated to Florida and settled in the village of Newnansville, Alachua County, whose future had been blighted a couple of years earlier by the decision to remove the county seat from Newnansville to Gainesville. On March 23, 1860, Dr. Williams announced his intention to settle permanently in Newnansville where he would occupy the office previously belonging to Dr. T.A. Bradford.[3]

With the coming of the War in 1861 Dr. Williams began to feel the pressure to offer his services to the Confederacy. On May 17, 1862, he appeared in Gainesville and enlisted for "three years, or the duration."[4] Notwithstanding his medical skills he was mustered in as a private and assigned to the 2nd Florida Cavalry but within the year he was given the medical rank of assistant surgeon and assigned to the medical staff for field service. By early 1863 he was placed on detached service as company surgeon for Co. F which could hardly have been considered a promotion. His record shows that he had been arrested for a minor offense and reduced to private but before the end of the year 1863 he was reinstated as company surgeon. His military service never took him out of Florida. He is said to have amputated the leg of a soldier without anesthesia following the Battle of Olustee.[5] He was with his company at Green Cove Springs when Gen. Lee surrendered at Appomattox. His unit surrendered to Union officers at Baldwin a day or so later. On May 17, exactly three years after enlistment, he received his parole.[6]

Dr. Williams returned to Newnansville to reenter practice. With organization of the Florida Medical Association in Jacksonville in 1874, he was among the first group to be elected to membership, having been nominated by his good friend and fellow-townsman, Dr. Thos. P. McHenry, one of the charter members. In the following year he made his only appearance at the Association's annual meeting, in this instance bearing the sad news of Dr. McHenry's death a few weeks earlier.[7] Although Dr. Williams continued his membership for some three or four years his name disappeared from the lists of the Association after 1879.

By 1880 Dr. Williams was devoting more time to farming and less to medicine. A booklet designed to promote the economic development of Alachua County in 1883 included the following: "Dr. Williams is the oldest physician in the town. His long residence here has given him a perfect knowledge of the best treatment for the diseases peculiar to this country. He has one of the largest and most beautiful orange groves and Peento peach orchards in this section."[8] Two years later a kindred publication included this: "Dr. J.A. Williams, E.D. Hodges and W.H. Geiger have succeeded well in truck farming. Dr. Williams is also the owner of a fine orange grove."[9] The 1880 census compiler gave no hint that Dr. Williams was a physician, designating him only as "farmer."[10]

Dr. Williams was twice married, first to an Alabama native, Florida A, prior to 1870.[11] There were no children. In 1872 he married Eliza Boston who survived him by many years, dying on May 12, 1918[12] To this union were born ninc children, but only four lived to adulthood.[13] Several members of the Williams family are buried in Newnansville Cemetery.

1. Records of the short-lived Savannah Medical College, Savannah, Ga., preserved in Georgia Historical Society, show him to have been a resident of Liberty County, Georgia. This is verified by the Liberty County Census Schedule, 1850, which shows him, age 13, living in the household of his mother and stepfather, Benjamin Dorsey.

2. The Medical College list of graduates for 1856 includes "J.A. Williams, Liberty Co., Ga."

3. Newnansville *Florida Dispatch*, May 11, 1860. This notice was first printed in the issue of March 23, not extant.

4. NA, Service Records, CSA, M 251, Roll 12.

5. Webster Merritt, "Physicians and Medicine in Early Alachua County and Gainesville, Florida," *Journal Florida*

Medical Association, XXXVII, No. 1, July 1950, 301.

6. See n. 4, above.
7. *Proceedings, Florida Medical Association*, 1874, 1875.
8. Carl Webber, *The Eden of the South*, N.Y., 1883, p. 69.
9. Wanton S. Webb, *Webb's Historical, Industrial and Biographical Florida*, N.Y., 1885, I, 27.
10. U.S. Census, 1880, Alachua County, Florida, p. 35.
11. Ibid., 1870, item 3719.
12. Dr. Williams on November 28, 1895. Dates of his birth and death from gravestone, Newnansville Cemetery, Alachua County, as are those of Mrs. Williams.
13. Gainesville *Daily Sun*, May 16, 1918, obituary notice. Surviving children were: Jas. A. Williams, of Alachua; Mrs. Bob Frederick, Jacksonville; Herbert Williams, Gainesville, and Mrs. S.R. Springer, Atlanta.

Williams, Jesse Kendrick, Marion County, 1805-1874

In spite of his prominence as a wealthy planter and physician in rural Marion County little is known of the life of Dr. Williams. He was born in North Carolina but moved to Georgia when still a young man, presumably practicing medicine there. His wife and four children were natives of Georgia.[1] On coming to Florida about 1851, Dr. Williams purchased land in the northwestern part of Marion County, a few miles east of Williston and slightly south of the Alachua County line near the settlement of Wacahoota[2] where he spent the rest of his life as farmer and medical practitioner. He died at his home on July 3, 1874. The Ocala *East Florida Banner* gave only a brief notice of his passing: "Dr. Jesse Williams, an old and esteemed citizen of this county, died at his residence near Wacahoota on the 3rd, inst. in the 70th year of his age."[3]

Even less is known of Mrs. Williams. Her gravestone in the Williams family cemetery bears the following inscription: "Mrs. A.B. Williams, Died Sept. 15, 1859, Aged 40."

1. Although Mrs. Williams' name does not appear in any Florida census—she came to Florida after 1850 and died in 1859—the four Williams children, two daughters and two sons, are listed. The elder daughter, Annie E., 17, in 1860, later married Dr. Elhanan C. Pasley and they had one daughter, Amanda. The younger daughter, Emma, aged 12 in 1860, married William A. Hammond, a farmer from South Carolina who settled near Flemington, a few miles south of the Williams plantation. Two children were born to this union. Mrs. Hammond died in 1836. The elder son, Thomas, aged 10 in 1860, is listed as a carpenter in the census of 1870 and in the 1880 schedule as farmer. The younger son, Retis Joseph, became a physician.
2. The Williams home, long since destroyed by fire, was located a short distance from the Alachua County line in the northwest corner of Marion County. Nearby is the Williams family cemetery, known as Oak Vale, where some 18 members of the Williams family are buried.
3. Ocala *East Florida Banner*, July 11, 1874.

Williams, L.R., Jefferson County, 1860

The Jefferson County Census of 1860 lists Dr. Williams as physician living in the home of fellow-physician, James Lawrence Palmer in Monticello. He was 26 years of age. His real property was valued at $750, his personal property at $4,250. Nothing further is known of Dr. Williams.[1]

1. U.S. Census, 1860, Jefferson County, Florida, p. 822, item 147.

Williams, Retis Joseph, Marion County, 1851-1927

Very little is known of the medical practice of Dr. Williams who spent the greater part of his life in the northwest part of Marion County. The family lands were located in what is known as the Wacahoota community. He was born in Georgia, son of Dr. Jesse Kendrick Williams, who moved with his family to Florida just prior to the Civil War.[1] He was doubtless the namesake of an uncle, Retis J. Williams, listed in the Marion County Census of 1880 as a farmer, aged 71.[2] At an unknown date Dr. Williams married a Scottish girl, named Mary. To this marriage were born three children: Hugh Emmet, Mabelle, and Thomas. Mrs. Williams died in 1892, the Doctor in 1927. Both are buried in the Oak Vale Cemetery near the site of the old Williams homestead.[4]

1. U.S. Census, 1860, Marion County, Florida, item 410. Dr. Retis J. Williams was the youngest of four children of Dr. Jesse Kendrick Williams.
2. U.S. Census, 1880, Marion County, Florida, p. 34.
3. Ibid.
4. Special Florida Census, 1885, Marion County, p. 47. The Oak Vale Cemetery is located in the northwest corner of Marion County near the Alachua County line on Road 335, off State Road 121.

Williams, Samuel R., Jefferson County, 1834

Dr. Williams was born in Florida, probably Jefferson County, about 1834.[1] He is presumed to have prepared for his profession at the Medical College of the University of Louisville, Kentucky. By the mid-1850s he was living in Waukeenah, Jefferson County, where he was a partner of Dr. James L. Palmer,[2] also a Louisville graduate. He shared a house with Dr. Palmer and his wife Caledonia. As slavery became a burning issue about mid-century, Dr. Williams became increasingly involved in Jefferson County politics. At a meeting of county Democrats in Monticello in March 1860,[3] he was one of three delegates selected to attend the State Democratic meeting in Quincy on April 7.

Meanwhile it was increasingly apparent that the conflict generated by the slavery issue was a distinct probability. As the summer of 1860 drew on, Brigadier General Daniel B. Bird of the Second Brigade, Florida Militia, appointed Dr. Williams as surgeon to the Brigade with the rank of Captain.[4]

In 1862, with the conflict having reached a critical stage, Dr. Williams exchanged his militia role for a commission in the Confederate Army with the rank of Assistant Surgeon, Field and Staff, with the Fifth Battalion, Florida Cavalry. He moved into Virginia in 1864 as Assistant Medical Officer and Inspector of Hospitals in the Richmond area. Late that year he was stationed at Riccoe's Bluff, a fairly important supply base on the Apalachicola River, a few miles south of present-day Blountstown in Liberty County.[5]

At the end of the War, Dr. Williams returned to Jefferson County and resumed medical prctice.

The Hillsborough County Census of 1870 lists Dr. Williams as a resident of Tampa, a medical practitioner at the age of 35. He was shown to have been married in the meantime to Laura, three years his junior, and a native of Florida.[6] There is no further information on Dr. Williams.

1. This date of birth is an extrapolation from the Census of 1860 which gives his age as 26.
2. Jerrell Shofner, *History of Jefferson County*, Tallahassee, 1976, p. 241. See also Theresa Yaeger Palmer, *The Palmer Physicians*, 1966.

3. Monticello *The Family Friend*, April 7, 1860.
4. Ibid., September 1, 1860.
5. NA, Service Records, CSA, Fifth Florida Battalion, Cavalry.
6. U.S. Census, 1870, Hillsborough County, Florida, p. 137.

Williams, W.M., Jefferson County, 1867

Dr. Williams, who practiced for a short time in Jefferson County, is known only because the death of his son, Napoleon Bonaparte Williams, on August 14, 1867, at the age of nine, was mentioned in the Tallahassee *Sentinel* of September 2.[1] A sentimental poem in the style of the times followed the obituary. Nothing further is known of Dr. Williams and his wife, Geneva.

1. Tallahassee *Sentinel*, September 2, 1867. A search through the censuses of 1860 and 1867 revealed no further information on the family.

Williamson, Robert, Apalachicola, 1860

Dr. Williamson, a native of Scotland, is listed in the Franklin County Census of 1860 as a practitioner of medicine, presumably in Apalachicola. He was 45 years of age and lived in the home of a local merchant, George E. Prosser. As was true of many mid-19th century physicians who tried their luck in Franklin County, Dr. Williamson tarried there for only a short time before moving on.[1] Nothing further is known of him.

1. U.S. Census, 1860, Franklin County, Florida, p. 424.

Willis, Byrd Charles, Tallahassee and Pensacola, 1781-1846

It has never been satisfactorily shown that Col. Byrd Charles Willis was a medical practitioner in Florida, although the title "Doctor" has occasionally been assigned to him. He may indeed have been a physician in his native Fredericksburg, Virginia, prior to moving to Florida in 1825. Dr. Henry E. Palmer stated that he occupied a house on Monroe Street in Tallahassee from which he carried on a medical practice for a few years.[1] He was a firm supporter of Andrew Jackson in the presidential election of 1828 and as a reward Jackson appointed him Naval Agent at Pensacola to which he moved.[2]

Col. Willis, as he is designated in genealogical studies of the Willis Family, was born into Virginia aristocracy.[3] He was the son of Col. Lewis Willis by his second wife, Ann Carter, the date of his birth being August 29, 1881. At the age of 19 he married Mary Lewis, granddaughter of George Washington's sister, Bettie. To this marriage were born nine children, most notably Lewis who practiced medicine in Florida and Catherine Dangerfield, who was the wife of Atchison Gray, after whose death and her move to Florida became the wife of Prince Achille Murat.[4] Mrs. Willis died on October 7, 1834, at the age of 52.[5] Two years later Col. Willis returned to Fredericksburg and spent the remainder of his life at the Willis plantation, *Willis Hill*, overlooking the town. He died there on October 1, 1846, at the age of 65.[6]

As a public figure Col. Willis was undistinguished. He joined the Army with the rank of captain in the Infantry and participated in the War of 1812. His civil service appointment in Pensacola ended with the expiration of Jackson's second term in 1836. By his own admission he had shown little zest for "book-learning," nor did he seem to care much for business enterprise. He wrote: "I was idle. . .fond of fox-hunting, racing and convivial parties. . .cared not for plantation duties."[7]

1. Henry E. Palmer, "Physicians of Early Tallahassee and Vicinity," *Apalachee*, Tallahassee, 1934, p. 30.
2. Byrd Charles Willis and Richard Henry Willis, *A Sketch of the Willis Family of Virginia*, Richmond, Whittet and Shepperson, 1898, p. 63. Into this work Richard Henry Willis has incorporated the genealogical notes by Col. Byrd Charles Willis in which he emerges as a genial, charitable member of the aristocracy, a devoted husband and father, but lacking professional skills or business acumen.
3. Ibid., p. 65.
4. Ibid., pp. 73-74. See also Alfred J. Hanna, *A Prince in Their Midst*, Norman, University of Oklahoma Press, 1946, passim.
5. Willis and Willis, *Sketch*, p. 88.
6. *National Intelligencer*, October 13, 1846. Copy from Fredericksburg (Va.) *Herald*.
7. Willis and Willis, *Sketch*, p. 63.

Willis, Lewis, Tallahassee and Pensacola, 1801-1835

Dr. Willis, native of Fredricksburg, Virginia,[1] arrived in Tallahassee late in 1825 accompanied by his father, Byrd C. Willis, his sister, Catherine Dangerfield Willis Gray, a young widow who would later become the wife of Prince Achille Murat, and several younger Willis children. Dr. Willis had received his medical degree from the University of Pennsylvania Department of Medicine in the spring of 1825.[2] His credentials, socially and professionally, were impeccable. He was the great-grandson of Major Lewis Willis and Bettie Washington Lewis, sister of George Washington. Other close relatives included members of the Madison and Byrd families. So Dr. Willis settled comfortably into the little community of transplanted Virginia aristocrats who had migrated to Leon County.

Dr. Willis announced his professional services on March 24, 1826, to the citizens of Tallahassee and vicinity.[3] A few days later he joined four other Tallahassee physicians[4] in drawing up a schedule of fees which they had agreed to charge for their various medical and surgical services. In January 1828 he was named to the Territorial Medical Board established by the Legislative Council on December 31, 1827, and approved by Governor William P. Duval on January 6, 1828.[5] The Board was charged with the responsibility for examining applicants seeking licenses to practice medicine in the Territory and succeeded the less-than-satisfactory system, dating from 1824, which placed the final decision on who should practice in the hands of county judges.

Dr. Willis appears to have been a respected and popular member of the Tallahassee medical faculty. Nevertheless in the summer of 1827 he elected to move to Pensacola where his father had gone and on August 30 announced the opening of his office "at the residence of the late Col. George Walton."[6] His move was possibly motivated by the presence in Tallahassee of at least six other practicing physicians.[7] His sojourn in Pensacola was brief, however, for in early 1828 he was once again residing in Tallahassee.[8]

Dr. Willis made his sole venture into the arena of local politics in 1829 when he ran unsuccessfully for one of Leon County's two seats in the Legislative Council. It was an eight-man contest which resulted in the election of Dr. Isaac W. Mitchell and Thomas Brown, both Tallahassee residents.[9]

In 1832 Dr. Willis joined his brother-in-law, Dr. James Henry Randolph, in a professional partnership.[10] Dr. Randolph, some eight years younger, was a graduate of the University of Pennsylvania, having received his M.D. in 1831. The partnership endured until 1835 and was terminated when Dr. Willis once more moved to Pensacola.

An unkind fate stalked two of Dr. Willis' three marriages. His first wife was Lucia Hackley, daughter of Richard S. Hackley of Norfolk, Virginia, their marriage ceremony having taken place on October 25, 1827, at Rambler's Rest, the residence of the bride's uncle, Robert J. Hackley near Tallahassee.[11] She died on April 14, 1829, while on a visit in the home of her father-in-law, Bryd C. Willis in Pensacola. She left an infant son, christened Byrd.[12] On December 24, 1831, Dr. Willis married Harriet Fluker, daughter of Thomas Eston Randolph, and sister of his medical partner, Dr. James Henry Randolph.[13] This union ended tragically when Mrs. Willis died the following year after the stillbirth of a child.[14] On January 30, 1834, Dr. Willis married Esther Savage, a native of Maryland's Eastern Shore and relative of the prominent Hayward family of Maryland and Tallahassee.[15] To this marriage was born a son, Thomas Hayward, who with his mother and half-brother, Byrd, survived Dr. Willis.

Early in 1835 Dr. Willis once more established his practice in Pensacola where his parents had lived for several years. In June of that year he offered his services to the citizens of the community.[16] Once more tragedy struck. While attempting to cross the Grand Lagoon west of the entrance to Pensacola Bay on horseback, the animal got beyond his depth; the doctor was swept into the water and drowned. His body was found a short time later in six feet of water only 40 yards from Foster's Island. This sad event occurred on October 3, 1835, when Dr. Willis was 34 years of age.[17,18]

1. *William and Mary College Quarterly*, VI, No. 4, April 1898, pp. 204-214. For Conokete information on the Willis Family see Byrd Charles Willis and Richard Henry Willis, *The Willis Family of Virginia*, Richmond, Whittet and Shepperson, 1898.
2. Archives, University of Pennsylvania, Lists of Matriculants and Graduates.
3. Tallahassee *Intelligencer*, March 24, 1826.
4. Ibid., April 14, 1826.
5. *Acts, Florida Legislative Council*, 6th Session, 1827-28, Tallahassee, 1828, pp. 46-49.
6. Pensacola *Gazette*, September 7, 1827; 1st printing, August 30, 1827.
7. Other Tallahassee physicians at that time were Isaac W. Mitchell and William D. Price.
8. Jerrell H. Shofner, *History of Jefferson County*, Tallahassee, 1976, p. 60. When Robert Gamble's wife gave birth to a child at Waukenah in 1828, the attending physician was Dr. Willis who came from Tallahassee.
9. Tallahassee *Florida Advocate*, June 13, 1829.
10. Tallahassee *Floridian*, January 17, 1832; ibid., January 11, 1834.
11. Pensacola *Gazette*, November 16, 1827.
12. See note 1, supra. See also Magnolia *Advertiser*, May 15, 1829.
13. Tallahassee *Floridian*, December 27, 1831.
14. "The Florida Randolphs," Randolph Whitfield and John Chipman, comps. mimeographed, P.K. Yonge Library of Florida History, p. 62.
15. Tallahassee *Floridian*, February 1, 1834.
16. Pensacola *Gazette*, June 13, 1835.
17. Ibid., October 10, 1835.
18. The two sons of Dr. Willis continued to live in Pensacola. In 1847 the elder son, Byrd, married Lucy Barclay and they had three sons, George, Lewis and Byrd. The second son, Thomas Hayward, became a physician. He was killed accidentally by a stray bullet while watching a street fight. See Willis and Willis, *The Willis family*, p. 68.

Wilson, Benjamin Rush, Brevard County, 1835-1913

Dr. Wilson,[1] one of the most beloved and public-spirited physicians ever to practice in Florida, was born in the little village of Gainestown, Clarke County,

Alabama,[2] on March 27, 1835. Nothing is known of his early education or medical training but he is thought to have entered the profession by way of the apprenticeship system, although it is possible that he attended for a term the Medical College of Alabama in Mobile, 50 miles from the place of his birth. After only a few years of professional practice and with the Civil War already under way he offered his services to an Alabama unit of the Confederate Army, serving as surgeon until the end of the conflict. Upon his return to civilian status he ran for the Alabama legislature, serving for two terms before moving to Florida in 1870.

Dr. Wilson was twice married, the first time prior to the Civil War but it ended tragically when his wife was killed in a gasoline stove explosion. To that marriage was born one daughter who became Mrs. J.W. Rogers, some of whose descendents still live in Alabama. In 1876 he married Ethland B. Feaster of LaGrange, a village near Indian River, some five miles north of Titusville where Dr. Wilson had settled. The couple lived in LaGrange for about six years before moving to Titusville. They had 10 children, eight of whom survived their father.[3] Dr. Wilson died on July 19, 1913, after two months of declining health which forced him to discontinue medical practice as well as other activities. Mrs. Wilson survived him by four years, dying on August 8, 1917.[4]

In addition to compassionate attention to numerous patients which endeared him to many citizens of Brevard County, Dr. Wilson's concern for civic matters was noteworthy. His eulogist wrote: "No physician has ever been loved more, neither will his place be filled by any one person. He was ever ready to relieve suffering humanity and always took a stand for the right and good of the town."

Dr. Wilson served Titusville as Mayor for 13 years, ultimately declining re-election when his health failed. For seven years he was County Judge, "filling both offices with dignity and credit." He was known as the "father of the city water works," having pressed constantly for installation of a safe and adequate system. The first pump was started by Dr. Wilson's own hand, and for years it was labeled "Dr. Wilson."

A Mason throughout much of his adult life and Past Master of Indian River Lodge, No. 90, Dr. Wilson was accorded the Masonic funeral ritual and buried in the LaGrange Cemetery.

1. A lengthy obituary for Dr. Wilson appeared in the Titusville *East Coast Advocate* of July 25, 1913, from which much of the biographical material of the present sketch was taken.

2. Gainestown, a mere village lying near the west bank of the Alabama River, about 50 miles north of Mobile, exists today with a population of less than a hundred.

3. The surviving children, as listed in the Brevard County Census of 1900 were: Julian P., 22, a druggist; Trezvant B., 20; Leonidas S., 16; Jeannette B., 12; Ethel, 10; Benjamin R., Jr., 7; Helen, 5; and Vivian, 3.

4. Gravestone of Mrs. Wilson in the LaGrange Cemetery.

Wilson, Francis C., Chipley, 1842-1921

Due in some degree to his wandering nature which led him hither and yon, Dr. Wilson remains a somewhat obscure figure. His parents, both Virginians, moved to Alabama about 1840 and Francis or Frank was born in 1842. Of his youth and education, general and professional, nothing is presently known. Since he is not listed among the graduates of any of the better-known medical schools of the South it is assumed that he was trained for his profession as an apprentice to a qualified practitioner.

With the outbreak of the Civil War in 1861, Dr. Wilson, then 19 years of age, volunteered for military service and was assigned to Company C, Eleventh Alabama Infantry Regiment, in which he is thought to have served for the duration of the War.

Shortly after the War Dr. Wilson moved to Florida and settled in Washington County. He married Elizabeth and there the two eldest of his numerous children were born.[1] In 1871 the family moved to Mississippi where four additional children were born. They were, in order of birth, Francis Jr. and Perry (twins), William and Dora, aged 15, 12 and 10 respectively.[2] From there the Wilsons went to British Honduras, City of Belize, in the late 1870s, remaining there for about seven years before returning to Chipley. Meanwhile Mrs. Wilson had died and Dr. Wilson had married a lady known only as Kate L.[3] She was a Georgian by birth, having been born there in 1864. Census data indicate that she was the mother of two sons, only the younger one, John J., still living in 1900.

For the last 25 years of his life Dr. Wilson seems to have lived free of wanderlust, choosing to remain in Chipley. In addition to medical practice his income derived from rental property.[3] On July 27, 1914, he was appointed postmaster of Chipley by President Woodrow Wilson and held this position until September 23, 1919, when he was replaced by James A. Douglas.[4]

Notwithstanding his apparent restlessness and search for "greener pastures," Dr. Wilson, in his later years, settled contentedly into the life of a country doctor in Chipley. He appears to have enjoyed a good practice. In the *Transactions of the Florida Medical Association,* he was listed as a member in good standing during the first decade of the 20th century, although he never attended an annual meeting. He was, however, a faithful and active member of the Washington County Medical Society from the time of its inception, having been its Secretary in 1904.

Dr. Wilson died in Chipley in 1921. The fact that his membership in the State Association was discontinued in 1913 would indicate that he became physically incapacitated and probably ceased to practice. He was 79.

1. The greater part of our knowledge of Dr. Wilson is derived from the Special Florida Census of 1885, Washington County; the United States Census, Washington County, Florida, 1900; ibid. 1910, and *Transactions of the Florida Medical Association.* The Special Florida Census of 1885, Washington County, lists 10 Wilson children, ranging in age from 18 years to six months. Included were two sets of twins; Francis C., Jr. and Perry B., aged 16, and Archibald and Julian, aged eight, the latter set having been born in Belize. The Census of 1900 indicates that the youngest Wilson child, John J., was born in Georgia in 1886.

2. The second Mrs. Wilson, Kate L., gave her age in 1900 as 36, her marriage as having occurred in 1892. She was the mother of two.

3. Dr. Wilson was the owner of a building in Chipley which was destroyed by a devastating fire which consumed the business portion of the town on May 14, 1898. See Elba Wilson Carswell, *Tempestuous Triangle; Historical Notes on Washington County, Florida,* Chipley, Florida, 1908, p. 207.

4. U.S. Post Office Dept., Record of Appointments of Postmasters, 1832-1971, Film M841, Roll 21.

Wilson, George Pinckney, Ocala, 1858-1862

Only meager information concerning the career of Dr. Wilson has been located. He is known to have arrived in Ocala from his native South Carolina in late 1858 or early 1859 but his sojourn was brief. The Marion County Census of 1860 lists him as a resident of the Ocala Hotel, E.J. Harris, Proprietor. He was 24 years of age.[1] Soon after arrival he joined Dr. Hilton D. Jones in a professional partnership. Dr. Jones had recently returned from a tour of duty in the Third Seminole War. In January 1860, this association was terminated.[2] Dr. Wilson enlisted in the Confederate Army on April 30, 1862, receiving appointment as Assistant Surgeon, Field and Staff, in the First Florida Cavalry Regiment. He remained in this capacity until March 1863, when he was transferred to an Alabama military unit. According to an Ocala historian he lost his life in combat.[3]

1. U.S. Census, 1860, Marion County, Florida, item 35. The Harris Hotel, later to be called Ocala House, was for years Ocala's main hostelry.

2. Ocala *Home Companion*, January 10, 1860.

3. Eloise Robinson Ott, "Ocala Prior to 1868," *Florida Historical Quarterly*, October, 1927, p. 103. In putting together this sketch the Alabama military record of Dr. Wilson has not been consulted.

Wilson, John Thomas Jefferson, Gadsden, Jackson and Leon Counties, 1802-1860

After examination of the available data on the career of Dr. Wilson, the man remains something of an enigma. Obviously well educated, intelligent, and at least in the antebellum years a man of property and good social standing, he nevertheless seldom emerges as a public figure, professionally, politically or socially.

Born in Barnwell District, South Carolina[1], about 1802[2] of landowning parents, he is assumed to have gained an early education in local schools and served a medical apprenticeship in the office of a local physician. In the fall of 1820[3] he enrolled in the Medical Department of Transylvania College in Lexington, Kentucky, which had opened in the fall of 1817 only to close after a single session as the result of faculty dissension. After a year's lapse it reopened and with appointment of two or three outstanding teachers, notably Daniel Drake and Benjamin W. Dudley, it immediately gained an enviable reputation.[4] Dr. Wilson was thus exposed to stimulating instructors. He was graduated Doctor of Medicine in the spring of 1823, having submitted a thesis bearing the title, "On Organic Sympathy." Seemingly fascinated with the challenge of medical learning he enrolled for an additional year as a postdoctoral student.[5]

Soon after completing his studies Dr. Wilson departed for Florida, settling in the northeastern part of Gadsden County. It is assumed that he began actual practice. Four years later he purchased four tracts of land amounting to about one half section in an area said to have contained some of the best farmland in the county.[6] In 1833 his successful ventures were verified when he was one of the chief investors in the Union Bank of Florida, having purchased 150 shares at $100 per share.[7] This purchase, combined with the earlier purchase of land, indicates that he had become a person of more than average means.

During these golden years Dr. Wilson was also an active medical practitioner. As early as 1827 he was a doctor of sufficient reputation to receive a legislative appointment to the Medical Board of the Territory at the legislative session that year.[8]

For reasons quite unknown Dr. Wilson moved to Jackson County at some time in the late 1830s. The census enumerator found him there in 1840.[9] Meanwhile he had married Mary Ann, a native of Georgia, known only by her Christian name. By 1840 three children had been born, Samuel W., Thomas, and Sarah. Before the end of the decade of the 1840s, however, the Wilsons had made another move, this time to Tallahassee.

As an established physician in Tallahassee Dr. Wilson became acquainted in the summer of 1848 with Dr. Cornelius C. Van Wyck, lately arrived in the city after serving one term as Professor of Surgery at the Frankin Medical College of Philadelphia, an institution which survived for only four years, 1847 to 1852. The two men formed a professional partnership for practice locally and in the surrounding area. Of greater interest but less significance, however, was their effort to launch a program for the instruction of young men considering entering the medical profession. They advertised their willingness to receive "a limited number of Office Students...who will be supplied with Books, Plates, and Anatomical and other Preparations." These students would be taught "according to the mode pursued in the large Northern cities...to compound and dispense Medicine, and will be instructed in the minor everyday duties of the Surgeon...Bleeding, Cupping, Bandaging, etc..." They were emboldened to add: "Perhaps no Private Office in any American city will afford a greater variety of new and approved remedies, or present more practical facilities for students." They went even further to suggest the establishment, as soon as possible, of an Infirmary for the reception of both surgical and medical patients, in which students would have the opportunity of practically studying diseases. Nothing came of the plan, however.[10]

The Census of 1850 lists Dr. Wilson as a resident of Tallahassee and owner of property valued at only $2,500. His slaves numbered 15.[11] Ten years later, however, he was living on his plantation on Lake Jackson, northwest of Tallahassee, where his neighbors included other members of the landed gentry such as the Bradfords, Hollands and Branchs. His property, real and personal, was valued at $35,000; he owned 25 slaves. He was designated only as "Planter."[12]

No date of death for Dr. Wilson has been discovered, although it is assumed that since he did not appear in the census of 1870 he had died before that date. As for the Wilson children, very little is known. Samuel W. became a teacher and is listed in the 1860 census as such. In 1866 he married Sarah V. Walker, also of Leon County.[13] Thomas managed the family lands. Sarah was married to H. Corley in June 1858.[14] Thomas was also married in 1866. Although the Confederate Army records are not totally reliable, it appears that the third son, Benjamin, enlisted in the Confederate cause in April 1861 at the age of 18 and was assigned to Company E, 1st Florida Infantry Regiment.[15]

It is clear that in his later years Dr. Wilson gradually relinquished medical practice and with the help of his maturing sons turned to the management of his plantation. It is probable that, as was true of many Southern landowners, the War and Reconstruction dealt him a severe blow economically and psychologically.[16]

1. Archieves, Transylvania University, Lists of Matriculants and Graduates.
2. This date is an extrapolation from census data.
3. See note 1, supra.
4. John H. Ellis, *Medicine in Kentucky*, Lexington, University of Kentucky Press, 1977, pp. 8-11.
5. See note 1, supra.
6. The Daniel F. McNeil Map of Gadsden County, 1824, gives the location of a Wilson homestead, thought to be that of Dr. Wilson. See Miles Kenan Womack Jr., *Gadsden: A Florida County in Word and Picture*, Quincy, 1976, p. 323.

7. Ibid., p. 33. Of the 32 purchasers of stock by Gadsden residents only four purchased more shares than did Dr. Wilson.

8. *Acts, Florida Legislative Council*, 7th Session, 1828, pp. 258-60.

9. U.S. Census, 1840, Jackson County, Florida, p. 190.

10. Tallahassee *Floridian*, July 22, 1848. The notice of the planned medical instructional facility also appeared in the Jacksonville *News*, August 19, 1848. It is not known exactly when Dr. Wilson moved to Tallahassee. The earliest known reference to his presence there is the notice in the Tallahassee *Floridian* of December 6, 1845. Here is printed a letter to him from a source in Savannah in response to his request for a supply of vaccine for smallpox. He had apparently asked R.R. Cuyler of Savannah to obtain a supply not only for himself but for other Tallahassee physicians as well.

11. U.S. Census, 1850, Leon County, Florida, p. 42. The property value seems inaccurate.

12. U.S. Census, 1860, Leon County, Florida, p. 69.

13. Florida Duke Varick and Sarah V. Walker, comps., *Gadsden County, Florida, Marriages, 1849-1976*, Quincy, 1980, p. 81.

14. Ibid.

15. NA, Service Records, CSA, M251, Roll 30.

16. This assumption is borne out by the fact that in the several cemetery surveys of Leon County no gravestone for any member of the Wilson family has been located.

Wilson, Robert S.R., Tallahassee, 1826

Dr. Wilson was born in Fayette County, Kentucky, about 1804. The records of Transylvania University in Lexington indicate that he was a third year student in its medical school in 1824-25. Presumably with his degree in hand, he appeared in Tallahassee in the spring of 1826 announcing to the people that his professional services were available to those who might require them.[1] On April 14 he joined other Tallahassee physicians in publishing a list of fees for their various services. The notice stated that the published fees had been agreed upon at a meeting of physicians of Leon and Gadsden Counties on March 25, 1826.[2] Since no further evidence of his presence in Florida has been located, it is assumed that he did not long remain in the state.

1. Tallahassee *Florida Intelligencer*, April 28, 1826. The issue of April 7, in which the notice first appeared, is not extant.

2. Ibid.

Wilson, Samuel W., Gadsden County, 1829

Dr. Wilson, son of physician, John T.J. Wilson, a resident of Leon County, was born in Florida in 1829. Of his early education nothing is known, although there is some indication it was of a classical type. He apparently served an apprenticeship under the guidance of his father. The census of 1860 lists him as a resident in the home of Samuel Parkhill, a prominent landowner near Tallahassee.[1] His occupation at that time is shown to have been "teacher."

Although Dr. Wilson was of an age to have served in the Army of the Confederacy, there is no record of his having done so. This leads to the speculation that he may have had a physical infirmity which rendered him unfit for military service.

Dr. Wilson married Sarah V. Walker[2] on September 4, 1866, and they had three daughters, Ada, Eula and Eva, whose ages were 11, eight and two respectively in 1880.[3]

In his later years Dr. Wilson apparently discontinued medical practice or at most pursued it on a limited scale. The Special Florida Census of 1885 indicates that he was more farmer than physician, although his land holdings were modest:

35 total acres of which only seven acres were under cultivation. His livestock were valued at $110. His household included his wife, three daughters and mother-in-law, Mrs. Penelope Walker.[4] He obviously did not achieve the level of success attained by his father who had been a successful physician and civic leader (one of the first commissioners of the Town of Quincy).[5]

1. See Leon County Census, 1850, p. 76, item 130.
2. Florida Duke Varick and Phyllis Rose Smith, compilers, *Gadsden County Florida Marriage Records*, Quincy, 1980, p. 81.
3. U.S. Census, 1880, Gadsden County, Florida, p. 76.
4. Special Census, Florida, 1885, Dist. No. 2, p. 7.
5. J. Randall Stanley, *History of Gadsden County*, Quincy, Gadsden County Historical Commission, 1945, p. 32.

Wilson, William S., Marianna, 1829-1868

Dr. Wilson was born in Gadsden County about 1829. Before entering the Medical College of South Carolina in 1850 he studied in Quincy under the preceptorate of Dr. J.L. Shields, one of the county's most successful physicians.[1] Receiving his medical degree in 1851 he settled in Marianna and continued to live there until his death in 1868.[2]

Dr. Wilson was twice married, first to Laura Robinson,[3] daughter of the Reverend Jesse Robinson, who inherited the Big Spring Plantation from his wealthy father, William H. Robinson, and second to Ann,[4] daughter of Jacob Robinson. She was a first cousin of the first Mrs. Wilson.

Only occasional references to Dr. Wilson are preserved in Jackson County records. It is recorded that in 1854 he joined Dr. Ethelbert Philips in performing a postmortem examination of a slave, the property of one Benjamin A. Dickens, for which service the General Assembly of Florida had authorized a payment of $25 for each physician.[5]

Dr. Charles A. Hentz, for a time a Marianna physician, in his recollections of his medical colleagues, remembered Dr. Wilson as follows:[6]

> Dr. William Wilson was doing the most practice; a very deserving, steady young man; who made up for the lack of extraordinary ability by a calm and dignified bearing in the sick room; and not talking too much; we were very good friends and got along nicely with each other, there was no professional jealousy between us.

Dr. Hentz recalled an embarrassing professional situation relating to his attendance upon the wife of Gen. Jesse J. Finley at the time of her accouchement. A few days after the event he dropped in to check on Mrs. Finley's condition only to find her in considerable pain and being attended by Dr. Wilson! Writing of the incident many years later Dr. Hentz seemed to recall General Finley's embarrassed but unconvincing explanation with amusement.[7]

1. *CMMCSSC*, Charleston, 1924, List, p. 123. This date of birth is an extrapolation from the 1860 Census giving his age as 31.
2. J. Randall Stanley, *History of Jackson County*, Marianna, 1950, p. 251. Marianna's first telephone exchange was housed in a building erected by Dr. Wilson in which his offices had been located.
3. Ibid., p. 20.
4. Ibid., p. 60. She had previously been the wife of John Gray Roulhac Jr., who died in 1857.
5. *Acts and Resolutions, General Assembly of Florida*, 7th Session 1854, p. 91.
6. Charles A. Hentz, Autobiography (unpublished), microfilm of transcription in P.K. Yonge Library of Florida History, I, 276.
7. Ibid., pp. 279-80.

Wilson, Young Thomas Strong, Jefferson County, 1821-1855

Almost no information has emerged concerning the medical career of Young Thomas Strong Wilson, a mid-19th century practitioner in Jefferson County. He was born in Newberry District, South Carolina, in 1821, the only son of James R. and Emaline (Knight) Wilson, and grandson of Thomas and Mary Wilson, who were among the early settlers in Newberry District.[1] It is unlikely that Dr. Wilson ever attended any established medical school but it is probable that he studied medicine in the office of a Newberry physician. It is reasonable to assume that he served an apprenticeship under his uncle, Dr. Thomas Wilson Boozer, himself an 1843 graduate of the Medical College of the State of South Carolina.[2]

Dr. Wilson is known to have practiced in Laurens District, South Carolina, for a year or so before moving to Florida. In 1845 he married Mary Ann Caroline Dean. Their two elder children were born in South Carolina, a daughter, Landen in 1846, and Hoye, a son, in 1847. Census data suggests that they arrived in Jefferson County, about 1848, their third child, a daughter, Fleta, having been born there.[3] A fourth child was born in the early 1850s.

Dr. Wilson's professional life was tragically brief. He is thought to have died about 1855; then his widow and the four children returned to her native Laurens District where she died two years later, in 1857.

1. The genealogical information relating to Dr. Wilson, provided by his great-grandson, Woodrow J. Dickson, of Brea, California, is gratefully acknowledged.
2. Charleston *Mercury*, March 18, 1843. His thesis, "Infantile Convulsions."
3. U.S. Census, 1850, Jefferson County, Florida, p. 44.

Wiltam, Samuel A., Key West, 1850

Dr. Wiltam, a native of Maine, was one of several physicians attracted to Key West during the antebellum period. He came to Florida from Ohio where he had met and married a woman some nine years his junior known as "E.V." Their first child, a daughter named Audrey, was born in Ohio in 1840. Soon thereafter the family moved to Mississippi where a second daughter, Mary, was born. It appears that the Wiltams arrived in Key West about 1849, remaining there until about 1859. No further information about them has emerged, although they are thought to have remained in Florida until the late 1850s.[1]

1. All that is presently known of the Wiltam Family is derived from the Monroe County Census of 1850, page 5.

Winn, Benjamin Franklin, Leon County, 1785-1832

Dr. Winn,[1] about whose origin nothing is presently known, is thought to have arrived in Florida about 1831 in search of a benign climate which, it was hoped, would bring about a cure for his serious ailment diagnosed as dropsy. Accompanied by his wife, Mary C., and son, Thomas, he settled at Ft. St. Marks when that area was still a part of Leon County. The move availed him nothing, however, his death coming on December 3, 1832, at age 40. Mrs. Winn arranged for his burial in the Skipper Cemetery located half a mile east of the Chaires crossroads and only a few hundred feet north of Highway 27. They also erected a monument to his memory.

Since no further information relating to Mrs. Winn and her son has been found, it is assumed that they departed the state a short time later.

1. The Tallahassee *Floridian*, December 29, 1832. Obit.

Winn, Thomas B., Leon County, 1838

Dr. Winn made a brief and somewhat dismal appearance on the Leon County scene about 1838. A resident of a remote part of the county, he suffered the loss of his wife, Mary Ann, on August 25, 1837. She was a victim of yellow fever, dying at the age of 24.[1] In March the following year he announced his candidacy for election to the State Constitutional Convention in St. Joseph on December 3. The election drew 15 nominees for the eight positions. Dr. Winn came in last.[2] Nothing further is known of this unfortunate man. He had apparently left the state prior to 1840.

1. Tallahassee *Floridian*, September 2, 1835.
2. The winners were George T. Ward, Samuel Parkhill, James D. Westcott Jr., Leslie A. Thompson, John Taylor, Thomas Brown, Leigh Read, and William Wyatt. See F.W. Hoskins, "The St. Joseph Convention," *Florida Historical Quarterly*, XVI, No. 1, p. 42.

Wirt, Henry Grattan, Jefferson County, 1818-1850

During the first two decades of its territorial period Florida with its cheap land and seemingly unlimited opportunities lured innumerable families from Virginia and the Carolinas into its comparatively unknown wilderness. Some had achieved wealth and social position in their native states. The names Eppes, Randolph, Gamble, Randle and Bradford are representative. To this list might be added the Wirts whose American founder was a Swiss immigrant of the late 18th century, Jacob Wirt. Jacob's son, William (1772-1834), endowed with exceptional intelligence, a penetrating intellect and enormous capacity for work, had by the turn of the 19th century established himself in the top ranks of the legal profession and was destined to become one of America's most distinguished attorney generals.[1] In 1802 he married Elizabeth Gamble, daughter of Col. Robert Gamble, a wealthy Richmond merchant. To this union were born 12 children of whom at least five died before reaching adulthood.

The youngest of the Wirt children was Henry Grattan, born in Richmond in 1818. His early education was closely supervised by his father[2] who without employing unduly rigorous discipline instilled in the minds of his children a respect for and love of learning. William Wirt himself had a lifelong passion for Latin classics. Upon his death, when young Henry was only 16, Mrs. Wirt moved to Florida and settled on lands which had some years earlier been purchased by her husband. These consisted of two tracts, one parcel of 1,200 acres at the south end of Lake Miccosukee, the other a large tract about four miles southwest of Monticello known as Wirtland.[3]

In 1839 Henry Wirt enrolled in the University of Maryland School of Medicine where in the spring of 1841 he was graduated with the M.D. degree.[4] He elected to return to Florida to enter practice. In the meantime, another Virginia-born physician, Benjamin Waller Taylor, had established his practice in Monticello and was able to persuade young Dr. Wirt to join him there, perhaps through misrepresentation of the opportunities awaiting a young physician and probably with the intimation that he would himself be retiring soon.[5] At any rate, Dr. Wirt went to Monticello only to have his expectations unfulfilled. Dr. Taylor decided to continue practice while Dr. Wirt had difficulty earning a living, a situation which caused some bitterness on his part. In order to eke out an existence he lived in his office and undertook to instruct young medical apprentices. Things took a turn for the better in 1843 when Thomas Palmer, eldest son of Martin Palmer, became his apprentice. Dr. Wirt subsequently moved into the Palmer household where he lived "not as a boarder but as a member of the family." He lived there until his marriage on January 2, 1844, to Harriet Louisa Anderson, a widow and sister-in-law of J. George Anderson, of the well-known cotton factorage of Coe, Anderson & Co.[6]

Dr. Wirt and his bride rented a house owned by Benjamin Johnson for which, says Prof. Shofner, they paid $100 per year. Johnson, a well-to-do Jefferson County plantation owner, became a valuable medical client of Dr. Wirt, entrusting to him the care of his family and slaves.[7] Three children were born to the Wirts, Elizabeth, born 1845; William, in 1847 and died as an infant, and Letitia Breckenridge, born 1849.[8]

By 1848 Dr. Wirt's health, never robust, began to fail. A chronic bronchial ailment gradually became acute. Unable to conduct his practice which had greatly increased in volume he invited young Dr. John L. Call to become his partner. Their association was publicly announced on August 4.[9] It was an ill-fated arrangement, however. Within a year Dr. Wirt's condition had so worsened that he was forced to give up practice and return to the family estate of Wirtland where he died on June 26, 1850.[10] Eight weeks earlier on May 1 his friend and companion in practice, Dr. Call, had died suddenly in Monticello. About a year after his death Mrs. Wirt married a third husband, William Girardeau, a Monticello school teacher.

1. William Wirt, friend and associate of many of the most famous public figures of his times such as John Marshall, Thomas Jefferson, James Madison and James Monroe, and participant in famous court cases such as Fletcher vs. Peck, McCulloch vs. Maryland, the Dartmouth College Case, and the trial of Aaron Burr (prosecution attorney), was James Monroe's attorney general throughout his two terms (1817-1825). Born in Maryland, he spent most of his professional life in Virginia, particularly as a lawyer in Richmond. He was also an author of note, having produced the first full-length biography of Patrick Henry. See John P. Kennedy, *Memoirs of the Life of William Wirt*, 2 vols., Philadelphia, 1850; also *Dictionary of American Biography*, XX, 418-421, sketch by Thomas P. Abernethy. The vast collection of Wirt papers is in the possession of the Maryland Historical Society, Baltimore.

2. Kennedy, *Memoirs*, contains numerous letters in which Wirt expressed his thoughts and philosophy of education as well as his paternal affection and tenderness.

3. WPA, "History of Jefferson County," unpublished mimeograph copy, p. 10. In the later 1820s William Wirt had joined several of his Virginia friends in acquisition of land in Leon and Jefferson Counties. He envisioned establishment of a utopian settlement modeled after the much publicized experiment of Robert Owen in Lanarkshire, Scotland. The abortive effort to accomplish this was launched in1833 and entrusted to Wirt's son-in-law, Louis Goldsborough, a naval officer. It is described in Kennedy, *Memoirs*, II, 335.

4. Eugene F. Cordell, *University of Maryland, School of Medicine*, 1807-90, Baltimore, 1891, p. 205.

5. Jerrell H. Shofner, *History of Jefferson County*, Tallahassee, 1976, pp. 61-64.

6. Tallahassee *Florida Sentinel*, January 9, 1844.

7. Shofner, *History*.

8. "Records, St. John's Episcopal Church, Tallahassee, Fla., 1832-1880." Typescript, pp. 15, 17. The daughter Elizabeth was married on June 11, 1867, to James McCutcheon.

9. Tallahassee *Floridian and Journal*, August 5, 1848.

10. Tallahassee *Sentinel*, July 2, 1850.

11. Shofner, *History*, p. 202. See also U.S. Census, 1850, Jefferson County, Florida, p. 3.

Wood, Robert Crooke, Ft. Brooke, Tampa Bay, 1799-1869

The Florida career of Dr. Wood was brief but significant, spanning approximately two years he spent as post surgeon at Ft. Brooke, Tampa Bay, during the Second Seminole War. He was born at Newport, Rhode Island, on September 23, 1799, the son of Major John Wood who commanded the defenses at Newport during the War of 1812. Dr. Wood was a graduate of Columbia College Department of Medicine (later to become the Columbia University College of Physicians and Surgeons) in the class of 1821.[1] After about four years of private practice he entered the Medical Department, United States Army, as assistant surgeon, his commission dating from May 28, 1825.[2] He was assigned to the Fifth Infantry Regiment.

In the general reorganization of the Army in 1828, a Lieutenant Colonel Zachary Taylor was assigned to Ft. Snelling, a remote outpost in the Louisiana Purchase on the Mississippi River, which still exists within the city limits of Minneapolis, Minnesota. At about the same date, Dr. Wood was assigned to the post as the medical officer.

It was a mark of Colonel Taylor's intelligence that he recognized the inadequacy of his own formal education and determined that his children should enjoy the best available educational opportunities. He therefore sent them away for a good portion of each year, usually to live with relatives, where they may receive proper education. They did, however, spend some time with their parents at the varous army posts. It was at Ft. Snelling that the eldest Taylor child, Ann Mackall, attracted the attention of Dr. Wood, who had been sent to Ft. Snelling in 1828. She was a charming 17-year-old girl who had been educated in Kentucky under the guidance of relatives. A courtship developed but before marriage plans developed Colonel Taylor was transferred to Prairie du Chien, some 200 miles down the Mississippi where he was to establish Ft. Crawford. In late 1829 Dr. Wood took leave from Ft. Snelling, made his way to Ft. Crawford where he married Ann Taylor, obviously with the blessing of the Colonel and Mrs. Taylor.[3]

The doctor and his bride returned to Ft. Snelling where they lived for the next six years and where their sons, John Taylor and Robert Crooke, were born on August 13, 1830 and April 4, 1832 respectfully.[4] Dr. Wood was assigned to Ft. Crawford in 1835 doubtless at the request of Colonel Taylor. Meanwhile he had been promoted to the rank of surgeon. At Prairie du Chien two daughters were born to the Woods, Blandina Dudley on January 9, 1834, and Sarah Knox on November 21, 1835.[5]

In early fall, 1837, Dr. Wood was ordered to prepare for transfer to Florida where the Second Seminole War, which had begun in late 1835, was not going well. Colonel Taylor was already making preparations for a major campaign designed to destroy the Indian strength lodged north of Lake Okeechobee between the Kissimmee and Peace Rivers. Before the attack could be launched, however, he was brought down by an attack of fever endemic to the area. He was quite ill for several days. It is said that his life was saved by the constant attention of his son-in-law and the gentle nursing care of Mrs. Taylor and Mrs. Wood.[6] The families of both Taylor and Wood had quarters at recently-reactivated Fort Brooke on Tampa Bay. The campaign finally got under way in mid-December, culminating in the Battle of Okeechobee, in which Colonel Taylor distinguished himself and was rewarded by promotion to the rank of brigadier general.[7]

Dr. Wood continued to serve as the medical officer in Taylor's command until both were removed in 1840. The doctor then joined General Taylor at his new command at Baton Rouge, Louisiana, arriving there, it is thought, in December 1840.

The last 29 years of Dr. Wood's life were spent at various military installations outside Florida. He was with General Taylor in the Mexican War, after which he is thought to have served in Washington. Near the beginning of the Civil War he was raised to the rank of assistant surgeon general with the nominal military rank of colonel. For his gallantry and meritorious service during the War he was brevetted brigadier general,[8] effective March 13, 1865. Apparently weary of the arduous life of an army physician he retired on February 22, 1869. He was probably in declining health at the time; he died in New York City four weeks later on March 28, 1869.[9]

1. *General Zachary Taylor, The Louisiana President of the United States.* This publication of the Louisiana State Museum was published in New Orleans on August 5, 1937. See pages 45-51, for genealogical information of President Taylor and his descendants.

2. Heitman, op. cit.

3. Brainerd Dyer, *Zachary Taylor*, Baton Rouge, LSU Press, 1946, p. 96.

4. See note 1 above.

5. Ibid.

6. Dyer, *Zachary Taylor*, p. 123.

7. For a carefully documented account of the Battle of Okeechobee and Taylor's role therein see John K. Mahon, *History of the Second Seminole War*, Gainesville, University of Florida Press, 1967, p. 226.

8. The chronology of Dr. Wood's advancement from assistant surgeon to brevet brigadier general is found in Francis B. Heitman, *Historical Register and Dictionary of the United States Army, 1789-1903*, Vol. I, Washington, Government Printing Office, 1903.

9. Heitman, Hist. Reg.

Woodley, Willis L., Gadsden, Jackson and Franklin Counties, 1840s

Dr. Woodley, whose origin and earlier years are unknown, arrived in Florida in late 1841, settling in Gadsden County where he found lodging in the home of Philip Blount, a farmer of more than average means. He announced his services to the residents of Gadsden and adjoining counties on April 6, 1841.[1] He remained in the county for about four years, appearing occasionally at public functions such as the Fourth of July celebration at Liberty Church in 1843 at which he offered a toast to John C. Calhoun.[2]

By early 1846 Dr. Woodley had moved to adjoining Jackson County where he married a propertied widow, Mrs. Sarah L. Scott, that year. He appears to have remained there for about three years before moving to Apalachicola. On March 15, 1849, he announced to the people of the community that he was offering his services to the public. He reassured the prospective clients that he had been "constantly engaged during the last twenty-three years in the practice of medicine in North Carolina, Virginia, Alabama and Florida," and that "he flatters himself that he is familiar with the character and modes of treatment of the prevailing diseases of this section." He could be found at any hour at his office opposite the barber shop.[3] Given his peripatetic behavior, it is not surprising that he had left the state prior to the census enumeration of 1850.

1. Tallahassee *Floridian*, December 25, 1841. He is designated M.D.

2. Tallahassee *Florida Sentinel*, July 11, 1843.
3. Apalachicola *Commercial Advertiser*, March 15, 1849

Worcester, Olive Estelle, Lake County, 1858-1926

Dr. Worcester, the first properly qualified woman to practice medicine in Florida, was born in Iowa on June 15, 1858. She was the older of the two daughters of Horace Westley and Mary Jane Bradford Worcester. Both parents were natives of upstate New York, the father having been born in Ticonderoga, the mother in nearby Crown Point.[1] They moved to Iowa as homesteaders in the early 1850s settling on land some five miles west of Cedar Rapids. The Worcesters were apparently a family of above average cultivation. Their younger daughter, Orpha, became an artist, a calling which she followed throughout most of her life. She was particularly gifted in watercolor paintings of Florida wildflowers. Several of her painted are hung in Lake-Sumter Community College in Leesburg. Olive chose medicine, enrolling in the Northwestern University Woman's College of Medicine, Chicago, in 1880 and graduating in 1882. The Worcester family moved to Florida about 1885, purchasing a tract of land in the northeast corner of what is now Lake County but which prior to 1887 was in Sumter County. They were located near the village of Conant,[2] where the father resumed farming and Dr. Worcester began medical practice.

Soon after arriving in Florida Dr. Worcester was accepted for membership in the Marion County Medical Society. She doubtless soon discovered that she was better qualified for her profession than many of those practicing at that time in central Florida. In April 1890 the Florida Medical Asociation held its annual meeting in Ocala. In one of the early sessions the Credentials Committee gave its report, which included the recommendation that 14 "gentlemen" be admitted to membership in the State Association. It is probable that there were some members present who were not aware that one of the gentlemen was indeed a lady, Dr. Worcester. All 14 were accepted.[3] The following day, April 9, Dr. Worcester was among the members selected to attend the annual meeting of the American Medical Association.[4]

In 1892 the Florida Medical Assocation held its annual meeting in Key West, arranging, however, to spend a day and night in Havana, Cuba, upon the invitation of the Havana Medical Society. There Dr. Worcester read a paper, "A Report of a Case of Diphtheria," which was immediately referred to the Committee on Publications.

The Association met in Pensacola in 1893 but due to remoteness of the town and difficulty of travel, the attendance was sparse. Dr. Worcester was among the absentees, nor was she present at the meeting the following year in Tampa. She had paid her dues and was in good standing, however. Meanwhile she had been added to the Committee on the Diseases of Children.[5]

In 1896 the Association met in Sanford. A delegate from the Marion County Society reported: "We have suspended during the year for non-payment of dues William M. Ellis, M.D., and expelled one, O.E. Worcester, M.D., for conduct unbecoming a medical practitioner." Her offense was not specified. She was not present at the meeting. Meanwhile the Committee on Ethics had taken her case under consideration. She had paid her dues and was in good standing. Although she was not present she had sent an affadavit explaining that her absence was due to sickness, and requesting that her case be suspended until the next meeting of the Association.[6]

At the 1897 meeting in Palatka, the Ethics Committee offered its report which was signed by only two members. The third member, Dr. James M. Jackson, of Bronson, explaining his refusal to sign the report, said that his action was based on disagreement with the findings of the Committee in reference to Dr. O.E. Worcester and his inability to thoroughly examine the case. It was further reported that "the consideration of the report and the adjustment of several matters therein, notably the cases of Drs. O.E. Worcester of Conant, W.B. Rush of Oakland, N.A. Williams of Dade City, and Theodore Turnbull of Monticello, provoked protracted discussion."[7] It appears clear that Dr. Jackson had serious doubts about the action taken by the Association with respect to Dr. Worcester.

Later in the session the Ethics Committee made the following report:[8]

> In the case of Dr. Worcester's appeal from the action of the Marion County Medical Society, we recommend that the case be remanded to the Marion County Medical Society for adjustment. If the Association wishes to hear the evidence upon which we base such a recommendation, the Committee has on hand enough evidence to consume several hours of your time, having read the most unprofitable, unelevating character sketches ever collected. We will only add that we believed that we have evidence, now before the Marion County Medical Society, which would doubtless have changed their action...evidence which we believe best for all parties concerned to leave in the hands of the Committee, to be forgotten as soon as possible.

Thus the Association, possibly fearful of provoking a schism within its ranks, failed to pursue a course of action which should have cleared Dr. Worcester's name.

It appears from the records of the 1897 meeting that there was dissenting opinion among Association members concerning the penalty imposed on Dr. Worcester. The condition under which she might be reinstated was set forth in a resolution: "That Dr. Worcester be informed that she must reinstate herself with the Marion County Medical Society, and failing that...before the next meeting of the Association she be requested to hand in her resignation to the Florida Medical Association."[9] She was apparently unwilling or unable to do this. At the meeting of the Association in Jacksonville in 1898 her resignation was presented to the Association.[10]

Dr. Worcester made no further effort to be reinstated to either the state or county organization. She did not cease to practice, however. Meanwhile she was married to Conant landowner, Chester M. Swan, continuing to live and practice medicine until her death on December 29, 1926.[11]

The author gratefully acknowledges the assistance of Miriam W. Johnson and Margaret Elmore, both of the Lake County Historical Society, Tavares, in the preparation of this sketch. It should also be stated that important vital information on Dr. Worcester is found in her death certificate on file in the Florida Bureau of Vital Statistics, Jacksonville.

1. Ticonderoga and Crown Point, near the Hudson River in Essex County, are only about seven miles apart.
2. The village of Conant, located in northern Sumter County just south of the Marion County line until 1887. After formation of Lake County from parts of Orange and Sumter Counties, it found itself in the northwest corner of Lake. It was named for Sherman Conant, an engineer who supervised construction of the Florida Southern Railroad. The nearest post office is now Lady Lake. Conant had its own post office from 1884 until 1919. Both Conant and the railroad have ceased to exist.
3. *Proceedings, Florida Medical Association,* (Hereinafter referred to as *Proc., FMA*) 1890, p. 8.

4. Ibid., p. 14.
5. Proc., FMA, 1894.
6. Proc., FMA, 1896, p. 11. Dr. R.P. Islar, Secretary of the Society, read the report. See also p. 24.
7. Proc., FMA, 1897, pp. 4607.
8. Ibid., pp. 46-47.
9. Ibid., p. 49.
10. Proc., FMA, p. 11.
11. It is apparent that notwithstanding the questionable treatment she had received at the hands of the Marion County Medical Society, Dr. Worcester never lost favor with the people of Conant and Lady Lake. Professor William T. Kennedy, in his account of Conant wrote: "Here Dr. Olive Estelle Worcester practiced for over forty years, covering all the trains between Fruitland Park and East Lake, the Oklawaha River and Oxford." Professor William T. Kennedy, *History of Lake County Florida*, St. Augustine, Florida, The Record Company, 1929, p. 15.

Wright, Charles, Jackson County, 1870

Dr. Wright, a practicing physician in Jackson County about 1870, remains a very obscure figure. He is known only through the Census schedule of 1870. He was 30 years of age, living alone, and owning property valued at a mere $10.[1] Nothing is known of his educational background, nor of his career subsequent to 1870. Professor Jerrell Shofner in his *Jackson County, Florida, A History* only says of him, "Other medical doctors included...C.C. Wright." It may be surmised that he returned to his native State of Georgia to spend the latter years of his life.

1. U.S. Census, 1870, Jackson County, p. 5.

Wylly, King, Orange County, 1849-1895

Although the career of Dr. Wylly does not fit into the time frame of the present study, having arrived in Florida in the 1870s, he merits mention in any catalogue of physicians practicing in Florida in the 19th century.[1] He was a highly esteemed physician, possessing a sharp intellect and an adventurous spirit. Born in Savannah in 1849, the son of George W. Wylly, he arrived in Florida shortly after the Civil War. His father had purchased fairly large acreage in the vicinity of Orlando and soon became one of the leading citrus growers of the area. Prior to arrival of the family in Orange County young King had attended the University of Virginia from which he was graduated in 1869.[2]

Driven by a lust for travel Dr. Wylly did not immediately launch his professional career. Instead he became concerned with the turn of events in the Franco-Prussian War at a time when the tide was turning in favor of the Germans. He hurried away to France to offer his professional services to the army. When that conflict ended in 1871, Dr. Wylly is presumed to have returned to Florida and launched his practice in Orange County. A few years later, probably in 1890, he was easily persuaded to join a group of friends on a trip to Egypt and Arabia, serving as their physician, probably with expenses paid.[3]

A year or so after returning to Orlando Dr. Wylly built a home at the corner of Orange Avenue and Jackson Street where he finally settled into serious professional practice. Accordings to local scholars the house stood there well into the 20th century only to be demolished in the 1820s to make way for a six-story office building.[4]

At some point in his career, probably in the early 1880s, Dr. Wylly moved to Sanford where he appears to have become a popular and trusted physician.[5] The Florida Medical Association held its annual meeting there in 1885 and he became a member.[6] His presence was immediately felt. Dr. F.H. Caldwell of Sanford read the list of those proposed for membership. Dr. Wylly was forthwith chosen as one of the Florida delegates to attend the next meeting of the American Medical Association. The following year he was present at the Palatka meeting where he was appointed to the Committee on Medical Education.[7]

Henceforth Dr. Wylly's attendance at the annual meetings of the Association was irregular. He was not present in St. Augustine in 1887 but his dues were paid. The following year he was present at the Gainesville meeting where he paid his dues and was appointed to the Committee on Ethics. He also proposed that the Association meet in the following year at Key West, a motion which was promptly adopted notwithstanding the remoteness of the town. The 1889 meeting was a memorable one in that Dr. Joseph Y. Porter was there to present his plan for establishment of a State Board of Health. To Dr. Porter's proposal Dr. Wylly offered a couple of minor changes which were readily agreed upon. In the early 1890s Dr. Wylly discontinaued payment of his dues to the Association. In the *Proceedings* of 1896 he was not listed as a member, an omission which suggests that he was in failing health. He was not present at the meeting in Gainesville in 1895 nor was he present at the Sanford meeting the following year.

No further information on Dr. Wylly has emerged. He is presumed to have lived out his life in Orange County, probably in Sanford. The date of his death has not been discovered.

1. Eve Bacon, *Orlando: A Centennial History*, Chuluota, 1975, pp. 194-195.
2. University of Virginia, *General Catalog, Roster of Students, Medical Department*, Charlottesville, 1880, p. 51.
3. Bacon, op. cit.
4. Ibid.
5. Proceedings, *Florida Medical Association*, 1874 to Present. Pertinent issues consulted.
6. The U.S. Census, Orange County, Florida, 1880, includes some interesting data relating to the Wylly Family. Here Dr. Wylly's father, George W. Wylly, is shown to have been 64 years of age and married for the second time. His present wife, Alzina, aged 40, was a native of Ohio. Their daughter, Naomi was three years of age. Included in the household were Mrs. Wylly's two sons by her previous marriage: Lyman, aged 16, and Chester, aged 12.
7. *Proceedings, Florida Medical Association*, 1874 to Present.

Wynn, Thomas B., Leon County, late 1830s

The earliest known indication that Dr. Wynn practiced medicine in Florida is the obituary of his wife, Mary Ann, who died in Leon County on August 25, 1837. She was 24 years of age and was reported to have been a victim of "congestive fever."[1] Nothing is known of Dr. Wynn's birthplace, youth or medical education. He is thought, however, to have been born in Gadsden County, where the Wynn family was one of prominence. It is probable that his father was Thomas Wynn who died in July 1837.[2]

As the Florida Territory prepared for a Constitutional Convention to be held in St. Joseph in early December 1838, Dr. Wynn was among the first to announce his candidacy for a seat at the Convention, stating his intention on March 24 of that year.[3] By June, however, there were 20 candidates for the eight seats allotted to Leon County. Dr. Wynn was one of the 20. Only 15 were nominated. Dr. Wynn had received the least number of votes and thus was eliminated.[4]

Whether from chargin at his dismal showing or for other reasons quite unknown, Dr. Wynn soon left the Territory.[5]

It may be that the Dr. Benjamin Winn, who died in St. Marks on December 2, 1872, and was buried in the Skipper Cemetery just east of the Chaires Crossroads, was the same person as the subject of the present sketch. The date of his birth, 1826, further supports the speculation.

1. Tallahassee *Floridian*, September 2, 1837.
2. Ibid., July 22, 1837.
3. Ibid., March 24, 1838.
4. Ibid., June 22, 1838.
5. Dr. Wynn's name does not appear in subsequent censuses for Florida.

Yarbrough, William, Jackson County, 1807-1870

Dr. Yarbrough (Yarborough) was born in South Carolina about 1807 and is thought to have been trained in the apprenticeship system which in the early 19th century was the avenue by which many practitioners made their way into the medical profession. When still a young man he migrated to Georgia about 1839 where he married Sarah and their three oldest childen were born: Gibson, William, and George.[1] About 1845 he left Georgia, crossed over into Florida, settling in rural Jackson County in a community known as Port Jackson, located a short distance north of the confluence of the Chattahoochee and Flint Rivers.

Dr. Yarbrough apparently was of moderate means having owned 10 slaves in 1850 and total property valued at $4,300. He continued to practice medicine in later life but appears to have divided his time between practice and farming as was characteristic of so many physicians in the antebellum period. As economic pressures on the cotton growers of the South began to mount about 1850 a meeting of representative planters was called for Macon on October 27, 1851. Previously the growers of Jackson County met in Marianna in September to choose their representatives and Dr. Yarbrough was among the 38 delegates.[2]

Dr. Charles A. Hentz, the well-known practitioner of Jackson and Gadsden Counties, recalling his brief period of practice at Port Jackson, remembered Dr. Yarbrough as "elderly" in 1849 and as "an old practitioner in the neighborhood, and a very sensible one, though uneducated, having attended a case with me." The two men had worked together in an attempt to treat a certain Mrs. Skipper suffering from a severe emotional or mental disturbance.[3]

Ten children are known to have been born to Dr. and Mrs. Yarbrough. They were in order of birth, Gibson, William, George, Sarah, John B., Jesse C. (male), Fleetwood, P.B., Charles and Andrew, and in 1860 ranged in age from 20 to three.[4]

With the outbreak of war in 1861, five sons volunteered for service. George, John and William are known to have served in the Confederate Army. They were members of Company B, 15th Florida Calvalry Regiment, commanded by Captain Richard L. Smith.[5]

Dr. Yarbrough died prior to 1870. The date of his death and place of his burial have not been determined. Two sons were buried in the Collins Chapel Cemetery northwest of Malone.

1. U.S. Census, 1850, Jackson County, Florida, p. 291; ibid., 1860, p. 49.
2. Tallahassee *Sentinel*, September 30, 1851.
3. Charles A. Hentz, "Autobiography," I, 164. In this instance a filmed transcription of the manuscript has been consulted, the original being among the MSS of the Southern Collection, Library, University of North Carolina, Chapel Hill. Dr. Hentz was by no means reluctant to express opinions on his numerous medical colleagues, some of whom he thought incompentent or even immoral.
4. See note 1, supra.
5. Confederate Records, 15th Florida Regiment, National Archives, Washington.

Yon, Jesse, Calhoun County, ante 1870

Records provide only a brief glimpse of Dr. Yon who practiced medicine for only a short while in Calhoun County. His post office, however, was Bristol which, subsequent to the formation of Liberty County in 1855, was in that county. Dr. Yon is believed to have "read" medicine in the office of a local physician prior to entering practice. About 1858 he married and his wife is known only as Sarah E. They had a son, William J., who is presumed to have died in early childhood. Later, about 1861, a second son, Braxton, was born.[1]

Dr. Yon died prior to 1870. The Census of that year lists Mrs. Yon, aged 30, and son, Braxton, aged nine.[2]

1. The Yons were a prolific family. The censuses of Calhoun and Liberty Counties of 1850 and subsequent years contain abundant evidence. It is unfortunate that so few historical records of the two counties have survived. See U.S. Census, 1860, Calhoun County, Florida, p. 128.

2. U.S. Census, 1870, Calhoun County, Florida, p. 295. In this instance Mrs. Yon's post office is listed as Marianna.

Yonge, Philip, Gadsden County, 1808-1834

Dr. Yonge, the eldest son of Henry Yonge by his second wife, Ann Cox, of Charles County, Maryland, was born near St. Augustine, Spanish East Florida, on August 23, 1808, one of 13 children. The elder Yonge had purchased land several miles south of the city after having moved there from Nassau in 1803. He had not prospered, however, and during Philip's childhood and youth the family made several moves seeking a better situation for the support of the rapidly growing family.[1] They settled briefly in Magnolia near Green Cove Springs, Amelia Island, Ormond, Savannah and Athens before locating on the Ochlockonee River east of Quincy. It is obvious that young Philip's education was frequently interrupted and probably fragmented.[2]

In spite of such difficulties Philip was able to serve an apprenticeship in medicine and in the fall of 1828 gain acceptance into the Medical College of the State of South Carolina, Charleston. On March 19 two years later he was graduated Doctor of Medicine, having submitted a doctoral thesis titled, "Rheumatism."[3]

Soon after receiving his degree Dr. Yonge returned to Quincy and began practice. Meanwhile he married Margaret Giles, a cousin, by whom he had a daughter, Annabella, born in 1831. His sojourn in Quincy was brief. By 1833 "he was practicing somewhere in Georgia." In that year he was visited by his father, who wrote: "I was gratified to find them very comfortably situated and Philip in good practice."[4]

But life for Dr. Yonge was short. He died in Thomaston, Georgia, in 1834, at the age of 26.[5] The cause of death is unknown.

1. The greater part of the present sketch is drawn from Edward Yonge, *The Yonges of Caynton, Edgmond, Shropshire*, Victoria, British Columbia, Canada, 1969, pp. 185-189; 191-192.

2. Ibid. By his second wife Henry Yonge had 13 children.

3. Charleston *Courier*, March 20, 1830.

4. Ibid.

5. Ibid.

Young, Edward R., Jefferson County, 1860

Dr. Young, a native of Georgia, was a graduate of the Medical College of Georgia, Augusta, in the class of 1859.[1] Soon after receiving his degree he moved to Jefferson County where his mother Elizabeth, brother C.H., and other members of the family had settled earlier.[2] With the outbreak of war in 1861 Dr. Young is thought to have returned to his native state and presumably served in one of Georgia's military units. The Young family was one of above average means, owning property valued at about $30,000 in 1860. Their slaves numbered 38. As far as is known Dr. Young never returned to practice in Florida after the war.

1. Medical Department, University of Georgia, Augusta, "List of Graduates From 1829 to 1891," Augusta, 1890, p. 27.

2. The family included the mother, aged 64; C.H. Young, farmer, aged 37; A.M. Young wife of C.H., aged 31 and born in Florida; and M.H. Young, presumably the sister of Dr. Young. There was also the overseer. U.S. Census, Jefferson County, Florida, 1860, p. 17.

INDEX

THE AUTHOR

Eugene Ashby Hammond, Ph.D., was born in Rowland, Robeson County, North Carolina, of Scotch-Presbyterians who settled there in the late 1700s. After completing Rowland High School, he enrolled at the University of North Carolina and was graduated with a Bachelor of Arts degree in 1936. He completed his Ph.D. degree in 1941 after submitting a dissertation entitled "The Medical Profession in England in the late Middle Ages." He was strongly influenced by two UNC historians, Drs. Loren McKinney and Josiah Cox Russell, both medievalists.

Dr. Hammond accepted a position at the University of Florida in 1942 but after six months his tenure was interrupted by World War II. He enlisted in the Army Air Corps and was commissioned a second lieutenant. He served in Europe and was posted to places of great interest to a medieval historian: Oxford, Chartres and Nuremburg.

Dr. Hammond returned to the University of Florida in 1946 where he taught in the history and social science departments. He again had time to focus on his primary area of interest: medieval medicine. He received several grants that supported his work in London at the Library of the British Museum and the Wellcome Historical Medical Library. While at the Wellcome, he was introduced to the Englishman, Charles Talbott, who also had a keen interest in medieval medicine. In 1965, *The Medical Practitioners in Medieval England* was published by Wellcome, coauthored by Hammond and Talbott.

When he moved to Florida in the 1940s, Dr. Hammond began to research and write about communities and individuals of the state. His articles included one on Sanibel Island and another on "The Spanish Fisheries of Charlotte Harbor." After publication of his first book, Dr. Hammond combined his interest in Florida history and medical history and began to search for information about physicians of 19th Century Florida. His investigations took him all over the state, and to Savannah, Charleston and New Orleans, as well. Many newspaper people, local historians and county clerks were of great assistance as he ferreted out names and biographical data about the region's early doctors. Of course, the archives and the staff of the P. K. Yonge Library of Florida History were instrumental in his work. Never quite satisfied that he had identified all of the appropriate individuals, Dr. Hammond continued gathering information through the late 1980s.

Dr. Hammond retired from the University of Florida, a Professor Emeritus, in 1978. Although he is no longer actively engaged in historical research, Dr. Hammond visits the P. K. Yonge Library of Florida History at least once a week. He lives in Gainesville with Margaret, his wife of 44 years, near daughter Peggy and family.